Religion and HIV and AIDS

Religion and HIV and AIDS

Charting the Terrain

Edited by Beverley Haddad

UKZN PRESS UNIVERSITY OF KwaZulu-Natal PRESS

Published in 2011 by University of KwaZulu-Natal Press
Private Bag X01
Scottsville 3209
South Africa
Email: books@ukzn.ac.za
Website: www.ukznpress.co.za

ISBN: 978-1-86914-207-0

Managing editor: Sally Hines
Editor: Christopher Merrett
Typesetter: Patricia Comrie
Proofreader: Juliet Haw
Indexer: Stacie Gibson
Cover design: Flying Ant Designs
Cover photograph: The Bigger Picture / Ruiters

Printed and bound by Interpak Books, Pietermaritzburg

Contents

Foreword

Robin Root and Alan Whiteside *

June 2011 marked an anniversary but not a celebration. It was 30 years since HIV was first identified, in the United States. Today, the epidemiological epicentre of HIV infection and AIDS is southern Africa, where 5.3 million individuals in South Africa alone are currently infected. In neighbouring Swaziland, an estimated 49 per cent of women aged 25–29 are HIV positive. Outside of Africa, in Russia and Ukraine in particular, there is a rapid spread among drug users, and while the prevalence rates are relatively low in China and India, the absolute numbers are significant. In all these places, as it has throughout human history, religion plays critical and complex roles in shaping how societies respond to threats to their socio-moral order. With respect to HIV and AIDS, religion, broadly conceived, may impact on individual risk perception, community reactions to HIV positive persons, and macro policy making. Yet only recently has the study of religion and HIV and AIDS drawn sustained scholarly attention.

There is consensus among many experts that the United Nations Millennium Development Goals set for 2015 are unlikely to be met. HIV and AIDS has imperilled a range of demographic and economic indicators. Life expectancy has plummeted; infant and maternal mortality rates have risen; and economic and population growth has slowed as a result of widespread morbidity and mortality. HIV and AIDS is rampant among young to middle-aged adults. Its risks and

---

* Robin Root, MPH, PhD, is a medical anthropologist and Associate Professor in the Department of Sociology and Anthropology at Baruch College, City University of New York. She has been researching social aspects of HIV and AIDS in Swaziland since 2005.

Alan Whiteside, DEcon, is the director of the Health Economics and HIV/AIDS Research Division at the University of KwaZulu-Natal. He has been working on issues relating to HIV and AIDS since 1987.

impact are exacerbated by food insecurity, material poverty and gender inequalities, with women bearing a disproportionate risk of infection and burden of care. The question thus arises: how are the challenges of HIV and AIDS to be met and human development supported under such conditions?

As a medical anthropologist and health economist, respectively, we are honoured to write this foreword. KwaZulu-Natal is the hardest hit province in South Africa, and the Collaborative for HIV and AIDS, Religion and Theology (CHART) research centre, located at the University of KwaZulu-Natal, has pioneered research on religion and HIV and AIDS in ways that demonstrate the importance of a multi-disciplinary and culturally situated approach to addressing the epidemic. CHART's collaborations with practitioners in the field who co-produce this knowledge is perhaps the most distinguishing feature of this edited volume. Each chapter is organised as a dialogue between academic and practitioner, recognising that with HIV and AIDS, true advancement in scholarship and health programming requires the synergistic expertise and experience of both.

In partnership with the African Religious Health Assets Programme (ARHAP), co-ordinated out of the University of Cape Town, CHART has helped to develop an emergent theory of religious health assets (RHA). RHA offers a conceptual framework for examining the 'tangible' and 'intangible' aspects of religious organisations, networks and practices that may be enacted to improve public health in sub-Saharan Africa. Such innovations in this area are critical to next-generation questions regarding HIV and AIDS. Until recently, the deeply embedded roles that religion(s) play in the everyday lives of individuals and communities affected by HIV and AIDS have been little explored. The politics of religious engagement arguably have distracted many researchers and policy makers from setting a scholarly – rather than a political – agenda. The latter has included debates over the faith-based clauses of the United States Presidential Emergency Plan for AIDS Relief and 'Abstain, Be faithful, and Condomise' (ABC) interventions, especially in evaluating the Uganda 'success'. Moreover, religion *vis-à-vis* HIV and AIDS often connotes, with unfortunate empirical evidence, the stigmatising effects that religious orthodoxies have perpetrated towards particular social groups on the basis of sexual behaviours or a person's HIV positive status.

But these are not the only markers of the history and current significance of religion and HIV and AIDS in Africa. Theologians were among the first to articulate the challenges that HIV and AIDS suffering poses for a new ethics of involvement with the real life implications of HIV and AIDS. Reverend Canon

Gideon Byamugisha, a Ugandan theologian, and, in 1992, the first religious leader in Africa to openly declare his HIV positive status, has been at the forefront of advancing human rights for individuals with HIV and AIDS. In conventional public health networks, the significance of his disclosure and subsequent formation of a continent-wide African Network of Religious Leaders Living With or Affected by HIV or AIDS (ANERELA), may be overlooked. Caring for AIDS 'widows' and 'orphans' is tremendously important and an activity many African churches have long undertaken. More recently, some church-run entities can be said to have 'scaled up' their responses to HIV and AIDS while national and international health agencies have 'scaled back'. The Shiselweni Reformed Church Home-Based Care organisation in Swaziland aims to address a host of HIV-related concerns, such as safe disclosure, ART uptake and adherence, and stigma reduction. By speaking constructively about HIV and AIDS in public and private settings, in biomedical and Christian terms, the group's 800 volunteer care givers are transforming HIV discourses and practices in ways that conventional biomedical approaches have not, and, arguably, could not.

However, to frame these observations as a religion versus science debate would be to miss the point entirely. The study of religion and HIV and AIDS shares with its clinical counterpart a concern for the human as well as the social body; for understanding the threats that may imperil each; and for mobilising the resources to protect both. Examining these intersections, this timely volume is essential, and inspiring, reading at a critical juncture when international agencies, national governments, local communities and academic-practitioners must do more with ever-dwindling material resources.

Abbreviations

AACC	All Africa Council of Churches
ABC	Abstain, Be faithful, Condomise
ACET	AIDS Care Education and Training
AEA	Association of Evangelicals in Africa
AIC	African Indigenous Church
AINA	Asian Inter-Faith Network on AIDS
AMAN	Asian Muslim Action Network
ANERELA	African Network of Religious Leaders Living With or Affected by HIV or AIDS
ANHERTHA	African Network of Higher Education and Research in Theology, HIV and AIDS
ARHAP	African Religious Health Assets Programme
ART	anti-retroviral treatment
ARV	anti-retroviral
ASEAN	Association of South East Asian Nations
ATR	African Traditional Religion
CAFOD	Catholic Agency for Overseas Development
CAPA	Council of Anglican Provinces of Africa
CCA	Christian Conference of Asia
CHART	Collaborative for HIV and AIDS, Religion and Theology
CIALIS	Comité Islamique des Actions de Lutte Contre le SIDA
CLAI	Latin American Council of Churches
CNCLS	Comité National Catholique de Lutte Contre le SIDA
CNELS	Comité National des Évangéliques pour la Lutte Contre le SIDA
CPE	clinical pastoral education
CRAN	Council of Religious AIDS Network
EAA	Ecumenical Advocacy Alliance
ECAP	ESSA Christian AIDS Programme

EFSA	Ecumenical Foundation in Southern Africa
EHAIA	Ecumenical HIV and AIDS Initiative in Africa
EKD	Evangelische Kirche in Deutschland
ELCAP	Evangelical Lutheran AIDS Programme
ELCRN	Evangelical Lutheran Church of the Republic of Namibia
EMS	Evangelisches Missionwerk Südwestdeutschland
EMW	Evangelisches Missionswerk in Deutschland
EPN	Ecumenical Pharmaceutical Network
ESEAT	Ecumenical Symposium of Eastern Africa Theologians
ESSA	Evangelical Seminary of Southern Africa
FACT	Family AIDS Caring Trust
FBO	faith-based organisation
FOCAGIFO	Friends of Canon Gideon Foundation
FOCCISA	Federation of Christian Churches in Southern Africa
GFATM	Global Fund to Fight HIV and AIDS, TB and Malaria
GNP+	Global Network of People Living With HIV
HAART	highly active anti-retroviral therapy
HEARD	Health Economics and HIV/AIDS Research Division
ICASA	International Conference on AIDS and Sexually-Transmitted Illnesses in Africa
IMAU	Islamic Medical Association of Uganda
INERELA	International Network of Religious Leaders Living With or Affected by HIV or AIDS
KABP	knowledge, attitudes, behaviour, practices
LGBTI	lesbian, gay, bisexual, transgender and inter-sex people
LUCSA	Lutheran Community in South Africa
LWF	Lutheran World Federation
MAP	Medical Assistance Program
MSF	Médecins Sans Frontières
NGO	non-governmental organisation
OAIC	Organisation of African Independent Churches
OVC	orphan and vulnerable children
PACSA	Pietermaritzburg Agency for Christian Social Awareness
PEP	post-exposure prophylaxis
PEPFAR	President's Emergency Program for AIDS Relief
PHC	primary health care

PLWAS	people living with AIDS
PMTCT	prevention of mother-to-child transmission
SACBC	Southern African Catholic Bishops' Conference
SAMS	Southern African Missiological Society
SAVE	Safer practices, Available medical and nutritional interventions, Voluntary but regular counselling and testing, Empowerment
SECAM	Symposium of Episcopal Conferences of Africa and Madagascar
SIM	Serving in Mission
SORAT	School of Religion and Theology, University of KwaZulu-Natal
STD	sexually-transmitted disease
STI	sexually-transmitted infection
UELCI	United Evangelical Lutheran Churches of India
UEM	United Evangelical Mission
UMG	Ugandan Martyrs Guild
UN	United Nations
UNAIDS	Joint United Nations Program on HIV and AIDS
UNDP	United Nations Development Programme
UNDPI	United Nations Department of Public Information
UNESCO	United Nations Education, Science and Cultural Organisation
UNICEF	United Nations Children's Fund
UNISA	University of South Africa
USAID	United States Agency for International Development
VCT	voluntary counselling and testing
WCC	World Council of Churches
WHO	World Health Organisation
WOFAK	Women Fighting AIDS in Kenya
YMCA	Young Men's Christian Association
YWCA	Young Women's Christian Association
ZINGO	Zambia Inter-Faith Networking Group in HIV and AIDS

Cartography of HIV and AIDS, Religion and Theology

An overview

Beverley Haddad

INTRODUCTION

Peter Piot, then executive director of the Joint United Nations Program on HIV and AIDS (UNAIDS), opened the Seventeenth International AIDS Conference in Mexico City on 3 August 2008 with these words:

> This conference takes place as we enter a new phase in confronting aids [*sic*]. A new phase because we now have results on a large scale. For the first time, fewer people are dying of aids and fewer people are becoming infected with HIV. For the first time we have empirical evidence that our brilliant coalition can move mountains. A unique and diverse coalition present here in this auditorium. This is cause for encouragement. But not cause for complacency, nor for declaring victory. Because the end of aids is nowhere in sight. Every day, almost three times as many people become newly infected with HIV as those who start taking antiretroviral treatment.[1]

Piot went on to argue that the coalition of people engaged in mitigating the epidemic needed to be broadened to ensure that all sectors of society were involved in 'combination prevention'.[2] This approach, which includes activists and academics from within the medical and social science fields, needs, says Piot, to take seriously localised epidemics that require specific contextual activities. In reminding the audience that the coalition of role players needed to be broadened, I as an activist-intellectual working in the field of religion and theology had no doubt that he meant to include religious leaders. Indeed, Piot identifies five reasons why religious organisations and faith communities have a role to play in the epidemic. Religion, he argues, continues to play a pivotal role in society and when there are crisis events such as the HIV epidemic, people look to religious leaders to 'explain what is happening, and to provide a framework for dealing with it'. Second, religious institutions have played an important educative role through centuries of history, meeting their constituencies once a week, 'a feat rarely attained by activists, academics, or politicians'. Third, suggests Piot, the HIV and AIDS epidemic raises issues related to disease as divine retribution or grace, sin, sexuality and taboos. Therefore, theologians 'need to ask what this means for their traditions, and what their traditions mean for AIDS'. Fourth, Piot asserts that 'forty percent of all AIDS care is provided by religious groups'. Last, many people living with HIV have strong religious beliefs and look to God and their faith community for support and comfort.[3] Piot's assertions are certainly true of the African continent.

It is for these reasons that religious role players are increasingly been drawn into multi-sectoral responses to HIV prevention by international agencies such as UNAIDS.[4] However, in Africa, coalitions are also necessary across the traditional divide of the academic and the activist, across divides of scholarly pursuit and the practice of actual work, to which Piot alluded. Such coalitions are necessary because in attempts to engage prevention of HIV and the mitigation of the impact of the epidemic, these divides are blurred. In a continent where 72 per cent of all AIDS-related deaths occur,[5] scholarly pursuit without actual engagement with the practice of working in affected communities is ethically untenable.

COLLABORATIVE FOR HIV AND AIDS, RELIGION AND THEOLOGY

It is for the above reason that the establishment of the Collaborative for HIV and AIDS, Religion and Theology (CHART) is of particular significance. CHART was founded in 2007 in the School of Religion and Theology (SORAT) at the University of KwaZulu-Natal by a small group of academics and practitioners.[6] Academics from a range of different religious and theological disciplines were already engaged in their own research and the supervision of postgraduate research in the interface between religion, theology and HIV. Much of this research was, and continues to be, carried out in conjunction with the community-based research centres and their field workers attached to SORAT, the Ujamaa Centre for Community Development and Research and the Sinomlando Centre for Oral History and Memory Work in Africa. The practitioners attached to these centres continue to benefit from the ongoing theological reflection on their work, while this symbiotic relationship means that research being conducted is ethically rooted in the lived experience of people with HIV.

CHART is an attempt to draw together academics and practitioners working in the field of HIV and AIDS, religion and theology, recognising that HIV and AIDS is a major public health crisis affecting society at large and impacting on faith communities. Importantly, its establishment is also recognition that because religious institutions and belief systems play both a positive and negative role in the impact of the epidemic, they must be drawn into collaboration with the other key role players. The epidemic, as Piot suggested, raises challenging issues such as sin, innocent suffering, exclusion, stigma and meaning and these are questions that call forth thoughtful theological reflection. The establishment of CHART, however, was also a response to the fact that despite the abundance of HIV- and AIDS-related faith documents, and the multiplication of databases, networks and forums, many policy makers and social scientists still do not understand the role that religious institutions and faith-based organisations play in the prevention of HIV and the mitigation of the epidemic.

CARTOGRAPHY OF HIV AND AIDS, RELIGION AND THEOLOGY PROJECT

To this end, a key project was initiated entitled the Cartography of HIV and AIDS, Religion and Theology. This project has sought first to compile a bibliographic database of published literature on the interface between religion, theology, HIV and AIDS. The bibliographic database is an ongoing project of CHART offered to researchers and activists via the worldwide web.[7] To date, it contains over 2 000 references and is partially annotated. A second aspect of the project is to analyse critically this body of work. This arose out of recognition that it is irresponsible to pursue research in this interface without assessing what has already been accomplished in different contexts and across an array of different religious disciplines. Future research needs can only be mapped from a realistic picture of existing research. To this end, researchers were recruited to survey and analyse various sub-sections within three major categories: religious and theological disciplines; health categories; and social categories. This framework was constructed heuristically as an attempt to investigate the intersection between religion and HIV and AIDS.

A third reason for the establishment of the project was to provide an opportunity to widen collaborative relationships and to form a coalition that straddled the academic-activist divide. In the religion and HIV project, it is the voices of those who are HIV positive, as well as those who work in communities, that need to be recovered and recognised in setting the agenda for any future research. In recognising this need, a research workshop was held in Durban in October 2008 to which academics and activists, and those who are openly living with HIV, were invited. The project also intentionally broadened the collaborative to include those from different contexts and continents. At the workshop, the researchers presented their analytical reflections with responses from activists and those living with HIV. The workshop thus provided the opportunity for the broad-based coalition within the religious network to which Piot alluded, as participants together shaped the discourse by their collaborative engagement. This book is a product of the project.

The chapters in this book presuppose the HIV epidemic to be a justice issue that is deeply political. Many of the authors demonstrate this political commitment through the careful and deliberate manner in which they frame HIV and AIDS discourse in their chapters and responses. UNAIDS has argued that because language shapes beliefs and may influence behaviours, considered use of appropriate language has the power to strengthen the response to HIV and AIDS.[8] It is with this understanding that the authors have adopted the guidelines offered by UNAIDS and in some instances made clear their deliberate use of terminology. Furthermore, while there are personal moral considerations in religious narratives that speak to the epidemic, these moral considerations need to take seriously its structural dimension.

In the analytical work of this book there was an attempt to be inclusive of all religions but there is an emphasis on Christianity and Islam as publications from these two major religions are more readily available. There is also a substantial focus on sub-Saharan Africa. Given the severity of HIV incidence in this part of the world, as well as the strongly religious dimension to life on the continent, it is not surprising that this is where the bulk of published work on the intersection between HIV and religion emanates. In exploring this intersection, it was also recognised that the published literature included in the bibliography is written from two perspectives: scholars of religion and theology; and medical and social scientists with an interest in religion. This became evident in the analysis of the literature.

There were many ways in which this book could have been constructed. As was indicated earlier, in conceptualising the project three major areas of intersection with HIV and AIDS were identified: religious and theological disciplines; health categories; and social categories. In the early stages of the project these three categories were each then sub-divided into five sub-sections. Initially, within the religious and theological disciplines the areas identified were biblical and other sacred texts; religious history; systematic theology; practical theology; and comparative ethics. Later, missiology was added to this framework. The health category was sub-divided into areas of prevention; treatment; care and support; stigma and discrimination; and cultural practices. The social category was sub-divided into areas of poverty; gender violence and masculinities; migration; orphaned and vulnerable children; and policy and public discourse. This framework was constructed heuristically as an attempt to investigate the intersection between religion and HIV and AIDS.

Of the sub-categories identified, the areas of practical theology, treatment, poverty and migration were not specifically addressed in formal presentations at the workshop. Through deliberations at the workshop, the additional areas of sexuality and spirituality were identified as major omissions in the project. A decision was taken to sub-divide the area of policy and public discourse into first, a chapter on how religion has engaged with policy and practice in the area of medicine and health; and second, a chapter highlighting the public statements made on HIV and AIDS by religious leaders. The issue of treatment, it was decided, would be included in the first chapter on policy and practice in the area of religion and medicine. Practical theology would be addressed in the chapter and response on care and support of people living with HIV. Thus the process of the workshop itself has contributed to the shaping of this book.

While other books, such as the *Encyclopedia of AIDS*,[9] deal with each of the major religions in turn, this one attempts to include the major religions in the analysis of each contribution. However, during workshop discussions, African Traditional Religion (ATR) was seen to be an exception as much of the practice of these religions is based on oral tradition rather than on sacred texts. Thus, a decision was taken to include a specific chapter on ATR that would complement those on culture and gender, and on masculinities.

SHAPE AND CONTENT OF THIS BOOK

This book includes analytical contributions by researchers, many of whom themselves straddle the academic-practitioner divide, and responses to them by practitioners, many of whom are also researchers. This unique format offers a comprehensive analytical survey of existing literature in particular religious areas of the interface with HIV which, importantly, have been shaped through dialogue with practitioners. The book concludes with the stories of four participants in the project who are living with HIV as a deliberate attempt to foreground their voices in this coalition.

Taking into account the discussions at the research workshop, the analytical survey work of this book has been divided into four parts. Part 1 consists of four chapters with responses that offer overviews of religious responses to the HIV and AIDS epidemic, including engagement with other key public and policy stakeholders. The first chapter, by Jill Olivier and Gillian Paterson, focuses on the intersection of the medical narrative with that of religion. It offers a brief overview of the history of religion-inspired medical responses to the epidemic before suggesting a theological and ethical rationale that religions claim for their medical work. The chapter continues by analysing the strengths and weaknesses of the involvement of religious sectors in prevention, care and support, and treatment; briefly explores the narratives on miraculous cures; and concludes by identifying the gaps in the literature survey and possible future work. It argues that there is insufficient 'nuanced work that acknowledges the differences in religion, or that compares religious and non-religious activities and organisations in the context of the HIV epidemic'. In responding to this chapter, Greg Manning, amongst other things, reminds the reader of the importance of the role of religious institutions in holding other stakeholders, such as government and health professionals, accountable for their actions in the epidemic. However, he also asserts that this multi-sectoral accountability needs to work hand in hand with multi-sectoral affirmation. This suggests that religious institutions need to be willing to take seriously the critique of their actions in the health sector by other stakeholders.

The second chapter in Part 1, by Philippe Denis, echoes some of the work of Olivier and Paterson but focuses on the history of the religious response to the epidemic more specifically in sub-Saharan Africa. He argues that religious discourses 'add meaning to the epidemic and mediate the prevention messaging'. Importantly, Denis shows how this discourse is not homogenous and suggests that the history of how religious institutions have dealt with the issue of sexuality, a key aspect of prevention messaging, is yet to be written. Denis also identifies studies that deal with the question of religious affiliation and HIV transmission and concludes that while religious affiliation might lead to behaviour change, much seems to depend on 'socialisation, religious experience, indoctrination and exclusion', all of which will vary over time within each religious grouping. The chapter also addresses the dilemmas of prevention faced by religious institutions, including the debate on the use of condoms and their historical role in treatment and care. Alison Munro, the respondent, identifies a number of key points made by Denis. These include questions about how little attention has been paid to the epidemic as a historical phenomenon; how religious institutions are defined and how religious beliefs and practices shape societal understanding of the epidemic; and the role of those beliefs and practices in the prevention and care efforts of religious institutions.

Jill Olivier's chapter, the third of Part 1, discusses how religious institutions are engaged in international policy on HIV and AIDS. By means of a brief history of the international policy context she shows how, initially, international health organisations were blind to religious institutions and how this attitude changed. In this critical discussion, Olivier helpfully addresses the ambiguous and shifting nature of the relationship between policy makers and religious institutions. She concludes the chapter by pointing out a way forward for future research. The potential assets of religion and religious institutions are an under-researched area, suggests Olivier, and there is a need for a far more nuanced and complex understanding of the religious sector. Bongi Zengele, in responding to Olivier, reminds readers that all too often policies are developed in arenas far from the lived experience of the HIV positive person. For HIV and AIDS policies to be meaningful there is a need for far greater involvement with those most affected by the epidemic. Zengele also suggests that while international policy makers need to draw on the assets of religious institutions, they also need to ensure that the policies in place hold the religious sector accountable for those of its practices and attitudes that are harmful to HIV positive people.

The final chapter in Part 1 is by Martha Frederiks. She analyses written public statements made by religious leaders and organisations, particularly as they pertain to the African context. The chapter begins by discussing statements made by international religious organisations residing outside the African context and attempts to document the regions from which these come. Through this analysis she shows that there are few statements emanating from the Middle East, western and central Europe, and North America. In discussing statements that emanate from Africa, she notes that the paucity of statements from within specific African contexts does not necessarily reflect the substantive activities that are taking place within religious institutions on the ground. Frederiks also tracks the shift in attitude from a focus on promiscuity with strong moral overtones in earlier statements, to a focus on the need for fidelity and abstinence. She also asserts that the prevailing discourses in these statements are those of morality, war and hope. Her chapter concludes by noting that public religious responses were slow in forthcoming in the early stages of the epidemic. Those that have since been made show little evidence of inter-faith collaboration. Therefore, there is a need for further research on the extent and nature of local inter-faith initiatives that address HIV and AIDS. In responding to Frederiks' chapter, Paula Clifford notes that 'the statements imply a practice that is far from being achieved'. Having said this, she asserts that it can and does happen that activities at a community level are often in advance of any official formulation by religious leaders. Therefore, she suggests that any assessment of the effectiveness of the response of religious organisations to HIV and AIDS cannot rely on an analysis of these statements alone but has to include the practical activities of faith communities at a local level.

Part 2 of this book includes four chapters and responses that focus on the intersection with HIV of religious and theological disciplines. The first chapter in this section is by Gerald West on sacred texts, particularly the Bible and the Qur'an. West, in this comprehensive analytical survey, argues that most religions embrace a theology of retribution undergirded by their sacred texts. In an attempt to counter this tradition, West then identifies in the literature what he terms redemptive readings of sacred texts within the HIV and AIDS context. Arguing for sacred texts as 'reservoirs of redemptive categories and concepts', West engages with a number of scholars from various religious traditions that use sacred texts in this precise way. He then goes on to demonstrate the way in which sacred texts have been appropriated and read both by people who are HIV positive and by scholars who read in solidarity with those living with HIV. The chapter concludes by showing that across religions there are signs of an emerging HIV hermeneutic that, while it differs from case to case, is generally inclusive and compassionate. Monica Jyotsna Melanchthon responds to West's chapter, affirming much of his analysis. She suggests that responses to HIV and AIDS often depend on the way in which the primacy and authority of the sacred text is understood to be binding on a faith community. Arguing for the need for religious pluralism, she suggests that 'the Bible no longer holds a privileged or pre-eminent place in a multi-scriptural society'. It is essential, therefore, that theologians take into account, in a range of contexts, 'the many sacred texts that have come to claim the allegiance of people in our world'.

Steve de Gruchy focuses the second chapter in Part 2 on the interface between HIV and systematic theology, particularly from within the Christian tradition. He argues that the very nature of the epidemic demands theological reflection and suggests that a variety of theological themes requiring clarity emerge out of the faith practices and responses to HIV by religious communities. These include stigma and discrimination, disease and healing, sexuality, gender issues, and questions of denial and responsibility. However, he notes that not only are theologians addressing these questions emerging from the epidemic, but the epidemic is forcing a shift in theological loci. In effect, HIV and AIDS are contributing to a new way of doing theology, particularly in Africa. Questions of suffering, hope, life and death, justice, and the nature of the church have become central to this emerging theological reflection on HIV and AIDS. De Gruchy further argues that this in turn has required that new models of education are necessary to ensure the efficacy of this theological work. In concluding, he notes a number of gaps, a key issue being how to bridge the theological work undertaken by those living with HIV and work being undertaken by scholars in the academy. He also notes the need for greater inter-religious dialogue at a theological level, including the discipline of ATR. The chapter concludes by suggesting that there are a number of themes that have received scant theological attention, namely sin, salvation, redemption and liberation. In responding, Jan Bjarne Sødal suggests that an overarching theme needing further discussion is that of human anthropology. He argues that whether we are dealing with the theological themes of suffering or sexuality, what is important is how we relate these issues to human life.

The third chapter in Part 2 is by Domoka Lucinda Manda. She discusses the early religious ethical discourse on HIV and AIDS, which focused almost solely on sexual morality and ethics. This discourse identified HIV infection as a result of sexual promiscuity and as a punishment from God. However, increasingly, she argues, there is a shift from this moralising discourse to a discourse that embraces an ethic of life. This shift embraces a sexual ethic that focuses on the goodness of sex and an emphasis on life in its fullness. Feminist ethics is shown to be an important aspect of this discussion along with an increasing focus in the literature on an ethic of community, care and compassion. However, Manda also demonstrates that the literature is beginning to move beyond this emphasis on care and compassion to questions of justice, although most of this ethical debate is taking place within Christianity and Islam, with little real engagement from other religions. In conclusion, she argues that 'there has been almost no reflection on our moral obligation to those who are HIV positive, nor on how those living with HIV are ethically engaging the epidemic'. This is an area that requires further research. Farid Esack responds to Manda's chapter specifically from a Muslim perspective. He argues that the Muslim response to HIV and AIDS can be characterised in the literature as following a trajectory of first, ignorance, indifference and silence; followed, second, by scorn; and third, by pity. However, we need to move to a trajectory of compassion, argues Esack. It is this compassion, embedded in an ethic of justice, which takes seriously relations of power. Esack, one of the key proponents of an ethic of compassion and justice, argues that religion does not, however, have an exclusive role in the epidemic: 'the path of exclusive options, either scientific or religious interventions, is long since discredited. Only a multi-faceted approach to disease and wellness that incorporates both personal transformation and socio-economic justice will offer humankind some hope in the face of this crisis, as well as future ones.'

Ute Hedrich's is the final chapter in Part 2. She suggests that the HIV and AIDS epidemic has posed new challenges to the field of missiology that offer 'a focal point for any new and further development of contextual understandings of missiology, including inter-faith perspectives'. While not focusing specifically on these inter-faith perspectives, she nonetheless shows that the Christian enterprise of mission has embraced the challenges of HIV and AIDS. This has been accomplished not so much through published literature but through conferences and gatherings of missiologists and mission agencies, including a series of study processes related to the epidemic and to mission agency policy. Hedrich argues that one of the gaps in the published literature is a lack of analysis of 'the different missiological traditions and influences that have led to the present understanding of sexuality and moral discourse as a response to the HIV epidemic'. In his response, Benson Okyere-Manu indicates a number of further processes that have been undertaken in the African context. He argues for their importance but suggests that there is a need for greater engagement with people living with HIV in order to break the conspiracy of silence that still persists.

Part 3 of the book includes four chapters and responses that address women, men and children within the African cultural context. To provide a specific analysis of this religio-cultural context, the opening chapter deals with ATR. Ezra Chitando shows how the literature has addressed the question of harmful cultural practices including, among others, polygyny, widow cleansing and hospitality.

Chitando also discusses aspects of the African world view that pose a challenge to the HIV and AIDS issue. They include fertility, dangerous masculinities, traditional healers and leaders, and witchcraft. There is, however, an emerging discourse, he argues, that suggests there are positive resources within ATR that can be drawn upon in the response to HIV and AIDS. Chitando concludes his contribution by identifying the gaps in the literature that require further research. These include the impact of HIV on African beliefs and practices such as death and dying, the emerging evidence for male circumcision as a prevention strategy, and an analysis of the ideological persuasions of authors publishing on HIV and ATR. Phumzile Zondi-Mabizela in her response indicates how important it was for her as a Christian Zulu woman living with HIV to reclaim her 'indigenous religious beliefs as part of the journey towards wholeness and healing'. Zondi-Mabizela provides an apologetic for cultural practices in the context of HIV and suggests additional cultural resources that could be used to mitigate the epidemic.

Nyokabi Kamau in her chapter helpfully discusses gendered cultural practices amidst poverty. She shows the strong emphasis in the literature on issues of sexuality and how they pervade the HIV and AIDS discourse in the African context. Cultural practices that have close associations with sexuality, such as puberty rites, are contested and need further discussion. In addition, suggests Kamau, 'the discourse of shame and blame as it pertains to religion and culture requires further research. While there is a growing body of literature, it remains an area of greatest challenge in the African continent and needs ongoing and sustained inquiry.' In responding to Kamau, Ezra Chitando reminds readers of two further points: that cultures are not static but dynamic; and that in the religious context of HIV in Africa there exists a deadly cocktail of sacred biblical tradition and culture that all too often reinforces harmful practices, particularly for women.

Adriaan van Klinken engages with the debate on gendered cultural practices. He does so, however, from the particular perspective of masculinity studies and discusses how men and masculinities in the context of HIV and AIDS are analysed and reflected upon from the religious perspective. In this discussion, he identifies three areas of focus: sexual decision making; sexual violence; and male sexuality, fertility and power. In addition, he addresses the literature that discusses the interface of religion and patriarchal masculinities. Arguing that hegemonic masculinities are increasingly being contested in the HIV and AIDS context, he shows how there is a growing body of work that suggests religious resources for their transformation. But, as Van Klinken shows, there is little emphasis in the literature on how this transformation can occur practically. He concludes his analysis by suggesting that all too often men are presented in the literature as 'one monolithic bloc dominating women and spreading HIV', and that this essentialising discourse does not take into account the plurality of masculinities. Furthermore, the emphasis on gender equality in the literature means 'that not much attention is paid to gender difference in the proposals to redefine masculinity'. In some contexts, Van Klinken argues, this may be a problem 'because in many cultural-religious constructions of masculinity and femininity, the biological differences between the sexes are marked by symbolic meanings that have social implications' and therefore cannot be ignored. There is thus a need for further reflection on 'how gender difference can be marked symbolically and socially in a way that promotes the values of solidarity, mutuality and companionship and leads to gender justice'. In responding to Van Klinken's chapter, Lilian Siwila concurs that the 'idea of engaging men in addressing the epidemic has meant a paradigm shift to a more holistic approach that does not simply see men as perpetrators but also as partners in mitigating HIV'. She suggests that men need to be engaged through sensitive readings of the sacred texts that offer more redemptive readings of hegemonic masculinities and enable men to be brought into the dialogue in a way that embraces their particular experiences.

The final chapter in Part 3 of the book focuses on children and is authored by Genevieve James. She argues for the importance of children as a sub-category in the discourse because of their marginalised status in the literature. She identifies a number of studies that focus on children and shows the varieties of methodology employed to address the challenges confronting children in the HIV and AIDS context. A key sub-theme in the literature is a focus on factors that render children vulnerable to HIV infection. These include violence and abuse, poverty and ways in which religious practice involving children is abusive and renders them vulnerable. James also shows the substantive body of literature that identifies the way in which children affected by the HIV and AIDS epidemic are being cared for through the services of religious organisations, and the positive theological reflection on children that motivates this work. In conclusion, James argues that in any further research, 'children should not be considered as a monolithic entity since they live within various cultural, religious, ethnic, geographical, political and socio-economic contexts'. Studies need to focus on particularities and also assess how HIV educational campaigns deal with the increasing rise of consumerism and its impact on children in various communities. Responding to the chapter by James, Bongi Zengele argues that the paucity of literature on children and HIV written from a religious and theological perspective indicates the neglect of children that she has witnessed in her experience as an activist and practitioner. She argues that all too often it is assumed, even in the religious community, that children will be cared for by the extended family when parents die. However, given the magnitude of the HIV crisis and the context of poverty, this is not always the case. As a result, children are often faced with neglect and various forms of abuse. There is, therefore, a need to strengthen aspects of theological education for religious leaders to include a greater emphasis on pastoral skills in working with children.

Part 4, the final section of this book, focuses on those who are HIV positive. It includes three chapters and responses on prevention, stigma, and care and support. The final chapter includes the personal stories of four participants at the research workshop who are HIV positive: Phumzile Zondi-Mabizela, Nokuthula Biyela, Faghmeda Miller and Johannes Petrus Mokgethi-Heath. It was decided to conclude with these stories, in what is otherwise a scholarly volume, as a reminder to practitioners and scholars alike that none of our scholarly pursuits or practical work can be carried out without engaging those for whom the HIV and AIDS epidemic has had the most impact.

The first chapter in Part 4 is by Greg Manning and he frames the analysis of literature on the interface of religion and HIV, using seven principles of prevention identified by UNAIDS.[10] He shows the complexity of the response of the religious sector to prevention efforts. Manning argues that religious and theological interaction with the framework suggests that 'theological input into the maturing of HIV prevention efforts needs to be well established in relationship with people who are demanding better approaches than that already available to them'. Furthermore, religious and theological efforts 'also need to be committed to supporting claims about HIV prevention with regular evaluation of the effectiveness of these claims'. Johannes Petrus Mokgethi-Heath in his response shows the inadequacies of the 'Abstain, Be faithful, Condomise' (ABC) prevention message. He outlines an alternative approach, 'Safer practices, Available medical interventions, Voluntary counselling and testing, and Empowerment' (SAVE) that deals with the complexities of the epidemic in a more holistic way.

The second chapter of Part 4, by Gillian Paterson, begins by mapping the history of the stigmatising discourse associated with the HIV and AIDS epidemic.

She argues that a vast body of work has emerged within the social sciences that conceptualises stigma and there is still a need for religious scholarship to engage with this work more comprehensively. Paterson identifies a number of recurring themes within the literature on HIV stigma from a religious and theological perspective. These themes include questions of truth and othering discourse, sex and sexuality, the human body, and economic and social marginalisation. She concludes by suggesting a number of areas that require further research. These include the 'need for an educated, inter-disciplinary conceptualisation of stigma'; multi-faceted research on personal experiences of stigma 'that offer a denser and more nuanced' understanding of situations of stigmatisation; a focus on the 'divisions that exist between specifically theological discourses'; what it means to be a compassionate community; and, most importantly, engagement with those living with HIV about the stigma they experience. In responding to Paterson's chapter, Gideon Byagumisha suggests four types of stigma that religious scholars need to understand better. These include, first, the individual, family and community fear of contagion that results in ostracism and rejection of the person who is HIV positive and can even lead to legislation that criminalises HIV infection; second, individual, family and community fear of death, which is intimately tied to religious values and belief systems; third, the individual, family and community connection of HIV with immorality and promiscuity that persists despite the number of studies that show the epidemic is also fuelled by a range of factors not directly related to issues of sexuality; and last, studies are necessary to address the question why being on anti-retroviral (ARV) medication is seen to be a sign of no faith in a God who heals.

Jill Olivier and Paula Clifford in their chapter analyse the body of literature that focuses on care and support of those who are HIV positive by the religious community. They maintain that much of this work takes place spontaneously at a community level and, it is often argued, is where religious organisations are most effective. But paradoxically, argue Olivier and Clifford, it is the area 'about which we know the least'. Having said this, the chapter then discusses the ethos of care that drives religious organisations; issues facing care givers at a community level; and finally the scope, scale and focus of care. The chapter concludes with a section on the special care offered by the religious response to HIV and AIDS. This tends to be holistic as it includes tangible assets such as material support as well as the intangible, which include faith, prayer and hope. In response, Edwina Ward suggests that a process such as clinical pastoral education enables the training of carers and pastoral workers to offer appropriate care and support. She also argues that too many of those involved in care giving work are volunteers and further research is needed to understand better their religious motivation to continue this work without remuneration. Ward concludes that the areas of spiritual care and the 'need for understanding of religious and cultural rituals' should be further developed to enhance the religious community care and support of those living with HIV.

AREAS IDENTIFIED FOR A FUTURE RESEARCH AGENDA

The Cartography of HIV and AIDS, Religion and Theology is an ambitious project. In seeking to map the published resources on the interface between religion and HIV and then carry out an analytical survey of this exercise there will, inevitably, be some who feel that large bodies of work have been neglected. This may well be true. A number of the authors of this book have indicated their awareness that the survey they have conducted has focused on texts that are written in English and the project still has to find ways of overcoming the obstacles to engaging with literature not written in the dominant language of the globalised world. Furthermore, many authors have also indicated their awareness that their survey has been dominated by Christian literature and literature from within the African context. It is this body of literature that is by far the largest and most accessible when dealing with the interface between religion and HIV. Again, this project needs to keep developing links across continents and religious backgrounds to give shape to a more comprehensive analysis of the role religion plays in the HIV and AIDS epidemic. This is particularly true as the epidemic grows outside Africa.

In attempting to summarise the areas needing further work from the analytical discussions of the authors of this book, a number of key themes emerge. It is not necessarily a comprehensive summary of each area identified but it is an attempt to identify broad trajectories of research that lie ahead as this project is taken further.

Need for greater inter-faith collaboration

An area that needs much greater attention in the response to HIV and AIDS is that of inter-faith collaborative efforts. Frederiks notes that there are almost no examples of inter-religious public statements. She goes on to add that there is a need for further research 'to explore whether there are local collaborative initiatives between Christians and Muslims and, if so, what forms these initiatives have taken'. West too asserts that 'more intentionally inter-faith work needs to be done in seeking to understand across faith communities how sacred texts function in constructing and deconstructing theologies of retribution'. Echoing these sentiments, De Gruchy suggests that from his analysis 'it is intriguing to see how little Christian theological reflection is done in dialogue with other major religious traditions'. This is no more obvious than in the missiological enterprise, which has focused little on an inter-faith component in the African context. So, Hedrich concludes her chapter by suggesting that 'scholars from Islam, Judaism, Hindusim, and African Traditional Religion should be communicating their various perspectives and missiological challenges. It is also necessary that in this inter-religious dialogue, questions of health, healing and sexuality be explored more fully.'

Need for greater focus on particularities of context and groupings

While there has been a particular focus on Africa in this book, much of the analytical work of the project has demonstrated the need for an even greater focus on particularities of contexts (within and outside Africa) and on particularities of groupings. This is true at a number of different levels. Frederiks has argued that questions of gender, poverty and culture need to be particularised in contexts rather than generalising their influence on the HIV and AIDS epidemic. Van Klinken has similarly argued that often 'men are represented as one monolithic bloc dominating women and spreading HIV'. He suggests that this essentialist discourse is unhelpful and there is a need for research to take into account 'the plurality of masculinities that are found in social, cultural and religious contexts'. Likewise, Kamau has identified the area of women's sexuality and James the area of children as categories that need to be particularised in the cultural and religious context. These authors argue that focusing on particularities of contexts and groupings will offer better programmatic and policy frameworks in response to the epidemic. However, particularising groupings and contexts is insufficient, suggests Chitando. There is also a need to conduct 'a more probing analysis of the various ideological categories of authors who have published on the intersection of these religions with the epidemic'. He argues that in the case of ATR, and even Islam, there are instances where discourses of religion and HIV have been framed 'against the backdrop of the idea of Western cultural imperialism' and there is therefore a need to defend religious traditions 'against images of backwardness and increasing vulnerability to HIV'. Paterson concurs and suggests that in 'the work that has been done on public discourses, little has been written about the divisions that exist between specifically theological discourses or the selective use of demographics to support particular discourses such as those of agency and of vulnerability'. She contends that there are negative cross currents existing within the religious community because of differing approaches to the response to HIV and AIDS between liberals and conservatives. There is, therefore, 'a need for small studies that enable reflection in rational and non-polemical ways about the cause and effect of differences that have their origin in clashes of discourse'.

Need for greater engagement with those living with HIV
Manda, in addressing the moral response of the religious community to the epidemic, has suggested that there has been 'almost no reflection on our moral obligation to those who are HIV positive, nor on how those living with HIV are ethically engaging the epidemic'. This sentiment is echoed in a variety of ways by a number of authors. Kamau believes that the discourse of shame and blame as it pertains to religion and culture 'remains an area of greatest challenge in the African continent and needs ongoing and sustained inquiry'. In discussing stigma, Paterson suggests that 'considerable rhetoric is expended on the need to engage with vulnerable and marginalised groups. However, there is little actual engagement with these groups in studies on stigma. Greater understanding is needed of the reasons, structural as well as religious, why religious groups find this so difficult.' Okyere-Manu suggests that the silence surrounding the epidemic will only be broken as people living with HIV are engaged to understand better the challenges with which they are contending. Zengele argues that this community engagement with HIV positive people, including children, is crucial to policy development. She suggests that further work is needed to bridge the gap between HIV policies and the people whose lives are greatly impacted by them.

Need for better understanding of the intangible assets of religion
Engaging people living with HIV in future research opens up the possibility of better understanding of what Olivier and Paterson speak about as the intangible assets of religion. They argue that this added value of religion is 'an area that is critically lacking in sensitive, in-depth research or theological reflection. This is accompanied by a critical lack of literature on how these intangible assets can be measured in order for them to move beyond the anecdotal and be recognised by

public health professionals and policy makers.' This includes building resilience in communities, offering support and hope, and the role religious organisations play 'in the intervention in public and private grief, for example, by providing mourning rituals'. In addition, Ward has called for a better understanding of spiritual care and the role that religious rituals play in support. Within the African context, ATR offers a range of religio-cultural resources that could be transformative of behaviours that contribute to the spread of HIV. Most noted is the African philosophy of *ubuntu*, which stresses the communal over the individual and is theorised with the field of comparative ethics (Manda), ATR (Chitando) and in transforming masculinities (Van Klinken). Zondi has further argued that 'there is still work to be done in reviewing, reclaiming and reviving some of the beliefs and teachings of ATRs, which could be positive resources in mitigating the HIV and AIDS epidemic'. Kamau develops this argument further by suggesting that there 'is a need to develop frameworks that can help us to understand and appreciate culture and tradition, yet are able to acknowledge the contested nature of its practice'.

Need for deeper theological reflection

In carrying out this task it is critical that the internal logic of belief systems within a particular symbolic universe or world view, and how they interact with HIV and AIDS, is understood. This is necessary for analysis of controversial debates such as that on miraculous cures and healing. Olivier and Paterson have shown that there is very limited research on this critical aspect of the intersection of religion and medicine. They argue that there is some literature that 'demonstrates cases where religious beliefs conflict with recommendations of health care providers in the treatment and care of people living with HIV'. Clearly there is a need for what Manning calls 'an accelerated process of evaluation of applied theologies in the context of HIV and AIDS'. Others have identified additional specific areas where deeper theological engagement is necessary, including policy (Olivier), discourse that has up until now focused on morality, war and hope (Frederiks), questions of death and dying (Chitando), resilience in children (Zengele), stigma as a theological concept (Paterson) and gender justice (Van Klinken). Not only should theological engagement become more sustained but it should be more systematic in its approach to the epidemic. De Gruchy has shown that while theologians have offered an insight or two on the epidemic, they then move on, 'leaving a rather chaotic theological patchwork'. He suggests that in future work it will be necessary 'for theologians to identify the key research frontiers and engage in sustained and systematic reflection, even if the content of this reflection speaks to dislocation and fragmentation'. De Gruchy also points to 'the ways in which [the epidemic] is calling forth entire new ways of doing theology, or even of conceiving of the theological task'. Similarly, West suggests that 'there is clear evidence that HIV and AIDS . . . is changing the theological landscape so significantly that sacred texts are being called to address this disease complex in ways that may alter how they are interpreted by religious communities'. But what has not taken place, De Gruchy argues, has been the sustained theological engagement between people living with HIV in community settings and scholars theologising in the academy.

Need to focus on the relationship between the religious and non-religious sectors

Olivier and Paterson, in their discussion on religion and medicine, argue that 'there is not enough nuanced work that acknowledges the differences in religion, or that compares religious and non-religious activities and organisations in the context of the HIV epidemic'. Manning has suggested that communication about HIV is related to the practice of evaluation and priority setting, in which all actors, be they state, commercial, community, professional, religious or academic, are accountable to each other for their words and actions. In his analysis of the religious sector in the prevention of HIV, he suggests that while there is descriptive work already carried out that identifies the roles played by this sector, this research 'does not establish these identified roles in relationship to other sectors of society'. He also argues that further work needs to be carried out to evaluate the claims made by the religious sector regarding the effectiveness of their prevention efforts in relation to other sectors. Olivier suggests that part of reaching an understanding of the efficacy of the religious response will only emerge once there is a better understanding of this sector by other stakeholders. Furthermore, she argues that there are 'few studies that contain content or process analyses of international and national HIV and AIDS policies addressing the role of religion and religious organisations; and this remains a critical area for future investigation'. Little is yet known about the varieties of religious assets or religious organisations and the work they do and even less about how these intersect with HIV and AIDS policy issues such as financing or economic impact. Therefore, there is a need for a 'comparative audit of HIV and AIDS policies; and how religion is addressed in different countries and on different policy issues'.

CONCLUSION

The role of religion, religious leaders and religious organisations in the epidemic has been contested within the scholarly discourse. This contestation is taken up by religious scholars themselves and by those outside the disciplines of religion and theology who have an interest in the role that religion plays in the HIV and AIDS epidemic. Clearly, as many of the chapters in this book attest, understanding the detailed nature of the role of religion still requires more nuanced investigation. Historians such as Denis argue in this book:

> By and large, the practice of religious institutions with regard to HIV and the manner in which the epidemic affected their operations and their identity remains undocumented. The task to be accomplished is enormous. Religious leaders, pastoral agents, workers in non-governmental organisations (NGOs) and ordinary believers involved in curbing the epidemic have to be interviewed, and minutes of meetings, annual reports, policy documents, sermon outlines and pamphlets produced in relation to HIV and AIDS, collected and analysed. It is only when this documentation is fully available, that a comprehensive history of HIV and AIDS and religion can be written.

That religion and religious actors play a crucial role in mitigating the HIV and AIDS epidemic is not contested. The nature of this role and the influence of religious beliefs and practices continue to be a source of ongoing study as the CHART cartography project so aptly demonstrates. What is of particular significance for this project is the growing body of work that focuses on the interface of religion and HIV by scholars outside religious and theological disciplines.

A significant recent contribution from within anthropological studies is a volume edited by Felicitas Becker and P. Wenzel Geissler. Contributors to it seek to understand 'religious commitment and practice as part of everyday life'.[11] Becker and Geissler, in their introduction, argue that religion is 'bound up with the wider experience of suffering within which the epidemic is set, and with other non-religious narratives and practices through which people address the experience of HIV/AIDS'.[12] That religious experience is bound up with the broader socio-cultural context has been undeniably revealed through the HIV and AIDS epidemic; and this has brought religion more firmly on to the agenda of the social sciences. This is also demonstrated and documented in a special issue of *Africa Today*. The editors suggest that Christianity 'is becoming one of the most influential factors in the engagement of AIDS in some African countries'.[13]

In addition, there are several extensive studies that include a specific section on the role of religion or religious leaders in the epidemic. Using a social theory lens, a collection edited by Jean Baxen and Anders Breidlid explores not only the cultural and contextual practices within the epidemic, but also the methodological and epistemological orientation in HIV education. Included in this task is an investigation into the role played by religious leaders and traditional healers.[14] In a more focused study of women's vulnerabilities to HIV and AIDS, Linda Fuller devotes a section to the ambiguous role that religion plays in the lives of African women vulnerable to HIV and indicates the growing body of work exploring this intersection.[15] The central role played by religion in the lives of those who are HIV positive is again demonstrated by Corinne Squire, who includes a chapter on religious and moral narratives in her volume.[16] Personal accounts of religious experiences are presented in narrative form. They show poignantly how the non-religious is bound up with the religious in what Becker and Geissler term popular epidemiologies. That those who are HIV positive regard religious practice as part of everyday practice leaves those of us in the academy no choice but to engage directly with this voice and with each other in inter-faith and inter-disciplinary collaboration.

By intentionally combining a range of voices in a collaborative cartographic project our book provides resources for this task. It is the beginning of a process that takes us, collaboratively, further into uncharted terrain and provides a map to guide us.

NOTES

1. Peter Piot, 'Don't give up the fight'. Speech at the opening of the Seventeenth International AIDS Conference, Mexico City, 3 Aug. 2008. Available at http://www.data.unaids.org/pub/SpeechEXD/2008/20080803_sp_piot_en.pdf (accessed 14 Dec. 2009).
2. Combination prevention refers to an approach that embraces role players from all sectors of society and moves beyond a narrow focus on biomedical preventative measures.
3. Peter Piot, 'Foreword' in *Islam and AIDS: Between Scorn, Pity and Justice*, edited by Farid Esack and Sarah Chiddy (Oxford: Oneworld, 2009): xi–xii.
4. See Beverley Haddad, Jill Olivier and Steve de Gruchy, *The Potential and Perils of Partnership: Christian Religious Entities and Collaborative Stakeholders Responding to HIV and AIDS in Kenya, Malawi and the DRC* (Cape Town: African Religious Health Assets Programme, 2008).

5. UNAIDS, 'AIDS epidemic update'. Available at http://www.data.unaids.org/pub/Report/2009/2009_epidemic_update_en.pdf (accessed 14 Dec. 2009).

6. For more information, see the CHART website http://www.chart.ukzn.ac.za.

7. This bibliographic database is available on the CHART website www.chart.ukzn.ac.za. Many of the chapters in this volume refer directly to the contents of this database in the analytical survey work carried out by their authors.

8. UNAIDS, 'UNAIDS editors notes for authors'. Available at http://www.amicaall.org/publications/UNAIDSEditors%20Notes_060825.pdf (accessed 14 Dec. 2009).

9. Raymond A. Smith, *Encyclopedia of AIDS: A Social, Political, Cultural and Scientific Record of the HIV Epidemic* (London: Penguin, 2001).

10. UNAIDS, 'Intensifying HIV prevention: UNAIDS policy position paper' (2005). Available at http://www.data.unaids.org/publications/irc-pub06/jc1165-intensif_hiv-newstyle_en.pdf (accessed 19 Dec. 2009).

11. Felicitas Becker and P. Wenzel Geissler (eds), *Aids and Religious Practice in Africa* (Leiden: Brill, 2009): 2.

12. Becker and Geissler, *Aids and Religious Practice in Africa*: 3.

13. Ruth Prince, Philippe Denis and Rijk van Dijk, 'Engaging Christianities: Negotiating HIV/AIDS, health, and social relations in east and southern Africa'. *Africa Today* 54(1) 2009: v.

14. Aysha Hattas, 'Examining religious leaders' and traditional healers' responses to HIV/AIDS in a modern community' in *HIV/AIDS in Sub-Saharan Africa: Understanding the Implications of Culture and Context*, edited by Jean Baxen and Anders Breidlid (Cape Town: University of Cape Town Press, 2009): 47–59.

15. Linda K. Fuller, *African Women's Unique Vulnerabilities to HIV/AIDS: Communication Perspectives and Promises* (New York: Palgrave Macmillan, 2008): 81–7.

16. Corrine Squire, *HIV in South Africa: Talking About the Big Thing* (London: Routledge, 2007).

PART 1

Engaging the public realm

1

Religion and medicine
in the context of HIV and AIDS
A landscaping review

Jill Olivier and Gillian Paterson

INTRODUCTION

This chapter was conceived as a review of the literature on religion, health and healing in relation to HIV and AIDS. It proved to be an impossibly wide brief. Whenever we thought we had identified a core agenda for a discussion of health and healing, we found it fragmenting into a dozen different parts. This was appropriate since an integrated, holistic understanding of healing must have, among its building blocks, issues such as stigma, poverty, culture, sex and gender. Indeed, all the topics listed in the contents page of this book are related, in one way or another, to the healing of individuals, institutions or communities.

And yet somewhere in there a core of unexplored concerns existed. Could it be that in our eagerness to embrace this broader narrative of healing we were in fact ignoring the elephant in the room: the fact that there is still a core medical narrative, which is arguably the dominant international narrative, eating up human and financial resources, and devoted to the development of treatments, the search for a vaccine and for better prevention methods, the management of public health programmes, the deepening of epidemiological understandings, the training of health professionals and so on?

Fifty years ago, of course, it would have been assumed in Western cultures and their institutions that a study of health would focus on this agenda. The emphasis would have been very much on the curing of disease, or at least alleviation of symptoms of disease and the correction of disability, by trained professionals working within a target community. The discussion might have included doctors, surgeons, nurses, allied health professionals and midwives; hospitals, clinics and school health initiatives; immunisation, birth control and screening; radiology, rehabilitation, mental health and physiotherapy services. There might have been a passing mention of so-called alternative therapies such as acupuncture, for example, but ancient Eastern systems such as Chinese or ayurvedic medicine would hardly have appeared in this discussion, let alone the multitude of local, orally transmitted traditions of health and healing that exist throughout the world. This bias towards a medicalised view of healing, in which the person or community becomes invisible, is confirmed by the World Health Organisation's (WHO) 2008 publication, *Restoring Hope*. In the preface, Srdan Matic says 'Unfortunately, the history of public health and medicine is replete with examples of what happens when medicine is reduced to a technology, and when the dimension of care, of decent care, is forgotten or abandoned.'[1]

A landmark moment came in 1946, when the WHO's charter redefined health as 'a state of complete physical, mental and social well-being and not merely the absence of disease or infirmity'. Recently, the idea of spiritual well-being has been added to this list. This broader view of health was taken up by those who were concerned about the very limited definition of health reflected in the mindset described in the last paragraph. One of the outcomes of this was the influential alliance between WHO and the Christian Medical Commission of the World Council of Churches (WCC), which led ultimately to the Alma Ata Conference in 1978 and the birth of the primary health care (PHC) movement.

In most of this world, in spite of Alma Ata's powerful emphasis on the need for a people-centred, holistic approach to health, PHC continued to co-exist with the kinds of health-facility-based, disease-orientated, specialty-focused medicine described above. Rarely did it succeed in integrating the plethora of regional and local medical traditions coming from, for example, China, India, Brazil or the African continent. Nevertheless, the years since Alma Ata have seen a growing understanding of the need for holistic, inclusive appreciation of health and healing: a movement that has gained momentum from the challenges encountered in responding to the HIV epidemic.[2] This emphasis is explored from a theological and religious angle by writers such as Gunderson, who calls eloquently for a paradigm shift in the way health care is seen: that is, not as a war against disease and death but as a road to health and life.[3] In addressing the HIV epidemic, the material in the present book speaks strongly out of this re-conceptualisation.

But we should not, in our eagerness to promote this holistic view, be blind to the fact that the medical profession has a critical role to play in the response to HIV and AIDS. The idea that health care is the job of everyone can have dangerous consequences if it serves to undermine the credibility of evidence that belongs specifically to a scientific discourse. HIV is a virus and, although there is as yet no cure, a great deal is known about its transmission, treatment and prevention methods. As a result of disciplined, expert research and development, millions of people are living today. It is from science and medicine that this knowledge and these resources originate. Ignore this fact and the results may be a dangerous lack of respect for the evidence base provided by a specific biomedical discourse, plus a vacuum when it comes to developing criteria for evaluating programmatic effectiveness. It then becomes all too easy for religious leaders and others to undermine prevention and care programmes with misleading statements suggesting that HIV is a punishment for sin, or condoms are ineffective, while the promises of the miraculous cure movement may remain unchallenged and its claims not subjected to the kind of professional research that might either refute or substantiate them. When religious responses to the epidemic gain a reputation for having an anti-science, anti-evidence bias, it does harm to the credibility of our faith traditions and undermines the excellent work that many religious health organisations are doing.

In drawing up the framework for this chapter, an attempt has been made, as far as possible, to limit the focus to the intersection between religion, HIV and medicine:[4] that is, the core agenda of the people regarded as medical professionals, leaving the wider agenda to other contributors. In terms of nomenclature, the term health is used in its broadest sense; the term religion to encompass the spectrum of faith, spirituality, religio-cultural practices and institutional religion; the term religious organisation to encompass the myriad of religious entities such as faith-based organisations, community-based initiatives, institutional bodies, religious health facilities, congregations and networks;[5] and the term medicine to indicate the field of biomedical response, planning and research, at the level of both individual care and of public health.

Inevitably, the scope of this chapter is limited by the available literature, which is generally biased towards understandings coming from mainstream religions with international presence and infrastructure. There is also a bias towards material written in English and towards the African continent, which has borne the major burden of the epidemic. These biases reflect an existing imbalance, which is in need of correction, within the literature.

This investigation will then include the following:

- a brief history of religion-inspired medical responses to the epidemic;
- material relating to the theological and ethical rationale that religions claim for their medical work;
- the strengths and weaknesses this sector brings to the interface;
- a section on HIV and the idea of miraculous cures; and
- some suggestions on gaps and possible future work.

A BRIEF HISTORY OF RELIGION-INSPIRED MEDICAL RESPONSES

The body of literature addressing the religious response to the epidemic has its own history.[6] In the earliest stages of the epidemic, very little was written about religion or religious organisations. This invisibility was a result of a series of factors, including the secularisation and religion-blindness of the social sciences in general, and also the sense that religious attitudes were often unhelpful to HIV prevention messages. Then, in the late 1990s, literature began to emerge that noted anecdotally that religious organisations were responding significantly.[7] Little of this response had actually been documented and there was limited awareness among public health planners of religious organisations' involvement in health and HIV. The early years of the present century saw a surge in international interest in mapping the response of religious organisations to HIV and health, and the literature has expanded significantly in the last five years. Much of this new research identifies critical gaps and calls for urgent research and attention in every possible area of investigation.[8]

Generally speaking, religious organisations and individuals around the world have long been involved in medical and social care provision, especially in resource-poor settings.[9] In some countries, religious organisations represent a significant portion of the national health infrastructure. Some of this is a legacy of Western medical mission, which resulted, among other things, in the establishment of health facilities and infrastructure.[10] Similar cases can be seen across the world's religions, for example in the establishment of Islamic hospitals or Buddhist medical ashrams.[11]

Recent work has in some sense rediscovered this legacy. A landscaping study of religious organisations involved in health in sub-Saharan Africa estimated that they provide 25 to 70 per cent of health provision in sub-Saharan Africa. This ranged, for example, from Mali, a mainly Islamic country where there are relatively few religious organisations working in formal health services, to countries such as Zambia, home to a complex range of religious organisations involved in HIV and AIDS work from facility-based health providers to local organisations.[12]

There is great variation in the speed and intensity with which religious organisations responded to the HIV epidemic in different countries. For example, some religious organisations in Kenya perceive themselves to have been at the forefront of the national response in the early 1990s, while in a country such as the Democratic Republic of Congo, religious organisations are only now beginning to respond, having been faced with more pressing issues such as food and security.[13] In fact, several studies of African contexts have noted a boom in the number of organisations responding to the epidemic since around 2000, both in the birth of new organisations and in a programmatic shift by older, established religious bodies.[14] Benn notes that 'it is estimated that the Roman Catholic Church alone provides 25% of all HIV and AIDS care, including home based care and support of orphans'.[15] Despite the increased strain on operations and health systems in these resource-poor settings, it would appear that the religious response to HIV and AIDS is proliferating at a remarkable rate. Further research could establish whether this phenomenon is specific to the southern African context, whether it is the result of targeted funding or a needs-based community response, and what effect this is having on the HIV epidemic.[16]

Religious organisations have a tradition, often rooted in their scriptures and sacred texts, of dealing with disease holistically. This is confirmed by literature suggesting that 'religious responses range across the continuum of prevention, care and support, treatment and rights, and are often "holistic" in nature, focusing on the emotional and spiritual aspects of care as well as the physical'.[17] The word holistic here implies not just an understanding of health that embraces all its elements but also of the wide range of services provided by religious organisations.[18] The philosophy of PHC struck a chord with many religiously motivated health professionals. Grundmann notes how medical mission work shifted to a focus on primary care:

> [. . .] priorities were identified as promoting life in abundance (see John 10:10) and justice (shalom), both to be accomplished by focusing on the commonly neglected diseases of the poor . . . in concentrating on providing

primary health care for families and local communities, medical missions turned away from hospital-centred medical work reflecting the financial affluence of the technocratic, secular culture dominant in the West.[19]

It has also been noted that the responses of religious organisations to HIV and AIDS may not fit readily into accepted categories.[20] Birdsall, for example, observed that the AIDS-related work of religious organisations in South Africa is often embedded within broader portfolios, making it difficult to disentangle purely AIDS-related services from the total range of services provided. She notes that this may mean that their findings understate the actual scope of HIV and AIDS work being conducted.[21]

It is common for funding streams and policy makers to demand specific information about timelines, scope and so on. However, general statements about the history of religious involvement in the HIV epidemic are still provisional, with more gaps and uncertainties than clear trends. As Birdsall says, 'much remains to be understood about the nature, scale and scope of these [faith-based] contributions and the way in which they supplement and interface with more centralised responses to the HIV and AIDS crisis'.[22] There is also a lack of research on the comparative response of religious organisations and virtually no material that compares the response of a religious organisation with a similarly engaged non-governmental organisation (NGO). There is also little that compares the responses of different religious traditions in the same area of HIV intervention. While some studies have begun to engage leaders of different faiths together on their response to HIV and AIDS,[23] there is still little hard data available to balance this qualitative research. Existing data, also, sometimes needs to be treated with suspicion:[24]

> Much of the information on the involvement of religious organizations in HIV/AIDS-related care and support comes from leaders and advocates of such organizations. This information is often selective and self-congratulatory and does not allow for an impartial assessment . . . The volume and frequency of HIV/AIDS-related assistance provided by religious organizations, as well as the relative distribution of that assistance between members and non-members of religious organizations, generally remain unknown.[25]

THE THEOLOGICAL AND ETHICAL RATIONALE FOR MEDICAL WORK[26]

In all formal religions there is a belief that healing and the care of the sick and dying are an important part of what it means to be human. In Buddhist philosophy, for example, healing is part of a metaphysic that embraces principles of compassion and wisdom, willingness to serve, a duty to do no harm and a belief in the significance of death. Thus Buddhist responses have notably focused on the building of hospices for the sick and dying, and the care of destitute people.[27] In Hinduism, healing involves a balanced relationship between the self, the soul, the community and the environment; and a holistic view of community that includes a commitment to the relief of suffering.[28] Judaism has a rich tradition of healing based on the belief that life is a gift of God; and the ethical assumption that concern with health is, therefore, in the final analysis a preoccupation with how each one cares for the life God entrusts to him or to her.[29]

In Islam, health is not a separate entity but an essential component of peace, which includes peace at the levels of individual, family and society. In common with other religious traditions, Islam has no single theodicy of healing, although Mohammed's own prophetic understanding of health had a formative influence on early legal and medical texts. Nevertheless, medical care and healing ministries are extremely important aspects of Islamic scholarship and social organisation.[30] Islam considers personal health to be, after faith itself, the greatest blessing to have been given to human beings by God. Health, therefore, should be properly cared for, not just as a personal asset but also as an aspect of the Islamic imperative to be concerned for the community: a principle that extends to a concern for water, sanitation and other provisions that affect health.[31] Abdulaziz Sachedina provides a well-organised summary of the traditions of medicine and healing that Islam brings to the encounter with HIV and AIDS.[32]

The culture and ethics of Christianity have included a powerful tradition of being of service to others, especially those in need. Christian healing traditions go back to the healing acts of Jesus himself, the context of Jewish purity rules he encountered in his ministry and the 2 000-year-old history of Christian health care ministries.[33] These scriptural and moral imperatives became, over the years, the basis of a Christian commitment to mission hospitals and the infrastructure that grew from them.[34] Early in the HIV epidemic, Christian health professionals drew the parallel between the special care of Jesus for people with leprosy and for children and used this as a theological rationale for their own work. On the other hand, both Christian and Islamic theologies have strong and well-documented veins of moralism and exclusivity that have provided an opposing rationale to exclude individuals living with HIV and their families from the availability of care.

Independent churches are less likely than mainstream ones to run formal medical organisations. On the other hand, spiritual healing is characteristic of many African Independent Churches. These include those known in southern Africa as Zionist and also newer forms of local Pentecostal churches in all parts of the world. Here, faith itself may be the crucial factor in healing. In prioritising the individual's relationship to God, biomedical evidence about transmission, treatment and care may be ignored or treated as irrelevant.[35] Unhappily, though, the distinction between faith healing and traditional healing is not always made in the available literature, with some using these terms interchangeably (discussed later in this chapter). In fact, while practices may differ, narratives of healing and health play an important part in most traditions. Like African Traditional Religion (ATR), Zionists and neo-Pentecostals often stress healing, in thought and in practice.[36]

A good deal of work has been done on the issue of discourse in relation to HIV and AIDS. Gausset speaks of the stigmatising double discourse produced by the introduction of Western biomedical discourse into an African context.[37] Schmid, Maluleke and Seidel have applied discourse theory in illuminating ways to the question of what is said and done in religion-inspired situations.[38] At the global level, the dominant discourse on health and HIV and AIDS is not a religious but a biomedical one based on germ theory, contemporary public health thinking and institutionally-based interventions. This has co-existed, often uneasily, with discourses associated with mainstream religious traditions, where the meaning of health and the rationale for medical intervention may be driven by theological, spiritual and moral considerations. In many parts of the world, these grafted themselves on to those older traditions and beliefs regarding the sources of life, sickness, disease and death that co-exist in all cultures. These traditions and beliefs may provide discourses of suffering and healing that are not publicly articulated but are nevertheless more real at family and neighbourhood level than the biomedical discourses that underpin publicly promoted strategies of care and prevention, or the formal religious discourses that underpin the practice of mosque or temple, synagogue or church.

For this reason, in any one culture (or even individual) there may be three or more separate discourses of health and healing in operation: the least obvious one being the traditional discourse, which is often not written down, and may be hidden from outsiders.[39] In exploring this, the contribution of medical anthropologists has been crucial.[40] Cultures often have powerful theological, moral and philosophical understandings of healing; and of the significance of physical, mental and spiritual wholeness, which is not necessarily articulated in their formal religious expressions. These are extremely important in the context of HIV and AIDS because they can endorse traditions of compassion and respect for others or, conversely, of stigma and the exclusion of outsiders.

At the risk of generalising, there are three particularly dangerous paradigms to which religious discourses of HIV are prone: first, the hostility to evidence-based paradigms, which may actively undermine more mainstream, biomedically validated responses; second, the idea that sickness and suffering are a punishment for sin and therefore part of God's plan for humanity's betterment; and third, that they are the result of lack of faith. These points are returned to in the discussion of miraculous healing below.

The tendency of religious thinking in recent years has been in the direction of the more holistic view of medicine and health care outlined in the opening sections. The WCC health desk, and before it the Christian Medical Commission, have made a significant contribution to the literature on faith responses to HIV and AIDS.[41] They have combined this holistic understanding with advocacy for an evidence-based approach to prevention, care and treatment, especially in relation to community-based approaches. They have also recognised the need for recognition of cultural diversity in biomedical discourses, observing that a Western emphasis on individual choice, responsibility and agency fails to recognise the vulnerability and lack of agency that are the daily experience of much of the world's population.[42] Through its particular focus on developing countries, and its influential health journal *Contact*, the WCC has tried to expand the scope of religious, especially Christian, discourses of health and to address the wider, communal issues raised by a healing ministry committed to HIV prevention and care. This, however, has also led to some confusion, which is reflected in the literature, about the precise role of particular sectors and their relationship with one another in health and healing.

There is a growing body of literature that stresses the importance of indigenous faiths in the response to the epidemic. The majority of work on the theological, ethical and spiritual challenges of healing comes from mainstream religious traditions with international networks. However, particular understandings of health, healing and wholeness are embodied in the spiritualities and religious traditions of Native Americans, of tribal Indians, and the indigenous peoples of Australasia, Latin America and Africa. In these traditions, the discourses of health and healing may differ markedly from those associated with mainstream religion.[43] The ancestors, the forces of nature and fate may play a role in influencing health, producing disease and determining issues of life and death. Bewitching, rather than pathology, may be blamed for disease or infirmity; and witchcraft may be more trusted than medicine for the purpose of cure. Thus medical practice and health care delivery may find themselves sabotaged by beliefs that make perfect sense to the people who hold them and may indeed be motivating convictions but may appear to Western science to be a jumble of disorganised superstitions. Similar accusations have also, on occasion, been made against mainstream religions; only these are made more accessible by the fact that they are written down.[44] African theologians such as Emmanual Katongole, Musa W. Dube, Laurenti Magesa and Agbonkhianmeghe E. Orobator have stressed the importance of acknowledging this interface of beliefs in responding to the epidemic.[45] Peter Knox describes this situation of having feet in both camps: 'Of course, many South Africans exposed to modern reasoning and Western scientific method do not subscribe exclusively to the world-view of which the ancestors form part. But that does not prevent them from being motivated to perform some of the requirements of the cult.'[46]

The last five years have seen a definite increase in the recognition of African traditional medicine as a health system and of traditional healers as a professional body. This has largely been as a result of the HIV epidemic and the needs of those many Africans who do not (or cannot) utilise standard public health systems.[47] Traditional healers are increasingly being drawn into biomedical interventions or at least into greater rapport with public health and biomedical health systems and are increasingly involved in many different levels of HIV and AIDS intervention.[48]

The HIV epidemic has resulted in a growing number of writers becoming fascinated by these often hidden dimensions of belief systems, with researchers increasingly aware of the need for a multi-dimensional approach to issues of belief and meaning. Rather than approaching such issues from the viewpoint of different, externally definable discourses or belief systems, the African Religious Health Assets Programme (ARHAP) has suggested a more people-centred understanding based on the idea that all people and all communities exist in practice in plural health worlds; by which they mean people's conceptions of health 'as framed by the background store of inherited or socialised knowledge that defines their being in the world'.[49] Thus health is defined by good relationships with the family, community and the ancestors; and also the means to live well, together with absence of disease. Disease is similarly broadly defined and includes being bewitched or depressed, conflict with neighbours or family and social determinants such as poverty or poor land.[50]

It is mainly in sub-Saharan Africa that thinking about health worlds has been related specifically to HIV and AIDS. However, similar thinking underpins recent approaches to health care elsewhere in the world. It suggests the conviction that health interventions, everywhere 'whether "Western scientific", "traditional indigenous" or "religious" must be placed within a broader range of behaviours and practices that are holistically conceived'.[51] And many of those behaviours and understandings originate, at some level, from religious belief.

WHAT THIS SECTOR BRINGS TO THE INTERFACE

In the literature addressing the religious response, the reader will most frequently encounter a list of perceived strengths of religious organisations, making them desirable partners for expanded HIV and AIDS work. Religious organisations, it is said, have unique and extensive reach and access: they are found in all communities, particularly the inaccessible and rural; they have access to dedicated volunteers and educated leadership; they have unique credibility and acceptance in communities, and therefore a particular potential to change behaviour; and they have well-developed networks extending from international to grassroots communities.[52] Unfortunately, such claims are usually based not on tested research but on subjective opinion whose verification remains a critical area for further engagement. With that proviso, some of the key strengths and weaknesses that religions bring to the medical or public health sector's response are considered.

Prevention

Religion's role in risk perception and behaviour change has been contested and controversial.[53] However, religious organisations have a long history in the prevention of disease and most traditions contain religious teachings addressing health. Further, education is a primary task for religious organisations, with communities running educational services that range from schools for orphans and vulnerable children to the education of religious leaders and potential community health educators.[54] This makes health education a key area of engagement, including the provision of information on HIV, sex and health, usually as part of a whole package of life skills based training and knowledge. A mass of grey materials produced by religious organisations address pastoral education on HIV and AIDS, using appropriate religious language, anecdotes and theological explanations as an 'interpretative filter'.[55]

So far, the effectiveness or impact of such educative materials on a community or individual's health status remains unknown.[56] The provision of education services by religious organisations is poorly documented and we know little about the positive and negative health effects of religious involvement in education. Also, education can be an area of weakness when it mixes moralistic and conflicting religious messages with medical HIV information. For example, some literature blames religious health education for being a cause of risky behaviour.[57] Further, although religious leaders are in theory well positioned to promote healthy behaviour, they may also have difficulty in talking about sex and sexuality; or they may discourage the education of adolescents on reproductive health, or deliver moralising messages that lead to stigmatisation.[58]

In practice, it is characteristic of this body of literature that every strength or positive aspect is counterbalanced by the need for caution or scepticism. For example, does the promotion of sexual restraint lead to less risky behaviour? Some studies note that religions and religious values can promote the ideals of abstinence, delayed intercourse and fidelity.[59] Other literature notes that messages of abstinence and fidelity are based on messages of moral authority that have a stigmatising effect.[60] The effectiveness of abstinence and faithfulness programmes are increasingly being questioned in the light of actual experience: for example, the meaninglessness of such messages to married women who are faithful but are still considered a high-risk group.[61] Religion and religious values can also have a positive or negative effect on perceived risk and on risk behaviour in general.[62] Religious fatalism, suggesting that life is predetermined by God and that individuals are powerless to change what happens to them, has been found to influence uptake of HIV testing and other HIV prevention strategies negatively.[63]

Finally, some recent literature speaks of different levels of risk according to type of religious affiliation. Several studies suggest that affiliation to an Islamic community or faith correlates with a lower level of risk, the possible causes being lower alcohol consumption, male circumcision and strongly held religious values.[64] Some of the more conservative religious denominations seem to be associated with more effective protection,[65] while other studies suggest that Pentecostalism is more protective than mainline Christianity.[66] Again, not enough is known about these suggested differences to justify targeted prevention strategies.[67]

The most visible area of conflict between the biomedical and the religious sector has been the controversy over condoms. Authors from all spheres have vigorously entered this field – religious, theological, political, social and medical.[68] Shades of grey are not welcomed in this debate, in which religious practice or ideals that promote abstinence but oppose the use of condoms are often portrayed in direct opposition to biomedical prevention strategies.[69] 'Religious taboos on sexual education have been harassing AIDS prevention throughout Latin America. The confrontation between the condom and abstinence or fidelity has snapped closed any possibility for negotiating joint strategies. It has polarized political stances that clash public opinion and counterattack official efforts for AIDS prevention.'[70]

However, generalisations and public statements do not always reflect reality.[71] Some studies show that religious organisations and religious health professionals on the ground often do not act in accordance with the guidelines of their religious body.[72] The Catholic Church has borne the brunt of the condemnation for its stance against condoms, yet it is observed that this is a major subject of contention among Catholics themselves, with many Catholic ethicists arguing for the utilisation of condoms in certain situations.[73] In other literature the Catholic Church is lauded as one of the largest health and health education providers in the world and is acclaimed for its response to HIV and AIDS.[74] An interesting development is the area of condom use in the context of discordant couples as a potential gateway to shared perspectives and partnerships.[75]

Treatment

The area of treatment is a contentious one and the issue of miraculous healing is discussed in more detail below. However, there is a critical shortage of literature on the role of religion in conventional, biomedical treatment of AIDS. Relevant data is likely to be embedded within other surveys and evaluations and has not yet been separated out. Generally speaking, an increasing number of religious organisations are engaged in home-based care, primary health activities and the provision of anti-retrovirals (ARVs) and accompanying care.

There is also growing interest in the extent of the involvement of religious organisations and networks in pharmaceutical and drug provision, especially in relation to ARVs.[76] In a collaborative study with the WHO, the Ecumenical

Pharmaceutical Network (EPN) indicated that 'the population served by 15 faith-based drug distribution organizations in 10 sub-Saharan countries [served] 25–60% of those in need'.[77]

A small amount of the literature notes the impact of religion on decisions to disclose HIV positive status and then to seek treatment. Préau and others found that those who 'place importance on religion appear to have difficulties in disclosing their HIV positive status due to the associated stigma and fear of discrimination'.[78] The effects of HIV-related stigma can hinder help seeking for sexual health concerns and, in effect, prevent individuals from seeking treatment.[79]

To what degree should religious organisations be expected to become active in HIV treatment? The WHO became interested in religious organisations as part of their strategy to get ARV treatment to more people in developing countries.[80] Yet religious leaders at community level may protest that they lack medical training or capacity.[81] Other elements of treatment, such as support (or accompaniment), may be particularly suited to such religious communities or organisations.[82] One study of a Moravian anti-retroviral treatment (ART) programme in South Africa found that recipients preferred to receive their ARVs from a religious organisation, believing that the religious tradition and the level of care made the medication more valuable. The accompanying rituals, they said, enhanced the likelihood of adherence: 'You read [your Bible], pray and drink your pills'.[83] There are several other studies, including anecdotal evidence, that religious health facilities are preferred to state facilities because of a perceived better level of care based on faith.[84]

Care and support

The literature shows that religious organisations have a particular involvement in care and support. This ranges from facility-based health care of those living with HIV to a high level of involvement in community or home-based care of those infected and affected. The notion of caring for the sick or aged is found in all religious traditions, translating readily into the generation of networks of care, or caring, communities.[85] As Liebowitz notes:

> Carrying out some form of home care and visitation was another common activity of many [faith-based organisations] FBOs ... During such visits, those involved provide some or all of the following: care, moral/emotional/ spiritual support, food, and treatment. Most FBO leaders identify home

care and visitation programs as the ones in which congregation members have taken the most interest and in which they have participated the most fully.[86]

Home-based care has become a vital strategy in the international response to HIV and AIDS and one of the phenomena that has alerted international organisations to the contributions religion can make. It is especially valuable in areas that do not have adequate health care or support facilities. As yet, though, there has been little evaluation of the scale or nature of the religious community's impact in this area.[87] The care of orphans and vulnerable children is also a primary focus area of religious organisations in the HIV and AIDS arena.[88] It is an area in which religious organisations and communities are theologically comfortable and theologically driven, and to which they are well-suited.[89] The extent of less visible aspects of community care, such as more amorphous networks, community systems and supporting roles, is poorly documented and remains largely anecdotal.[90]

There is another key area of engagement, described here as religion and coping. Religion is frequently posited as a positive force that provides coping strategies and support for those infected and affected by HIV.[91] Several studies have:

> [. . .] documented the importance of spirituality, defined broadly as prayer, meditation, having faith in God and drawing one's strength from one's beliefs, on the psychological health of HIV-positive individuals. Research has also shown that people who are HIV positive who report greater engagement in spiritual activities report lower emotional distress, lower depression, greater optimism, and better psychological adaptation.[92]

Impacting on coping is the issue of hope and studies alternately express the positive and negative impact of religion on the sense of hope felt by those infected and affected by HIV.[93]

At a public health level, there is emerging evidence suggesting that religious organisations are particularly involved in the provision of psycho-social support to the HIV positive,[94] especially in locations where no other such support is available, and in the provision of end-of-life and bereavement support.[95] In sub-Saharan Africa, there are anecdotal reports of HIV-related funerals every weekend; and that religion and religious organisations play a critical role in the intervention in public and private grief, for example, by providing mourning rituals. Although this focus is well-known, the work of religions in this area is poorly documented:[96]

> Thus far, this has been mostly treated as a theological or psychological matter – but it can also be argued that it is relevant to public health. If a ritual provides comfort and understanding to a community, it might also have an effect on social networks and emotional and mental health. This might in turn affect health-seeking behaviour or choices.[97]

Religion has also been commended for its long-standing contribution to the end-of-life experience of AIDS patients, although the emphasis and character of end-of-life work varies between religions.[98] Palliative care is another area in which religious communities are often heavily involved, often through community-based spontaneous initiatives or individuals driven by a religious motive. In providing palliative care, religions have access to a range of strategies that encompass 'emotional, psychosocial, spiritual and environmental support and care in respect of those infected and affected by HIV and AIDS'.[99]

Other

We have so far skated over the literature that speaks of the value added of religious responses to HIV and AIDS: that is, the claim that the presence of religious elements or traditions actually enhances the quality of the response. There is a large body of literature that speaks, mostly anecdotally, of the extra something that religious organisations bring to the interface and it is on the basis of this value added that they are often seen as potentially positioned for greater involvement in the HIV epidemic. Examples are factors such as motivated and committed volunteers and workers, compassion, spirituality or faith, trust, hope, special care, resilience or durability.[100] For example, in the area of coping and end-of-life support discussed above, Taylor notes that 'many of the distinctive contributions of the church are intangibles, such as dignity for the dying or prayers with the sick, and so are difficult to monitor or evaluate'.[101]

This is an area that is critically lacking in sensitive, in-depth research or theological reflection. It is accompanied by a critical lack of literature on how these intangible assets can be measured in order for them to move beyond the anecdotal and be recognised by public health professionals and policy makers. Such research requires an understanding of the complexities of religion, combined with a familiarity with public health measures and standards.[102] It may make perfect sense to a religiously orientated reader to be told that an organisation believed its major impact was to bring hope to its community and 'create meaning in life'[103] but be foreign to a public health professional:

> Some aspects of religious health assets can – and should – be examined appropriately by public health [economic] analysis. However, other aspects of these assets need another frame of analysis to measure, evaluate and build strategies for enhancing such qualities as compassion, mutual support, honesty, prayer, and moral authority. These converge with economic measures when we seek to understand the performance and tenacity of leaders, employees, volunteers and the community linkages that are the key to the durability and effectiveness of religious assets.[104]

The intangibles that motivate religious organisations are sometimes also weaknesses, or may be points of contention in partnerships with governments and other civil society bodies. In Kenya some secular participants showed exasperation that religious organisations hired HIV programme staff because they were deemed to be good Christians rather than for their experience or skills.[105] Another example is that religious organisations are believed to be particularly weak in the area of documentation and the underlying skills that enable this type of activity.[106] Frustratingly for outsiders, this weakness may be claimed with pride, not as a matter of poor skills but as a key principle of their theological understanding of stewardship. They are responsible, they may say, to a higher power or they are too busy saving lives (as Jesus did), implementers and doers, not fillers-in of forms.[107] A further reason might be that religious organisations have often grown spontaneously from a combination of community need and religious imperative, lacking formal NGO status and the information or planning ability to deal with rapid growth into organisational status. Furthermore, while the unique ability to mobilise and inspire volunteers is frequently mentioned in the literature[108] – adding that these volunteers are motivated by such intangibles as a sense of vocation based on their religious traditions of caring – other literature considers that the heavy reliance of religious organisations on volunteers can also be regarded as a threat to the ultimate sustainability of their programmes.[109]

The issue of value added, while complex, is of critical concern to decision makers at all levels. Religious health organisations working in the area of HIV and

AIDS are coming under increasing strain as a result of financial constraints, the health workforce crisis and so on. Health-providing religious organisations are facing crises where their mission to serve the marginalised comes into direct conflict with financial survival:[110]

> This is a critical time in the history of these facility-based health providing FBOs – as they are being pushed to weigh their organizational culture and reason for being, against the realities of financial support and survival . . . it is a challenge that cuts to the heart of the religious-health landscape, arguing that if FBOs do have the unique strengths listed above, a 'value added', then now is the time to consider just what that value added is 'worth' and therefore, in what ways it is to be supported.[111]

HIV AND MIRACULOUS CURES

Finally, treading carefully, it is important to mention the growth, especially in Africa, of the complex phenomenon of miraculous healing in the context of HIV and AIDS. In the mid-1990s the HIV and AIDS agenda underwent a radical change in the wake of the new availability of ARV treatments. For over a decade, medical science had been failing to provide treatment but here, now, was a way to prevent people from becoming sick and dying.[112] This development continues to be a source of celebration and millions of lives have been transformed by it. One of its long-term effects, however, was to undermine some of the more integrated responses to the epidemic and to bring religion into the act by making it appear that apparently miraculous cures were not only possible, but validated by science.

In his State of the Union address of 2003, announcing the inauguration of the President's Emergency Programme for AIDS Relief (PEPFAR),[113] President George W. Bush proclaimed that we are now living in 'an age of miraculous medicine'. It was not a happy choice of words. Emmanuel Katongole comments:

> Said simply, this is an age and a culture of drugs. The primary way our age deals with issues of sickness and suffering is through medication . . . President Bush's remarks help us to see the (over)confidence and great expectations that an age of miraculous medicine sets us up for – expectations of dramatic, life-saving results. Slower, less dramatic, step-by-step methods not only now seem archaic; they are also dubbed irresponsible.[114]

In this situation, says Katongole, 'Christian ethics is easily reduced to a form of advocacy (focusing on issues of equity, access or distributive justice) with the wider considerations of human flourishing edited out of view'.[115] Another unintended consequence has been to lend credence to the kind of pseudo-science that allows so-called miraculous healers to produce magic cures in the name of religion; a phenomenon that has undermined attempts at evidence-based education in all parts of the world and reinforced existing prejudices against religious interventions.[116]

There is only limited research on this critical aspect and, as yet, little that successfully straddles the intersection of religion and medicine. Some literature demonstrates cases where religious beliefs conflict with recommendations of health care providers in the treatment and care of people living with HIV. For example, Ugandan researchers who were initiating ART in a cohort study found that a small percentage of HIV positive individuals discontinued therapy as a result of their belief that they had been spiritually healed and thus no longer needed therapy.[117]

The interaction between perceptions of healing or cure is complex, involving overlapping understandings of spirit, body and community. In a recent study in Malawi the participants were the leaders or managers of HIV and AIDS pro-grammes from religious organisations. The majority of this group said they understood healing to mean that 'God could heal people from HIV infection, and in fact had done so'.[118] However, from Zambia comes an anecdote about a local community, narrated by the pastor himself:

> As a pastor, we had a patient who was sick, a church member, and we prayed for her for two weeks, and each time there was no improvement. Until one time the spirit of God says, 'can you just ask, if she has eaten anything?' So I asked, 'Madam, have you eaten anything'. And she said, 'how can I get anything?' So the church decided to do something. In the afternoon they all went and bought her this and that, such as a bag of maize-meal. And the very next morning . . . she was healed! Hallelujah![119]

The community group laughed at this anecdote. And yet it does reflect the complex interaction of belief, faith and action, and warns us against the danger of taking a simplistic, one-sided view of either biomedical treatment or religious cure.

POSSIBLE FUTURE WORK

This review has explored a broad spectrum of issues and revealed a critical lack of knowledge about aspects of the religious response to HIV and AIDS. In particular, there is not enough nuanced work that acknowledges the differences in religion, or that compares religious and non-religious activities and organisations, in the context of the HIV epidemic. Every perceived strength of religious involvement in health, HIV and AIDS is balanced by caution. This is a result of a delicate historical relationship between religion and medicine; and because there is a critical lack of nuanced research work on all these issues. It has been easy, throughout this chapter, to pinpoint these gaps in research and in the literature; and it is true that there is much that we do not know or understand about the interface between religion and medicine in the context of HIV and AIDS. In any case, it is a field that is evolving so fast that what is true one day may well be superseded the next. In the light of the research that does exist, though, a number of important things are known.

Religious medical and health inputs constitute a valuable and sizeable dimension of the overall response to HIV and AIDS. For this reason, they are currently of interest to international organisations desperate to strengthen responses and searching for further capacity to enable them to do it. It would be most convenient for national and international planning if religious responses could be persuaded to fit tidily into its needs slot. This is to ignore the fact that religious understandings of medicine, health and healing are, in fact, different from secular ones, and the contribution they can most fruitfully make is also different. The burning question, which urgently needs answering, is this: just what are the treasures that religious health assets bring to the table? That is why the literature reviewed in this chapter is so important.

NOTES

1. Srdan Matic, 'Preface' in *Restoring Hope: Decent Care in the Midst of HIV and AIDS*, by Ted Karpf (Geneva: World Health Organisation, 2008): vii.
2. The term epidemic is used to indicate the broad HIV and AIDS pandemic or, more correctly, epidemics.
3. Gary Gunderson and Larry Pray, *Leading Causes of Life* (Memphis: Methodist LeBonheur Healthcare Center of Excellence in Faith and Health, 2006).
4. In practice there is so much overlap in the literature that this is barely achievable. However, we have endeavoured to reference fields of enquiry dealt with elsewhere without exploring them in detail.

5. See Jill Olivier, 'An FB-oh?: The etymology of the religious entity and its impact on our understanding of the intersection of religion and health in Africa'. Paper presented at ARHAP Conference: When Religion and Health Align: Mobilising Religious Health Assets for Transformation, Cape Town, 13–16 July 2009.

6. This is a summary. See Chapter 3 for a more complete discussion.

7. Jill Olivier, James R. Cochrane and Barbara Schmid, *ARHAP Literature Review: Working in a Bounded Field of Unknowing* (Cape Town: African Religious Health Assets Programme, 2006): 38–42.

8. Barbara Schmid et al., *The Contribution of Religious Entities to Health in Sub-Saharan Africa* (Cape Town: African Religious Health Assets Programme, 2008): 94.

9. Georges Tiendrebeogo and Michael Buykx, *Faith-Based Organisations and HIV/AIDS Prevention and Impact Mitigation in Africa* (Amsterdam: KIT Publishers, 2004).

10. Christoffer H. Grundmann, 'Mission and healing in historical perspective'. *International Bulletin of Missionary Research* 32(4) 2008: 185–6.

11. See Sara Woldehanna et al., *Faith in Action: Examining the Role of Faith-Based Organisations in Addressing HIV/AIDS: A Multi Country Key Informant Survey* (Washington, DC: Global Health Council, 2005).

12. Schmid et al., *The Contribution of Religious Entities to Health in Sub-Saharan Africa*: 49; Steve de Gruchy et al., *Appreciating Assets: The Contribution of Religion to Universal Access in Africa* (Cape Town: African Religious Health Assets Programme, 2006): 106–22.

13. Beverley Haddad, Jill Olivier and Steve de Gruchy, *The Potential and Perils of Partnership: Christian Religious Entities and Collaborative Stakeholders Responding to HIV and AIDS in Kenya, Malawi and the DRC* (Cape Town: Africa Religious Health Assets Programme, 2008): 110.

14. De Gruchy et al., *Appreciating Assets*: 125. Karen Birdsall, *Faith-Based Responses to HIV/AIDS in South Africa: An Analysis of the Activities of Faith-Based Organisations (FBOs) in the National HIV/AIDS Database* (Johannesburg: Centre for AIDS Development, Research and Evaluation, 2005): 8; Haddad, Olivier and De Gruchy, *The Potential and Perils of Partnership*: 28; Schmid et al., *The Contribution of Religious Entities to Health in Sub-Saharan Africa*: 52–72.

15. Christoph Benn, 'Why religious health assets matter' in *ARHAP: Assets and Agency Colloquium, Pietermaritzburg, South Africa, August 2003* (Cape Town: African Religious Health Assets Programme, 2003).

16. Haddad, Olivier and De Gruchy, *The Potential and Perils of Partnership*.

17. De Gruchy et al., *Appreciating Assets*: 22.

18. Olivier, Cochrane and Schmid, *ARHAP Literature Review*: 39–40.

19. Grundmann, 'Mission and healing in historical perspective': 187.

20. De Gruchy et al., *Appreciating Assets*: 22.

21. Birdsall, *Faith-Based Responses to HIV/AIDS in South Africa*: 20.

22. Birdsall, *Faith-Based Responses to HIV/AIDS in South Africa*: 3.

23. De Gruchy et al., *Appreciating Assets*; Haddad, Olivier and De Gruchy, *The Potential and Perils of Partnership*.

24. It would be a mistake to think that this hermeneutic of suspicion applies only to religious responses. See Chapter 3 in this book for a more complete explanation of the current status of such research.

25. Victor Agadjanian and Soma Sen, 'Promises and challenges of faith-based AIDS care and support in Mozambique'. *American Journal of Public Health* 97(2) 2007: 362.

26. The theological rationale relating to issues of care, which are of course critically relevant to this chapter, is discussed in detail in Chapter 15 on care in this book.

27. A useful website for resources on Buddhist philosophical approaches to health, and particularly to HIV and AIDS, is http://www.buddhanet.net/tib_heal.htm. UNICEF has produced excellent material on Buddhist responses to HIV and AIDS in Thailand, Vietnam and Cambodia.

28. *HIV/AIDS: The Human Dimension: Voices from the Hindu World* (Shanthi Ashram and WCRP). Available at http://www.shantiashram.org (accessed 22 Dec. 2009).

29. Johanna Stiebert, 'Does the Hebrew Bible have anything to tell us about HIV/AIDS?' in *HIV/AIDS and the Curriculum: Methods of Integrating HIV/AIDS in Theological Programmes*, edited by Musa W. Dube (Geneva: WCC Publications, 2003).

30. Non-formal materials include the excellent resource list from the work of the Islamic Medical Association of Uganda: for example, *AIDS Education Through Imams: A Spiritually Motivated Community Effort in Uganda* (Geneva: UNAIDS, 1999).

31. Mohammad Haytham Al Khayat, *The Right Path to Health: Health Education Through Religion: An Islamic Perspective* (Alexandria: WHO Regional Office for the Eastern Mediterranean, 1997).

32. Abdulaziz Sachedina, 'Afflicted by God?: Muslim perspectives on health and suffering' in *Islam and AIDS: Between Scorn, Pity and Justice,* edited by Farid Esack and Sarah Chiddy (Oxford: One World, 2009). In the UK, the African HIV Policy Network has recently launched a toolkit on HIV to be used within Muslim communities; see *Life and Knowledge* (London: AHPN, 2009).

33. The WCC Christian Medical Commission, and later its health desk, took an early lead in exploring the interface between Christian health services and Christian theologies of healing. The Ecumenical HIV and AIDS Initiative in Africa of the WCC series is an important contribution to theological reflection.

34. Schmid et al., *The Contribution of Religious Entities to Health in Sub-Saharan Africa*: 33.

35. Schmid et al., *The Contribution of Religious Entities to Health in Sub-Saharan Africa*: 34.

36. Olivier, Cochrane and Schmid, *ARHAP Literature Review*: 57.

37. Quentin Gausset, 'AIDS and cultural practices in Africa'. *Social Science and Medicine* 52(5) 2001: 509–18.

38. Barbara Schmid, 'AIDS discourses in the church: What we say and what we do'. *Journal of Theology for Southern Africa* 125 (2006): 91–103; Tinyiko Maluleke, 'African "Ruths", ruthless Africas: Reflections of an African Mordecai' in *Other Ways of Reading: African Women and the Bible*, edited by Musa W. Dube (Atlanta: Society of Biblical Literature, 2001); Gill Seidel, 'Thank God I said no to AIDS: On the changing discourse of AIDS in Uganda'. *Discourse and Society* 1(1) 1990: 61–84.

39. Gillian Paterson, *AIDS and the African Churches* (London: Christian Aid, 2001): 12.

40. Ralph Bolton and Gail Orozco, *The AIDS Bibliography: Studies in Anthropology and Related Fields* (American Anthropological Association, 1994).

41. *Facing AIDS: The Challenge, the Churches' Response* (Geneva: WCC, 1997). See in particular the chapter 'Pastoral care and the healing community'.

42. Gert Rüppell and Usha Jesudasan, *Healing as Empowerment: Discovering Grace in Community* (Geneva: WCC, 2005).

43. See Chapter 9 of this book.

44. The question of what is, or is not, written down is an important one for this literature survey.

45. Emmanual Katongole, 'Postmodern illusions and the challenge of African theology: The ecclesial tactics of resistance'. *Modern Theology* 16(2) 2000: 237–54; Musa W. Dube, *The HIV and AIDS Bible* (Scranton: Chicago University Press, 2008) – see in particular the chapter 'African women's hermeneutics and the HIV and AIDS apocalypse'; Laurenti Magesa, 'AIDS and survival in Africa: A tentative reflection' in *Moral and Ethical Issues in African Christianity: A Challenge for African Christianity*, edited by Jesse N.K. Mugambi and Anne Nasimiyu-Masiki (Nairobi: Acton Publishers, 1991); Laurenti Magesa, *African Religion: The Moral Traditions of Abundant Life* (Maryknoll: Orbis Books, 1997); Agbonkhianmeghe E. Orobator, 'Ethics of HIV/AIDS prevention: Paradigms of a new discourse from an African perspective' in *Applied Ethics in a World Church*, edited by Linda Hogan (Maryknoll: Orbis Books, 2008): 147–54.

46. Peter Knox, *AIDS, the Ancestors and Salvation: Local Beliefs in Christian Ministry to the Sick* (Nairobi: St Paul Publications, 2008): 226.

47. Jaco Homsy et al., 'Traditional health practitioners are key to scaling up comprehensive care for HIV/AIDS in sub-Saharan Africa'. *AIDS* 18(12) 2004: 1723–5.

48. Olivier, Cochrane and Schmid, *ARHAP Literature Review*: 57; Jo Wreford, *'We Can Help!' A Literature Review of Current Practice Involving Traditional African Healers in Biomedical HIV/AIDS Interventions in South Africa* (Cape Town: Centre for Social Science Research, University of Cape Town, 2005); Rachel King, *Collaboration with Traditional Healers in HIV/AIDS Prevention and Care in Sub-Saharan Africa: A Literature Review* (Geneva: UNAIDS, 2000); Edward C. Green, 'Involving healers'. *AIDS Action* 46(3) 1999.

49. See Paul Germond and James R. Cochrane, 'Healthworlds: Ontological, anthropological and epistemological challenges on the interface of religion and health' in *Reasons of Faith: Religion in Modern Public Life* (Johannesburg, Wits Institute for Social and Economic Research, 2005); Paul Germond and Sepetla Molapo, 'In search of Bophelo in a time of AIDS: Seeking a coherence of economies of health and economies of salvation'. *Journal of Theology for Southern Africa* 126 (2006): 27–47; Schmid et al., *The Contribution of Religious Entities to Health in Sub-Saharan Africa*: 34–5.

50. Olivier, Cochrane and Schmid, *ARHAP Literature Review*: 16.

51. Olivier, Cochrane and Schmid, *ARHAP Literature Review*: 56. Luke L. Pato, 'Being fully human: From the perspective of African culture and spirituality'. *Journal of Theology for Southern Africa* 97 (1997): 53–61.

52. Schmid et al., *The Contribution of Religious Entities to Health in Sub-Saharan Africa*, 84–5: Haddad, Olivier and De Gruchy, *The Potential and Perils of Partnership*: 25–6.

53. Lucy Keough and Katherine Marshall, *Faith Communities Engage the HIV/AIDS Crisis* (Washington, DC: Berkley Center, Georgetown University, 2007). Available at repository.berkleycenter.georgetown.edu/AIDS_final.pdf (accessed 22 Dec. 2009).

54. Olivier, Cochrane and Schmid, *ARHAP Literature Review*: 52; De Gruchy et al., *Appreciating Assets*; Haddad, Olivier and De Gruchy, *The Potential and Perils of Partnership*.

55. Olivier, Cochrane and Schmid, *ARHAP Literature Review*: 52. For examples of these materials see Sam Pick, *HIV/AIDS Our Greatest Challenge Yet!: The Road Ahead for the Church in South Africa* (Wellington: Lux Verbi, 2003); Daniela Gennrich (ed.), *The Church in an HIV+ World: A Practical Handbook* (Pietermaritzburg: Cluster, 2004).

56. Olivier, Cochrane and Schmid, *ARHAP Literature Review*: 52–3.

57. Olivier, Cochrane and Schmid, *ARHAP Literature Review*: 50; Victor Agadjanian, 'Gender, religious involvement, and HIV/AIDS prevention in Mozambique'. *Social Science and Medicine* 61(7) 2005: 1529.

58. Olivier, Cochrane and Schmid, *ARHAP Literature Review*: 50.

59. Jeremy Liebowitz, *The Impact of Faith-Based Organisations on HIV/AIDS Prevention and Mitigation in Africa* (Durban: Health Economics and HIV/AIDS Research Division, University of KwaZulu-Natal, 2002); Edward C. Green, 'The impact of religious health organisations in promoting HIV/AIDS prevention' in *The AIDS Crisis in Developing Countries*, edited by Edward C. Green (Westport: Praeger, 2003); Sarla Chand and Jacqui Patterson, *Faith-Based Models for Improving Maternal and Newborn Health* (Baltimore: USAID-ACCESS, 2007).

60. Olivier, Cochrane and Schmid, *ARHAP Literature Review*: 50.

61. Jonathan Cohen and Tony Tate, 'The less they know, the better: Abstinence-only HIV/AIDS programs in Uganda'. *Human Rights Watch* 17(4a) 2005; Daniel Low-Beer and Rand L. Stoneburner, *Behaviour and Communication Change in Reducing HIV: Is Uganda Unique?* (Johannesburg: Centre for AIDS Development, Research and Evaluation, 2004); Susheela Singh, Jacqueline E. Darroch and Akinrinola Bankole, *The Role of Behaviour Change in the Decline in HIV Prevalence in Uganda* (New York: Alan Guttmacher Institute, 2002).While it is certainly true to state that married women constitute a risk group, we have to point out that the danger is by no means restricted to married women or women per se.

62. Jenny Trinitapoli and Mark D. Regnerus, 'Religion and HIV risk behaviours among men: Initial results from a panel study in rural sub-Saharan Africa'. *Working Paper Series* 2004–5 (Austin: Population Research Center, University of Texas, 2005); Jenny Trinitapoli, 'Religious responses to AIDS in sub-Saharan Africa: An examination of religious congregations in rural Malawi'. *Review of Religious Research* 47(3) 2006: 253–70.

63. Suzanne Maman et al., 'The role of religion in HIV-positive women's disclosure experiences and coping strategies in Kinshasa, Democratic Republic of Congo'. *Social Science and Medicine* 68(5) 2009: 965–70.

64. Noah Kiwanuka et al., 'Religion, behaviours, and circumcision as determinants of HIV dynamics in rural Uganda'. *International Conference on AIDS* 11(2) 1996: 483; Sarah S. Gilbert, 'The influence of Islam on AIDS prevention among Senegalese university students'. *AIDS Education and Prevention* 20(5) 2008: 399–407.

65. See Emmanuel Lagarde et al., 'Religion and protective behaviours towards AIDS in rural Senegal'. *AIDS* 14(13) 2000: 2027–33; Baffour K. Takyi, 'Religion and women's health in Ghana: Insights into HIV/AIDS preventive and protective behavior'. *Social Science and Medicine* 56 (2003): 1221–34.

66. Kiwanuka et al., 'Religion, behaviours, and circumcision as determinants of HIV dynamics in rural Uganda': 483; Robert C. Garner, 'Religion in the AIDS crisis: Irrelevance, adversary or ally?' *AIDS Analysis Africa* 10 (1999): 6–7.

67. For further discussion see Chapter 2 of this book.

68. Gideon B. Byamugisha, *Am I My Brother's Keeper? Reflections on Genesis 4:9* (Kampala: Tricolour, 1998).

69. Maman et al., 'The role of religion in HIV-positive women's disclosure experiences and coping strategies in Kinshasa, Democratic Republic of Congo'; Byamugisha, *Am I My Brother's Keeper?*

70. G. Ornelas et al., 'Sex education for priests'. *International Conference on AIDS* 8(2) 1992: 435.

71. Byamugisha, *Am I My Brother's Keeper?*; Maureen Farrell, 'Condoms and AIDS prevention: A comparison of three faith-based organizations in Uganda'. *AIDS and Anthropology Bulletin* 15(3) 2003; Maureen Farrell, 'Condoning or condemning the condom: Lessons learned from Uganda'. *Sexual Health Exchange* 1(2004): 7–8.

72. De Gruchy et al., *Appreciating Assets*; Haddad, Olivier and De Gruchy, *The Potential and Perils of Partnership*; Olivier, Cochrane and Schmid, *ARHAP Literature Review*; Farrell, 'Condoning or condemning the condom'.

73. Jon D. Fuller and James F. Keenan, 'Introduction: At the end of the first generation of HIV prevention' in *Catholic Ethicists on HIV/AIDS Prevention*, edited by James F. Keenan et al. (New York: Continuum, 2000): 21–38.

74. Schmid et al., *The Contribution of Religious Entities to Health in Sub-Saharan Africa*: 90; Olivier, Cochrane and Schmid, *ARHAP Literature Review*: 34.

75. Haddad, Olivier and De Gruchy, *The Potential and Perils of Partnership*: 58, 83, 112; James F. Keenan et al. (eds), *Catholic Ethicists on HIV/AIDS Prevention*.

76. Schmid et al., *The Contribution of Religious Entities to Health in Sub-Saharan Africa*, 83; Ecumenical Pharmaceutical Network, available at http://www.epnetwork.org (accessed 20 Aug. 2008); Sophie Logez and Marthe Everard, *Multi-Country Study on Drug Supply and Distribution Activities of Faith-Based Supply Organisations in Sub-Saharan African Countries, 2003* (Nairobi: EPN and WHO, 2004).

77. *A Situational Analysis Study of the Faith Based Health Services Vis-a-Vis the Government Health Services* (Nairobi: Christian Health Association of Kenya and German Technical Cooperation, 2007).

78. Marie Préau et al., 'Disclosure and religion among people living with HIV/AIDS in France'. *AIDS Care* 20(5) 2008: 521.

79. Stephen Pearson and Panganai Makadzange, 'Help-seeking behaviour for sexual-health concerns: A qualitative study of men in Zimbabwe'. *Culture, Health and Sexuality* 10(4) 2008: 361.

80. De Gruchy et al., *Appreciating Assets*: 6–8.

81. Haddad, Olivier and De Gruchy, *The Potential and Perils of Partnership*.

82. See the work on accompaniment by Methodist le BonHeur Healthcare. Available at http://www.methodisthealth.org/portal/site/methodist/ (accessed 3 Dec. 2008).

83. Elizabeth Thomas et al., *Let us Embrace: The Role and Significance of an Integrated Faith-Based Initiative for HIV and AIDS* (Cape Town: African Religious Health Assets Programme, 2006): 44.

84. De Gruchy et al., *Appreciating Assets*: 75.

85. Olivier, Cochrane and Schmid, *ARHAP Literature Review*: 64. The focus here is specifically on care in relation to health care. See Chapter 15 in this book for further discussion on religious traditions of care and support.

86. Jeremy Liebowitz, *Faith-Based Organisations and HIV/AIDS in Uganda and KwaZulu-Natal* (Durban: Health Economics and HIV/AIDS Research Division, University of KwaZulu-Natal, 2004): 10.

87. Olivier, Cochrane and Schmid, *ARHAP Literature Review*: 64.

88. Olivier, Cochrane and Schmid, *ARHAP Literature Review*: 34, 40; Geoff Foster, *Study of the Response by Faith-Based Organisations to Orphans and Vulnerable Children: Preliminary Summary Report* (New York: World Conference of Religions for Peace and United Nations Children Fund, 2003).

89. Schmid et al., *The Contribution of Religious Entities to Health in Sub-Saharan Africa*: 82; Chand and Patterson, *Faith-Based Models for Improving Maternal and Newborn Health*: 3–4.

90. Schmid et al., *The Contribution of Religious Entities to Health in Sub-Saharan Africa*: 48.

91. Karolynn Siegel and Eric W. Schrimshaw, 'The perceived benefits of religious and spiritual coping among older adults living with HIV/AIDS'. *Journal for the Scientific Study of Religion* 41(1) 2002: 91–102; C. Jeff Jacobson et al., 'Religio-biography, coping, and meaning-making among persons with HIV/AIDS'. *Journal for the Scientific Study of Religion* 45(1) 2006: 39–56.

92. Maman et al., 'The role of religion in HIV-positive women's disclosure experiences and coping strategies in Kinshasa, Democratic Republic of Congo': 965.

93. Jill Olivier, 'Where does the Christian stand?: Considering a public discourse of hope in the context of HIV/AIDS in South Africa'. *Journal of Theology for Southern Africa* 126 (2006): 81–99; Olivier, Cochrane and Schmid, *ARHAP Literature Review*: 67.

94. Haddad, Olivier and De Gruchy, *The Potential and Perils of Partnership*: 54, 84, 99.

95. ZINGO, *Faith-Based Organizations' Responses to HIV/AIDS in Livingstone, Lusaka and Kitwe: Strategic Visioning for a Zambia Free of HIV/AIDS* (Lusaka: Zambia Interfaith Networking Group on HIV/AIDS and the National AIDS Council of Zambia, 2002); Thomas Cannell, 'Funerals and AIDS: Resilience and decline in KwaZulu-Natal'. *Journal of Theology for Southern Africa* 125 (2006): 21–37.

96. Olivier, Cochrane and Schmid, *ARHAP Literature Review*: 65–6.

97. Olivier, Cochrane and Schmid, *ARHAP Literature Review*: 65.

98. The emphasis and character of end-of-life work varies between religions.

99. ZINGO, *Faith-Based Organizations' Responses to HIV/AIDS in Livingstone, Lusaka and Kitwe*: 16.

100. Olivier, Cochrane and Schmid, *ARHAP Literature Review*: 66–8.

101. Nigel Taylor, *Working Together? Challenges and Opportunities for International Development Agencies and the Church in the Response to AIDS in Africa* (Teddington: Tearfund, 2006).

102. African Religious Health Assets Programme, available at http://www.arhap.uct.ac.za (accessed 14 Jan. 2009).

103. Christoph Benn, 'The influence of cultural and religious frameworks on the future course of the HIV/AIDS pandemic'. *Journal of Theology for Southern Africa* 113 (2002): 3–18.

104. Olivier, Cochrane and Schmid, *ARHAP Literature Review*: 66.

105. Haddad, Olivier and De Gruchy, *The Potential and Perils of Partnership*: 61.

106. Generalisation is problematic as there are some religious organisations with exemplary skills. However, these are seen as the exception to the general rule. Schmid et al., *The Contribution of Religious Entities to Health in Sub-Saharan Africa*: 86.

107. Schmid et al., *The Contribution of Religious Entities to Health in Sub-Saharan Africa*: 87.

108. Olivier et al., *ARHAP Literature Review*: 41; Tearfund, *Faith Untapped: Why Churches Can Play a Crucial Role in Tackling HIV and AIDS in Africa* (Teddington: Tearfund, 2006); Ritva Reinikka and Jakob Svensson, *Working for God?: Evaluating Service Delivery of Religious Not-For-Profit Health Care Providers in Uganda* (Washington, DC: World Bank, 2003).

109. Olivier, Cochrane and Schmid, *ARHAP Literature Review*: 64.

110. Schmid et al., *The Contribution of Religious Entities to Health in Sub-Saharan Africa*: 88.

111. Schmid et al., *The Contribution of Religious Entities to Health in Sub-Saharan Africa*: 88.

112. Peter Allen, *The Wages of Sin: Sex and Disease, Past and Present* (Chicago: University of Chicago Press, 2000).

113. PEPFAR supports many millions of people on ARV therapies. See http://www.pepfar.gov/ (accessed 21 May 2009).

114. Emmanual Katongole, 'AIDS, Africa and the "age of miraculous medicine": naming the silences' in *Applied Ethics in a World Church: The Padua Conference*, edited by Linda Hogan (Maryknoll: Orbis Books, 2008): 138.

115. Katongole, 'AIDS, Africa and the "age of miraculous medicine"': 139.

116. Musa Dube, 'Healing where there is no healing: Reading the miracles of healing in an AIDS context' in *Reading Communities, Reading Scripture*, edited by Gary A. Phillips and Nicole Wilkinson Duran (Harrisburg: Trinity, 2002): 121–33.

117. Jane Wanyama et al., 'Belief in divine healing can be a barrier to antiretroviral therapy adherence in Uganda'. *AIDS* 21(11) 2002: 1486–7.

118. Haddad, Olivier and De Gruchy, *The Potential and Perils of Partnership*: 89.

119. De Gruchy et al., *Appreciating Assets*: 68.

Practitioner response

Greg Manning

Injecting drug users in rural and urban India have shown that the pursuit of good health includes accessing informal as well as formal health care. It includes preventing new infections and new epidemics. It also includes transformational agendas, such as changing social attitudes, law reform and scientific discovery. Drug users prioritise urgent time frames, knowing that without constant support for their health seeking, each day holds a series of painful and life-threatening situations. The pragmatism and urgency of populations of drug users contrasts starkly with the visions of holiness and eternity that characterise the global identity of Evangelical Christians. In my work, these contrasting worlds meet in a shared and complicated struggle for community, justice and compassion.

In this response to the chapter by Olivier and Paterson, some issues I consider important in the delivery of medical services are highlighted. These relate to communication about HIV within religious networks, as well as between populations identified by belief, and other stakeholders in medical responses to HIV. Second, I advocate that the notion of mutuality be added to the analysis of this subject. In my religious tradition, the mandate for mutuality is succinctly stated: do to others as you would have them do to you. A similar sentiment can be found in most religions.

Issues in the delivery of medical services

Olivier and Paterson describe a level of religious involvement in health care that is of interest to activists, practitioners and health planners in scaling up towards universal access by the year 2010 of prevention, treatment, care and support services. The problem is that the reporting of religious work is dominated by self-congratulatory assessments and assertions about its own quality and importance. These assertions are sometimes difficult for allies to support robustly in contexts of health planning and budget formulation that are highly competitive.

Activists, practitioners and health planners communicate using specific models of health care, which enable ongoing cycles of critical evaluation for priority setting, quality control and accountability. More needs to be done to understand and communicate the processes of public critical evaluation that are compatible with religious identity. This will enable the assertions about the quality and importance of religious work to be better evaluated for more appropriate inclusion in health planning. The Ecumenical Advocacy Alliance's guide aims to support the establishment of collaborative relationships between the public health sector and faith-based organisations.[1] However, new collaborations may not be sustainable in the absence of strategies enabling multi-sectoral decision making, problem solving and conflict resolution.

The chapter begins by identifying the absence of a religious discourse enabling the accountable presence of religious groups in multi-sectoral communication about medical responses to HIV. It ends with the question: what are the treasures that religious health assets bring to the table? The authors locate their discussion of religious health assets in a discourse concerned with funding, from organisational survival to the global and national financing of medical responses to HIV. They conclude that if the inclusion and resourcing of religious health care within national models is a concern, then religious assets must be more clearly identified and effectively modelled.

Virtues, such as voluntary or sacrificial care and service, which have been the motivation behind much religious medical work, are now confronted by questions about how good they really are and what they are worth in a market economy. This more arbitrary, market-like context, in which the prices of virtue are being assessed, may explain to some extent the self-congratulatory assessments and assertions mentioned above.

The funding of medical services in HIV epidemics has placed even greater demands on religious communicators in relation to what it means to bear witness, to tell the truth and to respect the wisdom and authority of elders and traditions. Even beyond accountability for service delivery and financial practices, the pursuit of virtue is being defined in economic terms.

Concepts regarding what it means to be human were proposed as a rationale common to the medical work of all religions. Olivier and Paterson identify elements such as compassion, peace and wholeness, service, relationships and community, and responses to suffering as human behaviours and inclinations that motivate medical service provision. Beliefs about what it means to be male, female, sexually active, homosexual, or addicted to illicit drugs were not mentioned. These also motivate actions related to health and healing, and continue to complicate religious participation in responses to HIV and AIDS. These beliefs, among Evangelicals, find expression in efforts to heal society from promiscuity, heal men who have sex with men from homosexuality, or heal people using illicit drugs from drug addiction. Such ideas of healing are often mistakenly confused with HIV prevention.

In its exploration of 'the theological and ethical rationale that religions claim for their medical work', the chapter moves from specific religious postures and the confidence of scientific definitions to an acknowledgement that people live in plural health worlds. These include a blend of scientific and medical insight, mainstream religion, and local custom and belief. The authors comment that personal health in Islam is a blessing from God second only to faith itself. This observation suggests that there is something more important in both Christianity and Islam than physical health and healing. In both these religions, health and healing are signs of the greatness of Allah,[2] and God's power and presence in creation. Tangible health and healing are more likely to be the guiding priorities of people living with HIV and populations who are specifically vulnerable to HIV. This is one factor that makes these populations essential stakeholders in the design, delivery and evaluation of medical responses to HIV.

While religious communication is comfortable working with anecdotal evidence, I have highlighted above that in isolation from a scientific evidence base, it limits opportunities for sustainable collaborations, sharing of resources and opportunities for the affirmation of distinctive contributions. Despite these limitations, storytelling still has a role in increasing the quality, availability and accessibility of medical care.

The presence and impact of HIV in societies calls for urgent and effective responses. Miracles and some religious practices support urgency and the authors observe situations where spiritual and physical perspectives exist with separate identities, blended in clumsy and ungainly ways. I appreciate the examples, which blurred the distinctions between miracles and money, and between listening to God and listening to a sick person. Awkward encounters between sacred stories and human experiences from the past three decades provide a valuable body of creative insight into fields where there remain an enormous number of people urgently needing health care.

Storytelling raises awareness about the limitations of existing health care systems and barriers to access to effective treatment. This makes it foundational for advocacy and transformation. Its freedom from the constraints of health care models and services provides a medium for imagining better health care, including better diagnoses, better medicines and vaccines, and better services. The telling of sacred stories and the telling of stories about seeking health and healing related to HIV and AIDS belong together. When told together, they can help to see and say things we may not have seen or said before; and may not see or say if the stories are told in isolation from one another.

Adding mutuality to the analysis

However, Olivier and Paterson do not explore the religious capacity to participate in mutually accountable relationships with other sectors. Rather, they focus primarily on whether religions can define and substantiate their own claims. Evaluating how religions currently call communities and governments and industries to account are areas for further academic work. At a systemic level, the political, commercial and legislative power accessible to religions is not mentioned among the list of intangible assets. These, along with wealth itself, need to be part of the self-awareness of religions in the twenty-first century. At a community level, the concept of accountability is often burdened with disempowering or aggressive connotations. For example, people seeking treatment for sexually transmitted infections are faced with stigmatisation, rejection, law enforcement and violence in the name of accountability. There should be greater attention paid to maturing the processes used by religions to call others to account in ways that champion peace, justice and compassion; encourage courage and persistence in the face of power; and resist the temptation to use power to dominate and control.

Beliefs about health and healing affect investment in the future. Religious imagination is often concerned with healing society and restoring people to a fully human condition. Scientific medical discourse does not feature prominently in these visions of the future. Activist imagination offers detailed descriptions of what is not available or accessible to the activist population and seeks to turn those descriptions into reality.

Tuberculosis challenges the priority setting frameworks of the agendas of both treatment activist and religious health and healing. It remains the leading killer of people who are living with HIV and is an illness that disproportionately affects children and impoverished people. While access to life-saving treatment for tuberculosis has increased, there have been no substantial developments in diagnosis and treatment for decades. This is despite widespread religious health services, despite strong theological platforms for overcoming poverty and injustice, and despite flourishing developments in access to improving medical diagnosis and treatment of HIV infection, championed by people who are living with HIV. What are the gaps in both religious and activist frameworks that have allowed this situation to develop?

The chapter's concluding question – just what are the treasures that religious health assets bring to the table? – belongs alongside an equally important question: how can religions publicly recognise and affirm the assets brought to the table by sectors that are distinctively different or divergent from any particular religious stakeholder? Olivier and Paterson highlight the assertions made by religious groups, but do not recognise the way religious groups have responded to assertions by other stakeholders in health and healing. Mutual, multi-sectoral accountability and affirmation are imperatives that require further elaboration within religious thought and action related to health and healing in the HIV epidemic. Self-promotion is an inadequate communication strategy.

Furthermore, theological and religious platforms used to motivate health and healing need to be reviewed in the light of lessons learned from experiences of providing medical treatment to people living with HIV around the world. I want to conclude by expressing the need for an accelerated process of evaluation of applied theologies in the context of HIV and AIDS. Perhaps more interaction between theologians working in generalised epidemics and theologians working in concentrated epidemics such as HIV would broaden the spectrum of emerging wisdom and experience.

Olivier and Paterson made passing reference to a Christian rationale that was used early in the HIV epidemic; namely the relationship between Jesus and lepers. Leprosy narratives are still widely used in Christian thought as the entry points for addressing stigma that prevents access to medicine, health and healing.[3] The impact of subsequent decades of HIV and AIDS on this early rationale is not examined in the chapter. However, the leprosy narratives of the Bible may not support the movements proposed in this response. These narratives develop the character of Jesus and of the prophets, but I argue that we should develop our understanding and relationships with people seeking better health. In the Bible, responsibility to verify health rests with religious authorities. I argue that the verification of health in relation to HIV must refer to diagnosis and epidemiology. The leprosy narratives preserve a clear distinction between healer and health seeker. I claim that marginalised people care for each other in the absence of prophets and priests.

Those affirming the scale of health care offered by religious institutions must also affirm the health and healing practices of marginalised, stigmatised and suffering communities. Many of these communities will not change their identity upon securing health and healing, yet they deserve respect. I urge religious scholars and educators to invest more time and energy in building mutually affirming and mutually accountable societies.

Notes

1. Steven Lux and Kristine Greenaway, *Scaling Up Effective Partnerships: A Guide to Working with Faith-Based Organizations in the Response to HIV and AIDS* (Geneva: EAA, 2006).
2. For example, see Muslim apologist writing such as Harun Yahya, *Miracle of the Immune System* (Hillsboro: Goodwill Books, 2001).
3. For example, see Gillian Paterson, *Stigma in the Context of Development: A Christian Response to the HIV Epidemic* (London: Progressio, 2009); UNAIDS, *HIV and AIDS Related Stigma: A Framework for Theological Reflection: A Report of a Theological Workshop Focusing on HIV and AIDS-Related Stigma* (Geneva: UNAIDS, 2004); Wati Longchar (ed.), *Health, Healing and Wholeness: Asian Theological Perspectives on HIV and AIDS* (Jorhat, Assam: Eastern Theological College, 2005); Razouselie Lasetso (ed.), *Health and Life: Theological Reflections on HIV and AIDS* (Jorhat, Assam: Eastern Theological College, 2007).

2

HIV, AIDS and religion in sub-Saharan Africa
An historical survey

Philippe Denis

INTRODUCTION

This chapter examines the history of the relationship between religion and HIV
and AIDS in Africa since the onset of the epidemic. It is based on a survey of
studies dealing, often indirectly, with this theme. Despite the fact that the
epidemic will soon be 30 years old (more if one considers that cases of HIV
infection occurred before they were diagnosed correctly) little attention has been
paid to HIV and AIDS as an historical phenomenon. Even less research has been
carried out on religion in the history of the epidemic. There does not seem to be
a single author who dedicated a study specifically to this subject.

Three recent collections of essays on HIV and AIDS in Africa include comparative studies of earlier epidemics such as smallpox, syphilis and HIV.[1] Some of
the papers refer to religion, but only in passing.[2] Aspects of the history of the
HIV and AIDS epidemic have been studied by Mirko Grmek, Charles Rosenberg,
Virginia Berridge, and Randal Packard and Paul Epstein.[3] As far as Africa is
concerned, the major work is by John Iliffe who has sketched, in a descriptive
rather than an analytical way, the history of HIV and AIDS in sub-Saharan Africa.[4]
The history of the epidemic in South Africa has attracted the attention of
historians such as Howard Phillips and, more recently, Gerald Oppenheimer and
Ronald Bayer.[5] These authors, Iliffe in particular,[6] recognise the importance of
religion in the management of the epidemic but they do not dwell on it.

In HIV and AIDS research, the boundary between history and anthropology
is often blurred. References to history abound in the anthropological literature,
although rarely in an articulate manner. Elizabeth Colson, who conducted a
longitudinal study of a small locality in Zambia, is one of the few anthropologists

57

who consciously looked at the history of the epidemic in its relationship with religion.[7] Journal articles or chapters of books dealing specifically with religion and HIV and AIDS in Africa were rare in the early years of the epidemic but they have now started to multiply. There is the work of Baffour Takyi on Ghana; Daniel Jordan Smith on Nigeria; Marc-Eric Gruénais and Joseph Tonda on the Republic of Congo; Jeremy Liebowitz and Helen Epstein on Uganda; Galia Sabar-Friedman and Bill Black on Kenya; Marjorie Mbilinyi and Naomi Kaihula, and Hansjoerg Dilger on Tanzania; James Pfeiffer and Victor Agadjanian on Mozambique; Rob Garner, Adam Ashforth and Mark Krakauer on South Africa; and Frederick Klaits on Botswana.[8] Their ethnographic work is of great relevance for a history on HIV, AIDS and religion in Africa.

By and large, the practice of religious institutions with regard to HIV and the manner in which the epidemic affected their operations and identity remains undocumented. The task to be accomplished is enormous. Religious leaders, pastoral agents, workers in non-governmental organisations (NGOs) and ordinary believers involved in curbing the epidemic have to be interviewed; and minutes of meetings, annual reports, policy documents, sermon outlines and pamphlets produced in relation to HIV and AIDS collected and analysed. It will only be when this documentation is fully available that a comprehensive history of HIV and AIDS and religion can be written.

THE MULTI-LEVEL RESPONSE OF RELIGIOUS INSTITUTIONS

As a substitute for church-based organisation, which excluded non-Christian institutions, the phrase faith-based organisation (FBO) was coined by the United Nations Program on HIV and AIDS (UNAIDS) around 1997.[9] FBO is commonly used in development circles, especially in the United States, to distinguish religious-based from public and other non faith-based organisations. However, it is an ambiguous term. Depending on who uses it, it can refer to religious leadership structures, local congregations, or HIV and AIDS initiatives inspired by religious beliefs but not necessarily formally linked to religious institutions. The definition of an FBO, Jeremy Liebowitz noted, 'include[s] both places of worship and their members as well as any organization affiliated with or controlled by these houses of worship'. This means 'that both formal NGOs and informal groups within congregations may be active as organizations although the degree of religious influence may vary between formal non-profits and informal congregation-based groups'.[10] For the purpose of this discussion, the term religious institution, less equivocal than FBO, is used.

When analysing the responses of religious organisations to HIV and AIDS three types of response should be distinguished: from the leadership structures of religious institutions; from local congregations or assemblies; and from the formal or informal organisations created by religious institutions in the context of HIV and AIDS. The responses themselves can be divided into four categories: religious discourses on HIV and AIDS; effects of religious affiliation on HIV prevalence; HIV prevention; and AIDS treatment and care.

The leaders of religious institutions contribute in a significant manner to the public discourse on HIV and AIDS. As representatives and interpreters of religious beliefs they influence both policy making and popular attitudes. They define moral norms in matters such as condom use or pre-wedding HIV test requirements and articulate a religious response to the epidemic. Yet, their impact on the sexual behaviour of their members should not be overestimated. The bigger and more inclusive a religious institution, the less its members are likely to follow its teaching on sexual matters.[11] Likewise, it should not be presumed that a statement issued by a religious institution against stigma and discrimination will translate into attitude change in the congregation. The second component of religious institutions, the local congregation or assembly, is probably the most important for this discussion. It is at this level that progress is made, or not, in curbing the HIV epidemic through behaviour change, stigma reduction, higher levels of disclosure, and care, treatment and ongoing support to people living with HIV. A significant factor with regard to religious institutions is the faith and spirituality of their members. It is this that informs their response to the epidemic, either positively by fostering care and compassion or negatively by encouraging stigma and discrimination. At a third level, religious institutions create, or encourage their members to create, formal and informal HIV and AIDS organisations. These can be managed by the national headquarters of a religious body, by a local congregation or by a group of believers with no formal link to a religious institution. Unevenly spread, they are the visible face of the religious response to the epidemic. In no way, however, can they claim to represent their religious institution. In terms of behaviour and attitudes, members of local congregations can be completely at odds with the religious-based organisations operating in the same territory even if they practise the same religion.

Preventing the spread of a disease and mitigating its effects are two different things. Historically, religious institutions have been more effective in their attempts to provide care and support to the people infected or affected by the epidemic than in their prevention campaigns. In this chapter, two types of response are examined. There is, however, a third type of impact that is perhaps more important. The most durable effect of religion on the epidemic may lie less in what members do (or omit to do) in response to HIV and AIDS than the manner in which the beliefs and practices of this religion shape the societal understanding of the epidemic. It is to this type of impact that the chapter now turns.

RELIGIOUS DISCOURSES ON HIV AND AIDS

As French anthropologist Jean-Pierre Dozon observed, religious institutions and traditional healers significantly contribute to the 'networks of explanation' or 'signifying processes' at work during the epidemic because they are in close contact with the people affected by it. They add meaning to the epidemic and mediate the prevention messaging.[12] They influence not only what is said but what is not said.[13] Religious institutions shape the discourse on HIV and AIDS in two ways: they contribute to the perception of HIV infection as caused by individual behaviour; and they spread the idea that it is a moral problem. They both individualise and moralise the issue.

By and large religious institutions reflect and reinforce a common representation of HIV infection as the result of multiple instances of individual risky behaviour caused by lack of information and poor decision making. Since the onset of the epidemic in the early 1980s, policy makers and planners acted 'as though increased information would be sufficient to change complexly determined action and as though individuals could exercise control over the social and cultural constraints to prevention'.[14] This representation leaves aside socio-political and economic phenomena such as gender violence, wars, migration, social inequality and poverty that prevent individuals from exercising any real control over their sexual lives. In South Africa, for instance, there is evidence that migrant workers have been more susceptible to preventable illness than non-migrants and that the labour migrant system has played a decisive historical role in the shaping of the epidemic.[15]

During colonial times, and seemingly in British more than in French colonies,[16] religious authorities blamed loose morals, especially among women, for the spread of sexually transmitted infections (STIs).[17] Similar models of explanation are applied to the current HIV epidemic.[18] The dominant discourse is that HIV infection is a matter of individual responsibility.

Religion thus contributes significantly to the moralisation of HIV and AIDS discourse. In the most extreme form, it explains the disease as a punishment from

God. Because God is the cause of everything, it is assumed that God is also the cause of HIV. In ascribing HIV and AIDS to this theology, only the repentance of sinners removes the threat of the epidemic. Mainline churches have since abandoned this view but it continues to be held today in some Pentecostal and African independent churches.[19] There are many instances of Muslim leaders preaching that HIV and AIDS is a punishment of Allah.[20] According to Malik Badri, the widely read Muslim scholar, 'the general Islamic belief about the AIDS pandemic is that it is divine retribution for the immoral homosexual revolution of the West and its aping in other countries'. This belief, he adds, 'is firmly rooted in the Muslim mind because every child in his early school years has been thrilled by the Qur'anic story of the Prophet Lot . . . and what God did to his homosexual people'.[21]

But the moral discourse on HIV and AIDS can take more subtle forms. Most religious leaders would agree that God never wanted people to suffer from AIDS. Yet, for many of them it is the lack of adherence to God-given sexual norms that is the ultimate cause of the disease.[22] The same applies to Islam. In south-eastern Tanzania, mainstream Muslim and reformists 'all integrate AIDS into narratives of decline: of increasing distance from God, of running out of blessings, of rising ignorance or "westernisation"'.[23] As Catholic theologian Charles Ryan noted, it cannot be denied that religion has always taught that sexual activity is for married people only. The implication is that any HIV infected person must be somehow guilty of sexual misconduct:

> Recently I asked a group of seminarians and religious that I was teaching what was their first response when hearing that somebody was HIV positive. The chorused answer was: 'How did he get it?' Subsequently, when I was discussing with a group of priests how difficult I was finding it to stop students thinking in terms of guilt when confronting HIV and AIDS, they became very silent until one of them said: 'But are they [the HIV/AIDS sufferers] not guilty?'[24]

In his study of care and compassion in an African independent church in Botswana, Fred Klaits observed that with regard to HIV and AIDS the areas of prevention and care seem completely disconnected. The church made HIV infected people feel guilty but as soon as they became sick they gave them support, conveniently ignoring the reasons why they had become infected.[25] Full responsibility for moralising discourses and resulting social demobilisation cannot therefore be laid solely at the feet of biomedical policy makers. The discourses and policy are embedded in the public culture to which religious institutions contribute in a significant way.[26] Directly or indirectly, they feed moralistic discourses.

The discourse of religious institutions on HIV and AIDS, however, is far from homogenous. As Mbilinyi and Kaihula showed in Tanzania, the moral interpretation of the epidemic is the subject of debate among believers.[27] HIV and AIDS prompted a reflection on health, sexuality and disease that contributed, in some sectors at least, to a new understanding of the core beliefs of religious communities. The theologies of AIDS that emerged as a result of the epidemic did not only influence the religious responses but the religious institutions themselves. The traditional doctrines of God, sin and redemption were revisited. AIDS came to be seen as a gendered disease and that affected the self-understanding of religious institutions. Sex came out of the closet.[28]

This history remains largely unwritten. In South Africa, for instance, the first attempts to reflect theologically on HIV and AIDS go back to the early 1990s.[29] Since then publications on the theology and spirituality of HIV and AIDS have developed exponentially, with the epidemic placed in the curriculum of many theological institutions.[30] Building on the work of social scientists, theologians, religious HIV activists and, in some cases, religious leaders brought to the fore the socio-economic factors of HIV transmission.[31] A new, less moralising, ethical reflection on sexuality and the epidemic is emerging.

RELIGIOUS AFFILIATION AND HIV TRANSMISSION

Is religious affiliation a co-factor of HIV transmission? Curiously, few authors have addressed this issue. There is hardly a word on religion in Alan Whiteside and Tony Barnett's classic work, for instance.[32] There are a few scholars who have examined the correlation between Islam and HIV, which is thought to be negative. Data on differences of HIV prevalence among members of Christian denominations are less conclusive.

In his history of the epidemic in Africa, John Iliffe has claimed that the Islamic social order might have limited the transmission of the disease in the savannah region (Mali, Niger and Chad), a zone of very low HIV prevalence. Non-marital sex was to an unusual degree confined to sex workers and young, unmarried, circumcised men, where it was least likely to spread infection to the general population. Likewise, the restraint imposed by Muslim culture explained, according to him, the difference in HIV prevalence between the Muslim north in Nigeria and the centre and south-east, which was largely Christian. Another example was Casamance, the area with the highest prevalence rate in Senegal and also the one with the biggest Christian population.[33]

Peter Gray's study of HIV prevalence among Muslims brought somewhat different results. On the basis of multi-variate analysis of information obtained from several online demographic and HIV databases, he noted that in 38 sub-Saharan African countries with a minimum of one million inhabitants, the percentage of Muslims negatively predicted HIV national prevalence. However, in the second part of his work, based on a survey of eleven published studies containing data on HIV prevalence and religious affiliation, he observed that 'the data on risk factors associated with HIV portray a mixed picture with respect to any protective benefits following from adherence to Islamic codes'. The data, he further explained, 'clearly show that these rules are not followed by everyone, and in some cases do not appear to alter patterns of behaviour by comparison to non-Muslim members of the same population'. What then explained the lower rate of HIV prevalence in Muslim countries? According to Gray it was because Muslims seemed to have lower alcohol consumption, which might partly underlie differences in risky sexual behaviour, and higher rates of circumcision compared to non-Muslims. On the other hand, Islam's allowance for polygyny and discourage-ment of condom use would work against reduced sexual transmission of HIV.[34]

Gray's study is based on research conducted in Uganda, Kenya, Tanzania, Nigeria and Senegal. Other studies come to similar conclusions. In northern Sudan, a predominantly Muslim area, official statistics registered a steady increase of HIV prevalence and the state-run media projected the epidemic as an imminent threat. Despite authoritarian Islamist rule, Sudan went through a process of liberalisation, secularisation and greater exposure to world cultures.[35] In Ghana, Muslim women reported less behavioural change in response to the HIV epidemic than their Christian counterparts, according to an epidemiological survey.[36]

Turning to the Christian churches, a key question is whether HIV transmission depends on the type of church affiliation. The scarce studies taking up this question are based on dated fieldwork in South Africa, Zimbabwe, Ghana and Malawi and none is fully conclusive.[37] Despite their limitations, these studies are nevertheless useful to understand the dynamics at work among religious institutions in matters of prevention.

On the basis of 334 household visits and 78 in-depth interviews conducted in Edendale near Pietermaritzburg in 1997, Rob Garner, a British anthropologist who later became a child activist, concluded that among the four church types present in the area he surveyed – mainline, Pentecostal, Apostolic and Zionist – the Pentecostal recorded the lowest degree of extra- and premarital sex. Why should Pentecostal or Spirit-type churches be more able to change the behaviour of their followers than other denominations? Garner claimed that four factors allowed these churches to promote more significant behavioural change. According to him, the strength of the Pentecostals in the four categories of indoctrination, religious experience, exclusion and socialisation allowed them to change the behaviour of their followers. For example, indoctrination, defined as the 'methods and depths of the group's educational programme', described the extent to which a religious group might educate its members about a particular issue. Pentecostals spent much more time and energy educating their followers about the importance of avoiding pre- and extra-marital sex. Exclusion referred to the boundary between one religious group and another. According to Garner, the impact of mainline churches on sexual attitudes and behaviour was 'slight but not completely insignificant'. The youth group in the mainline church he visited in Edendale was not well established and 'although the church would theoretically oppose extra- and premarital sex, the youth [did] not receive much Bible teaching on this subject'.[38]

In a similar way Simon Gregson and his colleagues, who conducted a demographic survey in the Honde and Rusitu valleys in Manicaland, Zimbabwe between 1993 and 1995, suggested that members of spirit-type churches were less likely to become infected by HIV because of their distinctive patterns of sexual behaviour. Religious affiliation explained the different mortality patterns in the region:

> The recent HIV-associated rise in mortality is less evident in the demo-graphic data for Spirit-type churches in both areas. This could be because members of these churches are more likely than other people to follow church teachings on avoidance of pre-marital and extra-marital sex and are therefore at lower risk of acquiring HIV infection despite the potential for rapid transmission posed by the multiple partner aspect of polygynous marriage systems.[39]

Both studies pointed at religious affiliation as a factor of risk reduction but they differed on the type of church that had an impact on HIV transmission. For

Garner, the church type reporting the lowest rate of multiple sexual partnerships was the Pentecostal, a group, one should note, that constituted only four per cent of his sample.[40] In Edendale the members of the Apostolic and Zionist churches, two African Independent Churches (AICs) with different modes of organisation and levels of indigenisation, did not seem to practise less extra- and premarital sex than the members of the other churches. In Gregson's study, on the other hand, the Apostolic and Zionist churches seemed to be the most effective in regulating the sexual behaviour of their members.

In Malawi, Jenny Trinitapoli found fewer extra-marital affairs and sexually transmitted diseases (STDs) among Pentecostals than Catholics in the three rural districts she surveyed between 1997 and 2000 but no significant difference of risk of HIV transmission.[41]

Baffour Takyi's study, which is based on the 1998 Ghana Demographic Health Survey, only differentiates between Catholics, Protestants, other Christians, Muslims, and African Traditional Religion (ATR). Religion, according to this author, is a 'significant predictor of behaviour change' in Ghana. While 71.8 per cent of Protestant women and 68.7 per cent of Catholic women indicated changing at least one risk practice, only 52.3 per cent of the ATR women reported doing so. ATR women were less likely to report being involved with a single partner than the women from the other denominations. Unlike the other studies, the Pentecostals were not isolated as a group. It is not clear whether they were considered as Protestants or other Christians. The difference between these two groups, in any case, was not significant. Muslims were slightly less likely to change their behaviour than Christians.[42]

In conclusion, religious affiliation may lead to behaviour change in sub-Saharan Africa, and probably more in some Christian denominations, the Pentecostal churches in particular, than others. However, there is no set pattern. The members of a given religious group may report behaviour change in one country and no behaviour change in another. The difference probably lies in the degree of what Garner terms socialisation, religious experience, indoctrination and exclusion. They vary over time in each religious group.

THE DILEMMA OF PREVENTION

Religious institutions were among the first to run HIV prevention campaigns in Africa. Brochures funded by Oxfam in Britain were distributed in the Catholic archdiocese of Kinshasa as early as 1985.[43] Church-run prevention seminars for religious leaders were run in Tanzania in the 1980s.[44] In Uganda church leaders were invited on national AIDS committees as soon as they were established in the early 1990s.[45] In KwaZulu-Natal a Methodist minister, Neil Oosthuizen, opened the Hillcrest AIDS Centre in 1991.[46] Muslims were also active in public education. The Sultan of Sokoto became part of Nigeria's National AIDS Commission.[47] In Senegal the Muslim NGO, Jamra, supported the government's efforts to combat HIV and AIDS.[48]

On two issues, however, religious leaders, whether Christian, Muslim or African traditionalist, clashed head on with governments and health authorities in matters of HIV prevention: the use of condoms and sex education.[49]

Regarding condoms, the Christian churches adopted a very ambivalent attitude. Only one church, the Roman Catholic, formally condemned the use of condoms as a way of preventing HIV. But at the same time the Catholic bishops were divided. The Holy See took a hard line, as one could expect, followed by some national bishops' conferences. In July 2001 the Southern African Catholic Bishops' Conference (SACBC) declared in a statement that the 'widespread and indiscriminate promotion of condoms' was an 'immoral and misguided weapon in [the] battle against HIV/AIDS'.[50] At the meeting of the International Forum for Catholic Action held in Bujumbura in August 2002, Archbishop Simon Ntamwana, the president of the Catholic Bishops' Conference of Burundi, said that as far as the church was concerned, AIDS was and would remain 'a moral evil' and that the 'narcissism of condoms would not help at all'.[51] Other bishops remained silent, tacitly condoning the use of condoms. In their April 1996 *Message aux fidèles*, for instance, the Congolese bishops outlined the church's position on HIV and AIDS without saying a word on condoms.[52] In 2002 the Catholic Bishops' Conference of Chad ruled that, with regard to the use of condoms, 'the ultimate rule is our conscience'.[53] These statements echoed the argument made by a group of Catholic theologians at the time that condom distribution and needle exchange were morally licit as a means of HIV prevention since there was no other way to save lives.[54] On the ground, Catholic doctors, nurses, counsellors and representatives of donor organisations often promoted, if discreetly, the use of condoms.[55] Significantly it was a Catholic priest, Bernard Joinet, who pioneered the prevention campaign later known as ABC (Abstain, Be faithful, and Condomise) in Tanzania in 1994.[56]

The Protestant churches were equally divided on the issue of condom use. The top leadership of the Lutheran and Moravian churches in Rungwe, Tanzania, for instance, strongly condemned the use of condoms but the local church leaders abstained from denouncing them. In focus groups, members of the local congregations unambiguously distanced themselves from their church leadership on the issue of condoms.[57] The Anglican Church in Nigeria supported the use of condoms, as did some branches of the Lutheran Church and the All-African Conference of Churches.[58] Most Pentecostal church leaders vehemently denounced the use of condoms. In Uganda a Pentecostal pastor organised bonfires of condoms at Makerere University in 2004.[59]

The establishment of the President's Emergency Program for AIDS Relief (PEPFAR), a funding agency of the United States government, at the instigation of the evangelical right, in 2003 boosted the development of abstinence and faithfulness-only programmes in Africa for which no less than US$1 billion were earmarked. Well-funded, these programmes multiplied in Uganda and other eastern African countries after 2003.[60] With the change of majority in the United States Congress in 2006 and the election of Barack Obama in 2008, however, PEPFAR became more independent from the religious right and its emphasis on abstinence and faithfulness gave way to a more diversified approach to prevention. But the agency continued to include FBOs in its programmes. In this way, religious institutions have maintained their influence on US HIV prevention policies, including the use (or not) of condoms.

Muslim traditional leaders have also rejected the use of condoms. In 2008 a group of Muslim scholars launched a campaign against condoms in north-eastern Kenya on the grounds that they promoted immorality.[61] However, the issue has also brought division within the Muslim community. Malik Badri, for instance, has expressed the opinion that the use of condoms should be viewed within the general law of choosing between two evils: 'If we apply this rule, on which there is a general consensus among Muslims jurists', he commented, 'we could make the use of a condom obligatory for a fornicating Muslim who might expect HIV infection from his promiscuous practices.'[62]

Likewise, ministers of AICs and traditional leaders have been opposed to the use of condoms. In traditional African culture interference with fertility was seen as immoral.[63] In South Africa groups of traditionalist Zulu and Xhosa women advocated the renewal of virginity testing as a way of preventing HIV.[64]

The opposition of religious leaders to the use of condoms in HIV prevention is often considered, in biomedical circles and among activists, as proof of moral conservatism and insensitivity to the loss of human lives. The reality is more complicated. Religious traditionalists contend that by promoting abstinence until marriage and faithfulness, in other words no sex outside marriage, they do prevention work. The fear of exclusion may lead their members to stick to one partner and in this way avoid the risk of infection. In this sense, as Jeremy Liebowitz noted, stigma attached to the disease can be helpful.[65] However, the problem is that the enforcement of strict moral rules in religious institutions can produce the opposite effect. By equating HIV and AIDS with sexual promiscuity, religion can provide a context for stigmatising HIV positive people. Stigma as a social construct has a significant impact on the life experiences of individuals. It encourages denial and prevents those who are HIV positive from seeking support and care. Religious institutions, in other words, are caught in a dilemma. They have the duty to teach moral values in sexual matters and by doing so they may reduce risk behaviour, thus preventing the spread of HIV. But at the same time, their moral discourse can lead to stigma and discrimination, a phenomenon that contributes to the growth of the epidemic.

Daniel Jordan Smith, who studied the relationship between Christianity and AIDS-related beliefs and behaviours in south-eastern Nigeria, gave a vivid illustration of the double-sided effect of religion on HIV prevention. He found denial very common among the young men worshipping in the local Pentecostal congregations. This observation could have been made in many African countries:

> It was not only young migrant women's involvement in economically motivated sex, or men's participation in these relationships, that fell into the category of denial. Through the rumours, gossip, and occasional confessions that were heard commonly during fieldwork, it was clear that many young men (and some, but seemingly fewer, young women) were, in fact, cheating on their 'moral partners'. Some people had (secretly) more than one moral partner. And, commonly, the beginning of one relationship and the end of another relationship overlapped, so at least for a period of time, many people violated the supposed trust of their moral partnerships. Popular expectations about what a moral sexual relationship should be, shaped so powerfully in this population by Christian discourses, combined with the messy reality of what people's sexual relationships are really like, created a context in which the risk of HIV/AIDS is difficult for young migrants to confront. Religious interpretations of sex and of HIV/AIDS decrease the perceived need of condoms in moral partnerships, but

exacerbate the extent to which people must deny the relationships and the risk from relationships that do not fit the moral model.[66]

TREATMENT AND CARE

The response of religious institutions to HIV and AIDS in the field of care and treatment has been considerable. They have initiated, complemented or supported Western-based biomedical programmes throughout the continent. One can argue that, with the advent of the epidemic, religious institutions regained an aspect of the role they occupied in the medical field during the missionary era. In most African countries they became a necessary complement to the public health sector. Africa has a long history of co-operation between church and state in health matters, particularly in the British colonies.[67] In Zimbabwe, Andrew Fleming, the colony's medical officer, resorted to funding medical stations in reserves under missionary control as early as 1912.[68] Missionaries and traditional leaders were involved in STD awareness programmes in Nyasaland in the 1940s.[69] These examples could be multiplied.

The mainline churches, and particularly the Catholic Church, started their involvement in the treatment and care of those living with HIV in the late 1980s. The Pentecostal churches have only contributed to this effort in recent years but their importance is rapidly increasing. The epidemic, one could argue, has been important for religious institutions. It broadened their base and gave them a powerful tool for evangelisation. Two decades later, with increased funding and an extended network of grassroots organisations, religious institutions have become major role players in the field of HIV and AIDS.

It has been noted that within the Christian community, more Catholics and Protestants than evangelicals (or Pentecostals) developed HIV and AIDS programmes in the early years of the epidemic.[70] In Zambia, for example, NGOs and Christian churches played a critical role from the start in managing HIV prevention and care and addressing some of the limitations of government intervention.[71] In the late 1980s church-based groups from Zambia and Uganda pioneered hospital-based and community-based home care, two models of care that later spread to the rest of Africa. Precedents existed, in the treatment of tuberculosis and leprosy for instance, but with AIDS, home-based care underwent unparalleled development. One of the first, if not the first, extensive hospital-based home care programmes in Africa was developed by the Salvation Army Hospital of Chikatanka in Zambia in 1987. Similar programmes started in Lusaka and Kampala almost simultaneously. The first community-based home care programmes appeared in Uganda, Zambia and Zimbabwe shortly afterwards. Many of these had strong church links, like the Family AIDS Caring Trust (FACT) in Zimbabwe or the programme set up by the Catholic diocese of Ndola in Zambia. The largest home care organisation in southern Africa is Catholic AIDS Action, a Namibian organisation founded in 1998.[72] Women's support groups such as those established by the Moravian Church in Tanzania also provided care and support to people with AIDS-related illnesses.[73] In South Africa many volunteers working in home-based care organisations are Christians.[74] Furthermore, Christians have played a leading role in hospitals. The first HIV and AIDS clinic in KwaZulu-Natal was instituted at McCord Hospital, Durban, a hospital with a strong Christian tradition. Many of the doctors and nurses interviewed by Oppenheimer and Bayer for their oral history of HIV and AIDS in South Africa spoke of their Christian faith as a strong motivating factor.[75] Less studied, but equally important, was Muslim charitable work. In countries such as Nigeria or Senegal the most progressive leaders insisted that people living with HIV must be embraced within Islam's powerful charitable institutions.[76]

Religious institutions also played a pioneering role in the provision of anti-retroviral (ARV) treatment to HIV positive people, particularly in South Africa.[77] It was not until late 2003 that, after much controversy, the South African government finally agreed to plan a national ARV rollout. The first ARV programme in South Africa was initiated by Médecins Sans Frontières (MSF) and the health department of the Province of the Western Cape in Khayelitsha in February 2000.[78] Soon after this, the model was replicated at St Mary's Hospital, Mariannhill in KwaZulu-Natal and in the Masangane ARV Treatment Programme in the Eastern Cape, with the support of the Catholic and Moravian churches respectively. Since then ARV treatment has become one of the main projects of the SACBC AIDS Office.

Another area where religious institutions multiplied initiatives is orphan care. As early as 1993 the Salvation Army was running homes in Johannesburg for HIV infected or affected babies. In Uganda, Kitovu Hospital, a Catholic health care centre developed an extensive programme of community-based orphan care at the same time in Massaka province. This model was reproduced throughout Africa. 'The strength of religion in Africa,' Geoff Foster wrote, 'is fundamental to the resilience of its responses to orphans and vulnerable children. It is difficult to overemphasise the importance of faith on this continent where religion is ubiquitous.'[79]

The response of religious institutions, even those who accepted the biomedical model of health care, was not homogenous. In Rungwe, Tanzania, a study revealed that some Christian women refused care to their unfaithful husbands. Such behaviour, however, is not widespread.[80] More common was discrimination against the HIV positive. In the early 1990s some Protestant churches in Kenya refused to admit HIV positive people or to bury those who died from AIDS-related illnesses. A Catholic priest was reported as having refused to conduct funeral services for fear, he claimed, that 'the church might be seen to be encouraging the spread of the disease'.[81]

Two types of religious institution offer alternatives to allopathic medicine, sometimes, but not often, with the approval and support of Western-based health professionals. On one hand, there are traditional healers who propose a variety of herbal or animal-based remedies and seek the co-operation of the ancestral spirits. Such indigenous forms of alternative medicine exist in Ivory Coast, Botswana, Malawi and South Africa, to name only a few countries.[82] Some health care professionals see traditional medicine as part of holistic care, particularly in the field of mental health. Others regard it as obscurantist and denounce the fraudulent exploitation of the sick.[83] On the other hand, there are healing churches, a phenomenon already attested to in Kinshasa in the 1980s and in Brazzaville in the early 1990s, and which have continued to develop.[84] They suddenly changed the social and cultural landscape in Zambia during the 1990s and in Uganda in the early twenty-first century.[85] The argument of the leaders of these churches was very simple: God, being almighty, gave AIDS to those who deserved it but also had the power to heal those who believed in God. As a Pentecostal pastor from Brazzaville explained in 1992, 'We, the people of God, we have the faith. When the patient arrives, we do not care about AIDS. We lay hands on him in the name of Jesus. We know the cause of the disease is sin. If we put our trust in God, God will do everything.'[86]

CONCLUSION

It was only in recent years that public health specialists and policy makers realised that religion – Christianity in particular – can be an asset, and not necessarily a hindrance, in curbing the epidemic. But the debate is all but over. This survey shows that in sub-Saharan Africa religious institutions shape the common discourse on HIV and AIDS in a manner that is not always helpful. Promoting abstinence and faithfulness can have the unintended effect of encouraging denial, stigma and discrimination even though adherence to religious-based norms of sexual behaviour demonstrably reduces the risk of infection. Unfortunately, research on the relationship between HIV transmission and religious affiliation is too fragmented for any general statement to be made. It seems, however, that the Pentecostal churches may be more effective, at least in some areas, than the other churches in enforcing Christian norms of sexual behaviour. Whether the Islamic social order limits the transmission of the disease is debatable. Largely borne by mainline churches, the impact of religious institutions on the mitigation of HIV transmission is more visible, especially since the turn of the century. Christian initiatives in matters of care and treatment are spread all over Africa. In three areas – home-based care, orphan care and ARV treatment – religious institutions can be said to have made a significant contribution.[87]

NOTES

1. Charles Becker et al. (eds), *Vivre et Penser le SIDA en Afrique: Experiencing and Understanding AIDS in Africa* (Paris: Karthala, 1999); Philip W. Setel, Milton Lewis and Maryinez Lyons (eds), *Histories of Sexually Transmitted Diseases and HIV/AIDS in Sub-Saharan Africa* (Westport: Greenwood Press, 1999); Philippe Denis and Charles Becker (eds), *L'épidémie du sida en Afrique Subsaharienne: Regards Historiens* (Paris: Karthala, 2006). English translation available at http://www.refer.sn/rds/article.php3?id_article=245 (accessed 23 Dec. 2009).
2. Charles Becker and René Collignon, 'A history of sexually transmitted diseases and AIDS in Senegal: Difficulties in accounting for social logics in health policy' in *Histories of Sexually Transmitted Diseases and HIV/AIDS in Sub-Saharan Africa*, edited by Setel, Lewis and Lyons: 65–96; Wiseman Chijere Chirwa, 'Sexually transmitted diseases in colonial Malawi' in *Histories of Sexually Transmitted Diseases and HIV/AIDS in Sub-Saharan Africa*, edited by Setel, Lewis and Lyons: 143–66; Bryan T. Callahan and Virginia Bond, 'The social, cultural, and epidemiological history of sexually transmitted diseases in Zambia' in *Histories of Sexually Transmitted Diseases and HIV/AIDS in Sub-Saharan Africa*, edited by Setel, Lewis and Lyons: 167–93; Benedict Carton, 'Le silence et la honte comme objet d'histoire' in *L'épidémie du sida en Afrique Subsaharienne* edited by Denis and Becker: 107–39.
3. Mirko D. Grmek, *Histoire du sida: Début et Origine d'une Pandémie Actuelle* (Paris: Payot, 3rd ed., 1995); Charles E. Rosenberg, *Explaining Epidemics and Other Studies in the History of Medicine* (Cambridge: Cambridge University Press, 1992); Virginia Berridge, *AIDS in the UK: The Making of a Policy, 1981–1994* (New York: Oxford University Press, 1996); Randall M. Packard and Paul Epstein, 'Epidemiologists, social scientists, and the structure of social research on AIDS in Africa'. *Social Science and Medicine* 33(7) 1991: 771–94.
4. John Iliffe, *The African AIDS Epidemic: A History* (Oxford: James Currey, 2006).
5. Howard Phillips, 'AIDS in the context of South Africa's epidemic history: preliminary historical thoughts'. *South African Historical Journal* 45 (2001): 11–26; Gerald M. Oppenheimer

and Ronald Bayer, *Shattered Dreams?: An Oral History of the South African Epidemic* (Oxford: Oxford University Press, 2007).

6. Iliffe, *The African AIDS Epidemic*: 94–7.

7. Elizabeth Colson, 'En quête de guérison: l'épidémie de sida dans la vallée Gwembe' in *L'épidémie du sida en Afrique Subsaharienne*, edited by Denis and Becker: 141–64.

8. Baffour Takyi, 'Religion and women's health in Ghana: Insights into HIV/AIDS preventive and protective behaviour'. *Social Science and Medicine* 56 (2003): 1221–34; Daniel Jordan Smith, 'Youth, sin and sex in Nigeria: Christianity and HIV-related beliefs and behaviour among rural-urban migrants'. *Culture, Health and Sexuality* 6(5) 2004: 425–37; Marc-Eric Gruénais, 'La religion préserve-t-elle du sida?: des congrégations religieuses Congolaises face à la pandémie de l'infection par le VIH' in *Colloque International: Sciences Sociales et Sida en Afrique: Bilan et Perspectives, Communications* (Dakar: Codesria, 1996): 671–82; Joseph Tonda, 'Les spécialistes non médicaux Congolais et le problème de la connaissance scientifique du sida in *Vivre et Penser le Sida en Afrique*, edited by Becker et al., 631–44; Jeremy Liebowitz, *The Impact of Faith-Based Organizations on HIV/AIDS Prevention and Mitigation in Africa* (Durban: Health Economics and HIV/AIDS Research Division [HEARD], University of KwaZulu-Natal, 2002); Helen Epstein, *The Invisible Cure: Africa, the West, and the Fight against AIDS* (New York: Farrar, Straus and Giroux, 2007): 185–201; Galia Sabar-Freidman, 'AIDS prevention and the Church: Kenya: Mixed messages'. *AIDS and Society* 6(2) 1995: 4; Bill Black, 'HIV/AIDS and the Church: Kenyan religious leaders become partners in prevention'. *AIDScaptions* 4(1) 1997: 23–6; Marjorie Mbilinyi and Naomi Kaihula, 'Sinners and outsiders: The drama of AIDS in Rungwe' in *AIDS, Sexuality and Gender in Africa: Collective Strategies and Struggles in Tanzania and Zambia*, edited by Caroline Baylies and Janet Bujra (London: Routledge, 2000): 76-95; Hansjoerg Dilger, 'Living positHIVely in Tanzania: The global dynamics of AIDS and the meaning of religion for international and local AIDS work'. *Afrika Spectrum* 36(1) 2001: 73–90; Hansjoerg Dilger, 'Healing the wounds of modernity: Salvation, community and care in a neo-Pentecostal church in Dar es Salaam, Tanzania'. *Journal of Religion in Africa* 37(1) 2007: 59–83; Hansjoerg Dilger, 'We are all going to die: Kinship, belonging and the morality of HIV/AIDS-related illnesses and deaths in rural Tanzania'. *Anthropological Quarterly* 81(1) 2008: 207–32; James Pfeiffer, 'Condom social marketing, Pentecostalism, and structural adjustment in Mozambique: A clash of AIDS prevention messages'. *Medical Anthropology Quarterly* 18(1) 2004: 77–103; Victor Agadjanian, 'Gender, religious involvement, and HIV/AIDS prevention in Mozambique'. *Social Science and Medicine* 61(7) 2005: 1529–39; Victor Agadjanian and Soma Sen, 'Promises and challenges of faith-based AIDS care and support in Mozambique'. *American Journal of Public Health* 97(2) 2007: 362–6; Robert Garner, 'Safe sects: Dynamic religion and AIDS in South Africa'. *Journal of Modern African Studies* 38(1) 2000: 41–69; Adam Ashforth, *Witchcraft, Violence, and Democracy in South Africa* (Chicago: University of Chicago Press, 2006); Mark Krakauer and Jodie Newbery, 'Churches' responses to HIV/AIDS in two South African communities'. *Journal of the International Association of Physicians in AIDS Care* 6(1) 2007: 27–35; Frederick Klaits, 'Making a good death: AIDS and social belonging in an independent church in Gaborone'. *Botswana Notes and Records* 30 (1998): 101–19; Frederick Klaits, 'The widow in blue: Death and the morality of remembering in Botswana's time of AIDS'. *Africa* 75(1) 2005: 46–62.

9. Information kindly provided by Ted Karpf, partnerships officer at the WHO Department of HIV/AIDS.

10. Liebowitz, *The Impact of Faith-Based Organizations on HIV/AIDS Prevention and Mitigation in Africa*: 4.

11. Garner, 'Safe sects': 63.

12. Jean-Pierre Dozon, 'From the social and cultural appropriations of HIV/AIDS to necessary political appropriations: Some elements towards a synthesis' in *Vivre et Penser le Sida en Afrique*, edited by Becker et al.: 692.

13. Donald Messer, *Breaking the Conspiracy of Silence: Christian Churches and the Global AIDS Crisis* (Minneapolis: Augsburg Fortress, 2004); see also Barbara Schmid, 'AIDS discourses in the church: What we say and what we do'. *Journal of Theology for Southern Africa* 125 (2006): 91–103.

14. Brooke Grundfest Schoepf, 'AIDS, history and struggles over meaning' in *HIV and AIDS in Africa: Beyond Epidemiology*, edited by Ezekiel Kalipeni et al. (Oxford: Blackwell Publishing, 2004): 17.

15. Simonne Horwitz, 'Migrancy and HIV/AIDS: A historical perspective'. *South African Historical Journal* 45 (2001): 103–23.

16. Becker and Collignon, 'A history of sexually transmitted diseases and AIDS in Senegal': 74.

17. Maryinez Lyons, 'Medicine and morality: A review of responses to sexually transmitted diseases in Uganda in the twentieth century' in *Histories of Sexually Transmitted Diseases and HIV/AIDS in Sub-Saharan Africa*, edited by Setel, Lewis and Lyons: 101; Jock McCulloch, 'The management of venereal disease in a settler society: Colonial Zimbabwe, 1900 to 1930' in *Histories of Sexually Transmitted Diseases and HIV/AIDS in Sub-Saharan Africa*, edited by Setel, Lewis and Lyons: 209.

18. Phillips, 'AIDS in the context of South Africa's epidemic history': 11–26.

19. At a bishops' conference in the Lutheran Church of Tanzania in 1987, AIDS was still characterised as God's punishment of human beings: see Mbilinyi and Kaihula, 'Sinners and outsiders': 87. But leaders such as Archbishop Njongonkulu Ndungane, then Archbishop of the Anglican Church of Southern Africa, made public statements in 2004 that categorically refuted the idea that AIDS was a punishment from God. Available at http://www.iol.co.za/general/news/newsprint.php?art-id+qw1101911580359B232&sf (accessed 12 Oct. 2009). Iliffe, *The African AIDS Epidemic*: 94 quotes an AIC leader in Botswana who suggests that HIV and AIDS is 'a punishment sent by God, as Sodom and Gomorrah'.

20. For an example in Ethiopia, see Iliffe, *The African AIDS Epidemic*: 95.

21. Malik Badri, 'The AIDS crisis: An Islamic perspective' in *Islam and AIDS: Between Scorn, Pity and Justice*, edited by Farid Esack and Sarah Chiddy (Oxford: Oneworld, 2009): 39.

22. Gruénais, 'La religion préserve-t-elle du sida?': 674. See also Daniela Gennrich et al., *Churches and HIV/AIDS: Exploring How Local Churches Are Integrating HIV/AIDS in the Life and Ministries of the Church and How Those Most Directly Affected Experience These* (Pietermaritzburg: PACSA, 2004).

23. Felicity Becker, 'The virus and the scriptures: Muslims and AIDS in Tanzania'. *Journal of Religion in Africa* 37 (2007): 35.

24. Charles Ryan, 'HIV/AIDS and responsibility: the Catholic tradition' in *Responsibility in a Time of AIDS: A Pastoral Response by Catholic Theologians and AIDS Activists in Southern Africa*, edited by Stuart C. Bate (Pietermaritzburg: Cluster Publications, 2003): 6.

25. I am grateful to Fred Klaits, lecturing fellow at Duke University, for sharing his thoughts on this issue. See his unpublished paper 'Faith and the intersubjectivity of care in Botswana' from the Symposium on Religious Engagements with HIV/AIDS in Africa, Copenhagen, 28–29 Apr. 2008.

26. Schoepf, 'AIDS, history and struggles over meaning': 18.

27. In Rungwe, Tanzania, Mbilinyi and Kaihula found evidence of division among the members of the Lutheran Church: 'The moral crusade against AIDS was by no means greeted with unanimity. Divisions within churches and between elders/leaders and youthful members were evident, reflecting widening divisions in general society' (Mbilinyi and Kaihula, 'Sinners and outsiders': 87).

28. The phrase is from Gillian Paterson in Chapter 14 of this book.

29. Willem Saayman, 'AIDS, healing and culture in Africa: A Christian mission perspective'. *Journal of Theology for Southern Africa* 78 (1992): 29–42; Willem Saayman and Johan Kriel, *AIDS: The Leprosy of our Time?* (Johannesburg: Orion Publishers, 1992); Gunther Wittenberg, 'Counselling AIDS patients: Job as a paradigm'. *Journal of Theology for Southern Africa* 88 (1994): 61–8; Ronald Nicolson, 'AIDS: The ethical issue'. *Missionalia* 22(3) 1994: 227–44. The first comprehensive theology of AIDS is Ronald Nicolson's *God in AIDS?: A Theological Enquiry* (London: SCM, 1996).

30. See Musa Dube, *Methods of Integrating HIV/AIDS in Theological Programmes* (Geneva: WCC, 2003).

31. Ronald Nicolson, *HIV/AIDS: A Christian Response* (Pietermaritzburg, Cluster Publications, 1995): 39; James Keenan (ed.), *Catholic Ethicists on HIV/AIDS Prevention* (New York: Continuum, 2000): 14; Alison Munro, 'Responsibility: The prevention of HIV/AIDS' in *Responsibility in a Time of HIV/AIDS*, edited by Bate: 41–2; Philippe Denis, 'Sexuality and AIDS in South Africa'. *Journal of Theology for Southern Africa* 115 (2003): 63–77.

32. Tony Barnett and Alan Whiteside, *AIDS in the Twenty-First Century: Disease and Globalization* (New York: Palgrave, 2002).

33. Iliffe, *The African AIDS Epidemic*: 55–7.

34. Peter Gray, 'HIV and Islam: Is HIV prevalence lower among Muslims?' *Social Science and Medicine* 58(9) 2004: 1754–5.

35. Atta El-Battahani, 'AIDS and politics in Sudan: Some reflections' in *Vivre et Penser le Sida en Afrique: Experiencing and Understanding AIDS in Africa*, edited by Becker et al.; 301.

36. Takyi, 'Religion and women's health in Ghana': 1129.

37. Garner, 'Safe sects'; Simon Gregson et al. 'Apostles and Zionists: the influence of religion on demographic change in rural Zimbabwe'. *Population Studies* 53(2) 1999: 179–93; Takyi, 'Religion and women's health in Ghana'; Jenny Trinitapoli and Mark D. Regnerus, 'Religion and HIV risk behaviours among married men: Initial results from a study of rural sub-Saharan Africa'. *Journal for the Scientific Study of Religion* 45(4) 2006: 505–28.

38. Garner, 'Safe sects'; Liebowitz, *The Impact of Faith-Based Organizations on HIV/AIDS Prevention and Mitigation in Africa*: 14–15.

39. Gregson et al., 'Apostles and Zionists': 191–2.
40. Liebowitz, *The Impact of Faith-Based Organizations on HIV/AIDS Prevention and Mitigation in Africa*: 16.
41. Trinitapoli and Regnerus, 'Religion and HIV risk behaviours among married men': 520.
42. Takyi, 'Religion and women's health in Ghana': 1229–30.
43. Fieldnotes, Kinshasa, 1987 in Schoepf, 'AIDS, history and struggles over meaning': 21.
44. Philip Setel, 'Local histories of sexually transmitted diseases and AIDS in western and northern Tanzania' in *Histories of Sexually Transmitted Diseases and HIV/AIDS in Sub-Saharan Africa*, edited by Setel, Lewis and Lyons: 135.
45. James Putzel, 'Histoire d'une action d'état: la lutte contre le Sida en Ouganda et au Sénégal' in *L'épidémie du Sida en Afrique Subsaharienne*, edited by Denis and Becker: 258. Online English translation available at http://www.refer.sn/rds/IMG/pdf/16PUTZEL.pdf (accessed 29 Aug. 2008).
46. See http://www.hillHIV/AIDS.org.za (accessed 23 Aug. 2008).
47. Iliffe, *The African AIDS Epidemic*: 95.
48. Putzel, 'Histoire d'une action d'état': 259.
49. Iliffe, *The African AIDS Epidemic*: 96–7.
50. SACBC, *A Message of Hope from the Catholic Bishops to the People of God in South Africa, Botswana and Swaziland* (Pretoria: SACBC, 2001). On this document see Denis, 'Sexuality and AIDS in South Africa': 73.
51. Paul Kocheleff, 'Le Sida au Burundi et en Afrique du Sud: le vécu au quotidien' in *L'épidémie du Sida en Afrique Subsaharienne*, edited by Denis and Becker: 199. Online English translation available at http://www.refer.sn/rds/IMG/pdf/14KOCHELEFF.pdf (accessed 29 Aug. 2008).
52. Gruénais, 'La religion préserve-t-elle du sida?': 672.
53. Quoted in Munro, 'Responsibility': 39.
54. Jon D. Fuller and James F. Keenan, 'Introduction: At the end of the first generation of HIV prevention' in *Catholic Ethicists on HIV/AIDS Prevention*, edited by James Keenan (New York: Continuum, 2000): 21–38.
55. Iliffe, *The African AIDS Epidemic*: 96.
56. Mbilinyi and Kaihula, 'Sinners and outsiders': 90. See also Bernard Joinet, *Survivre Face au SIDA en Afrique* (Paris: Karthala, 1994).
57. Mbilinyi and Kaihula, 'Sinners and outsiders': 90.
58. Iliffe, *The African AIDS Epidemic*: 96.
59. Epstein, *The Invisible Cure*: 195–6.
60. Epstein, *The Invisible Cure*: 185–6.
61. Pius Kamau, 'Islam, condoms and AIDS'. *The Huffington Post*, 30 Aug. 2008. Available at http://www.huffingtonpost.com/pius-kamau/islam-condoms-and-aids_b_120418.html (accessed 30 Aug. 2008).
62. Badri, 'The AIDS crisis': 41.
63. Carton, 'Le silence et la honte comme objet d'histoire': 133.
64. Fiona Scorgie, 'Virginity testing and the politics of sexual responsibility: implications for AIDS intervention'. *African Studies* 61(1) 2001: 55–76.

65. Liebowitz, *The Impact of Faith-Based Organizations on HIV/AIDS Prevention and Mitigation in Africa*: 16.
66. Smith, 'Youth, sin and sex in Nigeria': 432.
67. Becker and Collignon, 'A history of sexually transmitted diseases and AIDS in Senegal': 77.
68. McCulloch, 'The management of venereal disease in a settler society': 199–200.
69. Chirwa, 'Sexually transmitted diseases in colonial Malawi': 157.
70. Epstein, *The Invisible Cure*: 185.
71. Callahan and Bond, 'The social, cultural, and epidemiological history of sexually transmitted diseases in Zambia': 186.
72. Iliffe, *The African AIDS Epidemic*: 108.
73. Mbilinyi and Kaihula, 'Sinners and outsiders': 38.
74. Katinka de Wet, 'Le volontariat associatif dans les soins à domicile pour les malades du Sida' in *Afflictions: L'Afrique du Sud de l'apartheid au Sida*, edited by Didier Fassin (Paris: Karthala, 2004): 185–6.
75. Oppenheimer and Bayer, *Shattered Dreams?*: 96, 110–13.
76. Rose Smart and Rob Fincham (eds), 'Study tour of AIDS programmes in Zambia, Uganda and Kenya, 3–17 October' quoted in Iliffe, *The African AIDS Epidemic*: 95.
77. Iliffe, *The African AIDS Epidemic*: 140–57.
78. MSF, *Providing HIV Services Including Antiretroviral Therapy at Primary Health Care Clinics in Resource-Poor Settings: The Experience from Khayelitsha* (Médecins Sans Frontières and Infectious Disease Epidemic Unit, School of Public Health and Family Medicine, University of Cape Town, 2003). Available at http://www.msf.org.za/docs/khayelitsha_2003.pdf (accessed 27 Aug. 2008).
79. Geoff Foster, 'Religion and responses to orphans in Africa' in *A Generation at Risk: The Global Impact of HIV/AIDS on Orphans and Vulnerable Child*ren, edited by Geoff Foster, Carol Levine and John Williamson (Cambridge: Cambridge University Press, 2005): 159.
80. Mbilinyi and Kaihula, 'Sinners and outsiders': 87.
81. Iliffe, *The African AIDS Epidemic*: 94.
82. Interviews, Abidjan, May 1997 quoted in Schoepf, 'AIDS, history and struggles over meaning'; 23; Iliffe, *The African AIDS Epidemic*: 95; Oppenheimer and Bayer, *Shattered Dreams?*: 106.
83. Oppenheimer and Bayer, *Shattered Dreams?*: 106–7.
84. Fieldnotes, Kinshasa, 1985–9 quoted in Schoepf, 'AIDS, history and struggles over meaning': 23; Tonda, 'Les spécialistes non médicaux Congolais et le problème de la connaissance scientifique du Sida', 634.
85. Colson, 'En quête de guérison': 156; Epstein, *The Invisible Cure*: 190–1.
86. Gruénais, 'La religion préserve-t-elle du Sida?': 675.
87. For further discussion see Chapter 1 of this book.

Practitioner response

Alison Munro

My institutional base is the SACBC AIDS Office and it against this backdrop that I respond to the chapter by Philippe Denis. Some of the major points he makes are used to frame my response.

Few authors have studied HIV and AIDS as an historical phenomenon and very few have paid attention to the role of religion in the epidemic.

Writings on HIV and AIDS, in my experience, have sometimes been pious rather than theological or historical. They have aimed to assist infected and affected people deal with HIV and AIDS rather than engaging members of religious institutions as a whole. The importance of religion in the management of the epidemic suggests something other than the long-standing medical model of intervention with its limited success; and something other than the socio-economic considerations that underpin the spread of HIV. About twenty years ago Ruben Sher, a pioneering AIDS medical specialist, emphasised the need to look at the social context, including religious, in which HIV and AIDS was unfolding. He called for a move away from the arrogance of the medical model which, while it claimed to address the problems, was in fact far from an understanding of the complexities of the epidemic.

The term faith-based organisation (FBO) is ambiguous and can include 'religious leadership structures, local congregations or AIDS initiatives inspired by religious beliefs . . .'

The use by Denis of the term religious institutions, covering a number of different responses, themselves divided into a number of categories, is to be welcomed. Over several years in HIV and AIDS work I have noted interesting interpretations of the meaning of church. There are three broad responses: some people see themselves as the church and responding in practical ways to the mission of Christ; others are more inclined to define the church as the hierarchy of leadership that is sometimes seen as lacking in its response to the epidemic; and a third group recognises the church as local and hierarchical, with everyone needing to get involved in responding to HIV and AIDS. There is certainly room for deepening understanding of ecclesiology and for moving beyond the technical approach suggested by the term FBO. Church teaching may on occasion be in conflict with ways in which people enact their faith and respond to the needs around them; and it may also on occasion be different from what an organisation, even one defined to all intents and purposes as an FBO, sees as its mandate. Denis is correct to suggest both that religious institutions have an influence on policies and attitudes and that they have less influence on society and on their own memberships regarding policies and practices than is sometimes believed.

The most durable effect of religion on the epidemic may lie less in what their members do (or omit to do) in response to HIV and AIDS than in the manner in which the beliefs and practices of this religion shape the societal understanding of the epidemic.'

Denis is making two points here: one that religion has something to say to broader society about HIV and AIDS and the other concerns how people live their lives and make choices. And so, for example, one may find generous responses to people infected with HIV based on people of faith living out the injunction to love God and neighbour. Conversely there may be evidence of stigma and discrimination shaped by particular interpretations of the beliefs of the faith concerned. The second point is that society, sometimes not accepting what religion is saying, discounts its interventions and teachings. Religious institutions are seen to hold a set of beliefs, promote certain teachings and act in certain ways that are not always borne out by historical reality.

Religious institutions 'shape the discourse on HIV and AIDS' by individualising and moralising it, reinforcing the common representation 'as the result of multiple instances of individual risky behaviour'.

The socio-economic conditions in which people live, part of what underlies the spread of HIV, are clearly structural rather than a matter of personal sin. Yet not enough attention is given to this by religious leaders and theologians. In the main, it seems that religion gets stuck in a moral discourse around individual behaviour. But is it only religion? I think not, as stigma, discrimination and denial in broader society all seem to attest.

'Regarding condoms, the Christian churches adopted a very ambivalent attitude' with bishops divided or silent, and people on the ground discreetly promoting their use.

Condom use is a contentious issue. The position in the SACBC AIDS Office is that people need to be informed about the efficacy of correct condom use. They also need to be informed about their particular church's position on abstinence and fidelity. People need to make their own choices and do, in fact, sometimes despite what they know. Condom use, or failure to use condoms, has very little, if anything, to do with what religious leaders have to say. People who choose to use condoms see them as helping to prevent HIV infection, regardless of religious beliefs and whether they are in faithful relationships or not. People who do not use condoms are more likely to think 'it won't happen to me', that there is no risk of infection, that it is against their cultural practice, or that sexual pleasure will be lessened, than to follow the directives of religious leaders.

Alison Munro

Religion, Christianity in particular, can be an asset in curbing the HIV and AIDS epidemic but religious institutions sometimes shape the discourse on HIV and AIDS in unhelpful ways.

While I agree that sometimes religious institutions shape the discourse in unhelpful ways, it is also true that their memberships shape alternative discourses that are often not heard. People presenting for treatment meet others in the same situation and are often happy to go to religious sites precisely because they offer spiritual resources. In my experience, some believe they get better because Roman Catholics pray over the drugs before they distribute them.

Undoubtedly, more debate is needed about the role of religious institutions in the epidemic and in particular a more comprehensive written history of their engagement and response. What is clear, though, is that religion plays an important role, not always understood and appreciated by its membership or by society, in curbing the epidemic. Were the response of religious organisations to be removed from the total equation, the world's response to HIV and AIDS would look very different.

3

Religion and policy on HIV and AIDS

A rapidly shifting landscape

Jill Olivier

INTRODUCTION

Attitudes towards religion and religious organisations appear to have shifted dramatically in the last decade and continue to evolve, changing the context in which HIV and AIDS policy is developed and practised.[1] Trying to understand this shift means engaging with a sprawling body of literature on religion, policy, HIV and AIDS which defies systematic review. Nevertheless, working alongside the companion chapter in this book that focuses on the policy statements of religious organisations,[2] this chapter seeks to focus more narrowly on the landscape of the international policy context in which the interaction of religion, HIV and AIDS is played out. It considers some of the main themes that have emerged in the documentation relating to the international policy environment relating to religion, HIV and AIDS and provides historical perspective to the shift in attitude towards religious organisations that has occurred in the last ten years.

This is an unwieldy body of literature with little focus, and much that is partially relevant. There are few studies that contain content or process analyses of international and national HIV and AIDS policies addressing the role of religion and religious organisations and this remains a critical area for future investigation. This review pulls together a variety of policy statements, briefs, research reports and a smaller number of academic articles. The scope is further limited by the nature of available literature, which is biased towards material in English about Africa.[3] This landscaping review does not claim to be comprehensive, nor was a systematic analysis of all international and national HIV and AIDS policies carried out. Furthermore, it does not address some of the classic concerns of HIV and AIDS policy work, and is rather focused on the context and attitudes that emerge at the intersection of religion, policy, HIV and AIDS.

Given these limitations, the following are considered: a brief history of the international policy context and attitudes towards religion and religious organisations in the HIV and AIDS arena; the research trends that have emerged as a result, including some of the complexities that have implications for HIV and AIDS policy work; and finally, some summary conclusions and cautions for the way forward.

A BRIEF HISTORY OF THE INTERNATIONAL POLICY CONTEXT

In the early stages of the epidemic, the attitude of international health organisations and their HIV- and AIDS-related policy was largely blind to religious organisations and their work in health.[4] As one review of literature on religion and health says:

> It is generally accepted that religious entities have long engaged in health-related activities such as providing educational interventions and caring for individuals affected by disease. In many locations around the world, such religious entities have been in the forefront or alone in the struggles to ameliorate suffering and provide support, and have often been doing so with little attention or documentation from public health authorities.[5]

This invisibility of religious organisations to the view of public health and policy makers had evolved as a result of several factors. One was the influence of forms of secularism that treat religion as derivative, secondary or private. In the academy, for example, as secularisation models began to dominate, the social sciences largely become religion-blind, with religion becoming a subset of culture, or other economic, anthropological or sociological categories;[6] and religious organisations similarly a subset of non-governmental organisations (NGOs) or civil society. Another factor was the secular nature of public health and biomedicine. Although religious organisations had been involved in the primary health care movement that grew out of the Alma Ata Conference in 1978, it had ultimately developed a secular ideology.[7] At a public health level, these factors resulted in the health work of religious organisations becoming largely invisible and unaligned with other national health systems and resources.[8]

Of course, in many circles in the early stages of the epidemic, religion was not only invisible but was also viewed with narrow-eyed suspicion. Many negative health impacts and outcomes had been identified with religion and in the case of the HIV and AIDS epidemic, 'many people who worked in HIV prevention believed religious leaders and organizations were intrinsically antagonistic to what they were trying to accomplish'.[9] The Joint United Nations Program on HIV/ AIDS (UNAIDS) took it a step further and named opposition from religious authorities as 'perhaps the greatest obstacle to AIDS prevention activities in many countries'.[10] This was not limited to the African continent, as 'religious taboos on sexual education have been harassing AIDS prevention throughout Latin America. The confrontation between the condom and abstinence or fidelity has snapped closed any possibility for negotiating joint strategies. It has polarized political stances that clash public opinion and counterattack official efforts for AIDS prevention.'[11]

However, by 2000 this attitude had largely begun to change. This is not to say that the context had shifted to a blindly positive attitude towards religion or religious organisations. Concerns and frustrations linger today, for example, towards the detrimental effect of some religious leaders on HIV prevention strategies, the fear that religious organisations may use public funds for proselytising, or 'concern that ideological considerations are replacing sound empirical evidence of effectiveness in delivering health services'.[12] Such issues continue to call into question the credentials of religious organisations to deliver HIV and AIDS services or intervention. The following has been noted:

> There has been a recent boom of interest in the potential of religious entities in establishing effective HIV and AIDS interventions. This interest usually reflects a strongly positive attitude towards working with religious entities and simultaneously some cautionary note, based on perceptions of the potential negative effects of religious messages.[13]

As this statement demonstrates, it is apparent from the literature of the late 1990s and early 2000s that a significant shift in attitude had occurred. Increasingly, statements were made regarding the potential role of religious organisations in the fight against HIV and AIDS and, even more strongly, that religious organisations might well be 'pivotal to the success of prevention and care efforts' globally.[14] Such statements were not only emerging from large-scale religious organisations or those that were traditionally sympathetic to the role of the religious sector. Even international health organisations were expressing a desire for increased integration of the work of religious organisations within the international response against HIV and AIDS.[15] For example, the World Health Organisation (WHO) stated in 2004: 'Faith-based organizations have a crucial role to play in the widespread uptake of HIV/AIDS treatments ... [they] could be brought into treatment scale-up in order to combine their comparative advantages.'[16] The United Nations Children's Fund (UNICEF) started to look at religious organisations as sites of support for child-headed households as well as for the care of people living with HIV.[17] The United States Agency for International Development (USAID) stated in its new 2002 policy on HIV prevention that religious organisations should be engaged in its fight against HIV and AIDS and established a Center for Faith-Based and Community Initiatives in the same year 'to create a level playing field for faith-based and community groups to compete for USAID programs'.[18] Another obvious example and catalyst is the United States President's Emergency Program for AIDS Relief (PEPFAR), launched in 2002, which profiled religious organisations, acknowledged the concept of spiritual care and entailed particular funding in relation to religious activities.[19] The Global Fund to Fight HIV/AIDS, TB and Malaria (GFATM) and the World Bank are also examples of agencies that took the decision to channel funds for health programmes to religious organisations as this was seen as a reliable and efficient means to impact on health crises.[20] McFarland and Cochrane point out that 'the global public health policy community ... has discovered religious organizations ... and increasingly looks at them as allies in the delivery of health services and the accomplishment of global targets'.[21]

Another theme found in the documentation of this period, and which continues today, is the frequent appearance of statements listing the unique and intrinsic strengths that religious organisations are said to exhibit and that can be utilised to curb the epidemic. For example, these strengths might be that religious organisations have extensive infrastructure, reach and access; are found in inaccessible and rural areas; have access to dedicated volunteers and educated leadership; have unique credibility and acceptance in communities; have well-developed networks extending from international to grassroots communities; and have particular resilience and staying power.[22] This is discussed in more detail below but it is important to note that such statements are largely anecdotal, not based on analytical research.

There is little literature that analyses this general shift in attitude. All that can be done here is to suggest some of the factors emerging from the literature that seem to have inspired this change in opinion. First, there has been general acknowledgement that the secularisation thesis is faulty and that, even in developed nations, religion remains a critical part of people's interaction with health and disease:

> Adding impetus to this renewed focus on religion is the realisation that, globally, religion is making a comeback into public life. The secularisation thesis has been shown to be flawed, and under the influence of epidemics such as HIV/AIDS, diseases are now being more readily seen and studied as epidemics of society – in which factors such as religious worldviews and motivations challenge our understanding just as much as the biomedical quandary does. Biomedicine cannot be expected to have all the answers . . . In practice, this gives academic researchers a new mandate to move beyond the secular-focused and departmentally-divided training of modern academics and to begin more actively to pursue a complex understanding of health and society – notably through the sometimes uncomfortable lens of religion.[23]

As this extract suggests, in the context of HIV and AIDS, it became apparent early in the epidemic that religion might be an important cultural constraint pertinent to policy formation.[24] This merged with a broader realisation that to comprehend an individual or community response to HIV and AIDS, an understanding of their religion and its interaction with health is critical. There has similarly been an increased interest in the role of traditional religion and practitioners are increasingly being drawn into HIV and AIDS work.[25]

The complexity of the HIV and AIDS epidemic had driven forward the perspective of disease as requiring intervention at all levels of society, in particular a multi-sectoral response encouraging partnership at all levels. Multi-sectoral collaboration has become one of the key strategies worldwide and national plans are now almost always multi-sectoral in design.[26] As UNAIDS stated in 2001, 'partnerships of key social groups, government service providers, non-governmental organizations, people living with HIV/AIDS, community-based groups and religious organizations are the basis of successful strategies addressing HIV/AIDS'.[27] It is reasonable to assume that the idea of a multi-sectoral response has also increased collaboration with religious organisations and made them more prominent to international decision makers seeking new avenues.[28] Furthermore, in countries such as Senegal, Uganda and Thailand early involvement of religious leaders in the planning and implementation of national AIDS strategies had seen some apparently positive changes in the course of the epidemic.[29] In fact, Uganda's success in combating HIV and AIDS is frequently attributed to the multi-sectoral approach that was taken and in particular to the inclusion of faith-based groups.[30] Although attribution is never straightforward in these cases, they did represent some very early positive thinking towards the involvement of religious organisations in HIV and AIDS.

At a different level there is another, more prosaic, set of reasons that possibly influenced this shift in attitude. In the face of the myriad resource constraints, governments, international organisations and decision makers were casting further afield than was customary in search of untapped resources. Governments and international organisations, under pressure to meet development goals on in-creasingly limited resources, became more interested in the potential capacity of religious organisations and communities to become involved in HIV and AIDS interventions.[31]

These resource constraints are reflected in the literature on the HIV and AIDS epidemic from a health systems perspective: they 'are most fragile in the countries and regions of the world where the disease burden is greatest'.[32] Many of these countries, which have historically weak and dysfunctional health systems, are coming under further pressure from a wide complex of health crises in general and HIV and AIDS in particular.[33] In Africa, for example, 'the desire to scale up distribution of ARVs . . . has brought the fragile state of health system resources – infrastructure, financial and human – into sharp relief'.[34] In 2002 Parry noted that 'FBOs are increasingly being asked to back up and support previously functioning health care systems'.[35] Increasingly, it was noted that in many countries, religious communities owned substantial amounts of national health infrastructure; and in some places, such as post-conflict situations, religious organisations provided the only functioning health service available.[36] More specific to the epidemic, several studies began to attempt to quantify the role of religious organisations in the HIV and AIDS arena. For example, the WHO stated in 2004 that faith-based organisations (FBOs) 'account for around 20% of the total number of agencies working to combat HIV/AIDS'.[37] Based on this concept of untapped resources, the religious sector began to be called the hidden giant.[38] Tearfund, for example, stated that 'this hidden force is Africa's churches – and they are already the front line of care for millions of people. They receive little recognition, virtually no outside funding or partnerships, and so their potential remains largely untapped.'[39]

It is likely that such factors – increased attention paid to the implications of religion for health, a multi-sectoral approach and the search for new resources in an increasingly resource-constrained environment – contributed to a shift in attitude towards religious organisations. In the sections that follow, some of the results and implications of this in the context of HIV and AIDS policy will be considered.

THE QUANDARY RELIGION POSES TO POLICY FORMULATION

On the heels of this shift in attitude came the realisation that frighteningly little was known about these religious organisations.[40] Indeed, the body of literature on religion, health, HIV and AIDS that could inform policy is famously incomplete in every area of investigation.[41] This observation was made not only of religious organisations in Africa but also on an international scale. As Luker says, 'although [churches] are major institutions in Papua New Guinea and other Pacific Island countries, very little secular analysis of their contemporary social capacities and roles is available'.[42] It is this secular analysis that was missing: analytical assessments of religious organisations and their activities that could be utilised to inform HIV and AIDS-related policy.[43] Literature on religious organisations and their in-volvement in HIV and AIDS was missing not only in the public health arena but it appeared that the religious sector was also lacking knowledge of its own responses and resources.[44] There has subsequently been a flurry of research in this area, sponsored not only by religious organisations but also by international health and development organisations such as UNICEF, WHO and the Bill and Melinda Gates Foundation.[45] In fact, there has been a recent surge of mapping, research and reporting on the intersection of religion and health, HIV and AIDS in particular.

One development, building on the idea that religious organisations held un-tapped resources and potential, has been the idea that religious communities and organisations hold religious health assets that could potentially be leveraged for better health.[46] They range from so-called tangible assets such as health facilities, clinics, hospitals or community groups to intangible assets such as motivated and committed volunteers, compassion, faith, trust, hope or resilience.[47] There have been challenges to the research of both tangible and intangible religious health assets. As the African Religious Health Assets Programme (ARHAP) notes, 'the potential that many assume for mobilizing religious health assets and bringing them to scale is only beginning to be systematically studied . . . However, no one has a remotely complete picture of this resource, to say nothing of the broader range of health promoting religious assets.'[48] The investigation of so-called intangible assets, including the intrinsic strengths of religious organisations mentioned above, necessitates the design of new and more sophisticated methods of research. For example, some studies have begun to engage with those previously anecdotal strengths of religious organisations already mentioned, such as commitment, reach or trust, seeking to assess not only the tangible assets but also the intrinsic something that makes them unique.[49] However:

> [. . .] most criteria and categories used to study religion look for something quantitatively measurable and 'objectively' present . . . What is largely missing from most studies . . . is the dimension of religion that is 'internal' to faith based communities or organisations, an element that explains their motivations, commitments, attitudes, actions and relational or associational strengths on the basis of their own self-understandings and world-views. This dimension is harder to take into account . . . particularly in any way that makes for easy identification, replicability and generalization . . . However, the magnitude of the HIV/AIDS epidemic has already forced decision makers to try to engage all aspects of these assets . . . This necessarily complex approach makes demands on all aspects of religious health assets, including those traditionally countable and those that are obviously necessary . . . but difficult to quantify.[50]

This extract demonstrates some of the complexities of producing data on religion that can lead to evidence-based and socially appropriate HIV and AIDS policies. It also hints at the fact that international and national action has, by necessity, run ahead of systematic knowledge of these religious health assets. An indication of this is the huge increase in the number of religious organisations responding to HIV and AIDS noted in several countries since around 2000. This boom is likely, in part, a response to an increase of support to them.[51] Yet this action runs ahead of our knowledge of the nature, scope and scale of religious organisations, not to mention their unique characteristics that may demand specific strategy.

The 1998 UNAIDS planning process stressed religion as an important social issue in HIV and AIDS strategy development, saying that the situation analysis team in any given country may note:

[. . .] the major religions and their stated attitudes towards sexual and other risk behaviours; state and social attitudes towards different religious groups; signs that people do not always conform to the professed principles of their religion; the influence of religious leaders on government; and traditions of social support and service provision within each religious community.[52]

National strategic planning on HIV and AIDS should therefore deal with the specific religious-health context in each country. However, despite this recommendation from UNAIDS, an informal assessment of currently available national HIV and AIDS strategy documents shows that this rarely occurs. Generally speaking, national HIV and AIDS strategic policies can be rated on a spectrum based on the way they deal with their religious context. At the one end are policies that do not mention religion at all;[53] then policies that mention religious organisations only as part of a listing of civil society bodies; then policies that mention religious organisations as part of civil society and also briefly mention religion as a cultural constraint to HIV and AIDS strategies. Finally, at the opposite end of the spectrum are policies that attempt to engage with contextualised religion and religious organisations in a more comprehensive manner.[54] This rough assessment suggests that there are far more policies that fall into the first part of the spectrum than into the latter. However, there has been no comprehensive assessment of these policy documents, so it is not possible to make any conclusions as to why certain countries address religion in their national strategy documents while others do not. Previously it has been mentioned that the data on religious organisations working in HIV and AIDS is famously incomplete and diverse; particularly lacking are national-scale surveys of religious assets and activities that could inform such national-scale strategic planning around HIV and AIDS.[55] It is possible that some of these national strategy planners have backed away from including a contextualised understanding of religion and religious organisations because the underlying evidence-based knowledge is missing, or because adding a contextualised understanding of religion would make an already complex issue unmanageable. There clearly remain a series of important areas for future research, one of which is the question of the interface or lack thereof between national and international policy on HIV and AIDS. As a literature review on religion and health notes:

[. . .] if religious institutions are not visible or recognized by the right people, are not properly understood and evaluated, then they ultimately will not be recognized through health policy – and no manner of 'increased interest' will draw them fully in to equal partnership in the public health system or mobilize the resources on the scale that is necessary to deal better with the health crises we face.[56]

This discussion has hinted at the current context, a situation where the demands of engagement with the epidemic seem to be running ahead of knowledge about religious organisations, and where there is both enthusiasm and lingering resistance to the involvement of religious organisations in HIV and AIDS. In the following three sub-sections, a few of the main concerns being brought to light as a result of the current interest and research on religion in the context of HIV and AIDS are considered, specifically those that have implications for policy. The three main areas of interest are: the difficulties inherent in generalisation about religion and religious organisations in policy documentation; the issue of collaboration and involvement of religious leaders and organisations in policy development; and some emerging concerns about the instrumental view of religion as a resource for national and international responses to HIV and AIDS.

Generalising about religion and religious organisations

As mentioned above, the current knowledge of religious health assets does not yet allow for easy identification, replicability or the generalisation sometimes necessary for policy work. Just as early generalisations about stereotypic moralist religious leaders disapproving of condoms was proved not to describe all religious leaders appropriately,[57] so too current discourses in HIV and AIDS policy documents (that speak of religion, the religious sector or religious organisations) are being shown to be problematic in the light of recent literature demonstrating the huge variations in religion, religious-health practices and religious organisations in the context of HIV and AIDS.[58]

A number of mapping studies have emerged as a result of the renewed interest in religious organisations and their response to HIV and AIDS. Mapping is seen as a way to make the invisible visible, first locating religious organisations and then assessing their potential.[59] Such studies have tended to discover a number of religious organisations working on HIV and AIDS that had not previously been known. Interestingly, what has also emerged in these studies is a mass of smaller community-based religious programmes and initiatives. They are often not recognisable NGOs or health facilities, difficult to assess and varying considerably, but frequently responding to need and involved in such activities as support of home-based care.[60] As Foster says:

> Despite some negative perceptions of their role and impact, faith-based organizations (FBOs) . . . have developed experience in addressing the multidimensional impact of AIDS and its particular impact on children. Religious organizations are prevalent throughout Africa . . . Yet most faith-based responses are small scale and remain undocumented. It is difficult to measure their cumulative impact compared to the more visible project responses of development agencies. Consequently, FBO HIV/AIDS activities remain undersupported.[61]

Mapping studies have also suggested that religious organisations are often fluid in nature, adapting to needs around them and shifting in focus, making it particularly difficult to categorise their type or activities.[62] All this speaks to the difficulty of classifying religious organisations and their response to HIV and AIDS.[63] It is important 'for policy-makers [to] heed important differences among these institutions when devising ways to harness this potential'.[64] Yet it is also critical that these layers of complexity and consideration do not become so onerous that those involved in policy and strategy formulation shy away from addressing religion at all.

The Malawian national HIV/AIDS policy falls into the end of the spectrum of policies that make a strong effort to recognise the importance of contextualised religion. The policy shows an awareness of the Malawian context, recognising that culture and religion have a strong influence on the lifestyle and choices of its citizens and that there is great diversity in religion, resulting in a wide range of practices, 'some of which are detrimental both to development and to an effective HIV/AIDS prevention programme'.[65]

As mentioned earlier, the HIV and AIDS epidemic has reinforced the understanding that individuals and communities commonly utilise different health frameworks, often simultaneously, be they biomedical, traditional or religious.[66] The issue of healing in the context of HIV and AIDS is one issue where these multiple perspectives come to the fore; and some religious interpretations frequently operate in direct opposition to government and medical strategies, and even more critically, HIV and AIDS policy.[67] This is demonstrated by a news report in 2008:

A pastor in southern Malawi recently hit the headlines when he told five HIV-positive people in his church to stop taking antiretroviral (ARV) medication because they had been treated by prayer . . . the government has drawn up legislation, currently before parliament, to muzzle anyone claiming they can cure AIDS.[68]

In fact, the national strategy already provides some direction on this. In the section on religious and cultural practices and services it states:

Rationale: Religious groups have an important role to play in promoting behaviours that reduce the risk of HIV infection, such as abstinence before and faithfulness within marriage, and the use of VCT [voluntary counselling and testing] prior to marriage and during marriage reconciliations (after divorce or separation). These groups can also provide care and support for PLWAs [people living with AIDS]. However, certain religious practices, such as refusal to seek medical care and treatment or belief in miracle cures, increase vulnerability to HIV infection.

Policy statements: Government, through the NAC [National AIDS Council], undertakes to do the following: work closely with religious leaders to facilitate the provision of accurate HIV-related prevention information and education, as well as care and support for PLWAs; sensitize religious leaders to HIV/AIDS and discourage them from making false claims of miracle HIV/AIDS cures.[69]

What is of interest to this discussion was the reading of this piece of policy by a group of key religious leaders and managers of religious HIV and AIDS programmes demonstrated during a collaborative research study.[70] When asked to comment on this national policy document it became clear that there were conflicting perceptions of the meaning of miracle cures and a discussion on healing ensued. The majority of the group expressed an understanding of healing to mean that 'God could heal people from HIV infection, and in fact had done so'.[71] Yet this group also expressed an unwillingness to engage the policy document critically, saying that they were satisfied and would not like it to be changed, even though it seemed to stand in direct opposition to their stated personal beliefs. Whatever the issues of power at play, or what emerges in the daily practice and management of HIV and AIDS programmes, they remain obscure. This is not the place for further analysis but this example does demonstrate some of the complexities at play with religious individuals and organisations reading and experiencing HIV and AIDS policy. The enforcement of further government legislation against false claims of miracle cure would prove to be another area needing investigation. More broadly, it shows some of the complexities faced by policy makers, who are perhaps more comfortably located in the biomedical paradigm.[72]

Critically, this also calls for careful theological engagement with HIV and AIDS policy. As Horowitz suggests, 'the human confrontation with the AIDS epidemic is at rock bottom a matter of values [rather] than of policies'.[73] Tiendrebeogo says that 'whilst religious organisations have a wide reach, influence and capacity to mobilise communities to respond to HIV/AIDS, their responses have lagged behind the challenges and their policies have shied away from conflicts with theological concepts'.[74] Yet it is just such theological conflict that is happening on the ground on a daily basis. It is perhaps then necessary for calls for a more relevant theological response to HIV and AIDS[75] to demand a more vigorous theological engagement with HIV and AIDS policy.

Collaboration and agency of religious organisations in HIV and AIDS policy

The example cited above raises another issue of concern – the degree of collaboration or involvement of religious leaders in policy formulation and development. At a broad, international level religious leaders appear to be increasingly involved in collaboration on HIV and AIDS. In 2002 then World Bank President James Wolfensohn said that 'half the work in education and health in sub-Saharan Africa is done by the church . . . but they don't talk to each other, and they don't talk to us'.[76] However, it seems that much has changed in the last few years under the influence of the multi-sectoral demands of the epidemic and riding the wave of new enthusiasm towards religious organisations. Tiendrebeogo notes that religious organisations and leaders contributed to the United Nations General Assembly Special Session on HIV and AIDS and considers this an indication of their increased engagement at the highest level.[77] Although it seems that religious leaders are increasingly being invited to multi-sectoral policy discussions:

> [. . .] little academic research has been undertaken as to the influence of religious leaders on the health-relating policies and consultations that they do attend or advocate for . . . while there are news articles delineating who

is at meetings, and sound bites from religious leaders, there is little academic material on religious leaders' influence on public health policy.[78]

In 2008 the United Nations High-Level Meeting on HIV and AIDS ended with civil society groups, including religious organisations, objecting to the lack of true partnership with governments: 'The involvement of civil society in official national delegations must be effective, not just tokenistic . . . real partnership between donors, governments, civil society, UN agencies and affected populations requires a balance of power in making decisions.'[79]

Of course, it was not too long ago that religious organisations were seen as the main obstruction to national collaborative efforts. For example, in 1998 Pisani said that 'the fear of offending powerful religious constituencies has created gridlock in some national governments, and for good reason. Conservative lobbies have shown that they can obstruct everything from family life education to condom promotion if they choose.'[80] It is also apparent that at a national level, collaboration has been easier on some HIV- and AIDS-related issues than on others. For example, the area of orphan and vulnerable children (OVC) has been a primary focus of religious organisations and one in which they are theologically comfortable,[81] while sexuality remains an area of tension. Taylor notes that 'this lack of trust and understanding can have serious implications in terms of co-ordination and planning around national and local strategies for responses to AIDS'.[82] ARHAP research suggests that at a national level, two main avenues for collaboration between religious organisations and governments around HIV and AIDS are utilised:

> The first is governments' collaboration with religious health [service] sectors such as national faith-based health networks or the Christian health associations – most commonly managed through Ministries of Health. The second is governments' collaboration with religious entities that are perceived to be part of 'civil society' – this relationship managed [on the governments' side] through national AIDS Commissions or Councils and multi-sectoral committees . . . Several pieces of secondary literature call for religious entities to be increasingly accountable to governments . . . However, a review of progress on the Three Ones found that civil society is not an equal partner – particularly when it comes to reviewing and updating national plans – and that people with HIV, women's groups and FBOs are particularly under-involved.[83]

Mandi lays out the main challenges of collaboration between religious organisations and government as being:

> [. . .] lack of co-ordination among FBOs when lobbying since they usually approach governments independently and not as a united front; FBOs do not have adequate lobbying or negotiating powers; there is a lack of trust between governments and FBOs; FBOs fear that if they partner with governments, they will be absorbed and lose their identities; governments view FBOs as direct competitors rather than partners.[84]

This lack of co-ordination among religious organisations appears to be critical. The formulation of a multi-sectoral national strategic plan usually results in the government seeking a representative of the religious sector of that country or region.[85] However, as mentioned above, in most countries the religious sector is a mosaic of different organisations and religious bodies:

> Much health policy in the world is governed by the modern conception of the nation-state. Within this framework, governance largely proceeds through bureaucracies best suited to dealing with organizations or groups in terms of their public presence. Religion, however, is not always construed in terms of visible institutions, let alone representative ones. There are often no clear representative structures or visible institutions given over specifically to religion as if it were an independent social reality or sector. This directly affects how policies play out in real contexts, and may explain why they often fail.[86]

Recent research on collaboration between religion and governments on HIV and AIDS in Kenya, Malawi and the Democratic Republic of Congo (DRC) found that in all three countries representation was highly problematic. Even when there was an inter-faith HIV and AIDS co-ordinating body in place (with the government assuming it was collaborating with the entire religious sector through this mechanism), most participating religious organisations felt that they were not properly represented or participating with government at a national level. Furthermore, this research also showed that although national HIV and AIDS policies claimed to have been participatory processes, involving religious leaders, most participants felt that their organisations had not been adequately involved.[87]

Not only is the religious sector in any given country usually fragmented but it is often the scene of difference and institutional rivalry. Agadjanian and Sen say that 'while seeking to enlist the help of religious organisations in providing this and other types of HIV/AIDS-related assistance, policymakers should take into account doctrinal and organizational differences among religious denominations, as well as their perpetual (and often bitter) ideological and organizational competition'.[88] Collaboration between religious groups has historically often been marred by suspicion and disassociation.[89] While there are signs that the HIV and AIDS epidemic has pushed some religious organisations into working together,[90] and 'collaboration is often possible on AIDS even in situations of significant inter-religious tension and conflict',[91] inter-religious tensions and competition are still dominant factors in international politics and communities today.[92] All these factors make for a fragile collaborative environment around HIV and AIDS policy.

Untapped assets and potentials: The dangers of an instrumental approach

Another implication of the shift in attitude and policy context focuses on the discourse that names religious organisations an untapped resource in the battle against HIV and AIDS. While there is little specific literature published on this as yet, there are growing murmurs that it has sometimes evolved into an instrumental view of religious organisations and the assets they hold. That is, there is concern that religious organisations are being given renewed attention because of a need for their resources, rather than for a genuine reciprocal desire for partnership.

Some of these fears could stem from the unfortunately frequent use of the term exploit in this discourse of untapped resources. For example, the World Bank says: 'The role of African faith-based organisations in combating HIV and AIDS is widely recognised as having growing significance but, at the same time, one which is not fully exploited, given the influence and reach of FBOs in African societies.'[93] The Zambian national HIV and AIDS strategy similarly states a primary objective as being 'to fully exploit the potential of faith-based organisations in the fight against HIV/AIDS'.[94] This discourse of exploitation is felt by religious leaders working with HIV and AIDS in a variety of ways. For example, in the research on collaboration, religious leaders expressed concern that they felt used by the ad hoc way they were being drawn into government HIV and AIDS programmes. They also spoke strongly of the feeling of being exploited by some international donors who sought to use their religious communities and programmes to raise funds or complete their own agendas.[95]

Following the international shift in attitude, religious organisations have in some sense become the current flavour of the month in the HIV and AIDS arena. Paterson warns that religious organisations have begun to be seen as:

> [. . .] a bottomless pit of volunteers, and we need to think about that. FBOs have felt good about being drawn in, and are suddenly part of the solution, but do we want to be regarded in this instrumental way, and we should be thinking through the values we want to bring to the table.[96]

As this says, more careful consideration is needed about the current attitude towards religious organisations. Part of this consideration must be a more nuanced assessment of religious health assets and the different kinds of support they require:

> This largely instrumental approach is contrary to . . . that of an asset-based community approach . . . The priorities in global health primarily driven by organizations and institutions external to a country do not necessarily reflect the priorities of communities or even of countries. They are most often developed by those in the dominant North responding to needs in the South as perceived by the North and as assessed by 'objective' evidence. This usually ignores the rich, deeply textured forms of evidence drawn from case studies that take the form of narrative more often than statistics.[97]

Religious organisations are also feeling the pressures of resource-constrained environments, failing health systems, workforce crises and the other impacts of HIV and AIDS that threaten their sustainability despite the assets they may hold.[98] Agadjanian and Sen conclude their study of religious organisations involved in HIV and AIDS with the following:

> Our analysis suggests, therefore, that the potential of religious organisations in the fight against HIV/AIDS in southern Mozambique [a typical sub-Saharan setting] exists, but this potential is underutilized . . . Because the material and financial resources of most religious organizations in sub-Saharan Africa are unlikely to improve substantially, the efforts of policy-makers should focus on the socio-psychological and organizational obstacles faced by these organizations.[99]

While it does seem that religious organisations may have some particular assets and strengths, this suggests that specific strategies are needed to support them, especially in resource-constrained environments.

CONCLUSIONS AND THE WAY FORWARD

This landscaping review has crossed a broad territory, laying out the changing international context and shifting attitudes towards religious organisations in the context of HIV and AIDS, and a few of the complexities of policy engagement at national and international levels. It is clear that despite a surge in interest and research there remains a significant amount of work to be done.

A great deal of partnership building is still needed if religious organisations and communities are to have agency to participate more fully with HIV and AIDS policy. New methods of collaboration and communication are needed, with strategies for unconfrontational dialogue on HIV and AIDS policy even in the face of myriad meanings given to policy issues (such as in the Malawian example). Some recent studies have emphasised the need for religious health literacy, particularly in the context of HIV and AIDS work: for religious leaders and those working in religious organisations to gain a better understanding of health concerns; and for health workers and decision makers to gain a better understanding of religion and how it interacts with health. This is intended to enhance tolerance and dialogue at the interface of religion, health, HIV and AIDS.[100]

Little is yet known about the varieties of religious assets or religious organisations and the work they do; and even less about how they intersect with HIV and AIDS policy issues such as financing or economic impact. There is a desperate need for a comparative audit of HIV and AIDS policies, and how religion is addressed in different countries and on different policy issues. Not enough is known to begin to generalise about religion at a national and international policy level. Critically, new methods and discourse are needed to be able to appreciate the nuances and complexities of the religious sector and its formations and still be able to speak more generally on HIV and AIDS policy work. Analysis of policy practice is needed (including theological engagement) to ensure that when religion does get into these policies it is done in a sensitive and useful manner. If 'policies that are not appropriately rooted in local realities, commonly give rise to apathy, passivity or resistance at local level [and perhaps beyond]',[101] then there is even more urgency to this work, to take what is being learned about religion, religious organisations and their interaction with the epidemic and translate it into evidence-based and socially appropriate policy.

This review has discussed a shift in attitude towards religious organisations over the last decade but in this fast-evolving field tomorrow may bring a sea change. It has been noted that in the context of HIV and AIDS the religious community have often lagged 'behind new trends that they could be leading'.[102] Perhaps this is the moment for both religious communities and those in public health to utilise this new environment proactively, appreciate difference and engage against HIV and AIDS together.

NOTES

1. In this chapter the term health is used in its broadest sense; epidemic to (more accurately) indicate the HIV and AIDS pandemic or epidemics; religion to encompass the spectrum of faith, spirituality, religio-cultural practices and institutional religion; religious organisation to encompass a myriad of entities such as faith-based organisations, community-based organisations, institutional bodies, religious health facilities, congregations and networks; and international health organisations to encompass a range of international entities such as health and development agencies, bilateral bodies or funding agencies. See Jill Olivier, 'An FB-oh?: the etymology of the religious entity and its impact on our understanding of the intersection of religion and health in Africa'. Paper presented at ARHAP Conference: When Religion and Health Align: Mobilising Religious Health Assets for Transformation, Cape Town, 13–16 July 2009.
2. See Chapter 4 in this book.
3. These biases reflect an imbalance in the literature that needs correcting.
4. Of course, it would be going too far to say that all religious organisations had been completely invisible as there are international organisations (such as UNICEF and USAID) that have had long-term relationships with religious organisations. This, however, is not the norm; nor does it appear that religious organisations were considered to be any different from secular organisations at this time.
5. Jill Olivier, James R. Cochrane and Barbara Schmid, *ARHAP Literature Review: Working in a Bounded Field of Unknowing* (Cape Town: African Religious Health Assets Programme, 2006): 38.
6. Olivier, Cochrane and Schmid, *ARHAP Literature Review*: 6; Peter L. Berger (ed.), *The Desecularization of the World: Resurgent Religion and World Politics* (Washington, DC: Ethics and Public Policy Centre, 1999); José Casanova, *Public Religions in the Modern World* (Chicago: University of Chicago Press, 1994).
7. See Chapter 1 in this book for more on this.
8. Barbara Schmid et al., *The Contribution of Religious Entities to Health in Sub-Saharan Africa* (Cape Town: African Religious Health Assets Programme, 2008): 92; Steve de Gruchy et al.,

Appreciating Assets: The Contribution of Religion to Universal Access in Africa (Cape Town: African Religious Health Assets Programme, 2006).

9. Edward C. Green, *Faith-Based Organizations: Contributions to HIV Prevention* (Washington, DC: US Agency for International Development and the Harvard Center for Population and Development Studies, 2003): 4.

10. Elisabeth Pisani, *Acting Early to Prevent AIDS: The Case of Senegal* (Geneva: Joint United Nations Programme for HIV/AIDS, 1999).

11. G. Ornelas et al., 'Sex education for priests'. *International Conference on AIDS* 8(2) 1992: 435.

12. *Faith in Action: Examining the Role of Faith-Based Organisations in Addressing HIV/AIDS: A Multi Country Key Informant Survey*, edited by Sara Woldehanna et al. (Washington, DC: Global Health Council, 2005): 12–13; Jeremy Liebowitz, *The Impact of Faith-Based Organisations on HIV/AIDS Prevention and Mitigation in Africa* (Durban: Health Economics and HIV/AIDS Research Division, University of KwaZulu-Natal, 2002).

13. Beverley Haddad, Jill Olivier and Steve de Gruchy, *The Potential and Perils of Partnership: Christian Religious Entities and Collaborative Stakeholders Responding to HIV and AIDS in Kenya, Malawi and the DRC* (Cape Town: Africa Religious Health Assets Programme, 2008): 13; Karen Birdsall and Kevin Kelly, *Pioneers, Partners, Providers: The Dynamics of Civil Society and AIDS Funding in Southern Africa* (Johannesburg: Centre for AIDS Development, Research and Evaluation and the Open Society Initiative for Southern Africa, 2007); Nigel Taylor, *Faith and AIDS: A Review for the Update of Taking Action* (London: Consortium on AIDS and International Development, 2007).

14. Magdalena Martínez and Anna Dulaney, *Religious-Based Initiatives* (Arlington: Family Health International/AIDSCAP, 1997); Christian Aid, *God's Children are Dying of HIV: Interfaith Dialogue and HIV* (London: Christian Aid, 2004); Geoff Foster, *Study of the Response by Faith-Based Organisations to Orphans and Vulnerable Children: Preliminary Summary Report* (New York: World Conference of Religions for Peace and United Nations Children Fund, 2003).

15. Woldehanna et al., *Faith in Action*: 12.

16. WHO, *World Health Report 2004: Changing History* (Geneva: World Health Organisation, 2004): 46.

17. UNICEF, 'Sharing common goals: UNICEF, faith-based organizations and children' (December 2004). Available at http://www.unicef.org/media/media_4537.html (accessed 23 Jan. 2009).

18. USAID, 'USAID's work with faith and community-based organisations' available at http://www.usaid.gov/our_work/global_health/aids/TechAreas/community/fbocbofactsheet.html (accessed 23 Jan. 2009).

19. PEPFAR, *The President's Emergency Plan for AIDS Relief: US Five-Year Global HIV/AIDS Strategy* (Washington, DC: Office of the United States Global AIDS Coordinator, 2004). Available at http://www.pepfar.gov/partners/ (accessed 21 Mar. 2009); Jo Renee Formicola, Mary Segers and Paul Weber, *Faith-Based Initiatives and the Bush Administration: The Good, the Bad and the Ugly* (Lanham: Rowman and Littlefield, 2003).

20. Nigel Taylor, *Many Clouds, Little Rain?: The Global Fund and Local Faith-Based Responses to HIV and AIDS* (Teddington: Tearfund, 2005); Nigel Taylor, *The Warriors and the Faithful: The World Bank MAP and Local Faith-Based Initiatives in the Fight against HIV and AIDS* (Teddington:

Tearfund, 2005). Nigel Taylor, *Working Together?: Challenges and Opportunities for International Development Agencies and the Church in the Response to AIDS in Africa* (Teddington: Tearfund, 2006).

21. Deborah A. McFarland and James R. Cochrane, 'The agency of religious health assets in strengthening health systems'. Paper presented at Ethics and Africa Conference, Cape Town, April 2006: 3.

22. Summaries of these statements can be found in Schmid et al., *The Contribution of Religious Entities to Health in Sub-Saharan Africa*: 84–5 or Haddad, Olivier and De Gruchy, *The Potential and Perils of Partnership*: 25–6. Some examples of such documents are: *Global Assessment of Faith-Based Organizations' Access to Resources for HIV and AIDS Response* (Tübingen: German Institute for Medical Mission, 2005); World Bank, *HIV/ AIDS Workshop for Faith-Based Organisations and National AIDS Councils, Accra, Ghana, January 2004: Concept Note* (Washington, DC: World Bank, 2004); Susan Parry, *Responses of the Faith-Based Organisations to HIV/AIDS in Sub-Saharan Africa* (Geneva: World Council of Churches and Ecumenical HIV/AIDS Initiative in Africa, 2003); Taylor, *Many Clouds, Little Rain?*; Taylor, *The Warriors and the Faithful*; Taylor, *Working Together?*.

23. Olivier, Cochrane and Schmid, *ARHAP Literature Review*: 7.

24. Fiona Smyth, 'Cultural constraints on the delivery of HIV/AIDS prevention in Ireland'. *Social Science and Medicine* 46(6) 1998: 661–72.

25. See also Chapter 1 in this book for a more comprehensive discussion of the simultaneous use of multiple frameworks of reference, be they religious, biomedical or traditional, in the context of HIV and AIDS.

26. Birdsall and Kelly, *Pioneers, Partners, Providers*: 42.

27. UNAIDS, *The Global Strategy Framework on HIV/AIDS* (Geneva: Joint United Nations Program on HIV/AIDS, 2001): 6.

28. Haddad, Olivier and De Gruchy, *The Potential and Perils of Partnership*: 29–33.

29. Georges Tiendrebeogo, Michael Buykx and Nel van Beelen, 'Faith-based responses and opportunities for a multisectoral approach'. *Sexual Health Exchange* 1(1) 2004: 1–3.

30. Susheela Singh, Jacqueline E. Darroch and Akinrinola Bankole, *A Comprehensive and Creative Multisectoral Approach is the Reason for Uganda's Success in Combating HIV/AIDS* (New York: Alan Guttmacher Institute, 2002); Susheela Singh, Jacqueline E. Darroch and Akinrinola Bankole, *The Role of Behaviour Change in the Decline of HIV Prevention in Uganda* (New York: Alan Guttmacher Institute, 2004).

31. Some of the dangers of this perspective are discussed below. De Gruchy et al., *Appreciating Assets*; A. Green et al., 'A shared mission?: Changing relationships between government and church health services in Africa'. *International Journal of Health Planning and Management* 17(4) 2002: 333–53. Paul Jellinek, 'Faith in action: Building capacity for interfaith volunteer caregiving'. *Health Affairs* 20(3) 2001: 273–8.

32. McFarland and Cochrane, 'The agency of religious health assets in strengthening health systems': 2.

33. Chris Bateman, 'Health care workers cracking under HIV/AIDS workload'. *South African Medical Journal* 93 (2003): 734–6; Solly R. Benatar, 'Health care reform and the crisis of HIV and AIDS in South Africa'. *New England Journal of Medicine* 351(1) 2004: 81–93.

34. McFarland and Cochrane, 'The agency of religious health assets in strengthening health systems': 5.

35. Susan Parry, *Responses of the Churches to HIV/AIDS: Three Southern African Countries* (Harare: World Council of Churches, Ecumenical HIV/AIDS Initiative in Africa, Southern Africa Regional Office, 2002): 9.

36. For a review of such literature see Schmid et al., *The Contribution of Religious Entities to Health in Sub-Saharan Africa*: 46–95.

37. WHO, *World Health Report 2004*: 46; Olivier, Cochrane and Schmid, *ARHAP Literature Review*: 33–4.

38. Tara S. Hackney, 'The Invisible Giant: The Christian Health System' (MPH dissertation, Emory University, Atlanta, 2000).

39. Tearfund, *Faith Untapped: Why Churches Can Play a Crucial Role in Tackling HIV and AIDS in Africa* (Teddington: Tearfund, 2006): 11.

40. Schmid et al., *The Contribution of Religious Entities to Health in Sub-Saharan Africa*; De Gruchy et al., *Appreciating Assets*; Olivier, Cochrane and Schmid, *ARHAP Literature Review*.

41. Schmid et al., *The Contribution of Religious Entities to Health in Sub-Saharan Africa*: 48. See also Chapter 1 in this book.

42. Vicki Luker, 'Civil society, social capital and the churches: HIV/AIDS in Papua New Guinea' (Canberra: Australian National University, Feb. 2004).

43. This will be discussed in more detail below. Woldehanna et al., *Faith in Action*: 9; Byron R. Johnson, Ralph B. Tompkins and Derek Webb, *Objective Hope: Assessing the Effectiveness of Faith-Based Organizations: A Review of the Literature* (Philadelphia: Center for Research on Religion and Urban Civil Society, 2002).

44. Olivier, Cochrane and Schmid, *ARHAP Literature Review*: 35.

45. Foster, *Study of the Response by Faith-Based Organisations to Orphans and Vulnerable Children*; De Gruchy, *Appreciating Assets*; Schmid et al., *The Contribution of Religious Entities to Health in Sub-Saharan Africa*.

46. African Religious Health Assets Program, 'About ARHAP' available at http://www.arhap.uct.ac.za/about.php (accessed 24 May 2009).

47. Olivier, Cochrane and Schmid, *ARHAP Literature Review*: 66–8; De Gruchy et al., *Appreciating Assets*; Elizabeth Thomas et al., *Let Us Embrace: The Role and Significance of an Integrated Faith-based Initiative for HIV and AIDS* (Cape Town: African Religious Health Assets Programme, 2006).

48. African Religious Health Assets Program, 'About ARHAP'.

49. Thomas et al., *Let Us Embrace*; Ritva Reinikka and Jakob Svensson, *Working for God?: Evaluating Service Delivery of Religious Not-For-Profit Health Care Providers in Uganda* (Washington, DC: World Bank, 2003).

50. African Religious Health Assets Program, 'About ARHAP'.

51. See Chapter 1 in this book for more on this. Haddad, Olivier and De Gruchy, *The Potential and Perils of Partnership*: 28, 124; Schmid et al., *The Contribution of Religious Entities to Health in Sub-Saharan Africa*: 52–72; De Gruchy et al., *Appreciating Assets*: 125.

52. UNAIDS, *The Guide to the Strategic Planning Process for a National Response to HIV/AIDS* (Geneva: Joint United Nations Programme on HIV/AIDS, 1998): 18.

53. Or associated terms such as faith, spirituality and FBO.

54. See, for example (from those that barely mention religion, to a more comprehensive and contextualised treatment): Swaziland, *The National Multisectoral HIV and AIDS Policy: A Nation at War with AIDS* (Mbabane: Government of the Kingdom of Swaziland, June 2006); Kenya, *Kenya National HIV/AIDS Strategic Plan 2005/6-2009/10: A Call to Action* (Nairobi: National AIDS Control Council, Office of the President, 2005); Malawi, *National HIV/AIDS Policy: A Call for Renewed Action* (Lilongwe: Office of the President and Cabinet, National AIDS Commission, 2003).

55. Schmid et al., *The Contribution of Religious Entities to Health in Sub-Saharan Africa*: 46–95.

56. Olivier, Cochrane and Schmid, *ARHAP Literature Review*: 36–7.

57. Green, *Faith-Based Organizations*: 4.

58. Even in regions which seem to have one main religion, such as Christianity, there are a multitude of different traditions in that category.

59. De Gruchy, *Appreciating Assets*: 6–27.

60. Haddad, Olivier and De Gruchy, *The Potential and Perils of Partnership*; Schmid et al., *The Contribution of Religious Entities to Health in Sub-Saharan Africa*: 48; De Gruchy, *Appreciating Assets*.

61. Foster, *Study of the Response by Faith-Based Organisations to Orphans and Vulnerable Children*: 1.

62. Schmid et al., *The Contribution of Religious Entities to Health in Sub-Saharan Africa*: 50; Olivier, Cochrane and Schmid, *ARHAP Literature Review*: 40; Victor Agadjanian, 'Gender, religious involvement, and HIV/AIDS prevention in Mozambique'. *Social Science and Medicine* 61(7) 2005: 1529.

63. De Gruchy et al., *Appreciating Assets*, Chapter 2; Olivier, 'An FB-oh?': 1.

64. Olivier, Cochrane and Schmid, *ARHAP Literature Review*: 40; Agadjanian, 'Gender, religious involvement, and HIV/AIDS prevention in Mozambique'.

65. Malawi, *National HIV/AIDS Policy*: 72–3.

66. See Chapter 1 in this book for a more extensive discussion on this.

67. See Chapter 1 in this book, particularly the section on miraculous cure, for more discussion on this.

68. 'Malawi: faith can give comfort, but cannot cure AIDS'. *PlusNews*, 12 Mar. 2008. Available at http://www.plusnews.org/report.aspx?ReportID=77251 (accessed 23 Dec. 2009).

69. Malawi, *National HIV/AIDS Policy*: 71.

70. Haddad, Olivier and De Gruchy, *The Potential and Perils of Partnership*: Chapter 5.

71. Haddad, Olivier and De Gruchy, *The Potential and Perils of Partnership*: 89.

72. Schmid et al., *The Contribution of Religious Entities to Health in Sub-Saharan Africa*: 35.

73. Irving Louis Horowitz in Mark S. Kaplan, 'AIDS: Individualizing a social problem'. *Society* 27(2) 1990: 3.

74. Tiendrebeogo et al., 'Faith-based responses and opportunities for a multisectoral approach': 1–3.

75. Daniela Gennrich et al., *Churches and HIV/AIDS: Exploring How Local Churches Are Integrating HIV/AIDS in the Life and Ministries of the Church and How Those Most Directly Affected Experience These* (Pietermaritzburg: PACSA, 2004).

76. James Wolfensohn in Michael Kitchen, 'World must coordinate efforts, end waste, says Wolfensohn'. *UN Wire* (24 Oct. 2002).

77. Tiendrebeogo et al., 'Faith-based responses and opportunities for a multisectoral approach': 1–3.

78. Olivier, Cochrane and Schmid, *ARHAP Literature Review*: 41.

79. PlusNews, 'Greater involvement of civil society has been identified by the UN as a critical strategy to combat AIDS'. *PlusNews Report* 13 June 2008; Haddad, Olivier and De Gruchy, *The Potential and Perils of Partnership*: 29–30.

80. Pisani, *Acting Early to Prevent AIDS*: 12.

81. Foster, *Study of the Response by Faith-Based Organisations to Orphans and Vulnerable Children*.

82. Taylor, *Working Together?*: 6.

83. Haddad, Olivier and De Gruchy, *The Potential and Perils of Partnership*: 29.

84. F. Mandi, *Planning, Developing and Supporting the Faith-Based Health Workforce* (Nairobi: The Capacity Project and Medicus Mundi International, 2006).

85. Indeed, most of the policy documents briefly assessed stated that religious representatives had been involved in the process as part of civil society.

86. Olivier, Cochrane and Schmid, *ARHAP Literature Review*: 37.

87. Haddad, Olivier and De Gruchy, *The Potential and Perils of Partnership*. This is a brief summary of a more complex area. There are several different levels of collaboration in which religious organisations engage with government beyond the national level discussed here.

88. Victor Agadjanian and Soma Sen, 'Promises and challenges of faith-based AIDS care and support in Mozambique'. *American Journal of Public Health* 97(2) 2007: 366.

89. Schmid et al., *The Contribution of Religious Entities to Health in Sub-Saharan Africa*: 91.

90. Andrew Doupe, *Partnerships Between Churches and People Living with HIV/AIDS Organizations: Guidelines* (Geneva: World Council of Churches, 2005).

91. UNAIDS website, available at http://www.unaids.org (accessed 21 Jan. 2009).

92. Haddad, Olivier and De Gruchy, *The Potential and Perils of Partnership*; Schmid et al., *The Contribution of Religious Entities to Health in Sub-Saharan Africa*; De Gruchy, *Appreciating Assets*.

93. World Bank, *HIV/AIDS Workshop for Faith-Based Organisations and National AIDS Councils* Accra, Ghana, January 2004.

94. Zambia, *National HIV/AIDS/STI/TB Policy* (Lusaka: Ministry of Health, 2005): 22.

95. Haddad, Olivier and De Gruchy, *The Potential and Perils of Partnership*: 59, 91.

96. Gillian Paterson, CHART consultation, Durban, Oct. 2008.

97. McFarland and Cochrane, 'The agency of religious health assets in strengthening health systems': 3.

98. Schmid et al., *The Contribution of Religious Entities to Health in Sub-Saharan Africa*.

99. Agadjanian and Sen, 'Promises and challenges of faith-based AIDS care and support in Mozambique': 366.

100. De Gruchy, *Appreciating Assets*: 127; Haddad, Olivier and De Gruchy, *The Potential and Perils of Partnership*: 129.

101. Olivier, Cochrane and Schmid, *ARHAP Literature Review*: 37.

102. David Patient and Neil Orr, 'B in ABC: Strategic thinking communication initiative' (20 December 2004). Available at http://www.comminit.com. See also Tiendrebeogo et al., 'Faith-based responses and opportunities for a multisectoral approach': 1–3.

Practitioner response

Bongi Zengele

My response to Jill Olivier's chapter arises out of experience as an activist working with the Ujamaa Centre for Community Development and Research at the School of Religion and Theology, University of KwaZulu-Natal. My work as co-ordinator of the Solidarity Programme for People Living with HIV and AIDS enables me to engage regularly with those living with HIV.

Olivier has paid attention to the nature of the ever-changing context of HIV and AIDS and how this impacts upon religion and policy. From my experience, there is a gap between what is being published about HIV and what is actually experienced by those directly affected by the epidemic. People in communities mostly do not know how to engage with policy and policy makers. This raises the question as to who informs policy decisions. Engagement with people at a community level is often minimal and they are left out of decision-making processes that have a direct impact on their lives. This results in a gap between policy and the real life experience of people living with HIV. The challenge is to bridge this gap.

Too often, people living with HIV are separated from the rest of the community and a clear distinction is made between us and them. This attitude feeds into stigma attached to HIV. People diagnosed with HIV often go through various traumas, a major one being internal, or self-stigma. This is exacerbated by the fact that communities have coined their own terms to refer to HIV and AIDS, colloquialisms that are often not sensitive to persons living with HIV: for example, referring to HIV as *amagama amathathu*, or the BMW car as Z3. While these colloquial terms are demonstrations of community attempts to adjust to the epidemic, they unfortunately add to the labelling and stigma experienced by people living with HIV. In a Siyaphila support group meeting,[1] one member expressed her frustration strongly when she said: 'We are not statistics, we are people, we have lives and we want them to be taken seriously.' Behind every statistic there is a person who really matters and who is yearning to be recognised as a full citizen belonging in the community. All too often, statistics further alienate people from first-hand expressions of lived experience of HIV and AIDS. Yet, it is often statistics that inform HIV policies.

Olivier has outlined clearly how the historical background of HIV and AIDS, at both national and international level, impacts the way we are trying to deal with prevention. The human rights approach has limited the focus of prevention to an individual's right and responsibility. This emphasis on the individual contradicts Africa's communal way of living. There is a need to search for alternative ways of dealing with the mitigation of HIV that are more centred on community. Unfortunately, there are hidden agendas that exist in relationships between the North and South. Therefore, involvement in the epidemic by the international community needs to be viewed critically. All too often, the historical background to the early stages of the epidemic in the North still sets the agenda. The sub-Saharan African context calls for a particular policy framework as well as religious formulations that are sensitive and holistic in their approach to gender and sexuality. Acknowledging the religion and culture of the people of sub-Saharan Africa will pave the way for more balanced policies that take into account cultural diversity.

This is why it is important to adopt an approach that speaks to notions of existence expressed in phrases such as *umuntu ngumuntu ngabantu* (a person is a person because of other people)[2] where love, care and compassion form the basis of engagement. Attempts to deal with these life challenges should be viewed at a community level, using a community emancipation approach. Thus, a person directly affected is not necessarily isolated but forms an integral part of the solution to mitigate the epidemic that is impacting on the larger community.

As Olivier shows, the role of religion in the epidemic has been ambiguous. She cautions against making sweeping statements about the religious sector being an untapped resource that can be used to tackle HIV prevention. She argues that there is a need to identify the limitations that result from religious perspectives. The impact of judgemental and stigmatising attitudes is seen as a huge setback to prevention. Olivier clearly outlines how religious messages coincide with confrontation in the debate between condom use and abstinence or infidelity. While acknowledging the increasing number of FBOs that are engaging HIV and AIDS work, it is imperative to monitor how far religious values have an impact on attitudes towards people living with HIV. Engaging people of faith who are living with HIV sharpens awareness levels and assists in creating new, less stigmatising avenues. This can influence the role of religious organisations in the epidemic and they can then also become a helpful part of the policy-making process.

Olivier has observed that increasingly it became clear there was little known about religion and health. Furthermore, she argues that there was little or no attempt to analyse or assess religious organisations and their activities, which could then be utilised to inform HIV and AIDS policy. One of the major roles played by these organisations in the context of HIV and AIDS has been care and support. However, there is still a need to understand the positive impact that religion contributes towards developing and instilling resilience in the lives of people facing the challenges of the HIV and AIDS epidemic. I agree with Olivier that these intangible religious health assets are difficult to evaluate using secular tools. Internal motivation, commitment, sacrifices, giving of time and money, and faith are difficult to measure; yet they contribute a great deal to the ongoing care and support of the vulnerable in an HIV-affected society. How then should these values be quantified? This complex task is essential to HIV and AIDS policy work. The challenge here is to engage critically with theological questions arising out of the development of resilience, as well as from ongoing theological reflection on current HIV and AIDS policies.

Finally, in South Africa there is a clear divide between rural and urban life. Many more resources are located in the urban areas and this reality is reflected in the amount of HIV and

AIDS information and the availability of ARV treatment. This inequality impacts negatively on accessibility of treatment and basic HIV and AIDS information and education. So policy needs to address issues of equal access to resources at a community level and how resources can be harnessed to benefit all South Africans. In most rural areas people walk long distances to public health clinics. Many of these clinics do not have sufficient medicine needed by people who are ill, which poses a serious threat to people on ARV treatment. Adherence is central in dealing with HIV and there is a serious need for the scaling-up of support systems that will enable people to take treatment regularly and correctly. Interfering with treatment is detrimental to people's lives and there is a need for the creation of a concrete policy across the religious sector that advocates appropriate support for those on ARV treatment. Strict measures need to be in place to caution those within the religious sector that undermine ARV treatment because of a false belief that AIDS can be cured. Religious reasons for making such claims need to be interrogated and legal measures put in place that will bring an end to such activities.

Notes

1. Siyaphila is a network of support groups for people living with HIV in the Pietermaritzburg area of KwaZulu-Natal.
2. This is a direct translation from isiZulu and is related to the fact that you live for other people in community: when you suffer we all are suffering with you, we identify with you and your pain.

4

Statements by religious organisations on HIV and AIDS

Intersecting the public realm

Martha Frederiks

INTRODUCTION

'A tiger is roaring just outside – or already inside – our villages; not to act now will bring death and suffering.' With these words Asian church leaders concluded their statement on HIV, drawn up during a consultation convened by the Lutheran World Federation and the United Methodist Church on Batam Island, Indonesia in 2003. The statement reflects growing awareness among Asian religious leaders that at the beginning of the third millennium Asia has become one of the epicentres of HIV and the document presents a plan of action on how to counter the epidemic.[1] A statement issued by the Symposium of Episcopal Conferences of Africa and Madagascar (SECAM), the Roman Catholic bishops of Africa and Madagascar, in that same year is far less optimistic. Though the title underscores a discourse of hope, the text itself describes the bitter realities in sub-Saharan Africa, saying: 'Millions of lives have already been lost prematurely, whole families dismembered and untold numbers of children orphaned and/or infected by HIV.'[2] By 2003 the HIV epidemic in sub-Saharan Africa had developed into a pandemic with infection rates in some countries rising up to 30 per cent of the population. The tiger was, to use loosely the words of the Asian leaders, already in our villages, bringing death and suffering.

Since the early days of the epidemic in the 1980s religious leaders have addressed the issue and public statements called for compassion for those living with HIV. Often this was combined with moral teachings on abstinence from sex before marriage and faithfulness in marriage to prevent the further spread of

HIV. However, over the years, with the staggering increase in infection rates, the tone of statements changed: it became clear that HIV did not just affect people outside religious communities or people living promiscuous lives but also members of the religious community and its leadership.[3] The statements then began to focus on topics such as the stigmatisation of and discrimination against people who were HIV positive; the unequal distribution of wealth; groups particularly vulnerable to HIV; and advocacy for free medication.

This chapter investigates the public statements of religious organisations in addressing the HIV and AIDS epidemic. Its approach is twofold: it intends to map statements about HIV and AIDS, as well as analyse the types of discourse used to discuss them. An effort will also be made to detect core theological motives within the statements. The research question has been restricted in a number of ways.

First, it focuses on religious organisations. In this contribution the term religious organisations is used for religious communities (such as churches and mosques) or organisations that represent these communities at the national or international level (such as ecumenical and inter-faith networks). While para-church organisations, international church families and transnational networks (for example, the Conference of Anglican Bishops in Africa) are included, faith-based non-governmental organisations (NGOs) are not. Second, this contribution only investigates written statements and does not address the many verbal statements made by religious leaders and organisations. As the chapter strives to give a representative rather than a comprehensive overview of the statements of religious organisations, and as oral statements are extremely difficult to trace, this research limits itself to texts only. Third, the phenomenon of policy statements presumes strong centralised structures, where policy is developed nationally or internationally and implemented at the grassroots level. This structure is not representative of a large number of religious communities in Africa and elsewhere, be they Christian, Muslim or Traditional Religion. Many of these communities have a different organisational model and advocate the independence of local communities. In his Master's thesis, researching the churches' responses to AIDS in two communities in KwaZulu-Natal, Mark Krakauer has pointed out that church structures can be barriers to as well as enablers of comprehensive HIV and AIDS programmes. The more loosely organised the structures, the more difficult it becomes to develop co-ordinated programmes and translocal policies.[4] Hence, loosely organised communities tend not to issue policy statements.

Fourth, in an attempt to access material and prioritise it, the choice was made to focus on national and international documents, while being aware of the limitations this implies. Fifth, within the category of public statements of religious organisations most attention was paid to contributions pertaining to Africa. Nevertheless, a number of statements from other parts of the world are discussed. Despite the fact that by far the majority of people living with HIV are in sub-Saharan Africa, the epidemic is global. In South East Asia there is a substantial number of HIV infections in Vietnam, Indonesia, Pakistan, Thailand, Cambodia and Myanmar. In Oceania numbers are high in Papua New Guinea and some of the smaller Pacific Islands, as well as in Australia and New Zealand. In central and eastern Europe HIV is rapidly becoming a major issue in Russia and Ukraine.[5] In these areas HIV testing facilities are scarce and hence one can assume that the available figures represent the tip of the iceberg. Also, in western Europe the number of new HIV infections is increasing. The major mode of transmission is heterosexual contact and a substantial number of newly diagnosed cases have a direct link with the migration of peoples from countries with an HIV generalised epidemic.[6] This underscores again that in a globalised world, pretending that HIV and AIDS is mainly an African problem is delusory.

The overview below does not in any way claim to be comprehensive. It merely endeavours to indicate trends in policy statements and HIV discourses produced by religious organisations.

POLICY AND PUBLIC STATEMENTS FROM OUTSIDE AFRICA

Though the HIV and AIDS epidemic has affected Africa more than any other continent, it is nonetheless global. Hence, large international organisations such as the World Council of Churches (WCC),[7] the Lutheran World Federation (LWF),[8] the Reformed Ecumenical Council,[9] the Anglican Communion,[10] the World Evangelical Alliance,[11] the Council for World Mission[12] and the Young Women's Christian Association (YWCA)[13] have issued statements on HIV. In particular, the WCC has since the beginning of the epidemic in 1986 continuously demanded attention for the impact of HIV and AIDS on societies, leading to the launching of the Ecumenical Advocacy Alliance (EAA) in 2000 and the establishment of the Ecumenical HIV and AIDS Initiative in Africa (EHAIA) in 2002.

In many instances these organisations have, in co-operation with regional councils of churches, taken the lead in calling meetings for the religious leadership to reflect theologically on HIV. The WCC was instrumental in calling the 2002 meeting of the Asia Christian Council in Colombo, Sri Lanka; the 2004 Panama meeting of the Latin American Council of Churches; and the 2004 meeting of the Pacific Council of Churches in Nadi, Fiji, while the LWF facilitated the Latin American Regional Consultation in 2003 in Ciata la Mar, Venezuela and (with the United Evangelical Mission) the Asian Church Leadership Consultation on Batam Island, Indonesia in 2003. Often these meetings generated the first statements by religious organisations on HIV. While Africa is the area hardest hit by the epidemic, central Europe and South East Asia have more recently become focus areas.[14] In South East Asia, the first public statement on HIV issued by a Christian organisation was by the Christian Council of Asia, dating back to a 2001 meeting in Chang Mai, Thailand. Soon others followed, such as statements of the Catholic bishops in India in 2003 and Myanmar in 2003.[15] In recent years there have also been a number of meetings, often initiated or co-sponsored by the Joint United Nations Program on HIV and AIDS (UNAIDS), of Muslim, Buddhist and Hindu leaders to discuss the HIV and AIDS epidemic.[16] The emphasis in statements is often on education and information. The statement of the 2008 Indian Hindu leaders' meeting, for example, reads:

> We recognise the need to incorporate HIV information in appropriate ways into our discourses, our rituals, our festivals, our religious education and training of future leaders of our faith; pledge to work towards overcoming HIV in an inclusive manner and for this purpose, mobilize the human, spiritual, institutional and financial resources that our community possesses; dedicate ourselves to safeguard the rights of Hindus living with HIV and ensure their complete inclusion in familial, social, economic and religious life.[17]

It is striking that many of statements from South East Asia are inter-religious, joint declarations of Buddhist, Hindu, Muslim and Christian leaders that emphasise the importance of co-operation.[18] In countries like Thailand, Indonesia and India inter-faith networks on HIV and AIDS were established in which national church councils as well as the Catholic bishops' conferences co-operated with their Hindu, Buddhist and Islamic counterparts. In 2005 the Asian Inter-Faith Network on AIDS (AINA) was launched. AINA advocates inter-faith co-operation in various Asian countries and stimulates the establishment of national inter-faith networks. The network continues to meet on a regular basis, issuing statements that call attention to HIV-related topics such as the availability of anti-retrovirals (ARVs), human trafficking and orphans and vulnerable children.[19]

Considering the religious map of Asia, inter-faith co-operation in matters of HIV and AIDS is not surprising. Despite the fact that Asia is not the only plural religious region, with the exception of the Cairo Declaration from the Middle East,[20] this seems to be the only area that has produced inter-religious statements on the epidemic and actively supported inter-religious action by religious leaders. Whether the near absence of Islamic and inter-religious statements from, for example, Africa is a reflection of what actually happens at the grassroots level is difficult to say. This merits further research. Should this indeed be the case, with most efforts undertaken along religious and possibly even denominational lines, then there is a dire need for more co-operation at both the inter-religious and inter-denominational level.

In terms of content, most statements from Asia address the usual issues, calling for unconditional love and support for people with HIV, emphasising the need for education, prevention, care, advocacy and combating stigma. The Catholic and Muslim declarations stress the need for faithfulness and reject the use of condoms except for discordant couples.[21] Noteworthy is the Asian Muslim Network's appeal to use *zakat* (alms) for treatment and care programmes.[22] The urgency, and often despair, present in African statements (discussed later) seem absent in the Asian statements. They are, generally speaking, more optimistic, talking about 'a window of opportunity to reverse the epidemic',[23] 'reducing the HIV epidemic',[24] 'the solidarity extended by the world community', 'the encouraging signs of new drugs' and 'the great strides made in the field of healthcare'.[25] Though some of the statements point to the inter-relatedness of the epidemic and poverty, this does not seem to be a major issue in these declarations. They do, however, underscore the inter-relatedness of HIV and AIDS and issues of sexuality and gender: the point is made in many of the texts that there is a need to talk about sexuality more openly.[26] The documents reflect little or no awareness of, or introspection on, the question of whether existing religious teachings on sexuality and gender might contribute to the spread of HIV. Generally speaking, two issues give rise to self-criticism: the slowness of religious organisations to support people living with HIV; and their participation in, and slow condemnation of, stigmatisation.

The statements from Latin America differ substantially in content from those from Asia. In line with trends set by Latin American liberation theology in the

1970s, statements from Latin America show a profound awareness of the HIV and AIDS epidemic as a socio-economic issue. Declarations reflect on HIV and AIDS, therefore, in a socio-economic as well as a religious context.[27] An example from a statement by the Latin American Council of Churches (CLAI) reads:

> We are shocked to see that the statistics and the impact on and attitudes towards HIV/AIDS confirm that we live in a sick society that requires a complete and radical transformation before we can become a new people, new Churches and new societies and thereby show that we are on the path forward towards the Kingdom of God. The present social and historical context is controlled by dark forces that have an interest in hiding this serious epidemic. The growth of the neoliberal quest for profit and an economic model of globalisation which promotes the development of a market exclusively for those with purchasing power discriminates against and is insensitive to the needs of two thirds of the population of our continent, who remain exposed to misery and the risks of the epidemic . . . With profound concern, we recognise that the HIV/AIDS situation reveals the different faces of the church. On the one hand it reveals the face of indifference, where the church has met and heard the clamour of those who live and are affected by HIV/AIDS in its path, but has nevertheless passed by, like the priest in the parable of the Good Samaritan (Luke 10: 27–35).[28]

What is noteworthy about the above statement is the fact that it does not just point fingers at the problems in society that have contributed to HIV and AIDS, pretending that the church is not part of society. CLAI members seem to realise that the church and its teachings are part of the problem. In a statement for World AIDS Day 2004 this is elaborated upon with regard to gender relations: 'We want to reinforce positive male behaviour which challenges cultural, social and religious patterns of exclusion and vulnerability of women . . . we want to challenge gender norms which encourage men into risk-behaviours which have the sole objective of demonstrating their masculinity.'[29] Latin American statements address some of the underscoring issues of the epidemic.

Since 2004 a number of statements have been produced by orthodox churches in central and eastern Europe, in particular by the Russian Orthodox Church.[30] Orthodox statements emphasise the moral discourse with regard to HIV:

The HIV epidemic finds a nutrient both in the widely spread asocial and amoral forms of behaviour, such as indulgence in promiscuous sexual contacts and use of injected drugs. At the same time, the cases are not uncommon where the infection occurs because of negligence on the part of medical staff, as well as rape and adultery.[31]

Documents emphasise the link between the epidemic and 'sin and neglect of God-commanded moral norms and interests of neighbours'. Though the 2004 document of the Russian Orthodox Church emphasises that one 'should hate sin but love the sinner', it tends to associate being HIV positive with refutable and sinful behaviour, be it as active agents in contracting HIV or as victims of the behaviour of others, thus contributing to the stigmatisation of those living with HIV.

In the Pacific region, the Nadi Declaration (Fiji, 2004), a statement of the WCC's Pacific member churches, seems to be the only document by a religious organisation addressing HIV and AIDS. This is remarkable when one takes into account that Papua New Guinea and Fiji have rapidly increasing infection rates and that this might be the case for several other areas as well, though no figures are available. The 2004 Nadi Declaration is optimistic, stating that 'we can work to overcome HIV/AIDS'.[32] Whether this is naiveté or optimism based on facts, is difficult to say.

Also significant for this mapping exercise is an observation about areas and groups for which there are no documents. Apart from a few documents from South East Asia, most statements are either Christian only, or inter-faith based with a strong representation of Christian voices. Most telling is the minimal number of statements from the Middle East, western and central Europe and North America. Despite the fact that the WCC and theologians such as Musa Dube have reiterated again and again that the epidemic affects the whole church – 'the church, the body of Christ has AIDS'[33] – this is not reflected in or taken up by statements or policy documents from Western churches or other religious organisations. Though many Western churches are to some extent involved in the HIV epidemic in sub-Saharan Africa through aid, support and research, this seems to be understood as a matter of assisting partners in the South to deal with HIV and AIDS. An example from the statement of the Church of Norway in 2001 underscores this point. Though it begins by emphasising that HIV has spread around the globe, the text continues, 'Every available means must be mobilized to give our fellow human beings, who are smitten by, or in danger of being smitten by, HIV/AIDS hope for the future. Together *we* can give *them* back *their* hope' [author's italics].[34] Though laudable in the sense that the Church of Norway is one of the few Western churches to make an official statement on HIV and AIDS, and no doubt well-intended, it stays within the stigmatising 'we-they' discourse that was strongly criticised by the 2006 WCC statement on the church's compassionate response to HIV and AIDS. Point 18 of this statement says: 'In a very real sense, we are all living with HIV and AIDS. We separate ourselves from God and from God's love if we speak of "them" and "us".'[35]

Emmanuel Katongole describes the involvement of Western churches regarding the epidemic as 'the church acting as an NGO'.[36] Despite the fact that many of the projects supported by Western churches and their funding agencies stress the inter-relatedness of HIV and poverty, this has not led to introspection amongst Western churches, questioning how they, by their present behaviour, contribute to the continuation of injustice and poverty and thus to the epidemic. Most statements from western Europe are from faith-based organisations such as Norwegian Church Aid,[37] and the United Evangelical Mission.[38] Statements of repentance by Western churches over the unjust division of resources in relation to HIV and AIDS seem non-existent.[39] The only logical conclusion would seem to be that many still consider the HIV and AIDS epidemic to be mainly an African problem. To use Katongole's words: 'Metaphorically speaking, one can say that the Western churches are yet to be infected by HIV/AIDS.'[40]

POLICY AND PUBLIC STATEMENTS FROM WITHIN AFRICA

When studying public statements by religious organisations in Africa, it is again noteworthy to see which groups have issued statements and which have rarely done so, or not at all. As early as 2001 a research team commissioned by the WCC and World Alliance of the Young Men's Christian Association (YMCA) to investigate the situation of HIV and AIDS in west Africa and the Christian response to it already signalled that there were relatively few Francophone or Lusophone statements by religious organisations.[41] Of 62 statements by the Roman Catholic bishops of Africa and Madagascar, only nine are from Francophone and two from Lusophone countries.[42] Apart from statements from the Roman Catholic Church, only one other Francophone church statement could be traced, from the Eglise du Christ de Mali, a church that also broadcast a series of radio programmes on HIV and the Christian faith in 2006.[43] Other materials produced by churches in

French-speaking areas are scarce.[44] The report of the WCC and YMCA team observes that most materials produced on HIV and AIDS are in English, thus excluding French- and Portuguese-speaking groups from accessing resources. In recent years, EHAIA has picked up on this concern and has produced materials in languages other than English.[45]

The low number of statements, however, does not necessarily reflect activities on the ground. In Burkina Faso the different faith communities have, since 2001, set up committees such as Comité National Catholique de Lutte Contre le SIDA (CNCLS), the Comité National des Évangéliques pour la Lutte Contre le SIDA (CNELS) and the Comité Islamique des Actions de Lutte Contre le SIDA (CIALIS) in attempts to curb the epidemic.[46] In Senegal there is the Alliance des Religieux et Experts Medicaux Contre le SIDA (established in 1999) within which Jamra, the national association of imams, together with Christian leaders and medical experts have developed sensitisation programmes and materials for the HIV context.[47]

There are very few statements from Islamic councils or Muslim brotherhoods such as the Tijaniyya, Qadariyya or the Murid. However, in the light of the above remarks, this does not necessarily imply that no action is taking place on the ground. But, as far as public statements are concerned, only the South African Muslim community seems to have consistently drawn attention to the epidemic. In 2000 this led to the establishment of the network Positive Muslims.[48] The 2001 report of the WCC and YMCA observes that in oral discussions amongst Muslim communities in west and central Africa there is a strong emphasis on HIV and AIDS as the 'result of disobedience to the laws of God which provoke his wrath',[49] but this attitude slowly seems to be changing. In Senegal the government has made a tacit agreement with religious leaders who will not openly condemn condom campaigns, provided these are not too aggressive and are embedded in a discourse of advice against premarital sex and promotion of fidelity within marriage.[50] In Ivory Coast imams have advised against the observation of Ramadan by people living with HIV as it adversely affects their health.[51] These are just a few examples indicating that Muslim religious leaders are beginning to be actively involved in HIV and AIDS campaigns. It would be a worthwhile field of research to assess HIV and AIDS initiatives developed by Islamic organisations at national and local level in various countries and whether materials on HIV and AIDS for predominantly Muslim environments entail specific requirements.[52]

A final observation on missing voices relates to the Association of Evangelicals in Africa (AEA). Its website pays no attention to the HIV and AIDS epidemic and statements on the epidemic are untraceable.[53] The only references to HIV amongst AEA official materials can be found in the 2008 AEA strategic review report, where HIV is mentioned as one of the health hazards threatening the continent.[54] Whether this means that the organisation has not tabled the issue is unclear. In 2008 the World Evangelical Alliance, of which the AEA is a member, published a statement stating that 'with brokenness we admit that we as Evangelical Christians have allowed stigmatisation and discrimination to characterise our relationships with people living with HIV'.[55] It will be interesting to see whether the global declaration will be instrumental in prioritising the HIV and AIDS epidemic on the agenda of the AEA.

The majority of African statements seem to come from within the Christian tradition: from churches and church-related organisations, particularly in southern and eastern Africa. International ecumenical organisations such as the All Africa Council of Churches (AACC), the WCC, LWF, EHAIA, the Episcopal Conferences of Africa and Madagascar, the Organisation of African Initiated Churches and the Anglican Communion (Africa Chapter) have contributed substantially to creating awareness through their statements on HIV and AIDS. The WCC has put immense effort into tabling the epidemic, not only in Africa but also in other parts of the world. As early as 1986, in its statement entitled 'AIDS and the churches', the executive committee of the WCC drew attention to the epidemic. Whereas WCC statements from 1986 and 1996 speak about the need for care and healing, the 2006 version is deeply marked by the fact that HIV and AIDS is an ongoing struggle that will affect the world for years to come. The 2006 document is strongly prescriptive. The word 'must' is reiterated, emphasising the obligations of churches and church leaders to take action. With its prescriptive tone the document stresses the gravity and urgency of the situation because 'despite all positive participation of churches, the epidemic still outstrips all efforts to overcome it'.[56]

The Roman Catholic Church has also been a key player, making statements on both HIV in general and on the African situation in particular. As early as 1987 Pope John Paul II spoke the much-quoted words: 'God loves all of you without distinction, without limits. He loves those of you who are sick, those suffering from AIDS . . . He loves all with an unconditional and everlasting love.'[57] However, when in 1988 a journalist enquired whether HIV was a punishment for homosexuals, his response was evasive, saying that it was not easy to know God's intentions. Some consider this a missed opportunity for the Pope to have clearly rejected any link between HIV and retribution theology.[58]

The Roman Catholic Church in Africa has also made itself clearly heard. As early as 1987 the Roman Catholic bishops of Kenya, Ghana and Zimbabwe made statements on HIV and AIDS.[59] Many of these early statements have a strong moral discourse, linking HIV to sexual promiscuity and emphasising fidelity and self-discipline. The 1987 statement of the Kenyan bishops is outrightly condemnatory:

> AIDS has cast a baleful shadow across, what was fancied to be, the beautiful lives of men and women emancipated after the sexual revolution . . . It would be wrong, theologically unsound, to think that this calamity is the work of an avenging God, punishing mankind for individual and collective sins. Certain actions will have certain consequences. Nature has its own law of retribution. When we misuse tobacco, drinks or drugs, the consequences are inevitable. So also AIDS is the necessary consequence of certain abuses. Promiscuity, it would seem, is at the bottom of the whole problem, the root-cause of the rapid spread of the disease in epidemic portions.[60]

Later statements, though reiterating the erosion of Christian values, avoid the direct connection between HIV and promiscuity and focus instead on the need for fidelity and abstinence. Also, the rejection of the use of condoms as a means to prevent HIV infection forms a recurrent theme in statements over the years.[61] While most of the statements address sexual behaviour and marital ethics, in some cases other dimensions of the epidemic are tabled. The statement of the Ugandan bishops from 1989 discusses the epidemic from a socio-economic perspective:

> Our country Uganda has for a long time fought against three main enemies, namely poverty, ignorance and disease, with varying degrees of success. But it is only in rare cases that all three enemies are intricately linked together in one; and such is the case now when we have AIDS in our midst.[62]

A decade later, the Roman Catholic bishops of Zambia underscored this link between poverty and HIV, a theme reiterated in the 2003 Dakar statement of SECAM: 'We have also come to realise that *poverty goes hand in hand with HIV and AIDS* ... Poverty facilitates the transmission of HIV, makes available treatment unaffordable, accelerates death from HIV-related illnesses and multiplies the social impact of the epidemic.'[63] In 1992 the Roman Catholic bishops of the Democratic Republic of Congo made a direct connection between the ongoing civil war and the spread of HIV, stating that 'if we are not able to establish the Rule of Law in our country, and then be able to combat ignorance, curable diseases and hunger, what chance do we have to triumph one day over AIDS?'[64]

The difference in tone between various statements is striking. The majority speak about morality and present action plans while some also explicitly lament the large numbers of people dead, infected, affected and orphaned. The odd one out is the Roman Catholic bishops' statement from Ivory Coast in 1997, which already anticipates the conquest of AIDS. Cardinal Agré says:

> I have this astonishing dream, of a day which I hope will come very soon when all those who marvel that they have vanquished the scourge of AIDS will shout a 'Eureka!' of final victory in an enormous concert of horns and drums. And I yearn to see, in this worldwide celebration, our authentic Black Africans taking part alongside Asians and Europeans and Americans; not on the sidelines as spectators or as consumers, but proud to have adorned the festivities with their flowers as they have added their own specific know-how to overcoming the foe. Is this not a beautiful path of hope![65]

All in all, the Roman Catholic statements are characterised by their focus on marital and sexual ethics, emphasising fidelity and self-discipline again and again. Many of them also outline action plans but much less so in comparison with the statements of ecumenical organisations and various national councils of churches. The statement of the Ugandan Roman Catholic bishops is unique in that it explicitly commends HIV positive people for their courage in disclosing their status and sharing their knowledge, thus saving the lives of others:

> I cannot fail to express my sincere gratitude to people living with HIV/ AIDS who have come out to share vital knowledge and information

through the testimonies of your life and your experiences. You have truly been heroes and heroines of the struggle to break the stigma on HIV/AIDS in this country giving us an opportunity to learn through your experiences.[66]

A refreshingly different document is the 2004 statement by the Organisation of African Independent Churches.[67] It stresses a number of cultural traits and traditional harmful practices that fuel HIV infection. For each, observations are supplemented with a resolution to work on these issues through particular and concrete action. It also confesses that understanding by the churches of human sexuality has been inadequate and that this has contributed to the epidemic, resulting in a resolution to work on further theological and cultural research and reflection in this area.

In the WCC/EHAIA documents, as well as those of the AACC, statements by the Anglican Communion Across Africa,[68] and the many statements produced by individual churches (in South Africa alone nearly twenty statements were produced during the period 2001–6)[69] the same policy issues are reiterated: the need for education, training, prevention, care and counselling, support, combat of stigma, treatment and advocacy.[70] The early documents focus on care, prevention and education; gradually stigma, advocacy and treatment were added over the years.[71] While the topics of poverty, culture and gender also feature, only a few of the documents do more than mention them and indicate that they contribute to the spread of HIV. Most statements are more practical than theological. Most refer briefly to biblical passages or core values of the Christian faith, with recurrent theological themes being equality and dignity (all are created equally and in the image of God), justice (God hearing the cry of his people), healing (Jesus as the great physician), compassion (Jesus weeping and empathising with those suffering) and solidarity (the church as the body of Christ infected with HIV). Considering that most statements are made by Christian organisations, the near absence of more profound biblical and theological reflections on the epidemic is noteworthy.

In analysing the documents, it seems that many copy from each other and there is little or no attention to contextual differences.[72] Considering the nature of the documents and the fact that they are exhortatory rather than analytical of concrete situations, this is understandable. Nevertheless, it would be worthwhile to investigate how issues of gender, poverty and culture influence the HIV and

AIDS epidemic in particular contexts, rather than generalising. Only by mapping the various contexts of the epidemic will it be possible to develop tailor-made policies and strategies of transformation.

DISCOURSE OF MORALITY, WAR AND HOPE

The fact that religious organisations engage in public policy discourse evokes a whole series of questions. The South African theologian Nico Koopman has the following queries: what is the exact role of religion in public discourse; does religion only provide a motivation and framework for debates on policy or does it have a unique contribution to make to the contents of the debate; what is the objective of statements made; what do religious organisations hope to achieve by making public statements; and how does religion negotiate between its vision and principles and the confines of implementing it in society?[73] These are intriguing questions for which there are no easy or clear-cut answers. It is without doubt, however, that when religious organisations enter the arena of public policy they wittingly or unwittingly contribute to the public perception of the topic discussed. Hence, utmost care is needed in the phrasing of statements because both the words chosen and the underlying theology implied shape public opinion.

A critical analysis of statements by religious organisations on HIV and AIDS leads to the conclusion that three types of discourse seem to dominate. They are related to morality, war and hope. All prove to be problematic when closely examined.

The discourse of morality and responsible individual behaviour is dominant in the Roman Catholic and Russian Orthodox Church statements, as well as in the statement of the World Evangelical Alliance. They emphasise the need for renewed teachings on Christian sexual ethics, strict marital fidelity, abstinence from premarital sex and self-discipline. Most of these documents, therefore, connect HIV to individual behaviour, despite the growing critique of this position. More and more authors point out that there is a direct link between social factors such as poverty, war and migration and a person's vulnerability to HIV. Behaviour, they underscore, is not always a matter of free choice.[74] The South African theologian Charles Ryan has also critiqued this discourse of morality. He has noted that though most religious organisations and churches nowadays formally avoid the notion that HIV is a punishment from God, the emphasis on moral discourse reinforces the idea that being HIV positive is the consequence of immoral sexual behaviour.[75]

As both Emmanuel Katongole and James Cochrane have recently pointed out, much of the discourse on HIV and AIDS takes place within a military vocabulary, within a discourse of war.[76] There is a fight or a war against HIV and AIDS, and people are invited to get involved to liberate the world from AIDS. Many statements from ecumenical organisations are characterised by this discourse. An example of a statement phrased in a predominantly military vocabulary is the 2001 AACC Dakar declaration on HIV and AIDS, which sets out to 'make the fight a top priority', 'mobilise workers', 'set up and equip units' and 'put mechanisms in place'. Also, the emphasis on technicalities vis-à-vis education, advocacy and ARVs can be considered to be part of this 'military' vocabulary. Katongole points out:

> The rhetoric of a 'war on AIDS' sustains the impression that HIV/AIDS is a temporary if serious nuisance that will eventually be overcome . . . The critical import of this observation is that a military metaphor assumes the legitimacy of, and in fact seeks to insure minimal disruption to, our current social, political, economic, and cultural arrangements.[77]

Katongole then goes on to argue that the epidemic should not be seen as an event in itself but as a sign of the much larger problem of global injustices in the realm of politics, economics and resources. A church, according to Katongole, that uses military vocabulary, perpetuates the 'externalist and interventionalist approach to HIV and AIDS' and avoids addressing the fundamental issues fuelling the epidemic. Similarly, Cochrane argues that adopting military discourse removes the agencies and assets of people on the ground, as it takes a negative starting point, disempowering people. He pleads for development work to begin with the assets and agencies of people (including their religious faith), arguing that people have resources, spiritual and otherwise, which can be mobilised to address HIV and AIDS.[78]

A third discourse evident from public statements is that of hope. Jill Olivier has pointed out that much of this has emerged as a counter-reaction to previous stigmatisation and 'othering'.[79] It permeates many of the statements studied thus far. The hope discourse emphasises the progress that has been made (ARVs, mobilisation of funds and so on); and that claiming their human dignity invites 'people living with HIV to come out of the shadow of despair, gloom and guilt and enter into a joyful hope and acceptance'.[80] Olivier points out that much of the public discourse on hope reinforces the polarisation between them, who need hope and human dignity, and us, who are not HIV positive. A quote from the Indian Catholic bishop's pastoral letter on World AIDS Day 2003 emphasises this point. The letter states:

> Let us help those people living with HIV to come out of the shadow of despair, gloom and guilt and enter into a joyful hope and acceptance. Those among us who are living with HIV/AIDS must not feel that they are alone and abandoned. We, who are their sisters and brothers, must walk in solidarity with them on their journey.[81]

Olivier observes that discourses of hope, when not carefully formulated, tend to exclude rather than include those living with HIV. She pointedly adds that hope in the Christian context is something different from mere optimism: it is a hope amidst despair, which faces the suffering, acts as a creational force and works towards a new future that includes all humankind, despite differences.[82]

SOME CONCLUSIONS AND OBSERVATIONS

It seems true to observe that, apart from a few noted exceptions from the WCC and African Roman Catholic bishops, official religious responses to HIV and AIDS were relatively slow to emerge. Most were issued from 2000 onwards. Those that have been issued tend to be generated by well-organised, hierarchically structured churches and ecumenical organisations. Furthermore, though statements on HIV and AIDS are produced around the world, the majority emerged out of Africa or address the African situation. Next to Africa, documents from Asia are the most prolific.

Many of the statements from outside Africa reveal that transnational ecumenical organisations like WCC and YWCA/YMCA have played a key role in stimulating churches and church-related organisations in their deliberations on the epidemic. Often, WCC and YWCA/YMCA were instrumental in bringing people together in workshops and conferences. By far the largest number of documents is of Christian origin. Asia seems to be the only region where leaders from other religious communities have gathered to address HIV and AIDS publicly. It seems necessary to explore further whether, and if so in which way, Islamic organisations in Africa are addressing the epidemic. It is noteworthy that in the documents studied, with the exception of Asia where AINA was established, there is little evidence of inter-faith co-operation. Where there is, inter-faith statements suggest substantial Christian involvement. For the African context, further research is needed to explore whether there are local collaborative initiatives between Christians and Muslims and, if so, what forms these initiatives have taken.

The majority of statements are in English. The scarcity of African Francophone contributions, especially from Protestant churches, is striking. So is the near absence of statements on HIV and AIDS from Western countries. This might be a sign that HIV and AIDS is still not considered to be a global issue but rather an illness that affects certain parts of the world. The documents do not clarify whether members of religious organisations from various parts of the world meet to exchange best practice and encourage one another.

As many of the documents are from groups that transcend the national level, they pay little attention to particular contexts and tend to address the HIV and AIDS epidemic generally. There is a need to map the particularities of HIV and AIDS in various contexts as well as a need to analyse whether strategies developed on the (inter)national level do in fact address the specific needs of each context.

Finally, the HIV and AIDS epidemic is discussed under various discourses in statements. The prevailing discourses are those of morality, war and hope, each being problematic in its own way. A close reading of these discourses suggests that there is still a profound need for further reflection – theological, religious and otherwise – on the epidemic.

NOTES

1. 'Covenant of life: Statement of the Asian Church Leadership consultation on HIV/AIDS'. Batam Island, 1–4 Dec. 2003.
2. SECAM, 'The Church in Africa in face of the HIV/AIDS epidemic: Our prayer is always full of hope in Catholic Bishops of Africa and Madagascar in *Speak Out on HIV and AIDS* (Nairobi: Paulines Publications Africa, 2004): 104.
3. For example, see INERELA+. Available at http://www.anerela.org/ (accessed 18 June 2009).
4. Mark Krakauer, 'Churches' Responses to AIDS in Two Communities in KwaZulu-Natal, South Africa' (M.Phil. thesis, Oxford University, 2004): 105.
5. *UNAIDS report* 2008; see also *Euro-AIDS report* 2006.
6. http://www.unAIDS.org/en/KnowledgeCentre/Resources/FeatureStories/archive/2007/20071015_European_meeting_discusses_migration_TB_and_HIV.asp (accessed 19 June 2009).
7. For documents by the WCC see http://www.oikoumene.org/en/resources/documents/wcc-programmes/justice-diakonia-and-responsibility-for-creation/ehaia/world-council-of-churches-statements-and-studies.html (accessed 5 June 2009). Examples are the 1986 executive

committee statement 'AIDS and the churches', the 1996 central committee statement 'The impact of HIV/AIDS and the churches' response' and the 2006 central committee statement 'Statement on the churches' compassionate response to HIV and AIDS'.

8. In 2002 the statement 'Compassion, conversion and care: Responding as churches to the HIV/AIDS pandemic, an action plan of the Lutheran World Federation' was issued. In 2003 the tenth LWF Assembly in Winnipeg dedicated part of its message to HIV and AIDS: section V 'Removing barriers that exclude'; section VI 'The Church's ministry of healing'; and section VII 'Justice and healing in families'.

9. In 2005, during its Utrecht Assembly, the Reformed Ecumenical Council issued the statement 'Towards a theology of hope in a time of AIDS'.

10. On 14 April 2002 the Anglican Communion issued the 'Report of the meeting of primates of the Anglican Communion: Appendix III statement . . . on HIV/AIDS ACNS 2961'. On 27 May 2003 the Anglican primates issued a 'Pastoral letter from the primates of the Anglican Communion'.

11. The 2008 Assembly of the World Evangelical Alliance adopted the statement 'Call to action on HIV'.

12. The Council for World Mission focused on the HIV epidemic in the 2003 'CMW Assembly statement, Ayr, Scotland 15–20 June 2003'.

13. The YWCA World Council at the 2003 Brisbane meeting issued the 'World Council resolution: Reproductive health and sexuality', while in 2004 the executive committee of the YWCA-World revisited the issue with 'Recommendations on HIV/AIDS adopted by the World Council executive committee'.

14. UNAIDS, 'Report on the global AIDS epidemic', Geneva, 2008.

15. Catholic Bishops of India, 'Pastoral letter from the Indian bishops on World AIDS Day 2003: The challenge to be His light today' (2003); Catholic Bishops of Myanmar, 'Pastoral letter on HIV/AIDS and the response of the church' (Dec. 2003); Asian Leaderships Consultation, 'Covenant of life' (Batam Island, Indonesia, Nov. 2003).

16. Already in 2003 Buddhist leaders from South East Asia had gathered in Bangkok to discuss HIV and AIDS. Available at http://www.aegis.com/news/afp/2003/AF030880.html (accessed 13 June 2009). In 2004 the Asian Muslim Action network issued a statement on HIV and AIDS. Available at http://www.oikoumene.org/en/resources/documents/wcc-programmes/justice-diakonia-and-responsibility-for-creation/ehaia/declarations-and-policy-statements-on-hivAIDS-by-churches-and-faith-based-organisations.html (accessed 14 Nov. 2008). In Oct. 2008 there was Buddhist leaders' meeting in Ho Chi Minh City, Vietnam. Available at http://vietnamnews.vnagency.com.vn/showarticle.php?num=06SOC271008 (accessed 19 June 2009), while in June 2008 Indian Hindu leaders had met in Bangalore, India. Available at http://www.unAIDS.org/en/KnowledgeCentre/Resources/FeatureStories/archive/2008/20080618_hindu_faith_leaders_AIDS_response.asp (accessed 15 June 2009).

17. 'Declaration on HIV and AIDS, Hindu leaders' caucus, June 1–2 2008, Bangalore'. Available at http://www.cabsa.co.za/newsite/DisplayPage.asp?Id=402 (accessed 19 June 2009).

18. 'For we are neighbours'. Statement from the Inter-Faith AIDS Conference, Bangkok, 2003; International Inter-Faith Conference on Prevention and Control of HIV/AIDS, Delhi, 2004; Muslim Workshop on HIV/AIDS, Asian Muslim Network, Bangkok, 2004.

19. For the 2008 meeting see http://www.globalministries.org/news/eap/reclaiming-rights.html (accessed 19 June 2009).

20. 'Cairo declaration of religious leaders in the Arab states in response to the HIV/AIDS epidemic', Cairo, Dec. 2004. This was a declaration of Christian and Muslim leaders.

21. Muslim Workshop on HIV/AIDS, Bangkok, 2004; Catholic Bishops of India, 'Pastoral letter from the Indian bishops on World AIDS Day 2003'; Catholic Bishops of Myanmar, 'Pastoral letter on HIV/AIDS and the response of the church'.

22. Muslim Workshop on HIV/AIDS, Bangkok, 2004.

23. 'Report of the WCC-CCA consultation on an ecumenical agenda to combat HIV/AIDS in South Asia', Colombo, 2002.

24. Muslim Workshop on HIV/AIDS, Bangkok, 2004.

25. 'Consultation on HIV/AIDS: a challenge for religious response'. Christian Conference of Asia statement, Chiang Mai, Thailand, 2001.

26. Catholic Bishops of India, 'Pastoral letter from the Indian bishops on World AIDS Day 2003'; Catholic Bishops of Myanmar, 'Pastoral letter on HIV/AIDS and the response of the church'.

27. C. Benn, 'The influence of cultural and religious frameworks on the future course of the HIV/AIDS pandemic'. *Journal of Theology for Southern Africa* 113 (2003): 3–18; E. Chitando, *Acting with Hope* (Geneva: WCC Publications, 2007).

28. The Church and HIV/AIDS in Latin America and the Caribbean: Regional Meeting Facilitated by the Latin American Council of Churches and Supported by the World Council of Churches, Panama, 2004.

29. CLAI, 'Message from churches, organizations and programmes on World AIDS Day 2004: Women, Girls and HIV/AIDS' (2004). Available at www.oikoumene.org/en/resources/documents/other-ecumenical-bodies/church-statements-on-hivaids/latin-american-regional-meeting.html.

30. 'Memorandum of intention: Strategy consultation on churches and HIV/AIDS in central and eastern Europe', St Petersburg, 2003; 'A message, urging love and tolerance for those suffering from AIDS/HIV', Romanian Orthodox Church, 2004; 'Concept of the Russian Orthodox Church's participation in overcoming the spreading of HIV/AIDS and work with people living with HIV/AIDS', Moscow, 2004.

31. 'Concept of the Russian Orthodox Church's participation in overcoming the spreading of HIV/AIDS and work with people living with HIV/AIDS'.

32. Available at www.oikoumene.org/.../nadi-declaration-by-wcc-pacific-member-churches. html.

33. Musa Dube, 'Theological challenges: proclaiming fullness of life in the HIV/AIDS and global economic era'. *International Review of Mission* 91(363) 2003: 539.

34. Church of Norway Bishops' Conference, 'The global HIV/AIDS epidemic', 2001.

35. 'Statement on the churches' compassionate response to HIV and AIDS', WCC Central Committee Final Report of Public Issues Committee, section 18. Available at http://www.oikoumene.org/en/resources/documents/central-committee/geneva-2006/reports-and-documents/final-report-of-the-public-issues-committee-adopted.html#c10110 (accessed 20 June 2009).

36. Emmanuel Katongole, 'AIDS in Africa: The church and the politics of interruption' in *Heil und Befreiung in Afrika: die Kirchen vor der Missionarischen Herausforderung durch HIV/AIDS*, edited by F.X. D'Sa and J. Lohmayer (Würzburg: Echter, 2007): 170.
37. Norwegian Church Aid, 'HIV/AIDS: A policy statement', 29 Sep. 2003.
38. United Evangelical Mission, 'Anti HIV/AIDS programme policy', UEM General Assembly, Manila, Oct. 2004). See also Christian HIV and AIDS Alliance at www.chaa.info (accessed 20 June 2009).
39. The 1998 statement of the National Church Council of the Evangelical Lutheran Church in Canada entitled 'A public statement of pastoral concern for those living with HIV/AIDS' seems an exception. Though not openly stating the *Mitschuldigkeit*, the statement highlights the direct relation between economic injustice, poverty and HIV and AIDS and pleads for a prophetic ministry to eliminate poverty.
40. Katongole, 'AIDS in Africa': 175.
41. J. Savee Kokoe, Y.A. Akolatse and K. Tatagan-Agbi, 'Churches and the HIV/AIDS pandemic: Analysis of the situation in 10 west/central African countries: Report presented to WCC and World Alliance of the YMCA, March 2001': 10. Available at http://www.wcc-coe.org/wcc/what/mission/aids-study-e.pdf.
42. Catholic Bishops of Africa and Madagascar, *Speak Out on HIV and AIDS*.
43. http://www.egliseduchristaumali.org/chemin_verite.htm (accessed 19 Sep. 2008).
44. Kokoe, Akolatse and Tatagan-Agbi, 'Churches and the HIV/AIDS pandemic': 10.
45. See http://www.oikoumene.org/en/resources/documents/wcc-programmes/justice-diakonia-and-responsibility-for-creation/ehaia/material-in-african-languages.html (accessed 20 June 2009).
46. http://www.lefaso.net/spip.php?page=impression&id_article=18047 (accessed 19 June 2009).
47. S.S. Gilbert, 'The influence of Islam on HIV prevention among Senegalese university students'. *AIDS Education and Prevention* 20(5) 2008: 399–407. Available at http://ipsnews.net/new_nota.asp?idnews=24549 (accessed 20 June 2009).
48. http://www.positivemuslims.org.za.
49. Kokoe, Akolatse and Tatagan-Agbi, 'Churches and the HIV/AIDS pandemic': 9. See also observations made by religious leaders of the South African Muslim community: A. Kayem Ahmad, 'Developing a theology of compassion: Muslim attitudes towards people living with HIV and AIDS in South Africa'. *Arisa: Annual Review of Islam in South Africa* 2000/3 [no page numbers]; Amina Wadud strongly rejects the *zina* (fornication) discourse and advocates looking more critically at Islamic perceptions of sexuality and gender relations; A. Wadud, 'Muslims, Islam and AIDS: Thoughts on the Second International Muslim Religious Leaders Consultation on HIV/AIDS, Malaysia, 2003'. Available at http://www.crescentlife.com/wellness/muslims,_islam_and_AIDS.htm (accessed 19 June 2009).
50. http://ipsnews.net/new_nota.asp?idnews=24549 (accessed 20 June 2009).
51. http://www.corridor-sida.org/spip.php?breve134 (accessed 21 June 2009).
52. The LWF produced materials for the Mauritanian, predominantly Muslim, context. See *Lutheran World Federation Information* 2005(11): 9.
53. http://www.aeafrica.org/.
54. http://www.aeafrica.org/news/news_view.htm?no=61&num=1 (accessed 18 June 2009).

55. WEA, 'HIV: A call to action', General Assembly, Thailand, 2008. This statement was prepared and affirmed by the Micah Challenge leadership and then forwarded and accepted by the General Assembly.

56. http://www.oikoumene.org/en/resources/documents/central-committee/geneva-2006/reports-and-documents/final-report-of-the-public-issues-committee-adopted.html#c10110 (accessed 10 June 2009).

57. R. Vitillo, 'Reaching out to those with HIV/AIDS' in *John Paul II: A Light for the World: Essays and Reflections on the Papacy of John Paul II*, by K. Anna and M.A. Walsh (Lanham: Sheed and Ward, 2003): 142.

58. http://www.gaytoday.com/garchive/viewpoint.071700vi.htm (accessed 15 June 2009).

59. Catholic Bishops of Africa and Madagascar, *Speak Out on HIV and AIDS*: 11–15.

60. 'The challenge of AIDS' (Kenya, 1987) in Catholic Bishops of Africa and Madagascar, *Speak Out on HIV and AIDS*: 11.

61. 'Communiqué' (Ghana, 1987, 1989, 1994 and 2001); 'AIDS and our moral responsibility' (Zimbabwe, 1987); 'Pastoral statement on AIDS' (SACBC, 1990); 'The family is the basic unit of society' (Zimbabwe, 1994); 'The prevention of AIDS' (Mauritius, 2000); 'Not to use condoms' (Nigeria, 2001); 'Letter on HIV/AIDS' (South Africa, 2001); and 'May the light of Christ enlighten your life' (Mozambique, 2003) all in Catholic Bishops of Africa and Madagascar, *Speak Out on HIV and AIDS*.

62. 'AIDS in our midst' (Uganda, 1989) in Catholic Bishops of Africa and Madagascar, *Speak Out on HIV and AIDS*: 18.

63. 'The missionary family' (Zambia, 1999) in Catholic Bishops of Africa and Madagascar, *Speak Out on HIV and AIDS*, 57; 'The Church in Africa in face of the HIV/AIDS pandemic' (SECAM, 2003) in Catholic Bishops of Africa and Madagascar, *Speak out on HIV and AIDS*: 106 (italics in the original).

64. 'World AIDS Day' (Zaire, 1992) in Catholic Bishops of Africa and Madagascar, *Speak Out on HIV and AIDS*: 38.

65. 'The Church and AIDS: facts, commitment' (Ivory Coast, 1997) in Catholic Bishops of Africa and Madagascar, *Speak Out on HIV and AIDS*: 51.

66. 'Strategic plan for HIV/AIDS activities 2001–2006' (Uganda, 2001) in Catholic Bishops of Africa and Madagascar, *Speak Out on HIV and AIDS*: 77.

67. 'OAIC HIV/AIDS Pretoria declaration 2004', Continental HIV and AIDS Conference: Critical Solidarity in the Face of HIV and AIDS.

68. For example, the All Africa Anglican AIDS Planning Framework, 'Our vision, our hope' (Johannesburg, 2001); Council of Anglican Provinces in Africa, 'Statement from CAPA AIDS board meeting' (Nairobi 2002); 'National HIV/AIDS strategic planning and policy development workshop communiqué' (Church of Nigeria, Anglican Communion, 2003).

69. http://www.cabsa.co.za/newsite/DisplayPage.asp?Id=27 (accessed 17 June 2009).

70. EHAIA, 'The ecumenical response to HIV/AIDS in Africa: Plan of action' (Nairobi, 2001).

71. See, for example, the 2006 appeal of the WCC for universal access to treatment. Available at http://www.oikoumene.org/en/events-sections/cc2006/news-media/news/display-single-english-news/article/1722/hiv-and-AIDS-wcc-asks-f.html (accessed 15 June 2009).

72. H. Dilger, '"Living positHIVely in Tanzania": The global dynamics of AIDS and the meaning of religion for international and local AIDS work'. *Afrika Spectrum* 36(1) 2001; 73–90; Kokoe, Akolatse and Tatagan-Agbi, 'Churches and the HIV/AIDS pandemic': 9.

73. N. Koopman, 'Churches and public policy discourse in South Africa', 26 May 2008. Available at http://www.csu.edu.au/special/accc/about/gnpt/papers/ (accessed 15 June 2009).

74. E.M. Zulu, F.N-A. Dodoo and A.C. Ezeh, 'Urbanization, poverty and sex: Roots of risky sexual behaviors in slum settlements in Nairobi, Kenya' in *HIV and AIDS in Africa: Beyond Epidemiology*, edited by E. Kalipeni et al. (Oxford: Blackwell, 2004): 167–74; S. Gillespie (ed.), *AIDS, Poverty, and Hunger. Challenges and Responses* (Washington, DC: International Food Policy Research Institute, 2006).

75. C.P. Ryan, 'AIDS and responsibility: the Catholic tradition' in *Responsibility in a Time of AIDS: A Pastoral Response by Catholic Theologians and AIDS Activists in Southern Africa*, edited by S.C. Bate (Pietermaritzburg: Cluster Publications, 2003): 4–5.

76. Katongole, 'AIDS in Africa': 176–7; J.R. Cochrane, 'Seeing healthworlds differently'. *Religion and Theology* 14 (2007): 6–8.

77. Katongole, 'AIDS in Africa': 169.

78. Cochrane, 'Seeing healthworlds differently': 21–4.

79. J. Olivier, 'Where does the Christian stand?: Considering a public discourse on hope in the context of HIV/AIDS in South Africa'. *Journal of Theology for Southern Africa* 126 (2006): 81–97.

80. 'The Nadi Declaration: A statement of the World Council of Churches Pacific member churches on HIV/AIDS, 2004'; 'Message from churches, organizations and programmes on World AIDS Day 2004: Women, girls and HIV/AIDS', Latin America, 2004; Indian Catholic Bishops, 'Pastoral letter for World AIDS Day 2003: The challenge to be His light', 1 Dec. 2003.

81. Indian Catholic Bishops, 'Pastoral letter for World AIDS Day 2003'.

82. Olivier, 'Where does the Christian stand?': 97.

Practitioner response

Paula Clifford

As a Christian organisation accountable to the churches in the United Kingdom and Ireland, Christian Aid finds natural partners for its work in both local churches and those in the South. Our long-established work on HIV and AIDS has clearly demonstrated to us the great value of the work of churches, particularly in sub-Saharan Africa, in tackling the crisis. At their best, they form natural networks for communicating vital information on prevention and offering care and support; and they can have a formidable voice when it comes to campaigning and advocacy. Yet few people would pretend that statements from religious organisations, whatever their regional and denominational origin, make gripping reading. All too often one has the impression that a statement on a social justice issue is more about a church seeking to justify itself and somehow prove its concern for the problems of today's world, rather than indicating a willing identification with people who are poor and marginalised. So Martha Frederiks has had a peculiarly thankless task in gathering such statements and giving them coherence.

What is of particular interest regarding the public statements of religious organisations is the motivation that lies behind them and the language used. For the most part, of course, one can do little more than hazard a guess at why an organisation may have made a particular statement at a specific time. What is probably true, however, is that statements from countries where HIV incidence is low have a rather different motivation from those being generated from countries where the incidence rate is high and continues to rise at an alarming rate. In both cases, though, the language is remarkably similar.

Reading Frederiks' chapter, and through my own research, I am struck by how much these statements focus not so much on people living with HIV as on what others might gain from the process. For example, a statement in 1993 by the Catholic Bishops' Conference of the Philippines says: 'For us, an encounter with people infected with HIV/AIDS should be a moment of grace – an opportunity for us to be Christ's compassionate presence to them as well as to experience His presence in them.'[1]

To see other people's suffering as an opportunity for personal spiritual growth is unacceptable even if, as I suspect, its origin is motivated by a desire to remove stigma by making a theological statement. Ten years later, in July 2003, the Methodist Church of Great Britain declared that 'AIDS is the new apartheid' and issued this call to action: 'The Conference calls on all governments across the world to pressurise pharmaceutical companies and multi-national corporations to release cheap generic drugs to the millions suffering from HIV/AIDS.'[2]

Here, the Methodist Church of Great Britain, deservedly well-known for its social conscience, is issuing a practical and relevant call to action. But what are we to make of the language of a new apartheid? In this context, it evokes the image of separation, stressing the divide between those who can afford ARV treatment and those who cannot. Furthermore, this terminology is a reminder of a time when the church did take a principled stand and became part of the anti-apartheid movement that was ultimately successful in ending an apparently unstoppable evil in South Africa.

But often public statements are compromised by hidden agendas. For example, the worldwide Anglican Church has allowed its theological and ecclesiological agenda to be dominated by questions of sexuality, which has been hugely controversial. Thus, because of the long-standing association between HIV and gay men in the United Kingdom and elsewhere in western Europe, issues of sexuality have posed a challenge for those formulating statements on HIV. As a result, the issue has not been adequately addressed. This point is highlighted in the Church of England's 56-page report issued in response to the statement by the primates of the Anglican Communion in May 2003.[3] The response briefly notes that sex between men is the predominant form of transmission in Germany and the Netherlands and has a short piece on homosexuality and human rights.[4] The turmoil that the HIV epidemic was causing in gay communities at the time (not least in London, the place of publication of the report) is left unacknowledged.

One question that arises from the fairly wide definition of religious organisation that underlies Frederiks' work is the possible disparity between sentiments expressed by an organisation for whom HIV and AIDS is just one among many matters for concern, and those stated by leaders who have come together for the sole purpose of working together on HIV. For example, the Jakarta Declaration of Islamic Religious Leaders (1999)[5] lists a number of important, though general, concerns: the increase of HIV in the Association of South East Asian Nations (ASEAN) region and its possible economic consequences; the need for dissemination of information; and the role of Muslim leaders in the community. But their statement is nowhere near as radical as that published by a group of diverse participants at the pre-conference Muslim Workshop on HIV and AIDS before the Bangkok International AIDS Conference in 2004. Among other things, this called for support for people living with HIV to be provided within mosques and other religious establishments; and unconditional love and support to replace stigma and discrimination: 'It does not matter how one is infected but it does matter how one is affected.'[6]

As Frederiks has pointed out, earlier statements on HIV within Africa tended to be corrective and attribute blame. Later, there was a shift in focus to an emphasis on theology reflecting Christ-like love and acceptance. Typical of this is a statement prepared by the Southern African Catholic Bishops' Conference (SACBC) and other Catholic leaders following a conference at St Augustine College of South Africa: 'We must break the connection between guilt and HIV/ AIDS', it proclaimed. There was a certain acceptance of responsibility for failures in sex education ('the education of conscience') and an admission that 'Catholic messages about condoms have tended to confuse the issue since they are tied to teachings about contraception'. Instead, the statement declared, 'the goal is to defend oneself against a deadly disease'. The statement ended with a call for compassion, support and non-judgementalism, as well as a note on the importance of recognising traditional African healing strategies that are holistic and community-based.[7] This may suggest that the Roman Catholic Church, at least in southern Africa, has a slightly broader outlook than is implied in some of the statements surveyed by Frederiks.

However, with the notable exceptions of HIV-friendly churches, particularly in South Africa but also in such high-profile places of worship as St John's Cathedral in Hong Kong, there is an almost inevitable disconnection between the statements issued by religious organisations and their practice. While it is generally the case that the statements imply a practice that is far from being achieved, it can and does happen that activities at grassroots level are in advance of any official formulation by religious leaders. So, ideally, any assessment of the effectiveness of the response of religious organisations to HIV and AIDS must combine the two. In this, the work of Frederiks is an important contribution.

Notes

1. *AIDS Action* 47 (April–June 2000, Asia-Pacific ed.): 7.
2. *Methodist Conference News* 4 July 2003: 1. Available at http://www.methodist.org.uk/index.cfm?fuseaction=opentogod.content&cmid=617 (accessed 20 Aug. 2009).
3. Primates is a term used to include all archbishops in the worldwide Anglican Communion. The statement was entitled 'The body of Christ has AIDS'.
4. 'Telling the story: being positive about HIV/AIDS' (London: Mission and Public Affairs Council of the Church of England, Apr. 2004).
5. Runizar Roesin (ed.), *Islamic Approach on HIV/AIDS: Report on the First HIV/AIDS ASEAN Regional Workshop of Islamic Religious Leaders* (Jakarta: Indonesian Council of Ulama, 1999).
6. Asian Muslim Action Network, Asian Resource Foundation and Thai Muslim Network, 'Muslim Workshop on HIV/AIDS'. Available at http://www.oikoumene.org/resources/documents/other-ecumenical-bodies/church-statements-on-hivaids/09-07-04-muslim-workshop-on-hivaids.html (accessed 11 Dec. 2009).
7. 'Responsibility in a time of AIDS: a Catholic theological response to the pandemic'. *Newsletter of the Catholic Theological Society of Southern Africa*, 7 Feb. 2003. Available at www.uni-tuebingen.de/INSeCT/members/ctssa/newsletter01.pdf (accessed 20 Aug. 2009).

PART 2

Engaging the religious and theological realm

5

Sacred texts, particularly the Bible and the Qur'an, and HIV and AIDS

Charting the textual territory

Gerald West

INTRODUCTION

A mapping of the place of sacred texts in the terrain constructed by HIV and AIDS is important[1] because sacred texts themselves are so important to the millions of people who inhabit parts of the world most affected by HIV. It is important because sacred texts are often taken for granted, hovering in the background of our religious response to the epidemic. For example, the *Encyclopedia of AIDS*, though covering the realm of religion, has very little to offer on the place of sacred texts within religious responses to HIV and AIDS.[2]

A mapping of the place of sacred texts in their intersections with HIV and AIDS is important for another reason. Common to most, if not all, religions faced by HIV and AIDS is the search for a cause or intention. And the dominant religious response to HIV is that it is some kind of punishment or lesson from God, angels, ancestors or the universe. Whatever the religion, there is some form of theology of retribution: what you sow you will reap. More precisely, this agricultural metaphor and proverb has become inverted within most religions: what you reap is a good indication of what you must have sown. If you are HIV positive you must have done something to deserve it. So say our religious traditions.

THEOLOGIES OF RETRIBUTION

Christianity and Islam are perhaps the clearest on this kind of theology. For example, as the dominant religious traditions on the African continent, often in partnership with forms of African Religion, African Christianities and African Islam(s), they are fairly unambiguous about a theology of retribution in the context of HIV. Variant strands of theologies of retribution form the sub-stratum of these religious traditions and so it is not surprising that the advent of HIV has invoked this ideo-theological orientation. The term ideo-theological represents the dual, but dynamic and dialectic, contributions of both context (ideology) and sacred text (theology) to the formation of religious notions of retribution. Though somewhat clumsy, the term is a reminder of the socio-historical and religio-cultural dimensions of, for example, stigma and discrimination associated with HIV.[3]

In the case of each of these religious traditions their respective sacred texts have been understood to undergird ideo-theologies of retribution. In his extensive engagement with HIV and AIDS in Africa,[4] Ezra Chitando of the Ecumenical HIV and AIDS Initiative in Africa (EHAIA) begins by stating that 'One of the most significant aspects of the Christian heritage in Africa has been the centrality of the Bible'. The Bible, says Chitando, 'acts as a guide to belief and action', is used 'as a resource to meet all the exigencies of life', is held in high esteem, enables (in the vernacular) 'the democratization of God's revelation' (compared to African Religion's restriction of divine oracles to select individuals) and resonates with traditional African beliefs and practices (forming often unhealthy patriarchal alliances). Consequently, continues Chitando, the 'key role played by the Bible in Africa has major implications for the church's response to HIV and AIDS'.[5]

During the early stages of the epidemic, Chitando argues, 'the Bible was often read in ways that did not affirm life', with HIV/AIDS seen as the 'wages of sin' (Romans 6:23) and part of the Deuteronomistic pattern of retribution. He reflects that it was 'perhaps inevitable for the church to frame its initial response to the epidemic in existing theological vocabulary', in which HIV 'became a manifestation of humanity's sinfulness'; the epidemic 'was interpreted as fulfilling the curses cited in Deuteronomy 28:27, which include God sending incurable diseases to an apostate people'; 'HIV was read as a signifier that the end of the world was drawing near (Luke 21:5–28)'; and the 'failure to develop a vaccine to cure HIV has been taken by some as confirming God's punishment of a stubborn and sinful generation'. 'Theological rigidity and intellectual aridity have led to the church's failure to interpret HIV and AIDS as a critical turning point,' says Chitando, emphasising the theological dimension of this failure but implying, perhaps, its failure to re-read the Bible in the face of the reality 'of the questions that emerge from the cemeteries that are rapidly filling with the bodies of young people in Africa'.[6]

Similarly, Felicitas Becker examines how the Qur'an is used to engage with HIV and AIDS in Tanzania. Rejecting homogeneity in the Muslim engagement, she argues that 'caught between their scriptures, habits and conflicting information on HIV/AIDS in the public sphere, Muslims, like everybody else, muddle through'. Significantly, Becker notes that African religio-cultural practices that predate conversion to Islam in the Lindi region are invoked by Muslims to explain the prevalence of HIV. It is because, says one female informant, 'they are breaking the taboos, they are breaking the customs (*mila*) of the country of their elders'. Becker goes on to argue that religion and culture provide the preferential lens through which to understand and respond to the HIV and AIDS epidemic, for though medical science was considered 'a source of prescriptions much like religion, its prescriptions had neither the weight of the past nor that of the scriptures behind them, neither God nor *wazee*, elders'. She concludes that 'Vernacular and Qur'anic (as well as biblical) language have a force that biomedical explanations and recommendations cannot match'.[7]

With respect to the Qur'an, reformist groups tend to argue 'that adherence to the prescriptions of the Qur'an regarding sex would have prevented the whole pandemic'.[8] One particular informant, an old woman, the daughter of a *sheshe* who is herself well versed in the Qur'an, claimed:

> AIDS is written in the Qur'an. God has said 'if people forget my *aya* (Qur'an verses), I will send them a creature that will make them talk'. This is a Qur'an verse; if it wasn't so late and dark, I would look it up for you. Now you might think this creature would be a large animal that comes to tell people, listen, don't act like this, but no, it is an invisible bug. If you think about it carefully, you will understand.[9]

For this informant, the emergence of HIV was itself a reminder of the centrality of God's word, not as a set of ready-made truths but rather as a conservation partner among believers struggling 'to work out the import of the Scriptures on their present situation'. From another perspective, however, another informant, an elderly male who sold religious books, made the following distinction: while 'AIDS could never be mentioned' in the Qur'an, he stated that 'the medicine for

AIDS is written in the Qur'an', which is 'Do not fornicate. There is no other cure'.[10]

REDEMPTIVE READINGS OF SACRED TEXTS

Though a theology of retribution hovers over this informant's invocation of the Qur'an, curative sacred texts are also a feature of the African HIV landscape. For some, Becker observes, the Qur'an as tactile text is directly redemptive, with Qur'anic healers practising '"book" healing, *uganga wa kitabu*' where 'Qur'an surahs are worn as amulets or "drunk" by ingesting the ink used to write them'. These practices, she argues, not only 'resemble ones pursued by Sufis in other parts of the Muslim world, they can also be seen as a continuation of indigenous medicine'.[11]

Similarly, among the resources taken up by the Ugandan Martyrs Guild (UMG) in their crusades against the dramatic rise in witchcraft associated with AIDS-related deaths are Bibles:

> Before the UMG went on an 'operation' or 'crusade', they announced their plans in monthly papers and on the radio. They sent letters to the local council and to the police, and sometimes, when they feared fierce resistance they asked for police protection. The day before the operation they fasted; the night was spent in church singing and praying until their bodies were filled with the Holy Spirit. In addition, the 'weapons' to fight the enemy – Bible, plastic bottles filled with holy water, rosaries and crucifixes – were 'loaded' with the Holy Spirit to empower them and transform them into efficient instruments to fight evil.[12]

However, the focus in the remainder of this chapter is on the less tactile and more textual or scriptural dimensions of sacred scriptures. What follows is not exhaustive but it is representative of the available literature.

Invoking the shape of sacred scripture

In theological treatments of HIV and AIDS, sacred texts are invoked in a whole range of ways, often in general terms, with occasional citations to particular biblical texts but with no attempt to probe them in any detail. For example, in order to address the many challenges confronting Africa, including HIV and AIDS (though this is not discussed in any detail), Godwin Akper from Nigeria argues that the Bible 'provides the spectacles with which we see what God is doing in South Africa and Nigeria'.[13] A similar, but bolder and more systematic, invocation of the Bible in general can be found in the article by Russel Botman in which he locates a vision of hope for the city of Cape Town, 'beset by AIDS' among other ills, within a retelling of the biblical story using both narrative and socio-historical resources. In the face of narratives of fear, he affirms that 'the Bible has its own story to tell'.[14]

Similarly, while the Qur'an is invoked to demonstrate 'Allah's sole and exclusive ownership of creation' and that 'Allah created disease for human correction, purification, and/or expiation', 'the Islamic AIDS remedy' also begins with the Qur'an. This remedy, argues Muhammad Morra Abdul-Wahhab is 'a *shifa* (healing) of spiritual and physical disease for those who believe in it (Qur'an 17:82)'. The Qur'anic *shifa*, he goes on to explain, 'incorporates Allah's instructions to consume, in moderation, food and drink that is permissible and wholesome (Qur'an 2:168, 2:172–173, 5:990–991). Conjoined with healthful nutrition is *tahara* (cleanliness) of the body and spirit realized through ritual hygiene (Qur'an 4:43, 5:6) and *salat* (daily obligatory prayer) and *du'a* (informal supplication)'.[15]

Noting that while there has been 'a steady rise in reported AIDS cases in countries with predominant or large Muslim populations', some Muslims have argued, says Abdul-Wahhab, that this steady rise 'is lower than the "accelerative" rise in reported cases in the majority of non-Muslim countries'. 'This discourse', the author continues, 'constructs AIDS as a disorder of decadence that plagues non-Islamic formations, in particular the immoral West. AIDS is construed as one of Allah's "signs" to verify Islam's truth to non-Muslims'. He then cites from the Qur'an: 'We will show them our signs in the universe and in their own selves, until it becomes manifest to them that this (Qur'an) is the truth (Qur'an 41:53).'[16]

Anchoring theological arguments in specific sacred texts

Just as portions of sacred texts, or thematic trajectories within sacred texts, are used to buttress theologies of retribution, so selected segments of sacred texts are also used to anchor redemptive ideo-theological orientations in sacred scripture. For example, in her discussion of how the Christian faith might respond to 'the deplorable effects of stigma, because there is no place for stigma in the fulfilment of God's reign on earth', Denise Ackermann draws up a set of theological suggestions, all of which emanate from her hermeneutical point of departure, 'namely that Christians are charged with living out the values of the reign of God.

This means confronting the *sinful* nature of stigma squarely and then finding hope in our scriptures and our traditions for communicating God's grace, mercy and compassion in our actions in present times'.[17] She then offers fifteen theological observations, citing one or more biblical text in each to situate her suggestion within scripture. For example, she says, 'Stigma is sin; it is totally alien to the *nature of God*. Our God is a God who embraces all of creation, who so loved the world and all that is in it that God "gave His only son, so that everyone who believes in Him may not perish but have eternal life" (Jh. 3:16).'[18]

Sara Paasche-Orlow and David Rosenn make it clear that although 'there is no universally accepted mechanism for determining Jewish doctrine or practice', the Hebrew Bible and related rabbinic texts do shape both.[19] They continue:

> Jewish teachings on sickness and health strongly emphasize human responsibility for ministering to the physical, social, and spiritual needs of the sick, regardless of the type or source of their illness. Saving the life of a dangerously ill person is a religious duty (Leviticus 19:16, 25:36), which overrides nearly all other religious obligations. Rabbinic teaching equates one who saves a single life with one who saves an entire world (Mishnah *Sanhedrin* 4:5).[20]

Furthermore the Bible, argue Paasche-Orlow and Rosenn, presents God as:

> [. . .] the supreme healer (Exodus 15:26), but Jewish tradition rejects views that place responsibility for healing wholly in God's hands or that view any medical intervention as interference with God's will. Rather, based on the verse 'And he shall heal' (Exodus 21:19), the Talmud teaches that human beings are called into partnership with God to save lives and preserve health (Babylonian Talmud *Bava kamma* 85a).[21]

On the basis of these sacred texts, 'For Judaism . . . HIV/AIDS prevention and treatment is a basic religious obligation'.[22] In addition, 'Jewish law requires preventive care on the part of each person and avoidance of situations of risk to life and health (Deuteronomy 4:9 and Babylonian Talmud *Berakhot* 3b). Consequently, practising safer sex is a Jewish obligation'. Though Jewish law rejects the 'two primary means of contracting HIV, injecting drug use and male homosexual intercourse', the latter proscribed by the Bible directly (Leviticus 18:22; 20:13), all branches of Judaism believe 'that sickness must be battled and the sick attended to with compassion, regardless of the origin of their disease . . . the moral stature of the patient':[23]

> Although Jewish religious opinion is divided over the extent to which any disease, including AIDS, can be said to be a chastisement from God, it is agreed that illness presents a person with an opportunity to examine his or her actions and draw closer to God. Indeed, tradition teaches that God draws near to the sick, portraying the sustaining presence of God near the head of a sick person's bed (Psalms 41:4 and Babylonian Talmud *Nedarim* 40b).[24]

Sacred texts as reservoirs of redemptive categories and concepts

Sacred texts also act as a reservoir from which redemptive organising categories and concepts can be extracted or substantiated. So, for example, in discussing the importance of notions of human dignity and the image of God in engaging theologically with HIV and AIDS, Johan Bouwer turns to the biblical concept of honour in search of a biblical category roughly analogous to human dignity. As he states: 'Ample biblical evidence can be found of the notion of honour.'[25] 'Because of the danger of "human dignity" becoming an empty concept, given its foundational position in international charters and jurisdiction', he argues, the biblical concept of honour:

> [. . .] which actually encompasses that of 'dignity' and its necessary counterpart, self-respect, might offer a common basis for a religious discourse uniting Africa and the West in finding a common language that will help people to not only escape the stigma, but also to act upon the need for the eradication of this pandemic. In this discourse God is seen as a friend who has compassion, shows respect for human beings, is trustworthy and non-judgmental and is One who cares unconditionally.[26]

Using both literary and socio-historical analysis, Caitlin Yoshiko Buysse reflects on the two distinct notions of poverty in the Qur'an:

> Poverty (*faqr*) in the context of the Qur'an takes on two distinct meanings: a spiritual condition connected to the quest for closeness to God and an unjust physical condition imposed by some human beings on others.

Spiritual poverty is the desired state of the believer in relation to God; in this state the believer is in need of no one and nothing else but God. An unjust poverty, however, puts the human being in need of something other than God Himself, imposing an idolatrous hierarchy in which the individual is forced to submit to one other than God. It is only to God that humans should be poor and in need; anything else is oppression. God's call to all humanity to be maintainers of justice is an imperative not only to secure a just order on earth, but also, most importantly, to ensure that all humans are able to worship only God – to be only His servants – and to be free from any persons, structures, or circumstances that force an individual to be in need of anything other than God. It is to combat this form of unjust physical poverty that the Qur'anic principles of economic justice are intended.[27]

With this insightful and provocative distinction, the author provides an analysis of the Qur'an in which systemic socio-economic justice is foregrounded, not the more obvious emphasis on charity.[28] Indeed, the author argues that when the Qur'an speaks about charity, which it does 'most profusely', it 'needs to be understood as intrinsically connected to an ethos of systemic economic equity'. Her starting point is that 'the monotheism espoused by the Qur'an challenged both the polytheism and socio-economic order of seventh-century Arabia'. In other words, 'polytheism was the theological representation of a fragmented society that bred socio-economic inequalities'. This leads her into a detailed analysis of empire and its manufacture of systemic poverty in a context in which AIDS is, quoting Sanjay Basu, a 'symptom Empire'.[29]

In reflecting theologically on drug addiction and HIV from the perspective of Muslim, HIV positive addicts,[30] Laura McTighe identifies and appropriates four key concepts from the Qur'an for a theology of liberation. In a two-way dialogue with the Qur'an, she reflects on a number of key inter-related concepts for a theology of liberation, informed by the realities of HIV positive people themselves: *tawid* ('signifying the unity of God, creation, and humankind'), *taqwa* ('manifested as a lived concern and compassion for others [in] intentional collaboration with God'), *al-nas* ('establishing the unity of humanity as part of God's just and ethical order on earth') and *mustad'afun* ('appropriating the exhortation of the Qur'an to stand alongside the *mustad'afun* [the marginalised] in the face of socio-economic injustice, power imbalances, and arrogance [Q. 4:75], and to struggle actively for the establishment of justice [Q. 5:8]').[31] Indeed, the entire book in which this chapter is located is an attempt to appropriate and reconfigure the notion of justice within Islam, privileging structural over personal understandings.[32]

HIV positive people reading sacred texts

There is some literature on social sites in which there is a communal reading of sacred texts. Here, those who are themselves HIV positive are privileged in the reading process. At the height of the HIV and AIDS epidemic in the 1980s in the USA, 'the Metropolitan Community Church of San Francisco was the church at the center of the maelstrom. It was a place where many churched and unchurched gay men dying with AIDS found a home'. From within this pastoral community Jim Mitulski, the senior pastor, offers a reading of the book of Ezekiel 'from the social location of living with HIV', which 'has revealed treasures in the text that were previously invisible to me'. Indeed, he continues, 'The experience of living with HIV has been the greatest catalyst in my spiritual life since coming out as a gay man over twenty years ago.'[33]

Merging the past and the present, Mitulski asserts:

> The book of Ezekiel is about an exiled community moving from devastation to resurrection; it is the story of a community affected by HIV re-constructing its future. It is told by Ezekiel, a prophet who understands deeply the HIV experience and who sees visions of hope that sustain himself and his people through the most difficult challenge of their lives.[34]

He begins his HIV positive reading of Ezekiel by 'identifying characteristics of an HIV hermeneutic' and then applying this to Ezekiel 37:1–14. His hermeneutic starting point is that his 'intellectual and spiritual instincts' discern that 'the Bible, on some fundamental level, contains stories told by people with HIV for people with HIV and for the communities affected by it'. This HIV positive hermeneutic is shaped by the understandings of the HIV positive community. The experiences that shape their hermeneutic include an understanding of exile and estrangement from family and society, and an understanding of blame and shame. But their understandings also include 'the innate desire of the soul and the body to overcome adversity and to survive'.[35]

'These insights culled from the social location of living with HIV', argues Mitulski, 'can make the pages of the Bible come alive. They help us to see and tell our own story as part of divine revelation'. Having outlined this HIV positive hermeneutic, he then goes on to read Ezekiel, arguing that his 'HIV hermeneutic helps me to identify the many judgements against the exiles as the editorial encroachment of the religious impulse to blame the victim, just as today many churches attempt to minister to people with AIDS while condemning our sexuality'. In turning to Ezekiel 37, he argues that 'it is the depth of Ezekiel's suffering and grief that gives him the credibility to talk about resurrection'. He concludes his study by arguing that just as Ezekiel was told to prophesy to the whole house of Israel, so too people with HIV 'are called to prophesy to the whole church and the whole community', to warn the churches 'to listen to what God is doing in our midst', to call to account 'the churches that will perform our funerals but not our marriages'.[36]

Working more closely and carefully with the detail of biblical texts, a socially engaged biblical scholar from the USA, Ken Stone, notes with dismay a similar co-option of the Bible as part of a wider religious response to HIV in which those living with the virus are blamed. Citing Michael Clark's 'scripture-phobia', induced in him by the reality of his context where 'the Bible has been used, over and over again . . . as the ideological justification not only for excluding gay men and lesbians, but also for blaming the victims in the AIDS health crisis',[37] Stone goes on to acknowledge that 'it is not difficult to think of biblical passages which state or imply disaster and distress are divine responses to sinful activities formerly carried out by those who suffer'.[38] But Stone then proceeds to 'consider the possibility that certain lament psalms can be read in a manner that will encourage resistance to the attitudes towards AIDS that rightly trouble Clark'.[39]

In the readings of the Bible that most trouble Clark, those living with HIV 'are objects of speech, and their distress is focalized by someone other than the sufferer'; they are 'treated as objects of authoritative discourses'. It is against this reality that Stone sets out to 'queer' both the Bible and biblical interpretation, 'to reverse the discursive positioning that structures such readings, focusing not on biblical texts that speak *about* the person who suffers but rather on texts in which suffering is focalized by a speaking subject that is, itself, a suffering subject'. And, as Stone notes, biblical laments (and his focus is the Psalms) 'do not generally acquiesce to suffering, do not in most cases try to give it a positive interpretation. Rather, they complain about it; and this complaint offers readers a subject-position from which an end to suffering and distress can be actively pursued'. In short, 'many of the laments respond to suffering with *resistance*'.[40]

Working with similar attention to the detail of the Bible, and granting a similar epistemological privilege to those living with HIV, the Ujamaa Centre for Community Development and Research in Pietermaritzburg has worked in collaboration with what has become the Siyaphila (we are alive/well/positive) movement for more than a decade.[41] Central to the Ujamaa Centre's collaboration has been regular contextual Bible study, in which the resources of Siyaphila support groups and those of socially engaged biblical scholars and organic intellectuals are shared in the struggle to live positively. In these collaborative interpretive sites, gospel texts in which Jesus takes a clear stand with the stigmatised of his day against the religious authorities who discriminated against them (as in John 8:1–11) have been rediscovered and explored.[42] In addition to re-reading these familiar biblical texts, unfamiliar texts such as Job 3 have been engaged for the first time, leading into individual and communal lament and protest. It was discovered that Job provides resources for a debate between the dominant theology of its time, the theology of retribution, and an emerging theology that takes account of unjustifiable suffering, a theology of protest and lament.[43] Also explored were the various ways in which the Bible had become more fully owned by those who were HIV positive through the contextual Bible study process.[44] Finally, there has been reflection on what has been learned for others from the epistemologically privileged reading of those living with HIV, discerning, in particular, the importance of a recovery of lament in the midst of HIV and AIDS and recognising other expressions of lament in South African art and music.[45]

Scholars reading sacred texts in solidarity with those living with HIV

There is an extensive literature in which socially engaged scholars work with sacred texts in a structured and systematic manner. What marks this work is an overt interpretive method. Here there is nothing self-evident about the sacred text: meaning has to be constructed; it is not just found. Another feature of the examples used below is that the detail of the sacred text is appropriated from within a redemptive ideo-theological orientation, with most of scholars believing that the detail actually undergirds their ideo-theological convictions.

With sustained attention to the detail of sacred text, the African-American scholar Cheryl Anderson locates her reading of the Naaman story in 2 Kings 5:1–27 within the parameters of the epidemic in the African-American community. She offers three ways of engaging with this text: focusing in front of it (as real readers engage with the theological implications of the story); in it (identifying the narrative detail of the text); and behind it (deciding whether the story of Gehazi is integral to the narrative or a secondary addition). In so doing, she offers the community two sets of resources: namely, particular methodological perspectives and their respective contributions.[46]

Anderson recognises that an in-front-of-the-text reading 'provides a sense of comfort' for the African-American community in that 'a condition that is dreaded and feared can be healed'; with the typical parallel being drawn between AIDS and leprosy. However, she goes on to argue, the story of this healing miracle is also problematic: first, because 'it describes a cure at a time when no such cure exists for individuals living with AIDS'; and second, because 'the story has the tendency to tell outsiders that they should become like those in the dominant culture'.[47]

Anderson follows the detail of the narrative in identifying five boundaries that Namaan has to cross in order to be healed: age, class, gender, nationality and religion. As she deals with each of these, she conducts a dialogue about how it intersects with the African-American community in the context of HIV and AIDS. Behind the text, Anderson uses scholarly debates on whether the story of Gehazi (2 Kings 5:19b–27) is integral to the narrative, or a later Deuteronomistic addition, in which the healing of Naaman is located theologically within the logic of 'blessing and curses'. While Anderson accepts that 'Without a doubt, the blessings and curses formula exists in the biblical canon', this formula 'is not the only explanation of human suffering that the Bible offers'.[48]

Along similar lines to the work of Mitulski on Ezekiel discussed above, Dorothy B.E.A. Akoto, from Ghana, reads Ezekiel 37:1–14 in the context of HIV and AIDS. She provides a fairly detailed exegesis of this passage before she too concludes that Ezekiel speaks 'to a universal human experience'.[49] 'The task of prophetic ministry', she argues, 'is to nurture, nourish and evoke a consciousness and perception alternative to the consciousness and perception of the dominant culture around us'. Like many biblical scholars, she links Ezekiel with other biblical texts, such as Matthew 28:19a, Hosea 6:4, and Luke 4:18–19, locating the prophetic voice of Ezekiel within a larger canonical trajectory that 'advocates for the downtrodden and abused'. But notwithstanding this trajectory, she finds herself uncertain about whether she can affirm with Ezekiel in answer to God's question: 'Can these bones live?', namely, 'Lord, you know.' Such is the enormity of the change required in our society's response to HIV and AIDS that she is almost overwhelmed, uncertain even to invoke Ezekiel's cautious optimism.[50]

Ezra Chitando from Zimbabwe locates his analysis of Proverbs 31:10–31 within an overt recognition of the Bible's ambiguity in Africa. While the Bible is clearly a resource that the community draws on in the context of sickness, suffering and death, it 'is also the Bible that is used to sustain traditions and practices that suffocate African women. The coalescence of African and Israelite patriarchal traditions has left African women staring at the forces of subjugation and death'. This leads him into a re-reading of Proverbs 31:10–31. He begins by noting that the popularity of this poem 'in the Zimbabwean context probably emerges out of the common ideals between the culture out of which the poem emerges and the receiving culture'. However, he is 'convinced that the reality of HIV/AIDS in Zimbabwe calls for a re-reading of this poem' that goes beyond its traditional patriarchal reception. The good wife must protect herself from infection but she is also more vulnerable because she has to resort to risky economic practices in order to feed her family; she must 'acquire the relevant information relating to HIV/AIDS' in order to empower herself; she must interrogate the ideology of patriarchy that insists she is the major care giver. In sum, 'there is a need to emphasise alternative relationships within families and communities'.[51]

Working too with an overtly ambiguous Bible, Musa Dube from Botswana uses a post-colonial feminist narrative perspective to read Mark 5:21–43.[52] Her focus is primarily methodological, exploring how we read a Bible so deeply implicated in colonialism and patriarchy. She admits that she has 'no particular formula to give' but continues by saying that what she definitely does know is that it is 'a fitting duty for all of us who live in the HIV/AIDS era and who read for healing and liberation' to keep asking and working towards how to 'walk and empathize with those who are invaded by HIV/AIDS and pronounce hope and life in the midst of despair and death'.[53]

In another essay, Dube offers a literary and sociological reading of the parable of the widow seeking justice in Luke 18:1–8, moving to and fro between the biblical text and the contexts of African women. In particular, she explores the vulnerability of widows to HIV infection and argues that, like this woman, we must refuse to be patient, waiting for the powerful to be ready to grant us justice. We must insist on justice now, affirming 'a God who is unfailingly in solidarity with the oppressed and exploited'.[54]

Malebogo Kgalemang, also from Botswana, reflects on John 9, which may become a pivotal biblical text in the context of HIV and AIDS stigmatisation.[55]

After an extensive discussion of the dimensions of HIV and AIDS stigma, she does a narrative analysis of John 9, concluding that it 'is a deconstructionist text that directly asserts that there is no relationship between sin and suffering/disease – God is not responsible for the HIV+'.[56]

Within the general context of preventing HIV infection and the specific context of virginity testing in KwaZulu-Natal, Patricia Bruce examines a number of aspects of virginity. She locates notions of virginity in their ancient and contemporary, socio-historical contexts before discussing the New Testament, particularly Paul's understanding, in depth.[57] She provides a detailed analysis of 1 Corinthians 7, concluding that the perspective here is that of males but that Paul was not seeking to control women: 'Paul was obviously open to the possibility of women not marrying and, in fact, believed that it was the better option in the circumstances (7:34).' This view, she continues, 'would give women an unusual choice in their context but it was not a choice based on a low view of women, the body or marriage. It was seen as a gift (7:7)'. She acknowledges, however, that after his death and due to his mythic apostolic status 'Paul's words were subsequently used to oppress virgins who were subjected to strict controls in the third and fourth centuries'. She concludes that 'because women were so closely controlled in ancient times, it is interesting that no real importance was attached to examining the hymen as a physical marker indicating virginity although it was known, at least to some, in both the Jewish and Roman worlds'. 'Contemporary Zulu culture,' she notes, returning to her starting point, 'is once again beginning to attach significance to physical indicators of virginity, as Western culture once did. As we have seen, this is based on negative perceptions of women and the belief that women, who now lead less overtly supervised lives, are out of control.' The church must be cautious, she argues, in using the context of HIV and AIDS to affirm such practices.[58]

Even hypothetical biblical texts have been appropriated by those seeking biblical detail in the quest for redemptive readings. Beginning with an argument for Q as a wisdom gospel for the members of the earliest church, the Nigerian scholar Ukachukwu Manus goes on to locate his analysis within an African context substantially shaped by HIV and AIDS. He finds resources in Q with which African congregations might be admonished to imitate Jesus by leading more prudent lives. He concludes that Q 'draws attention to the relevance of being wiser in the choices we make in the use of human sexuality in the era of the HIV and AIDS epidemic'.[59]

While biblical scholars have worked with an array of texts in some depth, the book of Job has received, without doubt, the most sustained attention in the context of HIV and AIDS from African scholars. While a few of these more structured and systematic engagements with the detail of the book of Job have adopted the voice of the compliant and patient Job of the prologue (and perhaps the epilogue), there is a growing body of work that amplifies the voice of the irreverent and resisting Job of the poetic cycles.

Leaning in the direction of the former, Patrick Adeso from Nigeria affirms that 'like Job, the African does not give up', even when confronted with 'another fatal scourge', that of HIV and AIDS. 'Like Job', the African 'seeks for meaning, life and growth from his sufferings'. His work affirms that even if we cannot understand the meaning of any particular suffering, nevertheless we may 'trust and depend on God for his help and salvation'. In searching out the similarities 'between Job and the African faced with suffering', Adeso identifies Job 42:1–6 as the 'summit passage of the book'. According to his analysis, this literary unit ends with 'personal confession and repentance', which is why Adeso is able to read this final speech by Job as Job's submission to God 'in all wisdom, knowledge and understanding', notwithstanding Job's earlier subtle attempts 'in calling Yahweh to account'. Adeso appropriates a Job who 'seeks for meaning, life and even growth from his suffering' and in so doing constrains suffering Africa to do likewise.[60]

Not so the South African biblical scholar Sarojini Nadar: '*Barak* [curse] God and die!', she declares. Though her initial appropriation point is also in the prologue, she reminds us that lament, protest and resistance have their origin in the book with the voice of Job's wife who both prefigures and prepares the way for the poetic Job. Locating her analysis against the backdrop of ideo-theological orientations of retribution from the Ancient Near East and Ancient Israel, Nadar argues that the challenge that faces us as biblical scholars is 'to find those alternative voices in the Bible'. She finds such a voice in the voice of Job's wife, a voice that has a long history of ambivalent interpretations. Reading her voice as redemptive, a voice that questions the logic of the received wisdom about retribution, Nadar identifies the question of Job's wife as 'integral to the central question that the narrative as a whole raises'. She too identifies 42:7 as a key moment in the drama of the book of Job, with God directly vindicating Job's speech about God, and indirectly vindicating Job's wife 'because Job does what his wife hints at – he begins the process of questioning his suffering in terms of his belief system'.[61]

In the early 1990s, before South Africa had begun to come to grips with HIV and AIDS, Gunther Wittenberg published an article on Job as a resource for counselling people living with HIV.[62] Wittenberg, like Nadar, identifies that a key contribution of the book of Job is that it explores 'how not to talk about God'. Job rejects, Wittenberg argues, 'a theology which places the responsibility for all suffering of the world on the suffering persons themselves in order to clear God of all blame'. But Wittenberg also draws attention to the book's contribution concerning 'how to talk to God'. Protest and lament are proper ways to talk to God against the backdrop of 'a theology which starts with abstract theological concepts but ignores the concrete life situation, suffering and hope of human beings'. 'To Job', Wittenberg contends, 'the God of the official theology is nothing other than a sadistic tyrant', and so he 'can only protest against this type of God'.[63]

The work of the Hebrew Bible scholar, Yehoshua Gitay, provides a similar appropriation of Job within the South African context of HIV and AIDS, in which he probes the question of who has the authority to determine morality and truth. His starting point is Job the dissident, who challenges the religious hermeneutical rules of his society, basing his dissidence on self-experience. Adopting the causal logic of his friends' arguments, Job uses his own experience to demonstrate that it is not his moral behaviour that has caused his suffering but the moral behaviour of God. The problem, argues Gitay, is that 'the friends' fault was to adapt a metaphysical theory "as it is" and accordingly deduct Job's specific instance as a confirmation of the theory without studying the particular event'. The tension in the book of Job is between individual self-knowledge and community theoretical-knowledge and while the reader's sympathy lies with Job, not the friends (who God also rebukes in Job 42:7), God does not entirely approve of Job's complaints. God's point, Gitay argues, is that while Job may have knowledge based on his experience, he does not have adequate knowledge to judge God. Job, by taking into account his actual experience, has done better than his friends, who have been too mechanical, basing their judgement on an existing paradigm, unable to take into account the new information which has the potential to shift their paradigm.[64]

Gitay then applies his reading of Job to the situation of HIV in South Africa during Thabo Mbeki's presidency. Is Mbeki, the AIDS dissident, like Job contending with the dominant paradigm? Are the media and the scientists like Job's friends, representatives of the communal status quo? With these provocative questions, Gitay opens up the space to ask the more, for him, fundamental questions: what are our sources of authority when it comes to HIV; and who possesses the appropriate knowledge? Questioning and contestation should not be dismissed, he argues, for they are constitutive of knowledge; but in the midst of the contending voices around HIV, Gitay calls for a recognition of the limits of our knowledge, for God 'is the only one who really knows'.[65]

In a creative fictive re-reading of Job, Madipoane Masenya, another South African biblical scholar, takes up the theme of unjust victims in her work with Job, trying to make sense via Job of African women's experience of HIV and AIDS.[66] The Job of Masenya's imaginative re-reading are the many married women, who 'though they remain faithful to their marriage partners, find that their partners are not faithful to them'. Their plight is similar to Job's.[67]

As indicated above, working with the Siyaphila network of support groups of people living with HIV, the Ujamaa Centre has offered some of the detail of the book of Job in the context of a communal and collaborative reading process. Juxtaposing the unfamiliar Job 3 with the familiar Job 1:21 has enabled an appropriation of lament, protest and resistance, which have then been legitimated by the frame provided by Job 42:7.[68] Local versions of Job 3 have also been gathered, discerning ways of working with the Bible and popular culture in the context of HIV from the perspective of those who are HIV positive.[69]

These reflections on the emergence of the book of Job as a resource for theologies of redemption is not exhaustive,[70] but it is representative of work being done in which the detail of particular biblical texts is used to destabilise and contend with the dominant ideo-theological orientations of retribution that claim some kind of scriptural authority. And those who work within the Christian tradition are not alone in using the detail of sacred texts to contend for redemption in the midst of retribution. The recent collection of essays by Farid Esack and Sarah Chiddy contains a number of contributions in which similar moves are made.[71]

It contains examples in which various levels of sacred text (whether the Qur'an, the Sunnah or Shari'ah) are interrogated, problematised and re-read. So, for example, in working towards an Islamic theology of compassion, Mohammad Hashim Kamali attempts 'to ascertain a Shari'ah perspective on AIDS' by considering the subject of *darar* (harm or injury), which ranks 'among the most prominent of the one hundred legal maxims that appear in the introductory section of the Ottoman Mejelle, the civil code of the Ottoman Empire in the late nineteenth and early twentieth century's [sic] which still represents the most widely accepted codification of the Shari'ah'. The maxims on the subject of *darar* he considers provide a range of perspectives, supported by the Qur'an and the Sunnah, for a compassionate community-based campaign. Here, for example, there 'is no room whatsoever for prejudice and discrimination': people living with HIV 'are no different to other unwell people' and 'are all entitled to equal treatment, compassion, and service, without any reference to the origins and causes of their condition'.[72]

Tackling all three levels of Islamic sacred text, Scott Siraj al-Haqq Kugle and Sarah Chiddy consider the issue of homosexuality in the Qur'an, the Sunnah and Islamic law, but with a particular emphasis on the story of Lut (Lot). In this detailed and carefully argued essay, the authors provide a historical and critical analysis of homosexuality within Islam. Their starting point is a nuanced take on social constructivism and an affirmation, agreeing with Imam Ali (661), that the Qur'an 'does not speak with a tongue; it needs interpreters and interpreters are people'. The latter enables them to argue that the Qur'an itself affirms non-procreative sexual acts (Q. 2:223) and the creation and affirmation of variety in human beings (Q. 17:84). The Qur'an and the Prophet, they assert, know of 'men who are not attracted to women' but do not condemn them as such. However, after the Prophet's death, 'his community gradually reverted to overtly patriarchal norms of social organization, adopted from pre-Islamic Arab custom and from the Persian and Byzantine cultures which were conquered and absorbed'. The essay then seems to make a distinction between sexual orientation and sexual acts, arguing that what is actually condemned is male rape, as in the story of Lut. Where the Sunnah does contain material in which the Prophet is reported to curse men who engage in sodomy, they contest the authenticity of such hadith. They make a hermeneutical distinction, in other words, between hadith that reflect the actual words and example of the Prophet and hadith later attributed to the Prophet. When it comes to Islamic law, the notion of one Shari'ah is disputed, with the authors emphasising the diversity of Islamic jurisprudence. Again, they make the distinction between the emphasis of Muslim jurists on sexual acts rather than sexual orientation. This distinction leads into the final section of their essay in which they recount the stories of gay Muslims and signs of encouraging responses to them from the religious establishment. The essay concludes by returning to the story of Lut and arguing that 'the deeper message of Qur'anic verses about Lut is about the need for a prophetic ethic of care, to highlight the urgent need for the rich and those in power in any society to care for those who are vulnerable and marginal'.[73] 'Those who are obsessed with anal sex between men, an obsession with roots in patriarchal culture and not Islamic scripture', continues Kugle, miss the point of the Prophet Lut's story:

> Perhaps there are more ethical principles that the Muslim community can deduce from the story of Lut, once the story is freed from a narrow attention to sex acts. Lut was exemplary in revealing the challenge of hospitality, generosity, and protection of the vulnerable. He struggled with his community to get them to support the needy, the poor, and those who appeared as strangers. He challenged their arrogance, their inhuman exertion of power over vulnerable people, and their creation of a coercive system out of trade and economic relations. Is this not a more compelling reading of the story of the Prophet Lut in a time of AIDS?[74]

Engaging with perhaps the most problematic Islamic sacred text linked to HIV and AIDS, Nabilah Siddiquee examines a frequently cited hadith. 'In much of the Muslim literature and rhetoric that explains AIDS as a form of divine punishment brought upon those who have sexually transgressed', argues Siddiquee, 'one particular hadith consistently appears as authoritative support for this kind of divine retribution'. The hadith in question is translated as follows: '*Fâhishah* [abomination] has never appeared amongst any people, which they commit openly, but an epidemic or disease that they have never encountered before became widespread amongst them. (*Sunan Ibn Mâja, Kitâb al-fitan*, Hadith 4019).'[75]

Siddiquee begins her re-reading of this allegedly retributive text by situating it in its broader literary context, explaining that it 'is actually only the first of five parts of the hadith', a hadith that 'in its entirety raises a number of important questions of divine justice and "collateral damage" in Islam'. She systematically analyses this hadith, beginning with traditional hadith methodology. The first step is an analysis of the transmission of this hadith (*isnâd*) in order 'to verify the accuracy and authenticity of the text'. Her conclusion, in terms of accepted methodology, is that the transmission history of this hadith is problematic and that therefore 'it should be clear that the strength and authenticity of this *isnâd* is not unanimously accepted'. Next, she moves into hadith content analysis (*matn*).

Here she analyses the hadith in its entirety, in which the notion of *fâhishah*, left untranslated for now, is one of five cautionary statements (though its syntactic structure is somewhat different from the syntactic pattern shared by the other four). The second has to do with 'cheating in weighing', the third with 'unwillingness to pay *zakât*', the fourth with 'damaging the bond between God and his Prophet' and the fifth with 'leaders refusing to base laws on the Book of God'.[76]

In each case – and it is this that Siddiquee finds 'deeply problematic to the justice-seeking reader', so declaring her ideo-theological orientation – 'a form of divine collective punishment is promised in response to the crimes of a specific part of the population'. For example, 'if the crime of *fâhishah* is committed openly amongst a people, we know that it is impossible that every person in that community is engaged in the crime. Why is the divine response an epidemic or disease, something that will necessarily afflict those not guilty of *fâhishah* as well as those who are guilty?' Leaving this haunting question for the moment, she shifts her focus in order to delve more deeply into the precise meaning for *fâhishah*, given that 'it is the first part of the hadith that is usually cited, and that here it is the word *fâhishah* that is often interpreted to be sexual transgressions that lead to AIDS'.[77]

Turning to the use of this word in the Qur'an, she accepts that 'this transgression often refers to sexual transgression, in the context of the social norms of that time period, but not always'. Having historically contextualised the notion of sexual transgression, she then goes on to demonstrate that in the Qur'an the term *fâhishah* can and does have a number of non-sexual meanings, including, she argues, in the story of Lut (Lot).[78] Having clarified that the term *fâhishah* is plurivalent, she then returns to the deeply problematic notion of a God who punishes collectively, turning again to the Qur'an.

Her analysis of the numerous divine punishment stories in the Qur'an leads her to conclude that 'divine punishment *is* referred to in the text'.[79] However, closer analysis demonstrates that:

> [. . .] the difference between the punishment in the hadith and the punishments in the Lut story and other Prophetic stories in the Qur'an is that chastisement in the latter comes directly in response to rejection of a messenger. The moral justification for divine punishment comes not from 'negligence' or from the disbelief itself, but from 'reckless disregard' for the truth expressed by a prophet of God.[80]

Returning to the story of Lut, she shows that in this Qur'anic text 'God's retribution affects specifically the guilty, and that the innocent are saved from the punishment'. Furthermore, she adds:

> [. . .] the idea that the innocent suffer along with the guilty also conflicts with the ethic enshrined in the following verse: 'Who receiveth guidance, receiveth it for his own benefit: who goeth astray doth so to his own loss: No bearer of burdens can bear that burden of another: nor would We visit Our Wrath until We had sent an apostle [to give warning]' (al-Isra [17], 15).[81]

Notwithstanding such arguments, she shows how the first clause in this hadith has been used 'to establish a causal relationship between sexual transgression and the AIDS epidemic, in which the suffering persons living with HIV is a form of divine punishment in response to transgression'.[82] But, she asks in conclusion, 'Is there an alternative reading of the hadith? Is there a better way to employ it in the AIDS discourse?' Her answer is worth quoting:

> When the text is taken in its entirety, we can see that God establishes serious punishments for the powerful and the wealthy who disregard their responsibilities to the poor and the public in general. God threatens to punish those who fail to pay *zakât* to the poor, as well as the leaders who fail to consider the interests of the public when governing. One might even conclude that the warnings of punishment are meant to be symbolic ones, elucidating the importance of God-consciousness, ethical conduct, honesty in trade, paying the wealth tax, and responsible leadership. In this light, one might read the hadith as a serious defence of the rights of the underprivileged, emphasizing the social responsibilities of all. When we pause and recognize that persons living with HIV in many parts of the world are among the most marginalized and oppressed, we can see how these themes are relevant and could be better applied as we engage with the AIDS crisis.[83]

This example has been dealt with in depth because it demonstrates how interpretive methodology, and not only content, are at the core of redemptive readings of sacred texts in the context of HIV and AIDS. While Siddiquee stops short of contextualising or reading the texts of the Qur'an as rhetorical (rather than historical?), though she does mention this option, she makes very similar moves to the biblical scholars considered above.[84]

An HIV hermeneutic

Indeed, across religions and their sacred texts we see signs of an emerging HIV hermeneutic. Though the detail of the hermeneutic differs from case to case, there is an overall inclusive and compassionate shape. Guided by compassion and justice rather than fidelity to religious orthodoxy, an HIV hermeneutic wrestles with sacred text in diverse ways in order to grasp its redemptive detail and potential. Two additional examples will serve to illustrate this, one from Islam and another from Buddhism.

Malik Badri is one of the foremost modern prophets of HIV and AIDS as divine retribution.[85] In a recent essay, Badri focuses on the cultural clash between Western and Islamic perspectives on sex and sexuality. Drawing on the Qur'an and the hadith, he argues that 'the general Islamic belief about the AIDS pandemic is that it is divine retribution for the immoral homosexual revolution of the West and its aping in other countries'. The story of Lut and Sodom are specific examples, with the Qur'an clearly removing any possible ambiguity from the biblical narrative, declaring that 'the townsfolk of Sodom were the first people on earth to adopt a homosexual lifestyle (*Surah al-A'raf*, 7:80)'. However, notwithstanding that AIDS is a form of divine retribution, both to punish and to test, the overall purpose, argues Badri, is 'to ward off more serious future pains and agonies, to coerce the sinful to repent and secure God's forgiveness (*Al-Sajdah*, 32:21)'. Furthermore, Badri quite boldly offers an alternative position on the use of condoms, arguing that the dominant discourse which insists that their use 'should be totally eliminated from any Islamically oriented prevention program' is 'not rational, practical, or Islamic'. Recognising that there 'is unmistakable evidence that, if used properly, condoms can help reduce HIV transmission . . . the use of condoms can be viewed within the general law of Fiqh or jurisprudence of *ikhtiyar akhaff al-dararain*, or choosing the lesser of two evils'.[86]

If we apply this rule, on which there is general consensus among Muslim jurists', he argues:

> [. . .] we could make the use of a condom obligatory for a fornicating Muslim who might expect HIV infection from his promiscuous practice.

Fornication is a major evil, but endangering another person is definitely a much greater evil. According to Muslim jurists, there is a hierarchy of evils, and under duress one should choose the least harmful.

What is more, he continues, for 'a Muslim who fornicates there is still every possibility of repenting, and his earlier sins would be changed to good deeds, as the Holy Qur'an states'.[87]

Remaining within a conservative orthodox framework, Badri nevertheless is compelled by the reality of HIV to search for a hermeneutic that deals with this reality.[88] It is a small shift but signals perhaps the emergence of a more compassionate and less stigmatising hermeneutic.

Similarly, within Buddhism, the theological notion of karma has become problematised. The Council of Religious AIDS Networks (CRAN) includes on its website a number of articles on the intersection between Buddhism and HIV and AIDS.[89] Though the articles published there are more like unpublished papers than peer-reviewed articles, they do provide some suggestive analysis. Among the most provocative is the question posed by Roger Corless: does the virus have a Buddha nature? Prior to this question, he adopts a fairly orthodox position on karma, arguing that a 'true understanding of the Buddhist teaching on karma can give us back our dignity' in the context of HIV and AIDS, precisely because 'in its early usage, in the Vedas and their ritual commentaries, it had no moral implications'. Indeed, he continues, instead of speaking of cause and effect we should, in Buddhism, 'speak of an action as the karmic seed and the outcome of an action as the karmic fruit', reserving the word karma itself 'for the law which connects the seeds and the fruits'. 'The law of karma', he argues, 'is organic, not mechanical'. 'What this all comes down to', he concludes with reference to HIV:

> [. . .] is seeing the fruiting of karma as an opportunity to be grasped rather than a fate to be endured. In the case of finding that one is HIV+ we can use the Buddhist teaching on karma as a support for our practice. We recognize that it has happened for a reason, but we do not need to feel guilty or victimized, and we can exercise some control over how we deal with it, knowing that our actions will not be fruitless. A diagnosis of HIV cannot be good news, but it can be turned to good.[90]

Part of the response, Corless argues, may be directed towards the virus itself. So, 'however bizarre it might seem at first, it is appropriate for a Buddhist infected with HIV to have compassion towards the being that is surviving by destroying its host'. However, he continues, this does not mean that a person living with HIV 'should invite death by refusing therapy and allowing the virus to multiply unchecked', for 'only from the human rebirth is the attainment of Buddhahood possible. Only humans can effectively engage in all three practices of the Triple Training (ethical conduct, meditation, and Dharma study)'. 'For these reasons', he continues:

> [. . .] it is taught, the human rebirth is more fortunate than other rebirths. A virus rebirth, we may imagine, is one of the three unfortunate rebirths (the realms of animals, hungry ghosts, and hell-beings) and a virus is unlikely to be able to practice Dharma. It can only live out its karma, part of which is to be attacked and killed by the cells of the host's immune system or by a medicine. In these circumstances, we can speculate that killing the virus is not a failing of compassion. But, the killing should be done with regret.[91]

In his entry on Buddhism in the *Encyclopedia of AIDS*, however, he adopts a different and more distinctive HIV hermeneutic. The entry begins by stating that Buddhism 'teaches that life is pervaded by suffering'. It continues: 'The origin of suffering is not ascribed to a deity but to the working of karma, which causes people to act unskillfully, especially by clinging to what is by nature impermanent. Thus, if unskillful action causes suffering, then skillful action leads to liberation from suffering.'[92] While the article does not cite any sacred text,[93] it does indicate that in contexts like Thailand, 'where HIV is reaching alarming proportions, especially owing to the large population of female sex workers, Buddhism is often regarded as an institution that explains HIV/AIDS as the karmic result of immoral actions'. However, the article continues, some Buddhists emphasise instead 'Buddhism as a religion of compassion with a responsibility to help'. Some Buddhists have even gone as far as to suggest that HIV and AIDS might contribute to 'reframing Buddhism as open to the future, based on the notion of *mangala* (good omen) rather than the backward-looking notion of karma'.[94]

CONCLUSION

From the available literature,[95] it is clear that sacred texts occupy an important place in the landscape of HIV and AIDS. They have the capacity to stigmatise, discriminate and bring death; and they have the capacity to embrace, affirm and bring life. Because of their capacity to bring death and life, and because of their presence almost everywhere religion is discussed, sacred texts are particularly significant in the interface between religion and HIV and AIDS.

What is also clear, at least for the dominant religions in Africa, Christianity and Islam, is that sacred texts take on different forms in their appropriations. For some ordinary believers their sacred materiality is a resource; for those who represent institutional religion, the sacred texts both affirm and uphold orthodox teachings and offer some capacity to reach out beyond the constraints of orthodoxy in order to address the realities of HIV and AIDS; for socially engaged scholars the sacred texts do not have fixed single meaning or a dominant trajectory, so their meaning in the context of HIV and AIDS has to be contested.

But more intentionally, inter-faith work needs to be done in seeking to understand across faith communities how sacred texts function in constructing and deconstructing theologies of retribution. In this work it is critical that an emic perspective is prioritised, discerning the internal logic of particular belief systems and how sacred texts within a particular symbolic universe or world view interact with HIV and AIDS.

Among the collected resources in the CHART bibliography,[96] the vast majority are prescriptive: they take a position on what sacred texts should say in the context of HIV and AIDS. But there are also a number of items that are more descriptive, documenting and analysing what is being done across various sectors with sacred texts within the new realities brought about by HIV and AIDS. The descriptive task remains important, documenting what is being done with sacred texts in a host of particular cases.

In the vast majority of cases HIV and AIDS is associated, explicitly or implicitly, with some other distinctive feature of particular social locations such as gender and class. HIV and AIDS is not an isolated dimension of life from which to read the Bible or any other sacred text. It is integrally related to other aspects of life.

Perhaps the most significant distinction among the materials covered in this chapter is between published sources that take the Bible and other sacred texts to have a readily self-evident meaning, evoked in this instance by HIV and AIDS, and those that foreground method, refusing to take meaning for granted. The latter is where the in-depth work on the interface between HIV and AIDS and theology and life resides. Sacred texts have the capacity to become idols of death and the landscape of HIV and AIDS is literally strewn with its corpses. We must be overt not only about *what* we interpret them to say to the contexts of HIV and AIDS but also, and more importantly, *how* we interpret them.

Finally, there is clear evidence that HIV and AIDS, particularly in Africa but also elsewhere, is changing the theological landscape so significantly that sacred texts are being called to address this disease complex in ways that may alter how they are interpreted by religious communities.[97]

NOTES

1. Thanks to Clare Amos, Musa Dube, Martha Frederiks, Alissa Jones Nelson, Katharine Doob Sakenfeld, Ken Stone and Adriaan van Klinken for being dialogue partners in this project and for their help in gathering the resources listed in the Chart Bibliography, from which this chapter draws. Thanks to the many others who have indicated their support for this project.

2. Raymond A. Smith (ed.), *Encyclopedia of AIDS: A Social, Political, Cultural and Scientific Record of the HIV Epidemic* (Chicago: Fitzroy Dearborn, 1998).

3. Richard Parker and Peter Aggleton, 'HIV and AIDS-related stigma and discrimination: A conceptual framework and implications for action'. *Social Science and Medicine* 57 (2003): 13–24.

4. Ezra Chitando, *Living with Hope: African Churches and HIV/AIDS* (Vol. 1); and *Acting in Hope* (Vol. 2) (Geneva: WCC Publications, 2007).

5. Chitando, *Living with Hope*: 6, 7, 8.

6. Chitando, *Living with Hope*: 8, 21, 22.

7. Felicitas Becker, 'The virus and the Scriptures: Muslims and AIDS in Tanzania'. *Journal of Religion in Africa* 37 (2007): 18, 21, 23. See also Felicitas Becker and P. Wenzel Geissler, 'Introduction: Searching for pathways in a landscape of death: religion and AIDS in east Africa'. *Journal of Religion in Africa* 37 (1) 2007: 10.

8. Becker, 'The virus and the Scriptures': 26.

9. Becker, 'The virus and the Scriptures': 31.

10. Becker, 'The virus and the Scriptures': 33.

11. Becker, 'The virus and the Scriptures': 28.

12. Heike Behrend, 'The rise of occult powers: AIDS and the Roman Catholic Church in western Uganda'. *Journal of Religion in Africa* 37(1) 2007: 51.

13. Godwin I. Akper, 'A decade of democracy in South Africa and the vocation of the South African and Nigerian theologian at the beginning of a new millennium'. *Scriptura* 89 (2005): 476.

14. H.R. Botman, 'Turning the tide of the city: An ecumenical vision of hope'. *Nederduitse Gereformeerde Teologiese Tydskrif* 45(3–4) 2004: 515.

15. Muhammad Morra Abdul-Wahhab, 'Islam' in *Encyclopedia of AIDS* edited by Raymond A. Smith: 304.

16. Abdul-Wahhab, 'Islam': 304.

17. Denise M. Ackermann, 'Engaging stigma: An embodied theological response to HIV and AIDS: The challenge of HIV/AIDS to Christian theology'. *Scriptura* 89 (2005): 391.

18. Ackermann, 'Engaging stigma': 391. See also Adelia Carstens, 'Die voorstelling van VIGS-verwante stigma in 'n versameling gedigte deur Afrikaanssprekende hoërskoolleerders'. *Koers: Bulletin vir Christelike Wetenskap* 69(3) 2004: 411–30.

19. Sara Paasche-Orlow and David Rosenn, 'Judaism' in *Encyclopedia of AIDS* edited by Raymond A. Smith: 312.

20. Paasche-Orlow and Rosenn, 'Judaism': 312.

21. Paasche-Orlow and Rosenn, 'Judaism': 312.

22. Paasche-Orlow and Rosenn, 'Judaism': 312.

23. Paasche-Orlow and Rosenn, 'Judaism': 312.

24. Paasche-Orlow and Rosenn, 'Judaism': 312.

25. Johan Bouwer, 'Human dignity and HIV/AIDS'. *Scriptura* 95(2) 2007: 267.

26. Bouwer, 'Human dignity and HIV/AIDS': 268.

27. Caitlin Yoshiko Buysse, 'The Qur'an, poverty, and AIDS' in *Islam and AIDS: Between Scorn, Pity and Justice*, edited by Farid Esack and Sarah Chiddy (Oxford: Oneworld, 2009): 169.

28. For a similar analysis see Kabir Sanjay Bavikatte, 'Muslims, AIDS, and justice: Beyond personal indictment' in *Islam and AIDS*, edited by Esack and Chiddy: 186–95.

29. Buysse, 'The Qur'an, poverty, and AIDS': 170, 171, 179.

30. For a sociological analysis of injecting drug use and HIV in the Muslim world see Chris Byrnes, 'Injecting drug use, HIV, and AIDS in the Muslim World' in *Islam and AIDS*, edited by Esack and Chiddy: 196–210.

31. Laura McTighe, 'HIV, addiction, and justice: Toward a Qur'anic theology of liberation' in *Islam and AIDS*, edited by Esack and Chiddy: 215–16.

32. Esack and Chiddy (eds), *Islam and AIDS*.

33. James Mitulski, 'Ezekiel understands AIDS, AIDS understands Ezekiel: Or reading the Bible with HIV' in *Take Back the Word: A Queer Reading of the Bible*, edited by Robert E. Goss and Mona West (Cleveland: Pilgrim Press, 2000): 153.

34. Mitulski, 'Ezekiel understands AIDS, AIDS understands Ezekiel': 153.

35. Mitulski, 'Ezekiel understands AIDS, AIDS understands Ezekiel': 154.

36. Mitulski, 'Ezekiel understands AIDS, AIDS understands Ezekiel': 154, 155, 159.

37. Kenneth A. Stone, 'Safer text: Reading biblical laments in the age of AIDS'. *Theology and Sexuality* 10 (1999): 16. See J. Michael Clark, 'AIDS, death and God: Gay liberation theology and the problem of suffering'. *Journal of Pastoral Counselling* 21(1) 1986: 40–54; J. Michael Clark, 'Special considerations in pastoral care of gay persons with AIDS'. *Journal of Pastoral Counselling* 22(1) 1987: 32–45; J. Michael Clark, *Diary of a Southern Queen: An HIV+ Vision Quest* (Dallas: Monument Press, 1990).

38. Stone, 'Safer text': 16.

39. Stone, 'Safer text': 16–17.

40. Stone, 'Safer text': 20–1.

41. See in Chapter 16 the story of Nokuthula Biyela, a member of Siyaphila.

42. Gerald West, 'Reading the Bible in the light of HIV/AIDS in South Africa'. *The Ecumenical Review* 55(4) (2003): 335–44.

43. Gerald West, 'Reading Job "positively" in the context of HIV/AIDS in South Africa'. *Concilium* 4 (2004): 112–24.

44. Gerald West and Bongi Zengele, 'The medicine of God's word: What people living with HIV and AIDS want (and get) from the Bible'. *Journal of Theology for Southern Africa* 125 (2006): 51–63.

45. Gerald West, 'The poetry of Job as a resource for the articulation of embodied lament in the context of HIV and AIDS in South Africa' in *Lamentations in Ancient and Contemporary Cultural Contexts*, edited by Nancy C. Lee and Carleen Mandolfo (Atlanta: Society of Biblical Literature, 2008): 195–214. For another example, in which a biblical scholar reads both for and with those who are HIV positive, see Dorcas Olubanke Akintunde, 'The attitude of Jesus to the "anointing prostitute": A model for contemporary churches in the face of HIV/AIDS in Africa' in *African Women, HIV/AIDS and Faith Communities*, edited by Isabel Apawo Phiri, Beverley Haddad and Madipoane Masenya (Pietermaritzburg: Cluster Publications, 2003): 94–110.

46. Cheryl Barbara Anderson, 'Lessons on healing from Naaman (2 Kings 5:1–27): An African-American perspective' in *African Women, HIV/AIDS and Faith Communities*, edited by Phiri, Haddad and Masenya: 23–43. The Nigerian biblical scholar Adekunle Dada does something similar with the same narrative for his context: see Adekunle Dada, 'Rereading the Naaman story (2 Kings 5:1–27) in the context of stigmatization of people living with HIV and AIDS in Africa'. *Old Testament Essays* 20(3) 2007: 586–600.

47. Anderson, 'Lessons on healing from Naaman (2 Kings 5:1–27)': 28, 29.

48. Anderson, 'Lessons on healing from Naaman (2 Kings 5:1–27)': 31–5, 37.

49. Dorothy B.E.A. Akoto, 'Can these bones live?: Re-reading Ezekiel 37:1–14 in the HIV/AIDS context' in *Grant Me Justice!: HIV/AIDS and Gender Readings of the Bible*, edited by Musa W. Dube and Musimbi R.A. Kanyoro (Pietermaritzburg: Cluster Publications, 2004): 108.

50. Akoto, 'Can these bones live?': 108, 109.

51. Ezra Chitando, '"The good wife": A phenomenological re-reading of Proverbs 31:10–31 in the context of HIV/AIDS in Zimbabwe'. *Scriptura* 86 (2004): 152, 154, 155, 156, 157.

52. Musa W. Dube, 'Mark's healing stories in an AIDS context' in *Global Bible Commentary*, edited by Daniel M. Patte et al. (Nashville: Abingdon, 2004): 379–84; Musa W. Dube, 'Twenty-two years of bleeding and still the princess sings!' in *Grant Me Justice!*, edited by Dube and Kanyoro: 189–92.

53. Musa W. Dube, 'Talitha cum!: A postcolonial feminist and HIV/AIDS reading of Mark 5:21–43' in *Grant Me Justice!*, edited by Dube and Kanyoro: 137.

54. Musa W. Dube, 'Grant me justice: Towards gender-sensitive multi-sectoral HIV/AIDS readings of the Bible' in *Grant Me Justice!* edited by Dube and Kanyoro: 19.

55. Malebogo Kgalemang, 'John 9: Deconstructing the HIV/AIDS stigma' in *Grant Me Justice!* edited by Dube and Kanyoro: 141–68. This text is being used extensively by the Ujamaa Centre in its redemptive masculinities work: see www.ujamaa.org.za.

56. Kgalemang, 'John 9': 163.

57. Here she draws on another of her essays, in which she examines virginity in the Old Testament using current virginity testing rituals as her entry point. See Patricia F. Bruce, ' "The mother's cow": A study of Old Testament references to virginity in the context of HIV/AIDS in South Africa' in *African Women, HIV/AIDS and Faith Communities*, edited by Phiri, Haddad and Masenya: 44–70.

58. Patricia Bruce, 'Virginity: some master myths: A study of biblical and other ancient references to virginity in the context of HIV/AIDS in South Africa'. *Neotestamentica* 38(1) 2004: 23, 24, 25. But see Chitando, *Living with Hope*: 31–2.

59. Ukachukwu C. Manus, 'Jesus, prophet of the Sophia-God of the downtrodden: Rereading the Q-wisdom sayings in the context of HIV/AIDS pandemic in Africa' in *Sagesse Humaine et Sagesse Divine dans la Bible*, edited by Jean-Bosco Matand Bulembat (Nairobi: Panafrican Association of Catholic Exegetes, 2005): 169–79. See also Ukachukwu Chris Manus and Bolaji O. Bateye, 'The plight of HIV and AIDS persons in West Africa: A contextual re-reading of Mk 1:40–45 and parallels'. *Asia Journal of Theology* 20(1) 2006: 155–69.

60. Patrick Adeso, 'Suffering in Job and in an African perspective: Exegesis of Job 42:1–6' in *Sagesse Humaine et Sagesse Divine dans la Bible*, edited by Bulembat: 77, 79, 81, 82, 83. See also Ghislain Tshikendwa Matadi, *From Human Suffering to Human Hope: Reading the Book of Job from the African Context of Suffering in Times of HIV–AIDS* (Berkeley: Jesuit School of Theology, 2003); Ghislain Tshikendwa Matadi, *Suffering, Belief, Hope: The Wisdom of Job for an AIDS-Stricken Africa* (Nairobi: Paulines Publications Africa, 2007).

61. Sarojini Nadar, ' "*Barak* God and die!": Women, HIV and a theology of suffering' in *Grant Me Justice!*, edited by Dube and Kanyoro: 191, 193.

62. Gunter H. Wittenberg, 'Counselling AIDS patients: Job as a paradigm'. *Journal of Theology for Southern Africa* 88 (1994): 61–8. Some years later a student of Wittenberg's, Habakuki Lwendo from Tanzania, analysed the theology of retribution in the Old Testament (and in African Traditional Religion) and the way in which the book of Job engaged with this theology, relating both to the issues of counselling those living with HIV and AIDS: Habakuki Y. Lwendo, 'The Significance of the Doctrine of Retribution in Old Testament Job for Pastoral Counselling in AIDS' (Master's thesis, University of Natal, 2000).

63. Wittenberg, 'Counselling AIDS patients': 62, 64, 65.

64. Yehoshua Gitay, 'Rhetoric and its limitations: Job the dissident X'. *Journal of Northwest Semitic Languages* 29(2) 2003: 50, 51, 52, 56, 57.

65. Gitay, 'Rhetoric and its limitations': 58–62.

66. Madipoane (ngwana' Mphahlele) Masenya, 'Between unjust suffering and the "silent" God: Job and HIV/AIDS sufferers in South Africa'. *Missionalia* 29 (2001): 186–99. As Masenya acknowledges, other biblical scholars have used fictive techniques as a resource for re-reading Job: see Elsa Tamez, 'A letter to Job' in *New Eyes for Reading: Biblical and Theological Reflections by Women from the Third World*, edited by John S. Pobee and Bärbel von Wartenberg-Potter (Geneva: World Council of Churches, 1986): 50–2.

67. Masenya, 'Between unjust suffering and the "silent" God': 187.

68. Gerald O. West and Bongi Zengele, 'Reading Job "positively" in the context of HIV/AIDS in South Africa'. *Concilium* 4 (2004): 112–24.

69. Gerald O. West, 'The poetry of Job as a resource for the articulation of embodied lament in the context of HIV and AIDS in South Africa' in *Lamentations in Ancient and Contemporary Cultural Contexts*, edited by Nancy C. Lee and Carleen Mandolfo (Atlanta: Society of Biblical Literature, 2008): 195–214.

70. See, for example, the use of Job in the formation of an HIV-competent curriculum: Musa W. Dube, 'HIV and AIDS curriculum for theological institutions in Africa' in *African Women, HIV/AIDS and Faith Communities*, edited by Phiri, Haddad and Masenya (Pietermaritzburg: Cluster, 2003): 225.

71. Esack and Chiddy (eds), *Islam and AIDS*.

72. Mohammad Hashim Kamali, 'A Shari'ah perspective on AIDS' in *Islam and AIDS*: edited by Esack and Chiddy: 77, 83, 84.

73. Scott Siraj al-Haqq Kugle and Sarah Chiddy, 'AIDS, Muslims and homosexuality' in *Islam and AIDS*, edited by Esack and Chiddy: 141, 142, 143, 144, 145, 152. See also A. Jamal, 'The story of Lot and the Qur'an's perception of the morality of same-sex sexuality'. *Journal of Homosexuality* 41(1) 2001: 1–88.

74. Kugle and Chiddy, 'AIDS, Muslims and homosexuality': 152.

75. Nabilah Siddiquee, 'When *Fahishah* becomes widespread – AIDS and the Ibn Maja Hadith' in *Islam and AIDS*, edited by Esack and Chiddy: 58.

76. Siddiquee, 'When *Fahishah* becomes widespread': 59, 60, 65–6.

77. Siddiquee, 'When *Fahishah* becomes widespread': 66, 67.

78. Siddiquee, 'When *Fahishah* becomes widespread': 67–70.

79. Siddiquee, 'When *Fahishah* becomes widespread': 70.

80. Siddiquee, 'When *Fahishah* becomes widespread': 71.

81. Siddiquee, 'When *Fahishah* becomes widespread': 71.

82. Siddiquee, 'When *Fahishah* becomes widespread': 72.

83. Siddiquee, 'When *Fahishah* becomes widespread': 74.

84. Siddiquee, 'When *Fahishah* becomes widespread': 71. For the full range of hermeneutical options being discussed within Islamic liberation theology, particularly Islamic feminism, see Clara Koh, 'Gender justice, Islam and AIDS' in *Islam and AIDS*, edited by Esack and Chiddy: 96–101.

85. Malik Badri, *The AIDS Crisis: A Natural Product of Modernity's Sexual Revolution* (Kuala Lumpur: Meedena Books, 3rd ed., 2007); Malik Badri, 'The AIDS crisis: An Islamic perspective' in *Islam and AIDS*, edited by Esack and Chiddy: 28–42. See also Sindre Bangstad, 'AIDS and the wrath of God' in *Islam and AIDS*, edited by Esack and Chiddy: 43–58.

86. Badri, 'The AIDS crisis': 34, 39, 40, 41.

87. Badri, 'The AIDS crisis': 41.

88. Similarly, see also Abdulaziz Sachedina, 'Afflicted by God?: Muslim perspectives on health and suffering' in *Islam and AIDS*, edited by Esack and Chiddy: 13–27.

89. Council of Religious AIDS Networks, 'AIDS and religion in America'. Available at http://www.AIDSfaith.com. This site contains articles on a range of religions with a number, for example, on Judaism.

90. Roger Corless, 'A Buddhist understanding of HIV/AIDS'. Available at http://www.AIDSfaith.com/convocation/paper14.asp.

91. Corless, 'A Buddhist understanding of HIV/AIDS'.
92. Roger Corless, 'Buddhism' in *Encyclopedia of AIDS*, edited by Raymond A. Smith: 110.
93. In an article on resources within Hinduism to deal with disease, including HIV and AIDS, there is some reference to sacred texts, specifically the *Brihadâranyaka Upanishad*. However, this article offers a re-stating rather than a re-reading of sacred texts and concepts: see Varadaraja V. Raman, 'Some Hindu insights on a global ethic in the context of diseases and epidemics'. *Zygon* 38(1) 2003: 141–5. Similarly, see also Acharya Palaniswami, 'Hinduism' in *Encyclopedia of AIDS*, edited by Raymond A. Smith: 258–60.
94. Corless, 'Buddhism': 110.
95. The most obvious gap in this chapter is published work in languages other than English. The task remains to gather this work. See the suggestive work of Paula Clifford, *HIV in Asia: Cultural and Theological Perspectives* (London: Christian Aid, 2006).
96. CHART, *The Cartography of HIV and AIDS, Religion and Theology: A Partially Annotated Bibliography*, available at www.chart.ukzn.ac.za.
97. A similar point is made by Steve de Gruchy in the next chapter of this book.

Practitioner response

Monica Jyotsna Melanchthon

By turning to their own scriptural traditions, people respond to crises that envelop their daily lives. Similarly, those who are HIV positive seek local intellectual and cultural resources and the aid of sacred texts (or more generally their religion) to make sense of their suffering, looking for hope and comfort. In doing so, they challenge the disjuncture between values and behaviour of the faith community which remains a continuing dilemma, particularly with regard to determining the appropriate response to persons infected with HIV. For those who subscribe to traditional religious values, commitments to love and justice are often lost in condemning people living with HIV because of the linkages made between illness and sin. HIV and AIDS has been theologically and ethically problematised as an issue of immorality and sexual promiscuity, as the wages of sin and divine judgement. For some, AIDS is a lethal judgement of God on the sin, especially that of homosexuality. On the other hand, for those who subscribe to more liberal religious values, acceptance and understanding sometimes seem to overshadow a willingness to set boundaries around what is not acceptable moral behaviour. As has been clearly demonstrated in Gerald West's chapter, both parties use the sacred texts to argue their position.

What is evident in West's analysis is the fact that in formulating a theological response to HIV and AIDS, Christians and Muslims begin at different points and draw on a variety of sources. A conservative response to HIV and AIDS often rests on a particular way of understanding the authority and primacy of the sacred text. God's truth is what is written in the sacred text and binding on the believer. Not only select portions of the Bible and Qur'an, but also their totality, is understood to be against those living with HIV. If one adopts this approach, disagreeing with or contradicting what the Bible or Qur'an is interpreted to say proves impossible. The starting point thus determines how the scriptural tradition is interpreted and what the response to the epidemic ought to be.

West's chapter outlines the alternative approach, which recognises that the Bible and Qur'an are not independent from their interpreters. Sacred texts did not suddenly appear in a bound volume but result from centuries of conscientious religious persons seeking to understand and interpret God's will and way for humanity. Written in language different from our own, the Bible and the Qur'an have been conditioned by historical, social and scientific understandings distinct from those of the contemporary world. But the Bible and the Qur'an are foundational for Christian and Islamic faith and witness: their contents collectively constitute the sacred texts of faith communities. It is for this reason that these communities seek their guidance in considering life's challenges.

West shows, however, that there is a distinction between theologically determined readings and detailed readings of the sacred text. I agree that it is in the latter, in 'the in-depth work on the interface between HIV and AIDS and theology' that life and meaning resides but wonder if the former is possibly an essential step, a need, an immediate response evoked and necessitated by the intensity of the crisis. Most liberational readings and interpretations that came into being at the margins of society began with this engaged, but quick and easy, identification with the sufferer in the text. It is this recognition of a meaning that spoke to and resonated with the experience of suffering. The foregrounding of method and a questioning of meaning came much later in the development of the movement's articulation of its ideological stance. While the former type of interpretations may be questioned and critiqued by the engaged scholar, it still needs to be acknowledged that such readings do empower those who suffer, enabling them to cope and bring about some form of liberation and healing.

I offer one example from India. The National Lutheran Health and Medical Board of the United Evangelical Lutheran Churches of India (UELCI) published a book by Daniel Premkumar, a pastor and biblical scholar.[1] The book is essentially a selection of biblical passages that are said to contain guiding factors for the lives of people living with HIV. The passages were selected in response to questions and feelings expressed by Ronnie, a victim of the illness, for their ability to provide comfort, hope, strength and courage. They are interspersed with brief comments by Ronnie who shares what the text is saying to him. In a situation where pastoral care is either non-existent or limited, the Bible, Premkumar maintains, is 'the only handy companion the [people living with HIV] are certain to have with them till the end'.[2]

For those of us from India, any reading or interpretation of the text in the context of HIV and AIDS has to be carried out in association with gender, class and caste; and we also need to be particularly cognisant of the effect of religious views on sexual behaviour. Any systemic attempt to deal with the epidemic cannot overlook religion or the sacred text. Furthermore, any morally well-founded approach to religion and HIV and AIDS cannot overlook the fact of religious pluralism. The Bible no longer holds a privileged or pre-eminent place in a multi-scriptural society.[3] It is seen as one sacred narrative among many in human history and relativised, often without Christian consent. We may choose to deny this reality but it is essential that theologians take into account the many sacred texts that have come to claim the allegiance of people in our world. While West's chapter offers the reader an analysis of the trends in the utilisation and interpretation of sacred texts in addressing the HIV and AIDS epidemic, it does not address how charting the textual territory of sacred texts alongside each other might contribute to a response to the epidemic. It is by learning and understanding how other religious communities hear, read, interpret and appropriate their sacred texts that we all benefit. Any identifiable resonances between diverse scriptural traditions will enhance united action and mutual support and enable a religiously and culturally inclusive approach to religion and HIV.

The manner in which Islam invokes its sacred text, and the survey of Qur'anic material used to engage with HIV and AIDS in the chapter, highlights redemptive categories such as human dignity, socio-economic justice, care and compassion which are common to both the Qur'an and the Bible. This directs Muslims and Christians to work to eradicate the suffering of others, including, among other things, working to eliminate discrimination based on sexual orientation and on HIV status. The Islamic reading and wrestling with the story of Lot (Prophet Lut) is particularly insightful. A collaborative reading of common texts such as the story of Lot, or even a joint reflection on approaches to sacred texts, might break down prejudices between faith traditions and walls of separation.

HIV and AIDS is breaking down barriers in surprising ways, as a further example from India illustrates. The state of Andhra Pradesh in southern India has the highest HIV incidence in the country. Recently, Devahi Selina, a theologian and activist, described a community of people living with HIV in Guntur that sees itself as an HIV *kulam,* roughly translated as caste or sub-caste.[4] Even as she notes the danger of thinking in caste categories, she highlights the fact that this *kulam* is different because one's membership is not determined by birth or profession. It does not embrace or practise any of the characteristic features of caste affiliation. It is instead a community of HIV positive people who have transcended traditional caste identities and draw strength from and build upon their stigmatised identity. Solidarity has been forged on the basis of the common experience of alienation and rejection. It has enabled those from the dominant castes within the *kulam* to become sensitive to the disempowering and discriminating power of the caste system. They have also transcended religious identities and are appreciative of each other's liturgical and worship practices, with an emphasis on life in the here and now. While not certain if they engage in any joint reading of sacred texts, it seems that if equipped to do so, this would contribute further to their solidarity across traditional divides of caste and religion.

That Hinduism did not feature prominently in West's chapter did not come as a surprise. Unlike Judaism, Christianity and Islam, Hinduism is not a religion of the book. It is not a religion that requires the believer to read sacred texts. Hence, looking to these texts for guidance in matters such as illness is alien to the Hindu believer. Given the great diversity of its philosophical traditions it is difficult to identify a unified response to HIV and AIDS in Hinduism. The Hindu response is, therefore, most often surmised from an understanding of its traditions and moral values that include compassion and care for the sick and the elderly. Unlike churches, Hindu temples or priests do not offer health services or discuss personal problems. Instead, finding rituals of healing, and religious practices such as meditation and yoga, are emphasised.

However, there are signs of hope that there is a concerted effort from within Hinduism to respond to the HIV and AIDS epidemic. First, there is an historical precedent for a Hindu response to disease and suffering that can be seen in the many associations addressing the needs of people all over the Hindu world. Second, senior Hindu religious leaders are open to join the national effort to reverse the spread of HIV since they have acknowledged that 'Stigma around the disease can only be overcome if religious leaders speak about it openly'.[5] Further, it is acknowledged that most infected individuals are religious, that their religious beliefs provide them with the motivation to persevere in the face of numerous calamities and that religious and culturally sensitive interventions can play an important role in improving the mental health of these individuals.

Nonetheless, the analysis in the chapter resonates with the Indian experience and is a resource for the socially engaged Indian interpreter. Asia, and more particularly India where HIV incidence is growing at an alarming pace, have much to learn from the African experience. The church in a limited way and the many Christian non-governmental organisations are most certainly at the forefront of addressing the issue but they are far behind in reading and interpreting the Bible from the perspective of those living with HIV. One attempt is evidenced in the work of Indian ethicist Nalunnakkal who has developed an ethic of just care and table fellowship based on his reading of Luke 5 as a response to people living with HIV.[6]

In India, where culture and religion are central, the stigma of disease adds an extra burden to families and individuals living with HIV alongside other sources of stigma such as caste and poverty. Liberative readings of sacred texts that employ an HIV hermeneutic are urgently called for, as this task is still to be effectively addressed by all faith communities.

Notes

1. Daniel Premkumar, *Ronnie's Bible: Addressed to People Living with HIV/AIDS* (Chennai: NLHMB/UELCI, 2007).
2. Daniel Premkumar, *Ronnie's Bible*: 2.
3. Paul Rajashekar, 'Christian theology and inter-religious hermeneutics' in *Witnessing in Context: Essays in Honor of Eardley Mendis,* edited by George Zachariah and Monica Melanchthon (Tiruvalla: Christava Sahitya Samithi, 2007): 55.
4. Devahi Selina, 'Positive people: Seeking strength from stigma'. Paper presented at a Consultation on Mission at the Margins: Patterns, Protagonists and Perspectives: A Critical and Constructive Contribution to the Edinburgh 2010 Conference, Hyderabad, 24 Sep. 2009.
5. Sri Sri Ravi Shankar, founder of the Art of Living Foundation, quoted in 'Hindu faith leaders commit to AIDS response', a UNAIDS Knowledge Center story. Available at http://www.unaids.org/en/KnowledgeCentre/Resources/FeatureStories/archive/2008/20080618_hindu_faith_leaders_aids_response.asp (accessed 8 Dec. 2009).
6. George Mathew Nalunnakkal, *HIV/AIDS: A Challenge to Theological Education*, edited by Samson Prabhakar and George Mathew Nalunnakkal (Bangalore: BTESSC/SATHRI, 2004): 90.

6

Systematic theological reflection on HIV and AIDS

Mapping the terrain

Steve de Gruchy

INTRODUCTION

The first Christian theological writings on HIV and AIDS appeared in 1985.[1] Twenty-three years later, the December 2008 version of the Collaborative for HIV and AIDS, Religion and Theology (CHART) bibliography of academic material had 1 557 entries.[2] Of these, 175 or 11.2 per cent had something to do with systematic theology and form the focus of this chapter. Given that one of the key elements of the bibliography is to capture what has been written theologically about HIV and AIDS, this would seem to be a small percentage and it points to three important issues that need to be identified at the outset.

First, it is extremely difficult to separate issues of systematic theology from some other Christian theological disciplines, particularly biblical studies and practical theology. Doing so is often a matter of personal judgement, yet it is important to name this so as to define what is meant by systematic theology. In terms of biblical studies, there are a number of essays that speak of the need for a theological response to HIV and AIDS, and then work with one or a series of biblical passages.[3] This is noted specifically about the issue of suffering and the book of Job below. Likewise there are a number of essays that deal with practical theological issues to do with ministry to and with those living with HIV that of necessity use theological resources to respond to questions of stigma, guilt, compassion, inclusion and justice.[4] None of this work is illegitimate, and it is clearly theological in a broad sense, but in this chapter the focus is narrowed to systematic theology. Its working definition is the systematic reflection on the faith, involving reflection beyond one particular biblical tradition, and beyond application to one particular practical issue. Nevertheless, the constraints of a somewhat artificial division should be remembered.

Second, this small percentage is a pointer to just how little work has actually been undertaken to reflect on HIV and AIDS from the perspective of systematic theology. This is made even more stark considering that a good number of the entries in the bibliography that concern systematic theology are actually essays that call for such reflection rather than seek to offer it. Third, it is significant that of the approximately 175 entries on issues to do with systematic theology, 101 (57 per cent) are written from Africa and of these 56 (32 per cent) are from South Africa alone. As far as is known, the first two theological documents on HIV and AIDS were published in Africa in 1989,[5] out of a total of 36, and not one was from South Africa; so this represents a major theological outpouring in more recent years. These figures may well be skewed because of the fact that CHART, the facilitator of the bibliographic project, is located in South Africa. However, given that southern Africa is the epicentre of the epidemic, it is not surprising that South African theologians have given HIV and AIDS more attention than theologians from any other part of the world.

Turning to mapping the engagement between systematic theology and HIV and AIDS, it is important to note that Martha Frederiks has published a helpful survey essay that undertakes a similar task.[6] She has a broader focus on practical theology and biblical studies but this is restricted to Africa. Nevertheless, her concluding summary is a helpful overview of the material:

> Theologising in the context of HIV and Aids is a fairly recent development. The first publications appeared about two decades ago. They focused on sensitizing people towards HIV and Aids, on analysing the causes of its rapid spread and on identifying physical, cultural and socio-economic factors that contributed to the spread of the virus. However, reflections on HIV and Aids did not become a theological trend until about five years ago. Nowadays the market is inundated with material on Aids and theology. The majority of the publications come from Southern and Central Africa – areas where the epidemic has hit hardest – though there are noted exceptions such as writings from Cameroun and Nigeria. Also note-worthy is the significant contribution of women theologians to the reflection on [the] HIV and Aids problematic. This achievement can be attributed to the

activities of the Circle of Concerned African Women Theologians, who for a number of years now have geared the majority of their research towards stigma, gender and HIV/Aids.[7]

In seeking to make sense of the material at hand, it is helpful to map the terrain in five ways:

- the challenge to undertake theological reflection on key issues central to the praxis of the church in this time of HIV and AIDS;
- identification of these issues; then
- the prising open of traditional theological themes by the epidemic; and even
- the emergence of some entirely new ways of doing theology; and finally
- pointing to some of the vacant spaces on the map where the terrain has yet to be explored.

HIV AND AIDS DEMAND THEOLOGICAL REFLECTION

The first theme that emerges is that the experience of HIV and AIDS, its impact upon the church and the poor, and its lived reality for people of faith calls for theological reflection. Two reasons drive this concern. First, it emerges out of a sociological awareness that belief and doctrine are important elements in driving the epidemic. Christoff Benn, a medical doctor working with the Global Fund to Fight AIDS, Tuberculosis and Malaria[8] makes this point in his essay.[9] Similarly, Afe Adogame from Nigeria, writing in a psychology journal, points out that failing to understand the beliefs and doctrines, or in wider perspective, the world views of people, leads to a failure to take their reality seriously and so undermines the ability to respond to the epidemic.[10] Rob Garner, working outside Pietermaritzburg, South Africa, has noted what seems to be the positive impact of certain doctrines and beliefs upon members of some Pentecostal churches.[11] The same point is made by Johnny Ramirez-Johnson and Edwin L. Hernandez in their essay.[12]

Beverley Haddad has noted in her work how the lack of theological training is hindering pastors in African Initiated Churches from responding in adequate ways to the epidemic, leading to theologies of moral condemnation: everyone seems to know these do not work but nevertheless they continue to adhere to them.[13] Almost the same point is made by Tom Cannell and Norman Mudau in their reflection on funerals amongst Zulu communities in KwaZulu-Natal, South Africa:

The majority of the religious leaders in KwaZulu-Natal work out of indigenous African Christian churches without formal structures in place to educate clergy. As a result, many of these ministers lack the theological resources to address the scourge of AIDS in a constructive way. Instead they resort to condemning the infected, suggesting that God has punished them for their sinful behaviour.[14]

Given this, it is no surprise that there has been a strong investment in theological education around the HIV and AIDS epidemic in Africa. Musa Dube has led a range of interventions in this regard.[15] But others have also reflected on this, including Peter Mageto, Tinyiko Maluleke, Moji Ruele, Nyambura Njoroge and Neville Richardson.[16] They have pointed out the importance of developing an adequate HIV and AIDS-sensitive theological curriculum so that clergy are prepared for the challenges that they will face.[17] A good sign of the progress made on this front was the publication of a series of essays written by graduate students in Africa and edited by Edwina Ward and Gary Leonard.[18] This need to engage the curriculum has also been picked up by theological educators in India.[19]

The call for such a curriculum requires that theological resources are prepared and it is in this context that the ways in which HIV and AIDS demand theological reflection are seen. A number of scholars have engaged with this demand. In the 1990s the first works came from Europe and the USA.[20] Ron Nicolson was the first to produce a book in the African context in 1996.[21] Then, in 2000, the World Council of Churches (WCC) published a study document that provided a theological, ethical and human rights approach to HIV/AIDS as well as a practical outline of what faith organisations can do.[22]

A significant event was a workshop held in Namibia in December 2003, attended by 36 Christian theologians and hosted by the Joint United Nations Program on HIV and Aids (UNAIDS), the first time the United Nations had sponsored such a gathering. They focused on the issue of stigma but also sought to develop a framework to provide a useful basis for theological reflection in the contexts of theological education, church councils and synods, and pastoral formation. The document that emerged from the gathering:

> [. . .] represents the efforts to grapple with the serious and complex issues related to stigmatising and discriminatory reactions to HIV and AIDS, and to discern the values and beliefs that underlie a justice-based response to

such negative phenomena. The consultation identified a number of theological themes relevant to this task: God and Creation; Interpreting the Bible; Sin; Suffering and Lamentation; Covenantal Justice; Truth and Truth-telling; and The Church as a Healing, Inclusive and Accompanying Community.[23]

This report subsequently stimulated the publication in 2007 of a volume of collected essays edited by Robin Gill.[24] This volume specifically seeks to make known to the European and North American churches the theological reflection emerging in Africa. In the same year, Bénézet Bujo and Michael Czerny edited a volume from within the Catholic tradition that seeks to answer the questions: 'what does God and His [*sic*] Church help us to learn about AIDS?' and 'what does AIDS teach us about God, our world, the Church and ourselves?'[25]

It is important also to note that a number of theological journals focusing on southern Africa have dedicated volumes to the theme of HIV and AIDS.[26] Owing to a particular subsidy system in South Africa that rewards scholars for publishing in accredited journals, as well as the speed at which the HIV and AIDS epidemic is moving, it is here – rather than in books – that the most significant theological work in South Africa is to be found. It is here, for example, that Musa Dube and Tinyiko Maluleke have called for theologians to be engaged in the epidemic; Ernst Conradie has argued that HIV and AIDS challenges us to offer a plausible account of each aspect of the Christian faith; and the former Anglican Archbishop of Cape Town, Njongonkulu Ndungane has reflected on the challenge of HIV and AIDS to Christian theology.[27]

For various physiological, cultural and social reasons HIV impacts upon women in Africa far more than men. Thus, it is significant that perhaps the most sustained theological engagement with the epidemic comes from the Circle of Concerned African Women Theologians. Both the 2002 and 2007 Pan African Conferences of the Circle, as well as a range of books,[28] were dedicated to the issue. The volumes of collected essays, while not all strictly focused on systematic theology, nevertheless represent a very significant theological response to HIV and AIDS.[29] To this has been added a collection of Musa Dube's writings, which 'argues for a strong theological presence alongside current economic, social, and political efforts to quell this devastating disease'.[30]

HIV AND AIDS SEEK THEOLOGICAL CLARITY

If the first theme identified concerns the demand to undertake theological reflection on HIV and AIDS, the second concerns the particular issues that emerge from the church's praxis and ministry around which theological clarity is sought. It is a reminder of the inter-disciplinary nature of theological reflection around HIV and AIDS and how tricky it is to work with a notion of pure systematic theology in dealing with such an all embracing issue. It is possible to identify the following five clusters of issues, bearing in mind that because they emerge from the seamlessness of life, they are theoretical abstractions and not mutually exclusive.

Stigma and exclusion

Stigma and exclusion are probably the most theologised issues. It has already been noted that the UNAIDS meeting in Namibia in 2003 focused much of its energy on the issue of stigma. Gillian Paterson, working within the structures of the Ecumenical Advocacy Alliance and the World Council of Churches, has been in the forefront and put this issue firmly on the agenda.[31] Michael Burke has also contributed to this issue.[32] The issues of exclusion and inclusion, avoidance and love have been at the forefront of the Christian response to people living with HIV from at least as early as 1995, when Joseph Allen contributed an essay to the *Ecumenical Review*.[33] Janet Brown and H. Jurgens Hendriks capture this tension with their essay and Johan Bouwer has engaged with the theme of human dignity in the face of prejudice.[34] Harriet Deacon and Leickness Simbayi were commissioned by the Anglican Church of Southern Africa in 2006 to assess the nature and extent of stigma within their structures.[35] Philomena Mwaura has looked at how discrimination and stigma affect women in Kenyan society and what this means for the church, while Lilian Siwila has paradoxically examined how the ethics of hospitality can become a threat to women's lives.[36]

A sustained engagement on this theme has been the dialogue between the councils of churches in the five Nordic countries and the eleven councils of churches in southern Africa known as the Federation of Christian Churches in Southern Africa (FOCCISA).[37] The dialogue, which intentionally included people living with HIV, was published in two volumes. The first engages issues of sexuality, sin, stigma and discrimination, while the second offers resources for worship to build an inclusive church that is sensitive to the concerns of those living with HIV and AIDS.[38]

Conceptions of disease and healing

The HIV and AIDS epidemic has raised issues related to conceptions of disease and healing. Adam Chepkwony edited a text from a symposium of the Ecumenical Symposium of Eastern Africa Theologians (ESEAT),[39] which added to previous work done in the Asian context.[40] For churches for which healing is a key aspect of ministry, the inability to heal provokes a major crisis and leads to questions about what healing means. As Haddad captures it: 'We pray, but we cannot heal.'[41] A key research project based in South Africa, the African Religious Health Assets Programme (ARHAP), which has undertaken work for the World Health Organisation, the Gates Foundation and UNAIDS in the area of religion and HIV and AIDS, has also raised questions about the relationship of Christian faith and healing in an African context. James Cochrane has reflected on this as have Paul Germond and Sepetla Molapo with their creative work on *Bophelo*.[42] Steve de Gruchy has also drawn from his work in ARHAP, suggesting the concept of healing as a key category for theology and development in Africa today.[43]

Issues of sexuality

The third issue arising from church praxis with HIV and AIDS has related to issues of sexuality. Clearly the mode of transmission of the HI virus in sexual intercourse and the church's traditional squeamishness and conservative moralism regarding sex and sexuality has created a major crisis that requires theological reflection. The fact that the AIDS crisis began in the gay community in the USA led to much reflection in the 1990s on issues of sexuality within the context of homosexuality and homophobia. This is clearly demonstrated in the work of William D. Lindsey, Grace Jantzen and T.J. John.[44] In the African context, matters of HIV and sexuality are rooted in heterosexual practices. Philippe Denis has engaged with sexuality within the particular political, cultural and economic context of South Africa.[45] Michael Haspel argues:

> [. . .] that starting from biblical insights and Christian anthropology in the current situation a contextual theology addressing HIV/AIDS and a respective sexual ethic have to be developed which enables Christians to live responsibly in a time of HIV/AIDS without demonising sexuality. This, in turn, could contribute to the ethical discourse in civil society and thus foster the development of a public theology.[46]

Manoj Kurian has also dealt with this theme. He argues that faith communities tend to distance themselves from honest discussion about sexuality, believing that this encourages promiscuity and exemplifies a lack of morals. The effect of this is that the gift of sexuality 'can be perverted to oppress and humiliate'.[47] From an African feminist perspective, Fulata Moyo has picked up this theme and shown how the dominant male theologies of sexuality are oppressive to women in Africa in a time of HIV and AIDS.[48]

Gender issues

As has already been suggested, the work of the Circle of Concerned African Women Theologians has provided theological reflection on HIV and AIDS within the framework of patriarchy. They have addressed many issues from this perspective, including female genital mutilation; gender violence; harmful cultural practices both within and outside the church; and most recently a drive to find cultural practices which may enhance and promote life rather than deny it.[49] In terms of theological reflection on some specific gender issues there has been work on gender violence by Beverley Haddad and Denise Ackermann;[50] and gender equality by Miranda Pillay.[51] There has also been an effort to engage with issues of masculinity and HIV in Circle work. For example, the Pan-African Conference held in Yaounde, Cameroon, for the first time in Circle history invited men to participate and held a special panel on masculinities as well. There is a growing number of publications in this regard.[52]

Denial and responsibility

The final cluster of themes to emerge from church praxis has to do with denying the extent of the epidemic; and its opposite – taking responsibility for it. Emanuel Katongole's essay on suspicion and despair captured the mood that surrounded the church's response to the epidemic at the turn of the century:

> What is often ignored is that the AIDS epidemic is changing the kind of people we are. It has reinforced both Western stereotypes of Africa, and African suspicion of the West, and of the West's intentions in Africa. AIDS has also caused suspicion in the most intimate relations – the one you love can kill you. In a continent where many struggle for bare survival, this has led to hopelessness and despair that manifests itself in a nihilistic playfulness. Christian ethics has not even begun to deal with this.[53]

Tony Balcomb's is the only essay to engage with the question of denialism from a theological perspective.[54] Against this, the ethics of responsibility have been proposed. Such ethics are not about apportioning blame but about taking responsible action in the face of the epidemic.[55] Charles Ryan has engaged with this theme from a Catholic perspective.[56]

HIV AND AIDS SHAPE THEOLOGICAL LOCI

It is important to note that not only are theologians reflecting upon the particular issues emerging from the church's praxis with the HIV and AIDS epidemic but this praxis and reflection is in turn having an effect upon the traditional theological loci of the church. In other words, it is not just one-way traffic. There is a dialectic happening between HIV and AIDS on the one hand and theology on the other. Much like the way in which fundamental experiences of Auschwitz and Hiroshima have shaped theology in the North, it is likely that HIV and AIDS will have a profound effect upon theology in Africa. And this effect will not just be on those themes that have to do specifically with HIV and AIDS (as has been noted in the section above) but upon the wider understanding of Christian faith.[57] The experience of HIV and AIDS, in other words, raises deep questions about such matters as suffering, hope, justice, and the body of Christ. When this is over it is likely that people in Africa may believe in God in ways very different to those before 1980.

Suffering

It should not be surprising that a fundamental theological theme interrogated in the light of the experience of HIV and AIDS is that of suffering. Early, simplistic theological reflection tended to see this suffering as the result of individual sinful behaviour, in which the victims had no one to blame but themselves. Padigail Meskin's comment about this early theology captures the point: 'When the first cases of HIV/AIDS were diagnosed in the late 1970s, the attitude of most faith based communities, indeed of most people, was that those being infected had no one to blame but themselves, their lifestyle and their own choices. Out of this was developed the "Theology of Sin and Punishment", sometimes called "Victim Theology"'.[58]

It is likely that this kind of victim theology remains at the heart of much Christian response to HIV and AIDS. However, with the passing of time and growing evidence about the course of the epidemic, there has been greater reflection on questions of suffering. Justin Soongie's more recent essay on the suffering of what he calls innocent victims is representative of this:

> The suffering of innocent HIV/AIDS victims includes the pain of betrayal, depression from rejection, and the deprivation of life. The fundamentalist response blames the victim or insistently expects a miracle. The humanitarian response gives sympathy, but does not address root issues or provide a better coping strategy. However, the innocent suffering of Jesus illustrates the potential for the innocent suffering of the AIDS victim to have a salvific dimension.[59]

Yet there are no simple answers. Ernst Conradie asks the question on many people's lips in the light of the epidemic – where on earth is God? – and seeks to answer this in dialogue with various existing theodicies.[60] The book edited by Kenneth Overberg has a number of essays responding to the question of suffering and explores a number of responses.[61] Some theologians have taken the opportunity to engage with particular theological understandings of suffering: Paul Crowley, who has worked with the thought of Karl Rahner, argues that 'as an expression of radical realism and hope, [his] theology helps us find in the sorrow of AIDS an opening into the mystery of God'.[62]

It was noted at the start of this chapter how a number of scholarly reflections engage with a particular biblical text in order to reflect theologically on HIV and AIDS.[63] The book of Job is particularly significant in contributing to the theme of suffering. In the CHART bibliography no fewer than seventeen essays deal with Job, suffering and HIV and AIDS.[64] This theme of suffering represents the fundamental theological issue to emerge from HIV and AIDS, and it in turn calls forth a range of other themes as a response to suffering; namely, hope in a time of suffering, the possibilities of life in the midst of such death, justice for the victims, and the very meaning of being church in such a context.

Hope

Many of the theological reflections on HIV and AIDS begin with the context of suffering and then move on to the question of where people are to find sources of hope. Some, like Anne Bayley, have argued in a more general sense that the Christian faith is itself a source of hope,[65] while others have turned to stories of hope in the Bible and re-read them in the face of the epidemic. For example,

Musimbi Kanyoro speaks of the stories of Jesus' healing of women in the Gospels: 'The message here is clear, that nothing is impossible, not even death has a final say. Facing HIV and AIDS from a faith perspective means finding every possible thread of hope that will keep us from giving in and giving up on ourselves.'[66]

In a wider sense, in the face of the devastation caused by the epidemic, Thinandavha Mashau has proposed 'a theology of hope and accompaniment that seeks to stand in solidarity with those infected and affected by HIV and AIDS thereby providing them with hope that enables them to deal with the present as they wait eagerly for the future'.[67] A text that places the question of hope firmly on the agenda is by Tetsunao Yamamori, David Dageforde and Tina Bruner.[68] Jill Olivier has promoted a theology of hope in the context of HIV and AIDS.[69]

Perhaps the most sustained theological reflection on hope comes from Daniël Louw in his work on the theology of resurrection.[70] Here he argues that the theological loci of creation, incarnation and passion are not enough to handle the depth of the epidemic:

> It should be supplemented by a *theologia resurrectionis* which can act as a theological critique on all forms of human suffering, including the spiritual suffering of punishment, guilt, rejection and stigmatisation. Due to the resurrection as a divine act, death is dead. Stigmatisation as a form of 'death' (rejection) is deleted so that theology in itself, and therefore the pastoral ministry of the church, become a direct protest against all forms of human discrimination. Resurrection hope empowers people living with HIV (PLWH) to resist all forms of labelling and prejudice. It equips them with the courage to be, and to live a positive life.[71]

Life

Louw's point about a resurrection theology, one that posits life against death, leads naturally into theological reflections on life. In the face of the death that comes in the wake of HIV and AIDS, Michael Czerny has made the point:

> The Church does not face the AIDS pandemic simply as 'a problem to solve,' but listens instead to the Lord who says: 'I have come so that they may have life, and have it to the full.' This involves affirming people's

dignity and forming their morality, so as to have the courage to say 'No' to oneself for the sake of 'Yes' to life.[72]

This theme has been picked up as a central strand in the work of African women theologians.[73] In his Master's thesis for Utrecht University, Adriaan van Klinken reflects on the work of Isabel Phiri, Beverley Haddad and Fulata Moyo under the theme, 'Theologising life, even in the face of death'.[74]

A key recent text that takes forward the need to engage in theological reflection around the theme of affirming life, as well as taking seriously the critique of patriarchy, is Ezra Chitando's double volume.[75] While the second volume focuses on practical matters, including the importance of engaging with men around themes of patriarchy and masculinity, the first volume argues strongly that the theological approach of the African churches has been characterised by rigidity, exclusivity, discrimination and punishment, all of which have been life-denying. He offers some pointers towards a life-affirming theology that would enable the church to take seriously the reality of the deaths of so many young people in Africa.

Justice

In the midst of the suffering brought by HIV and AIDS, theologians have engaged not just with the themes of hope and life but have also raised questions of social ethics, reworking the prophetic tradition and its call for justice. The feminist theologian Lisa Cahill has made this the central pillar of her theological engagement with the epidemic, as has Margaret Farley.[76] This approach is picked up by Catholic moral theologians in a number of settings.[77] Steve de Gruchy has noted how the church often moves into modes of care and compassion while avoiding the more political and policy work around public health and the social structures that create the conditions in which people get sick.[78] Likewise Frits de Lange, drawing on the themes of the Kairos Document and the Belhar Confession, 'makes an appeal to the churches not only to accept their pastoral responsibilities vis-à-vis HIV/AIDS, but also their prophetic responsibilities in exposing factors that promote the spread of or aggravate the suffering caused by the disease, especially economic globalisation and gender inequality':[79]

> Justice is the central theme . . . At this moment in the history of HIV and
> AIDS, we know very well that poverty, ignorance and powerlessness

compromise many women particularly in Africa and increase their risk and vulnerability. We know that those women who have no access to medication die faster; while those who access and use medication and have care and good nutrition live longer. These facts define both the advocacy work as well as the operational work that we need to be involved in.[80]

Likewise, Kenneth Overberg, who edited a book on the theme of suffering, has followed this up with a call to action.[81] This is similar to a call found in the work of J.S. Dreyer and Elias Bongmba.[82] His central argument is that the theological motif of the image of God invites a prophetic critique of the social environment in which HIV and AIDS thrives and calls for a praxis of love and compassion.

Church

The fifth key theological area being reshaped by the reality of HIV and AIDS is ecclesiology, for the epidemic raises a deep theological question about what it means to be the People of God in the midst of all God's people who are sick, suffering, shunned and silenced.[83] The church is experienced by many who are HIV positive as an enemy, and yet it should be their friend.[84] Five themes have been raised around ecclesiology. The first is the fact that because of the reality and presence of church members who are HIV positive, the church itself is HIV positive; or as it has been provocatively said, the Body of Christ has AIDS.[85] Letty Russell has edited a book specifically on this theme.[86]

The second theme has to do with the fundamental issue of what it means to be the church. Neville Richardson has argued:

> The very nature and function of the church – what the church is and what it does – oblige the church to be active in responding to HIV/AIDS. The diaconal ministry of the church can be revived in the simple everyday care that ordinary Christians give to their neighbours in need. Contrary to some widely-held assumptions, the central and distinctive actions of the church – its worship and Eucharist – properly understood, highlight its duty to care.[87]

It is for this reason that De Lange has drawn from the tradition of the Belhar Confession the notion that the church needs again to be a confessing church, given the HIV and AIDS epidemic.[88]

The third theme concerns the transformation that needs to take place in order for the church to live up to this high vision. Patricia Hoffman spoke of the 'sleeping church' in the face of AIDS.[89] Van Wyngaard has noted that 'the churches must be transformed in the face of the HIV/AIDS crisis, in order that they themselves may become a force for transformation – bringing healing, hope, and accompaniment to all infected with and affected by HIV/AIDS'.[90] James Cochrane explores this theme and asks: 'Are the churches competent to understand and respond to the crisis represented by HIV and AIDS? What kind of ecclesial practice is required for an adequate response?' In response, his essay 'poses critical ecclesiological questions in relation to the potential of Christian communities and churches to contribute to the massive challenges posed by HIV and AIDS, ending with the proposal that a conception of "decent care" offers an important integrative paradigm for action'.[91]

The fourth ecclesiological theme picks up this challenge and points to examples of certain local churches that have embraced the crisis and become places of hope and life in the midst of death. Hansjörg Dilger has explored the ways in which a neo-Pentecostal church in urban Tanzania, the Full Gospel Bible Fellowship Church in Dar es Salaam, 'is becoming highly attractive to its followers because of the social, spiritual and economic perspectives that it offers, and particularly because of the networks of healing and support that it has established under the circumstances of urbanisation, structural reform programmes and the AIDS epidemic'.[92] Pamela Leong examines an African-American AIDS ministry in Los Angeles, noting how this congregation has been able to address the health, spiritual and social needs of its parishioners with an activist orientation without losing sight of its religious traditions:

> The reworking of dominant Christian ideology is exemplified in how the pastor has reframed the divine, in how he has incorporated psycho-therapeutic elements into religious rituals, in his method of exegesis, and in how he has reworked the sacred-profane divide. But as a separatist religious organization, this congregation also offers alternative and opposi-tional religious and social cultures, providing a familiar and empowering site for its members.[93]

The final theme picks up on ways in which an essential denial of dignity and respect to women in the church (particularly in Africa) with regard to, for example, issues around hospitality and care giving, is a contributing factor to the spread of HIV.[94] Denise Ackermann has argued that the churches have promoted gender inequality by their promotion of a gospel that discriminates against women and this in turn leads to the vulnerability of women to HIV infection.[95] Beverley Haddad has engaged on this theme, reflecting on the ways women have worked within the patriarchal church to respond to the impact of HIV and AIDS on the lives of their communities.[96]

HIV AND AIDS GENERATE THEOLOGICAL MODELS

We have noted above how the HIV and AIDS epidemic is forcing a re-think and re-shaping of some traditional theological loci. Fundamental theological themes such as suffering, hope, life, justice and ecclesiology are being reflected on in new ways in the light of the reality of social experience and the praxis of the church. In doing this, there have been creative attempts to re-work key theological traditions in the face of contemporary reality. Thus, Esther Kenge in her Master's thesis worked with the doctrine of social holiness in the Methodist Church and Paula Clifford has engaged with the thought of Karl Barth and Jurgen Moltmann.[97] There have been some contributions from Lutheran theologians seeking to work with ideas of the Law-Gospel dialectic with Georg Scriba's creative engagement with Martin Luther's response to the plague as an interesting case study in the modern retrieval of an historical tradition.[98] Montagu Murray has written on living standards, redemption from sin and HIV and AIDS from within the reformed tradition; Phillip Marshall has engaged with a range of theological themes from an evangelical perspective, and Danny Alan Bauer has written from the perspective of liberation theology.[99] Finally, Laurenti Magesa has also shown how African theological models can enable theology to take African culture seriously in responding to HIV and AIDS.[100]

However, perhaps the most fascinating impact of HIV and AIDS upon theology has been the ways in which it is calling forth entire new approaches to theology, or even of conceiving of the theological task. Piet Naudé suggests that the 'HIV/AIDS pandemic requires a fundamental reorientation of our theological reflection' but even he might be surprised at the range that this re-orientation has taken.[101] What is noticeable is that the experience of HIV and AIDS is not just calling for theological reflection around certain issues, nor is it just shaping certain key theological loci as the above three sections have suggested; it is providing a powerful laboratory in which entirely new ways of doing theology are being born.

First, local theologies, what Cochrane calls incipient theologies,[102] are being constructed all the time in the face of the new challenges brought by the epidemic. Hlongwana and Mkhize reflect on a support group whose members 'rationalise their HIV infection to enhance their coping abilities, using Christianity and the Bible in particular, as a reference'.[103] Felicitas Becker and P. Wenzel Geissler point to a similar theme in their introduction to a journal volume on the theme of religion and AIDS:

> The papers in this issue explore how Aids is understood and confronted through religious ideas and practices, and how these, in turn, are re-interpreted and changed by the experience of Aids. They reveal the creativity and innovations that continuously emerge in the everyday life of East Africans, between bodily and spiritual experiences, and between religious, medical, political and economic discourses. Countering simplified notions of causal effects of Aids on religion (or vice versa), the diversity of interpretations and practices inserts the epidemic into wider, and more open, frames of reference. It reveals East Africans' will and resourcefulness in their struggle to move ahead in spite of adversity, and goes against the generalised vision of doom widely associated with the African Aids epidemic.[104]

Moving into the academy, Denise Ackermann has spoken of an embodied theology to respond to issues of HIV and AIDS stigma.[105] This desire to root theological reflection in an embodied experience is reflected in a similar approach by Wendy S. Boring, John A. Geter and Stefano Penna.[106] Likewise, Christina Landman, in reflecting on issues of abuse in relationship to HIV and AIDS, has used Lisa Isherwood's notion of body theology:

> This article explores the faces of harmful religious discourses that render believers vulnerable to abuse. It furthermore describes how these discourses can be deconstructed to healthy religious discourses that empower believers against abuse and enhance their physical and emotional safety. The insights of Body Theology play an important role in describing this shift in religious discoursing . . . Body Theology acknowledges that a person has at least four bodies, thus religious discourses of safety explore the physical body as a site of resistance; the symbolic body as a site of relationship; the

political body as a site for sharing energy and not for exercising power; and the spiritual body as a site of recreation.[107]

In a separate essay she has examined what this might mean for older women living with HIV and AIDS.[108]

Given the emergence of HIV and AIDS within the gay community in the USA in the 1980s, it should be no surprise that work has been done on building a gay theology on the basis of the experience of the epidemic.[109] Michael Clark has been in the forefront of this.[110]

A third new way of reconceiving theology is one that is rooted in the discordant and fragmented nature of the experience of HIV and AIDS. Heidi Epstein has written on the feminist thinker Diamanda Galas 'whose theo-musical constructions of the AIDS crisis radically subvert the concept of stable identity'.[111] In a similar manner, Philip Hefner engages with the theme of fragments in promoting a theology of disease:

> Our ideas of disease try to explain it, and they aim at facilitating cures. In the process, they become entwined in sociocultural networks that have totalizing effects. Disease, however, counters this totalizing effect by revealing to us that our lives are fragments. Unless we engage this fragment character of disease and of our lives, we cannot properly understand disease or deal with it. HIV/AIDS clarifies these issues in an extraordinarily powerful fashion. Medical, legal, commercial, political, and institutional approaches to disease overlook the fragment character of disease in favour of totalizing world-views. A theology of disease is necessary in order to maintain the focus on fragments. Unless we recognize this fragment character, we do not really understand our lives, and we do not really understand either disease or healing.[112]

The theme of discordance and fragmentation is picked up in the final section of this chapter.

HIV AND AIDS REQUIRE THEOLOGICAL WORK

It should be clear from this survey that there is a great deal of creative theological work being undertaken in the context of HIV and AIDS, much of it in southern Africa. Some of the key ideas being reflected on, some of the creative insights emerging about Christian doctrine and a new resourcefulness about theological method have been noted.

In closing, it is necessary to draw attention to some of the gaps that appear in the work. Seven can be noted. The first four are methodological. At the beginning of the chapter it was suggested that one of the major reasons to work at HIV and AIDS from a systematic theology perspective was the struggle of local Christians and pastors to make sense of the epidemic. Another reason is that some of the 'bad' theologies being peddled stigmatise people living with HIV, leading to silence and denial and making their lives worse. At the same time, it is clear that crucial new and creative theological work is happening, even at grassroots level amongst people infected by HIV. Theological reflection and education has to happen somewhere in the dialogical space between the emerging theologies from below and the academy in which more disciplined theologies are being created; between theology with a small 't' and theology with a big 'T'. Little work has been done on what this means in the context of HIV and AIDS.

Second, it has been noted throughout this chapter that systematic theology is difficult to isolate from other Christian disciplines like practical theology and biblical studies. Likewise, insights from anthropology and the sociology and psychology of religion enable considered theological judgements. The sheer scope and breadth of the epidemic calls for a theological method that integrates these disciplines the academy serves to divorce. This methodological issue has yet to be seen on the agenda of systematic theology.

A third gap is the area of inter-religious dialogue. It is intriguing to see how little Christian theological reflection is done in dialogue with other major religious traditions. Because of the early impact of AIDS in North America there is some work by Jewish scholars, particularly Gad Freudenthal, and Azila Reisenberger has written about South African Jewish women and the epidemic.[113] Buddhist scholars have written on the theme of compassion;[114] and there is a growing corpus of literature on dialogue between Christian theology and African Traditional Religions around HIV and AIDS.[115]

Perhaps the most interesting dialogue would be with Muslim theologians because many of the same themes on which Christian theologians are reflecting are emerging in Islamic theology as it responds to the epidemic.[116] The dominant, conservative anti-Western position is represented by scholars like Malik Badri who blame HIV and AIDS on the decadent West.[117] Some Muslim scholars argue that this gives rise to a judgemental and moralistic position that is discriminatory towards people living with HIV and AIDS.[118] Because of this, the contextual experience of the crisis within Muslim communities is starting to shape new insights into the interpretation of sacred texts, and the themes of law and grace, justice, mercy and compassion.[119] This alternative voice is best represented by the South African organisation, Positive Muslims,[120] and has found expression in the book edited by Farid Esack and Sarah Chiddy.[121] Essays in this collection deal with themes of suffering, the wrath of God, compassion, gender justice, masculinity, homosexuality, drug use, justice and liberation.

A fourth methodological concern raised by this chapter is the striking fact that systematic theological reflection on HIV and AIDS is extremely unsystematic. An overview of the literature, as employed here, makes one aware of the shotgun approach that has been taken. Many theologians seem to have offered an insight or two on the epidemic and then moved on, leaving a rather chaotic theological patchwork. From a methodological standpoint it is surely necessary for theologians to identify the key research frontiers and engage in sustained and systematic reflection, even if the content of this reflection speaks to dislocation and fragmentation.

Turning to content, what is surprising is how little theological reflection has been done on the theme of sin. It is possible that because the dominant con-servative and discriminatory attitude towards HIV and AIDS has been couched in the language of sin and the judgement of God, theologians have shied away from this topic. Yet in many ways the issues that have been noted in this chapter to do with stigma and discrimination, gender violence, denial and injustice all suggest ways in which sin is manifest in the world.

The sixth gap is the fact that the major theological themes of salvation, redemption and liberation are not being engaged in a sustained way in the light of HIV and AIDS. Clearly this is the mirror image of the previous point, because salvation, redemption and liberation make sense in a context of sin. It may be that Christian theologians are struggling to find the redemptive side of HIV and AIDS but that admission itself would provide an important starting point for such reflection.[122]

Finally, it is clear that while much creative work has been done around HIV and AIDS from the perspective of embodied theologies, African women's theologies, gay theologies and feminist theologies, the emergence of a theology that enables us to hold together the all-encompassing nature of the epidemic, and its relationship to fundamental themes such as gender, poverty, globalisation, ecological crises, climate change, African identity, sexuality and racism has yet to be seen. But then again perhaps such an über-theology would itself miss something of the radical dislocation and fragmentation of the experience of those living with and dying because of the virus. Possibly a theology of an in-between-time is the most to be hoped for.

NOTES

1. As far as we can tell, the first theological works were by Eileen P. Flynn, *AIDS: A Catholic Call for Compassion* (Kansas City: Sheed and Ward, 1985); and Leon Howell, 'Churches and AIDS: Responsibilities in mission'. *Christianity and Crisis* 45 (9 Dec. 1985): 483–4.

2. CHART, *The Cartography of HIV and AIDS, Religion and Theology: A Partially Annotated Bibliography* (Pietermaritzburg: CHART). The current version of the bibliography is available at www.chart.ukzn.ac.za.

3. See, for example, Miranda Pillay, 'Luke 7:36–50: See this woman?: Toward a theology of gender equality in the context of HIV and AIDS: The challenge of HIV/AIDS to Christian theology'. *Scriptura* 89 (2005): 441–55; Sarojini Nadar, 'Re-reading Job in the midst of suffering in the HIV/AIDS era: How not to talk of God'. *Old Testament Essays* 16 (2003): 343–57; and Adekunle Dada, 'Rereading the Naaman story (2 Kings 5:1–7) in the context of stigmatization of people living with HIV and AIDS in Africa'. *Old Testament Essays* 20 (2007): 586–600.

4. See, for example, Dorcas Olubanke Akintunde, 'The attitude of Jesus to the "anointing prostitute": A model for contemporary churches in the face of HIV/AIDS in Africa' in *African Women, HIV/AIDS and Faith Communities*, edited by Isabel Apawo Phiri, Beverley Haddad and Madipoane Masenya (Pietermaritzburg: Cluster Pubications, 2003): 94–110; Keith August, 'A post-modern narrative approach to understanding the effect of HIV/AIDS on some families in Grabouw'. *Praktiese Teologie in Suid-Afrika* 18(3) 2003: 82–93; Stuart C. Bate, 'Differences in confessional advice in South Africa' in *Catholic Ethicists on HIV/AIDS Prevention*, edited by James F. Keenan et al. (New York: Continuum, 2000): 212–21; Damien Ridge et al., 'Like a prayer: The role of spirituality and religion for people living with HIV in the UK'. *Sociology of Health and Illness* 30(3) 2008: 413–28; Tshisamphiri A. Thugwana, 'Biblical Counselling to Sexually Active People with HIV/AIDS Within a Christian Perspective' (M.Th. dissertation, Potchefstroom University for Christian Higher Education, 2003); Newell J. Wert, 'The biblical and theological basis for risking compassion and care for AIDS patients' in *AIDS, Ethics and Religion: Embracing a World of Suffering*, edited by Kenneth R. Overberg (Maryknoll: Orbis, 1994): 231–42.

5. See Egidio Toccally, *About AIDS* (Nairobi: St Paul Publications Africa, 1989); Catholic Bishops of Uganda, 'Message on the AIDS epidemic to the clergy, the religious and all people of God, to men and women of good will: Peace and God's blessings'. *African Ecclesial Review* 31(5) 1989: 289.

6. Martha T. Frederiks, 'HIV and AIDS: mapping theological responses'. *Exchange: Journal of Missiological and Ecumenical Research* 37(1) 2008: 4–22.

7. Frederiks, 'HIV and AIDS': 22.

8. The Global Fund to Fight AIDS, Tuberculosis and Malaria is an international financing institution that supports large-scale prevention, treatment and care programmes against the three diseases in countries with the greatest need. See http://www.theglobalfund.org/ (accessed 11 Dec. 2009).

9. Christoph Benn, 'The influence of cultural and religious frameworks on the future course of the HIV/AIDS pandemic'. *Journal of Theology for Southern Africa* 113 (2002): 3–18.

10. Afe Adogame, 'HIV/AIDS support and African Pentecostalism: The case of the redeemed Christian Church of God'. *Journal of Health Psychology* 12(3) 2003: 475–84.

11. Rob Garner, 'AIDS and theologies of discipline'. *Bulletin for Contextual Theology in Africa* 7(1) 2000: 13–17; Rob C. Garner, 'Safe sects?: Dynamic religion and AIDS in South Africa'. *Journal of Modern African Studies* 38(1) 2000: 41–69.

12. Johnny Ramirez-Johnson and Edwin L. Hernandez, 'Holiness versus mercy: How theology both hinders and facilitates the Church's response to the HIV/AIDS pandemic'. *Andrews University Seminary Studies* 43(1) 2005: 101–12.

13. Beverley Haddad, 'We pray but we cannot heal: Theological challenges posed by the HIV/AIDS crisis'. *Journal of Theology for Southern Africa* 125 (2006): 80–90.

14. Thomas Cannell and Norman Mudau, 'The view from beside the coffin: AIDS funerals in South Africa'. *Yale Journal of Public Health* 3(2) 2006: 2.

15. Musa W. Dube (ed.), *HIV/AIDS and the Curriculum: Methods of Integrating HIV/AIDS in Theological Programmes* (Geneva: WCC Publications, 2003).

16. Peter Mageto, 'Beyond "victim theology": reconstructing theological education in an era of HIV/AIDS in Africa' in *Theological Education in Contemporary Africa,* edited by G. le Marquand and J. Galgalo (Eldoret: Zapf Chancery, 2004): 147–66; Tinyiko Sam Maluleke, 'Towards an HIV/AIDS-sensitive curriculum' in *HIV/AIDS and the Curriculum*, edited by Musa W. Dube: 59–76; Tinyiko Sam Maluleke, 'The challenge of HIV/AIDS for theological education in Africa: Towards an HIV/AIDS sensitive curriculum'. *Missionalia* 29(2) 2001: 125–43; Moji Ruele, 'Doing theology in the era of HIV/AIDS: A critical evaluation of the Theology and Religious Studies Department, University of Botswana'. *Missionalia* 29(2) 2001: 161–73; Nyambura Jane Njoroge, 'An ecumenical commitment transforming theological education in mission'. *International Review of Mission* 94 (2005): 248–62; R. Neville Richardson, 'HIV and AIDS in the theological curriculum?: Reflections on the HIV and AIDS Consultation for Theological Institutions in Eastern and Southern Africa, Nairobi, Kenya, June 2000'. *Bulletin for Contextual Theology in Africa* 7(1) 2000: 37–9.

17. See, for example, Charles Klagba and C. B. Peter (eds), *Into the Sunshine: Integrating HIV/AIDS into the Curriculum* (Eldoret: Zapf Chancery, 2005).

18. Edwina Ward and Gary S. D. Leonard, *A Theology of HIV & AIDS on Africa's East Coast: A Collection of Essays by Masters Students from Four African Academic Institutions* (Uppsala: Swedish Institute of Mission Research, 2005).

19. See Samson Prabhakar and George Mathew Nalunnakkal (eds), *HIV/AIDS: A Challenge to Theological Education* (Bangalore: BTESSC/SATHRI, 2004).

20. James Woodward, *Embracing the Chaos: Theological Responses to AIDS* (London: SPCK, 1990); Jon D. Fuller, *AIDS and the Church: A Stimulus to Our Theologizing* (Cambridge: Weston School of Theology, 1991).
21. Ronald Nicolson, *God in AIDS?: A Theological Enquiry* (London: SCM, 1996).
22. World Council of Churches, *Facing AIDS: The challenge, the Churches' Response: WCC Study Document* (Geneva: WCC Publications, 2000).
23. UNAIDS, *A Report of a Theological Workshop Focusing on HIV- and AIDS-related Stigma* (Geneva: UNAIDS, 2005). Annotation from CHART bibliography available at http://www.chart.ukzn.ac.za (accessed 10 Dec. 2009).
24. Robin Gill (ed.), *Reflecting Theologically on AIDS: A Global Challenge* (London: SCM, 2007).
25. Bénézet Bujo and Michael Czerny (eds), *AIDS in Africa: Theological Reflections* (Nairobi: Paulines Publications Africa, 2007).
26. *Bulletin for Contextual Theology* 7(1) 2000; *Missionalia* 29(2) 2001; *African Ecclesial Review* 46(1) 2004 and 47(4)–48(1) 2005–6; *Scriptura* 89 (2005); *Journal of Theology for Southern Africa* 125 (July 2006) and 126 (Nov. 2006); and *Journal of Religion in Africa/Religion en Afrique* 37(1) 2007.
27. Musa W. Dube and Tinyiko Sam Maluleke, 'HIV/AIDS as the new site of struggle: theological, biblical and religious perspectives'. *Missionalia* 29(2) 2001: 119–24; Ernst M. Conradie, 'HIV/AIDS and human suffering: Where on Earth is God?' *Scriptura* 89 (2005): 406–32; Njongonkulu Ndungane, 'The challenge of HIV/AIDS to Christian theology'. *Scriptura* 89 (2005): 385–95.
28. Isabel Apawo Phiri, Beverley Haddad and Madipoane Masenya (eds), *African Women, HIV/AIDS and Faith Communities* (Pietermaritzburg: Cluster Publications, 2003); Musa W. Dube and Musimbi R. A. Kanyoro (eds), *Grant Me Justice!: HIV/AIDS and Gender Readings of the Bible* (Pietermaritzburg: Cluster Publications, 2004); Isabel Apawo Phiri and Sarojini Nadar (eds), *African Women, Religion, and Health: Essays in Honour of Mercy Amba Ewudziwa Oduyoye* (Maryknoll: Orbis, 2006); Teressia M. Hinga et al. (eds), *Women, Religion and HIV/AIDS in Africa: Responding to Ethical and Theological Challenges* (Pietermaritzburg: Cluster Publications, 2008).
29. See also Madipoane Masenya, 'Killed by AIDS and buried by religion: African female bodies in crisis'. *Old Testament Essays* 19(2) 2006: 486–99.
30. Musa W. Dube, *The HIV and AIDS Bible: Some Selected Essays* (Scranton: University of Scranton Press, 2008).
31. See Chapter 14 of this book for a fuller discussion by Gillian Paterson of the stigma. Gillian Paterson, *AIDS Related Stigma: Thinking Outside the Box: The Theological Challenge* (Geneva: Ecumenical Advocacy Alliance and World Council of Churches, 2005); Gillian M. Paterson, *Love in a Time of AIDS* (Geneva: WCC Publications, 1995); Gillian M. Paterson, *Church, AIDS and Stigma* (Geneva: EAA, 2003); and Gillian M. Paterson, 'Who sinned?: AIDS-related stigma and the church' in *Applied Ethics in a World Church: The Padua Conference*, edited by Linda Hogan (Maryknoll: Orbis Books, 2008): 163–9.
32. Michael Burke, *A Theology of Stigma in a Time of HIV and AIDS* (West Pennant Hills: Michael and Jean Burke, 2006).

33. Joseph Allen, 'The Christian understanding of human relations: Resource for the churches' response to AIDS'. *Ecumenical Review* 47(3) 1995: 353–63.

34. Janet Brown and H. Jurgens Hendriks, 'The AIDS fulcrum: The church in Africa seesawing between alienation, estrangement, prejudice and love'. *Praktiese Teologie in Suid-Afrika* 19(2) 2004: 19–36; Johan Bouwer, 'Human dignity and HIV/AIDS'. *Scriptura* 95(2) 2007: 262–8.

35. Harriet Deacon and Leickness Simbayi (eds), *The Nature and Extent of HIV and AIDS Related Stigma in the Anglican Church of the Province of Southern Africa: A Qualitative Study* (Cape Town: Human Sciences Research Council, 2006).

36. Philomena N. Mwaura, 'Stigmatisation and discrimination of HIV/AIDS women in Kenya: A violation of human rights and its theological implications'. *Exchange: Journal of Missiological and Ecumenical Research* 37(1) 2008: 35–51; Lilian Siwila, 'Care-giving in times of HIV and AIDS, when hospitality is a threat to African women's lives: A gendered theological examination of the theology of hospitality'. *Journal of Constructive Theology* 13(1) 2007: 69–82.

37. For a short history of Nordic-FOCCISA co-operation, see Chapter 8 in this book.

38. Elizabeth Knox-Seith, *One Body: Volume 1 – North-South Reflections in the Face of HIV and AIDS; Volume 2 – AIDS and the Worshipping Community* (Oslo: Nordic FOCCISA Church Co-operation, 2005).

39. Adam Chepkwony (ed.), *Religion and Health in Africa: Reflections for Theology in the 21st Century* (Nairobi: Paulines Publications Africa, 2006).

40. See Wati A. Longchar (ed.), *Health, Healing and Wholeness: Asian Theological Perspectives on HIV/AIDS*. (Jorhat, Assam: Eastern Theological College, 2005); Razouselie Lasetso (ed.), *Health and Life: Theological Reflections on HIV and AIDS*. (Jorhat: Eastern Theological College, 2007).

41. Haddad, 'We pray but we cannot heal'.

42. James R. Cochrane, 'Of bodies, barriers, boundaries and bridges: Ecclesial practice in the face of HIV and AIDS'. *Journal of Theology for Southern Africa* 126 (2006): 7–26; Paul Germond and Sepetla Molapo, 'In search of Bophelo in a time of AIDS: Seeking a co-herence of economies of health and economies of salvation'. *Journal of Theology for Southern Africa* 126 (2006): 27–47.

43. Steve de Gruchy, 'Re-learning our mother tongue?: Theology in dialogue with public health'. *Religion and Theology: A Journal of Contemporary Religious Discourse* 14(1–2) 2007: 47–67.

44. William D. Lindsey, 'The AIDS crisis and the church: A time to heal'. *Theology and Sexuality* 2 (1995): 11–37; Grace Jantzen, 'AIDS, shame and suffering' in *Sexuality and the Sacred: Sources for Theological Reflection*, edited by James B. Nelson and Sandra P. Longfellow (Louisville: John Knox Press, 1994): 305–13; T.J. John, 'Sexuality, sin and disease: Theological and ethical issues posed by AIDS to the churches: reflections by a physician'. *Ecumenical Review* 47 (1995): 373–84.

45. Philippe Denis, 'Sexuality and AIDS in South Africa'. *Journal of Theology for Southern Africa* 115 (2003): 63–77.

46. Michael Haspel, 'Christian sexual ethics in a time of HIV/AIDS: A challenge for public theology'. *Verbum et Ecclesia* 25(2) 2004: 480.

47. Manoj Kurian, 'The HIV and AIDS pandemic'. *Ecumenical Review* 56(4) 2004: 432–6.

48. Fulata L. Moyo, 'The red and white beads and the Malawian women's sexual freedom' in *Cultural Practices and HIV/AIDS: African Women's Voice*, edited by Elizabeth Amoah, Dorcas

Akitunde and Dorothy Akoto (Accra: Sam-Woode, 2005): 66–75; Fulata L. Moyo, 'Sex, gender, power and HIV/AIDS in Malawi: Threats and challenges to women being church' in *On Being Church: African Women's Voices and Visions*, edited by Isabel Apawo Phiri and Sarojini Nadar: 127–45.

49. Constance Shisanya, 'Un-sexing the sexualised: implications of "celibate" Quaker widows on HIV and AIDS transmission in Nairobi, Kenya'. *Journal of Constructive Theology* 12(2) 2006: 45–64; Margaret Umeagudosu, 'An act of God?: The experiences of girl-children and women living with vesico-vaginal fistula in Northern Nigeria'. *Journal of Constructive Theology* 13(1) 2007: 57–67.

50. Beverley Haddad, 'Gender violence and HIV/AIDS: A deadly silence in the Church'. *Journal of Theology for Southern Africa* 114 (2002): 93–106; Denise M. Ackermann, '"Deep in the flesh": Women, bodies and HIV/AIDS: A feminist ethical perspective' in *Women, Religion and HIV/AIDS in Africa*, edited by Hinga et al.: 105–25.

51. Miranda N. Pillay, 'Re-reading New Testament texts: A resource for addressing gender inequality in the context of HIV and AIDS in South Africa' in *Heil und Befreiung in Afrika: Die Kirchen vor der Missionarischen Herausforderung durch HIV/AIDS*, edited by Francis X. D'sa and Jürgen Lohmayer (Würzburg: Echter, 2007): 138–55; Miranda N. Pillay, 'Luke 7:36–50: 441–55.

52. Julius Gathogo, 'The use of ancestral resources in combating HIV and AIDS: Mundurume's task'. *Journal of Constructive Theology* 13(1) 2007: 5–24. See also the special 'Masculinities' issue of the *Journal of Constructive Theology* 14(1) 2008.

53. Emmanuel M. Katongole, 'Christian ethics and AIDS in Africa today: Exploring the limits of a culture of suspicion and despair', *Missionalia* 29(2) 2001: 144.

54. Anthony Balcomb, 'Sex, sorcery, and stigma: Probing some no-go areas of the denial syndrome in the AIDS debate'. *Journal of Theology for Southern Africa* 125(2006): 104–14.

55. Stuart C. Bate (ed), *Responsibility in a Time of AIDS: A Pastoral Response by Catholic Theologians and AIDS Activists in Southern Africa* (Pietermaritzburg, Cluster Publications, 2003).

56. Charles Ryan, 'AIDS and responsibility: The Catholic tradition' in *Responsibility in a Time of AIDS*, edited by Bate: 2–18; Charles Ryan, 'AIDS and responsibility' in *Reflecting Theologically on AIDS: A Global Challenge*, edited by Robin Gill (London: SCM Press, 2007): 60–76.

57. This point is also made by Conradie in 'HIV/AIDS and human suffering'.

58. Padigail Meskin, 'The role of religious leaders and faith-based organisations in HIV/AIDS' in *HIV/AIDS in Africa: The Not So Silent Presence*, edited by Madhu Kasiram, Rubeena Partab and Babalwa Dano (Durban: Print Connection, 2006): 111.

59. Justin Ain Soongie, 'A theological reflection on the suffering of innocent AIDS victims'. *Melanesian Journal of Theology* 21(1) 2005: 92.

60. Conradie, 'HIV/AIDS and human suffering'.

61. Kenneth R. Overberg (ed.), *AIDS, Ethics and Religion: Embracing a World of Suffering* (Maryknoll: Orbis, 1994).

62. Paul G. Crowley, 'Rahner's Christian pessimism: a response to the sorrow of AIDS'. *Theological Studies* 58(2) 1997: 286.

63. For further discussion of the detailed reading of biblical texts, including the book of Job, in the light of the HIV and AIDS epidemic, see Chapter 5 of this book.

64. See for example Patrick Adeso, 'Suffering in Job and in an African perspective: Exegesis of Job 42:1–6' in *Sagesse Humaine et Sagesse Divine dans la Bible/Human Wisdom and Divine Wisdom in the Bible*, edited by Jean-Bosco Matand Bulembat (Nairobi: Pan-African Association of Catholic Exegetes, 2005): 77–83; Madipoane Masenya, 'Between unjust suffering and the silent God: Job and the HIV/AIDS sufferers in South Africa'. *Missionalia* 29(2) 2007: 186–99; Ghislain Tshikendwa Matadi, *Suffering, Belief, Hope: The Wisdom of Job for an AIDS-Stricken Africa* (Nairobi: Paulines Publications Africa, 2007); Sarojini Nadar, 'Re-reading Job in the midst of suffering in the HIV/AIDS era: How not to talk of God'. *Old Testament Essays* 16(2) 2003: 343–57; Gerald West, 'Reading Job positively in the context of HIV/AIDS in South Africa'. *Concilium* 4 (2004): 112–24; Gunter H. Wittenberg, 'Counselling AIDS patients: Job as a paradigm' in *Reflecting Theologically on AIDS: A Global Challenge*, edited by Robin Gill (London: SCM Press, 2007): 152–64.

65. Anne Bayley, *One New Humanity: The Challenge of AIDS* (London: SPCK, 1996).

66. Musimbi R.A. Kanyoro, 'Reading the Bible in the face of HIV and AIDS' in *Grant Me Justice!* edited by Dube and Kanyoro: xi.

67. Thinandavha D. Mashau, 'Where and when it hurts most: The theology of hope and accompaniment in the context of HIV and AIDS in marriage and family life'. *Exchange: Journal of Missiological and Ecumenical Research* 37(1) 2008: 23.

68. Tetsunao Yamamori, David Dageforde and Tina Bruner, *The Hope Factor: Engaging the Church in the HIV/AIDS Crisis* (Waynesboro: Authentic Media, 2003).

69. Jill Olivier, 'Where does the Christian stand?: Considering a public discourse of hope in the context of HIV/AIDS in South Africa'. *Journal of Theology for Southern Africa* 126 (2006): 81–99.

70. Daniël J. Louw, 'The HIV pandemic from the perspective of a theologia resurrectionis: Resurrection hope as a pastoral critique on the punishment and stigma paradigm'. *Journal of Theology for Southern Africa* 126 (2006): 100–14.

71. Louw, 'The HIV pandemic from the perspective of a theologia resurrectionis': 100.

72. Michael Czerny, 'AIDS: Africa's greatest threat since the slave trade'. *La Civiltà Cattolica* 3741 (6 May 2006): 1.

73. Musa W. Dube, 'Theological challenges: Proclaiming the fullness of life in the HIV/AIDS and global economic era'. *International Review of Mission* 91(363) 2002: 535–49; Isabel Apawo Phiri, 'Life-affirming African theological reflection on HIV and AIDS' in *AIDS*, edited by Regina Ammicht-Quinn and Hille Haker (London: SCM Press, 2007): 41–7; Mary Getui and Matthew M. Theuri (eds), *Quest for Abundant Life in Africa* (Nairobi: Acton Publishers, 2002).

74. Adriaan S. van Klinken, 'Theologising Life, Even in the Face of Death: A Study on the Reflections of Three African Women Theologians, Namely B. Haddad, I. A. Phiri and F. L. Moyo, on HIV/AIDS and Gender and its Relationship' (Masters dissertation in Theology, Utrecht University, 2006).

75. Ezra Chitando, *Living with Hope: African Churches and HIV/AIDS 1* (Geneva: WCC Publications, 2007); Ezra Chitando, *Acting in Hope: African Churches and HIV/AIDS 2* (Geneva: WCC Publications, 2007).

76. Lisa Sowle Cahill, 'AIDS, justice and the common good' in *Catholic Ethicists on HIV/AIDS Prevention*, edited by James F. Keenan et al. (London: Continuum, 2000): 282–93; Lisa Sowle

Cahill, 'AIDS, global justice, and Catholic social ethics'. *Concilium* 3 (2007): 91–101; Margaret A. Farley, *Just Love: A Framework for Christian Sexual Ethics* (New York: Continuum, 2006).

77. See James F. Keenan et al. (eds), *Catholic Ethicists on HIV/AIDS Prevention*; Michael J. Kelly, *HIV and AIDS: A Justice Perspective* (Lusaka: Jesuit Centre for Theological Reflection, 2006); and Mary Jo Iozzio et al. (eds), *Calling for Justice Throughout the World: Catholic Women Theologians on the HIV/AIDS Pandemic* (New York: Continuum, 2009).

78. Steve de Gruchy, 'Doing theology in a time of AIDS'. *Journal of Theology for Southern Africa* 125 (2006): 2–6.

79. Frits de Lange, 'Confessing and embodying justice: About being a confessing church vis-a-vis HIV/AIDS: Barmen en Belhar'. *Nederduitse Gereformeerde Teologiese Tydskrif* 47(1–2) 2006: 254–67.

80. Kanyoro, 'Reading the Bible in the face of HIV and AIDS': viii–x.

81. Kenneth R. Overberg, *Ethics and AIDS: Compassion and Justice in Global Crisis* (Lanham: Rowman and Littlefield, 2006).

82. J.S. Dreyer, 'Justice for the oppressed: The HIV/AIDS challenge' in *Divine Justice-Human Justice,* edited by J.S. Dreyer and J.A. van der Ven (Pretoria: Research Institute for Theology and Religion, UNISA, 2002): 85–112; Elias Kifon Bongmba, *Facing the Pandemic: The African Church and the Crisis of AIDS* (Waco: Baylor University Press, 2007).

83. See Agbonkhianmeghe E. Orobator, *From Crisis to Kairos: The Mission of the Church in the Time of HIV/AIDS, Refugees, and Poverty* (Nairobi: Paulines Publications Africa, 2005).

84. Allan H. Cadwallader (ed.), *AIDS: The Church as Enemy and Friend* (London: HarperCollins, 1992).

85. Kittredge Cherry and James Mitulski, 'We are the church alive, the church with AIDS'. *The Christian Century* 105 (27 Jan. 1988): 85–8.

86. Letty M. Russell (ed.), *The Church with AIDS: Renewal in the Midst of Crisis* (Louisville: John Knox Press, 1990).

87. Neville Richardson, 'A call for care: HIV/AIDS challenges the church'. *Journal of Theology for Southern Africa* 125(2006): 38–50.

88. De Lange, 'Confessing and embodying justice'.

89. Patricia L. Hoffman, *AIDS and the Sleeping Church* (Grand Rapids: Eerdmans, 1995).

90. Arnau van Wyngaard, 'Towards a theology of HIV/AIDS'. *Verbum et Ecclesia* 27(1) 2006: 265–90.

91. Cochrane, 'Of bodies, barriers, boundaries and bridges': 7.

92. Hansjörg Dilger, 'Healing the wounds of modernity: Salvation, community and care in a neo-Pentecostal church in Dar es Salaam, Tanzania'. *Journal of Religion in Africa – Religion en Afrique* 37(1) 2007: 59.

93. Pamela Leong, 'Religion, flesh, and blood: Re-creating religious culture in the context of HIV/AIDS'. *Sociology of Religion* 67(3) 2006: 295.

94. Fulata Moyo, 'When the telling itself is a taboo: The Phoebe practice'. *Journal for Constructive Theology* 9(2) 2003: 3–20; Fulata Moyo, 'Sex, gender, power and HIV/AIDS in Malawi'; Lilian Siwila, 'Care-giving in times of HIV and AIDS, when hospitality is a threat to African women's lives'; Kari Hartwig, 'Confronting religion, AIDS and gender in Tanzania: Church leaders at the crossroads'. *Journal of Constructive Theology* 12(2) 2006: 25–43.

95. Denise M. Ackermann, 'Tamar's cry: Re-reading an ancient text in the midst of an HIV and AIDS pandemic' in *Grant me justice!* edited by Dube and Kanyoro: 27–59.

96. Beverley Haddad, 'Reflections on the Church and HIV/AIDS'. *Theology Today* 62 (2005): 29–37; Beverley Haddad, 'Surviving the HIV and AIDS epidemic in South Africa: Women living and dying, theologising and being theologised'. *Journal of Theology for Southern Africa* 131 (2005): 47–57.

97. Esther Lubunga Kenge, 'The Doctrine of Social Holiness in the Free Methodist Church' (Masters dissertation, University of KwaZulu-Natal, 2007); Paula Clifford, *Theology and the HIV/AIDS Epidemic* (London: Christian Aid, 2004).

98. David R. Liefeld, *A Lutheran Response to AIDS: The Law Gospel Perspective* (Portland: Theological Research Exchange Network, 1992); Klaus Nürnberger, 'Theology of AIDS: A Lutheran/ Moravian case study'. *Scriptura* 81 (2002): 422–36; Georg Scriba, 'The 16th century plague and the present AIDS pandemic: A comparison of Martin Luther's reaction to the plague and the HIV/AIDS pandemic in southern Africa today'. *Journal of Theology for Southern Africa* 126 (2006): 66–80.

99. Montagu Murray, 'Lewenspeil, verlossing van sonde en MIV en VIGS in suider-Afrika: Gedagtes uit die gereformeerde tradisie'. *Hervormde Teologiese Studies* 61(4) 2005: 1299–320; Phillip Marshall, 'Toward a theology of HIV/AIDS'. *Evangelical Review of Theology* 29(2) 2005: 131–48; Danny Alan Bauer, 'Negotiating Cultural and Social Barriers Through Confrontation: The Textual Force of Liberation Theology and AIDS Rhetoric' (Ph.D. dissertation, New Mexico State University, 1997).

100. Laurenti Magesa, 'Taking culture seriously: Recognising the reality of African religion in Tanzania' in *Catholic Ethicists on HIV/AIDS Prevention*, edited by Keenan et al: 76–84.

101. Piet Naudé , '"It is your duty to be human": A few theological remarks amidst the HIV/ AIDS-crisis: The challenge of HIV/AIDS to Christian theology'. *Scriptura* 89 (2005): 433.

102. James Cochrane, *Circles of Dignity: Community Wisdom and Theological Reflection* (Augsburg: Fortress, 1999).

103. Khumbulani Hlongwana and Sibongile S. Mkhize, 'HIV/AIDS through the lens of Christianity: Perspectives from a South African urban support group'. *Journal of Social Aspects of HIV/AIDS* 4(1) 2007: 556.

104. Felicitas Becker and P. Wenzel Geissler, 'Introduction: Searching for pathways in a landscape of death: Religion and AIDS in East Africa'. *Journal of Religion in Africa – Religion en Afrique* 37(1) 2007: 1.

105. Denise M. Ackermann, 'Engaging stigma: An embodied theological response to HIV and AIDS: The challenge of HIV/AIDS to Christian theology'. *Scriptura* 89 (2005): 385–95.

106. Wendy S. Boring, John A. Geter and Stefano Penna, 'A maternal body and a body with AIDS: Theological reflections on carnal knowledge of the incarnate God'. *Theology and Sexuality* 10 (1999): 7–15.

107. Christina Landman, 'Religion as a means of preventing injury and promoting safety: Christian discourses on embodiment as safety discourses'. *African Safety Promotion* 5(2) 2007: 17.

108. Christina Landman, 'Theology for the older, female HIV-infected body'. *Exchange: Journal of Missiological and Ecumenical Research* 37(1) 2008: 52–67.

109. For example, James Alison, *Faith Beyond Resentment: Fragments Catholic and Gay* (London: Darton Longman and Todd, 2001).

110. Michael Clark, 'AIDS, death and God: Gay liberation theology and the problem of suffering'. *Journal of Pastoral Counselling* 22(1) 1986: 40–54; Ronald Long and Michael Clark, *AIDS, God, and Faith: Continuing the Dialogue on Constructing Gay Theology* (Las Colinas: Monument Press, 1992).

111. Heidi Epstein, 'Re-vamping the cross: Diamanda Galas's musical mnemonic of promiscuity'. *Theology and Sexuality* 15 (2001): 45.

112. Philip Hefner, 'The necessity for a theology of disease: Reflections on totalities and fragments'. *Zygon* 39(2) 2004: 487.

113. Gad Freudenthal, *AIDS in Jewish Thought and Law* (Hoboken: Ktav Publishing House, 1998); Azila Talit Reisenberger, 'South African Jewish women and HIV/AIDS' in *African Women, HIV/AIDS and Faith Communities*, edited by Phiri, Haddad and Masenya: 168–85.

114. Ann Boyd, Pinit Ratanakul and Attajenda Deepudong, 'Compassion as common good'. *Eubios: Journal of Asian and International Bioethics* 8 (1998): 34–7.

115. See, for example, Sipho Vitus Ncube, 'Towards a Theology of *Ukugula, Ukufa Nokuphumula Ngoxolo* (Sickness Unto Death and Rest in Peace) in Time of HIV-AIDS with a Special Reference to Zulu Concepts of *Ukubhula* (Divination) *Nokuthakatha* (Witchcraft)' (M.Th. dissertation, University of Natal, Pietermaritzburg, 2003); Gathogo, 'The use of ancestral resources in combating HIV and AIDS'; Augustine Musopole, *Spirituality, Sexuality and HIV/AIDS in Malawi: Theological Strategies for Behaviour Change* (Zomba: Kachere, 2007); Magesa, 'Taking culture seriously'.

116. See the overview in Ersilia Francesca, 'AIDS in contemporary Islamic ethical literature'. *Medicine and Law* 21(2) 2002: 381–94. Also see the discussion around the sacred texts of Islam and Christianity in Chapter 5 of this book.

117. Malik Badri, *The AIDS Crisis: An Islamic Sociocultural Perspective* (Kuala Lumpur: International Institute of Islamic Thought and Civilisation, 1997); Malik Badri, *The AIDS Crisis: A Natural Product of Modernity's Sexual Revolution* (Kuala Lumpur: Meedena Books, 3rd ed., 2007); Malik Badri, *AIDS Prevention: Failure in the North and Catastrophe in the South: A Solution* (Qualbert: Islamic Medical Association of South Africa, 2000).

118. See the overview in Ahmed Shams Madyan, 'Islamic institutions in Indonesia: failure of leadership in the fight against HIV'. *Nasir* 1(3) 2007.

119. See Ahmed Shams Madyan, 'Islamic Responses to HIV-AIDS: A Comparative Study on Malik Badri, Farid Esack and Indonesian Muslim Responses' (Dissertation, Gajah Mada University, Centre for Religious and Cross Cultural Studies in Indonesia, 2006).

120. Positive Muslims, *HIV, AIDS and Islam: Reflections Based on Compassion, Responsibility and Justice.* (Observatory: Positive Muslims, 2004).

121. Farid Esack and Sarah Chiddy, *Islam and AIDS: Between Scorn, Pity and Justice* (Oxford: Oneworld, 2009).

122. Steve de Gruchy, 'How then shall we be saved?: AIDS, community and redemption'. *Bulletin for Contextual Theology in Africa* 7(1) 2000: 18–20.

Practitioner response

Jan Bjarne Sødal

The chapter on the mapping of the terrain of systematic theology by Steve de Gruchy gives an excellent overview and analysis, identifies gaps in the literature and reflects on the inter-relatedness of issues and methodologies. This response arises primarily out of work with the One Body project[1] through which I have been exposed to church-related stigma and discrimination of people living with HIV. I shall briefly argue for some perspectives that seem to be missing from systematic theological reflection generally.

The published material arising out of the One Body project speaks about HIV and AIDS having 'become a mirror that reflects the injustice and inequalities, stigmatization and prejudices that already exist in society'.[2] For me, the epidemic also mirrors our theologies and enables us to see certain issues more clearly. De Gruchy's analysis begins a process whereby our theologies are being stripped of some of their destructive consequences.

Several of the particular issues that De Gruchy mentions, such as stigma and exclusion, disease and healing, gender, sexuality, suffering and hope emerge from what he calls the seamlessness of life. These issues point more and more to an area where too little has been done in relation to HIV; namely real theological work on anthropology. The HIV and AIDS epidemic is revealing all kinds of anthropologies actually lived out, acted upon and believed in within churches, acknowledged or not, with the Bible in our hands. The epidemic thus raises the question of what it means to be human.

In the material referred to in De Gruchy's chapter under the issue of sexuality, Michael Haspel argues 'that *starting* from biblical insight and *Christian anthropology* . . . a contextual theology addressing HIV/AIDS . . . and a respective sexual ethic have to be developed'.[3] Today's experience of HIV and AIDS has to inform, in the first instance, work on anthropology from a theological perspective. It is this prior reflection that can then give direction to theological work on other issues and to reading of the sacred texts.

The important question to ask in the HIV and AIDS context is: how do we understand human life in the light of creation and redemption? It is human life in all its complexity, lived out in vulnerable bodies, as women and men, faced with suffering and diseases, longing for healing, hope and life in all its fullness that needs to be addressed theologically. There is a danger that these different life-concerning issues are dealt with separately from one another. As a consequence, faith, lived experience, and what the church says and requires seem to contradict each other. Lived experience and the traditional teachings of the church become impossible to hold together.

Thus, deeper theological reflection is needed to understand life. We are created by God but where is all the complexity of life, full of contradictions, lived and experienced as it is individually and in community? This has to be listened to and taken into account. One of the major theological themes arising out of the workshop on stigma hosted by UNAIDS in 2003 is that of truth and truth telling.[4] Life needs to be spoken about truthfully.

Another aspect of reflecting on anthropology from a faith perspective is to take into account the multitude of life conditions, circumstances, expressions and situations. Man or woman, sick or healthy, disabled or not, straight or gay, adult or child – often people are valued differently according to who they are or their station in life. This reality has to be questioned in the light of the fact that people are, according to the Bible, created equally in the image of God.[5] This tenet of the Christian faith has important consequences for the way anthropology is reflected upon, and is an indictment against the stigmatisation and discrimination of those who are living with HIV.

Gender is an area where a Christian anthropology should have radical implications for the way men and women live. There is much excellent theological work on the power dynamics of gender relations, gender-based violence and harmful cultural practices, all of which are the practical consequences of gender inequality. However, Gillian Paterson pushes the discussion further as she sees gender injustices in relation to human value when she argues that the stigmatisation of women and girls implies a belief that they are in some way lesser human beings with fewer rights.[6] When the socialised gender roles of women and girls consistently mean a subordinate position, being submissive, not being respected, denied dignity – all of which open up the option of all forms of abuse – we are forced to rethink the nature of Christian anthropology. An area that has also not been addressed is the question of sexual orientation. More dynamic and constructive systematic theological work is needed on gender equality, sexual orientation and the deconstruction of roles that are not life-giving. It is this work that must continuously be in dialogue with, and critique other, aspects of reflection. This is to ensure that, first, there are no contradictions in thinking; and, second, that patriarchy and dominant masculinities, which are not helpful either in the private sphere of the family or in the public sphere of church leadership and life, are being addressed.

Sexuality is another area, highlighted by De Gruchy, of crucial importance to theological reflection. We are trapped between suggesting that sexuality is a gift from God (usually stated in abstract terms) and that sexuality is sinful. There is a need to be bolder in our attempts to understand sexuality theologically. This is a threatening, complicated, but yet attractive task. When dealing with HIV prevention there needs to be thorough engagement with issues of sexuality, including taboos, desire, lust, shame and sexual urges; and how these impact upon sexual encounters. But there is also a need to work on sexuality in relation to gender and power imbalances related to age and social status. Is sexuality a part of the *imagio dei*, the image of God? Or to put it differently, does sexuality and the physical union between two people have the potential to reflect the image of God in human beings? However, there is no freedom in a time of HIV and AIDS to discuss these questions openly while creating a moral climate of fear when focusing solely on abstinence and faithfulness. Often the enforcement of strict moral rules can produce the opposite effect and hamper attempts to discuss issues of sexuality in a healthy and open way.

This leads to the issue of sin, which De Gruchy also points out needs more theological work. Sin has in a damaging way been linked with sexuality and HIV, partly because of a lack of theological reflection, partly because of unhelpful theologies; or, in De Gruchy's words, bad theologies. These are disruptive as opposed to redemptive theologies, with the latter paralleling redemptive images of God. Disruptive theologies are not necessarily the result of a lack of theological resources or training. One can be well trained and practising theology at an academic level and still promote a theology that can make the lives of people living with HIV worse.

Douglas Hall has suggested that 'As long as the concept of sin is understood in moral and moralistic terms, it can only be a negative influence in our dealing with AIDS, and nearly everything else! It has to be understood ontologically, as broken relationship or relatedness, alienation, estrangement' from God, one another, the other, and the rest of creation.[7] In this understanding there is an essential belonging and relatedness within creation. Sin breaks this relatedness. It is destructive and it makes life worse for individuals, for communities, for humanity, and for the whole of creation.

Finally, De Gruchy mentions the lack of theological training in relation to HIV, which has resulted in work being done on developing curricula and resources for theological educational institutions. While this has been important, there is still an urgent need for theological resources developed for people who are working in local churches in lay leadership positions. These would include accessible and popular versions of sound and well-reflected theology in printed form and material to be used in training situations. Many are looking for ways to respond differently and positively to the epidemic but they just do not know how. But as De Gruchy suggests, people at the grassroots should not only be on the receiving end. There is an urgent challenge to move into a new and radical methodology that takes into account the theological reflection of both trained and grassroots theologians. There is a need to explore and develop 'the dialogical space between the emerging theologies from below and the academy', as De Gruchy suggests. But it is misleading to speak about theology with a big 'T' when referring to theology from the academy. I would argue that all theologies are theologies with a small 't'. All are poor attempts to grasp the truth that can never be fully formulated in words. If anything, this is the lesson we are learning through the crisis of the HIV epidemic.

Notes

1. The One Body project brings together FOCCISA and the Nordic European countries to fight stigma and discrimination in churches towards people living with HIV.
2. Elizabeth Knox-Seith, *One Body: Volume 1*: 5.
3. Michael Haspel, 'Christian sexual ethics in a time of HIV/AIDS: 480; author's emphasis.
4. UNAIDS. *A Report of a Theological Workshop Focusing on HIV- and AIDS-related Stigma*: 16.
5. Genesis 1:27.
6. See Chapter 14 by Gillian Paterson in this book.
7. Personal conversation with Douglas Hall, Sep. 2008.

Comparative ethics and HIV and AIDS
Interrogating the gaps

Domoka Lucinda Manda

INTRODUCTION

This chapter presents an analysis based on a survey of extant literature on comparative religious ethics and HIV and AIDS. A wide variety of literature exists in the field of religion and theology dealing with the issue of HIV and AIDS. From an ethical point of view, the focus is on sexual morality and ethics as prescribed by the major religions of the world. Despite the diversity in their teachings and practice, a common denominator can be distinguished in the early religious literature on the epidemic; namely that HIV and AIDS is a punishment from God and the only way to deal with the epidemic is to return to the moral way of life prescribed by the teachings of the major religions. However, more recently there has been a growing body of literature that attempts to probe and reflect theologically on approaches to HIV and AIDS in a way that seeks to emphasise life-promoting and life-affirming values. The guiding ethical values in this body of literature focus on relationality, inclusivity, love, care and compassion; and demonstrate an attempt on the part of world religions to remain contextually relevant. However, gaps in the published literature do exist and it is these that are identified in this chapter in order to point to a future research agenda on HIV and AIDS from an ethical perspective.

The first section deals with a survey of the literature on HIV and AIDS from the perspective of sexual morality and ethics. Common themes in religious literature on HIV and AIDS and ethics are noted. The second section pays attention to literature that offers theological reflection on various ethical responses to the epidemic, especially relating to treatment of people living with HIV. The third section provides suggestions to guide further research in the area of HIV and AIDS and comparative ethics.

EARLY RELIGIOUS ETHICAL DISCOURSE ON HIV AND AIDS

Discussion on religious ethics 'is often conducted by reference to moral rules which prohibit or mandate the performance of certain types of action'.[1] The major religions of the world have tended to adopt a rule-based approach in their attempts to provide ethical solutions to moral problems. Often the solution to moral challenges is a call to return to traditional religious values as prescribed (and interpreted) in the sacred texts. Thus, early ethical literature on HIV and AIDS written from a religious perspective initially focused almost solely on sexual morality and ethics. This focus was, arguably, influenced by early medical literature on HIV and AIDS, which stressed AIDS as a gay disease because many of the first reported cases were from within the gay community. As reports of HIV infection began to spread across the sexual-orientation divide, other explanations were sought. As a result, two recurring explanations are found in religious discourse on HIV and AIDS in the early period of the epidemic. The first stated that HIV and AIDS was a consequence of improper lifestyle and immoral sexual behaviour. The second stated that HIV and AIDS was a form of punishment from God or Allah. Throughout this discourse, notions of sin as a punishment for homosexuality continued to lurk in the background.

In essence, the literature moralised the epidemic with blame being accorded to those who were infected with HIV. As Loretta Kopelman points out: 'From the earliest awareness of HIV and AIDS, people, including patients, have viewed this disease as punishment for sin.' This, says Kopelman, created a 'punishment theory of disease' in which 'illness is divine punishment; it is inflicted on human beings for an offence, to give them a chance for rehabilitation, to warn them to become more virtuous, to demonstrate that the bad perish and the good thrive, or to show that some cosmic order requires the punishment of sin'.[2]

Similar sentiments are echoed in Islamic ethical literature on HIV and AIDS because according to a number of Muslim scholars, 'AIDS is a warning from God not to indulge in illicit conduct'.[3] As Ersilia Francesca notes:

Muslim ethical literature considers homosexual and extramarital relations as primary reasons for the spread of AIDS as well as contaminated syringes used by drug addicts. It is eager to prove that the illness is a direct consequence of the sexual promiscuity and perverted sexual contacts prevalent in Europe and America, and that the illness would not have existed in Muslim countries had the people not indulged in behaviour condemned by Islam.[4]

Malik Babikir Badri strongly endorses the view that HIV and AIDS in the Muslim world is a result of sexual immorality in the form of homosexual sex.[5] The problem has arisen, as Badri sees it, because of the appropriation of Western liberal sexual mores. His position on the issue of HIV and AIDS in the Muslim world is to condemn and chastise those who are infected. He outlines some Islamic principles governing sex and sexuality, the prohibition of homosexuality and the use of drugs and argues that:

> Regardless of where the Muslim AIDS activist or medical practitioner may find him or herself, any program that he or she engages in should not adopt an ethically non-judgmental attitude or stand which condones, or does not point out the immoral aspects of promiscuity, homosexuality, and drug and alcohol intake.[6]

Such explanations, as Kabir Sanjay Bavikatte states, 'view AIDS only in light of sexual morality and divine reprimand; even the innocent are part of God's larger plan of punishment. The operating equation is that sexual immorality causes punishment and suffering.' In essence:

> There are two recurring themes that have permeated orthodox Islamic discourse on AIDS since the early 1980s: AIDS is a curse from God to punish those who are engaged in immoral sexual behaviour; and the only way to deal effectively with the AIDS epidemic is to return to the moral way of life prescribed in the Qur'an as interpreted by Islamic orthodoxy.[7]

In short, an analysis of early Christian and Islamic ethical literature on HIV and AIDS demonstrates that the primary focus is on moralising the HIV epidemic and ascribing blame to those infected. As Charles Nzoika writes, HIV infection is 'seen as a form of punishment for behaviour that breaks social rules and moral judgment is passed through stereotyped beliefs regardless of the circumstances that lead to infection'.[8] HIV and AIDS was perceived as a shameful disease, which in turn led to stigma and discrimination.

In Hindu literature, the explanation that HIV and AIDS is a punishment from God is not that apparent. Instead, there is an emphasis on the behaviour of the individual. Varadaraja Raman suggests that according to Hinduism, not all diseases that afflict humankind are a result of some higher power but can be the result of humankind's own weakness. It thus follows that HIV infection is 'quite clearly a direct consequence of our excesses and transgressions'.[9] Therefore, the epidemic is a direct result of the inability of human beings to repress their carnal desires, especially in relation to sexual activities. So, although Hinduism does not seem to attribute HIV and AIDS directly to God as with early Islamic and Christian religious expressions on the subject, Hinduism does understand the epidemic as a direct consequence of improper sexual behaviour. Interestingly, Jewish scholar Norbert M. Samuelson condemns such causal links between homosexuality, sexual promiscuity and HIV and notes, 'even if there was a causal link between homosexuality and AIDS, the suggestion that the disease is a punishment for homosexuality is insidious, an example of "stupid" religion that is unrepresentative of the qualitatively best of Jewish (as well as Christian) theology'.[10]

The moral emphasis within early religious literature on HIV and AIDS has led to a theology of the damned that generates shame, guilt and blame towards people who are HIV positive. The world religions sent a moral message that reinforced the primacy of heterosexual, monogamous sexual relationships. As Philippe Denis notes: 'This message [. . .] appeal[s] to personal responsibility of the sexually active people to arrest the spread of the epidemic.'[11] However, it ignores the fact that most sexual relations today tend to take place outside the confines of the institution of marriage. Consequently, this traditional and conservative religious discourse has, in my view, failed to engage the complexity of the epidemic critically.

SHIFT FROM MORALISING TO AN ETHIC OF LIFE

Recently, there has been an increasing emphasis in the literature on ethical frameworks that promote and protect human life. Religious and global values that give birth to ethical principles and approaches that are life-giving and life-affirming are embraced and promoted. Emmanuel Katongole thus argues that the purpose of ethical discussion and reflection is in order for human beings to better 'understand ourselves and the sort of people we become as we make particular decisions and choices, even as these are responses to crises, anxieties, tensions within our everyday life struggles'.[12]

Armin Zimmerman argues for a shift in traditional sexual ethics to find new but authentic Christian responses to the challenges HIV and AIDS present. He discusses how the Christian Church should first alter its traditional view of sex as an act of procreation and rather see it as an expression of love; and, second, it should accept the reality that people will engage in sexual activity outside the confines of marriage. Thus, there should be the development of a new Christian sexual ethic that focuses not only on promoting safe sex but also on promoting values such as reciprocity, mutuality, respect, love, fidelity, trust and equality between the sexes. He concludes that when sex is understood as a loving activity that is based on these values, people will learn to behave responsibly towards each other.[13]

The meaning of behaving responsibly and promoting life is exemplified in the ongoing religious ethical reflection on the promotion of condom use. Zimmerman explores the church's position on condom use and challenges the traditional conservative approach, which states that 'it promotes promiscuity because it makes casual sex safer, or that it even creates the impression that the churches accept promiscuity'. He believes that from an ethical perspective, the church is obligated to preserve life. In the context of HIV and AIDS, promoting the use of condoms indicates that the church is fulfilling this role and, he argues, not to do so would be unethical.[14]

Mfutso-Bengo et al. argue that a risk-benefit analysis of the promotion of condom use in the context of HIV and AIDS is a challenge to religious institutions. Promoting abstinence and faithfulness, they argue, is not enough and there is case to be made for promoting condom use on the ethical grounds of 'choosing the lesser of two evils'.[15] Katongole also argues that the moral argument against condom use is no longer sufficient, especially in Africa where poverty and despair is a breeding ground for 'playful nihilism' and 'cynicism' because death through war and famine, let alone HIV and AIDS, is so prevalent. Given this context, a multi-dimensional approach to HIV prevention is necessary, including the use of condoms.[16]

It is African women scholars who have argued that deconstructing notions of gender is crucial for a multi-dimensional approach and call for a feminist ethical response. Teresia Mbari Hinga examines some of the ecclesiological and theological challenges within religion, especially as they affect women. She notes how, for instance, the hierarchical nature of religion and the theologies of marriage reinforce patriarchy and the submission of women. These theologies disempower women and deny them their moral agency. One appropriate ethical response to the epidemic, argues Hinga, is for religion to endorse and practise equality. Embracing the principle of equality would require a religious and theological response that places women at the centre of church life in order to transform society.[17]

Advocating equality is also emphasised by Denise Ackermann.[18] The continued inequality and inequity faced by women in society prompts her to ask how a Christian feminist ethic can assist the church in dealing with the epidemic in her midst. Her response to this question is based on a discussion on the significance and meaning attached to being the Body of Christ and the celebration of the Eucharist:

> The celebration of the Eucharist makes the Reign of God present to us in the form of Christ's body broken 'for us' and Christ's blood shed 'for us'. Christ invites us to the feast, and He is both the giver of the feast and the gift itself. In other words, the gift of the Reign of God is quite simply present in the person of Christ himself – Christ crucified and risen. Thus the communion meal mediates communion and true-life-giving relationship with the crucified one in the presence of the risen one. It becomes a foretaste of the messianic banquet of all human kind. It is the meal at which the bodies of all are welcome. In Christ's Body, the Eucharist is the sacrament of equality. Only self-exclusion can keep one away. At the communion table we are offered the consummate step in forging an ethic of right relationship, across our differences. 'We who are many are one body for we all partake of the one bread'. This visible, unifying, bodily practice of relationship with all its potential for healing is ours.[19]

Given that the church today is infected with HIV, Ackermann proposes the development of an ethic of resistance and affirmation based on 'the belief that the human person has inviolable worth that must be affirmed in the human community in actions of love and justice'.[20] The application of an ethic of resistance and affirmation results in upholding values such as dignity and respect for persons.

A further theo-ethical theme addressed in religious literature focusing on an ethic of life is that of the call for care, compassion and community. This is predicated on the idea of promoting common good. Neville Richardson reflects theologically on the moral obligation of Christians to respond to people living with HIV with love, compassion and care. Richardson embraces the idea that members of the church are part of a community, echoing Ackermann, as they gather to participate in worship and Eucharistic celebrations. Communal worship should be instrumental in challenging Christians to take responsibility for those in need, pain and suffering, not least those who are HIV positive.[21] Ronald Nicolson's seminal early work also raises the notion of an ethic of community. He suggests that the appropriate ethical response for Christians is to assist in caring for people living with HIV and a failure to do so would be a failure to love.[22]

An emphasis on community is also reflected in the writings of scholars of African Traditional Religion. Munyaradzi Felix Murove, an African ethicist, has written on the relationality that stems from an awareness of our common existence. He argues that the Shona concept of *ukama* (relationality) implies 'living virtuously in relationship with others in the community as well as in relationship with the ancestors'. This is similar to the ethic of *ubuntu*, which is based on humanness. Murove suggests that we take the concept of *ukama* and prefix *ubuntu*: 'we end up with a phrase – *ukama ubuntu* so as to imply that our humanness is indispensable from our relationality'. The ethical implication that arises is the moral obligation to care, because 'to be fully human is to belong to a wider community of existence'.[23] I have made a similar case for the African ethic of *ubuntu* in the promotion of women's health and well-being.[24] However, it must be noted that a number of African women theologians have criticised the ethic of *ubuntu*. They have argued that it is a harmful cultural resource that reinforces patriarchy and disempowers and denies women their moral agency by hindering their autonomy and independence. This is especially so when it comes to when and how sex takes place. For example, Fulata Moyo states that in traditional African life women are placed in a subordinate position because traditional African culture affirms and safeguards the power of men. In her view, African culture explicitly supports hierarchy, because men are respected as the head of the house and, because of this, husbands do not take into consideration women's dignity. She argues that *ubuntu*, as a cultural practice, reinforces the subordination of women because it is inherently hierarchical in nature – for instance, over respect for elders and ancestors. In her view *ubuntu* as an ethical concept cannot adequately address health issues facing African women.[25]

Ezra Chitando also analyses the phrase 'I am because we are', which embodies the concept of *ubuntu*. He, as with some women scholars, has reservations about the use of an *ubuntu* ethic and prefers to use the term solidarity.[26] He argues that solidarity can be used 'as a helpful resource for empowering men to adopt safer sexual practices, increase participation in caregiving and help to overcome stigma and discrimination'. Solidarity, as defined by Chitando, implies 'standing for, and standing with "the Other"'. According to Chitando, solidarity moves beyond the philosophy of *ubuntu* because 'most African philosophical reflections do not grapple with oppressive masculinities that lie behind these impressive concepts'. To illustrate his point he asks:

> How has it been possible for many African men to proclaim 'I am, because we are' and then proceed to engage in risky sexual behaviour in the context of HIV and AIDS? Or, to proclaim 'I am, because we are' and yet leave all the care-giving responsibilities of people living with AIDS to women?[27]

Thus, ethical discussions on relationality and humanness need to be addressed within the framework of justice leading to solidarity.

BEYOND COMPASSION TOWARDS THEOLOGIES OF JUSTICE

Reflection that moves beyond care and compassion to a focus on justice is an important task for religious scholars. The need to move away from compassion as an area of theo-ethical reflection is partly motivated by the associated negative connotations, such as pity. All too often, those that exercise compassion tend to do so from a position of superiority which, according to Farid Esack and Sarah Chiddy, 'ignores the heart of what makes us human: agency, the ability to take charge of and control our own lives'. They go on to add that 'compassion must simultaneously construct a discourse both of agency and of the rights of HIV positive persons'.[28]

In Islamic theo-ethical literature care and compassion are two recurring themes. In the context of HIV and AIDS, caring from Islamic perspectives requires that Muslims do not discriminate and judge harshly individuals who are HIV positive. Ethically speaking, this means that Muslims ought to exercise mercy and compassion towards those living with HIV despite their beliefs, race, ethnic affiliations, social status and wealth.[29] Numerous publications in Islamic studies demonstrate that ethical reflection is taking place as many Muslim scholars are beginning to appraise critically the sacred and legal sources in the light of the challenges the HIV and AIDS epidemic continues to present. In other words, a more contextual approach to Islam is being adopted in regard to how, for example, Shari'ah law and the Qur'an can contribute to the development of Islamic ethical principles, guidelines and approaches to a number of issues, such as access to health care and treatment, gender and poverty in the context of HIV and AIDS.

Mohammad Hashim Kamali discusses how Shari'ah law can contribute to the ethical discourse on HIV and AIDS.[30] He argues that there are general principles and guidelines in Islamic law with ethical implications that can be used to develop a theology and ethic of compassion. He identifies the principles of *darurah* (necessity) and *darar* (harm) and argues that in relation to HIV and AIDS, efforts towards eliminating harm that threatens the essential well-being of human life (illness caused by HIV) are a necessary moral obligation.[31] This theme of compassion is also developed by Kabir Sanjay Bavikatte. He tackles the issue of global structural injustices in the form of inequality between the rich and poor, between the developing and developed world, and between race and sex.[32] He attempts to develop an Islamic perspective on justice in the context of HIV and AIDS that is underscored by a theology of compassion. A central objective of his article is to begin to develop an Islamic liberation theology that seeks to apply to the epidemic Qur'anic precepts that oppose injustice.

A Qur'anic theology of liberation is also articulated by Laura McTighe. She offers insights into how the Qur'an can provide crucial ethical guidance needed for the construction and articulation of a sound liberation theology in the context of HIV and AIDS. She notes how the concepts of *tawhid*, *taqwa* (a consciousness of God), *al-nas* (humankind) and *mustad'afun* (the marginalised and oppressed) can be effectively applied to the guidance of social behaviour and action. The ethical implication of placing HIV and AIDS within the framework of *tawhid*, *taqwa*, *al-nas* and *mustad'afun* means that it is the moral responsibility of a Muslim who aims to pursue Allah's call for unity, piety and justice to stand in solidarity with those who are marginalised and oppressed by offering protection to the vulnerable.[33]

Scholars from other religious traditions have also attempted to provide theo-ethical reflection on the HIV and AIDS epidemic from a justice perspective. Mary E. Hunt emphasises the value of justice through an analysis of the positive and negative aspects of globalisation. She argues that one of the negative consequences of globalisation is that wealthy nations benefit more, while poor impoverished and resource-strapped nations continue to struggle to survive. In this context, Hunt suggests broadening religious ethical focus by confronting contemporary capitalism. This means making a stronger call for justice in the distribution of resources such as anti-retroviral treatment (ART). The confrontation of capitalism also raises ethical questions around profit making and corporate greed as exhibited by pharmaceutical companies who fail to exercise their moral responsibilities or obligations to those who are desperately ill and cannot afford ART.[34] Joseph Gaie also addresses this issue with reference to corporate responsibility and argues that it is the moral responsibility of companies to keep prices of medication low in their duty to alleviate pain, suffering and early death. He applies the Setswana concept of *botho* to argue that the corporate world has a responsibility to put human well-being above profit in dealing with the HIV and AIDS epidemic.[35]

CONCLUSION

In concluding this analytical review of the extant literature on religious ethics and HIV and AIDS, some observations are warranted. First, it is apparent that religious communities place much emphasis on serving the communities within which they operate. In the context of HIV and AIDS, this service is rendered largely through the provision of care and compassion. Providing care and exercising compassion are important values for Christian, Muslim, Hindu, Jewish and African religious life because they are inherent to what it means to be a good human being. Second, it has also been argued that an appropriate theo-ethical framework for the HIV and AIDS context needs to move beyond the care and compassion context to one of justice. While there are scholars who deal with the issue of justice, further ethical reflection from a religious perspective is required. Furthermore, I would also like to note that this review is dominated by the Christian discourse on HIV and AIDS. While the Islamic scholarly voice is beginning to make its presence felt, unfortunately voices from the Hindu, Jewish and African Traditional Religions are not strong. Finally, this critical review of the theo-ethical literature on HIV and AIDS suggests that reflection largely remains at the level of theory. There has been almost no reflection on our moral obligation to those who are HIV positive, nor on how those living with HIV are ethically engaging the epidemic. As we move into these areas of research, we might discover that we still have a great deal to learn.

NOTES

1. Baruch Brody, 'Religion and bioethics' in *A Companion to Bioethics*, edited by Helga Kuhse and Peter Singer (Oxford: Blackwell, 2001): 41.
2. Loretta Kopelman, 'If HIV and AIDS is punishment, who is bad?' in *Ethics and AIDS in Africa: The Challenge to Our Thinking*, edited by Anton A. van Niekerk and Loretta Kopelman, (Walnut Creek: Left Coast Press, 2008): 208, 210.
3. Ersilia Francesca, 'AIDS in contemporary Islamic ethical literature'. *Medicine and Law* 21 (2002): 381. Also see Kabir Sanjay Bavikatte, 'Muslims, AIDS, and justice: Beyond personal indictment' in *Islam and AIDS: Between Scorn, Pity and Justice*, edited by Farid Esack and Sarah Chiddy (Oxford: Oneworld, 2009): 186–95.
4. Francesca, 'AIDS in contemporary Islamic ethical literature': 383.
5. Malik Babikir Badri, *The AIDS Crisis: A Natural Product of Modernity's Sexual Revolution* (Kuala Lumpur: Medina Books, 3rd ed., 2000).
6. Malik Babikir Badri, 'The AIDS crisis: An Islamic perspective' in *Islam and AIDS*, edited by Esack and Chiddy: 30–1.
7. Kabir Sanjay Bavikatte, 'Muslims, AIDS, and justice': 186, 188.
8. Charles Nzoika, 'The social meanings of death from HIV and AIDS: An African interpretative view'. *Culture, Health and Sexuality* 2(1) 2000: 5.
9. Varadaraja Raman, 'Some Hindu insights on a global ethic in the context of diseases and epidemics'. *Zygon*, 39(1) 2003: 144.
10. Norbert M. Samuelson, 'Ethics of globalization and the AIDS crisis from a Jewish perspective'. *Zygon*. 38(1) 2003: 131.
11. Philippe Denis, 'Sexuality and AIDS in South Africa'. *Journal of Theology for Southern Africa* 115 (2003): 72.
12. Emmanuel Katangole, 'Christian ethics and AIDS in Africa today: Exploring the limits of a culture of suspicion and despair'. *Missionalia* 29(2) 2001: 145.
13. Armin Zimmerman, 'Towards a new Christian sexual ethic in the light of HIV/AIDS'. *International Review of Mission* 93(255) 2004: 267.
14. Zimmerman, 'Towards a new Christian sexual ethic': 267.
15. Joseph-Matthew Mfutso-Bengo, Eva-Maria Mfutso-Bengo and Francis Masiye, 'Ethical aspects of HIV/AIDS prevention strategies and control in Malawi'. *Theoretical Medicine and Bioethics* 29(5) 2008: 350.
16. Katongole, 'Christian ethics and AIDS in Africa today': 145.
17. Teresia Mbari Hinga, 'AIDS, religion and women in Africa: Theo-ethical challenges and imperatives' in *Women, Religion and HIV/AIDS in Africa: Responding to Ethical and Theological Challenges*, edited by Teresia M. Hinga et al. (Pietermaritzburg: Cluster Publications, 2008): 89, 90–3.
18. Denise Ackermann, 'Deep in the flesh: Women, bodies and HIV/AIDS: A feminist ethical perspective' in *Women, Religion and HIV/AIDS in Africa*, edited by Hinga et al.: 105–25.
19. Ackermann, 'Deep in the flesh': 121–2.
20. Ackermann, 'Deep in the flesh': 114.
21. Neville Richardson, 'A call for care: HIV and AIDS challenges the Church'. *Journal of Theology for Southern Africa* 125 (2006): 43, 45.

22. Ronald Nicolson, *AIDS: A Christian Response* (Pietermaritzburg: Cluster Publications, 1995): 18.

23. Munyaradzi Felix Murove, 'The empirical contradiction of globalisation: A quest for a relational ethical paradigm'. *Journal of Theology for Southern Africa* 121 (2005): 16.

24. Domoka L. Manda, 'The Importance of the African Ethic of Ubuntu and Africa's Traditional Healing Systems in Black South African Women's Health in the Context of HIV and AIDS' (Unpublished thesis, Pietermaritzburg: University of KwaZulu-Natal, 2008). Also see Sophia Chirongoma and Domoka L. Manda, '*Ubuntu* and women's health agency in contemporary South Africa' in *From Our Side: Emerging Perspectives on Development and Ethics*, edited by Steve de Gruchy, Nico Koopman and Sytse Strijbos (Amsterdam: Rozenburg, 2008): 189–208.

25. Fulata L. Moyo, 'Sex, gender, power and HIV/AIDS in Malawi: Threats and challenges to women' in *On Being Church: African Women's Voices and Visions*, edited by Isabel A. Phiri and Sarojini Nadar (Geneva: World Council of Churches, 2005): 130.

26. For a fuller discussion, see Chapters 9 and 11 of this book.

27. Ezra Chitando, 'Religious ethics, HIV and AIDS and masculinities in southern Africa' in *Persons in Community: African Ethics in a Global Culture*, edited by Ronald Nicolson (Pietermaritzburg: University of KwaZulu-Natal Press, 2008): 56, 57, 60.

28. Esack and Chiddy, *Islam and AIDS*: 6.

29. See G. Hussein Rassool, 'The crescent and Islam: Healing, nursing and the spiritual dimension: Some considerations towards an understanding of the Islamic perspectives on caring'. *Journal of Advanced Nursing* 32(6) 2000: 1476–84.

30. Mohammad Hashim Kamali, 'The Shari'ah and AIDS: Towards a theology of compassion' in *Islam and AIDS*, edited by Esack and Chiddy: 76–87. See also, Kate Henley Long, 'On sex, sin and silence: An Islamic theology of storytelling for AIDS awareness' in *Islam and AIDS*, edited by Esack and Chiddy: 154–68.

31. Kamali, 'The Shari'ah and AIDS': 76–86.

32. Bavikatte, 'Muslims, AIDS and justice': 186–95.

33. Laura McTighe, 'HIV, addiction, and justice: Toward a Qur'anic theology of liberation' in *Islam and AIDS*, edited by Esack and Chiddy: 215–16.

34. Mary E. Hunt, 'Globalisation and its discontents'. *Zygon* 39(2): 475–6.

35. Joseph B.R. Gaie, 'Moral issues and responsibilities regarding HIV/AIDS'. *Missionalia* 30(2) 2002: 283.

Practitioner response

Farid Esack

This response attempts to carry out three inter-related tasks: to comment on the chapter by Domoka Lucinda Manda; to do so from within my own context and experience; and to offer an alternative to the dominant Muslim response to HIV and AIDS – one rooted in compassion and justice. I am responding to Manda's chapter as an engaged scholar of Islam in general and, more specifically, in terms of its relationship to AIDS and people living with HIV. My broader terrains of engagement span the HIV and AIDS epidemic, Palestine solidarity, and environmental and gender justice. All of these shape the questions that accompany me in my wrestling with the Qur'an, which at times inspires and sustains me and at other times frustrates me. The immediate context in which this wrestling takes place is a Cape Town-based organisation, Positive Muslims, that I co-founded with Faghmeda Miller and Kayum Ahmad.[1] From this organisational base I observe and research Muslim responses to the epidemic and, as a progressive scholar of Islam, try to find and articulate alternative liberative responses to HIV and AIDS.

Manda's chapter is insightful, scholarly and engaging. From my own research I believe that the trajectory of the development of Muslim literature on HIV and AIDS largely follows the same pattern observed by her: from ignoring the disease to placing it entirely within a framework of moral ethics and then, as Manda points out, a morality confined to sexual moralism. The difficulty in locating material about Islam is due to the fact that the amount of literature dealing with Christianity is vastly greater than that dealing with Islam, or any other religion for that matter. Within the extant literature, I still want to note that Muslim literature in general takes a less charitable view of persons living with HIV than does Christian literature.

Despite the commonality between Muslims and Christians in this trajectory, it is crucial to understand an additional dimension to the way in which Muslims respond to the epidemic and the suspicion of those who do want to intervene from an ethical or human rights perspective. There is a larger context in which Muslims are responding to the epidemic. This is a context of globalisation; war; economic exploitation; invasion and occupation, sometimes manifesting itself in more crude ways such as military invasions and at other times through globalised culture popularised through transnational corporations such as McDonalds and Coca-Cola. This culture results in a general, guarded defensiveness towards everything viewed as Western. Those responding to the epidemic from human rights, sexual justice or gender justice approaches are then viewed as Trojan horses in a larger project to civilise the Muslim barbarian who dares to resist the empire. Given this context, it is necessary to observe that Muslim literature on HIV and AIDS follows a trajectory of ignorance, indifference, silence, scorn and pity.

In general Muslim literature on ethics, even more recent work, does not refer to HIV and AIDS at all. In some ways this reflects a lack of awareness of prevalence in the Muslim community, and in others it reflects conscious indifference. This arises out of a perception that speaking about the demon may cause it to come alive, while pretending it is not there will make it disappear.

When HIV and AIDS is mentioned, it is mostly presented as the justified price of sin. This is exemplified in the work of Malik Badri who refers to HIV as 'an angelic virus sent by God in the same way that angels were sent before time to destroy sinful communities'.[2] A third and growing response is a move away from simply pitying the AIDS sufferer to a more genuine empathy with the innocent victim, as well as a more reluctant pity for those who got what they deserved but who nevertheless need support.

However, it is necessary to move beyond pity. The dominant assumptions of narrow religious moralism and the perception of people on the margins of society as mere recipients of scorn or pity can, and should, be addressed. The challenge that emerges from the reality of HIV among Muslims is to develop an approach to Islam that takes the epidemic seriously and affirms the full humanity of all those living with the virus. The challenge is not only one of affirming the humanity of the HIV positive other but to do so in the awareness that one is doing so for oneself as an affirmation of one's own humanity. Furthermore, such compassion – literally one feeling or one pain – must simultaneously construct a discourse of agency and human rights for those Muslims who are HIV positive. Mere appeal for mercy and compassion towards the sick or diseased other is itself dehumanising for this simply transforms objects of medical surveillance (classification, examination, treatment, statistics and so on) into objects of theological surveillance (who plead mercy for the sins of the body almost as if the bearing of the disease is a public confession that, once made, will entitle the sufferer to public compassion).

A number of Muslims engaged in HIV intervention work now speak of a theology of compassion, a term first used in the literature of Positive Muslims in 2000 and subsequently in the material of the Malaysian AIDS Council.[3] Along with a growing awareness of the epidemic in the last few years, there has also been a marked increase in the number of Muslim voices arguing for a compassionate approach to those living with HIV. The most significant indication of the emergence of such an approach was the broad consensus reached at a United Nations Development Programme (UNDP) conference of religious leaders held in Cairo in 2004. The conference, with the theme 'Compassion in Action', issued a statement declaring that 'illness is one of God's tests; anyone may be afflicted by it according to God's sovereign choice.'[4] In our work within Positive Muslims, we have tried to underline the idea that while compassion is one of those innocent-sounding words, it is fairly consequential: the challenge to own the pain of another. For Muslims, compassion is not, or rather ought not to be, mere charity but also a profoundly theological concern. Given that each person is a carrier of the divine spirit infused in his or her being at the time of creation (Qur'an 15:29), there is 'that of God' in each one of us, and much of life ought to be about actualising this divine spirit. God is compassionate and if we are required to, in the words of the Prophet Muhammad, 'pattern ourselves on the character of God', then we must become compassionate and recognise the sacredness of self and other.

A theology of compassion and justice must also make the connections between compassion, on the one hand, and power, or more appropriately, a lack of, on the other. HIV is not an isolated entity. The epidemic is just as much about a crisis and collapse of all social security structures in society as it is about a crisis of the immune system in the body. In many ways, the actual illness is one tragic symptom of the major injustices of the world, particularly the growing gap between the rich and the poor. The context of our struggle to bring dignity to those living with HIV is part of a larger one where the obscured connections between disease and socio-economic conditions and processes are interrogated. A key question is thus: How do we work with those living with HIV to ensure that they remain or become the bearers of rights and conscious agents of change? Persons who are HIV positive are not victims who fell off the moral radar but persons effectively marginalised by structures of oppression around them.

We do not want to encourage a call for action on the basis of fear of a particular disease but out of concern for the way things stand in this world. We do want to encourage healthy practices in people but also ask for support for those who do not have the ability to freely make those choices in their lives. Our argument is not that people are dying and we could be next. Our argument, rather, is that people are living in ways in which they should not be forced to live and, as human beings, it is our duty to see to it that this situation changes. Most of the views expressed concerning Islam, Muslims and AIDS suggest that homosexuals, adulterers and fornicators who, influenced by the West, have neglected their faith (*din*) are now paying the price for their wayward ways. The return-to-faith solution ignores the impact of structural violence due to inequality and the lack of access to resources and when these issues are unaddressed, even the most fervent Islamic exhortations will still be of limited value.

An Islamic perspective on the HIV epidemic is not synonymous with adopting a religion or culture-specific approach. Addressing the question of religion and HIV makes no assumptions about an exclusive religious role. It is not being suggested that the answer lies solely in religion or in a behaviourist model of intervention that most religious organisations offer. The path of exclusive options, either scientific or religious interventions, is long since discredited. Only a multi-faceted approach to disease and wellness that incorporates both personal transformation and socio-economic justice will offer humankind some hope in the face of this crisis, as well as future ones.

Notes

1. See history of Positive Muslims at www.positivemuslims.org.za.
2. Badri, *The AIDS Crisis*: 128.

3. Abdul Kayum Ahmad, 'Developing a theology of compassion: Muslim attitudes towards people living with HIV' (2000). Available at http://web.uct.ac.za/depts/religion/documents/ARISA/2000_G_Kayum.pdf (accessed 20 Nov. 2009); Farid Esack, *Muslims Mapping AIDS: Mapping Muslim Organisational and Religious Responses* (Geneva: UNAIDS Positive Muslims, 2007): 38.

4. United Nations Development Programme, 'The Cairo Declaration of religious leaders in the Arab States in response to the HIV/AIDS epidemic, 23-12-2004' (Cairo: UNDP HIV/AIDS Regional Programme in the Arab States, 2005). Available at www.harpas.org/temp/Cairo%20Declaration_English.pdf (accessed 14 Dec. 2009).

8

Missiology and HIV and AIDS

Defining the contours

Ute Hedrich

INTRODUCTION

Although Christian mission is an old activity, missiology as a discipline is a relatively new field within Christian theology:

> The Protestant and Catholic 'awakening to world mission' since the end of the eighteenth century constitutes the historical background of the beginnings of missiology, founded as a branch of theology in the Protestant church in the nineteenth century and in the Catholic Church in the first half of the twentieth century.[1]

Some university faculties have departments of missiology, while others neglect or reject the study of missiology due to linkages between Christian mission and colonialism. But despite some critics, missiology has been established as a subject within theological disciplines, particularly in the northern hemisphere. It was the landmark work of David Bosch from South Africa that led others to question the shape of an African missiological perspective.[2] In fact, it was a missiological society from the southern hemisphere, the Southern African Missiological Society (SAMS) that offered the first missiological contribution to the discourse on HIV and AIDS.[3]

The HIV and AIDS epidemic has posed new challenges to this field and it can be argued that it might be a focal point for any new and further development of contextual understandings of missiology, including inter-faith perspectives. A recent publication in German describes responses of various religions to HIV and AIDS that offer potential for discussion between different religions on similar moral and ethical convictions that could in turn foster common projects.[4] This interesting collection deals with practical issues rather than a specific contribution to missiology. However, it certainly suggests possibilities for inter-faith dialogue on missiological issues.

The task of this chapter is to offer an analytical reflection on the published literature that intersects HIV and AIDS and the field of missiology.[5] Its emphasis will be on Christian missiology, in particular as expressed by mission-initiated Christianity. Classifying the findings, given the suggested limitations, the chapter is divided into five sections. The first deals with published contributions by missiologists on HIV and AIDS and the second considers the range of themes missiologists have addressed in relation to HIV and AIDS. The third section indicates the written contributions of some mission organisations in defining their response to the epidemic while the next attempts to show the developments and processes in mission and missiology, which are largely drawn from oral sources. Finally, questions are suggested that are yet to be addressed by missiologists in relation to HIV and AIDS.

MISSIOLOGISTS ON HIV AND AIDS

The 2001 volume of *Missionalia* addressed the HIV and AIDS epidemic. In the guest editorial Musa Dube and Tinyiko Maluleke suggest their intention to open up 'a brave, informed, creative and constructive discussion on HIV/AIDS issues'.[6] They boldly assert:

> Given the magnitude of the HIV/AIDS epidemic and its concentration in Africa and southern Africa in particular, we must ask ourselves whether our theology and religious studies departments have responded adequately. Can we say we have produced sufficient publications? Can we say we have organised enough conferences and workshops on HIV/ AIDS issues? . . . Different academic institutions and departments will answer these questions differently.[7]

A range of issues is dealt with. These include the need for curricula development given the *kairos* moment expressed in the HIV and AIDS crisis (Maluleke); ethics in a post-modern world facing HIV (Katongole); biblical responses to illness, health and healing (Siebert); a gendered reading of the book of Job (Masenya); the need for a practical theological response to people living with HIV (Kgosikwena); reports of field studies (Kealotswe; Njoroge); the memory-box project (Denis); and a gendered reflection on the media (Qakisa).[8] It must be pointed out, however, that although these papers were hosted by a journal of missiology, no specific contribution deals with the response of missiology departments or of mission organisations to HIV and AIDS. The intention as mentioned in the conclusion of the foreword was a different one:

> This special issue challenges African scholars to become socially engaged intellectuals, whose research and writing seek to contribute to the creation of a better and just society; whose intellectual activity contributes to the reduction of the spread of HIV/AIDS, to the delivery of quality care to the infected and affected, and to minimisation of the impact of HIV/AIDS in general.[9]

In an approach similar to that of the editorial committee of *Missionalia*, the Faculty of Catholic Theology of the Julius-Maximillian University of Würzburg formed a committee to prepare for a consultation on HIV and AIDS consisting mainly of experts from Catholic mission organisations and the organisation Action against AIDS.[10] An international call for papers was put out and a consultation held in October 2006. This was the first conference organised by a theological faculty, as all previous conferences or workshops in Germany were either prepared by mission organisations or non-governmental organisations (NGOs). These activities rarely had a clear theological focus. Papers from this consultation were published.[11]

The opening essay is by Cardinal Javier L. Barragán, who is based in Rome. In discussing HIV prevention, he quotes Pope Benedict XVI:

> The traditional teaching of the Church has proven to be the only fail-safe way to prevent the spread of HIV/AIDS. For this reason, 'the companionship, joy, happiness and peace which Christian marriage and fidelity provide, and the safeguard which chastity gives, must be continuously presented to the faithful, particularly the young'.[12]

At the conference, this presentation evoked a strong reaction with many feeling that Barragán was not in touch with the reality of the epidemic. There was much discussion, including contributions from Klaus Fleischer, Piet Rejier, Nyambura Njoroge and several other men and women from the business sector, from NGOs and the German Federal Ministry for Economic Co-operation and Development, which were published in the second section of the book.[13] These contributions countered Barragán's arguments with facts backed up by statistics as well as concrete analysis of specific life situations of people living with HIV. In the third section, the responses from churches in Namibia (Bishop Tomas Shivute), Botswana (Bishop Frank Nubuasah) and South Africa (Simone Lindörfer) are presented together with a response from Germany (Marco Moerschbacher).[14]

Lastly, theological reflections on the theme of the conference are outlined. Miranda Pillay suggests:

> [B]y addressing gender-power relations the church could strengthen its pro-active response to HIV/AIDS. For the Christian church, it is primarily a theological question, rooted in the rhetoric of moving from theology of hierarchy, of male headship, of power and dominion based on separateness, to a theology of community, mutuality and relationality.[15]

Emmanuel Katongole also addresses questions regarding the nature of the church. He argues that the HIV and AIDS epidemic 'is an invitation to rethink the very nature of the church as an interrupted and interrupting presence in the midst of Africa's ways of living, playing and working'. Furthermore, the epidemic forces the church to recognise her own woundedness, powerlessness and the struggle for life. The church thus becomes the place 'where a different way of being is nourished and made concretely visible'.[16]

The consultation and published proceedings indicate the complexity and diversity of approaches to mitigating the epidemic. The interpretation of the work and life of the church and her mission can be an approached from top down, as Barragán suggested, or understood in a much more egalitarian way, as was the case with the Katongole and Pillay contributions.

Jürgen Lohmayer analyses these two approaches and indicates the two different systems of thinking. He suggests that the first approach focuses on moral teaching as the centre of doing theology, while the second focuses on individuals in relation to their family and community. With his starting point shaped by liberation theology, Lohmayer emphasises the latter approach and indicates how this understanding shapes our perception of God. So, he argues, God is no longer seen as the guarantee for natural law and a moralistic order but, rather, God is understood as related to the praxis of Jesus Christ.[17]

Despite the difference in approach, the conference succeeded in its task of enabling scholars from different continents and denominations to share their life experiences in the context of HIV and AIDS. This kind of exercise is important if one is to conceptualise a contextual missiology, as mentioned earlier. The discipline of missiology was used to facilitate dialogue between, in this case, Europe and Africa. However, as with the volume of *Missionalia* discussed earlier, there is no overt missiological contribution in the book that presents an overview of the shape the response from missiology to HIV and AIDS should take. So, it is clear that while these initiatives by missiologists enabled the facilitation of discussion and dialogue, an overview of a missiological perspective is yet to be published.

While there might not be a comprehensive missiological response to HIV and AIDS, there are a number of ways in which missiologists are contributing to the discussion, or being challenged by others to contribute and add their views on certain questions arising out of the epidemic. One of these questions relates to health and healing. Historically, mission work was often linked to the delivery of primary health care, resulting in the founding of many institutes of medical mission.[18] So it has been understandable that the issue of HIV has continued to be an area of a global Christian response.

A number of study processes have been initiated, mainly under the umbrella of the World Council of Churches (WCC). In 2005 it organised, together with the Northelbian Centre for Mission and World Service in Breklum, Germany, a consultation on 'The global health situation and the mission of the church in the 21st century'. The proceedings of this consultation were published in a double volume of *International Review of Mission*.[19] An appeal was made in an open letter to the member churches of the WCC, to Christians involved in national government health ministries, as well as to delegates to the WCC Assembly in Porto Alegre in 2006:

> The state of the world's health is worsening, in particular in Africa, Eastern Europe and Central Asia. We feel a sense of urgency for churches, congregations, and individuals to take up the healing ministry in all its dimensions more seriously. We believe that the Church must reawaken and reorient itself to a health and healing ministry. We need a better theological understanding of the healing process in the different cultural contexts, which will allow us to re-energize and re-engage local congregations, churches and church-related organizations in the area of health care delivery. We feel strongly that churches and local congregations should redouble their efforts to eliminate stigma and discrimination and become healing agents for families and communities. We would recommend that

special attention is given to better address the churches' ministry of healing in relation to mental health, persons with disabilities, HIV and AIDS, and combating gender-based violence and child abuse. Therefore, in order to achieve these goals, we must scale up the efforts within the WCC and other stakeholders to reintegrate health concerns into our overall ecumenical agenda and engage in both an ecumenical and inter-religious dialogue, and together with secular entities. In promoting our holistic understanding of faith, health and healing, and a more equitable access to health and health-related services, we also advocate for the collection, development, adaptation, and dissemination of relevant resources, training and networking within both health and church bodies, local capacity building, outreach, and advocacy.[20]

In Africa, the work of the African Religious Health Assets Programme (ARHAP) is important in understanding the role of religious organisations in health and healing.[21] An analysis of this role was presented at the 2005 WCC consultation by James Cochrane, which showed the significant contribution made by religious institutions to health through the missionary enterprise in Africa.[22] Furthermore, there are discussions taking place within African Indigenous Churches (AICs) on healing and HIV. Obed N. Kealotswe shows clearly how two concepts of health and healing, Western and African, are opposed to each other. He refers to ongoing research on the role of clinics and hospitals versus that of the AICs who use the concept *diagelo* where 'a patient may not necessarily be healed of HIV/AIDS, but their health will improve and the life of the patient is prolonged'.[23] Clearly, further research on the role of healing within the AICs, and the contribution they make to mitigating the epidemic through their work, is much needed.

A further area that needs discussion is that of sexuality and sexual ethics. Some research has been carried out on the teaching of missionaries who advocated Victorian and/or Prussian sexual ethics and their resulting influence on family matters.[24] The power of this missionary enterprise and colonialism often went hand in hand with the establishment of a society established according to the values of the motherland and colonial church. While there is historical research that reflects on gender, moral teaching and the influence of socio-economic factors on sexual practice, there is little current research that roots these discussions in the current HIV crisis.

An attempt to address the impact of modernity on Africa in relation to sexuality is a book by Jean-Samuel Hendje Toya.[25] This offers critical reflection on the teaching and preaching churches in relation to the experiences of people living with HIV. Toya argues:

> The church is also slow to read and interpret the signs of the time. Sexuality and AIDS constitute an ineluctable factor in our time. The church cannot continue to read them only with glasses of chastity and faithfulness in the life as a couple. Very few people, even Christians, understand this message today in our society.[26]

Toya clearly indicates the need for the empowerment of women and uses missiological arguments for his acceptance of the use of condoms as a preventive measure.

Another example is the exciting collaborative Nordic–Federation of Christian Churches in Southern Africa (FOCCISA) project.[27] Human sexuality is discussed by scholars from Mozambique (Elias Zacarias Massicame), Zambia (Japhet Ndhlovu) and Norway and Denmark (Elisabeth Knox-Seith) and offers a contextual approach based on North-South dialogue.[28] This process began at a conference in Lusaka in 2004 and was carried on by a study group of pastors, general secretaries of councils of churches, scholars, people living with HIV and other invited specialists in the field from the four countries mentioned above. The two-volume publication arising out of this common study process deals with the challenges of HIV and AIDS as experienced and expressed through this diverse ecumenical encounter. The study process moves beyond the way in which policies are normally developed between mission and partner organisations. It clearly shows that through mutual dialogue, a new understanding of mission that responds to contextual needs is possible. Such an approach gives rise to the possibility of new ways of understanding partnerships that do not give mere lip service to so-called equal relationship and demonstrates a more egalitarian model of ecclesiology.

With these exceptions, this review of the literature clearly indicates that there are a number of gaps from a missiological point of view. There is a need to analyse the different missiological traditions and influences that have led to the present understanding of sexuality and moral discourse as a response to the HIV epidemic. Furthermore, there is a need for greater reflection on understanding the historical influences of mission on the teachings and moral understanding of sexuality and health and healing within specific contexts in Africa.

CONTRIBUTION OF CHURCH COUNCILS

The Commission of Sustainable Development of the Council of the Evangelical Church in Germany (EKD), the umbrella body of all Protestant churches in Germany, issued a document in 2007.[29] This marked a new, less moralistic, response to the epidemic. As Wolfgang Huber suggests in the introduction to the document, 'The last publication of the Council of the Evangelical Church in Germany (EKD) was called "AIDS: orientations and paths to danger" in 1988. Since then, however, the epidemic and its dramatic consequences have changed radically, making a new study necessary.'[30]

This new study process acknowledged the challenges and threats facing people living in sub-Saharan Africa, Asia, eastern Europe and Latin America. Therefore, the Committee on Sustainable Development was tasked to research and write a document dealing with questions of development, church aid, globalisation, and HIV and AIDS. The intention of the study process and resulting publication was to sharpen knowledge and understanding of these realities so as to sensitise mainly German churches and organisations. It was hoped that this process would build solidarity and effort, and encourage engagement in programmes lobbying for support to address pharmaceutical companies on the high costs of anti-retroviral treatment, as well as global political players around issues of poverty eradication.[31]

Appealing to the Christian tradition, Huber argued in the foreword to the document:

> Although the infection rate in Germany can be said to be very low in comparison to other parts of the world, that does not mean that HIV/AIDS is 'other people's' problem. This is particularly true from a Christian perspective, for the Church is a community in which, as members of the body of Jesus Christ, the healthy and the sick, those affected directly and indirectly by HIV/AIDS and people who are not sick themselves are accepted as being of equal value and equal dignity, and support one another in solidarity.[32]

What is noteworthy about this process is the fact that the German Church recognised its culpability in its relationship with churches in the South. And so it was asserted, 'In their struggle with the challenges posed by the epidemic, many churches around the world have recognized, with a measure of self-criticism that they have often been and sometimes still remain part of the problem.'[33] However, there is also evidence in the document of language that speaks of people living with HIV as 'them', a category that makes them other and potentially contradicts the message of the church needing to represent the one body of Jesus Christ, to be one community.[34]

This emphasis that embraces diversity and complexity and transcends regional and international boundaries lacking in the above publication is evident in the study process initiated by the WCC, published much earlier in 1997.[35]

MISSION ORGANISATIONS' POLICY ON HIV AND AIDS

In March 2008 the Evangelisches Missionswerk in Deutschland (EMW)[36] published a document stating:

> Mission organisations do not understand themselves firstly as funding agencies, but as partners connected to one another as a communion of churches. Mission organisations are in discussion with their brothers and sisters facing the same problems . . . Planning and evaluation of AIDS-programmes is important . . . In all our communication we have to reckon with the fact that HIV and AIDS is a sensitive issue which is difficult to tackle openly . . . The theological work on the issue is very important. Programmes should include theological (hermeneutical, educational) elements, taking seriously the proclamation and the mission of God's Word.[37]

This document suggests that HIV and AIDS programmes should be developed jointly by EMW and their partner organisations, which has often not been the case in the past. It offers a theological foundation, practical aspects of the establishment of a non-discriminatory environment, and suggestions about partnership with EMW. It is too early to establish the reception and the practical outcome of this document.

Even before publication of the EMW document, other mission organisations began processes aimed at common policy between them and their partners. One example is the document produced by the United Evangelical Mission (UEM) in Manila in 2004.[38] This UEM policy on HIV and AIDS was written collaboratively by members from Asia, Africa and Europe. Despite the diversity of people formulating this policy, it successfully addresses the wide range of experiences and divergent views on issues such as condom use as a preventative measure and acceptance of homosexuality.[39] Angelika Veddeler, co-ordinator of the UEM AIDS programme, has argued that this was only possible because much effort was spent on creating an atmosphere of mutual trust and dialogue that led to acceptance and support of one another within the 'family of this mission community'.[40] After publication of this policy, at the UEM general assembly in 2008 a decision was taken to mainstream HIV and AIDS in all programmes.

NEW PROCESSES AND RELATIONSHIPS WITHIN THE HIV CONTEXT

The HIV and AIDS epidemic is fundamentally changing and re-shaping relationships between mission and partner organisations, as the Nordic-FOCCISA project discussed earlier demonstrates. Many of these processes are not recorded in published literature but are nonetheless of note as they are profoundly changing patterns of communication.

In 2001 the Evangelical Lutheran AIDS Programme (ELCAP)[41] was established by the Evangelical Lutheran Church of the Republic of Namibia (ELCRN) in collaboration with the UEM HIV and AIDS programme. ELCAP, together with other Lutheran churches in Namibia, developed programmes that targeted HIV prevention amongst young people. Having received funding from the President's Emergency Program for AIDS Relief (PEPFAR), ELCAP was encouraged to emphasise the promotion of abstinence and the delay of sexual relations until marriage as the only prevention message offered to young people. Information on condoms and their promotion was discouraged. As a result of this, ELCAP and the ELCRN withdrew. UEM, a partner of ELCRN, supported this clear stand and raised monies on their behalf. ELCAP was thus able to organise its own youth awareness programme. The established relationship between the mission organisation and its partner was thus beneficial as they attempted to adopt a contextual approach to HIV prevention. Unfortunately, this is not always the case. Some member churches of the UEM in Tanzania have rejected such a stance to HIV prevention with young people, insisting on messages of abstinence until marriage.[42]

Another example of dialogue took place between two mission communities, UEM and Mission 21 based in Basel, Switzerland,[43] and their partner churches with a conference on 'Preaching in times of HIV and AIDS' in 2003. About 50 men and women, lay people and academic theologians, met in Tanzania with the specific intention of writing sermons in multi-cultural and mixed gender groups.

The book that arose out of this conference has been translated into French, Indonesian, Kiswahili and German.[44] This exchange offers a challenge to missiology to reflect on this kind of experience, perhaps analyse how preaching has changed, and ask whether old patterns of mission are a hindrance to creative and contextual responses to the HIV and AIDS epidemic.

A further contextual challenge, gender relations, has been brought on to the agenda of mission and partner organisations. This is illustrated by the example of a workshop in India organised by the Evangelisches Missionwerk Südwestdeutschland (EMS or Association of Churches and Missions in South Western Germany) together with their member churches and partners. The workshop focused on gender and HIV and AIDS and the proceedings were published in a booklet.[45] At its end, the relevance of the mission relationship is emphasised in a call for greater networking. It is suggested that such an HIV and AIDS network would be important for three reasons: first, to share information and experiences; second, to support one another in implementing appropriate projects and programmes; and third, for the sharing of theological understanding about HIV and AIDS and gender.[46]

A final example of new processes and mission relationships is a programme where churches and church institutions in Germany and southern Africa are working closely together with small and medium business enterprises. Within the programme entitled 'Church and Business against HIV and AIDS', HIV information, prevention, counselling and testing, and a network of support organisations are offered.[47] Through the assistance of German partners, South African and Namibian church organisations are able to gain access to the corporate business world. In this co-operative venture, churches and businesses are working together to overcome some of the difficulties faced by employers and those who are HIV positive. Experience has shown that employees are not willing to test for HIV for fear of information discussed during their counselling session and their HIV test results being passed on to management. Church leaders are drawn into this process, to encourage testing and also to facilitate the process of those who test HIV positive joining a support group. One business partner from Cape Town mentioned in a meeting in Germany recently: 'I never expected we can work on this level of corporate social responsibility with a church organisation as a partner, but now I am convinced that this is a good and productive partnership.'[48] This project seeks to reach people in the work environment and is a new form of mission born out of the challenge of HIV and AIDS. This, and other areas or spheres of new mission activities, have to be discussed and analysed within the field of missiology.

These examples demonstrate how the process of defining standards and resulting cultural conflicts tied to economic power must be described and analysed within missiology. In this way, missiology will be understood as an open process of dialogue leading to new and creative partnerships. Furthermore, a more contextual missiology needs to wrestle with the tension-filled arenas that exist between funding agencies and national churches living within the context of HIV.

CONCLUSION

As was suggested at the beginning of this chapter, mission activity began a long time ago. However, for it to remain relevant and contextual, addressing challenges such as HIV and AIDS, dialogue is constantly needed. An area that has not been discussed in this chapter is that of missiological inter-religious dialogue and what this means for a holistic approach to HIV and AIDS. Scholars from Islam, Judaism, Hindusim and African Traditional Religion should be communicating their various perspectives and missiological challenges. It is also necessary that in this inter-religious dialogue, questions of health, healing and sexuality be explored more fully. Given the history of moralistic teaching within all world religions, this remains a major challenge. Within the field of missiology, the past is reflected upon in order to understand the present and to challenge the future. Much of this work is yet to be done.

NOTES

1. Hans-Jürgen Findeis, 'Missiology' in *Dictionary of Mission*, edited by Karl Müller et al. (Maryknoll: Orbis, 1997): 299.
2. David Bosch, *Transforming Mission: Paradigm Shifts in Theology of Mission* (Maryknoll: Orbis, 1991); Willem Saayman, 'A South African perspective on transforming mission' in *Mission in Bold Humanity. David Bosch's Work Considered*, edited by Willem Saayman and Klippies Kritzinger (Maryknoll: Orbis, 1996): 40–52.
3. The Southern African Missiological Society was formed to further the study of, and research into, Christian mission and related topics in southern Africa. See http://www.missionalia. org.za/index.php?option=com_frontpage&Itemid=1. The published contributions are found in *Missionalia* 29(2) 2001.
4. Andre Gerth, Anna Noweck and Simone Rappel (eds), *Religionen im Kampf Gegen HIV/AIDS: Quellen, Spiritualität, Ethik [Religions Fighting Against HIV/AIDS: Sources, Spirituality, Ethics]* (München: Don Bosco Verlag, 2009).

5. I acknowledge with thanks the assistance of Marco Moerschbacher from the Missionswissen-schaftliches Institut in Aachen, Germany, for his analytical and editorial comments. I also want to thank the following people for their assistance with the literature review: Nico Botha (UNISA), Christoffer Grundmann (Valparaiso University, USA), Marco Moerschbacher (Institute for Missiology-Missionswissenschaftliches Institut, Aachen), Theo Sundermeier (Heidelberg, Germany) and Angelika Veddeler (United Evangelical Mission, Wuppertal, Germany).

6. Musa W. Dube and Tinyiko S. Maluleke, 'Guest editorial: HIV/AIDS as the new site of struggle: Theological, biblical and religious perspectives'. *Missionalia* 29(2) 2001: 119.

7. Dube and Maluleke, 'Guest editorial': 120.

8. Tinyiko S. Maluleke, 'The challenge of HIV/AIDS for theological education in Africa: Towards an HIV/AIDS sensitive curriculum'. *Missionalia* 29(2) 2001: 125–43; Emmanuel M. Katongole, 'Christian ethics and AIDS in Africa today: Exploring the limits of a culture of suspicion and despair'. *Missionalia* 29(2) 2001: 144–60; Johanna Siebert, 'Does the Hebrew Bible have anything to tell about HIV/AIDS?' *Missionalia* 29(2) 2001: 174–85; Madipoane Masenya, 'Between unjust suffering and the silent God: Job and HIV/AIDS sufferers in South Africa'. *Missionalia* 29(2) 2001: 186–99; Kagiso Billy Kgosikwena, 'Pastoral care and the dying process of people living with HIV/AIDS: Speaking of God in a crisis'. *Missionalia* 29(2) 2001: 200–19; Obed N. Kealotswe, 'Healing in the African independent churches in the era of AIDS in Botswana: A comparative study on the concept of *diagelo* and the care of home-based patients in Botswana'. *Missionalia* 29(2) 2001: 220–31; Nyambura J. Njoroge, 'Come now, let us reason together'. *Missionalia* 29(2) 2001: 232–57; Philippe Denis, 'Sharing family stories in times of AIDS'. *Missionalia* 29(2) 2001: 258–81; Mpine Qakisa, 'The media representation of women and HIV/AIDS: How it affects preventative messages'. *Missionalia* 29(2) 2001: 304–20.

9. Dube and Maluleke, 'Guest editorial': 124.

10. Action against AIDS is a body of churches (Protestant and Catholic), development agencies, NGOs and AIDS activist groups in Germany running campaigns, engaged in advocacy work and active in a committee on HIV and AIDS, ethics and theology. See http://www.aids-kampagne.de/english/index.html.

11. Francis D'Sa and Jürgen Lohmayer (eds), *Heil und Befreiung in Afrika: Die Kirchen vor der Missionarischen Herausforderung durch HIV/AIDS* (Würzburg: Echter Verlag, 2007). The book is also published in English as *Healing and Liberation in Africa: The Churches Confronted by the Missionary Challenge due to HIV/AIDS*.

12. 'Eccesia in Africa, 116: Address of His Holiness Benedict XVI to the Bishops of South Africa, Botswana, Swaziland, Namibia and Lesotho on their *limina Apostolorum* visit, Friday, 10 June, 2005', cited in Javier L. Barragán, 'Salvation and liberation in Africa: The mission of the churches challenged by HIV/AIDS' in *Heil und Befreiung in Afrika*, edited by D'Sa and Lohmayer: 19–20.

13. Klaus Fleischer, 'AIDS: Eine globale seuche von bestürzender dynamik [AIDS: A global epidemic of an alarming dynamic]' in *Heil und Befreiung in Afrika*, edited by D'Sa and Lohmayer: 33–45; Piet Rejier, 'Sozioökonomische auswirkungen von AIDS [Socio-economic consequences of AIDS]' in *Heil und Befreiung in Afrika*, edited by D'Sa and Lohmayer: 46–53;

Nyambura Njoroge, 'Resisting gender equality and injustice in the name of Jesus' in *Heil und Befreiung in Afrika*, edited by D'Sa and Lohmayer: 54–73.

14. Tomas Shivute, 'Pastoral positions: A response of the Evangelical Lutheran Church in Namibia' in *Heil und Befreiung in Afrika*, edited by D'Sa and Lohmayer: 109–14; Frank Nubuasah, 'Salvation and liberation in Africa: Pastoral reactions and challenges: Botswana' in *Heil und Befreiung in Afrika*, edited by D'Sa and Lohmayer: 123–32; Simone Lindörfer, 'Skizzen zur prävention von HIV aus der perspektive afrikanisch-feministischer befreiungstheologie [Outlines for preventing HIV from the perspective of African-feminist-liberation-theology]' in *Heil und Befreiung in Afrika*, edited by D'Sa and Lohmayer: 115–22; Marco Moerschbacher, '"Mit europäischen ohren": Rückmeldung zum referat von Bischof Frank Nubuasah [With European ears: Response to the contribution of Bischof Frank Nubuasah]' in *Heil und Befreiung in Afrika*, edited by D'Sa and Lohmayer: 133–7.

15. Miranda N. Pillay, 'Re-Reading New Testament texts: A resource for addressing gender inequality in the context of HIV and AIDS in South Africa' in *Heil und Befreiung in Afrika*, edited by D'Sa and Lohmayer: 152.

16. Emmanuel Katongole, 'Aids in Africa, the Church, and the politics of interruption' in *Heil und Befreiung in Afrika*, edited by D'Sa and Lohmayer: 182.

17. Jürgen Lohmayer, 'Missionarisch von AIDS sprechen: Die befreiung der theologie im zeichen des verschweigens von AIDS: Eine fundamentaltheologische option [Missionary talks about AIDS: The liberation of theology in the time of silencing AIDS: A fundamental theological option]' in *Heil und Befreiung in Afrika*, edited by D'Sa and Lohmayer: 207–8.

18. For example, the German Institute for Medical Mission (DIfäM) is celebrating 100 years of work around the world.

19. *International Review of Mission* 95(576–7) 2006.

20. *International Review of Mission* 95(576–7) 2006: 165.

21. For further information on ARHAP see http://www.arhap.uct.ac.za. ARHAP is a partner programme of the CHART process.

22. James R. Cochrane, 'Religion, public health and a church for the 21st century'. *International Review of Mission* 95(576–7) 2006: 59–72.

23. Kealotswe, 'Healing in the African Independent Churches in the era of AIDS in Botswana': 230.

24. For example, see Ursula Trüper, *Die Hottentottin: Das Kurze Leben der Zara Schmelen (ca. 1793–1831): Missionsgehilfin und Sprachpionierin in Südafrika* (Köln: Rüdiger Köppe Verlag, 2000); Fiona Bowie, Deborah Kirkwood and Shirey Ardener, *Women and Missions: Past and Present Anthropological and Historical Perceptions* (Oxford: Berg, 1993); Martha Mamozai, *Schwarze Frau, Weiße Herrin: Frauenleben in den Deutschen Kolonien* (Hamburg: Rororo, 1989); Brigitte Lau, 'A Critique of the Historical Sources and Historiography Relating to the Damaras in Pre-Colonial Namibia' (Research essay [BA], University of Cape Town, 1979).

25. Jean-Samuel Hendje Toya, *AIDS: African Perspective* (Dar-es-Salaam: Business Printers, n.d.). Toya was writing this book while working in Dar-es-Salaam as the regional co-ordinator for Africa of the United Evangelical Mission. Originally from Cameroon, he studied in France.

26. Toya, *AIDS*: 129.

27. This project is also discussed in Chapter 6 of this book.

28. Elisabeth Knox-Seith, *One Body: North-South Reflections in the Face of HIV and AIDS* (Copenhagen: Jønnson, 2005).

29. EKD, *For a Life with Dignity: The Global Threat of HIV/AIDS: Possible Courses of Action for the Church* (Hanover: Kirchenamt der EKD, 2007). The English version can be downloaded at http://www.ekd.de/english/56899.html.

30. Wolfgang Huber, *For a Life with Dignity*: 3. Available at http://www.ekd.de/english/ekdtext91_0.html (accessed 8 Aug. 2008).

31. EKD, *For a Life with Dignity*: 39–41.

32. EKD, *For a Life with Dignity*: 3.

33. EKD, *For a Life with Dignity*: 39.

34. EKD, *For a Life with Dignity*: 4.

35. WCC, *Facing AIDS: The Challenge of the Churches' Response*, (Geneva: WCC Publications, 1997).

36. EMW, the Association of Protestant Churches and Missions in Germany, is an umbrella organisation. Its members include the EKD, Protestant Free Churches, regional mission centres and departments and various mission associations and societies. See its website, available at http://www.emw-d.de/en.root/index.html.

37. EMW, *Gott Vertrauen: Unsere Verantwortung Angesichts von HIV und AIDS* [*Trust in God?: Our Responsibility in Facing HIV and AIDS*] (Hamburg: EMW Publications, 2008): 15–16. Available at http://www.emw-d.de/fix/files/Unsere_Verantwortung_%20angesichts_HIV_und_AIDS%20.2.pdf, translation by the author.

38. UEM is a communion of 34 churches from Africa, Asia and Europe, and the von Bodelschwingh Institution in Bethel, Germany: 'Emerging from the Rhenish Mission Society, founded in 1828, and the Bethel Mission, founded in 1886, which came together in 1971 to form what was known as the Vereinigte Evangelische Mission, the new international UEM has been in existence since 1996.' See http://www.vemission.org/en/who-are-we/ (accessed 15 Sep. 2008).

39. UEM, 'Anti HIV/Aids programme policy: 4. Available at http://www.vemission.org (accessed 15 Sep. 2008).

40. Conversation with the author, Sep. 2008.

41. See http://www.pepfar.gov/.

42. Conversation with Angelika Veddeler, co-ordinator of the UEM HIV and AIDS programme.

43. See http://www.mission-21.org/english/index.php?globo_count=1.

44. The proceedings of this conference were published under the title *God Breaks the Silence: Preaching in Times of Aids* (Wuppertal: United Evangelical Mission, 2005).

45. EMS, *Stop Gender Injustice and the Spread of HIV and AIDS* (Reutlingen: EMS, 2008). See www.ems-online.org.

46. EMS, *Stop Gender Injustice and the Spread of HIV and AIDS*: 26.

47. This project is a joint venture between the Global Business Coalition in South Africa and Namibia, the Lutheran Community in Southern Africa (LUCSA), and the Ecumenical Foundation in Southern Africa (EFSA).

48. Franz Peter Falke, CEO of the Falke Group (Germany-South Africa) at a public event hosted by the Chamber of Commerce and Industry in Mönchengladbach, Germany, 27 Aug. 2009.

Practitioner response

Benson Okyere-Manu

My response to the chapter by Ute Hedrich arises out of my experience of mission and HIV and AIDS from within the evangelical theological stream of Christianity. Hedrich did not specifically focus on this perspective in her chapter. There are a number of evangelical networks and conferences on HIV and AIDS in Africa that are important to any discussion on missiology and HIV and AIDS that I highlight in this response.

Given its missiological emphasis, the Medical Assistance Program (MAP) International seeks to provide health and hope to impoverished people throughout the world. In 1996 MAP International organised a consultation for theologians, pastors and academics[1] that resulted in the production of the first modules of a HIV and AIDS curriculum for theological institutions in Africa.[2] As a result of this consultation, a number of theological institutions in Africa began to incorporate HIV and AIDS into their programmes in order to educate the pastors they train and sensitise them to the issues faced by those who are HIV positive. This pioneering work of HIV modules undertaken by MAP International became the foundation for the WCC HIV and AIDS Curriculum for Theological Institutions in Africa.[3]

Serving in Mission (SIM)[4] is an international, inter-denominational Christian mission organisation that was one of the first to tackle the HIV and AIDS epidemic. With about 30 of its employees attending the Eleventh International Conference on AIDS and STDs in Africa in Lusaka in 1999, SIM initiated networking and strategy development around the epidemic, entitled 'Windows of Hope for HIV'. In addition to raising funds, SIM organises regular capacity building workshops and training for mission partners.

In early 2002 the Samaritan's Purse hosted an unprecedented global Christian conference on HIV and AIDS named 'Prescription for Hope' held in Washington, DC.[5] The purpose was to bring together churches, mission organisations and individual Christians involved in HIV and AIDS work from around the world. At the conference, Arthur Ammann, president of Global Strategies for HIV Prevention and Clinical Professor of Pediatrics at the Center for AIDS Prevention of the University of California, challenged the gathering on the growing global HIV incidence. His writings have become a key resource within the evangelical community and helped them to soften their stance against the use of condoms. The work of Samaritan's Purse has since focused its energy on strengthening the international Christian response to HIV and AIDS; to mobilise private, church, corporate and government resources; and to develop a unified plan to respond to HIV and AIDS.

The Micah Network is a global group of about 300 evangelical mission organisations, Christian relief, development and justice agencies. In September 2002 Micah organised an international conference in Chang Mai, Thailand, with the theme 'Integral Mission and HIV/

AIDS'. One of the major contributions of the conference was the setting up of a team of people to reflect on the conference papers and case studies and develop a theology of HIV.[6]

Initiated by Patrick Dixon,[7] a medical doctor from Uganda, AIDS Care Education and Training International was formed to help educate and train people at the grassroots in their response to HIV and AIDS. It organised an HIV and AIDS International conference in Uganda in 2005. This was an attempt to provide an opportunity for organisations and individuals to share good practices with each other. Three years later in Entebbe, Uganda, it once again organised a global forum. This brought together 200 leaders and supporters or partners in HIV and AIDS work from 35 nations. The gathering sought to set an agenda for HIV and AIDS work over the following five years.

In conclusion, Hedrich reflects on some of the processes within the field of missiology and missions seeking to address the HIV and AIDS epidemic. I have added to these reflections. What is of utmost importance, however, is the need for all research, conference resolutions and statements to be expressed in a language and medium that is accessible to ordinary people. In reflecting on the success of the 2000 World AIDS Conference in Durban that tackled the silence around HIV, Urban Jonsson[8] suggested the conference only broke what he calls the first wall of the conspiracy of silence at national and international levels. However, as much as this work is crucial, Jonsson points out that there is a second wall of silence, not as well defined but even more damaging: 'This "second wall of silence" includes the wall between government officials and communities; between politicians and voters; between communities and households; between households and households; between husband and wife; between parents and children; between teachers and students and between boyfriend and girlfriend.'[9]

This means that if missiology is to have an impact upon the HIV and AIDS epidemic, then there is a need for greater engagement with people at the grassroots level in order to break this second wall of silence.

Notes

1. Jim Johnson, then pastoral counselling lecturer at the Evangelical Seminary of Southern Africa (ESSA) in Pietermaritzburg, attended this consultation. As a result, he introduced a module on HIV and AIDS into the curriculum in 1997. This in turn led to the author helping to establish the ESSA Christian AIDS Programme (ECAP) in 1998.

2. P.W. Robinson, *Choosing Hope: Curriculum Modules and Pastoral Response to the HIV/AIDS Epidemic* (Nairobi: MAP International, 1996).

3. Musa Dube (ed.), *HIV/AIDS and the Curriculum: Methods for Integrating HIV/AIDS in Theological Programmes* (Geneva: WCC Publications, 2003).

4. See www.sim.org.

5. See http://samaritanspurse.org/index.php/pfth/.

6. See 'Towards a Christ-centred theology of HIV/AIDS'. Available at http://www.en.micahnetwork.org/content/download/1458/16343/file/Micha-towards a Christ-centred theology/.

7. Patrick Dixon has authored a number of books on AIDS including: *The Truth about AIDS* (Kingsway: ACET International, 2004). Available free at http://www.globalchange.com/Books/; *AIDS and Young People* (Kingsway: ACET International, 1989). Available at http://www.globalchange.com/Books/; and *AIDS and You* (Kingsway: ACET International, 2004).

8. Urban Jonsson, the UNICEF regional director for eastern and southern Africa in his address at the Conference of the European Parliamentarians for Africa in Nov. 2001 introduced the concept of first and second walls of silence around HIV.

9. Jeff Balch and Geertje Hollenberg (eds), *Parliament and the AIDS Budget: Resources for Community Empowerment: Report Containing the Contributions, Conclusions and Recommendations of the Fourth International Parliamentary Conference on HIV/AIDS* (Amsterdam: European Parliamentarians for Africa, 2002). Available at www.awepa.org.

PART 3

Engaging the socio-cultural realm

African Traditional Religions and HIV and AIDS

Exploring the boundaries

Ezra Chitando

INTRODUCTION

The role of religion in response to the HIV epidemic[1] has come under increasing scholarly scrutiny. There is growing awareness that religion is both part of the problem and part of the solution. Theologians, scholars of religion, anthropologists and other specialists have begun to examine the impact of religious beliefs and practices on the response to the epidemic. The dominant trend, however, has been to focus on the so-called world religions and how they have responded to HIV. By far the bulk of the literature is on the contribution of Christianity, Islam, Hinduism, Buddhism and other scriptural religions to the struggle against HIV.[2] The assumption is that sacred texts can be appropriated for values to minimise stigma and mobilise communities of faith to respond with compassion.[3]

Literature on the contribution of faith-based organisations[4] in responding to HIV has fallen into the trap of marginalising the contribution of African Traditional Religions (ATRs). Alternatively, when ATRs are referred to, emphasis has been on their negative impact or harmful cultural practices. This chapter seeks to analyse the literature on ATRs by examining the views of different scholars regarding their response to HIV. It also highlights the gaps that need to be filled if the full story of the indigenous religions of Africa's engagement with HIV is to be told.

AFRICAN TRADITIONAL RELIGIONS: THE DEBATE ON TERMINOLOGY

The academic study of religion places emphasis on accurate terminology in describing religious phenomena. This emerges from the realisation that the words used to characterise religious phenomena are often laden with meaning. Assumptions and biases are sometimes expressed in the terms adopted. When a religious group is classified as a sect or cult, for example, we are most likely saying that its beliefs and practices do not conform to the norm in society.[5] In actual fact, we are passing judgement regarding what is felt should be appropriate religion. The study of ATRs has grappled with the question of accurate terminology for some time. Each of the competing terms has its own advantages and disadvantages. As it is beyond the scope of this chapter to interrogate the various terms that have been used, only the contestation is highlighted.

The most popular term has been African Traditional Religions. It became popular in the 1960s as scholars sought to provide an umbrella term for diverse religious beliefs and practices across sub-Saharan Africa. It has been embraced by most African scholars as it evokes the notion of traditions that have been handed down from one generation to the other. While the term ATRs enjoys considerable currency, it has come under increasing scrutiny. Some critics charge that the term is an ideological invention, particularly when it is used in the singular.[6] Others insist that the notion of traditional is negative. It gives the misleading impression that ATRs belong to the remote past and one might therefore conclude falsely that they are of no relevance to current struggles. However, research shows that ATRs remain significant in the contemporary period.[7]

In view of the challenges facing the term African Traditional Religions, alternative labels have been put forward, such as Africism. According to the defenders of this alternative term, it would place the religions of Africa on a par with other world religions such as Hinduism. This proposal has not found enthusiastic support. The one label that is gaining popularity is African Indigenous Religions. The idea of indigenous religions appeals to many as it has political overtones. It speaks to the notion that the practitioners are the first peoples or original inhabitants of the land. Furthermore, it places the religions of Africa on a par with other indigenous religions.

Despite the contestation, the term African Traditional Religions is used in this chapter. The main reason relates to the currency that the term enjoys within the academic study of religion in Africa and globally, with most of the available scholarly literature on the subject using the term. Second, the focus of this chapter necessitates its adoption. The material that examines the interface between the religious beliefs and practices of Africa and the HIV epidemic uses the term and it is, therefore, prudent to retain it.

THE DISCOURSE ON HARMFUL CULTURAL PRACTICES

It is difficult to isolate the role of ATRs in the context of HIV, as many authors struggle to separate religion from culture.[8] While this challenge is not peculiar to ATRs, it is more pronounced in the case of the indigenous religions of Africa. As many researchers on ATRs have noted, religion is built into all aspects of life in Africa. It permeates all dimensions of existence. Although there is still a need to isolate the specifically religious aspects of life, it must be conceded that this is a difficult undertaking.[9] Consequently, it is important to cover literature in this chapter that relates to cultural practices with a bearing on HIV.

From the earliest writing on the topic, there has been keen interest on the possible impact of African beliefs and practices on the spread of HIV in the region. Non-governmental organisations (NGOs), activists and scholars have observed that some cultural practices increase the vulnerability to HIV of women especially, but also men. In particular, the Circle of Concerned African Women Theologians (the Circle) has sought to unravel harmful cultural practices in the context of HIV. Contributors contend that ATRs justify the persistence of these harmful beliefs and practices.

Before examining the various beliefs and practices to which the Circle has drawn attention in the era of HIV, it is important to appreciate the point that most contributors aver that it is patriarchy, informed and buttressed by ATRs, that has left women and girl children more vulnerable to HIV. Rigid gender roles that are supposed to have been handed down by God or the ancestors have disadvantaged women. Musa W. Dube, a biblical scholar from Botswana, contends that women's vulnerability to HIV is due to the roles that societies have assigned them. Dube argues:

> Due to their ascribed gender roles, women are highly vulnerable to infection; they bear the burden of caring for the infected; they carry the HIV/AIDS stigma and when infected they are less likely to have access to quality care. In all the four concerns of the HIV/AIDS epidemic (prevention, care, stigma and confronting social injustice) women are the hardest hit due to their gendered roles.[10]

One of the institutions singled out for criticism by the Circle and other writers is polygyny, often called polygamy in the literature. The practice where one man marries more than one wife, they observe, endangers all the women in the marriage if the man (or one of his wives) is not faithful or does not use condoms consistently and correctly. In one of the earliest Circle volumes, Musimbi Kanyoro, later to serve as a general co-ordinator of the Circle, raised her misgivings about polygamy.[11] The reality of HIV and AIDS has made the opposition to the institution even stronger. The South African biblical scholar, Madipoane Masenya argues that the canon of African culture subjects women to a subordinate status.[12]

Another cultural practice that has come under attack is levirate marriage or wife-inheritance. In some African cultures, a male relative of the deceased is expected to inherit the widow. He is supposed to provide protection and meet her sexual needs. Dora Rudo Mbuwayesango, a Zimbabwean biblical scholar, argues that practices like levirate marriage increase women's vulnerability to HIV. According to her:

> The traditional practices such as polygyny and levirate-like (wife-inheritance) marriage are now practised openly. These practices increase the vulnerability of women to HIV because there is more likelihood of infection of other members of the extended family by the inherited in the cases of polygyny and levirate-like marriages. An infected man does not only infect the widow if she is not yet infected, but the widow may already be infected and infect the inheritor who then infects his other wife or wives in the case of polygyny. In most cases the man chosen to inherit a widow is already married.[13]

Another harmful practice identified by Circle scholar-activists is that of widow cleansing. This practice, where a man is expected to have sex with a widow in order to set her free from the spirit of her deceased husband, has also caused an outcry in a time of HIV. Activists maintain that the practice violates the rights of the widow. Other contentious practices include female circumcision (also referred as genital cutting or mutilation in the literature) and early child marriage or the giving away of girl children for propitiation purposes. The *trokosi* practice in some Ghanaian communities has been cited as a further example:

> The *trokosi* is a young virgin given up by her family in propitiation for the sins committed against the gods by her ancestors. The young, innocent virgin becomes a slave-wife of a fetish priest, who is usually old enough to be her grand parent. He has children with her in a loveless relationship.[14]

A similar practice is found among the Shona people of Zimbabwe. It is believed that the spirit of a murdered man can only be compensated by the extended family of the perpetrator giving up a virgin to be married into the family of the deceased. Children's rights advocates and gender activists have highlighted the vulnerability of the girl child to HIV due to this *kuripa ngozi* (placating the avenging spirit) practice. Such practices have led critics to regard ATRs as retrogressive in the time of HIV.

While male African scholars of religion have celebrated the notion of hospitality in African cultures, some African women theologians have questioned the limits of hospitality. Critics have drawn attention to the challenges associated with the notion of hospitality when it is extended to women granting sexual favours to men. Lilian Siwila from Zambia argues that the concept of hospitality increases the vulnerability of women and girls to HIV, particularly when care giving is taken up only by women and girls.[15]

At this juncture, it is important to highlight the fact that the Circle's engagement with ATRs in the context of HIV has been largely to draw attention to the negative dimensions. While many male African theologians have sought to promote inculturation, that is, the appropriation of African culture in African Christianity and theology, Circle activists have been more critical of ATRs and cultures. Whereas male African theologians have tended to celebrate ATRs, Circle activists have applied a hermeneutic of suspicion. However, as is shown below, some Circle authors such as Dube have sought to highlight positive aspects of ATRs that are useful to the response to HIV.

THE AFRICAN TRADITIONAL WORLD VIEW AS A CHALLENGE TO HIV

Alongside the discourse on harmful cultural practices, various aspects of the traditional African world view have come under criticism for increasing vulnerability to HIV.

The African preoccupation with fertility has been singled out as a major stumbling block to HIV prevention. Prior to developments in anti-retroviral therapy, it was risky for an HIV positive woman to fall pregnant as there was a high probability that her baby would be infected. However, in the traditional African world view marriage is associated with children and therefore many HIV positive women have taken the risk in order to protect their marriages. Furthermore, some men and women engage in extra-marital affairs in an effort to have children.

This further exposes them to the risk of HIV.[16] Promoting condom use also becomes problematic in an environment where the emphasis is on expanding the clan.

As noted in the previous section, Circle activists have highlighted the negative impact of patriarchy in the era of HIV. ATRs and cultures tend to socialise men to be in charge and have power over women and children, a dimension shared with other religions of the world. Unfortunately, this has given rise to toxic and dangerous masculinities.[17] The phenomenon of multiple concurrent partnerships has been identified as a major driver of HIV.[18] Men who have multiple sexual partners appeal to indigenous religion and culture to support their behaviour.

Male dominance in the African world view is supported by numerous myths and sayings. The overall impression is that men were created to dominate and that male sexual pleasure is an absolute priority. Tabona Shoko, a Zimbabwean scholar of ATRs, notes that the ideology of masculinity has led some men to use aphrodisiacs as they believe that these will enhance their sexual performance.[19] The focus on sexual conquest endangers women and men in the context of HIV.

Condom use is also compromised by the idea that real men are not afraid of sexually transmitted infections and HIV. The socialisation of young boys to become fearless risk takers is a major challenge in the era of HIV. The negative attitude towards condoms and power over women frustrates prevention efforts.[20] It is in this context that attention to the need to challenge dangerous masculinities informed by religion and culture is growing. Gender activists are challenging traditional religious leaders to invest more resources in the transformation of masculinities.

Traditional healers have an important place in the study of ATRs. They are key sacred practitioners in these traditions and are believed to act as a conduit between the community and its departed elders. They are also believed to have powers to discern challenges to health and well-being and are endowed with spiritual power to defeat negative forces and restore health. However, their role has come under scrutiny in the time of HIV.

In most parts of southern Africa, traditional healers and religious leaders have been criticised for a number of reasons. First, they are held responsible for the myth that having sex with a virgin girl cures HIV and AIDS. The marked increase in the abuse of girls has been attributed to this myth. Traditional healers have been attacked for prescribing this solution to their desperate clients.[21] This myth has left girls vulnerable to HIV as some men believe in the efficacy of the traditional healers' prescription.

Second, some traditional religious leaders have also sought to revive the practice of virginity testing. They seek to reinforce traditional morality and expose cases of sexual abuse of minors.[22] However, critics point out that the practice violates children's rights. In addition, the handing out of virginity certificates increases the vulnerability of girls to abuse as they are marked out as virgins.[23] Patriarchal bias is written all over the practice. Boys are not examined for virginity and, furthermore, the responsibility of men in eliminating violence against women is glossed over.

The third reason why traditional healers have been attacked is for compromising anti-retroviral therapy by claiming to heal those living with HIV.[24] This has been a long-running controversy in different African contexts. To some extent the challenge lies in interpretation. In the traditional context, when the symptoms of an illness are reversed, one is therefore healed. However, Western biomedicine seeks to question the efficacy of traditional healers by subjecting their clients to HIV tests. Wotsuna Khamalwa from Uganda calls for collaboration between traditional healers and Western-trained doctors.[25]

It is, of course, debatable whether witchcraft must be included in discussions on ATRs. Doing so runs the risk of perpetuating negative images of these religions. However, there is some merit in including the theme as witchcraft stands in opposition to the forces of life and health that are promoted by the indigenous religions of Africa. In the specific case of HIV, witchcraft is regarded as aiding denial and minimising the reality of HIV. Witchcraft has been used to account for many deaths due to AIDS, thereby lulling communities into a dangerous complacency:

> Although many people know that AIDS is not caused directly by witchcraft, a witch can influence a man or a woman, for example, to drink too much beer so that he or she leaves all caution aside and has sex with a[n] HIV-positive person and so may contract the virus. In addition, those who are HIV-positive and their kin usually deny a diagnosis of AIDS and try to identify a witch or cannibal whose evil acts can be countered.[26]

The belief in witchcraft makes prevention efforts more difficult as some people may adopt fatalistic attitudes. In addition, treatment can become a challenge when a person living with HIV utilises the paradigm of witchcraft to explain his or her illness. They may resort to traditional healers or exorcism rituals and not undergo anti-retroviral therapy.

AFRICAN TRADITIONAL RELIGIONS AS A RESOURCE

The foregoing section has outlined some of the scholarly reflections on the status of ATRs in the response to HIV. The dominant trend has been to highlight the challenges posed by ATRs to effective responses to the epidemic. To be fair, the focus on the fault lines found in ATRs is not restricted to these religions. Researchers have also analysed how other religions, for example Christianity and Islam, are implicated in reinforcing stigma.[27] Nonetheless, as other scholars have sought to highlight progressive ideas in Christianity and Islam, so have some scholars drawn attention to the positive dimensions of ATRs.

It is critical that the discussion on the positive dimensions of ATRs in the struggle against HIV be put into proper context. First, there is an underlying conviction that the overwhelming focus on the negative aspects of ATRs perpetuates the negative images of them in the media and the academy. Books and encyclopaedias on world religions systematically leave out the indigenous religions of Africa. The marginalisation of Africa on racial, economic and political grounds implies the need for a hermeneutic of suspicion when examining the portrayal of ATRs in discourses on HIV and AIDS.

The most articulate and passionate scholars to draw on ATRs as a strategic resource in the response to HIV have noted the dominance of European and North American perspectives in discourses on the epidemic. They contend that the impact of colonialism and globalisation continues to prevent researchers and activists from appreciating the positive aspects of indigenous knowledge systems. Dube writes:

> The structural epistemology that assumes that the West/North holds the best answer for the whole world – civilization, progress, language, science, faith, its brand of democracy, medicine, law, education, environmental care, development, and freedom – was established in colonial times and continues today, informing the economic, political, and reproductive policies that are often recommended to all worldwide. The global approach to HIV & AIDS has been no different. Western categories of understanding and preventing HIV & AIDS became the standard approach in extremely

different contexts around the world. Twenty-four years after the first scientific discovery of HIV & AIDS, it is important to ask: what is lost when HIV & AIDS prevention proceeds without fully factoring in the AIR/s (African Indigenous Religion/s) worldview in African contexts?[28]

Given the challenges of race in southern Africa and the minimisation of ATRs due to Christianity, Dube's call for the need for more sensitivity to African cosmologies is understandable. Nokuzola Mndende, a South African scholar and practitioner of ATRs, is equally convinced that there are political and ideological factors at play in the research on religion and HIV. According to her, ATRs continue to be overlooked or presented negatively in discourses on HIV. Furthermore, they do not benefit from the funding available in this field. She further observes:

> The question that now arises is how could [*sic*] we even go to the discussion of the role that could [*sic*] be played by African Traditional Religion in decreasing HIV/AIDS infection when the religion itself is not recognised, yet a lot of research is done on its people from an outside perspective?[29]

The stance adopted by Dube and Mndende is supported by Rasebate I. Mokotso from Lesotho. Mokotso argues that there is a need for a solution to the epidemic to emerge from the most affected people. The hegemony of Eurocentrism needs to be challenged, he avers, by initiating dialogue with indigenous knowledge systems:

> The traditional belief in the supremacy of Western medicine and the conviction that Western-based science knowledge has the ability to provide solutions to all pertinent human problems has been challenged. Western behavioural principles such as individualism have been put to the test and beyond reasonable doubt were proved wrong. Western theories of health and disease could not adequately explain or give direction toward the resolution of [the] HIV and AIDS problem. The long held supremacy of Western knowledge production has been seriously undermined. In general, HIV and AIDS has demystified the hegemony of Eurocentrism.[30]

The views emerging from the scholars cited above call for greater openness and fairness towards the role of indigenous religions in responding to HIV. There is a growing awareness that ATRs do not only represent beliefs and practices that increase vulnerability to HIV. Rather, as with other religions, they do possess valuable beliefs and practices that have protected millions of their adherents from infection, as well as helping others to live with HIV.

The concept of *ubuntu* ('I am because you are'/oneness of humanity) has attracted the attention of African philosophers, theologians and other specialists. It places emphasis on solidarity and the notion of interdependence. It speaks to the African idea that an individual does not exist in isolation but is tied to other members of the community. *Ubuntu* has been celebrated as a distinctive concept that ATRs can bequeath to the global community as it struggles against HIV and AIDS-related stigma, as well as to promote care and support.[31]

The African concept of *ubuntu* has been utilised to challenge aggressive masculinities.[32] It is argued that if African men sincerely believe that the fate of women is tied to theirs, they need to do more to prevent their partners from getting infected with HIV. *Ubuntu* challenges men to care about the abuse of women and focuses on the idea that community members are responsible for the welfare of each other.[33] Furthermore, it has been adopted in HIV and AIDS discourses to counter stigma and discrimination and promote solidarity with people living with HIV.[34]

However, it is important to note that while many scholars have alluded to the importance of *ubuntu* in mobilising communities to respond to the epidemic, they have not always used the concept directly. One area where *ubuntu* has been appropriated practically is in the care of orphans and other vulnerable children. AIDS has orphaned millions of children in many parts of Africa.[35] The African focus on the extended family has ensured that many of these children are catered for.

Catholic theologian John Waliggo admits that there are some cultural practices that need to be abandoned in the face of HIV but contends that indigenous religions can be utilised to respond positively to the epidemic:

> We need to identify those many *genuine African values and practices*, which, when challenged by Christian teaching and modernity, they remain *positive, true, noble and capable of resisting* and eventually defeating this deadly epidemic.

Such values include, among many: Africa's *central concern for life*: transmitting, protecting, curing, healing life and making all sacrifices so that life may continue; the *family values* of educating children in the appreciation and proper use of their sexuality; the *community values* of caring for one another; the *medical and healing* values whereby everyone seeks an active role in saving life and the spiritual-religious values based on strong beliefs that only God is the ultimate source of all cure and healing, the Omnipotent Doctor of all ages, the unrivalled Inspirer of all effective medicines.[36]

Waliggo concludes that the most appropriate strategy is to retain positive beliefs and practices, transforming less harmful ones, and eliminating dangerous beliefs and practices altogether.[37]

Earlier, attention was drawn to the critique that ATRs promote patriarchy and harmful masculinities in the era of HIV. However, Desmond Lesajane, writing from within a South African context, argues that it is possible to retrieve the traditional masculine notion of *kgotla* (village council) and enrich it with more democratic values. This will give rise to sensitive and effective men at family, community and national levels. He writes:

> The concept of *kgotla*, entrenched in southern Africa culture, offers a model of management and communication within the family. A *kgotla* is a forum for discussion where all participants are equal, as symbolised by the circular seating arrangements. Decisions are made by consensus after everybody has had an opportunity to air their views. Reappropriating this concept will facilitate better interaction between fathers, children, mothers and other members of the family. A prerequisite for the concept to work today would be to open up the *kgotla* to women, and even children, as equal participants.[38]

Taking up the same theme, Julius Gathogo argues that the traditional ideals regarding masculinities among the Gikuyu in Kenya are relevant in the era of HIV and AIDS. He maintains that initiation rites sought to socialise the *Mundurume* (man) to be a fearless defender of his community and provide leadership. Gathogo holds that in this contemporary age, men must show the same qualities:

Thus, *Mundurume* (read, the African man) must, as in ancient times, respond decisively and play a leading role in the midst of the HIV and AIDS crisis that is rapidly engulfing Africa. They must be good soldiers of the community and protect the entire society of women, men and children against HIV and AIDS. This is the authentic maturity that is climaxed by the initiation, for which we all should crave.[39]

Writing from a Zimbabwean context, Sophia Chirongoma suggests that the traditional practice of *zunde ramambo* (chief's granary) whereby volunteers collect agricultural produce from every capable household is strategic in the time of HIV and AIDS. As a sacred practitioner in ATRs, the chief is expected to ensure the welfare of all the people within his territory. This practice has enabled communities to support their more vulnerable members, particularly orphans.[40]

Furthermore, although traditional healers have been criticised for promoting harmful myths and frustrating anti-retroviral therapy, other scholars have pointed out that such healers play an important role in the era of HIV. Adam K. arap Chepkwony from Kenya argues that there is a need to appreciate the contribution of traditional healers to health and well-being in their communities. He maintains that colonialism and Christianity have undermined the position of traditional healers and contends that ritual practices in indigenous religions have a healing dimension: 'Today, rituals heal diseases brought about by the pain of abuse, trauma of parental neglect or grief due to loss of a loved one, broken marriages, and HIV/AIDS'.[41]

AFRICAN TRADITIONAL RELIGIONS AND HIV: THE GAPS

The foregoing sections have drawn attention to the literature on ATRs and HIV. On the one hand, there are scholars who have raised the problematic dimensions of ATRs in the era of HIV, while others draw attention to the positive aspects. However, there is a need to look at sharp distinctions in scholars' arguments. Often, the same scholar will highlight the challenging aspects of ATRs while accepting their contribution to the struggle against the epidemic. Thus, for example, Dube challenges the patriarchal nature of ATRs in her work while also celebrating the concept of *botho/ubuntu*.[42]

Having examined the reflections on ATRs and HIV, it is helpful to draw attention to some of the key issues that have not benefited from scholarly analysis. It is vital that more research into the interface between ATRs and HIV be conducted as these religions provide the spiritual basis for most inhabitants of sub-Saharan Africa. How religions respond to HIV in the region will, to a very large extent, depend on how ATRs respond to HIV.

There is a tendency to regard religious/cultural beliefs and practices as static and unchanging. Religious ideologies tend to mask their fluidity by posing as permanent so that they are handed down from one generation to another. In reality, however, beliefs and practices are always undergoing change and transformation. The sheer impact of HIV and AIDS on communities suggests that there has to be a fundamental change in beliefs and practices in order to adapt to the crisis. Researchers need to discern how the HIV epidemic has forced gatekeepers to rethink indigenous beliefs and practices. In order to do this, a number of key questions need to be asked: what is the meaning of death when so many people are dying; have beliefs about witchcraft remained the same in the wake of the increase in the death rate; given that ATRs place emphasis on longevity, what is the impact of so many young people dying; how have communities developed alternative rituals in the face of dangerous cultural practices?

There is a growing emphasis on male circumcision as an HIV prevention strategy within biomedical studies.[43] However, few social science researchers have sought to explore the religious and cultural factors that inform male circumcision and implications for HIV prevention. There is a need for scholars of ATRs to provide contemporary descriptions of male circumcision and the underlying spiritual factors. This would enable activists to find entry points into HIV prevention efforts.

Attention has been drawn to the fact that a number of African scholars have sought to highlight both positive and negative aspects of ATRs in the response to HIV. However, what is still required is a more probing analysis of the various ideological categories of authors who have published on the intersection of these religions with the epidemic. This analysis could be useful in providing valuable insights into the way scholars have reacted to negative images of their religions in the face of HIV. For example, a study comparing Nokuzola Mndende's defence of ATRs and Malik Badri's defence of Islam in the time of HIV would be instructive in this regard.[44] They frame their discourses on religion and HIV against the backdrop of the idea of Western cultural imperialism and are at pains to defend their religious traditions against images of backwardness and increasing vulnerability to HIV. Undertaking ideological criticism would yield rich rewards for researchers studying publications on religion and HIV both in Africa and globally.

CONCLUSION

Although most of the surveyed publications on the role of religion and HIV have tended to focus on the contributions of the so-called literate or world religions, some authors have drawn attention to the importance of ATRs. However, the bulk of the literature to date has tended to concentrate on the negative impact of indigenous religions in relation to prevention, treatment and support. In particular, the writings of the Circle have focused on negative cultural practices that increase the vulnerability of women and girl children to HIV. This chapter has explored these different categories of writers and has noted some of the gaps in the available scholarly literature. There is no doubt that more work is required to ensure that the resources of indigenous religions of Africa are used more effectively in the response to the HIV epidemic.

NOTES

1. There is a growing tendency to refer to HIV to characterise the epidemic. This is also political: HIV must not be allowed to develop into AIDS in the era of anti-retroviral therapy.
2. See, for example, Steven Lux and Kristine Greenaway, *Scaling Up Effective Partnerships: A Guide to Working with Faith-Based Organisations in the Response to HIV and AIDS* (Geneva: Ecumenical Advocacy Alliance, 2006).
3. See, for example, Lovemore Togarasei, 'Fighting HIV and AIDS with the Bible: Towards HIV and AIDS biblical criticism' in *Mainstreaming HIV and AIDS in Theological Education: Experiences and Explorations*, edited by Ezra Chitando (Geneva: WCC Publications, 2008): 71–82. Also see Chapter 5 in this book.
4. As with many other popular concepts, the notion of faith-based organisations (FBOs) is a contested one. Critics feel that it brings together disparate phenomena under one umbrella. The idea of religious entities has been suggested as an alternative. However, due to the currency enjoyed by FBOs, it is used here.
5. Michael F.C. Bourdillon, *Religion and Society: A Text for Africa* (Gweru: Mambo Press, 1990): 159.
6. See, for example, Rosalind Shaw, 'The invention of "African Traditional Religion"'. *Religion* 20 (1990): 339–53.
7. See, for example, Jacob K. Olupona (ed.), *African Traditional Religions in Contemporary Society* (New York: Paragon House, 1991).
8. For further discussion see Chapter 10 of this book.
9. Ezra Chitando, 'A curse of the Western heritage?: Imagining religion in an African context'. *Journal for the Study of Religion* 10(2) 1997: 75–98.

10. Musa W. Dube, 'Grant me justice: Towards gender-sensitive multisectoral HIV/AIDS reading of the Bible' in *Grant Me Justice!: HIV/AIDS Gender Readings of the Bible*, edited by Musa W. Dube and Musimbi Kanyoro (Pietermaritzburg: Cluster Publications, 2004): 8.

11. Musimbi R.A. Kanyoro, 'Interpreting Old Testament polygamy through African women's eyes' in *The Will to Arise: Women, Tradition and the Church in Africa*, edited by Mercy A. Oduyoye and Musimbi R.A. Kanyoro (Maryknoll: Orbis Books, 1992): 87–100.

12. Madipoane Masenya (Ngwana' Mphahlele), 'Trapped between two "canons": African Christian women in the era of HIV/AIDS' in *African Women, HIV/AIDS and Faith Communities*, edited by Isabel Apawo Phiri, Beverley Haddad and Madipoane Masenya (Ngwana' Mphahlele) (Pietermaritzburg: Cluster Publications, 2003): 116.

13. Dora Rudo Mbuwayesango, 'Levirate marriage and HIV and AIDS in Zimbabwe: The story of Judah and Tamar (Genesis 38)'. *Journal of Constructive Theology* 13(2) 2007: 5–6.

14. Dorothy B.E.A. Akoto, 'Women and health in Ghana and the *trokosi* practice: An issue of women's and children's rights in 2 Kings 4:1–7' in *African Women, Religion, and Health: Essays in Honor of Mercy Amba Ewudziwa Oduyoye*, edited by Isabel Apawo Phiri and Sarojini Nadar (Maryknoll: Orbis Books, 2006): 103.

15. Lilian Siwila, 'Care-giving in times of HIV and AIDS: When hospitality is a threat to African women's lives: a gendered theological examination of the theology of hospitality'. *Journal of Constructive Theology* 13(1) 2007: 69–82.

16. See, for example, Chiropafadzo Moyo, 'A Karanga Perspective on Fertility and Barrenness as Blessing and Curse in 1 Samuel 1:1–2:10' (Doctor of Theology thesis, University of Stellenbosch, 2006).

17. For further discussion, see Chapter 11 of this book.

18. UNAIDS, *2008 Report on the Global AIDS Epidemic: Executive Summary* (Geneva: UNAIDS, 2008): 17.

19. Tabona Shoko, *Karanga Indigenous Religion in Zimbabwe: Health and Well-Being* (Aldershot: Ashgate, 2007): 21.

20. Akosua Adomako Ampofo and John Boateng, 'Multiple meanings of manhood among boys in Ghana' in *From Boys to Men: Social Constructions of Masculinity in Contemporary Society*, edited by T. Shefer et al. (Cape Town: UCT Press, 2007): 58.

21. Jo T. Wreford, *"We Can Help!": A Literature Review of Current Practice Involving Traditional African Healers in Biomedical HIV/AIDS Interventions in South Africa* (Cape Town: Centre for Social Science Research, University of Cape Town, 2005): 27–8.

22. Liz Walker, Graeme Reid and Morna Cornell, *Waiting to Happen: HIV/AIDS in South Africa: The Bigger Picture* (Cape Town: Double Storey, 2004): 47.

23. Letetia van der Poll, 'Formulating an appropriate legal response to dry sex and virginity testing within the discourse on sexuality and human rights in Africa'. Paper presented at the Fourth Conference of the International Association for the Study of Sexuality, Culture and Society 'Sex and Secrecy', Johannesburg, University of the Witwatersrand, 22–25 June, 2003: 5.

24. K. Rowe et al., 'Adherence to TB preventative therapy for HIV-positive patients in rural South Africa: Implications for antiretroviral delivery in resource-poor settings'. *International Journal of Tuberculosis and Lung Disease* 9(3) 2005: 266.

25. Wotsuna Khamalwa, 'Religion, traditional healers and the AIDS epidemic in Uganda' in *Religion and Health in Africa: Reflections for Theology in the 21st Century*, edited by Adam K. arap Chepkwony (Nairobi: Paulines Publications Africa, 2006): 82–95.

26. Heike Behrend, 'The rise of occult powers, AIDS and the Roman Catholic Church in western Uganda'. *Journal of Religion in Africa* 37(2007): 46.

27. See Chapter 14 of this book.

28. Musa W. Dube, '*Adinkra!*: Four hearts joined together: On becoming healing-teachers of African indigenous religion/s in HIV & AIDS prevention' in *African Women, Religion, and Health*, edited by Phiri and Nadar: 134.

29. Nokuzola Mndende, 'Religion and AIDS in Africa: African Traditional Religion response'. Paper read at the Conference on Prolonging Life, Challenging Religion, 15–17 April 2009, Justo Mwale College, Lusaka: 2.

30. Rasebate I. Mokotso, 'The challenges of HIV and AIDS on the hegemony of Eurocentric Christianity: The context of Lesotho'. *Lesotho Journal of Theology* 1(1) 2008: 54.

31. See, for example, Joseph B.R. Gaie, 'Ethics of breaking stigma: African, biblical and theological perspectives' in *Into the Sunshine: Integrating HIV/AIDS into the Ethics Curriculum*, edited by Charles Klagba and C.B. Peter (Eldoret: Zapf Chancery for Ecumenical HIV/AIDS Initiative in Africa, 2005): 91–111.

32. This discussion is also addressed in Chapter 7 of this book.

33. Ezra Chitando, *Living With Hope: African Churches and HIV/AIDS: Volume 1* (Geneva: WCC Publications, 2007): 58.

34. See, for instance, Fhumulani M. Mulaudzi, 'Comments on the XVI International HIV/AIDS Conference: An "ubuntu" perspective'. *Religion and Theology* 14(1–2) 2007: 108.

35. Benjamin Atwine, E. Cantor-Graae and Francis Bajunirwe, 'Psychological distress among AIDS orphans in rural Uganda'. *Social Science and Medicine* 61 (2005): 555.

36. John Waliggo, 'Inculturation and the HIV/AIDS pandemic in the AMECEA region'. *African Ecclesial Review* 47(4) 2007: 294.

37. Waliggo, 'Inculturation and the HIV/AIDS pandemic': 294–6.

38. Desmond Lesejane, 'Fatherhood from an African cultural perspective' in *Baba: Men and Fatherhood in South Africa*, edited by Linda Richter and Robert Morrell (Cape Town: Human Science Research Council, 2006): 180.

39. Julius Mutugi Gathogo, 'The use of ancestral resources in combating HIV and AIDS: *Mundurume*'s task'. *Journal of Constructive Theology* 13(1) 2007: 23.

40. Sophie Chirongoma, 'Women's rights and children's rights in the time of HIV and AIDS in Zimbabwe: An analysis of gender inequalities and its impact on people's health'. *Journal of Theology for Southern Africa* 126 (2006): 62.

41. Adam K. arap Chepkwony, 'Healing practices in Africa: Historical and theological considerations' in *Religion and Health in Africa: Reflections for the 21st Century*, edited by Adam K. arap Chepkwony (Nairobi: Paulines Publications Africa, 2006): 41.

42. Dube, '*Adinkra!*: 140–1.

43. See, for example, WHO/UNAIDS, *New Data on Male Circumcision and HIV Prevention: Policy and Programme Implications* (Geneva: WHO/UNAIDS, 2007). The report states that 'The research evidence that male circumcision is efficacious in reducing sexual transmission of

HIV from women to men is compelling' (p. 3). See also Stuart Rennie, Adamson S. Muula and Daniel Westreich, 'Male circumcision and HIV prevention: Ethical, medical and public health tradeoffs in low-income countries'. *Journal of Medical Ethics* 33(6) 2007: 357–61; Geoffrey Setswe, 'The snip: Male circumcision and HIV prevention'. *HSRC Review* 7(4) 2009, available at http://www.hsrc.ac.za/HSRC_Review_Article-170.phtml (accessed 10 Dec. 2009).

44. See, for example, Nokuzola Mndende, 'Religion and AIDS in Africa'; Malik Badri, 'The AIDS crisis: An Islamic perspective' in *Islam and AIDS: Between Scorn, Pity and Justice*, edited by Farid Esack and Sarah Chiddy (Oxford: Oneworld, 2009): 28–42.

Practitioner response

Phumzile Zondi-Mabizela

I am an activist openly living with HIV and also an ordained church leader and CEO of the KwaZulu-Natal Council of Churches in Pietermaritzburg. As much as I am committed to making sure that we strive for HIV-free churches and communities, the reality is that there are many people who are already living with HIV. I believe it is important to find creative resources and tools from different knowledge and belief systems in order to empower persons living with HIV to live long and fruitful lives.

In the offices of the KwaZulu-Natal Christian Council, there have been lively debates around the role of ATRs. In our attempts to strengthen our Men and Gender Programme in the Context of HIV and AIDS, we reviewed the positive elements of ATRs. Spearheaded by my colleague, Lucas Ngoetjana and assisted by students of the School of Politics, University of KwaZulu-Natal, we have focused on training men to be care givers in the HIV and AIDS context. Convincing them to recognise the importance of being carers, even though they are men, based on the values and teachings within Christianity and indigenous African beliefs was not an easy task. But, drawing on positive religious resources within these traditions, we constructed training workshops. To date, we have 45 fully committed men – pastors, traditional healers and community leaders who now serve as home-based carers.

In my own personal journey, it was important as a Christian Zulu woman to reclaim my indigenous religious beliefs as part of the journey towards wholeness and healing. The advent of Christianity brought along with it a serious identity crisis as our religions were not understood by the missionaries and thus rejected as pagan. When I was diagnosed as HIV positive, it resulted in an identity crisis. My reclaiming of core indigenous religious values was part of a process of rejecting feelings of non-importance and of non-belonging and so coming to accept my HIV positive status.

Chitando makes the important point that it is difficult to distinguish cultural from indigenous religious practice in ATRs. Here, the divine and the material are in constant interaction. Furthermore, within the cosmology of ATRs there is a continuum of life and death. Yet, when the HIV epidemic emerged in Africa, there was great emphasis on death and shame. I would like to suggest that these notions of the inter-relationship of the material and divine, as well as the continuum of life and death, could be important resources in the eradication of HIV and AIDS stigma and discrimination.

Chitando addressed the issue of harmful cultural practices comprehensively. The negative impact of practices such as patriarchy, polygamy, wife inheritance and widow-cleansing is evident in my work with women. However, some women will opt for polygamous marriages, as they feel polygamy is better than tolerating men who have multiple partners even when they are married to one wife. So it could be argued that it not the practice but rather the issue of secure and trusting relationships that needs to be emphasised in ensuring that women can negotiate safer sexual practices.

The issue of fertility, raised by Chitando, is important because of the pressure in traditional communities for women to have children that has made them vulnerable to HIV. However, the reasons why women choose to have children are more complex than Chitando suggests. Women themselves sometimes choose to have children and make informed decisions to take the risks involved because of their desire to become mothers. Also, in the South African context, out of financial desperation some choose to become mothers in order to access the child support grant offered by the government.[1] This is a form of survival for women and is not specifically linked to any traditional belief system.

There is a traditional cultural practice that has made both men and women vulnerable to HIV but which is not mentioned by Chitando, namely dry sex. Women have been forced to use dangerous drying agents, like herbs and bleach, in order to enhance the pleasures of the sexual experience of men. However, this has proved to be very dangerous for both men and women as it leads to tearing and provides easy access for the transmission of HIV.[2]

Chitando has shown both the positive and negative aspects of ATRs in the context of HIV. These two dimensions are present in all religions. It is important for academics, activists and practitioners to work together in research teams to identify positive religious resources that can be harnessed and used to improve the lives of HIV positive people. In the remainder of this response, therefore, I would like to highlight a few cultural practices not addressed by Chitando that could be used positively in tackling the epidemic.

In South Africa, at the beginning of 2009, there was an outcry against the revival of the culture of *ukuthwala* or *ukuthwalwa* which literally means being carried.[3] Traditionally, these were marriages that were arranged by men who were close to the woman with the intention of making sure that she married someone who had good genes, came from a good family and was relatively wealthy. The outcry in the media was a result of this practice being misappropriated and distorted. Older men were abducting girls as young as fourteen years old, then paying their parents to impregnate and so marry them. This of course increased the number of women who were infected with HIV in rural and poor households because their parents accepted payment in exchange for their daughters. However, if this practice were reintroduced appropriately, it could be an important religio-cultural resource for addressing the epidemic.

An example illustrates this point. In an unpublished paper, I discuss my experience of doing contextual Bible studies with rural women who were in arranged marriages that had begun with the cultural practice of *ukuthwalwa*. Women in these marriages claimed that they were accepted by their in-laws and were respected by their husbands. Because this was an arrangement between two families, the possibility of abuse and vulnerability to disease, they argued, were reduced.[4]

A further area of necessary exploration within ATRs is an understanding of the origin of sickness and disease. In many traditions, sickness and disease are as a result of a breakdown of communication between the living and the living dead, or ancestors. The Western emphasis on individual sin or wrongdoing is a foreign concept to the traditional African belief system. Therefore, if this emphasis on illness and disease as a communal concern is addressed, it offers possibilities for the reduction of stigma, rejection and discrimination, especially within families.

Finally, women are often viewed as the victims of gender inequality within traditional cultures but in reality the more senior they are within traditional cultures, the more power they have. In addressing issues faced by elderly women within the context of HIV, such as their vulnerability as carers of the sick and of children, their traditional respected role needs to be recovered and emphasised. While these practices offer potential resources, there is a need for further research into how they (and those mentioned by Chitando) can be appropriated in the globalised context of poverty. This is the major challenge faced by academics and practitioners alike.

In conclusion, it is clear from Chitando's important chapter that there is still work to be done in reviewing, reclaiming and reviving some of the beliefs and teachings of ATRs, which could be positive resources in mitigating the HIV and AIDS epidemic. As he suggests, much of the focus on negative aspects of indigenous beliefs and practices has emerged out of the scholarship of African women theologians. With the exception of Nokuzola Mndende's work, there has been little emphasis by women on the positive resources that ATRs offer. This gap in the literature survey needs to be filled with clear articulation by women living with HIV who have benefited from reclaiming indigenous tradition as part of their healing. This is true for me and, no doubt, for many other women. It is the voices of these women that need to set the agenda for any future research into ATRs and HIV.

Notes

1. Brenda Nkuna, 'Teenage mothers abuse state child grant'. *Cape Argus*, 29 Sep. 2008. This is a contested issue with some arguing that the anecdotal evidence suggesting that young girls fall pregnant in order to access the government child support grant is not supported by research. See, for example, Monde Makiwane and Eric Udjo, *Is the Child Support Grant Associated with an Increase in Teenage Fertility in South Africa?: Evidence from National Surveys and Administrative Data* (Pretoria: Human Sciences Research Council, 2006): 3.

2. Lisa Vetten and Kailash Bhana, *Violence, Vengeance and Gender: a Preliminary Investigation into the Links Between Violence Against Women and HIV/AIDS in South Africa* (Johannesburg: Centre for the Study of Violence and Reconciliation, 2001): 6.

3. See, for example, Pumza Fihlani, 'Stolen youth of SA's child brides'. *BBC News*, 14 Oct. 2009, available at http://www.news.bbc.co.uk/2/hi/africa/8303212.stm (accessed 10 Dec. 2009); 'Lusikisiki girl abducted in Kwa Ncele' Treatment Action Campaign, 17 June 2009. Available at http://www.tac.org.za/community/node/2611 (accessed 10 Dec. 2009).

4. Phumzile Zondi-Mabizela, 'Seducer, victim or agent: A gendered reading of Bathsheba's story (2 Samuel 11:1–27) in the context of HIV and AIDS'. Honours Research Project, School of Religion and Theology, University of KwaZulu-Natal, 2009.

10

African cultures and gender in the context of HIV and AIDS

Probing these practices

Nyokabi Kamau

INTRODUCTION

Culture can be defined as a people's way of life, including arts, beliefs and institutions passed on from one generation to another. The United Nations Educational, Scientific and Cultural Organisation (UNESCO) describes culture as taking diverse forms across time and space; encompassing different sets of distinctive spiritual, material, intellectual and emotional features that characterise a particular society or social group; and including value systems, traditions and beliefs.[1] For the purpose of this chapter, culture is understood to include indigenous religious beliefs and practices.[2]

In this era of HIV and AIDS, much has been said about African cultures having been eroded by Western cultures. Dortzbach, for example, argues that some good African cultural practices such as faithfulness to a spouse, avoiding sex before marriage and family care for the sick and orphaned have been abandoned and there is a need to restore them.[3] There are also debates, however, about cultural practices that are harmful and outdated, such as wife inheritance, female genital mutilation and sex cleansing; and it is argued that they should be abandoned.[4]

The culture of a people is usually demonstrated through social institutions such as religion and the family and includes rituals that mark birth, initiation, the beginning and end of war, planting, marriage, harvest and death, among others. It is through such practices and institutions that culture is upheld. In many African cultures, it is a common belief that good human conduct is rewarded by the spiritual world with abundant rainfall, plentiful harvests, offspring and general prosperity, while adverse conduct is punished with disease, epidemics, famine, drought and even death.[5] Given this reality, understanding people's culture has been deemed crucial in informing appropriate ways of handling the HIV and AIDS epidemic. How people deal with sexuality, gender relations, marriage, initiation, illness and death is central to both their interconnected cultural and religious practices.

It has been noted in the literature on HIV and AIDS that the highest infection rates are in those cultures where women have little power over their sexual behaviour.[6] It is argued that women are more vulnerable because of cultural norms that restrict their decision-making power over most areas of their lives, including lack of capacity to use protective measures against HIV and AIDS, added to the lack of accessibility of accurate and reliable information. Current statistics show that in some countries in sub-Saharan Africa for every infected man there are four infected women.[7] It is, therefore, important to understand the socio-cultural and economic factors that render women vulnerable to HIV infection.

This chapter critically analyses literature that deals with issues of African cultures and gender and seeks to chart areas for further research.

CULTURE AND GENDER

It has been increasingly recognised that HIV and AIDS is not just a health matter but also involves cultural, religious, political, economic and gender issues. The focus in this section of the chapter is on the intersection of gender and cultural issues. Discussions in the literature have shown gender to be a central aspect of sexuality and relations between men and women. This reality is central to any efforts related to prevention and management of HIV and AIDS.

In understanding HIV transmission and initiating appropriate programmes of action, it is crucial that the socially constructed aspects of relationships between men and women that underpin individual behaviour be understood. These include gender-based rules, norms and laws governing the broader social and institutional context. In most societies, gender relations continue to be characterised by an unequal balance of power between men and women, with women having fewer legal rights and less access to education, health services, training, income-generating activities and property. This situation affects both their access to information about HIV and AIDS and the steps that they can take to prevent its transmission.[8] Gender is a culture-specific construct indicating varying patterns in gender relations within different cultures. However, there is similarity in many African cultures in the gendered division of roles between men and women. Typically, it is men who make most of the important decisions in homes and in wider society while women remain responsible for the reproductive and productive roles within the household.[9] This gender imbalance is manifest in all sectors of society and, as a result, women experience the impact of the HIV and AIDS epidemic more severely than men, given the lack of power and control in many aspects of their lives.[10]

Analysis that engages this gendered power dynamic enables us to discern the impact that cultural constructs of feminine and masculine have on HIV transmission.[11] The cultural symbolisation of sexual difference has had a profound mark on human existence. While sexual differences form the basis for a particular distribution of social roles, most human activity classified as masculine or feminine is not naturally determined. Instead, these classifications are socially determined through processes of gender construction.[12] Gendered social systems establish stereotypes and different moral standards for women and men.

In most parts of the world, dominant gender systems deny women the right to a pleasurable sexuality, impose stereotypes and create double standards that divide women into those socially considered worthy of motherhood within the sanctified institution of marriage, and those expected to satisfy the sexual appetites of men and categorised as whores.[13] Good women should marry, be virgins at marriage, remain monogamous and be sexually naive in bed.[14] In some African cultures the deep-rooted tradition of female genital mutilation is practised to ensure the sexual satisfaction of men. Assitan Diallo, however, has noted from work in Mali that there are often inconsistent messages about women's sexuality. He observes that there is a shift between trying to control women's sexuality through sexual mutilation and encouraging women's sexual pleasure. Diallo's suggestion that there are practices for controlling women's sexuality while at the same time promoting women's sexual pleasure 'reveals a social context of gender inequality and resistance to change women's status in society'.[15]

Writing about gender and sexuality in Kenya, Nelson argues that the social and cultural position of women and their vulnerability to HIV infection needs to be theorised as an issue of power.[16] Research has shown that many married women are not in a position to negotiate safer sex with their husbands.[17] Joanne Manchester argues that marriage can be a principal risk factor for women.[18] The sad reality is that it is in marriage women may have the most difficulty negotiating safer sex, such as the use of a condom, as this implies a lack of trust. So, it can be argued that marriage may be unsafe for women since these relationships are not based on equality. As Noriene Kaleeba and Sunanda Ray state: 'For some women, even though they are married, there's no joking about sex. If there is going to be sex, you will just jump to bed. In such a situation you cannot just raise the subject [of condoms].'[19]

A study carried out in Tanzania and Zambia showed that women specifically avoided raising issues of condoms with their husbands for fear of violent retaliation. The study indicated that in Zambia fewer than 25 per cent agreed that a woman could refuse to have sex with her husband, even if he was known to be violent, unfaithful or HIV positive.[20] Writing about the Kenyan situation, Mumbi Machera also argues that many women cannot use contraceptives because of their husbands' fear that they may be unfaithful. Some men suffer from what Machera refers to as 'condom phobia' that suggests that using a condom with a wife is like 'begging for what belongs to you'.[21]

Musa Dube has further noted how the lack of control over their bodies renders women particularly vulnerable to HIV infection in contexts of poverty:

> [I]t has been documented that poverty is quite central to the spread of HIV/AIDS through its capacity to pull many threads of transmission . . . if poverty takes the lead in sponsoring HIV/AIDS, women are at the receiving end of the poverty driven epidemic due to gender constructions that distance them from property ownership, decision making and control over their own bodies.[22]

The role of poverty in fuelling the spread of HIV and AIDS has been documented by other scholars. John Illife observes that a study of over 2 500 workers conducted in Addis Ababa, Ethiopia in 1994 showed that while HIV infection in men was strongly associated with reported sexual behaviour and a past history of syphilis, among women it was associated with socio-demographic characteristics such as low income, low education and living alone.[23] This suggests that while men were likely to have become infected through voluntary risky sexual behaviour, the women were mostly driven to such behaviour by a need to make ends meet and survive. Similarly, Fulata Moyo observes that 'it is evident that HIV spreads more rapidly among women who have a lower social-economic status and little decision making power or education'.[24]

Lack of economic empowerment means that women's work always takes place in the private sphere of the home. Thus, scholars have observed that care giving amongst many African communities continues to be a gendered role ascribed to women.[25] Dorcas Akintunde observes that women within traditional Nigerian Yoruba society, as in other cultures, assume the main role of care giving as 'they not only bear life but they nurse, they cherish, they give warmth and they care for life because all humanity passes through their bodies'.[26] In relation to gender and care work, Dube also observes that women spend much time and energy at home 'washing, cleaning, changing, feeding and talking to the depressed patients'. This has a negative effect on their economic production as they can no longer attend to farms or businesses, or at best only for brief periods. This situation serves to deepen already existing poverty, or to make once economically stable women poor. In addition, as Dube notes, when it is the women themselves who are sick they are not likely to have someone care for them. Many widows also find themselves ejected from their marital homes and disinherited by their in-laws after nursing sick husbands, leading to serious poverty that further perpetuates vulnerability to infection.[27] This suggests that, socially and culturally, men's health is perceived to be of greater importance than that of women. The issues raised here form an area that needs further research and intervention.

Linked to the discussion on gender and care work is the need to acknowledge that social inequality between men and women also affects women's access to care and treatment. Dube, for example, observes that 'women living with HIV and AIDS, after having taken time off their economic activities to nurse sick spouses are unlikely to have sufficient money to buy ARVs for themselves'.[28] Research thus also needs to be carried out on how gender inequalities affect access to care and treatment.

Furthermore, Dube observes that stigma associated with HIV and AIDS is also gendered in many African cultures: disease and uncleanness are associated with women's bodies. She notes that 'in some Setswana cultures, STDs are referred to as ... women's diseases' and in many cases women are seen as the HIV transmitters and are accused of having sex with foreign men, thus bringing HIV into their homes.[29]

AFRICAN CULTURE, SEXUALITY AND HIV AND AIDS

One of the factors driving HIV and AIDS stigma is its sexual nature.[30] In order to understand the complexity of HIV and AIDS, it is important to look at the historical background to current attitudes about sexuality in Africa. Susan Hunter provides background to the origins of the shame that became associated with sex in Africa long before the HIV and AIDS epidemic. During colonial times, the British set up laws in the colonies that were tougher than those in their own country because they believed that perceived primitive practices required harsher enforcement.[31] Similarly, Sylvia Tamale notes that 'Africans were encouraged to reject their previous beliefs and values to adopt the "civilised ways" of the colonial masters'.[32] In the days of colonialism, according to Hunter, 'Victorians thought that tropical climates acted as breeding grounds for disease, inflamed passions and negated reason . . . primitive peoples, they believed, were simply more tolerant of filth and STDs because of their unrestrained sexuality, both symptoms of non-western and moral decay'.[33]

Charmaine Pereira, for example, notes that the notion of sexuality as bad or filthy is relatively new in Africa because it was introduced to Africans through colonialism and Christianity.[34] Among the Gikuyu of Kenya there were restrictions on sex before marriage for both men and women, with training on sexual matters offered to both boys and girls before they were initiated. A practice known as *ngwiko* – a form of sexual foreplay on the male and female genitalia – was allowed for young people to express their sexuality without penetration. During *ngwiko* the couple would share an intimate encounter with the woman's skirt tightly tied to her thighs to avoid possible penetration. The practice often took place with a number of young men and women in the same room as this strengthened peer pressure and minimised chances of full sexual intercourse.[35] The missionaries misunderstood *ngwiko*, branding it sinful. Anyone caught performing it would be punished.

Hence, Jomo Kenyatta has argued that much of the stigma currently associated with sex (at least among the Gikuyu) can be linked to colonialism and Christianity.[36] It is documented that the Gikuyu people's way of life was the most disrupted by colonial rule in Kenya.[37] Some have even suggested that the current subordinate status of women in sexual relationships among the Gikuyu can be linked to the stigma that Christianity associated with sex. This is because women found it difficult to talk about sex with their husbands as they would appear un-Christian, unschooled and backward.[38] Similarly, John Mbiti argues that traditionally sex was not viewed as an act of shame or immoral because it was normally performed according to specific rules of the African communities.[39]

Puberty and initiation rites

Initiation of young people to adulthood was practised throughout the continent with varying rites and rituals in pre-colonial Africa. One common factor, however, was the fact that communities always had a way of marking the shift from childhood to adulthood. The main aim of these initiation rites was to prepare young people for sex in marriage, parenthood and other leadership responsibilities. In the case of Kenya, almost all communities had some form of puberty rite usually performed for both boys and girls. Some involved male circumcision, female genital cut and, on rare occasions, for example among the Somalis, female genital mutilation. Others involved the removal of teeth or the killing of a lion by the young Maasai men as a sign of growing up. Nahasio Ndung'u points out that traditional African communities dealt with matters of sex, sexuality and family life during these puberty rites. In modern Africa puberty rites have become a private affair for most communities, especially with regard to girls' initiation, as this was the most condemned by Christianity and the fact that some practices, such as female genital cut, are illegal.[40] It has been on record in the media that many communities in Kenya still take their daughters for the cut but usually this is a secret affair. This secrecy sometimes means that the girls are in worse danger as they may not be cut under hygienic conditions. Anecdotal evidence suggests that many Kenyan parents still practise some form of female initiation and are opting to do it to girls as young as five years old because they cannot resist or report their parents to the authorities. This is an area that needs much more research and theological reflection in order to provide life-giving solutions in the context of HIV and AIDS.

Other puberty rites such as the elongation of the labia minora among the Baganda needs to be addressed. Sylvia Tamale explores some of the ways in which this practice infuses the cultural lives of Baganda women and discusses the erotic-textual constructions of Baganda women's bodies. She argues that the practice of elongating the labia minora served three main purposes:[41] first, enhancing the erotic experience of both the male and the female as they touched during foreplay or during mutual masturbation; second, elongated labia served as a kind of self-identifier for Baganda women (the stamp of legitimacy for a true Muganda woman and as many participants in Tamale's study indicated, a practice worth preserving); and third, a purely aesthetic function as several Baganda men interviewed suggested that they enjoyed looking at and fondling the stretched labia of a woman. Whether such practices need to be preserved and whether they would help to empower women in their negotiations for safer sex in the context of HIV and AIDS requires further research.

Similarly, Heike Becker argues that the practice of women's initiation known as *efundula* in Namibia is worth revisiting. According to Becker, this would provide an opportunity to rethink gender construction and how culture is also tied to the evocation of sexuality.[42] For researchers interested in understanding African sexuality in the context of HIV and AIDS, it would be useful to establish why these practices have persisted for so long. It would also be worthwhile to find out the role they can play in handling sexuality and gender issues in a way that would leave men and women better placed to face the epidemic, rather than to continue condemning them en masse.

The discussion on puberty rites has been controversial. Eunice Kamaara, for example, attributes prevalence of HIV in some African communities to initiation which, according to her, licenses young people to early and unprotected sex.[43] But others argue in support of puberty rites. In Ghana, for example, Brigid Sackey notes that there has been a concerted attempt by religious groups, chiefs, public officials and individuals to restore puberty rites, arguing that their abolition has created a vacuum in the moral lives of the youth, manifest in sexual laxity and associated problems of teenage pregnancy and the spread of sexually transmitted diseases (STDs), including HIV. According to Sackey, the moral laxity of Ghanaian youth has been caused by a lack of marking of puberty rites as traditionally carried out. While condemning harmful rites, for example female genital mutilation, incision, scarification, nudity and so forth, Sackey asserts that puberty rites are extremely beneficial and educative. In research on young girls in Accra, however, it was found that the majority thought initiation as it existed in the past was obnoxious, indecent and stressful. After lengthy discussions with the girls, the researcher observed that there were indeed some negative and cruel aspects of initiation but at the same time emphasised the positive and moral values inherent in the rites and their implications for managing the spread of HIV and other STDs. This led to more than 70 per cent of the participants in the study undergoing a kind of initiation devoid of nudity and cruelty. Sackey concludes that these girls came to understand that cultural values and practices of traditional Africa can be positive when adjusted to modern Africa.[44]

In my experience, modern forms of initiation of both girls and boys have also been embraced in Kenya where individuals and churches have started school holiday programmes at which teenage boys and girls receive sex education. In the case of boys, where male circumcision is now being actively encouraged, they undergo sex maturation talks and then go through the cut. In some cases the education is not directly connected to the cut. In the case of girls, these programmes are popularly referred to as initiation without a cut. In the review of literature for this chapter, I found no research that assessed the impact of these more recent programmes, so this would be an interesting area for research as the issue of sexuality and culture is so central to understanding and managing the spread of HIV.

Marriage and sex

Given the importance of marriage and family relationships in Africa, sexual practice within the marriage relationship must be interrogated in the context of HIV and AIDS. While marriage should be a source of protection for women, it has been found in many instances to be a source of oppression and pain. Studies increasingly show that married women are vulnerable to HIV infection because they are unable to insist on the use of condoms, as discussed earlier in the chapter.[45]

Sex within marriage should be a source of mutual pleasure and bonding rather than only a duty and a condition for procreation. This is often not the case because whereas men are given sexual freedom, women do not have the same freedom and many are at the mercy of their husbands and partners. A World Health Organisation report observed that although there are certain cultures in which casual sex is not tolerated for either of the partners in marriage, the more common picture is that women are expected to remain faithful to their husbands, while it seems acceptable for men to have multiple sex partners, whether official or otherwise.[46] The dominant ideology on femininity emphasises uncompromising loyalty and fidelity in marital relations.[47] Dhianaraj Chetty observes that in South Africa there is an expectation that married women should be faithful and compassionate to their HIV infected husbands while husbands are known to abandon infected wives.[48] These double standards create an environment where HIV thrives.

However, these double standards did not always apply to marital relations in pre-colonial Africa. Writing about the Gikuyu people of Kenya, Kenyatta notes that adultery was prohibited for both men and women. However, polygamy and an organised form of adultery were used as channels for men to deal with their sexual desires out of wedlock.[49] Men were free to marry as many women as their wealth could allow and, indeed, their other wives would normally suggest future brides. This gave women certain power to decide which other women would be their co-wives because if they did not approve of who was brought to the home, they would gang up against her, resulting in her leaving the homestead. My own mother was a wife in a polygamous marriage of nine wives and shared such an experience. Today, out-of-wedlock relationships are carried out in secret, leaving married women especially vulnerable as they have no control over their husbands' behaviour.[50]

Furthermore, in some communities, women could have sex with her husband's friends of the same age with the consent of her husband if they were staying overnight.[51] This practice was only acceptable if it was not secret, or the man and woman would be punished. In present-day Africa, wives and husbands do have sex outside marriage, but secretly. Even though it is mainly men who talk about their adulterous behaviour, women too are engaged in such behaviour but, due to societal restrictions on their sexuality, this is never openly discussed. Modern-day marriage seems to thrive on hypocrisy. Therefore, further research on sexual practice in marriage that takes seriously the agency of both men and women is sorely needed.

Widow cleansing and wife inheritance

Wife inheritance, where practised, was also blamed for increased HIV infections. In some communities in Kenya it is still a requirement that a woman is married off to a brother of her deceased spouse. Before this is done she first has to have sex with a professional inheritor who sleeps with all the widows in the village. A member of a women's NGO known as Women Fighting AIDS in Kenya (WOFAK), herself living with the virus, shared that when she lost her husband due to AIDS-related illness in 1999, she was required by the family to have sex with the village inheritor for cleansing and then she was to be inherited by her brother-in-law.[52] She disobeyed but this meant that she was excommunicated from her family and lost all the property of their rural home. This is a common experience for many women in Kenya across all classes.

In the context of HIV and AIDS, this practice of wife inheritance involving sexual intercourse has been severely criticised with proposals being made to offer support for widows and their children.[53] Yet many people cling to such practices and further research is needed on why people do so, especially in the HIV and AIDS context. Such research could help to inform how the positive aspects, such as providing economic support to women, could be retained while the more harmful aspects of the practice are modified or removed. Some of this work is being documented, for example the study by Julia Maxted in Zambia.[54] It showed that with time and adequate information communicated in language that people can easily understand, they do evaluate their practices and abandon those that are not beneficial or put them at risk.

RELIGION, SEXUALITY, SHAME AND BLAME

This chapter has, thus far, argued that in sub-Saharan Africa where HIV is mainly transmitted sexually, it is crucial to understand cultural norms that govern people's sexual behaviour. Most of these are underpinned by deep-rooted gendered power dynamics, as discussed earlier. What is being assumed in this discussion is that religion is inter-connected with gendered cultural practice.

According to Helen Jackson, the influence of religion and culture on sexual behaviour is complex at both individual and societal levels.[55] Agrippa Khathide argues that in South Africa there is a conspiracy of silence around sexuality that has been a major problem in mitigating the epidemic. Khathide points out that whenever there is discussion about sex one is told either that Africans do not talk about sex in public because they are Christians, or that it is not African to do so.[56] Nevertheless, it is necessary to talk about sexuality and sexual practices in the HIV and AIDS context.

Marjorie Mbilinyi and Naomi Kaihula, for example, note that in Zambia the so-called good people blame the problem of HIV and AIDS on sinners and outsiders:

> Christian and indigenous polarities of good and evil, holiness and sin, framed the dominant discourse through which HIV and AIDS was constructed in Rungwe ... Everyone associated AIDS with their own version of high risk groups; youth (male and female), sex workers, women traders and bar maids, outsiders (factory workers, truck drivers). The dominant discourse was that of people blaming others for the problem – women blaming men and vice versa, old blaming the youth, outsiders being blamed by insiders, young men blaming old men for infecting young girls leaving them no women to marry etc.[57]

Thus, issues of sexuality are infused with religious discourse that incorporates both Christian views of morality where the evil of the HIV and AIDS epidemic is seen as a product of an adulterous life;[58] and the indigenous African view that health and well-being is dependent on being good. As a result, a discourse of shame has emerged. In Kenya, for example, HIV infection is still associated with the promiscuity of women, resulting in greater stigmatisation of HIV positive women. When they try to access health benefits they are more likely to be treated with spite as bad mothers and deserving of HIV infection. As a result, many women do not seek help from health facilities.

My own work with senior university women confirmed this shame associated with HIV that makes it difficult for even professional women to come to terms with their HIV status and that of their relatives.[59] The issue of the stigma associated with HIV and the question of how one became infected is an enormous challenge for women and girls.[60] The denial of women's sexuality, as has already been discussed, and the social assumption that women must be pure, make it difficult to acknowledge sexual experience before marriage.[61]

The discourse of shame and blame as it pertains to religion and culture requires further research. While there is a growing body of literature, it remains an area of greatest challenge in the African continent and needs ongoing and sustained inquiry.

EVALUATIVE CONCLUSION

Richard Parker and Peter Aggleton argue that current research should move beyond behavioural and psychological models that have tended to dominate HIV and AIDS studies. While behavioural models have provided some insights and will continue to play a crucial role in a broader research and programmatic response to this epidemic, they need to be complemented by new ways of understanding and overcoming HIV and AIDS-related stigma, stigmatisation and discrimination. The issues raised in this chapter show clearly the need for new conceptualisations of both traditional and modern African culture. Conceptual studies have a crucial role to play in ensuring that existing knowledge is constantly reviewed for its adequacy and appropriateness in the light of changing needs and circumstances. They conclude by suggesting that there is a need for research that can lead to new categories of thinking, together with new ways for identifying priorities, to examine the social, cultural, political and economic determinants and consequences of stigmatisation and discrimination.[62] From the discussion in this chapter, it is clear that there is a need to conduct broad comparative research across the African continent. This will enable a better understanding of those religious and cultural aspects that cross geographical and ethnic boundaries that need new conceptualisation in order to offer more life-giving programmatic solutions.

Furthermore, research into issues of sexuality, particularly African women's sexuality in traditional and modern cultures, is required because it continues to be shrouded in silence. Gender inequalities are products of culture. It is imperative, therefore, that the starting point in any intervention or strategy should be consideration of how various aspects of a people's culture, including their religious beliefs, work for or against the interests of women. There is a need for a deeper analysis of traditional and modern initiation practices and the role they can play in de-stigmatising sexuality for both men and women. Future research should, therefore, investigate African sexuality beyond Christian, colonial and patriarchal discourses. It would be useful to establish which practices are worth preserving and those that need to be changed. Research needs to address questions such as: how can Africans hold on to what was useful in their cultures while still upholding what is helpful in modern situations; and what is the meaning of enculturation in the HIV and AIDS context?

Cultural values are deeply rooted and require sustained and careful examination. The HIV crisis offers an opportunity for culture to be challenged and to change when issues are understood and alternatives are explored. Cultural values that preserve life need to be emphasised and those that threaten life should be discarded. The paradox of cultural tradition is that it can assist in ending the spread of HIV, if handled well, but can also be the most fertile ground for disaster.[63] There is a need to develop frameworks that can help us to understand and appreciate culture and tradition, yet are able to acknowledge the contested nature of its practice.

NOTES

1. UNESCO, 'Universal Declaration on Cultural Diversity' (2001). Available at http://www. unesdoc. unesco.org/images/0012/001271/127160m.pdf.
2. It was argued in Chapter 9 of this book that cultural beliefs and practices were inseparable from indigenous religions.
3. Deborah Dortzbach (ed), *AIDS in Kenya: The Church's Challenge and the Lessons Learned: Challenge to Care* (Nairobi: MAP International, 1998): 11.
4. For further discussion on some of these practices see Chapter 9 of this book.

5. Jaap Breetvelt, *Theological Responses to HIV and Aids Pandemic* (Utrecht: Kerk in Actie, 2009): 7.

6. See, for example, Virginia Vliet, *The Politics of AIDS* in *Briefings*, edited by Peter Collins (London: Bowerdean, 1996); Nyokabi Kamau, *Aids, Gender and Sexuality: Experiences of Women in Kenyan Universities* (Eldoret: Zapf Chancery, 2009); and Catherine Campbell, *Letting Them Die: Why HIV/AIDS Prevention Programmes Fail* (Cape Town: International African Institute, 2003).

7. UNAIDS, 'Epidemic update, 2009'. Available at http://www.data.unaids.org/pub/Report/2009/2009_epidemic_update_en.pdf (accessed 8 Dec. 2009).

8. Commonwealth Secretariat, *Gender Mainstreaming in HIV/AIDS: Taking a Multisectoral Approach*, edited by Tina Johnson (London: Commonwealth Secretariat, 2002).

9. Caroline Moser, *Gender Planning and Development: Theory, Practice and Training* (London: Routledge, 1993).

10. Geeta Rao Gupta, Daniel Whelan and Keera Allendorf, *Integrating Gender into HIV and AIDS Programmes* (Washington, DC: WHO, 2003).

11. Luisa Ana Liguori and Marta Lamas, 'Gender, sexual citizenship and HIV/AIDS'. *Culture, Health and Sexuality*: 5(1) 2003: 87–90.

12. Voluntary Service Overseas. *Gendering Aids: Women, Men, Empowerment, Mobilization* (2003). Available at http://www.vso.org.uk/advocacy/hivaids_gender.htm: 9–11.

13. Marjorie Mbilinyi and Naomi Kaihula, 'Sinners and outsiders: The drama of Aids in Rungwe' in *Aids, Sexuality and Gender in Africa: Collective Strategies and Struggles in Tanzania and Zambia*, edited by Carolyn Baylies and Janet Bujra (London: Routledge, 2000): 78.

14. Timothy Njoya, *The Crisis of Explosive Masculinity* (Nairobi: Men for the Equality of Men and Women, 2008): xvii–xxv.

15. Assitan Diallo, 'Paradoxes of female sexuality in Mali: Of the practices of Magonmaka Abd Bolokoli-Kela' in *Re-Thinking Sexualities in Africa*, edited by Signe Arnfred (Uppsala: Nordic Africa Institute, 2004): 173, 188.

16. Nici Nelson, ' "Selling her kiosk": Kikuyu notions of sexuality and sex for sale in Mathare Valley, Kenya' in *The Cultural Construction of Sexuality*, edited by Pat Caplan (London: Tavistock Publications, 1987): 217–39.

17. Merge Berer and Sunanda Ray, *Women and HIV/AIDS: An International Resource Book* (London: Pandora, 1993).

18. Joanne Manchester, 'The HIV Epidemic in South Africa: Personal Views of Positive People' (MA dissertation, University of London Institute of Education, 2000).

19. Noriene Kaleeba and Sunanda Ray, *We Miss You All* (Harare: Women and AIDS Support Network, 1997): 60.

20. Commonwealth Secretariat, *Gender Mainstreaming in HIV /AIDS*: 48.

21. Mumbi Machera, ' "Opening a can of worms": A debate on female sexuality in the lecture theatre' in *Re-Thinking Sexualities in Africa*, edited by Arnfred: 167.

22. Musa W. Dube, 'Grant me justice: Towards multi-sectoral HIV/AIDS readings of the Bible' in *Grant Me Justice!: HIV/AIDS and Gender Readings of the Bible*, edited by Musa W. Dube and Musimbi Kanyoro (Pietermaritzburg: Cluster Publications, 2004): 8.

23. John Illife, *The African AIDS Epidemic: A History* (Athens: Ohio University Press, 2006): 31.

24. Fulata L. Moyo, 'Sex, gender, power and HIV/AIDS in Malawi: Threats and challenges to women being church' in *On Being Church: African Women's Voices and Visions*, edited by I.A. Phiri and S. Nadar (Geneva: WCC Publications, 2005): 127–37.

25. For further discussion see Chapter 11 of this book.

26. Dorcas O. Akintunde, 'Women as healers' in *African Women, Religion and Health: Essays in Honour of Mercy Amba Ewudziwa Oduyoye*, edited by I.A. Phiri and S. Nadar (Pietermaritzburg: Cluster Publications, 2006): 157.

27. Dube, 'Grant me justice': 10.

28. Dube, 'Grant me justice': 10.

29. Dube, 'Grant me justice': 11.

30. Catherine Campbell, Yugi Nair and Sbongile Maimane, 'AIDS stigma, sexual moralities and the policing of women and youth in South Africa'. *Feminist Review* 83 (2006): 132–8.

31. Susan Hunter, *Who Cares?: AIDS in Africa* (Basingstoke: Palgrave Macmillan, 2003): 168.

32. Sylvia Tamale, 'Eroticism, sensuality and "women's secrets" among the Baganda: a critical analysis'. *Feminist Africa* 5 (2005): 25.

33. Hunter, *Who Cares?*: 169.

34. Charmaine Pereira, 'Where angels fear to tread: Some thoughts on Patricia McFadden's "Sexual Pleasure as Feminist Choice"'. *Feminist Africa* 2 (2002): 62.

35. Jomo Kenyatta, *Facing Mount Kenya: The Tribal Life of the Gikuyu* (London: Secker and Warburg, 1938): 155–62.

36. Kenyatta, *Facing Mount Kenya*: 158–9.

37. Caroline Elkins, *Imperial Reckoning: The Untold Story of Britain's Gulag in Kenya* (New York: Henry Holt, 2005).

38. Signe Arnfred, 'African sexuality/sexuality in Africa: Tales and silences' in *Re-Thinking Sexualities in Africa*, edited by Arnfred: 18–27.

39. John Mbiti, *Introduction to African Religion* (London: Heinemann, 1975).

40. Nahasio W. Ndung'u, 'Quests for abundant life in Africa' in *Youth, Sexuality and AIDS*, edited by M. Getui and Mathew M. Theuri (Nairobi: Acton Publishers, 2000): 132.

41. Tamale, 'Eroticism, sensuality and "women's secrets" among the Baganda': 27.

42. Heike Becker, 'Efundula: Women's initiation, gender, sexual identities in colonial and post-colonial Namibia' in *Re-Thinking Sexualities in Africa*, edited by Arnfred: 36.

43. Eunice K. Kamaara, *Youth, Sexuality and HIV/AIDS: A Kenyan Experience* (Eldoret: AMECEA Publications, 2005).

44. Brigid M. Sackey, 'Cultural responses to the management of HIV/AIDS: The repackaging of puberty rites'. *Research Review* 17(2) 2001: 63, 65, 69.

45. Recent statistics show HIV infection is increasing in stable, low-risk groups. See UNAIDS, 'Epidemic update, 2009'. Available at http://www.data.unaids.org/pub/Report/2009/2009_epidemic_update_en.pdf (accessed 8 Dec. 2009).

46. World Health Organisation, *AIDS: Images of the Epidemic* (Geneva: WHO, 1994).

47. Gupta, Whelan and Allendorf, *Integrating Gender into HIV and AIDS Programmes*.

48. Dhianaraj Chetty, *Institutionalising the Response to HIV/AIDS in the South African University Sector: A Sauvca Analysis* (Pretoria: South African Universities Vice-Chancellors' Association, 2000): 45.

49. Kenyatta, *Facing Mount Kenya*: 181–2.

50. For a further critique of polygamy see the work of the Circle of Concerned African Theologians such as Musimbi R.A. Kanyoro, 'Interpreting Old Testament polygamy through African women's eyes' in *The Will to Arise: Women, Tradition and the Church in Africa*, edited by Mercy A. Oduyoye and Musimbi R.A. Kanyoro (Maryknoll: Orbis Books, 1992): 87–100.

51. Kenyatta, *Facing Mount Kenya*: 181, 184. For a critique of this and other such practices in the context of HIV and AIDS see Chapter 9 of this book.

52. Discussion with a group of students at St Paul's University, Limeru, Kenya, 2008.

53. Mae Alice Reggy-Mamo, 'Levitate customs and HIV & AIDS: A personal experience' in *Sexual Cultural Practices and HIV/AIDS Transmission in Nigeria*, edited by E. Amoah, D. Akitunde and D. Akoto (Accra: Sam-Woode, 2005): 45–65.

54. Julia Maxted, 'Mobilizing communities for HIV/AIDS prevention: Sociological perspectives'. Paper presented at UNAIDS/UNDP/SIDA Winter School, Johannesburg, July 2003.

55. Helen Jackson, *AIDS in Africa: Continent in Crisis* (Harare: SAfAIDS, 2002): 134–8.

56. Agrippa G. Khathide, 'Teaching and talking about sexuality: A means of combating HIV/ AIDS' in *HIV/AIDS and the Curriculum: Methods of Integrating HIV/AIDS in the Theological Programmes*, edited by Musa W. Dube (Geneva: WCC Publications, 2003): 1.

57. Mbilinyi and Kaihula, 'Sinners and outsiders': 85–6.

58. For a further discussion of the historical development of this morality discourse, see Chapter 2 of this book.

59. Kamau, *Aids, Gender and Sexuality*: 201–2.

60. For a further discussion on HIV stigma, see Chapter 14 of this book.

61. Kamau, *Aids, Gender and Sexuality*: 203–5.

62. Richard Parker and Peter Aggleton, 'HIV and AIDS related stigma and discrimination: A conceptual framework and implications for action'. *Social Science and Medicine* 57 (2003): 20, 24.

63. Peter K. Sarpong, 'The cultural practices influencing the spread of HIV/AIDS' in *AIDS and the African Church*, edited by Michael Czerny (Nairobi: Paulines Publications Africa, 2005): 43–8.

Practitioner response

Ezra Chitando

The chapter by Nyokabi Kamau has largely succeeded in drawing attention to the scholarly literature on this major theme of culture and gender in relation to the HIV and AIDS epidemic. In this response, I would like to suggest further themes that require attention.

The first theme is that of culture as a resource. One of the major challenges in the discussion on culture and HIV is the tendency to regard culture only in negative terms. Every culture has positive and negative traits. In the response to HIV, negative cultural beliefs and practices tend to receive emphasis. To a very large extent, the Circle of Concerned African Women Theologians has fallen into this trap of presenting only the negative traits of African culture in the struggle against the epidemic. The challenge lies in identifying positive cultural values, beliefs and practices that have enabled Africa to respond to the pandemic. In my experience with working with the Ecumenical HIV and AIDS Initiative in Africa (EHAIA), in most parts of the region we have encountered life-giving beliefs and practices. These include the transformation of culture in the face of HIV, including changing inheritance practices.

Second, it must be noted that culture does not serve everyone the same way. In fact, there are gatekeepers who interpret culture in particular ways and so there is a need for a hermeneutic of suspicion whenever references are made to culture. Who is speaking? Do they benefit from a particular interpretation of culture? What do they stand to lose if culture is transformed? In workshops across most parts of the region, EHAIA personnel have reported that young people appear more willing to experiment with new beliefs and practices. Elderly men, as well as men and women in positions of authority, tend to be more conservative in relation to the need to change culture. Further research needs to be undertaken on who speaks on behalf of particular cultural beliefs and practices.

Third, culture is not static but dynamic. What is new today will be granted traditional status in the near future. African cultures have borrowed and will continue to borrow from other cultures. There is, therefore, a need to identify the extent to which this presents a window of opportunity to transform African cultures in the face of HIV and AIDS.

Last, I would like to note that the marriage between biblical and African cultures is a deadly cocktail. At a workshop in Swaziland in November 2007, EHAIA staff (including me) were stunned when the majority of male participants argued that marital rape is a contradiction in terms. Both the Bible and Swazi culture confirm that such a phenomenon does not exist, they argued. There is need for further scholarly analysis of how certain forms of inculturation increase women's vulnerability to HIV. How do men abuse the Bible and culture to achieve specific objectives?

In conclusion, the discussion on culture and HIV and AIDS needs to recall the contestation over culture in missionary discourses. This has left male African theologians in a difficult situation. They feel that they should not join African women theologians in bashing African culture, even though they admit that the women theologians have raised valuable arguments. The struggle against HIV and AIDS is equally the struggle for the transformation of cultures across the world, so that they become life-giving.

11

Transforming masculinities towards gender justice in an era of HIV and AIDS

Plotting the pathways

Adriaan van Klinken

INTRODUCTION

In the context of the HIV and AIDS epidemic, men and masculinities have become contested. This is especially so in contexts where HIV is transmitted predominantly through heterosexual contact and men are criticised for spreading the virus and contributing to the impact of the epidemic on women's lives. This has given rise to investigations of masculinities as these are said to inform male behaviour. The intersection of men, masculinities and HIV and AIDS is studied, among others, from the perspective of religion and theology. This chapter seeks to survey the literature on this particular intersection. It further investigates how issues of men and masculinities are addressed, analysed and reflected upon in the context of HIV and AIDS from the perspective of religion and theology.

The chapter begins with an introduction to the concept of masculinity, briefly outlining how it has become central to the study of the HIV epidemic and how it is understood theoretically. In the following section the problematic aspects of masculinity in the context of HIV and AIDS are discussed, investigating in particular scholars' consideration of the role of religion. The subsequent section outlines how scholars imagine a transformation of masculinities, including the helpfulness of religious resources and the theological view from which these are explored. The chapter concludes with a few evaluative reflections.

But, before moving on to the first section, some introductory remarks have to be made on the body of literature to be discussed. First, studying men and masculinities in the context of HIV and AIDS and from the perspective of religion and theology is a very recent development. Therefore, the number of publications in this area is relatively small and the issues of interest are often only explored briefly. Second, most of the available publications focus on sub-Saharan Africa, and in particular southern Africa. Third, the body of literature is limited not only in terms of number and geographic focus but also in terms of religious scope. Most publications explore masculinities and HIV and AIDS in relation to Christianity, with only a few focusing on African Traditional Religions (ATRs) and Islam.

CONCEPT OF MASCULINITY

Masculinity as a concept has only recently emerged in studies on HIV and AIDS from the so-called gender perspective that increasingly became influential during the 1990s. Initially, this gender perspective focused on women, as they were said to be disproportionately infected by HIV, affected by stigma and discrimination and burdened with care.[1] Women's position with regard to the impact of the epidemic was often (and still is) described in terms of vulnerability and powerlessness. The subsequent intervention strategies are often aimed at the empowerment of women in order to realise gender equality. Over the past decade it has become increasingly recognised that not only women need to be empowered, but also men, in order transform gender relations.

Initially, men were considered simply as those in power who were the cause of women's vulnerability to HIV infection. However, the understanding of gender as two static and monolithic blocs of men and women is increasingly being critiqued. Currently, scholars of gender and HIV and AIDS call attention to differentiation and variability within gender categories, and for the agency of individuals.[2] With attention being paid to men's role in the gender dynamics of the HIV and AIDS epidemic, the concept of masculinity emerged. This concept has been utilised in the social sciences since the 1980s and was later also introduced to disciplines in the humanities. Although there is still some theoretical debate about the concept of masculinity, it is commonly understood as the social construction of male gender identities and of men's place in gender relations.[3]

Masculinity, as with gender, is regarded as a social construct. In gender theory, social constructionism is opposite to essentialism. The latter argues that there are some essential or natural features that characterise the categories of men and women. Social constructionism, in contrast, emphasises that these categories are attached to social and symbolic meanings, which are rooted in social structures and in cultural and religious ideologies.[4] This understanding opens up space to investigate how masculinity is constructed in relation to particular social factors, for example specific religious traditions. Precisely because of the fact that masculinity is constructed in connection with context-specific structures and relations, it has become common to speak about masculinities in the plural. It is argued that even in one context several masculinities co-exist, placing men in a dynamic male gender order of contesting understandings of what it means to be a man.[5] The theoretical concept of masculinity as a social construction and the insight that multiple masculinities are dynamic both acknowledge the possibility of intervention and change.[6] As will emerge from this chapter, this is crucial to the HIV and AIDS context. Finally, the idea of masculinity as a social construction may prevent blaming discourses that point to men as the cause of the HIV epidemic.[7] Without ignoring the responsibility of men for their behaviour, it is important to realise that the masculinities that inform critical male behaviours are often maintained by both men and women.

Significantly, the historical development outlined above can also be observed in the study of gender, masculinity and HIV and AIDS from the perspective of religion and theology. The Circle of Concerned African Women Theologians (the Circle), which has contributed significantly to opening up this field of study, is an example. Having addressed gender inequality and its consequences for women's lives in the context of HIV and AIDS for a number of years, the Circle invited male theologians to its 2007 pan-African conference on gender and HIV and AIDS for the first time and included a session on liberating masculinities.[8] This session challenged male theologians in Africa to work on a project on masculinities, gender and HIV.[9] Scholars in religion and theology who reflect on gender and masculinity in relation to HIV and AIDS largely subscribe to the social constructionist approach outlined above.

Adopting this social constructionist perspective, Ezra Chitando emphasises the importance of acknowledging men's socialisation into masculinities that maintain gender inequalities. He states that 'while being male is a biological factor, the process of expressing manhood is informed by social, cultural and religious factors'.[10] Hence, Chitando does not only offer a call to investigate how problematic masculinities are constructed but also how they can be transformed. Undertaking this challenge, he and other scholars point to religion as a factor contributing to both preservation and transformation of masculinities considered to be critical in the HIV and AIDS context.[11] This ambiguous role of religions is explored in the next two sections.

RELIGION AND CRITICAL MASCULINITIES

The reason why men and masculinities are addressed by scholars in religion and theology is that several critical aspects of dominant masculinities are believed to be informed by religious beliefs and practices. Chitando is one of the few male scholars in religion and theology in Africa who contributes significantly to the debate on masculinities. He denounces three aspects of dominant masculinities in southern Africa that are problematic in the HIV and AIDS context.[12] First, he points to particular constructions of male sexuality that lead men into risky sexual behaviours. This issue will be discussed below. Second, Chitando mentions the issue of care, observing that dominant masculinities dissuade men from engaging in the provision of care to people living with HIV. This observation is supported by women theologians who time and again mention that women are disproportionately burdened with the care of relatives living with HIV.[13] Although Chitando refers to cultural and religious factors that allow men to leave women and children to cope with the provision of care, he does not explore these factors in any detail. The third issue mentioned by Chitando is stigmatisation. He notes that dominant masculinities contribute to the stigmatisation of women living with HIV because they tend to portray women as the source of the disease. He observes:

> [M]asculinities play an important role in the spread of HIV in the region of southern Africa. Masculinities inform and facilitate the tendency by some men to have multiple sexual partners and not to use condoms, limit the participation of men in the provision of care for PLWHA [people living with HIV and AIDS] and contribute to the stigmatization of women.[14]

Chitando and other scholars explain these masculinities from patriarchal religious gender ideologies. These have informed the construction of masculinities that give rise to gender inequalities critical to the spread and impact of the epidemic. Before exploring these ideologies, attention is paid to an area of critical importance to the discussion, namely male sexuality. In this area, two issues have attracted particular attention: sexual decision making and sexual violence.

Sexual decision making

HIV in sub-Saharan Africa is often assumed to be transmitted predominantly through heterosexual intercourse.[15] Much attention has been paid to women's vulnerability in sexual relations and hence recently men's behaviour in sexual relationships has been the subject of scholarly investigation. African women theologians have constantly insisted that women are not in a position to insist on safe sex because of the dominance of men in sexual decision making. Fulata Moyo, for example, clearly states: 'Sexuality is about power for those who determine the what, when, where and how of sex, be it socio-economic and/or religio-cultural. In heterosexual relationships, those who have this power are men.'[16] She argues that this gendered structure of sexual decision making is informed by Christian as well as traditional religious sexual socialisation. Elaborating upon this, Moyo especially refers to female initiation rites in Malawi, both the traditional one (*chinamwali*) and the Christianised version (*chilangizo*) where women are taught to serve men's sexual needs, subordinating women's sexual life to that of men. This socialisation of women enables men to indulge in risky sexual behaviour.[17] It is significant to note that female initiation rites are organised by women who also provide sexual education to the young girls about to be initiated.[18] This raises the question as to how and why women contribute to the maintenance of unequal gender relations and patriarchal masculinities but unfortunately this issue is not discussed. Further, while Moyo discusses women's initiation into sexuality and womanhood as enabling men to engage in risky sexual behaviour, there is no reference to the way men are initiated into manhood and are educated on issues of sexuality in religio-cultural contexts. She does, however, suggest that cultural and Christian teaching about men as the head of the family contributes to a construction of masculinity and of gender relations in which sexual decision making is carried out by men.[19]

With Moyo, Madipoane Masenya also points to the notion of male headship as contributing to inequality in sexual decision making:

> The view that the headship of men is viewed as God-ordained assigns all authority and power to control to men. This includes the control of women's bodies. The understanding that a wife must be subject to her husband in everything (Ephesians 5:24) would thus also be understood to entail that she must always be willing to avail her body for her husband's sexual gratification.[20]

A similar observation has been made by Trad Godsey with regard to Islam, as he says that most Muslim men expect their wife to be sexually available as the husband pleases. He notices that this is often justified by religious authorities with reference to the Qur'an (Surah 2:223).[21] As with the Qur'an, the Bible is used to teach women to be sexually available to their husbands, asserts Isabel Phiri.[22] She indicates that religious authorities, in this case Christian churches, support this form of teaching and legitimise male dominance in sexual decision making. Some churches are even found to practise this in their institutional structures, as becomes apparent from Moyo's article on the so-called Phoebe practice. Here, women in a particular church are expected to show sexual hospitality to the male church leadership. While noting its importance to the discussion of this piece of research, it can be questioned whether this particular case legitimates Moyo's generalising conclusion that 'the Church sustains the same mentality [of men's sexual aggressiveness] using the Bible as a tool that justifies the objectification of women's bodies to serve men's sexual gluttony'.[23]

Sexual violence

Related to the issue of sexual decision making is that of sexual violence. This has been discussed predominantly from the perspective of women, especially by African women theologians. In their publications on HIV and AIDS they have addressed different forms of sexual violence: the strategic use of sexual violence as an instrument of war in the recent history of genocide and violence in countries like Rwanda and Congo;[24] sexual violence in formal or institutional relations such as at schools and in the workplace and churches;[25] and sexual violence in domestic spheres.[26] These women theologians, while addressing different contexts in which sexual violence takes place, all understand this violence in terms of power. Phiri states: 'At the centre of violence against women is a demonstration of who is in power.'[27] As with sexual decision making, sexual violence raises the issue of male domination in sexual relationships. Trying to explain situations of sexual violence, Tinyiko Maluleke and Sarojini Nadar point to what they call the unholy trinity of religion, culture and the subsequent power of gender socialisation as reinforcing a culture of violence against women.[28] With regard to the role of religion they note that sacred texts are often used by religious leaders to justify sexual violence. This is supported by Phiri in her work with faith communities on sexual violence where she found the belief that the man owns the woman in a marriage relationship. Phiri notes that this facilitates sexual violence because sex is used as a weapon of domination.[29] Likewise, Moyo points out that women are taught in church to keep silent about violence in marriage and again she explains this from the notion of male headship: 'As the head, the man deserves all the respect. Therefore anything that would lead to his losing respect should not be made known to others.'[30] Further, Maluleke and Nadar note that women do not receive support from their religious traditions in cases of violence.[31] This observation is confirmed by Beverley Haddad who points to the silence of churches on issues of violence against women and appeals for the breaking of this silence by calling men to account:

> The church can no longer assert to be the moral watchdog of society without challenging men to take responsibility for their sexual behaviour. Issues of gender violence, HIV/AIDS, and the links between the two cannot be dealt with without addressing men's abuse of power in relating to women, and dare I suggest without addressing the abuse of power within the structures of the church. One cannot theologise nor moralise while patriarchy continues unabated . . . Attitudinal and behaviour patterns of men in church communities have to change, and the onus is largely on the primarily male leadership to effect this change.[32]

So here patriarchy is presented as the source of men's abuse of power and churches are challenged to address this.

Male sexuality, fertility and power

As mentioned above, the literature on sexual decision making and sexual violence often points to issues of male dominance and men's power in sexuality issues. It is important to mention here the risk of generalisation as several publications tend to represent African men generally as being dominant, using violence and unable to control their sexuality. This approach echoes colonial and racist essentialising discourse on an African sexuality.[33] Nevertheless, several publications do deal with the question of why male sexuality tends to be expressed through dominance and power. Dealing with this question, Chitando points to the widespread understanding of a man as a sexual predator, meaning that men are possessed with virility and understand themselves as having uncontrollable sexual urges.[34] Likewise, Godefroid Kä Mana notes that masculinities in patriarchal cultures are characterised by power, potency and fertility. Hence, HIV prevention strategies, which often focus on sexual abstinence, marital fidelity and the use of condoms, are not successful because they are often experienced by men as a threat to their manhood.[35] These observations of Kä Mana are confirmed by Godsey with regard to Muslim masculinities (not particularly in Africa) where sex often serves as a confirmation of male power.[36] None of these authors, however, explores the way religious and cultural traditions inform these notions of male sexuality. Chitando briefly mentions that boys are highly valued in society because they are responsible for perpetuating their ancestral lineage.[37] The connection between sexuality, fertility and ancestry might be a good starting point to understand better the manifestations of male sexuality that have become problematic in contemporary Africa. Significantly, scholars of ATRs such as John Mbiti and Laurenti Magesa have explained the tradition of polygamy from this point of view.[38] They point out that polygamy is informed, among others, by the cultural-religious importance of transmitting the force of life and ensuring immortality. It would be interesting to explore the significance of these beliefs in the light of current understandings of male sexuality in contexts where formal polygamous relationships are no longer possible for socio-economic reasons.

Religion and patriarchal masculinities

From the discussion in the above section it appears that dominant masculinities are often explained through the lens of patriarchy. This is used to understand structural inequalities in the power relations between men and women. Scholars often point to religion as a factor in maintaining patriarchal gender relations. In Christianity the notion of the male headship has been criticised especially, as noted above. In Islam there exist dominant masculinities in which the husband possesses power and authority over his wife, as Godsey makes clear.[39] Indeed, religious gender ideologies generally tend to support patriarchy, whether it is in Islam, Christianity or ATRs.[40] The connection between religious traditions and patriarchy is a recurring theme in the literature.

However, I have some difficulty with the way patriarchy is conceptualised and the way in which the relationship between religion and patriarchal masculinities is explored. Most authors refer to patriarchy in a generalised way, with reference to African patriarchal culture, or similar overarching phrases. Not only can the suggestion of a singular African culture be questioned but also the monolithic understanding of patriarchy that arises from such discourse. This approach does not take into account the different ways in which masculinities are constructed, even within a patriarchal setting. Nor does it take into account the different ways in which men engage in patriarchal gender relations and how they understand themselves and behave in relation to other men, women and children. Therefore, a more complex conceptualisation of patriarchy is needed: while dominant masculinities may all be patriarchal, not all have the same extent of negative impact in the context of HIV and AIDS. As part of this investigation, the role of religion has to be explored and evaluated in a more complex way.

From my research in Christian churches in Zambia, I found that they reinforce patriarchal masculinities but yet define them in ways that might actually be helpful to HIV prevention.[41] These churches emphasise the concept of the man as the head of a marriage and family but use this concept to point out their related responsibilities in the areas of sexuality, relationships, marriage, the community and so forth. This indicates that religious gender ideologies in themselves, even when they inform patriarchal masculinities, are not necessarily negative in the context of HIV and AIDS. This view is supported by Phiri's observation that girls view male headship positively, as a weapon to help prevent sexual violence against women.[42]

But Chitando suggests that 'men have largely *abused* [emphasis mine] religious and cultural resources to continue engaging in risky sexual behaviour, while dangerously exposing their partners to HIV'.[43] He asserts that religions are misinterpreted and misapplied by men to legitimate negative behaviour, rather than religion directly legitimating this behaviour. This distinction calls for a more nuanced understanding and exploration of the role of religion in the construction of patriarchal masculinities and the way men engage them.

RELIGION AND THE TRANSFORMATION OF MASCULINITIES

As has become clear from the above discussion, hegemonic masculinities have become contested because they are said to contribute to the spread and impact of the HIV and AIDS epidemic. Hence, there is now a quest for the transformation of masculinities in order to overcome their negative aspects. Significantly, it is believed that religion can provide helpful resources for the transformation of masculinities. In as much as religion is used to reinforce problematic gender ideologies and masculinities, it is argued, religion can be used for transformation.

Religious resources for transformation

Imagining a transformation of masculinities, scholars draw on several religious and theological resources derived from Christianity, ATRs and Islam. Often, these resources are only briefly mentioned and without their meaning being explored in any depth.

Observe, for example, the work of Fulata Moyo, whose critical discussion on the notion of men as head of the family has been outlined above. She calls for a transformation of the concept of headship towards gender equality, and mutuality and companionship in marriage.[44] She mentions several religious notions to inform the call for such a transformation. First, she points to the creational notion that humanity, both male and female, is created in the image of God. For Moyo this means that both women and men deserve equal life and dignity. She not only draws on biblical texts but also on African creation myths in which the God-creator is often portrayed in gender-neutral or bi-gender terms, reinforcing the notion of the equality of men and women as co-bearers of the image of God.[45] Second, she briefly points to Jesus' liberation and life-giving mission in men's and women's sexuality but the meaning of this is not explored. Third, Moyo mentions the biblical notion of *agape* which she uses to argue for mutuality and companionship in marriage. This argument is aimed at preventing men from abusing their power and authority at the expense of women. Moyo briefly equates *agape* with the African traditional notion of *ubuntu* but at the same time she warns that *ubuntu* can easily be understood in a patriarchal way.[46]

The notion of *ubuntu* is central in the accounts of two other scholars, Musa Dube and Ezra Chitando. Dube mentions concepts from different indigenous groups that have similar meaning: *setho*, *isintu*, *chitu*, and *ubuntu*. These concepts, she argues, all refer to the central belief within ATRs that one can only be human by living within community, contributing to its well-being and harmony, and respecting others. According to Dube, this understanding is crucial to the struggle against HIV and AIDS because, among other reasons, it forces men to rethink their understanding of masculinity. Dube proposes a manhood that is characterised by the ethic of indigenous religions, which she describes as an ethic of 'earning respect by first giving it'.[47] In her view, the respect automatically paid to men in patriarchal cultures should rather become something that has to be earned by engagement in the well-being of the community and in healthy relationships with women and their families. A similar ethical ideal for masculinity is explored further by Chitando.[48] He suggests the notion of *ubuntu* as crucial for an African indigenous theology of HIV and AIDS.[49] In a recent publication, Chitando applies this specifically to the transformation of masculinities in the HIV context. Here he proposes the concept of solidarity, which he contrasts to the traditional religious notion of *ubuntu*. According to Chitando, solidarity means standing for, and with, the other. In relation to masculinities:

[S]olidarity implies the willingness of men to be self-emptying and to stand with women in the battle against HIV and AIDS. Solidarity calls for self-reflection on the part of men in southern Africa, so that they interrogate their position of power and show that they can identify with the cries of pain from women and children.[50]

Chitando points out that a masculinity of solidarity will push men to change their sexual ethics and not to engage in multiple sexual relations any longer. Further, men will be encouraged to participate in care giving to those living with HIV and overcome stigmatising attitudes. It is noteworthy that Chitando mentions that solidarity is related to, but goes beyond, *ubuntu* because the *ubuntu* philosophy is connected to a male-centred definition of community that leaves women and children at the margins. This corresponds with Moyo's reluctance to make *ubuntu* a central concept for the transformation of masculinities and gender relations, as noted above. In order to overcome the patriarchal overtones of *ubuntu*, Chitando suggests the ministry of Jesus, the one who always stood in solidarity with those at the margins, as the perfect model for solidarity.[51] In making this theoretical move, he corrects the tendency of men who approve the community ideal of *ubuntu* while at the same time not caring about the well-being of women and children. Chitando's reference to Jesus as the exemplary embodiment of solidarity indicates that he considers Jesus to be the role model for the transformation of masculinity. Unfortunately, he does not explore this in any great depth.

Africa Praying: A Handbook on HIV and AIDS Sensitive Sermon Guidelines and Liturgy includes a contribution in which Jesus is also proposed as a role model for manhood. The author, Cheryl Dibeela, draws from Mark 9:33–36 where Jesus rebukes the disciples when they are discussing which of them is the greatest. Dibeela points out that the question of greatness is irrelevant to Jesus because his concept of power is different from ours. Subsequently, Dibeela calls upon men to acknowledge that they have not used their power to prevent transmission or care for those living with HIV and challenges them to change their lives according to the standard set by Jesus.[52] While both Chitando and Dibeela present Jesus as an example for men, neither addresses the question of how Jesus, who in the Christian tradition is dissociated from sexuality and marriage, is to be a helpful model for the transformation of masculinities.[53] I therefore wonder if, in the HIV and AIDS context, where men's marital and sexual relations are so crucial to the discussion, another role model who directly addresses these relations would not be more constructive.

As Jesus is presented as a role model for men by Christian theologians, the Islamic scholar Trad Godsey presents Muhammad as the model for a transformative Muslim masculinity in the context of HIV and AIDS. Contrary to prevailing perceptions of Muhammad, according to Godsey the prophet is the ideal man. The particular notion that Godsey derives from Muhammad as crucial to a redefined Muslim masculinity is the aspect of vulnerability.[54] By being willing to be vulnerable and to show his weakness before his wife (or wives), the Prophet is said to encourage contemporary men to express their emotions rather than suppressing them through power, control and authority. According to Godsey, not only Muhammad but also the Qur'an supports this understanding of manhood, which contributes to equality in gender relations:

> The redefinition and reformation of masculinity in the Muslim world to allow manliness to be expressed as weakness and vulnerability has both a Qur'anic and Prophetic precedent. While the AIDS epidemic creates an urgency for change, the Qur'an and the *Sunnah* have always contained tools to reconstruct manhood in a way that achieves greater gender equity for men and women alike.[55]

While Godsey gives this positive account of Muhammad, Clara Koh in her article on gender justice and Islam argues that the Qur'an and the Islamic tradition are very ambiguous with regard to gender equality.[56] These contradictory views thus indicate that further exploration is needed to see how Muhammad can become a role model for Muslim men in the context of HIV and AIDS.

Practical implications of transformation

Although several scholars explore religious and theological resources that challenge or redefine masculinities, there is little reference to what this means in practice. Again, it is Chitando who explores some ways for churches to mobilise men and transform masculinities in the HIV context. In his opinion, when churches engage in the transformation of masculinities they have to address men on two fronts: inside and outside the church. According to Chitando, they should address masculinities within the church because there men are just as susceptible to patriarchy as those outside. Therefore, sermons should challenge men to embrace gender justice and new understandings of manhood should be developed in Sunday schools, youth groups and men's and women's organisations. According to Chitando, 'if all church departments were actively involved in the shaping of new ideals to manhood, society would be transformed in a radical way'. Chitando also considers the transformation of masculinities as an aspect of the church's mission in the context of HIV and AIDS: creative evangelism is needed to reach men at the worldly places where they are to be found. Churches 'need to sacralize such spaces and reach men'. Further, they also need to collaborate with men's organizations and non-governmental organisations that focus on men in order to reach them and transform masculinities.[57]

One way of addressing Chitando's need for the creative evangelism of men may be the use of the contextual Bible study method developed by the Ujamaa Centre for Community Development and Research at the School of Religion and Theology, University of KwaZulu-Natal.[58] This method could be used as a way of addressing, among others, issues of gender violence and HIV and AIDS in communities, and aiming at women's empowerment.[59] Recently the method has also been applied to involve men in the transformation of masculinities. Biblical texts are read and discussed using guiding questions about the male characters in the text and the type of masculinity they represent.[60] Questions are then offered that force the reader to question how these biblical texts may assist in correcting aspects of these dominant masculinities. In so doing, redemptive masculinities are recovered. The text on the rape of Tamar, 2 Samuel 13:1–22 is offered as helpful to the quest for alternative African masculinities. According to Gerald West, a contextual Bible study on this story produces a social space where dominant masculinities are disrupted and contradicted and where alternatives can be articulated that lead, potentially, to social transformation.[61]

A further resource is the liturgical handbook mentioned earlier that provides practical resources to address men and transform masculinities using sermons at Sunday services.[62] There are a number of essays in the volume that address this issue. Included are: examples of services on the boy child by Chitando and by Augustine Musopole; on men and their role in the community by Tinyiko Maluleke; and on men and the use of power by Dibeela.[63] Although these scholars do not explore the theology of masculinities extensively, they try to point to a way of being a man that is life-giving in the context of HIV and AIDS. This is done by addressing male power, pointing men to their responsibilities and emphasising the equality of women and men.

More of these practical resources are needed from different religious traditions to provide faith communities with materials that can be used when working with men to transform masculinities.

Gender justice as a theological horizon

In the above section, a number of diverse religious and theological notions are proposed by several scholars insisting on a transformation of negative aspects of masculinities. These various resources have one aspect in common: they are adopted within an ideology and theology of gender justice. Gender justice, therefore, can be considered as the horizon for the transformation of masculinities in the HIV and AIDS context.

While gender justice is often only referred to briefly, there are a few scholars who have elaborated upon this concept in more detail. Isabel Phiri and Musa Dube have developed a theology of gender justice in the context of HIV and AIDS from a Christian theological perspective while, recently, Farid Esack and Clara Koh have explored it from an Islamic perspective.[64] According to Phiri: 'African women theologians have argued that as long as there is gender injustice in Africa, HIV/AIDS will continue unabated.'[65] Resisting gender injustice, like other forms of injustice, is therefore a major challenge for these theologians.[66] Elaborating upon what gender justice means, Phiri suggests that the justice of God needs to be embodied in the male-female relationship. This will result in the liberation of all forms of oppression in these relations and in the promotion of responsibility, mutuality and acceptance of duties towards each other. Thus, gender justice is concerned with the humanity of both women and men and it claims the fullness of life for all human beings regardless of their gender. Theologically, Phiri relates the fullness of life to the mission of Jesus, which was to bring wholeness in people.[67] Further, the humanity of both women and men is grounded in the creation of human beings in the image of God.[68] For Phiri, ultimately gender justice is rooted in the character of God because the biblical God is a God of justice, and the practice of Christianity should reflect the character of God.[69] She notes that women theologians are working with God in the transformation of society and seek to construct new male and female identities that are empowering and inclusive for all of humanity. For Phiri, therefore, this engagement with justice occurs within an eschatological perspective as 'justice for all of humanity is not only important but it is necessary for the realization of the presence of God on earth'.[70]

Musa Dube explores the concept of gender justice from a biblical-theological perspective and provides a reading of the parable of Luke 18:1–8 in which the attitude of the unjust judge is compared with God as a just judge. She concludes:

The parable strongly assures us of a God who is unfailingly in solidarity with the oppressed and exploited. God is a God of justice, the parable underlines. It is this strong expression of God's solidarity with the oppressed and exploited that gives the women writers of this volume the courage to say, 'grant me justice'.[71]

Thus, as with Phiri, Dube understands justice as a characteristic of God. Further, she presents Jesus as the one who embodied this justice. Referring to several passages in the Gospel, Jesus is represented by Dube particularly as someone fighting for gender justice, a programme that should be followed by the Christian church.[72]

From the perspective of Islam, the need for gender justice in the context of HIV and AIDS has been emphasised by Farid Esack. He especially calls men to engage in the struggle for gender justice: 'All of us, particularly Muslim men, need to understand that justice is not just something that we demand from others. It is also something that we demand from ourselves, something that we may give in order that there may be greater justice.'[73] Hence, Esack calls on men to give up their power for the greater good of gender justice in the context of HIV and AIDS, regardless of whether Allah has sanctioned this male power or not. This latter issue is central in Islamic feminism. Clara Koh, evaluating the way Islamic feminists deal with the Qur'an in their quest for gender justice, suggests that the Qur'an is ambivalent with regard to gender justice and therefore cannot function as a helpful resource. She concludes her essay by stating that Islamic feminism should embrace a holistic understanding of gender justice because HIV and AIDS is embedded in multiple inequalities but she does not explore how the Qur'an or Islamic tradition may be helpful to this project.[74] She also does not point out an alternative way to argue for gender justice from an Islamic perspective. So, although there are some Muslim scholars who call for gender justice in the context of HIV and AIDS, there is almost no theologising in this regard.

EVALUATIVE AND REFLECTIVE CONCLUSION

In the introduction it was noted that the scholarly literature on men and masculinities in the context of HIV and AIDS from the perspective of religion and theology is relatively scarce. Indeed, the survey shows that the project of intersecting masculinities, HIV and AIDS, and religion is still in its early stages and needs further exploration. The literature, as discussed, clearly points out both the negative aspects of dominant masculinities and the need to overcome and transform them. It also makes clear that religious traditions and institutions play an ambiguous role in this area. On the one hand they reinforce or legitimate masculinities that appear to be negative in the context of HIV and AIDS while on the other they can be applied to raise awareness among men and to transform masculinities.

In the above section on the concept of masculinities, it has been mentioned that scholars in the area of gender and HIV increasingly pay attention to differentiation and variability within gender categories and argue for the agency of individuals in these categories. However, with regard to the field of religion there are still important challenges. Too often, men are represented as one monolithic bloc dominating women and spreading HIV. This essentialist discourse is similar to the way the concept of patriarchy is used, as was critiqued above. There is thus a lack of consideration of the plurality of masculinities that are found in social, cultural and religious contexts. Although this plurality is acknowledged in some of the literature, the differentiation among men and masculinities is yet to be explored by religious scholars. A negative outcome of this essentialising discourse is that it often generalises about men and male sexuality. Sometimes men are represented in a way that comes close to the racist representations of an African sexuality in earlier colonial discourses and a more sophisticated conceptual and methodological framework needs to be employed. When a concept such as patriarchy is used, its meaning has to be defined and attention has to be paid to the diversity of masculinities and gender relations. In addition, the question of how religion interferes with the constructions of masculinities needs further scholarly attention.

With regard to the transformation of masculinities, the urgent question is the nature of the hermeneutic. As explored above, gender justice functions as a theological horizon in the work of scholars from Christian and Islamic perspectives. However, the concept of gender justice is somewhat vague and needs further theological reflection. It was noted that if gender justice is about enhancing the life of men and women together, some masculinities that are labelled as patriarchal may be acceptable in certain contexts. They may even be helpful and constructive in the context of HIV and AIDS. However, when gender justice is understood as a radical call for equality of men and women, it does not leave space for a gender ideology that puts men in a primary position in relation to women.

Related to the question of how gender justice is understood is the issue of gender difference. The literature discussed in this chapter suggests notions such as solidarity, mutuality and companionship as a way to define gender relations and transform masculinities. Generally, these notions are mentioned in order to ensure gender relations are more equal. This is important, as the project to transform masculinities originates from the awareness that HIV and AIDS impacts women particularly as a result of gender inequality. The emphasis on gender equality, however, means that not much attention is paid to gender difference in the proposals to redefine masculinity. This may be a problem because in many cultural-religious constructions of masculinity and femininity, the biological differences between the sexes are marked by symbolic meanings that have social implications. These are often firmly rooted in the perception of both men and women; therefore gender difference cannot be neglected. The question, then, is how gender difference can be marked symbolically and socially in a way that promotes the values of solidarity, mutuality and companionship and leads to gender justice. This is a difficult challenge that needs further reflection.

This difficulty can be illustrated by the example of the concept of male headship. This cultural and religious concept marks the difference between men and women by declaring men to be the head in marriage and family relationships. From my research in churches in Zambia,[75] and from the literature discussed in this chapter, it appears that the notion of headship is central in religious constructions of masculinity. It has also been mentioned that the concept of male headship is said to facilitate male behaviour that is destructive in the context of HIV and AIDS. Yet it was also noted that the same concept can be applied in a way that is more constructive in the HIV context, despite the fact that the notion of male headship clearly fits into a patriarchal gender ideology. From a radical understanding of gender equality it has to be deconstructed. Criticising this notion, however, will probably result in men feeling threatened. Practically, it may be easier to respect this notion but redefine its meaning, and to point men to their related responsibilities. This is a possible way to transform masculinities and a few authors suggest that masculinities be transformed within the paradigm of male headship.[76] However, the question is whether the principle of gender justice allows for the concept of male headship at all. This concept not only marks gender difference but qualifies it in terms of headship (men) and submission (women) and therefore facilitates an unequal relationship between men and women. It raises the question whether the concept of headship should, for this reason, be rejected. If so, are there other religious and cultural concepts that define male gender identity without making a qualified difference between men and women? These are crucial questions that need to be addressed if masculinities are to be transformed.

To conclude, in the literature discussed here, many critical questions have been raised concerning the role of men and the significance of masculinities in the context of HIV and AIDS, and the way these are reinforced by religion. Furthermore, important steps to be taken to overcome the problems concerning men and masculinities revealed by the HIV epidemic are addressed. However, many issues need further analysis and exploration in order to understand and transform negative masculinities and realise gender justice.

NOTES

1. Carolyn Baylies and Janet Bujra (eds), *AIDS, Sexuality and Gender in Africa: Collective Strategies and Struggles in Tanzania and Zambia* (London: Routledge, 2000).
2. Hansjörg Dilger and Johanna Offe, 'Making the difference?: Structure, agency and culture in anthropological research on gender and Aids in Africa'. *Curare* 28(2–3) 2005: 274–5.
3. R.W. Connell, *Masculinities* (Berkeley: University of California Press, 2nd ed., 2005): 67ff. A similar understanding of the concept of masculinity is used in the emerging field of men's studies in religion, a concept introduced around the 1990s. See Stephen B. Boyd, W. Merle Longwood and Mark W. Muesse, 'Men, masculinity and the study of religion' in *Redeeming Men: Religion and Masculinities*, edited by Stephen B. Boyd, W. Merle Longwood and Mark W. Muesse (Louisville: Westminster John Knox Press, 1996): xviii–xxii.
4. Some social constructionist accounts of gender have an essentialist aspect as well. This has been critically mentioned by recent post-structuralist theories of gender. In the field of HIV and AIDS, however, social constructionism is the prevailing theoretical perspective on gender. For an overview and introduction to theories of gender see Rachel Alsop, Annette Fitzsimons and Kathleen Lennon, *Theorizing Gender* (Cambridge: Polity Press, 2002).
5. Connell, *Masculinities*: 76ff.
6. This possibility is acknowledged and explored, among others, in Reshma Sathiparsad, 'Masculinities in the era of HIV/Aids: The perspectives of rural male Zulu youth' in *From Boys to Men: Social Constructions of Masculinity in Contemporary Society*, edited by Tamara Shefer et al. (Cape Town: UCT Press, 2007): 191ff; Janet Bujra, 'Targeting men for a change: AIDS discourse and activism in Africa' in *Masculinities Matter!: Men, Gender and Development*, edited by Frances Cleaver (London: Zed Books, 2002): 218, 225.
7. Punima Mane and Peter Aggleton, 'Gender and HIV/AIDS: What do men have to do with it?' *Current Sociology* 49(6) 2001: 28.

8. Isabel Apawo Phiri, 'Major challenges for African women theologians in theological education (1989–2008)'. *International Review of Mission* 98(1) 2009: 116. For an introduction to the Circle's response to HIV and AIDS from a gender perspective see Isabel Apawo Phiri, 'African women of faith speak out in an HIV/AIDS era' in *African Women, HIV/AIDS and Faith Communities*, edited by Isabel Apawo Phiri, Beverley Haddad and Madipoane Masenya (Pietermaritzburg: Cluster Publications, 2003): 3–22.

9. The first outcome of this project is *Redemptive Masculinities: Religion, Men, Gender-Based Violence and HIV*, edited by Ezra Chitando (Geneva: WCC Publications, 2010).

10. Ezra Chitando, 'Religious ethics, HIV and AIDS and masculinities in southern Africa' in *Persons in Community: African Ethics in a Global Culture*, edited by Ronald Nicolson (Pietermaritzburg: University of KwaZulu-Natal Press, 2008): 51.

11. See Chapter 9 of this book where Chitando addresses the question of construction of masculinities from this point of view.

12. Chitando, 'Religious ethics, HIV and AIDS and masculinities in southern Africa': 52ff.

13. For example, see Musa W. Dube, 'Grant me justice: towards gender-sensitive multi-sectoral HIV/AIDS readings of the Bible' in *Grant Me Justice!: HIV/AIDS and Gender Readings of the Bible*, edited by Musa W. Dube and Musimbi R.A. Kanyoro (Pietermaritzburg: Cluster Publications, 2004): 10–11; Phiri, 'African women of faith speak out in an HIV/AIDS era': 15.

14. Chitando, 'Religious ethics, HIV and AIDS and masculinities in southern Africa': 55.

15. The silence on the homosexual transmission of the virus in the discourse on the HIV epidemic in Africa is mentioned by Marc Epprecht as 'a puzzling blindspot, a troubling silence, a strange consensus' which he explains from the general assumption of Africans as naturally heterosexual. See M. Epprecht, *Heterosexual Africa?: The History of an Idea from the Age of Exploration to the Age of AIDS* (Pietermaritzburg: University of KwaZulu-Natal Press, 2008), especially 16–17. The heterosexual assumption also characterises the literature surveyed in this chapter. This could probably be explained by the historical focus on the gendered (female) face of the epidemic, even in more recent discussions on masculinities. Yet the issue of homosexuality in relation to masculinities and HIV cannot continue to be ignored, particularly given the taboo of homosexuality in faith communities and the opposition to homosexuality by religious leaders.

16. Fulata Lusungu Moyo, 'Religion, spirituality and being a woman in Africa: Gender construction within the African religio-cultural experience'. *Agenda* 61 (2004): 73.

17. Fulata Lusungu Moyo, 'Sex, gender, power and HIV/AIDS in Malawi: Threats and challenges to women being church' in *On Being Church: African Women's Voices and Visions*, edited by Isabel Apawo Phiri and Sarojini Nadar (Geneva: WCC Publications, 2005): 130ff. See also Ezra Chitando, '"The good wife": A phenomenological re-reading of Proverbs 31:10–31 in the context of HIV/AIDS in Zimbabwe'. *Scriptura* 86 (2004): 151–9.

18. Fulata Lusungu Moyo, 'A Quest for Women's Sexual Empowerment Through Education in an HIV and AIDS Context' (Ph.D. thesis, Pietermaritzburg: University of KwaZulu-Natal, 2009): xiii.

19. Moyo, 'Sex, gender, power and HIV/AIDS in Malawi': 131, 133.

20. Madipoane Masenya, 'Trapped between two "canons": African-South African Christian women in the HIV/AIDS era' in *African Women, HIV/AIDS and Faith Communities*, edited by Phiri, Haddad and Masenya: 119.

21. Trad Godsey, 'The Muslim man and AIDS: Negotiating spaces for new conceptualizations of masculinity' in *Islam and AIDS: Between Scorn, Pity and Justice*, edited by Farid Esack and Sarah Chiddy (Oxford: Oneworld Publications, 2009): 133.

22. Isabel Apawo Phiri, 'Why does God allow our husbands to hurt us?: Overcoming violence against women'. *Journal of Theology for Southern Africa* 114 (2002): 25.

23. Fulata Lusungu Moyo, '"When the telling itself is a taboo": The Phoebe practice' in *On Being Church* edited by Phiri and Nadar: 193.

24. Anne Nkirote Kubai, 'Living in the shadow of genocide: Women and HIV/AIDS in Rwanda' in *Women, Religion and HIV/AIDS in Africa: Responding to Ethical and Theological Challenges*, edited by Teresia M. Hinga et al. (Pietermaritzburg: Cluster Publications, 2008): 49–74.

25. Ruth Muthei James, 'Factors that render the girl-child vulnerable to HIV/AIDS in Kenya' in *Women, Religion and HIV/AIDS in Africa*, edited by Hinga et al.: 14; Sophie Chirongoma, 'Women's and children's rights in the time of HIV and AIDS in Zimbabwe: An analysis of gender inequalities and its impact on people's health'. *Journal of Theology for Southern Africa* 126 (2006): 57; Pacificah Florence Okemwa, 'Maid in Nairobi in the age of HIV/AIDS: The plight of female domestic workers facing AIDS: cases from Kenya' in *Women, Religion and HIV/AIDS in Africa*, edited by Hinga et al.: 20–33; Beverley Haddad, 'Choosing to remain silent: links between gender violence, HIV/AIDS and the South African Church' in *African Women, HIV/AIDS and Faith Communities*, edited by Phiri, Haddad and Masenya: 160.

26. James, 'Factors that render the girl-child vulnerable to HIV/AIDS in Kenya': 13; Nyambura Jane Njoroge, 'Daughters and sons of Africa: Seeking life-giving and empowering leadership in the age of the HIV/AIDS pandemic' in *Women, Religion and HIV/AIDS in Africa*, edited by Hinga et al.: 185–7; Chirongoma, 'Women's and children's rights in the time of HIV and AIDS in Zimbabwe': 54–7; Phiri, 'Why does God allow our husbands to hurt us?': 19–30.

27. Phiri, 'African women of faith speak out in an HIV/AIDS era': 14.

28. Tinyiko Sam Maluleke and Sarojini Nadar, 'Breaking the covenant of violence against women'. *Journal of Theology for Southern Africa* 114(1) 2002: 5–17.

29. Phiri, 'Why does God allow our husbands to hurt us?': 24.

30. Moyo, 'Sex, gender, power and HIV/AIDS in Malawi': 133.

31. Maluleke and Nadar, 'Breaking the covenant of violence against women': 14.

32. Haddad, 'Choosing to remain silent': 155, 160.

33. These essentialising discourses on African sexuality are also discussed in Chapter 10 of this book.

34. Chitando, 'Religious ethics, HIV and AIDS and masculinities in southern Africa': 52–3.

35. Godefroid Kä Mana, 'Culture, societe et sciences humaines dans la lutte contre le VIH-SIDA en Afrique' in *Religion, Culture et VIH-SIDA en Afrique: Un Hommage au Docteur Jaap Breetvelt*, edited by Godefroid Kä Mana, Jean-Blaise Kenmogne and Helene Yinda (Yaounde: SHERPA, 2004): 70.

36. Godsey, 'The Muslim man and AIDS': 133.

37. Chitando, 'Religious ethics, HIV and AIDS and masculinities in southern Africa': 50.
38. Laurenti Magesa, *African Religion: The Moral Traditions of Abundant Life* (Maryknoll: Orbis Books, 1997): 136–40; John S. Mbiti, *African Religions and Philosophy* (London: Heinemann, 2nd ed., 1990): 138–41.
39. Godsey, 'The Muslim man and AIDS': 130.
40. See Chapter 9 of this book.
41. This research can be found in 'The Need for Circumcised Men: The Quest for Transformed Masculinities in African Christianity in the Context of the HIV Epidemic' (PhD thesis, Utrecht University, Utrecht, 2001). It involves case studies in two local churches to investigate how men in these communities are addressed and masculinities (re)defined against the background of the HIV epidemic. The churches are Regiment Parish and Northmead Assembly of God, both located in Lusaka, Zambia.
42. Isabel Apawo Phiri, 'A theological analysis of the voices of teenage girls on men's role in the fight against HIV/AIDS in KwaZulu-Natal, South Africa'. *Journal of Theology for Southern Africa* 120 (2004): 42.
43. Chitando, 'Religious ethics, HIV and AIDS and masculinities in southern Africa': 53.
44. Moyo, 'Sex, gender, power and HIV/AIDS in Malawi': 131ff.
45. Moyo, 'Religion, spirituality and being a woman in Africa': 74.
46. Moyo, 'Sex, gender, power and HIV/AIDS in Malawi': 135–6. This discussion is also addressed in Chapter 7 of this book.
47. Musa W. Dube, 'Adinkra!: Four hearts joined together on becoming healer-teachers of African indigenous religion/s in HIV and AIDS prevention' in *African Women, Religion, and Health: Essays in Honor of Mercy Amba Ewudziwa Oduyoye*, edited by Isabel Apawo Phiri and Sarojini Nadar (Maryknoll: Orbis, 2006): 140, 152.
48. Ezra Chitando's work in this regard is dealt with by Lucinda Manda in Chapter 7 of this book and in Chapter 9 by Chitando himself.
49. Ezra Chitando, *Living with Hope: African Churches and HIV/AIDS 1* (Geneva: WCC Publications, 2007): 56ff.
50. Chitando, 'Religious ethics, HIV and AIDS and masculinities in southern Africa': 56.
51. Chitando, 'Religious ethics, HIV and AIDS and masculinities in southern Africa': 57, 58–60.
52. Cheryl Dibeela, 'Men and the use of power' in *Africa Praying: A Handbook on HIV/AIDS Sensitive Sermon Guidelines and Liturgy*, edited by Musa W. Dube (Geneva: WCC Publications, 2003): 194.
53. For further discussion of this point, see Stephen D. Moore and Janice Capel Anderson (eds), *New Testament Masculinities* (Atlanta: Society of Biblical Literature, 2003).
54. Godsey, 'The Muslim man and AIDS': 125.
55. Godsey, 'The Muslim man and AIDS': 125.
56. Clara Koh, 'Gender justice, Islam and AIDS' in *Islam and AIDS,* edited by Esack and Chiddy: 88–104.
57. Ezra Chitando, *Acting in Hope: African Churches and HIV/AIDS 2* (Geneva: WCC Publications, 2007): 46–7, 49–52.
58. For a further discussion of the work of the Ujamaa Centre, see Chapter 5 of this book.

59. Gerald O. West and Phumzile Zondi-Mabizela, 'The Bible story that became a campaign: The Tamar Campaign in South Africa (and beyond)'. *Ministerial Formation* 103 (2004): 5–13.

60. Ujamaa Centre, *Redemptive Masculinities: A Series of Contextual Bible Studies*. Available at http:// www.sorat.ukzn.ac.za/ujamaa/redmasc.ppt (accessed 9 Apr. 2009).

61. Gerald West, 'The contribution of Tamar's story to the construction of alternative African masculinities' (unpublished paper).

62. Dube, *Africa Praying*.

63. Ezra Chitando, 'The boy child' in *Africa Praying*, edited by Dube: 171–3; Augustine Musopole, 'The boy child' in *Africa Praying*, edited by Dube: 169–71; Tinyiko Maluleke, 'Men and their role in the community' in *Africa Praying*, edited by Dube: 190–3; Dibeela, 'Men and the use of power': 193–5.

64. Isabel Apawo Phiri, 'Life in fullness: Gender justice: a perspective from Africa'. *Journal of Constructive Theology* 8(2) 2002: 79; Dube, 'Grant me justice'; Musa Dube, 'Grant me justice: Female and male equality in the New Testament'; *Journal of Religion and Theology in Namibia* 2 (2001): 82–115; Farid Esack, *HIV, AIDS and Islam: Reflections Based on Compassion, Responsibility and Justice* (Cape Town: Positive Muslims 2004): 50–1; Koh, 'Gender justice, Islam and AIDS'.

65. Phiri, 'Life in fullness': 79.

66. Nyambura Jane Njoroge, 'Resisting gender inequality and injustice in the name of Jesus' in *Heil und Befreiung in Afrika: Die Kirchen vor der Missionarischen Herausforderung durch HIV/AIDS*, edited by Francis X. D'Sa and Jürgen Lohmayer (Wurzburg: Echter, 2007): 54–73.

67. Phiri, 'Life in fullness': 78, 80.

68. Phiri, 'Life in fullness': 77; Phiri, 'Why does God allow our husbands to hurt us?': 26.

69. Phiri, 'Life in fullness': 77, 79.

70. Phiri, 'A theological analysis of the voices of teenage girls on men's role in the fight against HIV/AIDS in KwaZulu-Natal, South Africa': 44–5.

71. Dube, 'Grant me justice': 19.

72. Musa W. Dube, 'Jesus, prophecy and AIDS' in *Reflecting Theologically on AIDS: A Global Challenge*, edited by Robert Gill (London: SCM Press, 2007): 92–3; Musa W. Dube, 'Who do you say that I am?'. *Feminist Theology* 15(3) 2007: 360–5.

73. Esack, *HIV, AIDS and Islam*: 50.

74. Koh, 'Gender justice, Islam and AIDS': 96–101.

75. See note 41.

76. This is indicated in subtle ways. Fulata Moyo, for example, is very critical of the concept of male headship but yet she wonders 'how can the Church *transform* [this writer's emphasis] the concept of headship' rather than arguing that the concept should be removed completely (see Moyo, 'Sex, gender and power': 131). Isabel Phiri uncritically points out that girls consider male headship a weapon against sexual violence, which may suggest that she considers this a real option (see note 42). Patriarchy in general is discussed by Christopher Isike and Ufo Okeke Uzodike in 'Modernizing without Westernizing: Reinventing African patriarchies to combat the HIV and AIDS epidemic in Africa'. *Journal of Constructive Theology* 14(1) 2008: 3–20. They distinguish between old and new types of patriarchy in Africa and argue that the former should be re-valued as it provides men with a constructive and HIV preventive model of manhood.

Practitioner response

Lilian Siwila

The strategy of working towards the transformation of masculinities in order to achieve gender justice within the field of religion is becoming increasingly significant in addressing the HIV and AIDS epidemic. The question of men and masculinities has emerged as a contested issue in addressing HIV and AIDS. In many activist campaigns and scholarly works, men have been criticised for the spread of HIV. Religion and theology have offered limited practical strategies in dealing with men, although the work of African women theologians, as well as organisations such as the Ujamaa Centre for Community Development and Research, referred to by Van Klinken, is beginning to address this issue.[1]

In discussing masculinities, he argues that this is not a new theoretical discourse but its engagement with HIV and AIDS has recently been introduced. The idea of engaging men in addressing the epidemic has meant a paradigm shift to a more holistic approach that does not simply see men as perpetrators but also as partners in mitigating HIV. In order to achieve this, Van Klinken concurs with Zeferino Teka who suggests that it is important to emphasise both the positive and negative aspects of dominant masculinities.[2] This is helpful because it opens up space for men to understand their manhood without becoming defensive.

When discussing masculinities in the context of HIV and AIDS, I agree with Van Klinken that dominant masculinities are informed by religious beliefs and practices. In most Zambian ethnicities, men's emotions are not supposed to be expressed. For example, the Bemba will use such phrases as *shipa uli mwa ume, fisanga aba ume* (a man can overcome all hardship); and there is a Tonga proverb, *mulombwana munyati* (a man is a lion), asserting male power, might and victory. This reinforces Chitando's view, highlighted by Van Klinken, that ATRs do expect men to be strong and assertive. It means that they do not engage in care giving, regarded as work for women. In my experience, it is clear that the women are burdened with the load of providing care during times of illness in the family.[3]

Van Klinken also discusses the problem of sexuality, which he asserts is an issue of power and also related to the way men and women are socialised. An example is that of the headship of a man, power exercised through sexuality. At the centre of forming masculinities, especially in culturally determined settings, men are taught to use their power to prove their sexual authority while women are taught to submit to the sexual demands of their husbands. In order to be recognised as a man you have to be sexually active. Socialisation teaches that men are to lead and control, while women are to follow and obey. According to Van Klinken, these patriarchal masculinities tend to be protected by religious gendered ideologies. He, however, laments the over-generalisation of men as oppressors and suggests that this essentialist discourse is not helpful to the effort of transforming masculinities. But from my perspective it is important to continue to problematise and analyse patriarchy.

In Africa, central to discussions on gender, men and masculinities is an issue of culture from which dominant masculinities emerge. As Musimbi Kanyoro rightly suggests, Africans cannot live outside their culture, as culture informs who they are as Africans.[4] It is for this reason that I suggest that all methodology used in the transformation of masculinities should employ cultural hermeneutics, as outlined by Kanyoro, in order to address some of the historical and culturally embedded, wounded masculinities.[5] Mercy Oduyoye has observed that the theory of cultural hermeneutics has been used effectively by African women theologians in their effort to engage African culture and the Bible.[6] However, there is a need to be vigilant in identifying the ways in which culture influences men's behaviour both positively and negatively. It is, therefore, important that both the Bible and the Qur'an are engaged in a culturally sensitive manner in an attempt to transform masculinities to mitigate the HIV epidemic.

My own research and activist work has shown the importance of the socialisation process. I have realised just how much people's behaviour is informed by their childhood and family backgrounds. This is also true for me. I was born into a relatively large Zambian polygamous Tonga ethnic family. My grandfather, despite being a learned man, came from a culture that believed in educating only boys as girls were to be married off. As a result he continuously reminded the girls in the family that we were not meant to be highly educated because one day we would marry and remain at home to care for children. As for the boys in the family, he taught them the tough side of life and reminded them to be as fierce and brave as lions in facing the world. As a Christian family, we found the same message in the church. I was fortunate to be one of the girls who survived the storm of my grandfather. This was largely due to my mother, who refused to follow her father's teaching. She stressed that a good wife does not totally depend on her husband for everything (particularly not on his money) yet remains respectful. This, she told me, is only possible through hard work at school that would eventually lead to good employment.

The issue of men and masculinities should not end with scholarly debates. Initiatives are needed that meet men where they are and engage in dialogue with them. Van Klinken commends the Bible study work of the Ujamaa Centre that is attempting to deal with redeeming masculinities through readings of the sacred Christian text.[7] There is a need for more inter-religious readings of the sacred texts, including the Qur'an, around issues of masculinities.

All work towards gender justice needs to be collaborative. Kanyoro poses the following challenge:

The feminist analysis of patriarchy sometimes approaches women's oppression by pointing to men as the oppressors. This approach is a nonstarter in Africa. While African women acknowledge men's role in oppression, they do not throw stones . . . moreover when dealing with cultural matters there is need for collective solidarity.[8]

In this collective solidarity, men need to become full participants in naming oppressive behaviours that perpetuate women's vulnerability to HIV and so become role models for future generations in building a humane society where gender justice prevails.

Notes

1. Pietermaritzburg Agency for Christian Social Awareness has produced a documentary 'Men and masculinity'. See http://www.promundo.org.br/Pesquisa/Young%20Men%20SubSaharan_Web.pdf.
2. Zeferino Teka, 'Male honour and HIV and AIDS as a gendered pandemic: An African male reflection on how man can be effectively engaged toward a positive male response'. *Journal of Constructive Theology* 14(1) 2008: 21–33.
3. Lilian Siwila, 'Care-giving in times of HIV and AIDS, when hospitality is a threat to African women's lives: a gendered theological examination of the theology of hospitality'. *Journal of Constructive Theology* 13(1) 2007: 69–82.
4. Musimbi Kanyoro, *Introducing Feminist Cultural Hermeneutics: An African Perspective* (Sheffield: Sheffield Academic Press, 2002): 14.
5. The term wounded masculinities is used to point to those masculinities that have been imposed on men as part of the socialisation process that deny men their true humanity and suggest, for example, that they should not cry or should be sexually aggressive.
6. Mercy Amba Oduyoye, *Introducing African Women's Theologies* (Sheffield: Sheffield Academic Press, 2001).
7. Ujamaa Centre, 'Redemptive Masculinities: A Series of Contextual Bible Studies'. Available at http://www.sorat.ukzn.ac.za/ujamaa/redmasc.ppt (accessed 20 July 2009).
8. Musimbi Kanyoro, 'Cultural hermeneutics: an African contribution' in *Other Ways of Reading: African Women and the Bible*, edited by Musa Dube (Geneva: WCC Publications, 2001): 106.

12

Children seldom seen and heard
Identifying the religious HIV and AIDS discourse

Genevieve James

INTRODUCTION

Children remain one of the most marginalised groups in academic discourse. Within the field of religion and theology they continue to receive lip service at best, or at worst are completely ignored. A review of the literature on the intersection of HIV, religion and theology, and children reveals a stark deficit. This is the case in spite of the proliferation of resources in the general area of HIV and AIDS and religion. The plights and voices of children register almost no concern on the agenda of researchers.[1] The United Nations Children's Fund (UNICEF) produced a report in 2006 on the state of the world's children and aptly subtitled it 'excluded and invisible'.[2] In this chapter it is argued that there is a lack of recognition and understanding of the consequences of HIV and AIDS for children within the field of religion and theology.

Given the unhelpful propensity for researchers to group the marginalised together, the separation of children as a distinct research priority is crucial. All too often there is a tendency to place women and children in the same research category. As Thorne rightly observes, 'in some ideological constructions, women are likened to children. In other constructions women are closely and unreflectively tied to children'.[3] He thus proposes a conceptual autonomy in order to facilitate knowledge production of the specific experiences of women and of children.

For the purpose of this chapter, children are regarded as eighteen years old and younger. The interface between children and HIV and AIDS in religion and theology is its primary focus. Having surveyed the available literature, themes are drawn out, gaps in the knowledge produced are identified and areas for further research are suggested. The literature survey is limited to English publications and cannot claim to be complete. Although many contexts are reflected in this study, a considerable sum of the literature gathered is located in the South African context and written from a Christian perspective. This is due to the significance of South Africa as a prime social and theological space in the encounter with HIV and AIDS and children because it is regarded as the epicentre of the epidemic.[4]

NATURE OF THE SURVEYED LITERATURE

Peter Okaalet, Ignatius Swart and Hannelie Yates, Daniel Smith and Jakobus M. Vorster have focused on the interface between HIV and AIDS, children, and religion and theology.[5] Their work provides status reports on children and theological reflection from contexts within the African continent. Research conducted by Mirolyn Naidoo and Bongi Zengele is located within a theology and development framework.[6]

The contribution of feminist theologians includes that of Sophie Chirongoma, Beverley Haddad and Isabel Phiri.[7] Their articles advocate for children's rights and include a strong discourse of empowerment, liberation and survival through giving knowledge, voice, and agency to children.

Statistical information abounds with publications providing wide-ranging information. Arnau van Wyngaard approximated the number of orphans under the age of fifteen who have lost their mothers or both parents to AIDS-related illnesses as seven million by the year 2000 and the expectation was that by 2010 this number would have doubled.[8] In the same age demographic, Frank Dimmock attributes the death of one in six children to AIDS-related illness and one in seven new HIV infections with the majority of infections caused by mother-to-child transmission.[9] Even more chilling is the report by Vorster that globally every minute a child under fifteen dies of an AIDS-related illness and every minute another child becomes HIV positive.[10] Okaalet suggests that in central and west Africa, only one per cent of pregnant women receive anti-retrovirals to prevent mother-to-child transmission.[11] Of course, the problem with statistical information, as Wyngaard points out, is that it swiftly becomes obsolete.[12] Also problematic is the fact that many children are not tested for the presence of the HI virus and as a result are statistically excluded. Further to this, the widespread under-reporting of children who are raped and subsequently become HIV positive contributes to the unreliability of statistics.

After an examination of the literature it became apparent that certain themes were common to reflections on HIV and AIDS and children. These are summarised with associated sub-themes in the following conceptual framework:

Children and HIV and AIDS in Religion and Theology		
Stakeholders/Actors	**Contributing factors to children's vulnerability to HIV and AIDS**	**Theology**
• Faith-based organisations • Faith communities • Individual's research responses	• Poverty • Sexual abuse • Gender violence and inequality • Moral-risk discourse • Masculinity • Education • Mother to child transmission	• Hope • Image of God • Human dignity • Jesus' special regard for and appreciation of children • The mandate to care for the vulnerable • Liturgy/Bible studies

Methodological issues

The methodologies used in the surveyed literature range from pilot study findings, as in the report by Philippe Denis and Nokhaya Makiwane on the memory box project, to Zamani Maqoko and Yolanda Dreyer's participatory research on the issue of child-headed households.[13]

In the field of practical theology, Julian Müller strongly advocates the use of a narrative approach. He gives an example of doing practical theology by using the narratives of children, providing seven methodological guidelines he calls movements, together with literary resources for each of them. Müller points to the importance of context and action field, or habitus, in the narrative approach. A specific context is described; in-context experiences are listened to; interpretations of experiences are made, described and developed in collaboration with co-researchers; experiences are described as continually informed by traditions of interpretation; religious and spiritual aspects are reflected upon, especially regarding God's presence as it is understood and experienced; experience is thickened through interdisciplinary investigation; and alternative interpretations pointing beyond the local community are developed. He unequivocally states that he is 'not writing a practical theology with reference to HIV/AIDS, but a practical theology developed out of HIV/AIDS'.[14]

Müller further promotes a narrative approach to exploring the lives of children who have been orphaned through the epidemic by doing ongoing research with his postgraduate students. He and Amanda Richter have studied the bereavement stories of three children. They suggest that it is important to consider carefully the distinctiveness of each story of bereavement 'since the narrative approach focuses on the personal meanings that people assign to specific events in their lives and how they tell the story of these meanings, reality is furthermore defined by the stories people live by and therefore tell one another'.[15]

Richter and Müller create the opportunity for these unique stories to be heard as opposed to being 'silenced by the wave of bereavement in the wake of countless deaths worldwide as a result of HIV and AIDS infection'. According to them, 'all children love stories and there is no better way to get children to open up and tell their own stories than by using the stories they know and love'.[16]

A further collaboration by Müller with student Juanita Loubser explores the poverty contexts of children living with HIV: they are 'often overlooked as regards their spiritual needs'. Loubser and Müller discover what they call 'truly amazing alternative narratives of hope and love' amidst 'pain and sorrow'.[17]

FACTORS CONTRIBUTING TO CHILDREN'S VULNERABILITY TO HIV AND AIDS

A further sub-theme in the surveyed literature is the nature of children's vulnerability. Within this sub-theme are a number of factors that make children vulnerable to HIV infection.

Violence and abuse

In Zimbabwe, Chirongoma describes how adolescent girls experience sexual harassment and victimisation from male schoolteachers who increase their vulnerability to HIV given the disturbing rate of infection among teachers.[18] In South Africa, Haddad notes that 'rape is not confined to women (young and old), but extends to the rape of very young girl children'.[19] Quoting a study by medical anthropologist, Suzanne Leclerc-Madlala, she notes that there is:

[A] steady increase in the number of HIV positive African female children between the ages of five and fourteen in the past few years. The only likely explanation from their point of view was that men with AIDS were raping or having sex with virgin girls . . . Thus it would appear that not only is girl child rape used as a preventative measure, but a myth has emerged within communities that sex with a girl child will cure the disease. Horrendous stories which confirm this view – from rural as well as urban areas – are slowly being documented.[20]

In both studies, the girl child is under threat of abuse and subsequent HIV infection. Therefore, while it is appropriate to stress that HIV and AIDS is a gender concern, as feminist theologians have done, it is necessary to add that the epidemic is a critical concern for the female child. It should be said, however, that while the gender of the child is important, it is inappropriate to disregard the implications of the category of child. There is much work still to be done in the area of the abuse of boy children.

Poverty

Yet another contributing factor to the vulnerability of children to HIV is the issue of poverty. Poverty is intrinsically linked to the untimely death of thousands of children. In addition, poverty leads to several social ills, including child labour which continues, despite increasing attention paid by scholars and activists.[21] Across the world entire industries are being fuelled by child labour. Researchers indicate that HIV and AIDS leave children exposed to appalling abuses of human rights as a result of poverty. Loubser and Müller describe some of these abuses as follows: 'The struggle of poverty reinforces malevolent people to use this disastrous situation as bait to exploit the young girl sexually . . . Young girls are often coerced, raped or enticed into sex by someone older, stronger or richer than themselves.'[22]

Furthermore, situations of poverty contribute to the occurrence of child-headed households where one or both parents have succumbed to death and children are left to fend for themselves. Moqoko and Dreyer ask serious questions with regard to the failure of adults and pastors to care for children in the context of HIV and AIDS:

The problem addressed . . . is how the devastation of HIV/AIDS causes young, under-aged orphans to have to function as heads of households. The question is whether pastoral care – that of the pastor and that of the entire faith community – has failed, especially in African communities where 'ubuntu' added a cultural incentive to care for the needy and destitute. Pastoral questions arising are: where are those uncles, aunts and grandmothers who cared so unconditionally for such children in the past? Why are these orphans not with older caregivers? Is the caring ministry failing today because of HIV/AIDS? [23]

Religious abuse

A disturbing and explicit link between children, religion, and HIV and AIDS that deserves special mention is the Devadasi system practised in India. Long quotes are included here since the description of the Devadasi system is crucial for an understanding of this link. The introductory statement to a website dedicated to the system offers the following:

> This site is dedicated to the thousands of Devadasis (the name signifies servant of god) who have been forced into prostitution in the name of religion in India. The Devadasis are dedicated to gods and then the priests claim first rights to them, and later on everyone else. They are courtesans in god's court. A Devadasi cannot belong to any one particular husband (generally the Indian ideas of marriage are that daughters are transferable property gifted to husbands), instead she is a common property! In other words, the Devadasi system is a 'system of votive offering of girls to the deities in Brahmanic temples'. [24]

Elizabeth Joy further describes the shameful situation of socially marginalised girl children in India and provides a direct link between the Devadasi system and HIV and AIDS:

> Prostitution in many cases takes place in the name of God and under traditional religious sanction. Due to STDs and the HIV/AIDS pandemic, more and more young girls are being pushed into prostitution as the customers prefer them to the older girls/women. Some practices within the Devadasi system, which is concentrated in the Karnataka, Andhra Pradesh, and Maharashtra border belt, as well as some Mathamma practices in Tamil Nadu in the southern part of India, have dedicated young girls from a very early age into a forced and religiously sanctioned prostitution,

ruining the lives of many young girl-children. They are dedicated to Gods
and Goddesses in order to fulfil promises made to the deity for favours
related to the health of individual or family members . . . the family gives in
to declarations made during religious celebrations that the particular Deity
wants a specific girl to be dedicated. These are manipulations that fulfil the
lust of the uppercaste landlords who are bent on having these young girls
at an age of 12–16. The young girls are later sent to urban areas to be
commercial sex-workers. This situation increases their vulnerability to
HIV/AIDS in a country which has unofficially crossed 1% of the total
population of 1033.4 million.[25]

In the Christian context G. Duncan bewails the system of discipline in the
reformed traditions that target girls as recipients of church discipline, in the case
of teen-pregnancies, for example, even when there are mitigating circumstances
such as rape and incest.[26] The extent to which religious ritual and blind devotion
across many cultures have contributed to the injury, ill health and even the death
of children is a crucial area of further research.

POSITIVE RELIGIOUS RESPONSE TO CHILDREN AND HIV AND AIDS

In a 2003 study Geoff Foster explores faith-based interventions in six countries,
namely Kenya, Malawi, Uganda, Mozambique, Namibia and Swaziland. According
to Foster, the number of local congregations is estimated to be in excess of 150
000. He describes the responses of faith-based organisations (FBOs) as small
scale and largely undocumented and under-supported on the basis that it is
difficult 'to measure their combined impact compared to the more visible project
responses of development agencies'.[27]

In the context of Botswana, Musa Dube speaks of efforts on behalf of
children and young people that are 'yet to be coordinated and intensified'.[28]
Okaalet confirms this view and describes the role of the church and other
religious organisations as unique due to their 'established history and grounding
in affected communities'. In this regard, Okaalet calls for new standards of co-
operation and collaboration amongst FBOs for the advantage of children.[29]

Foster has also written on the religious response to orphans in Africa, offering
a brief overview of the response of the major religions – Christianity, Islam and
Hinduism – to orphans affected by the HIV and AIDS epidemic. He refers to the

teachings of the sacred texts, the Bible, Sura, Vedas and the Bahai scriptures and shows how they substantiate these religions' social concern for orphans.[30] These texts are not interrogated in any great detail as Foster writes from a paediatrics and child health and development perspective, rather than as a religious scholar.

In discussing those who care for and as act as advocates for children, Foster includes local congregations where individuals act in a 'basic community level religious gathering' and religious co-ordinating bodies that organise, support and supervise the work of local congregations, including initiating new HIV projects.[31] According to Foster, FBOs:

> [. . .] have continued to respond in the face of conflict, natural disaster, political oppression, and disease . . . [they] address the universal need for community and spiritual life, endure for the long term when others tire, drop out or shift energies to other crises . . . [they] are considered one of the few external sources of support for orphans outside of the extended family.[32]

While Foster offers these positive remarks about the actions of FBOs, he is also critical of religious action, stating that it is often characterised by lack of knowledge, co-ordination and partnership among organisations at different levels. In addition, FBOs have failed to incorporate HIV prevention activities and are unwilling to support risk reduction strategies in their initiatives.[33]

THEOLOGICAL THEMES ADDRESSED IN THE LITERATURE

Vorster asserts that 'certain biblical doctrines reflect this high value of the child'. He speaks of a covenantal family where children are 'faced with a mysterious multifaceted relation with their parents. This relationship is more than blood or parental love: it has a spiritual dimension'.[34] For Vorster, having children is regarded as an important gift or blessing and therefore there are special obligations that need to be considered. Foster describes children as belonging to a community and suggests 'it takes a village to raise a child' and 'the child of the mother is the one in the womb but once it is born everybody will play with it'.[35] The involvement of the community in raising children orphaned by the epidemic is a crucial and under-researched area in religion and theology.

Hope is a key health asset in the often pessimistic arena of HIV and AIDS.[36] Chirongoma discusses the role of Christianity and the Shona religion in inspiring hope through intentional collaborations in a Zimbabwean district.[37] Anthropologists have considered the theme of hope in the study of young people in the context of HIV and AIDS.[38] Similarly, researchers in Brazil focus on religion and hope as a means of coping for young mothers with children who are living with HIV. They argue that the primary contribution of religion is the creation of social and emotional support, as well as an understanding of life experiences through faith.[39] This area of hope is a major contribution that religion and theology can make to the study of children and HIV and AIDS. A much greater emphasis is needed in future research.

According to Linthicum, in the biblical text the prophet Isaiah's vision is for 'the city to be a place of health and the church has the responsibility to work for the longevity and healthcare of its inhabitants'.[40] Despite the unprecedented rate of urbanisation in Africa and explosive urban growth in several global contexts, there has been little work carried out in the field of religion and theology on children in an urban context. Orphan is the word given to a child who has lost parents, yet in many languages there still is no word to describe parents who have lost their children as this goes against the natural order. In today's world it has become common for parents to bury their children. According to Wyngaard, between 60 and 80 per cent of infected children acquire HIV before and during the birth process.[41] Children also die of opportunistic diseases brought about by HIV and AIDS. Longevity is a serious issue for children across the world.

Clifford Odimegwu adds:

> [. . .] religious practices of attending religious services frequently, daily exercises of Bible reading and prayer, evangelisation measured by preaching and distribution of religious leaflets and tracts, are critical religious indicators that affect adolescent sexual debut, attitudes to premarital sexual activity, and engagement in current sexual behaviour.[42]

According to Odimegwu, it would appear that belonging to and participation in religious activities contribute to a delay of sexual activity and thus religious activity could contribute to longevity at an individual level.[43] The social collective mobilisation of religion towards longevity in urban contexts needs to be a focus of research and these claims of Odimegwu substantiated.

CREATIVE RESOURCES FOR FAITH COMMUNITIES

In recognition of the present and potential role of faith communities and in answer to the call for tools and resources from the religious sector, UNICEF, the World Conference of Religions for Peace and the Joint United Nations Programme on HIV/AIDS (UNAIDS) collaborated to produce a workbook.[44] This is based on sources from diverse religious groups and has been tested and reviewed by religious leaders in Africa and Asia as well as representatives from global FBOs and networks. The workbook is designed to appeal to religious leaders with minimal training and includes information on HIV and AIDS under categories such as 'how to prevent HIV infection', 'mother-to-child transmission' and 'what you can do'.

There is also a variety of congregational and youth resources with specific reference to children and HIV and AIDS. Hip hop is a genre in the popular music industry that is often disparaged as violent, sexist and consumerist. With lyrics such as 'I like girls, they like me, I want to be faithful but I can't keep my hands out the cookie jar',[45] popular hip hop, often imported from the West, hardly contributes to a sense of critical consciousness among the youth. Despite the bad rap given to hip hop, a unique and creative appropriation of the hip hop style is evolving in a South African township church, the J.L. Zwane Centre in Gugulethu, Cape Town. According to Zoe Hussain, the church informally known as the HIV church (people did not want to be seen to be associated with it) has initiated a music programme called the Siyaya AIDS programme. This seeks to encourage young people from disadvantaged backgrounds 'to reach and educate their peers about HIV and AIDS'.[46]

Yet another innovative project called the Memory Box Programme specifically responds to the emotional needs of children and seeks to promote resilience in children whose lives have been traumatised by HIV and AIDS.[47]

Dube helpfully offers liturgies and Bible studies for children and young people.[48] Tinyiko Maluleke, in an important Bible study on the disregard of the child Jesus, describes what he calls the over-theologised Jesus:

> He is the Alfa and the Omega. King of Kings. The Risen Lord. The Son of Man, the Messiah, the Christ, Saviour and Lord of Lords. These are the titles we use for Jesus. We sing, pray and worship Him as such. Rightfully so; because for us He is indeed Lord and Saviour. But how often do we pause to think that Jesus Christ was once a child?[49]

In addition to the need for more of these liturgies, there is also a need for qualitative research on the use of existing liturgies in specific communities with children. Furthermore, liturgies created by children themselves have largely been ignored in the field of religion and theology.

Another under-researched area is the use of sacred texts, especially those developed for children. For example, there is a multitude of publications on the Bible and violence against women but rarely are the stories of certain abused women in the Bible recognised as abused children. The story of the rape of Tamar in 2 Samuel 13 is actually the story of the rape of a child yet this story is primarily viewed as, and reflected on, as a story of the rape of a woman. Elsewhere I have discussed how this text is proving to be a valuable resource for raising the awareness of children about their bodies as private and special and not for abuse by known or unknown predators.[50]

A further area of necessary research is on contextualised programmes for children that amplify their agency in different socio-economic and educational contexts. Much more context-specific research in the areas covered in this chapter is necessary. As stated at the outset, it is important that children should not be considered as a monolithic entity since they live within various cultural, religious, ethnic, geographical, political and socio-economic contexts. In some parts of the world the spirit of individualism and consumerism has turned children into disrespectful, unsatisfied, easily bored consumers who have the right to be pleased whether at home, school or church. Some children engage in sex on demand in school and at home and create new, more dangerous sexual exploits to keep themselves entertained. Internet and cellphone technology enables children to capture group sex acts and distribute them for the viewing pleasure of their peers. How do children in a consumerist age understand and protect themselves from an often distorted need to please and entertain their friends? HIV educational campaigns need to take this into account and the religious community must not ignore this dimension in research on children and HIV and AIDS.

CONCLUSION

As was suggested at the beginning of this chapter, children remain one of the most marginalised groups in religious and theological discourse. The time has come for this situation to change. This sentiment is echoed by Stephan de Beer who suggests that 'children should be more central on the agenda of theological education and reflection'. He asks the following essential question:

Why is it that so little is said or done about children by the most prominent theologians of our world? There is a theological silence that needs to be overcome. Pastors need to take the lead in placing children on congregational agendas and in integrating children meaningfully into worship services and other events of the church. They need to affirm childcare workers much more as key members of the ministry team. They need to invest in the development of effective and knowledgeable child-care workers.[51]

Frank Mokoro asks a similar question: 'How can the church be so silent about the plight of children? Theological colleges rarely conduct research on these issues or organise symposiums to highlight the plight of these powerless children in the midst of the very crude generation in which they are trapped.'[52]

However, it would be beneficial for research to be undertaken beyond the customary sites of statistics and status reports to include the voices of children and their own theology. As Thorne states: 'Conceptualizing children as victims does reveal these harsh realities, but that view – when it fails to acknowledge children's worlds of meaning and their capacities for action and survival – also distorts.' Virtually all studies of children have been done by adults and while children assist in the research, they should be in 'central positions of knowledge creation'. This is the greatest need with regard to research on children, HIV and AIDS, religion and theology. While children are interviewed, observed, monitored, interpreted, taught and trained, the voice of children is channelled through the priorities (or lack) of methodologies and charity of adults. Thorne laments that 'our ways of thinking about children reflect adult interests and limits understanding of children's experience and actions'.[53] The alternative is indeed revolutionary – the research agenda and empowerment of children by children.

NOTES

1. The word plights is deliberately used since it is inappropriate to assume that there is one unifying plight that connects children geographically, ethnically or socio-economically.
2. UNICEF, 'The state of the world's children: excluded and invisible' (2006). Available at http://www.unicef.org/sowc06/pdfs/sowc06_fullreport.pdf (accessed Aug. 2008).
3. B. Thorne, "Revisioning women and social change: Where are all the children gone?'. *Gender and Society* 1(1) 1987: 104.

4. J. Sachs, 'South Africa as the epicentre of HIV/AIDS: Vital political legacies and current debates'. Available at http://www.tc.columbia.edu/cICE/archives/3.1/31sachs.pdf (accessed Aug. 2008). India is another country gaining wide attention due to increasing rates of HIV and AIDS.

5. P. Okaalet, 'Some religious responses to HIV/AIDS and children in Africa'. *Religion and Theology* 14 (2007): 94–104; I. Swart and H. Yates, 'The rights of children: A new agenda for practical theology in South Africa'. *Religion and Theology* 13 (2006): 314–40; D. Smith, 'Youth, sin and sex in Nigeria: Christianity and HIV/AIDS-related beliefs and behaviour among rural-urban migrants'. *Culture, Health and Sexuality* 6(5) 2004: 425–37; Jakobus Vorster, 'Protecting the most vulnerable'. *Ecumenical Review* 59(2–3) 2007: 346–62.

6. M. Naidoo, 'Orphaned and Vulnerable Children: A Development Challenge to the Christian Community in Pietermaritzburg' (Master's thesis, University of KwaZulu-Natal, 2007); B. Zengele, 'The Images of God as Perceived by Abandoned Children: An Exploratory Study into the Spiritual Development of Children' (Master's thesis, University of KwaZulu-Natal, 2006).

7. S. Chirongoma, 'Women's and children's rights in the time of HIV and AIDS in Zimbabwe: An analysis of gender inequalities and its impact on people's health'. *Journal of Theology for South Africa* 126 (2006): 48–65; B. Haddad, 'Gender violence and HIV/AIDS: A deadly silence in the church'. *Journal of Theology for South Africa* 114 (2002): 93–106; I. Phiri, 'A theological analysis of the voices of teenage girls on men's role in the fight against HIV/AIDS in KwaZulu-Natal, South Africa'. *Journal of Theology in Southern Africa* 20 (2004): 34–45.

8. A. Wyngaard, 'Towards a theology of HIV/AIDS'. *RFC Focus* 6(1–2) 2006: 51–75.

9. F. Dimmock, *Africa's Children: A Church Response to Children's Issues in Sub-Saharan Africa* (Louisville: Presbyterian Church, 2007).

10. Vorster, 'Protecting the most vulnerable': 349.

11. Okaalet, 'Some religious responses to HIV/AIDS and children in Africa': 94.

12. Wyngaard, 'Towards a theology of HIV/AIDS': 51.

13. P. Denis and N. Makiwane, 'Stories of love, pain and courage: Aids orphans and memory boxes in KwaZulu-Natal, South Africa'. *Journal of the Oral History Society* 31(2) 2003: 66–74; Z. Maqoko and Y. Dreyer, 'Child-headed households because of the trauma surrounding HIV/AIDS'. *Hervormde Teologiese Studies* 63(2) 2007: 717–31.

14. Julian Müller, 'HIV/AIDS, narrative practical theology and postfoundationalism: The emergence of a new story'. *Hervormde Teologiese Studies* 60 (1–2) 2004: 296, 301–4.

15. Amanda Richter and Julian Müller, 'The forgotten children of Africa: Voicing HIV and Aids orphans' stories of bereavement: a narrative approach'. *Hervormde Teologiese Studies* 61 (3) 2005): 1002.

16. Richter and Müller, 'The forgotten children of Africa': 999, 1002.

17. J. Loubser and J. Müller, 'Spiritual narratives of female adolescent orphans affected by HIV and AIDS and poverty'. *Practical Theology in South Africa* 22 (1) 2007: 84, 86.

18. Chirongoma, 'Women's and children's rights in the time of HIV and AIDS in Zimbabwe'.

19. Haddad, 'Gender violence and HIV/AIDS': 97.

20. Haddad, 'Gender violence and HIV/AIDS': 97.

21. Vorster, 'Protecting the most vulnerable': 348. See also Sinenhlanhla Ngwenya, 'From Womb to Work: A Theological Reflection of Child Labour in Zimbabwe' (M.Th. Thesis, University of KwaZulu-Natal, 2009).

22. Loubser and Müller, 'Spiritual narratives of female adolescent orphans affected by HIV and AIDS and poverty': 88.

23. Maqoko and Dreyer, 'Child-headed households because of the trauma surrounding HIV/AIDS': 730.

24. Samantha Chattoraj, 'The Devadassi system'. Available at http://weswa.org/devadasi.htm (accessed Aug. 2008).

25. E. Joy, 'The healing of the woman with haemorrhage and Talitha Cum as models for dalit liberation' in *Talitha Cum!: The Grace of Solidarity in a Globalized World*, edited by M. Degiglio-Bellemare and M. Gabriela (Geneva: World Student Christian Federation, 2004): 76.

26. G.A. Duncan, 'Church discipline: *Semper reformanda* in a time and space warp?' Inaugural address, University of Pretoria, Apr. 2009.

27. Geoff Foster, *Study of the Response by Faith-Based Organisations to Orphans and Vulnerable Children: Preliminary Summary Report* (New York: World Conference of Religions for Peace and United Nations Children's Fund, 2003): 2. For further discussion of this work and the role of religious organisations in orphan care, see Chapter 1 of this book.

28. Musa Dube, 'Fighting with God: children and HIV'. *Journal of Theology for South Africa* 114 (2002): 31–42.

29. Okaalet, 'Some religious responses to HIV/AIDS and children in Africa': 100, 102.

30. Geoff Foster, 'Religion and responses to orphans in Africa' in *A Generation at Risk: The Global Impact of HIV/AIDS on Orphans and Vulnerable Children*, edited by Geoff Foster, Carol Levine and John Williamson (New York: Cambridge University Press, 2005): 160–3.

31. Foster, 'Religion and responses to orphans in Africa': 165.

32. Foster, 'Religion and responses to orphans in Africa': 159, 167.

33. Foster, 'Religion and responses to orphans in Africa': 169, 170. The question of the response of religious organisations to caring for orphan and vulnerable children is also addressed in this book in Chapter 1.

34. Vorster, 'Protecting the most vulnerable': 352, 353.

35. Foster, *Study of the Response by Faith-Based Organisations to Orphans and Vulnerable Children*: 165.

36. M. Wills, 'Connection, action, and hope: An invitation to reclaim the spiritual in health care'. *Journal of Religion and Health* 46 (2007): 423–36. This is a discussion on the emergence of a spiritual dimension to health models and the role of hope in the healing and well-being of the ill.

37. Chirongoma, 'Women's and children's rights in the time of HIV and AIDS in Zimbabwe': 61.

38. D. Gibson and K. Nadeson, '"I have plans": scrutinizing the meaning, production and sustaining of hope in safe sexual practices among young men in Kayelitsha, Cape Town'. *Anthropology Southern Africa* 30 (1–2) (2007): 1–10.

39. R.A.R. Silva et al., 'Ways of coping with AIDS: Opinion of mothers with HIV children'. *Rev Latino-am Enfermagem* 16(2) 2008: 264.

40. Robert C. Linthicum, *City of God, City of Satan: A Biblical Theology of the Urban Church* (Grand Rapids: Harper-Collins, 1991): 165.

41. Wyngaard, 'Towards a theology of HIV/AIDS': 277.

42. Clifford Odimegwu, 'Influence of religion on adolescent sexual attitudes and behaviour among Nigerian university students: Affiliation or commitment?' *African Journal of Reproductive Health* 9(2) 2005: 137.

43. Odimegwu, 'Influence of religion on adolescent sexual attitudes and behaviour among Nigerian university students: 127.

44. UNICEF, *What Religious Leaders Can Do about HIV/AIDS: Actions for Children and Young People* (New York: UNICEF and World Conference of Religions for Peace, 2003).

45. See http://www.shexy.nl/lyrics/1047/gym-class-heroes-cookie-jar (accessed Aug. 2008).

46. Zoe Hussain, 'Hip hop and the HIV church' (Council for World Mission, 2008). Available at http://www.cwmission.org/features/hip-hop-and-the-hiv-church.html?Itemid=3 (accessed 8 Dec. 2009).

47. Denis and Makiwane, 'Stories of love, pain and courage': 66.

48. Musa Dube, *Africa Praying: A Handbook on HIV/AIDS Sensitive Sermon Guidelines and Liturgy* (Geneva: WCC Publications, 2004).

49. Tinyiko Maluleke, 'Defenseless baby Jesus in the midst of the defenseless children of the world'. Available at http://www.ukzn.ac.za/sorat/ujamaa/jesusmid.doc (accessed 15 Aug. 2008).

50. Genevieve James, 'Tell it like it is!: The case to include the story of the rape of Tamar in children's bibles as an awareness tool'. *Journal for Semitics* 16(2) 2007: 312–32.

51. S. de Beer, *Children, the City and the Bible* (Pretoria: TLF, 2004).

52. Frank Makoro, 'Caring for orphans in South Africa'. *Studies in World Christianity* 12(3) 2006: 193–234.

53. Thorne, 'Revisioning women and social change': 98, 102.

Practitioner response

Bongi Zengele

My response to the chapter by Genevieve James arises out of experience as an activist working with the Ujamaa Centre for Community Development and Research at the School of Religion and Theology, University of KwaZulu-Natal. My specific experience of working with children arises out of a Master's degree in Theology and Development and research carried out on images of God as perceived by children.[1]

James's contribution to this book raises serious concerns regarding the paucity of literature on the plight of children within the field of religion and theology. She makes us aware that children are seldom seen or heard; and are excluded and invisible. She rightly argues that there are untapped resources that can be utilised in facing the challenges confronting children in the present context of HIV and AIDS. Furthermore, James suggests that the notion of conceptual autonomy[2] is important for the facilitation of knowledge production using the specific experiences of children. But it is important that we move beyond doing research simply for the sake of accumulating knowledge. It is what we do with, and how we act on, the findings of research that remains the challenge.

While some work on children has been accomplished, there is still a need for further holistic responses to the plight of children infected and affected by HIV and AIDS. There is also a need to deconstruct the way society views children as belonging to the domain of the family. There are too many assumptions that, for example, families and extended families will take care of orphans when parents die. The magnitude of both poverty and the HIV crisis often means this is not always the case. Inevitably, directly and indirectly, children's needs are often under threat. Furthermore, the fact that families are the custodians of children does not necessarily ensure their well-being and safety because of the high rate of trauma, violence and abuse that takes place within the home. The death of a breadwinner gives rise to poverty and children are inevitably exposed to hunger. As a result more and more children run away from their homes: life tends to be unbearable and they are attracted by the potential for survival in the cities. Large numbers of children end up living on the streets of African cities. A city that has a rising number of children living on the streets demonstrates both the socio-economic crisis of the society as well as dysfunctional family life. These children are challenging core community values, indicating that communities cannot feed and care for their own children. What has gone wrong? James argues clearly that this is a direct result of the marginalisation of children.

The harsh reality remains that children are losing their parents and are cared for by either their grandparents or older siblings who are also children in need of guidance. Many children in our communities are in a constant state of grieving. They are exposed to multiple losses

315

ranging from parents and extended family members to the larger community of friends and neighbours. Some children are displaced many times as they are moved after each death in the family to stay with various relatives. They seldom make their own choices, nor are they consulted, but are simply moved from pillar to post because of the circumstances brought about by family deaths. It is important to remember that in all these circumstances children are vulnerable and exploited. So dealing with the needs of children is a matter of urgency.

James takes note of the contribution of FBOs to the plight of children. But there needs to be a much stronger emphasis on an advocacy approach to ensure that children's issues are dealt with from within a justice framework. It is important to open up channels of communication where conflict prevails and to challenge obstacles in the system that exposes children to secondary abuse.

In this present context there is a serious challenge to look for religious and theological resources to deal with a multi-faceted crisis posed by HIV and AIDS and its effect on children. It poses a deep challenge to our ethical understandings and approaches. Theologically speaking, the injunction from the biblical text, 'you shall not steal',[3] needs to be contextually interpreted in the current HIV and AIDS crisis. What about children resorting to petty crime as a result of their hunger? It is the context that renders children exposed and vulnerable to criminal acts.

James argues that children should be central to the agenda of theological education. There is also a need to focus on pastoral counselling that enhances resilience in children and seeks to heal and restore their multiple woundedness. This calls for a well-structured psycho-theological developmental approach. Religious and theological resources may not be sufficient to deal with deep-seated psycho-social problems experienced by children. These resources need to be complemented by participatory approaches that include children themselves, as well as the skills of child care workers and other experts in the field.

While it is true that this is a highly specialised field, this should not be a stumbling block to engaging a transformational approach to children. While theologians may feel ill-equipped to deal with issues pertaining to children, there are religious resources that have always been integral to the socialisation of children. One is prayer which, as my own work with children has shown, is crucial to their spiritual development and builds resilience.[4] Spiritual development needs to play a role in this present context where children are looking for meaning and should be nurtured by religious leaders. This is particularly true for children who are HIV positive. There is almost no research on what this means for children and how it shapes their understanding of the future. It is an area of much needed research.

Our present context is also an invitation to theologians to create new theologies that stem from lived experiences of children. These theologies will provoke a calling for a God who listens and speaks the language of children. They will reflect the often-hidden lamentations of children forced into sex work and other degrading acts that infringe their human rights because of circumstances beyond their control and understanding. These theologies will resonate with the unheard, silent screams of children who are sexually molested in the privacy of their homes. These theologies will create ways of responding to the loud silence around issues of masculinities that are unable to challenge and protect vulnerable children. These theologies will advocate transformative justice that evokes the nurturing nature of God.

The biblical text Luke 18:15–16 draws attention to the way children were treated by Jesus. When people brought children to him in order that he might touch them, his disciples spoke sternly to them. Jesus, seeing this, was indignant and said to them, 'Let the little children come to me, do not hinder them for the kingdom of God belongs to them'. In this text Jesus reflects unconditional love towards children and demonstrates the way they should be treated. This example counters the marginalisation of children that James has demonstrated in her chapter. It offers an alternative way of relating to children and provides a model of social transformation sensitive to the impact of HIV and AIDS in children and their communities. It also demonstrates that there are theological resources to be drawn upon in dealing with the well-being of children. This remains the challenge.

Notes

1. Bongi Zengele, 'Images of God as Perceived by Abandoned Children: Exploration Study into Spiritual Development of Children' (M.Th. thesis, University of KwaZulu-Natal, 2006).
2. Thorne, 'Revisioning women and social change': 104.
3. Exodus 20:15.
4. Zengele, 'Images of God as Perceived by Abandoned Children'.

PART 4

Engaging the communal realm

13

Religion and HIV prevention

Surveying the contestations

Greg Manning

INTRODUCTION

At an individual level, prevention is understood in terms of transmission of the human immuno-deficiency virus (HIV) from one person to another and how it can be blocked. Prevention at this level assumes that individuals are willing and able to convert knowledge about HIV into timely behaviours that effectively reduce the risks that might cause new infections. At a national and international level, HIV prevention refers to slowing down existing epidemics and stopping new ones. The effectiveness of HIV prevention is often measured using medical diagnosis and scientific modelling. However, the range of academic disciplines with a stake in the pursuit of effective HIV prevention is much broader than these two fields of inquiry.

The purpose of this chapter is to survey and analyse research conducted at the interface between HIV prevention and religion in order to support ongoing theological work that seeks to address individual, national and international concerns. The primary database for the literature survey used in this chapter is the December 2008 edition of the CHART bibliography.[1] Much important religious scholarship has not been acknowledged in this review. The work of Hindu and Jewish academics is obviously and regrettably absent, along with scholarship published in languages other than English.

In 2005 the Joint United Nations Program on HIV and AIDS (UNAIDS) adopted a strategy to intensify HIV prevention efforts around the world.[2] This strategy includes seven over-arching principles that provide the framework for the analysis in this chapter. For each of the seven principles for effective HIV prevention, related theological study is sought, with occasional reference to investments by social scientists and others in defining the presence of religion within the frame of HIV prevention. The material reviewed has itself defined some directions for further research. The following overview also allows for the identification of additional aspects of the UNAIDS principles not addressed by the theological work included in this survey.

PRINCIPLE 1

'HIV prevention programmes must be differentiated and locally adapted to the relevant epidemiological, economic, social and cultural contexts in which they are implemented.'[3]

A quick survey of the CHART bibliography suggests that the overt connection between HIV prevention and its context can become masked by the academic scholarship of sacred texts, traditions and beliefs. The word prevention appears in the titles of over 80 references in the CHART bibliography. That subset of titles links HIV prevention to African Traditional Religion (ATR), Afro-Brazilian religion, Buddhism, Christianity, Islam, Judaism and traditional African healers as well as to transcendence and spirituality. References are to places in Africa, Asia, Latin America, the Caribbean, the Middle East, the Pacific and the United States of America. The majority of studies with a strong theological focus are from within Christianity and Islam. It may be useful to make three observations regarding the context of the theological study of HIV prevention before considering the cultural, social, economic and epidemiological contexts.

Theological context

The interplay between the local and transglobal issues facing Catholics involved in HIV prevention is evident in the work of a group of Catholic ethicists who wrote on HIV prevention at the turn of the century. In addition to addressing issues recognised by theologians as fundamental in HIV prevention, they provide 'twenty-six cases from around the world highlighting the complexity of HIV prevention, illustrating the relevance of local issues and concerns, but demonstrating the ability of Catholic moral theological tradition to address HIV prevention'.[4]

The case studies regarding HIV prevention education, programming and multi-sectoral collaboration identify competing senses of responsibility and accountability felt by local Catholic actors toward their global church hierarchy and to 'fundamental moral issues' as well as toward the people in the specific context being considered.[5]

Specific interest in prevention in Islamic scholarship can be identified in the work of Malik Badri.[6] Badri's work is analysed by Ahmed Shams Madyan who explores its application to the context of Indonesia.[7] Madyan compares Badri's work with the contesting Islamic theology of Farid Esack. Esack has observed elsewhere that Islamic theology and authority is intrinsically contextual, saying that 'there are competing nexus of international and local religious leaderships and overlapping tendencies with most Muslims themselves only vaguely aware of the presence of other authority structures'. Esack goes on to say that even in places where there is a predominant, influential religious authority, 'local competing formations for religious authority must be factored into any intervention'.[8] Madyan's examination of the Indonesian religious decrees regarding HIV prevention indicates that, although articulated by local religious scholarship, they do not speak to the local epidemiological context. Instead, they address universal moral issues, independent of context.[9] This conclusion itself cannot be generalised. However, it provides a useful guideline in analysis. It illustrates that religious scholarship in a specific context does not necessarily mean that local religious scholarship addresses the local epidemiological context.

Within Christianity, too, there are many theological approaches and denominational authorities and structures articulating transglobal morality. Musa Dube interacts in the institutionally diffuse diversity of ecumenical Christian scholarship.[10] She and her colleagues have identified that the cultures of African Christianity are linked to ATR. The approach to ATR within this curriculum is different from that of the public health sector. The latter has focused attention on collaboration between the medical sector and traditional healers for the delivery of HIV prevention services such as treatment of sexually transmitted infections and condom promotion.[11] In contrast to this, the theological curriculum examines ATR in order for the students to understand the cultures of their own Christian communities as they mobilise for HIV prevention. The World Council of Churches (WCC) curriculum encourages theology from diverse denominational and cultural perspectives but is distinctively designed for Africa. Furthermore, it is built on a perspective that churches and their members are not exempt from the risks of HIV infection and therefore have a direct interest in designing and receiving truly effective HIV prevention programmes for themselves.[12]

Cultural context

The importance of ATR and culture to HIV prevention is well documented.[13] A recent development in debates on culture has been the focus on the role of male circumcision in HIV prevention. Scaling up the practice of male circumcision was recommended by the World Health Organisation (WHO) and UNAIDS in 2007 to reduce the risk of heterosexually acquired HIV infection in men in countries with high HIV prevalence and low rates of male circumcision.[14] The WCC curriculum, discussed above, addresses male circumcision both in relationship to debates regarding circumcision in the biblical text and its relationship to contemporary male sexuality in African contexts.[15] Male circumcision has a history as a divisive theological issue. In the WCC curriculum it is critiqued as a cultural practice that increases risky sexual behaviour, contrary to the WHO recommendations. However, it must be noted that the WCC curriculum was published before the WHO recommendation and does acknowledge ongoing studies into the role of male circumcision in HIV prevention. Religious education is thus challenged to keep pace with scientific developments in HIV prevention. It is challenged by both the developments themselves as well as by conflict between recommendations from the public health sector and from theological reflection on culture.

Social context

The social contexts in which HIV prevention programmes are implemented are often defined in studies into the knowledge, attitudes, behaviours and practices of geographically and demographically defined populations. These so-called KABP studies are based on a survey methodology and can have differing orientations. One of the earliest of these surveys is a national study sanctioned by Uganda's AIDS Control Programme.[16] It set out to create baseline data to inform culturally sensitive interventions. Some KABP studies inform the design of multi-sectoral collaboration for HIV prevention such as that between medical doctors and traditional healers or Muslim scholars.[17] Some explore diversity within and between religions and beliefs regarding sexual morality,[18] while others explore religious attitudes towards homosexuality and the causes of HIV infection.[19] KABP studies recognise that religions may influence the design of some HIV prevention efforts. Such studies are often designed and published independently of religious structures and theological analysis. This body of work is complementary to other religious work identified later in this literature survey.

Economic context

Michael Kelly has conducted research in Zambia that critiques the UNAIDS framework used in this chapter and offers an alternative conceptual framework for approaching HIV prevention. His framework includes the economic contexts of personal and national poverty; exploitative global economic structures; gender inequality; and stigma and discrimination. He endorses the human rights foundations of the UNAIDS approach to HIV prevention but objects to 'the rational, linear, individualistic approaches that have dogged the response to HIV transmission' that he sees as prevalent in the UNAIDS framework. Kelly's conceptual framework is interesting because he introduces key issues into the principles of HIV prevention. He considers migration and the movement of people in his observations of the economic context of HIV transmission and bases human rights assertions on the theological principle of justice. He affirms the longevity and scale of influence of Christian institutional presence and its role as service provider, teacher, prophet and ally in social change. He identifies that young people do not have sufficient voice in the design of HIV prevention.[20]

Kelly's analysis illustrates a problem facing theological approaches to HIV prevention. The evaluations of effective HIV prevention based on Kelly's work are moral judgements. Kelly himself perceives that the adoption of responsible sexual behaviour is essential in order to slow down the spread of HIV, though injustice prevents many people from this possibility. The Jesuit Centre for Theological Reflection, who commissioned the study, concluded: 'Addressing HIV/AIDS serves as an entry point and catalyst for addressing these broader issues. Briefly then, one can say that the more HIV/AIDS, the less justice – but the more justice, the less HIV/AIDS.'[21]

The effectiveness of HIV prevention, here, is evaluated according to moral indicators of responsible sexual behaviour and justice; not HIV status, prevalence, or measures of re-infection. The possibility that morally evaluated HIV prevention is an entry point to address other issues of interest to religious organisations may further fuel tensions associated with the accountability of religions in HIV prevention. This is addressed later in this survey.

Theology in generalised epidemics

The survey in this chapter is punctuated by studies relevant to the prevention of heterosexually transmitted HIV in sub-Saharan Africa. In order to acknowledge the global scope of the theme of HIV prevention and religion and theology, two observations are made regarding generalised epidemics (that is, countries where the HIV prevalence was estimated to be over one per cent in the adult population) outside Africa. In 2007 UNAIDS identified fifteen countries outside Africa experiencing generalised epidemics.[22] One was Thailand, where the main religion is Buddhism. The Buddhist Leadership Initiative utilised Buddhist teachings, beliefs and traditions to mobilise monks and nuns to participate in and support multi-sectoral HIV prevention efforts. This initiative, framed in Buddhist philosophy and language, enabled three primary responses for the nuns and monks involved in HIV prevention: caring for the sick; educating people how to prevent infection; and accepting and collaborating with other HIV prevention initiatives besides the specifically religious.[23]

The CHART bibliography identifies only one theological study emerging from the national generalised epidemics occurring outside Africa. This is the work of Mary McCarthy, who worked with the poetry of Maura Elaripe Mea, a woman living with HIV in Papua New Guinea, as a context to explore biblical themes of hope, suffering, and life and death. Mea's poetry draws attention to themes of gender inequality, discrimination against people living with HIV, and the right to life and dignity. McCarthy sees Mea's expression of suffering with her dying children to be an important interpretive perspective for reading the Bible and its application to awareness raising and challenging discrimination.[24]

Theology in concentrated epidemics

Concentrated epidemics are commonly found among groups of people who are already stigmatised within Christianity and Islam as sinners, regardless of their HIV status – sex workers, drug users and men who have sex with men. Besides drawing attention to specific populations, focusing on concentrated epidemics draws attention to a broader interface between HIV prevention and theology outside Africa.

The majority of citations in the CHART bibliography from countries where the national HIV prevalence is less than one per cent come from research conducted in the USA. My analysis suggests that the USA is the fourth most cited country in the titles contained in the CHART bibliography. Research from epidemics in the USA is predominantly about religion within specific contexts. Its prominent themes include work with African-Americans, drug users, homosexuals and women. The extensive study of the religious context of HIV prevention in the USA is not matched by extensive theological reflection on the same themes, with the exception of the study of homosexuality.

The CHART bibliography contains references to interfaces between homo-sexuality and religion in Africa, Asia, Australia, the Americas, the Caribbean, the

Middle East and the United Kingdom. Three issues warrant attention. First, theological study related to homosexuality that exists within specific religious traditions has been developed. For example, Vincent Genovesi offers an account of Catholic teaching on homosexuality, including a review of positions in relation to human rights and discrimination.[25] Donald Messer examines the contrasting approaches of Protestant scholars advocating for and against the inclusion of homosexuals in the life of the church.[26] Ersilia Francesca offers a review of Islamic ethical literature related to HIV and AIDS, including a review of differing views of homosexuality.[27] Second, there is a theological discourse in which the homosexual identity of researchers is important in the interpretation of sacred texts. This discourse can be identified by references to queer and gay studies. William Lindsey is another who has analysed the work of Catholic theologians on homosexuality, observing that gay voices were absent from theological attempts to develop a sexual ethic sensitive to homosexuality. He argues that the church is unable to see the essential humanity of homosexual people.[28] In 2008 the Global Theological Conversation of the Ecumenical Advocacy Alliance (EAA) on HIV prevention acknowledged the variety of populations and academic disciplines that had informed their understanding of the epidemic.[29] It is important to note that homosexuals (along with drug users and sex workers) were not acknowledged among those attributed with informing the theologians' understanding of HIV epidemics. Third, some theologians are linking women and homosexuals in their studies. Margaret Farley is motivated by the vulnerability of women in Africa to HIV infection due to gender injustice and tests her framework of justice in same sex relationships.[30] Denise Ackermann affirms that the biblical tradition of lamentation, utilised by both female and homosexual scholars, offers important theological approaches to all sectors of church communities for overcoming stigma, exclusion and injustice.[31]

In Africa, developments in the study of what has traditionally been called sex work in HIV prevention discourse are advancing: gender, poverty and sexuality have provided themes for theological study related to women involved in transactional or survival sex. In Zimbabwe, Sophie Chirongoma equates transactional sex to food for work and offers gender justice as the theological foundation for HIV prevention.[32] In Uganda, Jo Sadgrove examines the relationship between Pentecostal Christian theologies and social structures and sexual behaviour in a context where sexual activity is exchanged for material goods.[33] The thirteen references to sex work or prostitution in the CHART bibliography identify religious interfaces with HIV prevention in Egypt, India and Thailand, including references to Buddhism, Christianity, Hinduism and Islam. However, none of these studies are particularly theological in nature.

The CHART bibliography includes studies on drug use in Bangladesh, Malaysia, Iran, Saudi Arabia, Senegal and the USA.[34] These references are all assessments of contexts where people are vulnerable to HIV transmission through drug use and are affected predominantly by Islamic religious attitudes. Buddhist and Christian thought has been applied to specific local HIV prevention projects amongst drug users in the USA.[35] Christian theological approaches to HIV prevention amongst drug users have been articulated in epidemics in the United Kingdom and India. Tearfund's theological adviser, Dewi Hughes, published an affirmation of harm reduction directed at Christian medical practitioners in the United Kingdom. He perceives that Christians prefer to approach HIV prevention by trying to restore a moral context. Based on his study of Old Testament law, Jesus and biblical ethics, he argues that doctors, including Christian doctors, are responsible for the protection of people who are vulnerable to infection even in an 'anarchic moral context'.[36] In the context of the spread of HIV among injecting drug users in India, I have suggested that biblical support for HIV prevention itself will be established from the study of the context in which HIV spreads, rather than focusing on the risk behaviours of drug users. Based on this understanding, the actual practice of HIV prevention by Christians in response to its spread among drug users will depend upon how they see their own identity within that specific context.[37]

PRINCIPLE 2

'All HIV prevention efforts/programmes must have as their fundamental basis the promotion, protection and respect of human rights, including gender equality.'[38]

The Asian Muslim Action Network (AMAN) and the WCC both specifically name human rights as foundational in their understanding of HIV prevention and maintain an awareness of human rights in a broad range of specific contexts.[39] In 1996 the WCC advocated that churches promote the human rights of people living with HIV as well as those of other populations at risk, acknowledging this as necessary to prevent the spread of HIV.[40] The WCC also addresses issues of human rights within its theological curriculum on HIV and AIDS.[41] This curriculum deals with human rights in relation to stigma, discrimination and gender inequality in detail but also addresses the human rights of children and homosexuals more generally. In 2006 the WCC published a collection of articles advocating the rights of drug users, sex workers, displaced people and prisoners.[42] Illustrative of the context of this advocacy, the EAA has indicated that the Orthodox Church is being invited to collaborate with HIV prevention efforts among drug users in eastern Europe, despite the fact that human rights based strategies challenge their current religious teachings and theology.[43]

Some Christian scholars recognise the human rights discourse within the theological theme of justice. Musimbi Kanyoro identifies justice as the central theme in a collection of essays by the Circle of Concerned African Women Theologians. The essays use biblical models of resistance to injustice to address the failure to recognise the human rights of women. Kanyoro introduces the essays by stating that the Bible shows that people who are affected by injustice are vital to changing laws and cultures in order to achieve justice.[44]

The founding of the organisation Positive Muslims and its emphasis on a theology of compassion is linked to the emergence of progressive Islam in South Africa.[45] Omid Safi, a prominent scholar of progressive Islam, sees commitments to human rights emerging out of the pursuit of social justice with an emphasis on gender equality.[46] The theology of compassion emerges out of the theology of liberation developed in South Africa's anti-apartheid movement. Katherine Willson interprets the Qur'anic hermeneutical keys of this theology as compassion, responsibility and justice. She further argues that people who are marginalised or oppressed by society are essential participants in the interpretation of the Qur'an.[47]

Other theologians have expressed reservations regarding the application of human rights to HIV prevention. Mohammad Yousuf Bhat argues for the superiority of human accountability to divine law over human rights, based on his review of the right to life within Islamic teaching.[48] Jakobus Vorster reviews the 'international guidelines for HIV/AIDS and Human Rights' from a reformed Protestant ethical perspective. He endorses the role of the state in implementing pragmatic laws which prioritise the health of the community over the rights of individuals. While Vorster ascribes gender inequality to interpretations of religious texts, he does not integrate this inequality into his analysis of HIV testing and disclosure of HIV status.[49] Vorster's analysis of HIV and human rights does, however, offer a baseline for important further theological reflection on the prevention of mother-to-child transmission of HIV.

Justice – be it divine, social, or administered by state authorities – is the common foundational value underpinning theological approaches to the application of human rights to HIV prevention. In many traditions, existing conceptions of divine, state or social justice have not yet been applied to support the human rights of all people in HIV prevention. The interpretations of sacred texts by women take up a social critique that successfully establishes a context of social justice. Their work raises an important question as to whether a similar hermeneutical approach is acceptable for other marginalised groups such as homosexuals, drug users and young people.

PRINCIPLE 3

'HIV prevention actions must be evidence-informed, based on what is known and proven to be effective and investment to expand the evidence base should be strengthened.'[50]

References to accountability to the divine are associated with religious work that links itself to evidence-informed action for HIV prevention. For example, the policy stance of the organisation Islamic Relief states that 'First and foremost, Islamic relief is accountable to our creator in all it does'.[51] The Christian Global Theological Conversation of EAA, which is concerned with HIV prevention, notes that evidence-informed action is based upon a principle of accountability to fellow human beings but adds that 'accountability to God ... may be an important factor in motivating people [of faith] to become contributors to evidence-based responses'.[52]

The theme of truth within Christian thought is also linked to scientific research used as evidence to support or critique HIV prevention strategies. A gathering of theologians in Namibia in 2003 identified the theme of truth and truth telling as crucial to addressing HIV-related stigma. They argue that truth includes both fact and meaning and suggest that, in both science and theology, truth includes confident assertions and uncertain inquiry. The theologians also identify truthful education as an essential element of HIV prevention, yet acknowledge that the definition of what constitutes truthful education is a theological challenge, particularly in the education of young people.[53]

The interplay between truth of fact and truth of meaning is demonstrated in ambiguous and ambivalent religious approaches to education on the use of condoms.[54] Gideon Byamugisha defines two prominent questions asked about the role of condoms in HIV prevention as follows: 'One concerns the concepts of efficacy and effectiveness, the other concerns fear that making condoms available will encourage early sexual activity among adolescents (promiscuity) and extra marital sex among adults (adultery) – affairs which are immoral in front of God and society'.[55]

Christian Aid published a literature survey in 2003 to address the specific concern that 'sexual health and HIV education may lead to promiscuity'. This review of research on the relationship between education about sex and HIV and the sexual behaviour of young people led to the conclusion that sex and HIV education does not increase promiscuity.[56] Jon Fuller and James Keenan provide an overview of Catholic moral theology's approach to the same two questions regarding condoms identified by Byamugisha. They identify a consensus among moral theologians that condoms do have an acceptable role to play in HIV prevention and believe that this consensus provides an evidence base capable of influencing the decisions of their church leadership.[57] However, David Crawford and Luke Gormally are contemporary theologians who are not satisfied by the advocacy of moral theologians for the use of condoms to prevent HIV infection.[58] This discussion centres on promiscuity and illicit sexual activity resulting in an inquiry into the use of condoms for HIV prevention that focuses on the morality of individuals and the responsibilities of their teachers. It does not address the question of the effectiveness of condoms in preventing and slowing down epidemics.

The dramatic reduction in HIV prevalence in Uganda during the 1990s has been a subject of particular interest for people seeking to understand, design and implement HIV prevention strategies to slow down the spread of HIV in generalised epidemics. Based on observations from Uganda's experience, the US government made large financial investments in building the capacity of faith-based organisations (FBOs) to deliver HIV prevention services with the establishment of the President's Emergency Program for AIDS Relief (PEPFAR).[59] The strategy adopted was referred to as the ABC (Abstain, Be faithful, and Condomise) approach to HIV prevention.[60] With associated educational guidelines it is embraced by many FBOs.

The research of Edward Green was influential in defining the ABC strategy.[61] Green's work is used to advocate and defend the engagement of FBOs in HIV prevention in generalised epidemics. During the 1990s, Green generated research that was used to advocate the greater involvement of traditional medical practitioners in the treatment of sexually transmitted infections and the promotion of abstinence, fidelity and the use of condoms. During this time, he recognised the opposition of some FBOs to the use of condoms for HIV prevention. Green then outlined a role for FBOs in slowing down the spread of HIV in generalised epidemics through the promotion of abstinence and fidelity as ways of avoiding and reducing exposure to HIV infection.[62] As evidence, he gathered information about two issues: the participation of FBOs in national HIV prevention efforts that had already slowed down generalised HIV epidemics; and the limits of the effectiveness of condoms in HIV prevention.[63] Green's research supports claims that the existing Christian and Muslim teachings on abstinence and fidelity play important and accountable roles in preventing infection. It also defends religious groups that do not want to promote, support or resource condom use. Green describes his own work as providing suggestive evidence and advocates careful monitoring of FBOs in order to enable better evaluation of their work in HIV prevention.[64] Green's more recent research outlines his 'wish to bring fear appeals back into the AIDS discussion and into research agendas'. Fear arousal draws upon a perceived 'comparative advantage' of the existing theological evidence base.[65]

Gideon Byamugisha, however, would argue that this discussion on the ABC approach must keep theological reflection in relationship with other scientific disciplines. He precedes his comments about the effectiveness and morality of condoms with information and reflections on teaching about marriage in achieving abstinence and fidelity. In Green's work, this information and reflection is absent, while reminders about the limits of the effectiveness of condoms are always present. Further, Byamugisha makes the observation that what is lawful is not always safe, and what is safe is not always lawful.[66] In doing so, he has defined an area for further theological inquiry, which addresses the gap identified earlier under the principle of human rights. He challenges the belief that lawfulness or justice can always be equated with HIV prevention and indicates that the unreflective application of even theologically established laws to HIV prevention (such as marriage) can nurture a 'risk increasing environment'.[67] Byamugisha's direction for future theological work on HIV prevention is that churches 'redeem sexuality from theological and historical distortions and inadequacies'.[68]

As is suggested in this section, for Christians and Muslims engagement with HIV prevention must have as its fundamental basis a means of accountability to the divine. These means of accountability – sacred texts, theology, history, missiology, ethics and culture – are addressed in this book. In addition, this chapter has argued that religious organisational structures are also a means of accountability. Accountability to human stakeholders in HIV prevention is identified later in this chapter as a weakness of religious HIV prevention efforts. If religious responses are to be taken seriously, then religious organisations need to engage in their prevention efforts in a more systematic way in order to support the multi-sectoral collaboration addressed under the next principle.

PRINCIPLE 4

'HIV prevention programmes must be comprehensive in scope, using the full range of policy and programmatic interventions known to be effective.'[69]

In expanding this principle, UNAIDS states that comprehensive HIV prevention should use a number of multi-sectoral approaches, including poverty reduction and sexual and reproductive health in order to reduce vulnerability as well as the risk and impact of HIV infection.[70] These same elements of a comprehensive approach to HIV prevention are asserted without qualification by the Catholic Agency for Overseas Development (CAFOD) arguing it is working from a platform that is both scientifically valid and based on sound theological principles and suggesting that it is accountable to both God and human beings. It asserts that multi-sectoral approaches are crucial to effective HIV prevention programming because most programmes will not address each of the elements necessary for effective HIV prevention.[71]

Interest in a comprehensive approach to HIV prevention is demonstrated in the EAA project, Global Theological Conversation, already referred to a number of times in this chapter.[72] Five of the seven contributors to the volume directly affirm that there are multiple approaches to and roles in HIV prevention and that the latter must address vulnerability as well as risk.[73] Three of the contributions – by Margaret Farley, Peter Okaalet, and Lisandro Orlov – identify roles that should be undertaken by Christian churches in HIV prevention. Farley explores aspects of a prophetic role and acknowledges the themes of human rights and responsibilities, local differentiation and accountability to God.[74] Okaalet highlights educational roles, including education to assist in making choices as well as theological education to strengthen religious institutional capacity over the long term.[75] Orlov draws attention to the role of the church in facilitating the spread of HIV and the need to engage governments and structures that produce inequality, including poverty.[76]

The study of the roles of religious organisations in HIV prevention offers an analytical starting point. There are 25 titles in the CHART bibliography that specifically claim to explore the subject of the role of religious organisations in HIV prevention. This material reveals a body of work that concentrates on the attitudes and practices of Christian organisations and all but four of these are located in Africa. It adds to the KABP studies identified in reference to the social context of HIV prevention earlier in the chapter but is distinct from and complementary to them. While most of the KABP studies are published in journals not identified as religious, this body of work tends to be accessible through publishers with religious identities. The material that focuses on the study of roles serves to identify the part that religious communities play in the spectrum of HIV prevention initiatives but does not establish these identified roles in relation to other sectors of society.

There are exceptions within Christian scholarship where steps have been taken to move beyond the articulation of the church's own role in HIV prevention to building institutional capacity for multi-sectoral partnership. The EAA has published a guide to be used by groups who may want to collaborate with FBOs.[77] This guide sees respect, understanding and trust of religious organisations by other partners to be important in the success of collaborative efforts. A complementary guide has been developed for people who identify themselves as church-based and applies the process of dialogue (involving people with different points of view) to issues that have proven to be obstacles for Christian engagement in effective HIV prevention.[78] Within Catholic ethics, the principle of co-operation has been applied to enable multi-sectoral collaboration on controversial HIV prevention efforts involving condom promotion; needle and syringe exchange programmes; HIV prevention with gay men; and participation in local and national programmes. The edited volume by Keenan includes local case studies from the USA and India.[79] Robert Vitillo, another Catholic scholar, has also outlined a co-operative process used by the Catholic Bishops Conference of India.[80]

Theological articulation of roles and responsibilities in HIV prevention is weighted inconsistently. Prominent attention has been given to the responsibilities of individuals and governments in preventing the transmission of HIV along with the roles of religious organisations and leaders. The responsibilities of religions in relation to epidemics and the valuable roles of people outside religious account-ability frameworks deserve further theological attention.

PRINCIPLE 5

'HIV prevention is for life; therefore, both delivery of existing interventions as well as research and development of new technologies require a long-term and sustained effort, recognizing that results will only be seen over the longer term and need to be maintained'.[81]

The principle of sustained effort in HIV prevention can be seen in the development of human resources and institutional capacity, specifically in the involvement and education of religious leaders and the development of sexuality education. The education of religious leaders has been a strategy for building the human resource and institutional capacity for large networks of Buddhist, Christian and Muslim religious leaders in Africa and Asia to enable them to participate effectively in HIV prevention. The Islamic Medical Association of Uganda (IMAU) has engaged in educational efforts with male and female Muslim leaders.[82] The Sangha Metta Project developed a multi-sectoral training programme for Buddhist monks, nuns and other Buddhist leaders in South East Asia.[83] Musa Dube and Wati Longchar have outlined foundations for the introduction of an HIV and AIDS curriculum in theological education in Africa and Asia.[84] The work of IMAU and Sangha Metta aimed to enable multi-sectoral collaboration, while the frameworks of Dube and Longchar aim to enable the development of Christian theological thought. Theological focus on sexuality is one of the foundations advocated by both Dube in Africa and Longchar in Asia to build institutional capacity through Christian theological education in order to engage in effective HIV prevention.

In Asia, the development of theological education related to HIV and AIDS also acknowledges a history of silence on the subject of human sexuality, as does Agrippa Khathide in Africa.[85] This silence is based on existing theological perceptions and local cultural experience.[86] Writing on silence in specifically Asian contexts, Donald Messer also addresses the themes of culture, youth, homosexuality, poverty and sexuality, and sexual violence against women and children. This claim by theological educators that there is a silence in teaching on sexuality speaks into a context where religious teaching is held up as effective in motivating sexual expression that is advantageous to HIV prevention – abstinence before marriage and fidelity within marriage.[87]

The WCC curriculum focusing on Africa devotes one of its ten modules to 'Human sexuality and HIV and AIDS'. In addition to teaching about abstinence and fidelity, this module explores additional subjects such as cultural issues affecting sexuality, sexuality and young people, masturbation, sexual violence against women and children, homosexuality, and poverty and sexuality.[88] The 'Guidelines for comprehensive sexuality education in the context of church theological training institutions' that preceded the WCC curriculum begin by claiming that they are part of the strengthening of Christian institutional capacity to address problems in discussing sexuality.[89] They conclude that young people should be involved in the development of the sexuality education programme. While there is some evidence in the CHART bibliography of young people engaged in the development and delivery of sexuality education programmes,[90] they are less obvious in the development of theology. One exception is the work of Isabel Phiri who draws upon a justice and gender perspective to analyse theologically the writings of girls about the roles of men in HIV prevention.[91]

There is urgency in developing effective HIV prevention for young people that moves beyond mere instruction on sexuality. Okaalet speaks of handing values on to young people.[92] Further study is needed on theological processes available to young people to awaken values that will guide effective HIV prevention.

PRINCIPLE 6

'HIV prevention programming must be at a coverage, scale and intensity that is enough to make a critical difference.'[93]

The concept of coverage is a measurable target-setting instrument on the agenda of the WHO programme of universal access to prevention, care, treatment and support.[94] Although coverage is not a theological theme, it intersects with the issue of accountability because of its concern with the overall planning and monitoring cycles of HIV prevention activities. The Catholic Medical Missions Board commissioned a key informant study on the role of FBOs in HIV epidemics in six countries. One of the questions the study posed was: 'what is the perceived accountability of FBO programmes in terms of basis for programming and empirical assessment of programme effectiveness?' It concluded:

> FBO strategies and programmes are perceived to be based on a varying mix of religious philosophy and empiricism. Science is not thought to be generally ignored, but the message is often tailored to be consistent with moral beliefs. This weakens the efforts and accountability of FBOs in the view of some informants.[95]

Sectors investing in HIV prevention among stigmatised populations recognise that religious organisations can influence these efforts whether or not an intervention is going to be effective.[96] But the extensive reach of religious organisations is perceived by national and international planners to be important for coverage, scale and intensity in order to slow down HIV epidemics.[97] PEPFAR has commented: 'Faith-based organizations remain an underutilized resource for expanding the reach of quality services.'[98]

When included in the large-scale HIV prevention initiatives of USAID, the role Christian and Muslim organisations play in efforts to delay the age of sexual debut in individuals, reduce the number of sexual partners, and provide reproductive health care is acknowledged.[99] It has also been demonstrated that African traditional medical practitioners influence people's sexual behaviour as well as provide widespread prevention and treatment services for sexually-transmitted infections (STIs).[100] The role of Buddhist monks and nuns in the large-scale Sangha Metta Project is to create an enabling environment for HIV prevention activities by 'leading lay people to accept and care for HIV positive people'.[101]

Adopting the role of service providers in the scaling up of HIV prevention does not always demand the development of sound theological understandings. This is because the roles of religious organisations may be defined and funded according to the compatibility between the application of their existing theology and what is deemed necessary and pragmatic for large-scale, centrally co-ordinated HIV prevention strategies. Dube reminds theologians that ABC strategies are crippled by gender inequality.[102] Her theological approach to HIV prevention is a transformative agenda towards the development and use of women-controlled prevention strategies, similar to those theologians whose strategies are based in a commitment to justice. Farley, in discussing prophetic discourse in the EAA's Global Theological Conversation, acknowledges the biblical tradition of divinely ordained social critique while also questioning prophetic discourse's 'usefulness as a primary form of advocacy regarding HIV prevention'.[103] Her application of prophetic discourse to HIV prevention highlights three issues: first, the contexts of injustice under critique should be understood in detail; second, the manner of prophetic discourse should offer hope, call for dialogue rather than silence other voices, include concrete actions in response to the critique, and be deeply affected by people who are most affected by HIV; and third, the content of prophetic discourse should articulate grief, be multi-cultural and address sexuality according to considerations of justice.[104]

Additional questions about theological affirmations of the goodness and importance of religious engagement with or against HIV prevention are raised by other contributors – Orlov, Adrian Thatcher and Johannes Petrus Heath – to the EAA Global Theological Conversation about HIV prevention.[105] These questions indicate that the practice of HIV prevention needs to be learnt and is not inherent. They offer directions for learning from mistakes made in the process of applying existing theologies to HIV epidemics.

PRINCIPLE 7

'Community participation of those for whom HIV prevention programmes are planned is critical for their impact.'[106]

At the turn of the century, Fuller and Keenan identified a movement away from theologically validating HIV prevention itself to a focus on the social problems that inhibit HIV prevention measures.[107] Farid Esack suggests that between 2000 and 2006 there was 'a significant increase in the willingness of Muslim organizations and religious leaderships to acknowledge the reality of HIV & AIDS in the Muslim world'.[108] These observations suggest that community participation by religious groups may be understood in two historical periods, either side of the turn of the century.

There are at least five prominent cases of community participation in the design of HIV prevention with a religious identity and supportive theology that can be traced back to the 1980s. These include: collaboration between the IMAU and Muslim leaders; publications of the WCC; Catholic scholarship and experience in HIV prevention; studies by women about women in Africa; and theological reflection by gay men in the USA. This list identifies two different movements: the mobilisation of formal religious establishments (such as IMAU, WCC or Catholic scholars); and the assertion by identifiable sub-populations that they belonged in HIV prevention planning. Theological perspectives offered by women in Africa and gay men in the USA were assertions of identity and humanity in the face of injustice and suffering, including vulnerability to HIV infection.

The turn of century saw intensified political commitment to HIV prevention and an increased academic interest in the involvement of religious leaders. The CHART bibliography contains 62 references to religious leaders from five religions in over seventeen countries with 52 of these references published since the year 2000. A new type of religious leadership emerged in the twenty-first century –

the leadership of people with religious identities and who are living with HIV. The organisation Positive Muslims was formed in 2000 and insisted on a new approach to HIV prevention with a specifically Muslim orientation.[109] The theology of compassion promoted by Positive Muslims has a greater emphasis on people who were already living with HIV in both the development of its theology and in its understanding of HIV prevention. The emergence and assertions of the African Network of Religious Leaders Living With or Affected by HIV or AIDS (ANERELA) promoted an alternative HIV prevention model called SAVE (Safer practice; Available medical interventions; Voluntary counselling and testing; and Empowerment).[110] SAVE emerged from a critique of the ABC model of HIV prevention led by people who are living with HIV, suggesting that it is stigmatising of HIV positive people.[111]

The principle of community mobilisation is itself an over-arching principle of HIV prevention. All theological traditions must consider which hermeneutical approaches can support the application of the principle of community mobilisation in their epidemiological context, in addition to embracing the opportunity for their own mobilisation.

CONCLUSION

While the above seven principles have been addressed individually, in the practice of HIV prevention they need to be applied simultaneously. This chapter indicates that religious and theological discourse related to HIV prevention is finding immediate application in a wide variety of situations. It takes place within a public examination of the simultaneous connectedness of people to God, and to other people, regardless of belief. Belief, however, is important as it affects identity and relationships in pluralistic contexts. The formation and practice of religious belief in HIV prevention has been identified in relation to theological themes of justice and human sexuality.

The analysis in this chapter has not sought to alter or enhance the UNAIDS conceptual framework upon which it is based. However, this is not to suggest that this framework cannot be improved. What the above interaction with the framework does suggest is that theological input into the maturing of HIV prevention efforts needs to be well established in relationship with people who are demanding better approaches than that already available to them. Religious and theological efforts also need to be committed to supporting claims about HIV prevention with regular evaluation of their effectiveness.

NOTES

1. Available at http:// www.chart.ukzn.ac.za (accessed 3 Jan. 2009).
2. UNAIDS, 'Intensifying HIV prevention: UNAIDS policy position paper' (2005).
3. UNAIDS, 'Intensifying HIV prevention': 17.
4. James Keenan et al. (eds), *Catholic Ethicists on HIV/AIDS Prevention* (New York: Continuum, 2000): 14.
5. Keenan et al., *Catholic Ethicists on HIV/AIDS Prevention*: 14.
6. Malik Badri, *AIDS Prevention: Failure in the North and Catastrophe in the South: A solution.* (Qualbert: Islamic Medical Association of South Africa, 2000).
7. Ahmed Shams Madyan, *Islamic Responses to HIV-AIDS: A Comparative Study on Malik Badri, Farid Esack and Indonesian Muslim Responses* (Yogyakarta: Gajah Mada University, 2006).
8. Farid Esack, *Muslims Mapping AIDS: Mapping Muslim Organisational and Religious Responses* (Cape Town: UNAIDS/Positive Muslims, 2007): 4.
9. Ahmed Shams Madyan, 'Institutions in Indonesia: failure of leadership in the fight against HIV'. *Nasir* 1(3) 2007: 4–5.
10. Musa Dube (ed.), *HIV and AIDS Curriculum for Theological Education by Extension in Africa and 10 HIV and AIDS Modules* (Geneva: World Council of Churches Publications, 2007).
11. Rachel King, *Collaborating with Traditional Healers for HIV Prevention and Care in Sub-Saharan Africa: Suggestions for Programme Managers and Field Workers* (Geneva: UNAIDS, 2006). Available at http:// data.unaids.org/Publications/IRC-pub07/JC967-TradHealers_en.pdf (accessed 15 Dec. 2009).
12. Dube (ed.), *HIV and AIDS Curriculum for Theological Education by Extension in Africa and 10 HIV and AIDS Modules: Introduction.*
13. See Chapter 9 in this book.
14. WHO, 'Operational guidance for scaling up male circumcision services for HIV prevention' (2008): 8.
15. Peter Ngure, 'Module 2: Human sexuality and HIV and AIDS': 79; and Musa Dube, 'Module 4: Reading the New Testament in the HIV and AIDS contexts': 80–6 in *HIV and AIDS Curriculum for Theological Education by Extension in Africa and 10 HIV and AIDS Modules*, edited by Dube.
16. E. Ankrah et al., *AIDS in Uganda: Analysis of the Social Dimensions of the Epidemic* (Kampala: Makerere University, 1989).
17. For example, see V.G. Chipfakacha, 'STD/HIV/AIDS knowledge, beliefs, practices and experiences of traditional healers in Botswana'. *AIDS Care* 9(4) 1997: 417–25; R. al-Owaish et al., 'Knowledge, attitudes, beliefs and practices about HIV/AIDS in Kuwait'. *AIDS Education and Prevention* 11(2) 1999: 163–73.
18. For example, see Lester Coleman and Adrienne Testa, 'Sexual health knowledge, attitudes and behaviours: Variations among a religiously diverse sample of young people in London, UK'. *Ethnicity and Health* 13(1) 2008: 55–72; Victor Agadjanian, 'Gender, religious involvement and HIV/AIDS prevention in Mozambique'. *Social Science and Medicine* 61(7) 2005: 1529–39.
19. For example, see L. Nicholas and K. Durrheim, 'Religiosity, AIDS and sexuality knowledge, attitudes, beliefs and practices of black South African first-year university students'. *Psychological Reports* 77(3) 1995: 1328–30; K. Hendrickx et al., 'Sexual behaviour of second generation

Moroccan immigrants balancing between traditional attitudes and safe sex'. *Patient Education and Counselling* 47(2) 2002: 89–94; S. Kalichman and L. Sambeyi, 'Traditional beliefs about the cause of AIDS and AIDS-related stigma in South Africa'. *AIDS Care* 16(5) 2004: 572–80.

20. Michael Kelly, *HIV and AIDS: A Justice Perspective* (Lusaka: Jesuit Centre for Theological Reflection 2006): 4, 7, 41, 59–62, 63, 64.

21. Kelly, *HIV and AIDS*: xxiii.

22. UNAIDS, *Report on the Global AIDS Epidemic* (2008).

23. UNICEF, *The Buddhist Leadership Initiative* (Bangkok: MUNICEF East Asia Pacific Regional Office, 2003): 3-5.

24. Mary McCarthy, 'Hope of living'. *Melanesian Journal of Theology* 21(1) 2005: 65–7.

25. Vincent Genovesi, *In Pursuit of Love: Catholic Morality and Human Sexuality* (Collegeville: Liturgical Press, 1996).

26. Donald E. Messer, 'Homosexuality and ecclesiology' in *Vision and Supervision: A Sourcebook of Significant Documents of the Council of Bishops of The United Methodist Church 1968–2002*, edited by James K. Mathews and William B. Oden (Nashville: Abingdon Press, 2003): 168–87.

27. Ersilia Francesca, 'AIDS in contemporary Islamic ethical literature'. *Medicine and Law* 21(2) 2002: 381–94.

28. William Lindsey, 'The AIDS crisis and the church: a time to heal'. *Theology and Sexuality* 1(11) 1995: 13–14.

29. Gillian Paterson (ed.), *HIV Prevention: A Global Theological Conversation* (Geneva: EAA, 2009): 2.

30. Margaret Farley, *Just Love: A Framework for Christian Sexual Ethics* (New York: Continuum, 2006).

31. Denise Ackermann, 'Stigma: implications for the theological agenda' in *A Report of a Theological Workshop Focusing on HIV- and AIDS-Related Stigma* (Windhoek: UNAIDS, 2005): 46–50.

32. Sophie Chirongoma, 'Women's and children's rights in Zimbabwe: An analysis of gender inequalities and its impact on people's health with special emphasis on HIV/AIDS'. *Journal of Theology for Southern Africa* 126 (2006): 48–65.

33. Jo Sadgrove, 'Keeping up appearances: Sex and religion amongst university students in Uganda'. *Journal of Religion in Africa* 37(1) 2007: 116–44.

34. L. Gibney et al., 'Behavioural risk factors for HIV/AIDS in a low-prevalence Muslim nation: Bangladesh'. *International Journal of STD and AIDS* 10(3) 1999: 186–94; C.S. Todd et al., 'Emerging HIV epidemics in Muslim countries: assessment of different cultural responses to harm reduction and implications for HIV control'. *Current HIV/AIDS Reports* 4(4) 2007: 151–7; Tariq Madani et al., 'Epidemiology of the human immunodeficiency virus in Saudi Arabia: 18-year surveillance results and prevention from an Islamic perspective'. *BMC Infectious Diseases* 4(1) 2004: 25; S. Gilbert, 'The influence of Islam on AIDS prevention among Senegalese university students'. *AIDS Education and Prevention* 20(5) 2008: 399–407; K. Ghalib and L. Peralta, 'AIDS and Islam in America'. *Journal of the Association for Academic Minority Physicians* 13(2) 2002: 48–52; Madyan, 'Institutions in Indonesia': 4.

35. For example, A. Margolin et al., 'A controlled study of a spirituality-focused intervention for increasing motivation for HIV prevention among drug users'. *AIDS Education and Prevention* 18(4) 2006: 311–22; Cassandra Collins, David Whiters and Ronald Braithwaite, 'The SAVED SISTA Project: a faith-based HIV prevention programme for black women in addiction recovery'. *American Journal of Health Studies* 22(2) 2007: 76–82.

36. Dewi Hughes, 'Friend of "sinners"?' *Triple Helix* Easter 2009: 15.

37. Greg Manning, 'The reduction of law-related harm: a biblical affirmation of HIV prevention'. *Zadok Perspectives* 76 (2002): 17.

38. UNAIDS, 'Intensifying HIV prevention': 17.

39. Asian Muslim Action Network, *Muslim Responses to HIV and AIDS: Case Studies, Key Issues and Ways Forward* (Bangkok: AMAN 2004), 38–59; WCC, *Facing AIDS: Education in the Context of Vulnerability to HIV/AIDS* (Geneva: WCC Publications, 1999); Dube (ed.), *HIV and AIDS Curriculum for Theological Education by Extension in Africa and 10 HIV and AIDS Modules*; WCC, 'HIV prevention: current issues, new technologies'. *Contact* 182 (2006).

40. WCC, *Facing AIDS*.

41. Dube (ed.), *HIV and AIDS Curriculum for Theological Education by Extension in Africa and 10 HIV and AIDS Modules*.

42. WCC, 'HIV prevention'.

43. Steven Lux and Kristine Greenaway, *Scaling Up Effective Partnerships: A Guide to Working with Faith-Based Organizations in the Response to HIV and AIDS* (Geneva: EAA, 2006): 55.

44. Musimbi Kanyoro, 'Reading the Bible in the face of HIV and AIDS' in *Grant Me Justice!: HIV/AIDS and Gender Readings of the Bible*, edited by Musimbi Kanyoro and Musa Dube (Pietermaritzburg, Cluster Publications, 2004): viii.

45. Katherine Willson, 'Breaking the Silence: South African Muslim Responses to HIV/AIDS and a Theology of Compassion' (Honours dissertation, College of William and Mary, 2007): 2. See also http://www.positivemuslims.org.za (accessed 11 Feb. 2009).

46. Omid Safi, *Progressive Muslims: On Justice, Gender and Pluralism* (Oxford: Oneworld, 2003): 48.

47. Willson, *Breaking the Silence*: 64–9.

48. Mohammad Yousuf Bhat, 'Right to life in Islam: A historical analytical study'. *Hamdard Islamicus* 27(1) 2004: 63–70.

49. J.M. Vorster, 'HIV/AIDS and human rights'. *Ecumenical Review* 55(4) (2003): 353, 357.

50. UNAIDS, 'Intensifying HIV prevention': 17.

51. Islamic Relief, *A Draft Policy Stance on HIV/AIDS* (Birmingham: Islamic Relief Worldwide, 2008): 6.

52. Paterson, *HIV Prevention*: 3.

53. UNAIDS, *A Report of a Theological Workshop Focusing on HIV- and AIDS-Related Stigma* (Windhoek: UNAIDS, 2005): 16.

54. For further discussion on ambivalence towards condom use, see Chapter 2 of this book.

55. Gideon Byamugisha, *Breaking the Silence on HIV/AIDS in Africa* (Kampala: Friends of Gideon Foundation, 2000): 45.

56. Mary Garvey, *Dying to Learn: Young People, HIV and the Churches* (London: Christian Aid, 2003): 7, 13.

57. John Fuller and James Keenan, 'At the end of the first generation of HIV prevention' in *Catholic Ethicists on HIV/AIDS Prevention*, edited by Keenan et al.: 21–8.

58. David Crawford, 'Conjugal love, condoms and HIV/AIDS'. *International Catholic Review* 33(3) 2006: 505–12; Luke Gormally, 'Marriage and the prophylactic use of condoms'. *National Catholic Bioethics Quarterly* 5(4) 2005: 735–49.

59. PEPFAR, *The President's Emergency Plan for AIDS Relief: Community and Faith-Based Organizations* (2005): 1. Available at http://www.state.gov/documents/organization/54420.pdf (accessed 15 Dec. 2009).

60. PEPFAR, *ABC Guidance #1 For United States Government In-Country Staff and Implementing Partners Applying the ABC Approach To Preventing Sexually-Transmitted HIV Infections Within The President's Emergency Plan for AIDS Relief* (2005). Available at http://www.state.gov/documents/organization/57241.pdf (accessed 15 Dec. 2009).

61. E.C. Green et al., *Evidence That Demands Action: Comparing Risk Avoidance and Risk Reduction Strategies for HIV Prevention* (Austin: Medical Institute for Sexual Health, 2004); W.H. Mosley, 'The ABCs of HIV/AIDS prevention: seeking the evidence and telling the truth'. *CCIH Forum* 13(2003): 2–10.

62. Edward Green, 'Impact of religious organisations'. Revised version of paper presented at 'Challenges for the Church: AIDS, Malaria and TB' Conference organised by Christian Connections for International Health, Arlington, 25–26 May 2001: 9.

63. Green, 'Impact of religious organisations': 2–8; Green, *Evidence That Demands Action*: 11.

64. Green, 'Impact of religious organisations': 10.

65. Edward Green and Kim Witte, 'Can fear arousal in public health campaigns contribute to the decline of HIV prevalence?'. *Journal of Health Communication* 11 (2006): 255–7.

66. Byamugisha, *Breaking the Silence on HIV/AIDS in Africa*: 16, 41–4, 62.

67. Gideon Byamugisha, 'Risk increasing context or individual behaviour?' in *HIV Prevention*, edited by Paterson: 90–9.

68. Byamugisha, *Breaking the Silence on HIV/AIDS in Africa*: 19.

69. UNAIDS, 'Intensifying HIV prevention': 17.

70. UNAIDS, 'Intensifying HIV prevention': 19–20.

71. A.M. Smith et al., *HIV Prevention from the Perspective of a Faith-Based Development Agency* (London: CAFOD, 2004): 4, 5.

72. Paterson, *HIV Prevention*.

73. Byamugisha, 'Risk increasing context or individual behaviour?': 90–9; Margaret Farley, 'Prophetic discourse in a time of AIDS': 57–68. Johannes Petrus Heath, 'The need for comprehensive, multi-faceted interventions': 69–77; Peter Okaalet, 'Behaviour change and the role of the church: Towards reducing and eliminating risk': 78–89; Lisandro Orlov, 'Social change and the role of the church: The people's resources for understanding and reducing vulnerability': 121–32 – all in *HIV Prevention*, edited by Paterson.

74. Farley, 'Discourse in a time of AIDS': 57–9, 68.

75. Okaalet, 'Behaviour change and the role of the church': 83–7.

76. Orlov, 'Social change and the role of the church': 123, 130.

77. Lux and Greenaway, *Scaling Up Effective Partnerships*.

78. Sara Speicher and Janice Wilson, *Exploring Solutions: How to Talk about HIV Prevention in the Church* (Geneva: EAA, 2007).

79. Keenan et al. (eds), *Catholic Ethicists on HIV/AIDS Prevention.*

80. Robert Vitillo, *The Catholic Church Response to HIV in India* (New York: CMMB, 2008).

81. UNAIDS, 'Intensifying HIV prevention': 17.

82. IMAU, *AIDS Education Through Imams: A Spiritually Motivated Community Effort in Uganda* (Geneva: UNAIDS, 1998).

83. Lawrence Maund, *A Buddhist Approach to HIV Prevention and AIDS Care: A Training Manual for Monks, Nuns and Other Buddhist Leaders* (Bangkok: UNICEF East Asia and Pacific Regional Office, 2006).

84. Dube (ed.), *HIV and AIDS Curriculum for Theological Education by Extension in Africa and 10 HIV and AIDS Modules*; Wati Longchar, 'HIV and AIDS pandemic: A call for a paradigm shift in theological education in Asia' in *Health and Life: Theological Reflections on HIV and AIDS*, edited by Razouselie Lasetso (Jorhat: Eastern Theological College, 2007): 101–33.

85. Agrippa Khathide, 'Teaching and talking about our sexuality: A means of combating HIV/AIDS' in *HIV/AIDS and the Curriculum: Methods of Integrating HIV/AIDS in Theological Programmes*, edited by Musa Dube (Geneva: WCC Publications, 2003): 1–9.

86. Longchar, 'HIV and AIDS pandemic'; Donald Messer, *Breaking the Conspiracy of Silence: Christian Churches and the Global AIDS Crisis* (Minneapolis: Augsburg Fortress, 2004).

87. Mosley, 'The ABCs of HIV/AIDS prevention': 2–10.

88. Ngure, 'Module 2: Human sexuality and HIV and AIDS'.

89. Byamugisha, *Breaking the Silence on HIV/AIDS in Africa*: 56–63.

90. See, for example, Rob Pattman and Megan Cockerill, 'Christian women and men from Durban: Peer sex educators in the making'. *International Journal of Inclusive Education* 11(4) 2007: 501–17; Sadgrove, 'Keeping up appearances': 116–44.

91. Isobel Phiri, 'A theological analysis of the voices of teenage girls on men's role in the fight against HIV/AIDS in KwaZulu-Natal, South Africa'. *Journal of Theology for Southern Africa* 120 (2004): 34–5.

92. Peter Okaalet, 'Behaviour change and the role of the church': 84.

93. UNAIDS, 'Intensifying HIV prevention': 17.

94. WHO, 'Proceedings for a technical meeting for the development of a framework for universal access to HIV/AIDS prevention, care, treatment and support in the health sector' (Geneva: WHO, 18–20 Oct. 2005).

95. S. Woldehanna et al., *Faith In Action: Examining the Role of Faith-Based Organizations in Addressing HIV/AIDS: A Multi-Country Key Informant Survey* (Washington, DC: Global Health Council, 2005): 10.

96. Global HIV Prevention Working Group, *Bringing HIV Prevention to Scale: An Urgent Global Priority* (2007): 24. Available at http://www.globalhivprevention.org.

97. For further discussion see Chapter 1 of this book.

98. *The President's Emergency Plan for AIDS Relief: Community and Faith-Based Organisations* (Washington, DC: Office of the United States Global AIDS Co-ordinator, 2005): 1. Available at http://www.state.gov/documents/organizations/54420.pdf.

99. E.C. Green, 'The impact of religious organizations in promoting HIV/AIDS prevention'. *CCIH Forum* 11(2001): 1–9.

100. King, *Collaborating with Traditional Healers for HIV Prevention and Care in Sub-Saharan Africa*: 9.

101. UNICEF, *The Buddhist Leadership Initiative*.

102. Musa Dube, 'Grant me justice: Towards gender-sensitive multi-sectoral HIV/AIDS readings of the Bible' in *Grant Me Justice!*, edited by Dube and Kanyoro: 3–24.

103. Farley, 'Prophetic discourse in a time of AIDS': 58.

104. Farley, 'Prophetic discourse in a time of AIDS': 59–68.

105. Orlov, 'Social change and the role of the church': 121–32; Adrian Thatcher, 'The virus and the Bible: How living with HIV helps the church to read it' in *HIV Prevention*, edited by Paterson: 100–12; Heath, 'The need for comprehensive, multi-faceted interventions': 69–77.

106. UNAIDS, 'Intensifying HIV prevention': 17.

107. Fuller and Keenan, 'At the end of the first generation of HIV prevention'.

108. Esack, *Muslims Mapping AIDS*: 4.

109. Abdul Kayum Ahmed, 'Developing a theology of compassion: Muslim attitudes towards people living with HIV/AIDS in South Africa'. *Annual Review of Islam in South Africa* 3 (2000): 1–10.

110. See http://www.anerela.org (accessed 11 Feb. 2009). For a fuller discussion, see the response to this chapter.

111. Heath, 'The need for comprehensive, multi-faceted interventions': 69–77.

Practitioner response

Johannes Petrus Mokgethi-Heath

HIV prevention is really very simple, or so I have been told. One needs to start by declaring HIV a notifiable disease. From here it is then simple to control the further spread of HIV. By instituting mandatory testing we can bring the problem under control. We certainly have the technical know-how to identify an immune response to HIV as well as the virus itself and can then isolate people identified as being HIV positive. I am not 100 per cent sure where one would isolate over 30 million people; whether we should be placed in concentration camps outside every town and city; whether this should be done by individual nations, perhaps continentally; or whether one should identify a certain land mass (maybe even the moon) as a location to move and then isolate people.

Considering this line of thinking, do not for one second think that it has not been and is not being acted upon in one form or another. The Cuban response to HIV was precisely this: mandatory testing, concentration camps and an entirely controlled epidemic, or so it is said. Various countries around the world have at various times instituted immigration or travel regulations to keep people living with HIV out and control the epidemic. Among these are the USA (until very recently), China, Russia and Australia. Even South Africa has legislation demanding that people seeking employment in the mining sector must undergo HIV testing before applying successfully for a post in South Africa.

Countries are not alone in operating on the hypothesis of limiting contact and keeping the contaminated out. I remember all too well my first encounter with HIV. It was in an ethics class while I was still in the Anglican diocese of Johannesburg. A young woman had approached a priest in the diocese for marriage to her fiancé. Already in 1990 he had taken the bold step of declaring his HIV+ status to the priest before the marriage. The position of the church was that the marriage could not take place as consummating the marriage would be tantamount to murder or suicide. A licence was eventually granted for the marriage on condition that it was not consummated. The same happens in far less explicit ways every day. Subtle messages of exclusion of the promiscuous, men who have sex with men, sex workers, injecting drug users are given in faith communities. Exclusion of those most at risk means reducing the risk of contamination.

What Manning has successfully illustrated in his chapter is that just a medical solution to HIV will never be possible or tolerated. From the secular perspective this has been couched in the language of human rights. In religious communities this is referred to as justice. What this should, and does, do is immediately force us to focus on how we can more compassionately and humanely approach HIV prevention. What should become immediately evident is that in

HIV prevention, people living with HIV are not the enemy but, rather, should be seen as valuable allies in halting its spread. Groups like the Global Network of People Living with HIV (GNP+) speak of positive prevention as both the duty and contribution of those living with HIV. In this model the person living with HIV makes the conscious decision that it stops immediately. It does not matter how the person came to live with HIV, the chain of transmission must stop now. For this to be effected within religious communities there needs to be an enabling environment in which people living with HIV not only feel welcome but are supported into positive living.

However, asking religious communities to intensify teaching on HIV prevention usually solicits intensification of moral teaching. In most cases all this really serves to do is lull people into a false sense of security – invulnerability. As I have suggested elsewhere, ANERELA argued that one of the main problems with HIV prevention is that it tends to focus on sex, sex and sex again. As Manning suggests, sexuality is not something that religious groups find easy to talk about. As a result, when they adopt the ABC approach to prevention they use it in such a way that there is a descending order of acceptability. What this approach seems to say when used by religious groups is: '**A**bstain, since no sex is the best sex; or if you can't abstain, then at least **B**e faithful; if you refuse to be faithful then at least have the decency to use a **C**ondom.'[1] In practice there is a variety of problems with the ABC approach. First, it intensifies that stigma round HIV and AIDS by focusing only on sex; and second, it leads people into a false sense of security since the message becomes: 'As long as you are in a faithful relationship you have no need to worry – you are safe from HIV.' Sadly this is not the case as statistics show that HIV infection is growing amongst married women.[2] Byamugisha has stressed that there is a major difference between risky behaviour and a risky environment. What this essentially means is that if you find yourself in an environment with a high HIV prevalence, behaviour that in other circumstances would have been considered safe suddenly take on new risk. Therefore, if you focus only on one element in the transmission chain without giving full information about all factors, people are given misinformation and are not able to judge the risk for themselves.[3] Furthermore, as already suggested, if the aim is to prevent HIV transmission then it is pointless to speak about being faithful in a sexual relationship until after people have learned the importance of knowing each other's HIV status.[4] Only then is it possible for them to make informed decisions as to how best to protect themselves and those they love.

It is for these reasons that ANERELA developed the SAVE approach to HIV prevention. This stands for four key principles:[5]

S = Safer practice
When speaking about safer practices all avenues of HIV transmission are addressed. Factors that reduce the risk of HIV transmission would include prevention of mother-to-child transmission (PMTCT); post-exposure prophylaxis (PEP); abstinence, but also the delay of sexual début; mutual fidelity within a committed relationship; the use of vaginal microbicides; needle exchange; oral substitution therapy; male circumcision;

use of condoms; clean and safe blood for transfusion; and sterile implements, not just for hospital or clinic-based surgery but also for cultural scarification.

A = Available medical interventions

One of the most effective prevention methods is the use of anti-retroviral (ARV) therapies. This is because where the viral load of the person living with HIV is reduced to undetectable, the chances of transmission drop to less than 1:25 000. But this is not the only medical intervention. There is a need for effective treatment of opportunistic infections and also all other STIs. In addition to this, good nutrition may be regarded as a medical intervention. Medical interventions also include the crucial, and seldom provided, access to all necessary blood tests. Without adequate monitoring of the efficacy of ARVs through viral load tests, a person could have developed an undetected drug resistance, compromising not only their own health but also the health of their sexual partner. The availability of viral load tests for babies is also important. The majority of babies dying from HIV die before they are two years old because the diagnostic tool most commonly used is the CD4 test, which cannot determine whether a baby is HIV positive until the infant is 18 months old. With a viral load test this can be done at birth.

V = Voluntary counselling and testing (VCT)

It is crucial that all people know their HIV status. We need to move from AIDS friendly congregations to congregations that know their HIV status. Whether this happens through VCT or provider-initiated testing is less important than getting people to know their status.

E = Empowerment

One of the single biggest challenges faced in increasing the impact of HIV prevention messages is the limited capacity of many people to respond. For example, it is no good telling a woman to use protection in her sexual relationship if she is not also helped to overcome clearly defined gender inequalities in her domestic, religious or cultural environment that prevent her from doing so. Further, most information about HIV prevention comes in written form when in many areas there are still high levels of illiteracy and, even when people can read, many of the publications use stigmatising, misleading or often incorrect language.

By definition, applying a holistic prevention approach such as SAVE involves challenging many of the deep-rooted prejudices and exclusivist approaches lived, if not defined, by many religious communities. Holistic prevention must respond to the needs of people involved in the transmission chain in any given community or country. It must meet them where they are, rather than where we would be comfortable to have them. This will mean finding ways of acknowledging prejudices, examining how they interfere with effective prevention, and investigating ways of effectively countering this.

Successful HIV prevention must respond from a justice perspective, actively enable people living with HIV to find safe spaces within religious communities, engage people living with HIV in the work of prevention and further address specific needs related to the modes of transmission prevalent in the community, society or country concerned. This broad statement implicitly includes care and support, addressing stigma, discrimination and specific vulnerabilities, and engaging religious communities to respond positively to these challenges.

Notes

1. Heath, 'The need for comprehensive, multi-faceted interventions': 70.
2. Recent statistics show HIV infection is increasing in stable, low-risk groups. See UNAIDS, 'Epidemic update, 2009'. Available at http://data.unaids.org/pub/Report/2009/2009_epidemic_update_en.pdf: 29–30 (accessed 8 Dec. 2009).
3. Byamugisha, 'Risk increasing context or individual behaviour?': 90–9.
4. Heath, 'The need for comprehensive, multi-faceted interventions': 70.
5. This explanation of the principles of the SAVE approach were first published in Heath, 'The need for comprehensive, multi-faceted interventions': 71–2.

14

HIV, AIDS and stigma
Discerning the silences

Gillian Paterson

INTRODUCTION

Ten years have passed since the sabotaging effect of stigma on global, national and local responses to the HIV epidemic became widely recognised. Stigma is an obstacle to care, treatment, prevention and practical assistance for orphans and other children affected by the epidemic. Because of stigma, or because of fear of stigma, people who are infected or affected are likely to deny the impact of HIV on their lives and to ignore the necessity to seek help or change behaviour. Individual denial is mirrored by a more general tendency to hide from the notion that one's own society, community or institution is affected, a silence that can be fatal to prevention efforts. Self-stigma and shame associated with HIV causes more suffering than the sickness, often making people fear knowing that they are HIV-infected more than they fear death. Carers often observe in the death of patients that it is the shame, rather than illness, that kills.

This suggests that at the outset, three crucial points need to be made about stigma. The first is that, to some extent, all the other issues discussed in this book could be viewed through the lens of stigma because this factor affects every aspect of the experience of and response to the epidemic. The second is that stigma is often connected with religion and to deeply held convictions about the nature of God, how we should live, and what the nature of religious institutions should be. This introduces a third, related insight: that making rules about discrimination and the use of language is not, on its own, enough.[1] Stigma also needs to be addressed theologically and ethically, and at the local level of religious communities. In 2001 the World Council of Churches (WCC) convened a meeting of African church leaders in Nairobi that came to the following conclusion:

> Our tendency to exclude others, our interpretation of the scriptures, and
> our theology of sin have all combined to promote the stigmatisation,
> exclusion and suffering of people with HIV or AIDS. This has undermined
> the effectiveness of care, education and prevention efforts and inflicted
> additional suffering on those already affected by HIV . . . For the churches,
> the most powerful contribution we can make to combating HIV trans-
> mission is the eradication of stigma and discrimination.[2]

In mapping the bibliographic material, therefore, the theology researcher is
confronted with complex and multi-faceted challenges. Stigma is not primarily a
theological concept, although it has theological and ethical implications; and
theological thinking may be a subconscious driver of discriminatory structures,
attitudes or actions.[3] Further, people tend to be blind to the stigmatising beliefs
and attitudes they themselves hold, or which are common to their social, cultural
or institutional context. It is easy to perceive other people's beliefs and attitudes as
stigmatising. One's own, by contrast, tend to look natural or self-evidently true
(for example, one's beliefs about gender roles or sexual orientation). This
undermines the validity of some of the stigma measuring tools available, which
tend to involve some kind of self-assessment process.[4] Also, despite the recent
emphasis on AIDS-related stigma, there has been relatively little research into the
interface between stigma and ecclesiology. This is partly because it involves asking
painful and challenging questions; partly because it is threatening to individuals
and institutions to have to question the beliefs and attitudes around which
personal or institutional identities are constructed; and partly because stigma is a
complex issue that impacts on so many aspects of life and faith that do not, at
first sight, appear to be connected with HIV or AIDS.[5]

This map of the available bibliographic material on stigma, therefore, starts
by mapping the journey itself and proposing a process.[6] There should not be a
rush to explore these theological and ethical dimensions without first reflecting
on the experience of individuals who have personally experienced HIV- or AIDS-
related stigma directed at them or a loved one. Second, it is important to challenge
the assumption that there can be universal answers, or that what works in one
context can be applied in another. Third, there needs to be a conceptualisation of
stigma dense enough to take into account conceptualisations that come from the
secular, empirical disciplines. Last, the recurring themes in the literature need to
be noted. Each of them will be dealt with in turn in the chapter, which concludes

with a section that looks at some of the more obvious gaps that exist in the literature and the research that still needs to be carried out.

EXPERIENCE OF INDIVIDUALS

The reality of stigma is most powerfully appreciated through the personal, embodied stories of individuals or groups who have been (or are) its victims.[7] These stories are often painfully physical ones.[8] Gideon Byamugisha, Noerine Kaleeba, Edwin Cameron and the writers represented in Kiran Desai's work all have moving stories to tell of HIV- and AIDS-related stigma and how it is overcome.[9] In addition, stories of HIV-related stigma appear regularly in the material produced by advocacy or development organisations and on websites such as the Af-AIDS family and AIDS_Asia.[10] Such stories are indispensable in demonstrating the damaging effect of stigma and play an important role in motivating people to act. However, as a basis for theological and ethical reflection, they should be treated with caution. This discourse often does not move beyond simplistic interpretations; and one should be wary of accounts of stigma that seem to be full of heroes (the stigmatised) and villains (the stigmatisers).

It is time consuming to research the more nuanced stories that seek to engage with what is going on between, and within the hearts and minds of, the individuals involved; or to identify with what actually motivates or terrifies a particular individual or group. Because of the private, often unacknowledged, nature of stigmatising attitudes there is a need for profound and searching conversations with the individuals concerned. This has been my experience in developing case studies nuanced and detailed enough to do justice to those involved. Harriet Deacon makes the same point in her study of AIDS-related stigma in the Anglican Church of the Province of Southern Africa.[11]

UNIVERSAL VERSUS AND THE CONTEXTUAL

Although the experience of HIV is predominantly a personal or communal one, the most influential voices in the dialogue are global, underpinned by global statistics, setting global priorities and influencing global financial initiatives. At the same time, early local constructions of HIV and AIDS (the gay plague that emerged in the USA in the 1980s) have had a profound influence on the history of the epidemic. The four Hs by which the epidemic was initially defined are telling: homosexuals, heroin addicts, Haitians and (w)hores. Thus from the beginning, stigma and fear of stigma, racism and fear of racism have defined and motivated public health responses, religious attitudes and the campaigning groups that burst into life in the context of the epidemic.

This history has led to a growing belief, especially in the South, that the dominant priorities set by global players are in fact Western ones inappropriate to non-Western contexts. African writers, in particular, have commented on the stigmatising, often downright racist, constructions applied to the epidemic on this continent; and the damaging effects of assuming that Western models of response are appropriate for African contexts. Journals such as *New African* have argued this case for over a decade.[12] Today in Africa the calls for contextually relevant constructions of the epidemic that do not stigmatise African voices, meanings and solutions are emerging from theologians as well as from public health and social policy strategists.[13] It is, therefore, ironic that protesting voices have recently and increasingly been heard from Asia and Latin America, complaining in their turn that African constructions of the epidemic are now regarded as the norm with African solutions assumed to be transferable, unaltered, to other contexts.

Against this complex background, claims to certainty, to one-size-fits-all solutions or to having the right answer must be greeted with scepticism. We need to adopt a hermeneutic of suspicion when encountering the stigmatisation (on whatever grounds) of alternative views and those who hold them, or the dismissal of contextual realities that may seem to conflict with the current global orthodoxy.

CONCEPTUALISING STIGMA

In recent years, partly in response to the HIV epidemic, a large bibliography on stigma has emerged from empirical disciplines such as medicine, sociology, anthropology, psychology and the theory of institutions. A religious and theological approach to stigma must take these theoretical conceptualisations seriously.[14] For example, Erving Goffman's seminal text on stigma was first published in 1963.[15] More recently, political, psychological and sociological thinking has come together in Bruce Link and Jo Phelan's important work and that of Harriet Deacon.[16]

Anthropologist Mary Douglas and others illuminate the cultural processes that lead to discrimination and exclusion and also the role of religion in reinforcing them. Douglas's approach is helpful in understanding, for example, issues of gender, sexuality, sin pollution and body taboo, all of which are central to any study of AIDS-related stigma.[17] In addition, it provides a denser understanding of the cultural and political contexts for stigmatising and exclusionary patterns of behaviour and also the relationship between context, meaning and belief.[18] Douglas and others offer important insights into the role of religion in reinforcing cultural norms and taboos, endowing them with universal validity and rooting them in relationships with the invisible, supernatural world of gods and ancestors, which may also be the gateway to the longed-for hereafter. Douglas's work is of particular interest to Christian theologians and ethicists because she remains convinced that the Christian message presents a real challenge to the deadly cocktail of body-sin-pollution that still provides a subconscious underpinning for much moral thinking.[19] Margaret Farley turns to Paul Ricoeur's work on sin, guilt and defilement to support her analysis of the role of taboo in the development of moral thinking.[20]

Recent work on scapegoating has provided further important insights into the ways in which stigma operates within societies and the reasons why it is so difficult to dislodge. René Girard suggests that without an understanding of the dynamic of scapegoating, Christian theology is not capable of working out what is going on when it talks about othering, stigmatisation and exclusion. Girard believes that the life, death and resurrection of Christ constitute the ultimate no to scapegoating.[21] There are a number of other important theological reflections on these themes. They include William Countryman's exploration of the biblical implications of Mary Douglas's work and James G. Williams's assessment of the biblical implications of Girard's work on scapegoating.[22]

RECURRING THEMES IN THE LITERATURE ON STIGMA

As argued earlier in the chapter, contexts and cultures are different: caution is needed in making judgements about one context that are based on the lessons of another. Nevertheless, there are a number of issues that recur in the literature on HIV and stigma. Among them are truth, sexuality and sin, the human body, and economic and social marginalisation.

Truth and discourse

The success of prevention and care programmes depends on people facing reality in terms of the help they need and the risks they choose to take. Prevention strategies are unlikely to succeed where there is denial, where reality is stigmatised, or where the messages given out by the dominant voices seem to bear no relation to individual realities.[23] Public education and practical interventions must not be based on politically or religiously motivated constructions that seek to generate fear, conceal truths or demonise particular social, ethnic or sexual groups.[24] Religion is particularly prone to such concealment. For example, prevention messages or youth education strategies may be based on an assumption that everybody's lives reflect the traditional religious ideal of monogamous marriage; whereas in fact this may be a context in which polygamy or concurrent sexual relationships are the norm, even among clergy.[25] This discussion is revived in the section on sex and sexuality.

Here, reference is made to interesting work on truth and discourse. It is informative to analyse the different discourses operating in any given situation and the discourse theory of Paul Ricoeur is useful.[26] He argues that discourse shapes reality and gives direction and language to the narrative within which we are living, including the characters in it. Paul Bové goes further. Discourse, says Bové, actually produces knowledge and thus makes possible the 'disciplines and institutions which, in turn, sustain and distribute these discourses'.[27]

In Britain, the main discourses currently influencing the public response to the epidemic might be described as biomedical, conservative-moral and liberal human rights, each assuming a world view that may well not be shared by others. The result is a political and value divide that people react to without conceptualising it and which may subconsciously undermine theological and ethical conversations where, for example, discourses of agency come into conflict with discourses of vulnerability.[28] There is also a growing body of work on HIV and discourse in southern Africa, exemplified in the work of Barbara Schmid and Gill Seidel.[29]

Considerations of discourse are particularly important because of what Ricoeur calls the 'self-universalising tendency of discourse'.[30] This tendency can lead people to assume that their own frame of reference is the only one rationally possible to hold: the only reason everybody does not hold it is because they do not understand. Because one's own discourse has the moral high ground, it becomes inevitable that one will make ethical and possibly stigmatising judgements about people who see things differently. Where the majority discourse is, for instance, a conservative religious one, this has an othering and stigmatising effect on people who are operating within a different discourse or frame of reference. This concept of othering is becoming increasingly important in psychological and sociological studies, especially those related to ethnicity, gender and sexuality.[31] More research is needed on the concept of othering in the context of communities brought together by religious belief or commitment.

355

In relation to HIV, a particularly stigmatising discourse (which also undermines evidence-based prevention messages) is the one generated by miraculous healers and their followers implying that healing is possible and that if it does not work for you, then it is your own fault for lacking faith.[32] Having some understanding of discourse analysis would help to build bridges over the many political and ideological divides that affect the world of HIV and AIDS.

Theologians reflecting on the epidemic are called to risk engaging with truth in this multi-faceted way in the awareness that this is profoundly unsettling to lovers of certainty and can easily be dismissed as post-modern relativism. Rowan Williams makes the case that one cannot combine theological certainty with theological integrity, insisting that all theological statements must allow the possibility of response.[33]

Sex and sexuality

In November 2001 African church leaders meeting in Nairobi stated: 'Our difficulty in addressing issues of sex and sexuality has often made it painful for us to engage, in any honest and realistic way, with issues of sex education and HIV prevention.'[34]

While gender justice is a necessary, indeed a non-negotiable, component of a sexual ethic, the two issues (sex and gender) are actually different in kind.[35] All cultures have taboos around sex and sexuality, which (because sex is the commonest way in which HIV is transmitted) contribute to the silence and denial mentioned in the section on truth.[36] Religion tends to reinforce those taboos rather than resist them. Thus, the conflict between the private and the public, especially over sexual issues, has become a stumbling block to the ability of religious organisations to engage with HIV-related stigma. As Michel Foucault points out, what actually happens between real people is the secret that is not spoken about, especially by Christians.[37] This is not a new discovery. Augustine of Hippo wrote of 'the lust which lords it over the unchaste, has to be mastered by the chaste, and yet is to be blushed at by the chaste and the unchaste'.[38] Nonetheless, there are biblical texts that provide examples of deeply private sexual experience. As Dietrich Bonhoeffer puts it: 'It is a good thing that [the Song of Songs] is included in the Bible, as a protest against those who believe that Christianity stands for the restraint of passion.'[39]

Accordingly, the epidemic has given birth to theological and ethical literature. Catholic moral theologian Kevin Kelly is among those who have observed that

the epidemic is challenging the world community 'to change our ways by...
formulating a satisfactory person-respecting sexual ethic'.[40] For him, the experience
of HIV and AIDS has acted as a lens through which justice and development
issues have become issues of survival with resulting ethical implications. African
women theologians have broken with cultural taboos to talk about sex and
sexuality from a woman's perspective.[41] Increasingly, work is being done on the
stigmatisation of sex and its lethal effect. The belief that sex is sinful leads readily
to the judgement that HIV is punishment for sin. Farley's work is a long-awaited
recent addition to the bibliography on sex in a time of HIV and AIDS.[42] Sex, it
seems, is coming out of the closet.

One interesting Christian study on stigma was a two-year process that took
place between the councils of churches in the five Nordic countries and the
eleven councils of churches in southern Africa (Nordic-FOCCISA).[43] Participants
from different contexts were struggling with issues of sex and sin. In the course
of this process, many differences of opinion emerged between participants from
the North and South. One area of agreement, however, was the incompatibility
of God and sex.

> It is often thought, particularly – but not only – by religious people, that
> sex belongs to the 'dark' side of human existence. At one end of the
> spectrum of human existence stands God, who is light. At the other,
> hemmed in by guilt, shame and taboo, is sex. In Western society, there has
> been a reaction away from this view. Sex seems to have become so freely
> available and so openly discussed that it has become quite difficult to
> admit that one doesn't want it or finds it difficult. The vulnerable, fragile,
> uncertain quality of sexuality seems to have been banished. While this
> reaction against moralistic views is healthy, its unintended by-product is a
> culture of sexuality in which sex has completely lost its connection with
> faith, ethics, or even – at times – with human relationship. So sex and
> God are still at the opposite ends of the spectrum, and it is difficult to find
> the rainbow that will bridge it.[44]

In our day, some of the most virulent responses to the epidemic have been
triggered not by heterosexually transmitted HIV but by links with homosexuality
and men having sex with men. In 1987, US Senator Jesse Helms stated: 'The only
way to stop AIDS is to stop the disgusting and immoral activities that continue to

spread the disease'. Tele-evangelist Jerry Falwell claimed in the spring of 1987 that 'AIDS is a lethal judgement of God on the sin of homosexuality, and it is also a judgement of God on America for endorsing this vulgar, perverted life-style'.[45] These examples both come from the USA but the stigmatisation of sexual activity between men is to be found everywhere, leading many religious and political leaders to reinforce existing taboos by denying the existence of homo-sexuality in their societies and institutions.

In this regard, there are useful insights from legal texts. Martha Nussbaum asks the question: 'should laws be based on social conventions about what is (or what lawmakers experience as) disgusting?' She argues: 'We should beware of these emotions – associated in troubling ways with a desire to hide our humanity. The thought content of disgust embodies magical ideas of contamination, and impossible aspirations to purity that are just not in line with human life as we know it.'[46]

The important thing about Nussbaum's analysis is her suggestion that the pathological reserve about sexual issues represents a desire to hide our humanity. But the law, and the ethical principles it enshrines, are about human life as we know it. There is nothing wrong with modesty, reserve and the wish for privacy in one's personal life, provided these are not mechanisms for concealing real injustices, abuses, scenarios of oppression and sources of disease transmission. Nussbaum, as with Farley, moves towards the normalisation of sex. Both suggest lowering the somewhat over-inflated terms in which discourses around sex and sexuality are sometimes couched; and learning to locate the context in which sexual encounters occur with the complex web of cultural expectations, familial pressures and social and economic relationships that, over much of the world, are part of the stable context of family or community life.

The human body

Connected to the discussion on sex and stigma is the ambivalence of religious tradition towards the human body, especially the bodies of women. As Susan Sontag points out, the Judaeo-Christian voice has been powerful and not neutral in the struggle for the 'the rhetorical ownership of illness . . . the age-old, seemingly inexorable process whereby diseases acquire meanings (by coming to stand for our deepest fears) and inflict stigma'.[47] The very origin of the word stigma suggests a brand that is burned into the flesh, thus stigmatising the body indelibly and forever. As the Jewish theologian Etty Hillesum put it: 'It is difficult to be on equally good terms with God and your body.'[48]

Metaphorical constructions, of course, relate to societal taboos as much as to religious ones. But for those who ascribe to monotheistic religion, given the sexual connotations of HIV they translate readily into the language of the struggle against sin. This struggle turns the body into a war zone with disease as the metaphorical punishment for losing the battle. Further, the association with sin was axiomatic to the meaning of pollution. An example from the biblical text, '"Who sinned, this man or his parents, that he was born blind?" asked the disciples'.[49] The response of Jesus clearly indicates that he was at least as concerned with the re-integration of the sick person into the community (the removal of stigma) as he was with the removal of the bodily signs and symptoms of disorder.[50] This suggests that associations between sin and disease, blame and pollution were at least as strong then as they are today. However, while it is important to retrieve what is helpful and positive in religious tradition, it should be combined with an effort to take a contextual view of its negative aspects.[51]

Christian feminist theologies, with their strong emphasis on the importance of embodiment, have done much to raise awareness of the body stigmatisation that is present in Christian tradition.[52] Kim Power and Caroline Bynum provide insights into the ways in which women, and also men, have resisted the body negativity of their cultures.[53]

Economic and social marginalisation

Epidemiological historians such as Charles Rosenberg have mapped the progress of infectious disease epidemics.[54] Because HIV is an infectious virus, societies find it necessary to put the blame for it on others. The virus has to be seen as coming not from within our society but from outside. For this reason, as in the case of syphilis, one repeatedly hears about the entry from outside of HIV into a culture and the need to document the foreign source of these origins. Sontag and Peter Allen both describe this scenario.[55]

Those who are viewed as being economically or socially marginalised in any society are also, often, those most at risk of acquiring HIV infection. These include injecting drug users who share needles; those who make a living out of sex work; men who have sex with men in homophobic societies; heads of families forced to migrate for employment and those at home who await them; and women and girls engaging in sex with older or richer men in order to support their children, their families or their school fees. The association of HIV with these marginalised groups reinforces the link between disease and sin. By this association, if you have leprosy, syphilis or AIDS, then you must have deserved it. Moreover, since the condition is in many cases presumed to be their own fault, it does not merit the sympathetic, supportive, humanitarian response that other catastrophes such as natural disasters attract. Donald Messer cites several surveys of church leaders' attitudes that reveal a majority belief that the epidemic is a punishment from God.[56]

Where marginalised groups are concerned, effective theological responses have depended on activist movements. For example, in the early years, HIV and AIDS took on almost iconic meanings for some gay men.[57] Feminist theologians and biblical scholars have shown how the marginalisation and vulnerability of women has resulted in their stigmatisation.[58] Stigmatisation of women and girls implies a belief that they are in some way lesser human beings with fewer rights than men and boys, especially in terms of property ownership, income control and the right to co-determine the terms of sexual encounters. Biblical scholars have used women in the Bible, such as Tamar, the woman who was bleeding or the woman who anointed Jesus with oil to highlight their stigma and vulnerability.[59]

Groups that are often absent from studies include children affected by the epidemic, people who make their living through commercial sex and injecting drug users.[60]

GAPS IN RESEARCH ON HIV AND AIDS AND STIGMA

Addressing the gaps in the research is an enormous task, so in this final section discussion is confined to a few issues that seem to be of particular significance.

There is a need for an educated, inter-disciplinary conceptualisation of stigma that can provide a secure base for theological reflection. A more adequate working definition is also needed. The global stand-off between so-called liberal and so-called conservative approaches is reflected in the politics of funding and in the negative cross currents that exist within the religious community and elsewhere. There is a need for small studies that enable reflection in rational and non-polemical ways about the cause and effect of differences that have their origin in clashes of discourse.

Personal accounts of HIV are often over-simplistic and morally naïve. There is a need for case studies that offer a denser and more nuanced understanding of what is going on in situations of stigmatisation in which all those concerned have the chance to articulate their thoughts and fears, and have them taken seriously. In religious organisations, in particular, there is a disconnection between what happens in theory and what people actually do or believe in their private lives. This is, in effect, a stigmatisation of reality. A stigma tool, which engages with this disconnection as well as with individual attitudes, is sorely needed.

In the work that has been done on public discourses, little has been written about the divisions that exist between specifically theological discourses or the selective use of demographics to support particular discourses such as those of agency and of vulnerability. Religious discourses of compassion may be well-meaning but they are often deeply stigmatising. More work is needed on the issue of compassion, including what it means to be a compassionate community.[61]

Considerable rhetoric is expended on the need to engage with vulnerable and marginalised groups. However, there is little actual engagement with these groups in studies on stigma. Greater understanding is needed of the reasons, structural as well as religious, why religious groups find this so difficult.

While this agenda may seem burdensome, it is necessary to remember that we have come a long way over the past decade in our understanding of stigma and willingness to learn from that understanding. This progress should spur us on to accomplish the task that still lies ahead.

NOTES

1. While HIV stigma is often discussed in conjunction with discrimination, for the purpose of this chapter comments are confined to the issue of stigma. As sociologists, lawyers and psychologists have pointed out, stigma and discrimination are not the same thing. Discrimination is to do with what happens between people and can be legislated against; stigma is to do with what happens inside people's hearts and minds, which cannot be changed through legislation, although situations can be encouraged in which change becomes more likely. See Bruce Link and Jo Phelan, 'Conceptualizing stigma'. *Annual Review of Sociology* 27 (2001): 363–85; Harriet Deacon et al., *Understanding HIV/AIDS Stigma: A Theoretical and Methodological Analysis* (Cape Town: HSRC Publications, 2005).

2. World Council of Churches, *The Ecumenical Response to HIV/AIDS in Africa: Plan of Action* (Geneva: WCC, 2001): 3.

3. Gill Sayce, writing on stigma and disability, says: 'Influence the beliefs of people who have the power to discriminate, and support those prepared to promote positive change... Stimulate open debate about different experiences of discrimination. Make inclusion happen, because inclusion challenges attitudes and behaviours. Most importantly, address power.' (Gill Sayce, 'Beyond good intentions: Making anti-discrimination strategies work'. *Disability and Society* 18 (2003): 625–42.

361

4. International Centre for Research on Women has developed well-respected stigma measurement toolkits, available at www.icrw.org/docs/2006_stigmasynthesis.pdf (accessed 30 Apr. 2009); International AIDS Society, 'Stigma Measurement: HIV/AIDS Stigma and Discrimination (S&D) Framework' is a concrete data collection offering tools and resources that can be adapted for use in relation to HIV- or AIDS-related stigma; Futures Group International Policy Project, 'HIV/AIDS Stigma Indicators: A Tool Measuring the Progress of HIV Stigma'. Available at www.popline.org/docs/1528/278926.html (accessed 30 Apr. 2009); Policy Project South Africa, Centre for the Study of AIDS, '*A Tool for Measuring the Progress of HIV/AIDS Stigma Mitigation*'. Available at www.csa.za.org/filemanager/download/ 67/Stigma%20Indicators.pdf (accessed 30 Apr. 2009).

5. Nordic-FOCCISA, *One Body: North-South Reflections in the Face of HIV and AIDS*, (Oslo: Christian Council of Norway, 2006); Harriet Deacon and L. Simbayi, *The Nature and Extent of HIV and AIDS Related Stigma in the Anglican Church of the Province of Southern Africa: A Quantitative Study* (Cape Town: HSRC, 2006); D. Gennrich et al., *Gender, Poverty and HIV/ AIDS* (Pietermaritzburg: PACSA, 2005).

6. Grateful thanks to Harriet Deacon, Donald Messer and Nyambura Njoroge for their contributions to the bibliography for this chapter and also to Gary Leonard for all his bibliographic assistance.

7. See Chapter 16 in this book for the personal stories of four people living with HIV.

8. Understanding of HIV-related stigma is further enlarged by powerful personal accounts of individuals living with stigmatised conditions other than HIV or AIDS. For example: Mercy A. Oduyoye, 'A coming home to myself: the childless woman in the West African space' in *Liberating Eschatology: Essays in Honour of Letty M. Russell*, edited by Margaret Farley and Sheila Jones (Louisville: Westminster John Knox Press, 1999): 103–20; Nancy L. Eisland *The Disabled God: Towards a Liberatory Theology of Disability* (Nashville: Abingdon Press, 1995); Robert Murphy, *The Body Silent* (New York: Henry Holt, 1987); James Alison, *Faith Beyond Resentment: Fragments Catholic and Gay* (London: Darton Longman and Todd, 2001); Maya Angelou, *I Know Why the Caged Bird Sings* (New York: Random House, 1969).

9. Gideon Byamugisha, *What Can I Do?: The HIV Ministry of Gideon Byamugisha* (London: Strategies of Hope, 2008); Noerine Kaleeba with Sunanda Ray, *We Miss You All: AIDS in the Family* (Pretoria: SafAIDS, 2nd ed., 2002); Edwin Cameron, *Witness to AIDS* (Cape Town, Tafelberg, 2005); Kiran Desai et al, *AIDS Sutra: Untold Stories from India* (London: Random House, 2008).

10. Af-AIDS@eforums.healthdev.org; AIDS_Asia@yahoo.com.

11. For example, the one that appears in Gillian Paterson, 'Who sinned?: AIDS-related stigma and the church' in *Applied Ethics in a World Church*, edited by Linda Hogan (Maryknoll: Orbis, 2008): 163–9; Deacon and Simbayi, *The Nature and Extent of HIV and AIDS related stigma in the Anglican Church of the Province of Southern Africa*.

12. See Raymond Downing's readable and passionate account, *As They See It: The Development of the African AIDS Discourse* (London: Adonis and Abbey, 2005).

13. See Emmanuel Katongole, 'Postmodern illusions and the challenge of African theology: The ecclesial tactics of resistance'. *Modern Theology* 16(2) 2000: 237–54; Paul Chummar, 'HIV/ AIDS in Africa: An urgent task for an inculturated theological ethics' in *Applied Ethics in a*

World Church, edited by Hogan: 155–62; Adbonkhianmeghe Orobator, 'Ethics of HIV/AIDS prevention: Paradigms of new response from an African Perspective' in *Applied Ethics in a World Church*, edited by Hogan: 147–54.

14. In my attempt to do so, I have suggested ten principles in conceptualising stigma: Gillian Paterson, *AIDS Related Stigma: Thinking Outside the Box: The Theological Challenge* (Geneva: EAA, 2005): 3–5.

15. Erving Goffman, *Stigma: Notes on the Management of Spoiled Identity* (New Jersey: Prentice Hall, 1963).

16. Link and Phelan, 'Conceptualizing stigma'; Deacon et al, *Understanding HIV/AIDS Stigma.*

17. Mary Douglas, *Purity and Danger: An Analysis of the Concepts of Pollution and Taboo*, (London: Routledge, 1966).

18. Mary Douglas, *Natural Symbols: Explorations in Cosmology* (New York: Vintage Books, 1973).

19. Douglas, *Purity and Danger.*

20. Margaret Farley, *Just Love: A Framework for Christian Sexual Ethics* (New York: Continuum, 2006): 177–8; Paul Ricoeur, *The Symbolism of Evil* (Boston: Beacon Press, 1969).

21. This powerful theory is discussed at length in René Girard, *The Scapegoat* (Baltimore: Johns Hopkins University Press, 1986).

22. William Countryman, *Dirt, Greed and Sex: Sexual Ethics in the New Testament and Their Implications for Today* (Minneapolis: Fortress Press, 1988); James G. Williams, *The Bible, Violence and the Sacred: Liberation from the Myth of Sanctioned Violence* (San Francisco: Harper Collins, 1991).

23. A recent process supported by the EAA saw theologians from different continents and faith traditions coming together to find common ground to address issues of HIV prevention. See Gillian Paterson (ed.), *HIV Prevention: A Global Theological Conversation* (Geneva: EAA, 2009).

24. In a controversial recent book, Elizabeth Pisani addresses the realities of HIV in the context of South East Asian cities and argues that a greater level of realism, openness and non-judgemental truth telling is needed, as well as deeper humility among so-called experts. Elizabeth Pisani, *The Wisdom of Whores: Bureaucrats, Brothels and the Business of AIDS* (London: Granta Books, 2008).

25. See Helen Epstein's *The Invisible Cure: Africa, the West and the Fight Against AIDS* (New York: Farrar, Strauss and Giroux, 2007).

26. Paul Ricoeur, *From Text to Action: Essays in Hermeneutics* (Evanston: Northwestern University Press, 1991).

27. Paul Bové, 'Discourse' in *Critical Terms for Literary Study*, edited by F. Lentricchia and T. McLaughlin (Chicago: University of Chicago Press, 1995): 50–65.

28. This dynamic is explored further in Gillian Paterson, 'The discourses of AIDS in Britain' in *Calling for Justice Throughout the World: Catholic Women Writing about HIV and AIDS*, edited by Mary Jo Iozzo (New York: Continuum, 2009): 113–18.

29. Barbara Schmid, 'AIDS discourses in the church: What we say and what we do'. *Journal of Theology for Southern Africa* 125 (2006): 91–103; Gill Seidel, 'Competing discourses of HIV/AIDS in sub-Saharan Africa: Discourses of rights and empowerment vs discourses of control and exclusion'. *Social Science and Medicine* 36 (1993): 175–94.

30. Paul Ricoeur, *From Text to Action*: 150.

31. Catherine Campbell, 'I have an evil child in my house'. *American Journal of Public Health* 95(5) (2005): 808–15; Edouardo Terren, 'Religion and the ties that bind: Rethinking the rhetoric of othering'. *Journal for the Study of Religions and Ideologies* 2(8) 2004: 13–22.

32. For a more detailed discussion of this issue, see Chapter 1 in this book.

33. Rowan Williams, *Christian Theology* (Oxford: Blackwell, 2000).

34. World Council of Churches, *The Ecumenical Response to HIV/AIDS in Africa: Plan of Action* (Geneva: WCC, 2001). This document and the meeting that produced it can be seen as a watershed in understanding the role of stigma in undermining responses to the epidemic.

35. For further discussion, see Chapter 10 in this book.

36. See also Kate Long, 'On sex, sin and silence' in *Islam and AIDS: Between Scorn, Pity and Justice* edited by Farid Esack and Sarah Chiddy (Oxford: Oneworld Publications, 2009): 154–68.

37. Michel Foucault, *The History of Sexuality: An Introduction*, translated by R. Hurley (London: Penguin, 1978): 35.

38. Augustine of Hippo, *De Nuptiis et Concupiscentia ii* (Vienna: Austrian Academy of Sciences Corpus Scriptorum Ecclesiasticorum Latinorum): 59. Available at www.fourthcentury.com/csel-on-internet/.

39. Dietrich Bonhoeffer, *Letters and Papers from Prison* (London: SCM Press, 1953): 100.

40. Kevin Kelly, *New Directions in Sexual Ethics: Moral Theology and the Challenge of AIDS* (London: Geoffrey Chapman, 1998): 11.

41. See, for example, Fulata Lusungu Moyo, 'Sex, gender, power and HIV/AIDS in Malawi: Threats and challenges to women being church' in *On Being Church: African Women's Voices and Visions*, edited by Isabel Apawo Phiri and Sarojini Nadar (Geneva: WCC Publications, 2005); and Chapter 10 in this book.

42. Farley, *Just Love*.

43. Nordic-FOCCISA, *One Body: North-South Reflections in the Face of HIV and AIDS* and *One Body: AIDS and the Worshipping Community* (Oslo: Christian Council of Norway, 2006): 19. See Chapter 6 in this book.

44. Nordic-FOCCISA, *One Body: North-South Reflections in the Face of HIV and AIDS*: 19.

45. Patrick Buchanan, 'AIDS and moral bankruptcy'. *New York Post*, 2 Dec. 1987: 23.

46. Martha Nussbaum, *Hiding from Humanity: Disgust, Shame and the Law* (Princeton: Princeton University Press, 2004): 14.

47. Susan Sontag, *AIDS and its Metaphors* (London: Penguin, 1991): 179.

48. Ettie Hillesum, *An Interrupted Life* (New York: Washington Square Press, 1981): 34.

49. John 9:2.

50. See Alison's study of John 9 in *Faith Beyond Resentment*: 3–26.

51. See, Countryman, *Dirt, Greed and Sex*; Peter Brown, *The Body in Society: Men, Women and Sexual Renunciation in Early Christianity* (New York: Columbia University Press, 1988); Rowan Williams, *Silence and Honey Cakes: The Wisdom of the Desert* (Oxford: Lion Hudson, 2003).

52. Denise M. Ackermann, 'Engaging stigma: An embodied theological response to HIV and AIDS: the challenge of HIV/AIDS to Christian theology'. *Scriptura* 89 (2005): 385–95.

53. Kim Power, *Veiled Desire: Augustine's Writings on Women* (London: Darton, Longman and Todd, 1995); Caroline Bynum, *Holy Feast, Holy Fast: The Religious Significance of Food to Medieval Women* (Berkeley: University of California Press, 1987).

54. Charles Rosenberg, *Explaining Epidemics* (Cambridge: Cambridge University Press, 1992).

55. Sontag, *AIDS and its Metaphors*; Peter Allen, *The Wages of Sin: Sex and Disease, Past and Present* (Chicago: University of Chicago Press, 2000).

56. Donald Messer, *Breaking the Conspiracy of Silence: Christian Churches and the Global AIDS Crisis* (Minneapolis: Fortress Press, 2004). This issue in the South African context is debated in the following publications: PACSA, *Churches and HIV and AIDS: Exploring How Local Churches Are Integrating HIV/AIDS in the Life and Ministries of the Church and How Those Most Directly Affected Experience These* (Pietermaritzburg: PACSA, 2004); Beverley Haddad, '"We pray but we cannot heal": Theological challenges posed by the HIV/AIDS crisis'. *Journal of Theology for Southern Africa* 125 (2006): 80–90.

57. See Peter Allen, *The Wages of Sin*: 119ff.

58. See, for example, Johanna Stiebert, 'Women's sexuality and stigma in Genesis and the Prophets' in *Grant Me Justice!: HIV/AIDS and Gender Readings of the Bible*, edited by Musa W. Dube and Musimbi R.A. Kanyoro (Pietermaritzburg: Cluster Publications, 2004): 80–96.

59. Denise M. Ackermann, 'Tamar's cry: Re-reading an ancient text in the midst of the HIV and AIDS pandemic' in *Grant Me Justice!*, edited by Dube and Kanyoro: 27–59; Musa W. Dube, 'Twenty-two years of bleeding and still the princess sings!' in *Grant Me Justice!*, edited by Dube and Kanyoro: 186–99; Dorcas Olubanke Akintunde, 'The attitude of Jesus to the "anointing prostitute": A model for contemporary churches in the face of HIV/AIDS in Africa' in *African Women, HIV/AIDS and Faith Communities*, edited by Isabel Apawo Phiri, Beverley Haddad and Madipoane Masenya (Pietermaritzburg: Cluster Publications, 2003): 94–110.

60. For further discussion see Chapter 12 in this book.

61. Recent work of Muslim scholars has explored traditions of compassion and pity in Islam. For example, Mohammed Hashim Kamali, 'The Shari'ah and AIDS: Towards a theology of compassion' in *Islam and AIDS*, edited by Esack and Chiddy: 76–87.

Practitioner response

Gideon Byamugisha

Gillian Paterson's chapter rightly identifies stigma as an obstacle to care, treatment, prevention and practical assistance for orphans and other vulnerable children affected by HIV and AIDS; as a major contributor to the spread of HIV; as having layers at individual, family, local community, national and global levels that generate corresponding denial and discrimination at each level; as having its roots in profound beliefs about the nature of God, how people should behave, and what kind of institution the church should be; and as not being researched enough, particularly in relation to its interface with theology, ecclesiology, spirituality and doctrine.

The chapter also gives more insight into the complexity of dislodging stigma from our midst by focusing on the anthropological habit and dynamic of scapegoating and reflections by various authors on the subject. In addition, it reveals the recurring themes of truth, gender, sex, economic and social marginalisation and the ambivalence of religious traditions in relation to the human body.

The themes highlighted in the chapter that merit further research in our work in the community include HIV- and AIDS-related stigma such as shame, denial, discrimination, inaction and mis-action. This includes the way current messages and communication strategies on HIV prevention within the faith sector further exacerbate this problem; the interface between irrational fear and stigma; the gap between what people read about in their sacred texts, sing about in their religious communities and pray about in worship services, and what they actually practise in their personal, family and community lives in relation to theological themes such as love and hate, fear and courage, despair and hope, affirmation and rejection.

In the communities in which we live and work, we still experience four types of stigma that theology researchers could help us to understand and confront better. As a religious leader living with HIV, I have identified these as follows.

Individuals known, believed or rumoured to be HIV positive are feared, despised, loathed and ridiculed as sources and reservoirs of HIV infection and as malicious actors in the cruel game of infection, transmission, sickness and death. Many community members, political leaders, policy framers and legislators do not hide their feelings that preferably HIV positive people should be withdrawn from society by resort to tough laws that criminalise both HIV infection and transmission.

Despite growing knowledge about HIV progression, care, treatment and impact mitigation, many community members and people living with HIV themselves still equate HIV infection with a quick and inevitable death. Some people within families and communities where HIV positive people live do not see why they should marry, be fed, cared for, treated, have school fees paid, be promoted at the work place, be given a scholarship for further studies, or given a job demanding responsibility. This is because in their eyes people will die soon anyway. Further research is needed about why these attitudes persist and their interface with religious beliefs, views and opinions.

Despite increasing knowledge about the different modes of HIV transmission and the difference between what is right and what is safe, the difference between refusing to change and failing to change, or that between risky behaviours and risky environments, in many people's minds AIDS is still a disease that one gets after doing bad, unacceptable, unfaithful or unlawful things either in sexual matters or in drug use. We need to understand why this is still the case. It is important also to understand why positive HIV status is still known or labelled as a condition of individuals, groups of people, families, communities, nations and continents with questionable morals and character. It is also important to understand the religious agenda behind this persistent, but inaccurate, way of looking at the HIV and AIDS epidemic.

'You are what you confess' some of our religious leaders and spiritual advisors warn us. 'If you declare with your mouth and heart that you are HIV positive, that is indeed what you will remain – HIV positive. On the other hand if you declare with your mouth and heart that you are HIV negative in Jesus' name; you claim instant healing and become HIV negative. No need for ARVs. Initiating or remaining on ARVs is a testimony to your little faith (or lack of faith) in a God of miracles and wonders'. As a result of this attitude, people who are HIV positive are stigmatised as second- or third-class citizens in spiritual and faith matters. This is even worse for religious leaders known or believed to be HIV positive and on ARVs. Further research is needed to understand how best to confront and neutralise this type and source of stigma.

15

Religious community care and support in the context of HIV and AIDS

Outlining the contours

Jill Olivier and Paula Clifford

INTRODUCTION

There is a core paradox embedded in the literature addressing the religious response to HIV and AIDS, which is most obvious when focusing on the subset of literature on care and support. Simply stated, this paradox emerges on the heels of the realisation that the area of greatest potential strength of the religious sector is also the area about which we know the least.

In the last decade, increasing attention has been given to the religious response to the HIV and AIDS epidemic. Much of the emergent literature has a combined focus on HIV- and AIDS-related health care (usually delivered through health facilities such as hospitals and clinics) and the more diffuse care and support activities (from primary health care activities such as home-based care to visiting and food parcels). It is, in fact, difficult to separate out this literature, although it is clear that more is known about the religious facility-based care activities than those that occur at a community level:

> [. . .] while the larger, facility-based entities such as hospitals are (sometimes) visible on public health maps, the mass of smaller non-facility based programmes and initiatives are rarely visible . . . Even the national religious co-ordinating bodies are often oblivious of their own congregations' initiatives at a local level . . . For example, some congregations provide home-based care and support services as part of their basic day-to-day efforts, often offering regular emotional, spiritual and practical support. These efforts are frequently not recognized.[1]

It is on this less distinct local level, where community and family care and support services are enacted, that this literature landscaping is focused. The review therefore begins with an acknowledgement of the absence of foundational information on which any substantial argument can be made. We speak here, then, not of what little we know about the response of religious health facilities providing care in the context of HIV and AIDS,[2] but the less acknowledged, yet equally important, layer of care and support activities that occur at community family levels. These activities, while clearly tied into facility-based health care, are much more difficult to assess and track.

There are further fundamental difficulties to this task. The information on community-level care activities is dispersed across a range of materials addressing not only HIV and AIDS but also a slew of primary health care issues; and the literature that is focused on HIV and AIDS generally does not make a clear distinction between primary and secondary care activities.[3] It is also difficult to separate out care from support activities. Different subsets of literature define these in a variety of ways and, as will be discussed below, religious activities frequently include a holistic spectrum that seamlessly combines prevention, treatment, care and support.[4] Indeed, religious organisations often refuse to make a clear distinction between HIV- and AIDS-related care and support activities.[5] Furthermore, even care is defined differently: for some it is a set of defined activities such as home-based care and treatment-related support, while for others it is a spectrum of activities ranging from visits to food parcels or transport. As discussed below, different religious traditions tend to describe care in particular ways. Generally, there are also 'deep differences in language, vocabulary, concepts and frameworks . . . [where the] fundamental terms "prevention," "treatment," "care and support" as well as "spiritual encouragement," "knowledge giving," and "moral formation" have very different meanings in religious and public health settings'.[6] This literature landscaping, therefore, begins with an inherent instability as well as several large gaps in knowledge. Further imbalance is caused by the heavy emphasis towards African, Christian-focused and English-language literature.

Nevertheless, the intention of this review, to focus on religious community-level care and support in the context of HIV and AIDS, remains a worthwhile endeavour. For, as is explored below, if it is considered that the greatest (potential) strength possibly lies in its community-level caring and support activities (where religious communities and organisations have reach, access, trust or support), then the continued lack of knowledge of these activities becomes increasingly dangerous and limiting to a contextualised and adequate response.

Therefore, a broad understanding of the concept of care (or more correctly care and support) is deliberately taken to include activities such as home-based care, palliative care, care of orphans and vulnerable children, care of families and widows, care of people living with HIV and AIDS, treatment support, material support, spiritual support, pastoral education and psycho-social support, as well as a range of other caring and supportive activities. This clearly goes beyond a narrower, public health oriented definition of public health care but also includes the HIV- and AIDS-related activities embedded within family planning, child and maternal health, health education and reproductive health services. What binds these concerns together is a focus on care at the local, family and community level. An in-depth analysis of cross-over areas, addressed elsewhere in this book,[7] is avoided although they are clearly tied into this spectrum of community-level care.

In this review, the broad ethos that drives religious communities into caring activities is first considered, followed by a brief description of different kinds of community carers (caring actors). This is followed by a consideration of the limited information about the scope, scale and focus of community caring activities as well as some of the clusters of activities named in the literature as being of particular import. Finally, there is discussion of some of the broad ideas prevalent in the literature about specific kinds of religiously motivated and instituted care (such as compassionate care) as well as some concerns raised by this powerful caring agenda.

AN ETHOS OF CARE: DRIVEN TO CARE

Many authors writing on religion, HIV and AIDS have noted the strong ethos of care that infuses most of the world's religions. This can be articulated differently, for example, as compassionate care or a mission to serve.[8] In Christian doctrine there are several discourses: for example, being of service to others or works of mercy that have led to a strong emphasis on care and support in the context of HIV and AIDS.[9] In 2001 a major international conference for churches and church-related organisations set out a plan of action to provide care and support for those impacted on by the epidemic.[10] The emphasis here, as elsewhere, was on the community rather than the church, with the aim being to build 'a movement of care that originates from communities'.[11]

Another example can be seen through Islamic law which mandates that individuals actively care for others: 'there is a strong current of mercy in Islam, which applies to anyone in distress, even sinners and criminals. Hence, men having sex with men *should* be able to expect compassionate care when they are taken ill.' The Qur'an also enjoins believers to visit the sick or bereaved, or to provide support through the giving of alms (Zakah).[12] At a community level, however, the literature describes fewer institutionalised care responses to HIV and AIDS in Muslim communities. Some authors, for example, have indicated that there are few formal Muslim health care institutions or support groups for people living with HIV and suggest that 'most Muslim activities, even those concerned with care and support for PLWHA, are most concerned with influencing behaviour'.[13] However, it should be noted that such statements are based on particular definitions of community care and it must be acknowledged that fewer care-focused entities does not necessarily equal less care at a community level; just different kinds of care.[14]

Of course, there are theologically constituted obstacles to care as well, particularly in the context of HIV and AIDS. Much has been written about the stigmatisation of people living with HIV who have not felt the care of their local communities and congregations (discussed in more detail below).[15] Nevertheless, despite the stories of stigmatisation and exclusion, based on the broad literature addressing the religious response to the epidemic it would be fair to conclude that such negative observations are far outweighed by the scope and scale of community-level care of people infected and affected by HIV and AIDS. What is known of the scope, scale and nature of these activities is considered below, but first what is said about the different kinds of community carers is looked at.

COMMUNITY-LEVEL CARERS

There is some literature on religiously associated or motivated individuals who provide care and support at a community level. The most obvious are the health professionals often associated with religious health facilities. While there are varying statistics on these, it should be noted that this health workforce is in crisis in many countries, particularly in Africa, both as a direct result of the epidemic and because of the lack of capacity. For example, qualified staff and health workers are moving to other locations and there has also been a significant reduction in the numbers of international mission staff.[16]

Religious leaders are frequently described as community carers and a large body of literature emphasises the role of religious leaders in pastoral care in the context of HIV and AIDS.[17] For example, definitions of Christian pastoral care are surveyed by Buffel, who argues that pastoral care for people living with HIV must be both contextual and liberating.[18] This argument stems from what the author sees as failure by the church to live up to its true nature as the body of Christ. This has implications for care and support and Buffel's contention is that traditional pastoral care has failed to meet the needs of people living with HIV. So he calls for the church to reclaim its true nature, while at the same time acknowledging that it is important to see the individual as part of a network of relationships within the wider community.[19]

There is also some significant interest in pastoral care through education observed in a body of literature that describes and motivates for the education of congregations, community, and religious leadership about HIV and AIDS as a caring activity. These publications have a characteristically religious slant specific to their audience and describe local theologies and curricula for pastoral care through HIV and AIDS education.[20]

Another cluster of community carers are addressed in the literature as volunteers. This is obviously a broad, and sometimes less useful, label that encompasses a range of activities paid and unpaid. Much of the literature describes the volunteer networks available to religious communities as a potential asset: for example, 'churches have the most valuable item needed for an effective outreach, they have volunteers'.[21] However, there are fewer studies that specifically measure the current scope, scale and motivation of such volunteers and it is generally agreed that little is known of the actual extent of this resource. A study by Tearfund resorted to what they called matchbox maths to estimate that there are over five million volunteers from Christian communities in Africa, resulting in accumulative work valued at £2.5 billion per year.[22] Furthermore, volunteerism is an increasingly difficult aspect to assess, not least because of the rapidly evolving descriptors of volunteer actors that range from caring community members who provide their time and care for free, to partially subsidised volunteers and fully reimbursed community health workers.

Even less is known about the internal, religious-specific aspects that motivate or sustain volunteers in comparison with individuals who are not religiously motivated.[23] Motives for undertaking this care work are clearly complex. For example, a study based in a poor area of Malawi speaks of volunteers, who 'lost their altruistic heart' once it became clear that they would receive no reward for their services.[24] Another example of this complexity comes from a study of a Moravian HIV and AIDS programme that articulated its volunteer activities in Christian terms but ultimately decided that it was unsustainable to base care activities on volunteers who are unemployed and have no income:

> [. . .] formerly they used unemployed volunteers, paying them a rather large stipend to cover travel and expenses; now they offer part-time coordinators who have other jobs (e.g. a parish pastor) an . . . allowance, employ six treatment assistants . . . and previously unemployed care workers on a sliding scale . . . In addition, teachers who work as volunteers get an . . . allowance to cover cell phone airtime and travel.[25]

Therefore, while much of the literature suggests that religious motivation offers different reimbursement criteria,[26] in fact religious care activities are faced with many of the same problems that exist in non-religious programmes using volunteers. This is a critical area for further research.

Importantly, much of the literature on the religious response to HIV and AIDS notes that many of these care activities are 'initiated proactively by community members who "see a need", which means that health responses often emerge well in advance of any systematic effort from outside to organize, train or resource them'.[27] Many of these spontaneous caring activities have no commonly recognisable form or name. For example, a mapping of religious activities and entities engaged in HIV and AIDS care in Lesotho found a range of care and support activities that had spontaneously begun from within religious communities and which were deeply religious in character:

> In communities where access to healthcare services and facilities is beyond the financial reach of ordinary Basotho there has been a dramatic upsurge of local community support groups. Self-initiated, deeply religious, though not formally linked to any religious structure, they are identified as among the most important health providers in these communities.[28]

In Lesotho, these groups were deeply religious (yet represented various religions and were independent of any specific church); comprised a majority of female members; were self-funded and used their own resources to feed, clothe, hospitalise and medicate patients; and were mostly self-initiated groups functioning independently of public health care facilities and religious networks. For example, one carer describes the development of their community support group: 'We've seen a lot of teenagers die. We asked how we can prevent this death . . . When we first met we were three . . . then the group was ten. We went from house to house getting patients.'[29]

Through participatory research with the broader community, researchers discovered that these support groups were rated the most highly as proactive and addressing the health of the community, ranking higher even than churches or orphanages in their level of compassionate care. This research report concluded that 'the dramatic increase of support groups in rural areas can be attributed to several factors; these include: (i) increased HIV/AIDS infection, (ii) economic constraints preventing community members from accessing formal healthcare services, and (iii) the stressed economic situation of small local churches, preventing an effective religious response to HIV/AIDS'.[30]

This is one example of many but describes the complexity of measuring and understanding a community care response to HIV and AIDS and the range of actors providing care in such communities. The community support groups in this example were spontaneously mobilised by individuals motivated by a concern for the health of their community and expressed as a religious motivation to care. Although these appeared to 'operate outside the formal "church" structures they understand themselves to be fundamentally religious. Their perceptions of and compassion for community members derives from an innate sense of community service, love and compassion.'[31]

Moving to a different context, another example can be seen in the development of a Congregational Health Network around a multi-billion-dollar hospital system in Memphis, Tennessee. Here a network has been developed that seeks to integrate the community care activities that emerge from within congregations, community health organisations and the hospital system. The carers engaged in this network include community health workers, congregational health liaison persons, religious leaders, hospital navigators, as well as doctors, nurses and public health practitioners.[32] While HIV and AIDS is not a main driver in this community, it is present and a lived reality of many of those being cared for. This care network is not described in any further detail here, the main point being that community care relating to HIV and AIDS occurs in vastly different contexts through a range of actors carrying different descriptive labels.[33] We are as yet poorly equipped with proper typologies or investigative frameworks to understand these actions and actors, and this remains a critical area for further investigation. Before continuing to a discussion of the scope and scale of community care activities, it is first necessary to consider two cross-over concerns expressed in the literature: first, the gendered nature of community care activities; and second, the importance of caring for the carers.

Gendered care

The available literature broadly proclaims that whether in Lesotho or Memphis, women carry out the bulk of community care activities in relation to HIV and AIDS and bear the burden of care giving.[34] Steinitz describes them as 'mostly women, mostly middle-aged, and invariably motivated by their faith and desire to help their neighbour in need'.[35] A different study by Tearfund identifies church volunteer care givers as predominantly women aged between 25 and 50.[36]

The need for proper training and recognition of the work of volunteer care givers is highlighted by Arnau van Wyngaard in a study with one small Christian congregation in Swaziland. During the training process for care givers, the organisers were amazed that a number of men volunteered to join them, a highly unusual development in a male-dominated society.[37] A Christian study from Mozambique outlines an intriguing clue about different approaches to care on gendered lines, noting that 'women were more likely than men to report providing assistance to congregation members, and the reverse was true for assistance provided to non-members'.[38] Nonetheless, the overwhelming majority of literature indicates that the tangible care is typically provided by women.[39]

The slowness of some ordained male church leaders to respond to the HIV crisis is explored by Beverley Haddad, who concludes that they found themselves in 'a theological and pastoral impasse' because of the sheer complexity of the pastoral situation that confronted them. However, lay women in the same churches were concerned to learn about health care and to undertake proactive interventions to support people living with HIV in their community.[40] The work of Ezra Chitando confirms these gendered dynamics and he makes a telling point when noting that while men as policy makers have recommended the adoption of home-based care, it is women who have been tasked with providing it.[41] Philomena Mwaura describes the gendered nature of the task even more forthrightly as women having to engage in 'forced care-giving', and argues that this is a form of violation of their human rights.[42]

375

Caring for the carers

Another growing theme in the literature is the need for care of the carers. For example, exemplar religious care programmes engaged in HIV and AIDS were noted by community members to be the ones that take good care of the carers. In Zambia, one such exemplar organisation identified by the community explained: 'At [St Francis HBC] we have a strict policy of taking care of our carers . . . it is not a job, it has to be something you want to do as a vocation . . . caring for the carers is very important . . . these carers are ecumenical, and many have been with [us] for eleven years.'[43]

Another study of a care initiative in South Africa notes that many, if not most, of the women receiving treatment and care were themselves carers for household members who had been chronically ill or died:

> Not surprisingly, depression was found in many women and this was linked to their own self rated health . . . It is within this context that the role of faith needs to be understood. Religion was reported as playing a major role in the well-being of over two thirds of the respondents as it offered them hope for the future, helped them to survive as well as giving meaning.[44]

What is important here is to recognise the complex layering of care activities and actors, particularly in communities where the carers can, even simultaneously, be those cared for.

De la Porte writes of care givers shaping their identity through the work that they do and being changed by it.[45] If this is the case, then the issue of caring for those care givers is crucially important as they work through situations that may well lead to them being stigmatised themselves. 'Caregivers experience special pressures, because they have to be there for a loved one or client who is desperately ill, and most attention is usually directed at the sick person in a home.'[46] The conclusion that follows from this is that there is a need for all organisations, including religious groups, to support their care givers. Daniela Gennrich suggests this should take the form of prayer, visiting and regular meetings for debriefing and confidential discussion of particular problems.[47] Regular meetings, including a meal and prayer together, have also been suggested as effective strategies in providing support for carers.[48] While there is a rapidly growing literature proposing strategies for assisting with the coping and resilience of carers, there is little literature that addresses religious-specific strategies for caring for the carers.[49] Finally, the incidence of HIV infection in older people, particularly women, is still not sufficiently well recognised.[50] And since it is the older generation who bear the main burden of caring for infected members of their families or for orphaned children, it is imperative that the needs of older women are recognised and met. Older people are more likely to have a positive engagement with local religious institutions and so their responsibility in this regard is crucial.[51] There is, though, little evidence of this responsibility being acknowledged.

SCOPE, SCALE AND FOCUS OF COMMUNITY CARE AND SUPPORT ACTIVITIES

As suggested earlier, the extent of less visible aspects of community care, such as more amorphous networks, community systems and supporting roles, is poorly documented and remains largely anecdotal.[52] Having said this, an attempt is made to report on some of the broader statements being made before engaging in closer thematic analysis.

First, in those studies that have asked religious organisations and communities about their range of HIV- and AIDS-related activities, it is clear that care and support is usually a primary activity, commonly placed ahead of prevention or treatment:[53]

> FBOs have displayed a number of strengths compared to government institutions and development NGOs. For example, they are clearly the most effective in service delivery in relation to care and support for people living with HIV/AIDS. Care and support is the Christian FBOs' strongest contribution to the struggle against HIV/AIDS in Sub-Saharan Africa.[54]

The focus of this care and support tends to be on two main areas: home-based care and the care and support of orphans and vulnerable children.[55] For example, a study of Christian religious organisations engaged in HIV and AIDS in Kenya and Malawi found this to be true and a broad reading of the literature suggests that orphans and vulnerable children appear to be the client group most served by religious organisations.[56] Furthermore, it has been suggested that the care of children is an area in which most religious traditions seem theologically more driven and comfortable.[57]

Of course, home-based care has emerged as an important aspect of engagement with the epidemic generally, especially in resource-poor settings such as sub-Saharan Africa: 'Extremely poor roads and general lack of transport in many areas severely limit health care access and services; religiously sponsored home-based care groups have become a critical resource in providing health services and material support to those in rural areas'.[58] Logically it then follows that this has become an important aspect, particularly for those carers based in local communities.[59] At the risk of repetition, while there is a growing public health literature on home-based care generally there is little that evaluates the scale or nature of the religious sector's contribution.

Little is known of the religious constituency of these carers and caring activities. Several studies have suggested that HIV and AIDS community care and support activities do not seem to be intentionally restricted to caring for those in one's own faith group, although in practice this does sometimes occur.[60] For example, in Kenya and Malawi it was found that although the Christian religious organisations that were questioned were in principle and policy committed to working with all people, in reality their work was mainly with those of the same faith. As one participant said: 'We do not discriminate but at the end of the day we work mainly with Christians, even though we do not discriminate.'[61]

Although it might be difficult to generalise about the scale of community care activities, several statements have been made to that effect. For example, Benn notes: 'It is estimated that the Roman Catholic Church alone provides 25% of all HIV and AIDS care, including home based care and support of orphans.'[62] While broad conclusions about the scale of community care worldwide clearly cannot be made, it is still possible to suggest that these activities have been growing rapidly over the last decade, given that there has been a boom in the religious response to HIV and AIDS at all levels.[63]

However, it is also clear that resources and support, national and international, are becoming increasingly scarce, particularly donor-supported care. It is also uncertain just how far such donor funding and support has trickled down to the community level. 'Although national and international funding seems to be available, allocation and fund raising at the local and individual organizational level is proving uncertain. This raises questions about the sustainability of most care and support initiatives in poor and remote settings.'[64] It is possible, or likely, that spontaneous community care activities have been forced to fill these growing care gaps, another area of necessary research engagement.

Religious care and support activities tend to be embedded within a holistic range of services.[65] They are also frequently described through a particular religious framework as addressing the emotional, communal and spiritual aspects of care, as well as the physical.[66] A holistic approach to care, is of course not limited to religious communities or carers: indeed, secular palliative care or nursing strategies follow many of the same principles. However, in the literature addressing the religious response to HIV and AIDS, the holistic nature of the care provided is strongly emphasised and described as a particular strength of these organisations.[67]

What emerges from the literature is a strong argument that the physical acts of HIV- and AIDS-related care and support activities provided by religious communities and organisations at a community level are deeply infused with spiritual elements, also described as pastoral or psycho-social. Such spiritually infused care is expressed in the literature in a number of different ways.

One area in which this focus on holistic blending of physical acts of care with the spiritual or religious ritual can be most clearly seen is the literature addressing care and support activities around death. Palliative care is clearly an area in which religious communities are often heavily involved. In providing palliative care, religions are said to access strategies that encompass 'emotional, psychosocial, spiritual and environmental support and care in respect of those infected and affected by HIV and AIDS'.[68]

The literature addressing the religious response has a further emphasis on aspects of community care related to the public expression of, and coping with, death and bereavement. 'It has been recognised that in the HIV/AIDS crisis, a substantial number of [religious entities] are offering support to family during illness, bereavement and funeral arrangements.'[69] In the case of community care and support responses, this goes beyond the palliative care of the individual to public facilitation of and sharing in grief and lament:

Religions and [religious entities] play a crucial role in the intervention in public and private grief. For example, religions provide mourning or lamenting rituals in face of mass grief and tragedy. While this has been mostly treated as a theological or psychological matter it can also be argued that it is relevant to public health. If a ritual provides comfort and understanding to a community, it might also have an effect on social networks and emotional and mental health. This might in turn affect health-seeking behaviour or choices.[70]

In the light of experiences from Botswana, Frederick Klaits looks at how survivors remember the circumstances surrounding death and alludes to the role of church members in offering material support, prayer support and companionship. Remembering here is seen as a way of maintaining love in the face of widespread death and dying.[71] More work is needed to understand how religious roles and rituals can be seen and supported as caring activities.

Another trend in the literature is for community care in the context of HIV and AIDS to be expressed in terms of the family. This has not yet been adequately linked to the broader literature that addresses the impact of the epidemic on the family.[72] Some authors have suggested that religious groups, such as a local congregation, could function as a family or a large-scale support group. This has both positive and negative implications, depending on the theological persuasions of the group. In an examination of neo-Pentecostalism within Christianity, Hansjörg Dilger observes that 'the church plays an important role in integrating its members into a tightly-knit spiritual community thereby countering – and at the same time reinforcing – processes of social and familial disruption that characterise their members' experiences in the context of urban hardships and the AIDS epidemic'.[73]

Dilger draws attention to small neighbourhood churches, each with 20 to 30 members that form a spiritual family and provide help and support to its members. The advantages of this are, as admitted by some of its members, counteracted by the familial conflicts that result between the saved and their relatives outside the church.[74] Magezi also contends that the church should embody the metaphor of family with its members responsible for caring for one another.[75] In the African context, for example, the notion of the extended family is seen as supporting a ministry of home-based care that is nonetheless acted out within a faith community.

A SPECIAL KIND OF CARE
So far, this review has avoided speaking too strongly of the comparative advantage, or value added, of religious caring activities in comparison with so-called secular activities. This is partially because this is a highly contentious issue and not enough is yet known about the comparative care of religious organisations or by

religiously motivated individuals to be able to support any such statement.[76] Nevertheless, it would be remiss of us not to note that much of the literature addressing the community care responses to HIV and AIDS describes religious care as holding some kind of comparative advantage. The strongest examples are those in which those who are cared for profess some kind of preference for religiously motivated and instituted care. Saying, for example, 'the difference is that the care done by church organizations is done with care, compassion and love, with encouragement – but in government hospitals, people just do it for money – no compassion, love or care' is just one example of many where an element of special care has been attributed to religious interventions.[77] This element of special care is also sometimes described as religiously and therefore culturally appropriate care. For example, Olsen describes the effectiveness of love and attention for their patients on the part of nurses, through 'appropriate spiritual and holistic nursing interventions'.[78] Another related example comes from the small amount of literature that describes carers as motivated and sustained in their caring activities as a result of internal religious resources. For example, Tiendrebeogo and Buykx suggest that volunteer Christian home-based care givers are 'more motivated than their secular colleagues' due to a shared value system and conclude that religious organisations 'offer a special advantage in care and support in their capacity for spiritual care'.[79] There is insufficient space to get too far into this discussion, the short answer being that there is not enough comparative research available to ratify such statements.[80] However, it is necessary to point out the large literature suggesting that religious care and support is a different kind of care.

Agadjanian and Sen describe religious care as being offered in two broad categories: psychological support (prayer, advice and encouragement) and tangible support (money, food, transportation and personal physical care).[81] Several other authors and commentators address this differently: for example, some speak of tangible and intangible aspects of care.[82] It would thus appear that one cross-over argument is that the basis of a special kind of care is care that combines tangible and intangible factors: physical (tangible) care and support that is infused with religious (spiritual, pastoral or psycho-social) factors.

Care that addresses the whole person is valued. For example, a study on a Moravian HIV and AIDS programme in South Africa showed that it was the 'integration of care across the continuum of activities' that was valued by programme participants, 'providing a continuum of care that includes both tangible and intangible assets, thus integrating the particular strengths of the allopathic health system with those of the faith community and thereby contributing to a much more comprehensive response to health and illness'.[83] In a research study conducted for the World Health Organisation in Zambia and Lesotho, researchers found that it was the interweaving of tangible care (for example, home-based care initiatives and food support) with intangible factors (compassion and hope) that gave particular strength to certain HIV and AIDS care initiatives. Activities that did this were most often considered to be exemplars by local communities.[84]

Another example of the weaving of tangible and intangible aspects can be seen in the discourse of a compassionate care threaded throughout much of the HIV and AIDS literature addressing the religious response. Compassionate care is differently described in the literature: for example, as the ideal care of people living with HIV without stigma, as a genuine support of people in mourning, as home-based care, or as a kind of pastoral response to HIV and AIDS that teaches families and communities.[85] Different religious traditions have a variety of theologies behind the descriptor compassionate care. In the Christian tradition, for example, a shared religious value system might include an understanding of God as caring and compassionate. Bouwer argues that God is understood to be a compassionate friend who is characterised as trustworthy and non-judgemental and, therefore, cares unconditionally. This understanding is founded on the notion of human dignity, which derives from the notion that humankind is made in God's image. Bouwer finds that the metaphor of God as friend creates confidence in the trustworthiness of God in difficult times, and culminates in compassion and care.[86]

In the Islamic tradition, a growing number of publications reflect concern about HIV on the part of Muslim leaders and acceptance that there are increasing numbers of people living with HIV in their faith communities. Positive Muslims, an influential community organisation in South Africa, urges a compassionate and responsible approach, reflecting the Islamic view of justice.[87] The scriptural basis for such an approach is made abundantly clear, leading to the conclusion that Muslims should reflect prophetic mercy in their commitment to care giving.[88]

The potential of congregations to offer compassionate care is spelt out in a comment from Peru cited by Nussbaum, where the church community is described as 'a home for the homeless and marginalised; a place where they can find people who can accompany them in their ordeal; a place where they can find compassion and love; a place where they can contribute in the midst of their suffering'.[89] Examining the progress made by faith communities, Keogh and Marshall identify care and compassion as distinctive features of faith-based programmes, which they argue outweigh any past tendency to insist on retribution for so-called sinful behaviour.[90] There are abundant other examples of expressions of the necessity for an attitude and action of compassionate care in the context of HIV and AIDS through a range of religious lenses. Again, it is the combination of tangible and intangible factors that is seen to provide particular strength.

In the research carried out in Zambia, the most significant religious response was described by several communities to be compassionate care infused with spiritual encouragement.

> When focusing on [religious entities] we have found that it is their ability to integrate these tangible and intangible factors that gives them 'strength'. It is perceived that to make a contribution to health and wellbeing, 'spiritual encouragement' needs to find an expression in 'compassionate care', but likewise, such caring outside of a 'spiritual' framework loses its strength. Thus, in Zambia, church-initiated home-based care groups are seen as the most important [religious entities] contributing to health and wellbeing, while in Lesotho it is community-based support groups – with a strong religious flavor – which are significant.[91]

THE (DIS)COMFORTS OF CARE

We have described above some of the suggested strengths of a religiously motivated or instituted community care response to HIV and AIDS. And many authors have noted that religious communities have great assets and potential for care. As Foster notes, 'there are more than a quarter of a million congregations in the AIDS belt of East and Southern Africa alone – more than enough to support the region's 12 million orphans. Kenya alone has 80,000 congregations: if each cared for 20 orphans, all the country's 1.6 million orphans would be supported'.[92] However, there are also several concerns and suggested weaknesses. Some have already been mentioned above. In resource-poor settings, the increased demands for care and support in already strained communities are hazardous. Even the unleveraged potential assets of religious communities become strained under the increased burden and spontaneous community responses are endangered. It has been noted elsewhere that an increasingly instrumental response towards religious communities is potentially dangerous.[93] Failing health systems in some areas also put an increasing burden on primary health care, and on local and community-level care networks and resources. The research on religious collaboration on HIV and AIDS in Kenya, for example, showed that while participant organisations were mainly focused on home-based care and care of orphans and vulnerable children, a concern was expressed about their capacity: 'We have been abandoned with the children . . . we do not have the resources . . . we are overwhelmed . . . we have no choice . . . there is no one else [to do this work].'[94] It is clear that the epidemic is placing increasing burdens on already strained community resources in many countries. This strain is translated into dwindling religious resources – if not the intangible assets, then certainly the tangible ones – often threatening their sustainability.

Another concern is that many religious communities appear to focus on caring initiatives to the detriment of other HIV and AIDS activities such as prevention or advocacy.[95] We are reminded of this by Steve de Gruchy, who noted:

> [R]eligious actors have to accept responsibility for engaging in social life – for taking on the tasks in the field of public health. While religious actors seem comfortable with the traditional roles of care and compassion once people are sick, there has to be a responsibility for preventative issues . . . This will also mean accepting political responsibility, as these issues draw one immediately into the field of policy and power.[96]

Religious community care initiatives have also been accused of sometimes taking on a lone-gun approach, forgoing co-operation with others and resulting in the duplication of care services.[97] The need for co-operative relationships at a community level (outside the immediate local religious group) is highlighted by various authors.[98] This may involve training care givers or obtaining financial and material assistance.[99] At a local level, however, this is not always possible and all too often, where religious organisations are encouraged to work together, questions of prestige and boosting membership come into play.[100] The improvement of local co-operative networks is urgently required in order to provide sustainable community care.[101]

It is clear that the religious response to HIV and AIDS has sometimes contained an ambivalent and even antagonistic attitude towards people living with

HIV. However, there is a strong emphasis in the literature on the need to move on from a negative judgemental approach to positive 'embracing of the other'.[102] Care in this context is seen as an expression against stigmatisation, visibly working in local communities. A study in Malawi documented how a perception of the church as cold and unloving was changed through the work of church volunteers offering home-based care: 'For the church, to leave the buildings and go and suffer with the people where they live, provides the opportunity to reclaim its struggle for human dignity, righteousness and justice'.[103]

CONCLUSION

In the beginning of this review a core paradox embedded in the literature addressing the religious response to HIV and AIDS was introduced. Simply stated, this paradox is based on the realisation that the area of greatest potential strength of the religious sector (community-level care and support) is also the area about which the least is known. Much of the reason for this is, as has been suggested, that many religious community care responses are spontaneously initiated. Religious organisations and community care activities are also commonly said to be fluid and adaptive to the needs of the communities in which they are based. This diversity and fluidity make it particularly important that 'policy-makers heed important differences among these institutions when devising ways to harness this potential'.[104] This certainly calls for more intelligent and creative donor responses, as Christoph Benn says: 'Many excellent community based initiatives have been started by committed Christians who are trying to serve their communities. In the future, it will be important that churches identify, recognize and support these initiatives. This might demand a high degree of flexibility and willingness to accept innovation.'[105]

However, preceding such a demand for flexibility and the acceptance of innovation there must, by necessity, be an earlier step: a much greater effort into investigating this layer of community-level care and support activities, a potentially powerful presence and activity of which we still know frustratingly little.

NOTES

1. Barbara Schmid et al., *The Contribution of Religious Entities to Health in Sub-Saharan Africa* (Cape Town: African Religious Health Assets Programme, 2008): 50.

2. See Chapter 1 of this book for more in-depth discussion of this point.

3. See Karen Birdsall, *Faith-Based Responses to HIV/AIDS in South Africa: An Analysis of the Activities of Faith-Based Organisations (FBOs) in the National HIV/AIDS Database* (Johannesburg: Centre for AIDS Development, Research and Evaluation, 2005).

4. See Jill Olivier, James R. Cochrane and Barbara Schmid, *ARHAP Literature Review: Working in a Bounded Field of Unknowing* (Cape Town: African Religious Health Assets Programme, 2006): 39–40.

5. See Beverley Haddad, Jill Olivier and Steve de Gruchy, *The Potential and Perils of Partnership: Christian Religious Entities and Collaborative Stakeholders Responding to HIV and AIDS in Kenya, Malawi and the DRC* (Cape Town: Africa Religious Health Assets Programme, 2008): 52.

6. Steve de Gruchy et al. *Appreciating Assets: The Contribution of Religion to Universal Access in Africa* (Cape Town: African Religious Health Assets Programme, 2006): 127.

7. For example, the care of children discussed in Chapter 12 of this book.

8. In Chapter 1 of this book, a summary is provided of some of the theological drivers in different religious traditions that translate into engagement in healing and care activities.

9. See H. Jurgen Hendriks, J.C. Erasmus and G.C. Mans, 'Congregations as providers of social service and HIV/AIDS care'. *Dutch Reformed Theological Journal* 45(2) 2004: 391; Georges Tiendrebeogo and Michael Buykx, *Faith-Based Organisations and HIV/AIDS Prevention and Impact Mitigation in Africa* (Amsterdam: KIT Publishers, 2004): 28.

10. Global Consultation on the Ecumenical Response to the Challenge of HIV/AIDS in Africa, 'Ecumenical response to HIV/AIDS in Africa: plan of action' (Nairobi, 2001).

11. Stan Nussbaum (ed.), *The Contribution of Christian Congregations to the Battle with HIV/AIDS at the Community Level* (Oxford: Global Mapping International, 2005); Global Consultation on the Ecumenical Response to the Challenge of HIV/AIDS in Africa, 'Ecumenical response to HIV/AIDS in Africa': 6.

12. Tiendrebeogo and Buykx, *Faith-Based Organisations and HIV/AIDS Prevention and Impact Mitigation in Africa*: 34.

13. See Schmid et al., *The Contribution of Religious Entities to Health in Sub-Saharan Africa*; Tiendrebeogo and Buykx, *Faith-Based Organisations and HIV/AIDS Prevention and Impact Mitigation in Africa*: 34.

14. Put differently, the failure here is the frame of investigation rather than the Islamic community care response to HIV and AIDS. Not enough is known to make conclusions about comparative levels of general community care in different religious traditions.

15. See also Chapter 14 in this book.

16. See Schmid et al., *The Contribution of Religious Entities to Health in Sub-Saharan Africa*: 85.

17. See Olivier, Cochrane and Schmid, *ARHAP Literature Review*: 61–3.

18. O. Andries Buffel, 'Pastoral care to people living with HIV/AIDS: A pastoral response that is contextual and liberating'. *Practical Theology in South Africa* 21(1) 2006: 1–18.

19. Buffel, 'Pastoral care to people living with HIV/AIDS': 11.

20. Olivier, Cochrane and Schmid, *ARHAP Literature Review*: 61–3.

21. Raphaela Handler in Susan Parry, *Responses of the Churches to HIV/AIDS: Three Southern African Countries* (Harare: WCC, 2002).

22. Nigel Taylor, *Working Together?: Challenges and Opportunities for International Development Agencies and the Church in the Response to AIDS in Africa* (Teddington: Tearfund, 2006).

23. See Olivier, Cochrane and Schmid, *ARHAP Literature Review*: 41; Tearfund, *Faith Untapped: Why Churches Can Play a Crucial Role in Tackling HIV and AIDS in Africa* (Teddington: Tearfund, 2006); Ritva Reinikka and Jakob Svensson, *Working for God?: Evaluating Service Delivery of Religious Not-For-Profit Health Care Providers in Uganda* (Washington, DC: World Bank, 2003).

24. J. Brown and H.J. Hendriks, 'Understanding HIV/AIDS through the dark lens of poverty'. *DEEL* 45(2) 2004: 403–15.

25. Elizabeth Thomas et al., *Let Us Embrace: The Role and Significance of an Integrated Faith-Based Initiative for HIV and AIDS* (Cape Town: African Religious Health Assets Programme, 2006): 28.

26. Reinikka and Svensson, *Working for God?* is one of the few studies that addresses this head on.

27. Olivier, Cochrane and Schmid, *ARHAP Literature Review*: 41.

28. De Gruchy et al., *Appreciating Assets*: 118.

29. De Gruchy et al., *Appreciating Assets*: 119.

30. De Gruchy et al., *Appreciating Assets*: 119.

31. De Gruchy et al., *Appreciating Assets*: 119.

32. See Teresa Cutts, 'Religious health assets mapping in Memphis'. Paper from MS Conference Leadership Training 'Shall You Be Healed?', Southaven, 29–30 Jan. 2008.

33. Because the bulk of the literature addresses the African continent, the review of such literature can also get caught up in this emphasis and descriptive frameworks particular to Africa.

34. For further discussion, see Chapter 9 of this book.

35. Lucy Y. Steinitz, 'Meeting the challenge with God on our side: Churches and faith-based organizations confront the AIDS pandemic in Namibia'. *International Review of Mission* 95(376–7) 2006: 101.

36. Tearfund, *Faith Untapped*.

37. A. van Wyngaard, 'On becoming the hands and feet of Christ in an AIDS-ridden community in Swaziland: A story of hope'. *Verbum et Ecclesia* 27(3) 2006: 1104.

38. Victor Agadjanian and Soma Sen, 'Promises and challenges of faith-based AIDS care and support in Mozambique'. *American Journal of Public Health* 97(2) 2007: 362.

39. Olivier, Cochrane and Schmid, *ARHAP Literature Review*.

40. Beverley Haddad, 'Surviving the HIV and AIDS epidemic in South Africa: Women living and dying, theologising and being theologised'. *Journal of Theology for Southern Africa* 131 (2008): 53.

41. Ezra Chitando, '"The good wife": A phenomenological re-reading of Proverbs 31:10–31 in the context of HIV/AIDS in Zimbabwe'. *Scriptura* 86 (2004), 151–9; Ezra Chitando, *Living with Hope: African Churches and HIV/AIDS* (Geneva: WCC Publications, 2007).

42. Philomena Njeri Mwaura, 'Stigmatization and discrimination of HIV/AIDS women in Kenya: A violation of human rights and its theological implications'. *Exchange* 37 (2008):

35–51. See also Julian C. Müller and Sunette Pienaar, 'Stories about care: women in a historically disadvantaged community infected and/or affected by HIV/AIDS'. *Hervormde Teologiese Studies* 60 (2004): 1029–47.

43. De Gruchy et al., *Appreciating Assets*.

44. Thomas et al., *Let Us Embrace*: 24.

45. André E. de la Porte, 'Towards conscious caring in the landscape of action as reflected in the unheard care stories of AIDS home-based carers'. *Practical Theology in SA* 18(3) 2003: 121–32.

46. Daniela Gennrich, *Churches and HIV/AIDS: Exploring How Local Churches are Integrating HIV/AIDS in the Life and Ministries of the Church* (Pietermaritzburg: PACSA, 2005): 27.

47. Gennrich, *Churches and HIV/AIDS*: 27.

48. Van Wyngaard, 'On becoming the hands and feet of Christ in an AIDS-ridden community in Swaziland': 1105–6.

49. See Corinne Strydom and C.C. Wessels, 'A group work programme to support and empower non-professional caregivers of people living with AIDS'. *Health SA Gesondheid* 11(4) 2006: 3–21; Steinitz, 'Meeting the challenge with God on our side': 101–2; Richards, for example, considers the power of private prayer in creating a positive state of mind in otherwise stressed care givers. See T. Anne Richards et al., 'Subjective experiences of prayer among women who care for children with HIV'. *Journal of Religion and Health* 42(3) 2003: 201–19.

50. See Christina Landman, 'A theology for the older, female HIV-infected body'. *Exchange* 37(1) 2008: 52–67.

51. Jaco Hoffman, 'Older persons as carriers of AIDS: The untold stories of older persons infected with HIV/AIDS and the implications for care'. *Practical Theology in SA* 18(3) 2003: 20–39.

52. See Schmid et al., *The Contribution of Religious Entities to Health in Sub-Saharan Africa*: 48.

53. See De Gruchy et al., *Appreciating Assets;* Haddad, Olivier and De Gruchy, *The Potential and Perils of Partnership*.

54. Tiendrebeogo and Buykx, *Faith-Based Organisations and HIV/AIDS Prevention and Impact Mitigation in Africa*: 47.

55. UNICEF, *The Role of Faith-Based Organisations in Providing Support to Orphans and Vulnerable Children in Africa* (New York: UNICEF and World Conference of Religions for Peace, 2003); H. Young, *More than Words?: Action for Orphans and Vulnerable Children in Africa: Monitoring Progress Towards the UN Declaration of Commitment on HIV/AIDS* (Milton Keynes: World Vision, 2005).

56. Olivier, Cochrane and Schmid, *ARHAP Literature Review*: 40; Tiendrebeogo and Buykx, *Faith-Based Organisations and HIV/AIDS Prevention and Impact Mitigation in Africa*: 29.

57. Olivier, Cochrane and Schmid, *ARHAP Literature Review*: 34, 40; Geoff Foster, *Study of the Response by Faith-Based Organisations to Orphans and Vulnerable Children: Preliminary Summary Report* (New York: World Conference of Religions for Peace and UNICEF, 2003). An interesting study is one of a Moravian HIV and AIDS project consciously based on a theology of justice, which translates into keeping parents alive through anti-retroviral treatment rather than focusing on care for their orphaned children (see Thomas et al., *Let Us Embrace*: 17).

58. In this discussion of home-based care we mean the broad range of activities including, but not limited to, palliative care; De Gruchy et al., *Appreciating Assets*.

59. See Tiendrebeogo and Buykx, *Faith-Based Organisations and HIV/AIDS Prevention and Impact Mitigation in Africa*: 28.

60. See Schmid et al., *The Contribution of Religious Entities to Health in Sub-Saharan Africa*: 52–72.

61. Haddad, Olivier and De Gruchy, *The Potential and Perils of Partnership*: 53.

62. Christoph Benn, 'The influence of cultural and religious frameworks on the future course of the HIV/AIDS pandemic'. *Journal of Theology for Southern Africa* 113 (2002): 21.

63. See De Gruchy et al., *Appreciating Assets*; Haddad, Olivier and De Gruchy, *The Potential and Perils of Partnership*.

64. Tiendrebeogo and Buykx, *Faith-Based Organisations and HIV/AIDS Prevention and Impact Mitigation in Africa*.

65. This was discussed in greater depth in Chapter 1 of this book.

66. De Gruchy et al., *Appreciating Assets*: 22.

67. See Olivier, Cochrane and Schmid, *ARHAP Literature Review*: 39–40.

68. See ZINGO, *Faith-based Organizations' Responses to HIV/AIDS in Livingstone, Lusaka and Kitwe, Zambia: Strategic Visioning for a Zambia Free of HIV/AIDS* (Lusaka: Zambia Interfaith Networking Group on HIV/AIDS and National AIDS Council of Zambia, 2002): 16.

69. Olivier, Cochrane and Schmid, *ARHAP Literature Review*; ZINGO, *Faith-based Organizations' Responses to HIV/AIDS in Livingstone, Lusaka and Kitwe, Zambia*.

70. Olivier, Cochrane and Schmid, *ARHAP Literature Review*: 65–6; Thomas Cannell, 'Funerals and AIDS: Resilience and decline in KwaZulu-Natal'. *Journal of Theology for Southern Africa* 125 (2006): 21–37.

71. Frederick Klaits, 'The widow in blue: death and the morality of remembering in Botswana's time of AIDS'. *Africa* 75(1) 2005: 48.

72. See Olivier, Cochrane and Schmid, *ARHAP Literature Review*.

73. Hansjörg Dilger, 'Healing the wounds of modernity: salvation, community and care in a neo-Pentecostal church in Dar es Salaam, Tanzania'. *Journal of Religion in Africa* 37 (2007): 72.

74. Dilger, 'Healing the wounds of modernity': 73.

75. Vhumani Magezi, 'Life Beyond Infection: Home-Based Pastoral Care to People With HIV-Positive Status Within a Context of Poverty' (D.Th. dissertation, University of Stellenbosch, 2005): 109–10.

76. See Jill Olivier, 'Exploring discourses of comparative advantage: Valuing and evaluating HIV/AIDS-engaged religious entities in sub-Saharan Africa'. Unpublished paper presented at the Conference on Religion Shaping Development, Birmingham, 21–23 July 2010.

77. De Gruchy et al., *Appreciating Assets*: 88. See also Reinikka and Svensson, *Working for God?*; Thomas et al, *Let Us Embrace*.

78. Norman C. Olsen, 'Reflections on faith and healing'. *Journal of the Association of Nurses in AIDS Care* 14(5) 2003: 73.

79. Tiendrebeogo and Buykx, *Faith-Based Organisations and HIV/AIDS Prevention and Impact Mitigation in Africa*: 28; Reinikka and Svensson, *Working for God?*; Thomas et al., *Let Us Embrace*.

80. See Olivier, 'Exploring discourses of comparative advantage'.

81. Interestingly, Agadjanian and Sen find that psychological support is reported more often than tangible support. They suggest that the latter tends to be co-ordinated by the leaders of religious congregations, sometimes with considerations of status coming into play (Agadjanian and Sen, 'Promises and challenges of faith-based AIDS care and support in Mozambique': 364).

82. See De Gruchy et al., *Appreciating Assets*.

83. Thomas et al., *Let Us Embrace*: 62–3.

84. Another way of describing care would be that it utilises a combination of performative and affective dimensions of religious community life. See Thomas et al., *Let Us Embrace*: 49.

85. See Tiendrebeogo and Buykx, *Faith-Based Organisations and HIV/AIDS Prevention and Impact Mitigation in Africa*: 46.

86. Johan Bouwer, 'Human dignity and HIV/AIDS'. *Scriptura* 95 (2007): 264, 268.

87. See http://www.positivemuslims.org.za.

88. See Positive Muslims, *HIV, AIDS and Islam: Reflections Based on Compassion, Responsibility and Justice* (Cape Town: Positive Muslims: 2004).

89. Nussbaum (ed.), *The Contribution of Christian Congregations to the Battle with HIV/AIDS at the Community Level*: 32.

90. Lucy Keogh and Katherine Marshall, *Faith Communities Engage in the HIV/AIDS Crisis: Lessons Learned and Paths Forward* (Washington: Centre for Religion, Peace and World Affairs, Georgetown University, 2007): 21–4.

91. De Gruchy et al., *Appreciating Assets*: 126.

92. Tearfund, *Faith Untapped*.

93. See Chapters 1 and 3 of this book.

94. Haddad, Olivier and De Gruchy, *The Potential and Perils of Partnership*: 52.

95. See Tiendrebeogo and Buykx, *Faith-Based Organisations and HIV/AIDS Prevention and Impact Mitigation in Africa*. FBO care and support activities need to be complemented by public health activities that support prevention: De Gruchy et al., *Appreciating Assets*: 80; Nussbaum (ed.), *The Contribution of Christian Congregations to the Battle with HIV/AIDS at the Community Level*: 24. This is, of course, an argument that must be made carefully as there are many groups and individuals who are powerfully engaged in both prevention and advocacy. See Keogh and Marshall, *Faith Communities Engage in the HIV/AIDS Crisis*: 25.

96. Steve de Gruchy, 'Like housework in the economy: The hidden ubiquity of religion in African wellbeing'. Presented at Religion and Health Connection Luncheon of the Inter-Faith Health Program of Rollins School of Public Health. Emory University, Atlanta, 2006.

97. Feiruz Surur and Mirgissa Kaba, 'The role of religious leaders in HIV/AIDS prevention, control and patient care and support: a pilot project in Jimma Zone'. *Northeast African Studies* 7(2) 2000: 59–80.

98. Hendriks, Erasmus and Mans, 'Congregations as providers of social service and HIV/AIDS care': 380–402; Klaus Nürnberger, 'Theology of AIDS: a Lutheran/Moravian case study'. *Scriptura* 81 (2002): 422–36.

99. Nussbaum (ed.), *The Contribution of Christian Congregations to the Battle with HIV/AIDS at the Community Level*: 38–9.

100. Agadjanian and Sen, 'Promises and challenges of faith-based AIDS care and support in Mozambique': 365.
101. See Haddad, Olivier and De Gruchy, *The Potential and Perils of Partnership*; Nürnberger, 'Theology of AIDS': 433; Makna Men, 'HIV/AIDS in Cambodia: Stigmatization, Isolation and the Intervention of Buddhist Monks' (M.A. thesis, Brown University, 2005).
102. World Council of Churches, *Facing AIDS: The Challenge, the Churches' Response* (Geneva: WCC Publications, 1997): 29.
103. Brown and Hendriks, 'Understanding HIV/AIDS through the dark lens of poverty': 403–15; Zamani Maqoko and Yolanda Dreyer, 'Child-headed households because of the trauma surrounding HIV/AIDS'. *Hervormde Teologiese Studies* 63(2) 2007: 729.
104. Victor Agadjanian, 'Gender, religious involvement, and HIV/AIDS prevention in Mozambique'. *Social Science and Medicine* 61(7) 2005: 1529–39.
105. Christoph Benn, *Does Faith Contribute to Healing?: Scientific Evidence for a Correlation Between Spirituality and Health* (Tübingen: German Institute for Medical Mission, 2001): 49.

Practitioner response

Edwina Ward

My response to the chapter by Jill Olivier and Paula Clifford arises out of experience in clinical pastoral education (CPE),[1] research in theological education and HIV and AIDS, in working with the African Network of Higher Education and Research in Theology, HIV and AIDS (ANHERTHA) and extensive teaching in the area of pastoral care and counselling. In the context of HIV and AIDS, training, education and recognition is lacking with regard to care giving. What is required is training in the counselling skills of listening, empathy, holistic caring, and ability to show compassion and offer meaning and purpose in life to those they care for. All of these skills are learned within the CPE process.

Much of what has been written on care giving in Africa does not seem to give sufficient recognition to, and appreciation for, the work of community-based volunteers.[2] Many of the care givers are older women. Many rely on their own pensions to bring up grandchildren and to feed large families, many are prevailed upon by the church to care for neighbours and fellow congregational members, and most are untrained and unskilled in the care and support they need when working with those affected by the epidemic. The community-based carers undergo many stressful situations, live in fear that they too may be stigmatised, and as volunteers receive no monetary recognition for their work.

Many care givers also lack support, both material and emotional, from religious organisations and it is these care givers who themselves need support and care when they are under pressure from coping with those who are HIV positive. When a care giver is confident and can adequately demonstrate the skills required to cope with daily activities, then burnout and lack of self-esteem are less likely. Quoting Lucy Steinitz, Barbara Schmid suggests that 'faith plays a huge role in people's response to HIV'[3] and, I would argue, it is this faith that keeps many community home-based care givers from total exhaustion.

Very often, community carers are volunteers in need of training and mutual support. Exploited in their services, they are the first to experience burnout because they feel inadequate in their work. In a recent study, Mfazo Madondo writes pointedly about the hurdles in volunteering. He states that 'people fail to see the significance of volunteering. For example, there is lack of trust in the volunteers by the community in general . . . lack of resources . . . such as gloves and nappies . . . in addition there is little support in the form of counselling, or what is called caring for the carers.'[4]

Madondo suggests that the future of volunteering will depend on the relationship between the government and religious organisations.[5] As was suggested by Olivier and Clifford, the motivation of individuals to be involved in care giving varies. According to Leila Patel: 'The idea of giving oneself for the benefit of others is not a new phenomenon; it can be traced to different epochs and has been expressed in different forms over the ages.'[6] But Madondo shows that many volunteers are hoping that in time they will receive employment or at least some remuneration.[7] This is an area where further research is necessary as the questions still remain: why do volunteers continue to give so much of their time and resources without remuneration; what role does faith play in driving their commitment to this service?

Professional care givers, such as nurses, are trained to save life and much of medical training has to do with finding a cure for illness. In the case of chronic illness and end-of-life care, this may no longer be possible. In my own experience, it is the nursing staff who are losing hope amidst the HIV and AIDS epidemic. Nursing sisters tell us in CPE that each day brings very few stories of hope. When they arrive at work they are confronted with children, mothers and patients who are dying, and they have no way of relieving them. Emotional and spiritual support in the form of prayer, comfort and compassion to both staff and patients is sorely needed.

We read in the work of Victor Frankl that meaning in life is what all seek even if we are at the end stages of life.[8] It has long been recognised that in addition to the physical and psychological aspects of patients with terminal illness, they will suffer existential distress as well. This shows that people who are desperately ill need to have answers that deal with issues concerning the meaning of life, the fear of death and the separation from loved ones.[9] These concerns seem greater in the experience of HIV and AIDS because of the stigma and judgement that is still part of people's lives. In the process of CPE, many find that people cope with their suffering when they find meaning in it. Spirituality or a relationship with God can give meaning and purpose to people's lives, sufferings and illness. It is important to note that patients who are spiritually active have less fear of death and less guilt about their illness.[10] Training of care givers is necessary if people who are suffering are to be given end-of-life care measures that include the existential domain, giving meaning in life and capacity for self-transcendence.[11]

There is, therefore, a need for further research in the area of spirituality and care. With so many people close to death we have yet to look at the spiritual needs of the dying. How are care givers to be trained for this task? Who will these care givers be and what skills do they require? At the root of spiritual care is compassion, being present to the patients in the midst of suffering.[12] This level of humanity provides hope and comfort and gives them an opportunity to find a sense of meaning, resolution and even peace in their last days. Those who undergo CPE are taught to be aware of their own values, beliefs and attitudes, particularly toward their own mortality. Moreover, they are taught to work with patients of different religious backgrounds or spiritual beliefs. The area of spiritual care and the need for understanding of religious and cultural rituals is underplayed in the area of care and support.

Notes

1. CPE is established in all continents and is a multi-cultural and inter-faith experience. It is a method and standard of training for ministry within a clinical environment. The focus is not on textbooks and lectures but upon disciplined and supervised reflection on real life experiences with people who are suffering and in

crisis – those called the living human document. Out of intense involvement with persons in need, and the feedback from peers and supervisors, students develop a new awareness of themselves as persons and of the needs of those to whom they minister. While most of the training is based in hospitals and hospices, the learning and growth can be applied to any pastoral situation – to home-based caring, prison visiting, counselling, youth work and caring for those affected and infected by HIV and AIDS.

2. This description is used by Helene Perold, René Carapinha and Salah Elzein Mohamed, *Five-Country Study on Service and Volunteering in Southern Africa: South Africa Country Report* (Johannesburg: Volunteer and Service Enquiry Southern Africa, 2006).

3. Barbara Schmid, 'What value does religion add to health services?' in *Collection of Concept Papers: ARHAP Conference, Monkey Valley, South Africa* (Cape Town: ARHAP, 2007): 27.

4. Mfazo C. Madondo, 'An Emerging Form of Church?: Community-Based Volunteers in HIV and AIDS Work as a Religious Health Asset' (M.Th. dissertation, University of KwaZulu-Natal, 2009).

5. Madondo, 'An Emerging Form of Church?'.

6. Leila Patel, 'Theoretical perspectives on the political economy of civic service' in *Service Enquiry: Service in the 21st Century,* edited by H. Perold, S. Stroud and M. Sherraden (Johannesburg: Global Service Institute and Volunteer and Service Enquiry Southern Africa, 2003): 89.

7. Madondo, 'An Emerging Form of Church?'.

8. Victor Frankl, *Man's Search for Meaning* (New York: Simon and Schuster, 1984); Victor Frankl, *The Will to Meaning* (London: Souvenir Press, 1971).

9. G. Fitchett and G. Handzo, 'Spiritual assessment, screening and intervention' in *Psycho-oncology,* edited by Jimmie C. Holland et al. (New York: Oxford University Press, 1998): 790–808.

10. L.C. Kaldijian, 'End-of-life decisions in HIV patients: The role of spiritual beliefs'. *AIDS* 12 (1998): 103–7.

11. John Patton, 'The "holy complexity" of the clinical: Some reflections on pastoral supervision and theology'. *Journal of Supervision and Training in Ministry* 13 (1991): 234–5.

12. Edwina Ward, 'Listening with the heart: The ministry of presence'. *Theologia Viatorum* 31(1) 2007: 136.

16

Stories of hope
Navigating HIV pathways of life

PHUMZILE ZONDI-MABIZELA

I was fortunate to be diagnosed with HIV when I was already empowered with information and knew that it was not a death sentence. I was diagnosed in 1999 after applying for life-insurance cover. I did not get any pre-test counselling and if it were not for prior knowledge about HIV, I would have been even more devastated.

My results were sent directly to my doctor two weeks after the test. That was the longest two weeks of my life. If it was not for my faith, I would not have survived. It took a long time for me to be able to share my status with other people, except for a few friends who supported me from the outset. Disclosure was a long journey because I had to be ready to deal with the different responses from people. I openly started talking about my status in public meetings in 2001. It was even more difficult for me to share my status with my family, especially my mother, and I only informed her after a year. I spent a long time preparing my children first before sharing my status with them. I had to make sure that they were not left with the fear of losing their only parent because I was a single parent when I was diagnosed.

I was fortunate because I was still very healthy when I was diagnosed. Therefore, I knew that I would live positively for a long time. I met my husband in 2001 and in 2002 we were blessed with a healthy baby girl. This is one area that is often problematic for women: they assume that HIV takes away their right to become mothers. I have used my own story to encourage other women who are living with HIV not to give up hope.

I equipped myself with as much information on the latest research and developments on HIV and AIDS as I could. I realised that HIV is a manageable condition and one can live for a long time with it. I also learned that in the North with all the available interventions, including anti-retrovirals (ARVs), it was treated like any other chronic disease. This has given me power and control over my health as opposed to viewing myself as a victim.

As a church leader, I have used every opportunity to challenge the church to develop positive responses to HIV in collaboration with others who are HIV positive. Being a member of the African Network of Religious Leaders Living With or Personally Affected by HIV or AIDS (ANERELA) has empowered me with many skills I have shared on many platforms all over the world. My theological studies and my past work with the Ujamaa Centre for Community Development and Research has also provided me with ammunition to openly discredit and reject negative interpretations of the Bible that are used to discriminate against people living with HIV.

I started taking ARVs in June 2006. My CD4 count had come right down to 146. Fortunately, because I have medical insurance I did not have to wait to go on treatment and realised that being financially independent empowers one to make decisions and access resources timeously. I started off by thinking of all the horror stories I had heard about ARVs but eventually chose to be positive and believe that God wants me to live. I was convinced that ARVs didn't have much of a choice but to work for me. The challenge for those living with HIV and the affected is to defy all the negative teachings and beliefs about HIV and AIDS, and claim life in abundance through Christ.

Taking ARVs comes with new challenges and I had to deal with a range of side effects. I struggled for the first two weeks but after that learned to manage the side effects. One example of taking things into one's own hands was when I struggled with peripheral neuropathy, which is one of the side effects. I went to three different doctors and none of them knew what was wrong with me. I then did my own research on the Internet and found out what the condition is called, what causes it and how it can be treated. I went back to my doctor armed with this information and only after that was I given the correct medication to treat the condition.

I have also benefited from talking to other people who have lived with HIV for much longer than I. When I come across challenges that are not that easy to deal with, I consult other empowered people living with HIV and usually they openly share their experiences and information. This has enriched my life as I

396

now know a lot more than I would have, had I not openly sought other people who are going through the same experiences.

I have not directly experienced any stigma and discrimination. I also have not allowed my life to be controlled by fear and shame. This is a choice I make on a daily basis to live my life to the best of my ability without worrying about other people's responses. When I was pregnant I knew for a fact that people felt that I was irresponsible but I made it a point to remind people of my right as a woman living with HIV to be a mother.

I took it upon myself to educate people that HIV does not take away one's sexuality but what is important is practising safer sex all the time. In order to promote holistic prevention strategies, it has been important for me to talk about the importance of the condom, with which most churches have problems. The reality is that condoms can save people's lives, including mine as a married woman.

Before my diagnosis I was only a gender activist, mostly concerned about the rights of women. But my diagnosis reshaped my life story. I became aware of all the injustices meted out against those who are HIV positive. The saddest part of it all for me has been the indifference of the church. The church has taken too long to develop positive theologies that promote acceptance and support for those who are HIV positive. Some churches have been very good at caring for the sick and dying but have not done enough to support those who are still healthy but struggle with issues like stigma and discrimination.

My journey with HIV has not been a smooth and easy one but it makes me a better person each day and has helped me to come to terms with my mortality. HIV has also taught me to be grateful for every day that is given to me and I always try my best to inspire and encourage others who may be struggling with difficult conditions or situations.

FAGHMEDA MILLER

I became infected with HIV in 1994 while married to my Malawian husband and living in Malawi. I discovered only after his death that I, like him, was infected. The first thing that went through my mind when they told me that I am HIV positive was the shame I had brought on my family.

I therefore decided to keep this information to myself. After all, I thought, it would not be long till I died. Death, however, did not come. No one told me that there is a difference between being HIV positive and having AIDS. So I went back to the hospital looking for answers and was told that I can live a long productive life being HIV positive if I take good care of myself. I received counselling on a regular basis and slowly built up enough confidence, acceptance and courage to live.

My life and attitude as well as my personality changed. I had a mission and purpose to become a spokesperson for Muslims living with HIV. I decided to disclose my status on a community radio station. It was met with mixed feelings as well as denial and often people state that as a Muslim one could never contract this disease. However, nothing anyone has said or done can stop me from talking openly about my HIV status. It has been a long and often lonely road for me but I will never give up. I believe that eventually the Muslim community's eyes will open, their attitude will change and they will come to see the need for HIV awareness through education programmes in our society.

Since being diagnosed, I have had three dreams and am fortunate to say that after living with HIV for the past fifteen years I have mostly achieved these. After many years of struggle, my dream of starting a support group for Muslims living with HIV was realised. I am so grateful for everyone who stood by me and supported me in getting the group going. I decided to disclose my status not only for myself but also for all other HIV positive Muslims who suffer discrimination, stigmatisation and disrespect in our community. I have seen many HIV positive people die and often it would feel like a part of me was dying too but my will to survive and live positively is strong.

I do not just help run the support group in our organisation, Positive Muslims, but also do home counselling and awareness programmes in different communities. Often people in my community do not want me to talk about the hardships and rejections suffered in the first few years after disclosing my status. Perhaps this is from feeling guilty. But what they do not know is this that I am fighting harder to change the mindset and behaviour of people, to allow those who want to disclose to have easier acceptance in society than I have had. Today I no longer believe that HIV and AIDS is a curse from God as some religious leaders led me to believe. In fact, I see it as a blessing as it has given me an avenue to help others, no matter the obstacles, and I appreciate life as I have never before.

My second dream was to write a book about my past fifteen years as an HIV positive woman. Though completed, it has not yet been published but I feel the time is not right for this. My third dream was to fulfil my holy pilgrimage to Mecca and this I completed with pride, showing that you can achieve anything you set your mind to, regardless of your HIV status.

In addition to the above, I have also done several television programmes locally and internationally, appeared in various magazines, newspapers, pamphlets and documentaries and on radio stations in Cape Town and Johannesburg. I have my own documentary 'The Malawian kiss' right on the top of my list. Yet I still feel that I have not achieved enough, to encourage people to talk openly about their status, even though one magazine referred to me as the woman 'setting the lead to save a nation'.

In the year 2000 I received the Femina Women of Courage Award and was nominated for Women That Made a Difference in their community. Despite this, I remain at the end of the day the shy woman my family knows best, her sole purpose being to be as outspoken as humanly possible about HIV and AIDS.

I always say that it is not the HI virus that is killing us but rather the stigma attached to it. The attitude of people is killing us quicker than the disease itself. It is for this reason that I will continue to speak out and show that we can live positively.

NOKUTHULA BIYELA

I am 32 years old and live in Imbali, Pietermaritzburg. I am from a family of four: three sisters and one brother. My mother is a single parent and unemployed and as a result I was raised by my grandmother. I grew up as a typical township girl. I had fun and enjoyed music, went to church and attended township functions. Part of my responsibility was to work as a care giver for relatives' children and to care for my younger siblings. This meant that I learned caring and housework at an early age. I had to do all these duties for survival as there was minimal income to care for my siblings and other cousins while sharing my grandmother's house. I began my early education at St Nicholas Primary School in Edendale, walking for an hour every day from home in Imbali through Dambuza to Edendale. Then later I attended Georgetown High School. As a teenager I started dating and really had fun in a love relationship. Life was so good. Everything was exciting and there were no complications then.

In 1995, I was in grade 9 and had severe migraine headaches. I remember that I could not write the final-year mathematics exam paper because of my headache. In 1996 there was a big change in my life. My boyfriend moved to Durban to further his studies at Mangosuthu Technikon. I was so lonely most of the time and I really missed him. The headaches came back and I went to a clinic to check on the problem. Unfortunately, I was simply given headache tablets. I was so frustrated because I knew there was more to this headache and that they should refer me to a hospital. But this did not happen. When the headache tablets were finished, the pain remained. I really suffered that year.

In 1996, I completed high school and started looking for a job. This was very difficult as it was not easy to find one. My first job was at Steers Restaurant where I worked for three months before the contract was terminated. After that I looked for piece work in the city and this was very difficult. My grandmother's pension was unable to pay for tertiary education so I needed to look for jobs for survival but I was young and straight from school with no experience. Life was very demanding and challenging because deep down in my heart I wanted to help my grandmother as I saw that she was struggling. But I was inexperienced and young.

Life was very stressful and my headaches returned on and off. I suddenly remembered that three years earlier at school there were HIV and AIDS awareness campaigns that highlighted meningitis that resulted in chronic headaches. I was very scared that maybe this was my problem. So in 1997 I went for an HIV test. The clinic sister began with pre-test counselling that prepared me for the real news about my status. Then my blood was taken to the laboratory and after three weeks I came back for my results. This was a turning point of my life because the news was very bad and I was diagnosed with the HI virus. It came as a great shock to me as a young girl looking forward to a great future. I was devastated and asked many questions with no answers.

Fortunately, at that time I heard of a group that was newly formed for people living with HIV. I became interested as I really did not know what to do and joined this support group for people living with HIV called Siyaphila (*Siyaphila* means 'we are alive even though we are HIV positive'). This group was very helpful in that I learned about positive living and sharing life with other men and women living with HIV which assisted me in learning how to come to terms with my own struggles and challenges as a young woman living with HIV. Bible studies became a life-assuring anchor as I learned that I am loved by God even though I am HIV positive. This was a real message of hope as I thought of the stigma and curse that is often associated with us. Learning these ways of reading the Bible assisted in developing my personal relationship with God. Gradually, through ongoing care and support from members and co-ordinators of Siyaphila, I learned to accept my status and live positively with HIV.

My new life within the Siyaphila support group began with election as the administration officer. This meant I was dealing with registration of new members and upgrading old members as well as doing follow-up on defaulters. This gave me access to a larger pool and variety of members. At that time food parcels were made available for people in need. I learned a lot about myself, first that I needed to be grateful for little things I have as I was with people who shared their hardships with me, some of which were heavier than mine. Then later with the help of Bongi Zengele of the Ujamaa Centre, I learned how to write a funding proposal. This was very exciting and challenging at the same time, for it meant we were working at odd hours and under extreme pressure so as to meet deadlines. This did not compare with the joys of knowing that not a single proposal was rejected. We were accessing government funding from the Department of Health and also from the Southern African Catholic Bishops' Conference (SACBC) that enabled us to change people's lives. We worked as a team and faced challenges but dealing with them directly was very helpful as it contributed to our personal growth. It is not easy to work with people in general as there are many expectations. This is felt even more in the context of HIV and AIDS as there is minimal or no direct support going to people living with HIV. So the initiatives geared at helping are often overwhelmed by enormous demands and frustrations felt by communities infected and affected. Siyaphila is one of the rare organisations that is community-based and takes the needs of HIV positive people seriously. However, this creates demands from the recipients of services as they become frustrated if their needs are not met. Working with Siyaphila has taught me to respect life, to be kind to myself and the people I serve, and to appreciate life as a special gift from God.

In 2004 I was invited by the SACBC to attend ARV treatment literacy training in Johannesburg as part of preparing me to start programmes for Siyaphila. This particular training was facilitated by the Treatment Action Campaign. For the first time I learned about the possibility of women living with HIV becoming pregnant. This was a life-changing experience because I had felt the loss of not having a baby from the time I knew my HIV status. Now, hearing about this possibility brought new life to me as I dreamed of becoming a mother one day. My partner was thrilled at the news. So we contacted our family doctor and began preparing for a new life. A baby is regarded as a blessing from God and for the woman as confirmation of her womanhood. It was a time full of mixed emotions, not really believing that I could have a baby and yet excited at the thought of being a mother.

In 2005 I conceived and was very happy, as was my partner. Unfortunately, I had a miscarriage towards the end of the first trimester, which made me very sad. It felt like a dark cloud hovering over my life. I was devastated and asked myself what went wrong? I felt a deep sense of failure as a woman. The critical part was the fact that I was so careful and thought I had everything in order. I remember how I cried and did not want to be comforted. I never realised how I had bonded so deeply with my unborn baby. I remember how I could not sleep and when my friends came to see me I was not able to communicate my deepest pain and hurt. The tears were rolling over my face without stop. How could I lose something so precious? But the reality was that my baby was no more and I had to deal with my loss. My grandmother was very supportive and helped me to deal with this pain. My partner responded by promising that we were going to have another baby and that God would give to us again. He felt the pain of losing our unborn baby but had his own way of dealing with it.

In our second attempt to have a baby our family doctor put me on the HAART (highly active anti-retroviral therapy) programme for pregnant women. Three months later I conceived. The pregnancy went well and there were no complications. When the baby was due I went to hospital. I had a very difficult labour and the baby was distressed and lacked oxygen, which led to a C-section. My beautiful baby boy, Thobani, was born with cerebral palsy and epilepsy. This meant facing new challenges again. All my joy seemed to be accompanied with challenges. While celebrating the birth of my little angel, he comes with more challenges. I was happy to have a baby but sad because of his health condition. I was scared about how to deal with these challenges as I had never dealt with cerebral palsy and epilepsy before. I am a brave person: this I know because I have dealt with the major challenge of HIV in my life. But now I was really overwhelmed and confused and did not know what to do. I began questioning God – where are you in all this?

As Africans we tend to consult with our ancestors when we are in this position. Even though I observed all the cultural rituals as expected in our tradition, I am still lost. It seems as if there are no answers and I am rejected and forsaken. I am stuck and left in the dark even though I have done good things at home and supported my siblings as a breadwinner. I do not earn a lot of money but the little I get I share with my family. I belong to a church, pay my tithes and support all the initiatives as well as visiting the sick. I am conscious of the love of God in my life but fail to comprehend why he or she would allow so many challenges to affect my life. Is HIV not enough? This experience has really left me confused, angry and unsure of the future. The support from my partner, my grandmother and many wonderful friends has really been a stronghold for me. They have made it possible for me to wake up every morning with a new purpose and to face the day with its challenges.

My life with Thobani began as a tough one as I had to learn about cerebral palsy and epilepsy. I read and searched the Internet looking for information about his health condition. He attends weekly occupational therapy at Northdale hospital and the epilepsy clinic at Edendale hospital. This is my journey and I am asking for your prayers for God to continue raising my son. I am continually praying for a miracle in his life as I see him growing bigger and responding to my voice and the children around him. This reminds me that I have a treasure hidden in this baby of mine and I am convinced that he really is a beacon of hope in my life.

JOHANNES PETRUS MOKGETHI-HEATH

Dear God! What else can go wrong? Now Paul is losing his sight. The last number of years had been extremely turbulent. First, there was the painful divorce which ended my unhappy and loveless marriage. I had been moved to a new parish. I was blessed to have a very supportive bishop and church council but the emotional and spiritual upheaval was wreaking havoc with my life. I had poured myself anew into different areas of ministry, initiating an outreach programme to the street children in Hillbrow, the flat land I served as priest. In the process I had met Paul, a pastor serving in a gay and lesbian affirming congregation in Hillbrow and his ministry of service, quietly washing dishes for street children, had drawn me to him. Nine months after I had met Paul, he moved into the church house in which I was living. I was trapped between my theological understanding that homosexuality was against God's will and my personal knowledge of a homosexual orientation. As we co-habited in the rectory our friendship deepened into a relationship.

Now it was two and an half years later, 18 May 2000. The bishop had moved me from Hillbrow to Mayfair. Paul and I had lived happily together through this change in our lives. Ministry in the parish was going well but Paul was not well. He had been continually ill for weeks on end and now his sight was going. He could

403

no longer see well enough to read or even watch television. I suggested to Paul that it was time that we went to have an HIV test. We were both frightened but with Paul's illness and further weakening of his sight it was time. After contacting a mutual friend, we went to see a doctor to deal with our worst fears. The results came out on 20 May and were frightening. Not only were both Paul and I found to be HIV positive but for both of us immunity had been seriously compromised already. Our CD4 counts, measuring the white blood cells and thus the level of immunity, was just above 200 but our viral load, measuring the number of HI viruses per millilitre of blood, was well over 160 000 – basically AIDS defining. The doctor gave us the devastating news: 'If we can get you treatment, we might be able to look at another five, maybe six years. If we can't, I'm afraid you might have between six and eighteen months.' The irony of course was that Paul's eye condition had nothing to do with HIV. His continuous flu and self-medication had caused a temporary paralysis of his retina, which meant his eyes could not focus.

I was filled with a deep sorrow. Suddenly all I could think of was David, my son, who was then only five years old. He would grow up without his father. If I could not access ARVs, I might live until he was seven. If by some miracle I managed to get medication, then I might live until he was eleven or twelve. Then there was the challenge of getting medication. I was certainly on the church medical aid but Paul was not, as the rules of the diocese did not allow it. In addition there were the challenges about accessing ARVs from the church medical aid. How confidential was confidential? If I applied for ARVs, how long would it be before this information was communicated to the bishop and my churchwardens? And then there was the cost. Tentative investigations had revealed that if I accessed ARVs through the medical aid it might cover me for four to six months a year. There was just no way in which I would be able to afford my own top-up, let alone buying medication for Paul.

There was yet one more reality. My mother had died the previous October and as a family we were very much still in mourning. How do I bring my family the news that my doctor says without medication I might have a maximum of eighteen months to live? I had to find a way. At the time Baragwanath Hospital, the state hospital serving the greater Soweto area, was being used for various drug trials related to HIV. Conditions were very strict but our doctor had managed to get our names down on the list. What followed was a further two months of first screening and then waiting for the trial to start. Under this particular trial, they needed people with a CD4 count of around 200 (we qualified), drug naive (we were as far as HIV was concerned) and able to attend Baragwanath at least once a week (again we were able). Both Paul and I were shortlisted for the trial. Its objective was to see if the introduction of steroids at the beginning of HIV therapy would reduce the side effects and thus help people to stay on therapy. There were three control groups receiving three, four and five different ARV drugs respectively; and the test groups receiving the three, four or five drugs, but with a steroid added. Paul was selected to receive the three drugs and I received the five. Within 24 hours I was no longer able to keep food down. I lost weight rapidly and was getting progressively weaker. I could not cope with the stress of trying to live a life of silent shame and so I first went to speak to my father about my HIV status and then to my bishop.

My father heard me with compassion but asked me please to tell my sisters because this was not something he could bear alone. The bishop was supportive, assuring me that he wished to share many further years of ministry with me, but cautioned me not to share my status with anyone else. He was caught under the same stigma as I and sought to find a way of protecting my employment. All the time I was getting weaker. It was clear that the medication was not agreeing with me but at the same time my viral load was dropping dramatically. The medication was working but my body could not cope. Two weeks into the treatment I asked my sisters to rush me to casualty as I thought I had a bone or something stuck in my throat. There was nothing but my oesophagus had been torn as a result of constant vomiting. The advice from the doctor in casualty was to try to control my vomiting! Twenty-eight days after starting treatment I had to take the difficult decision to stop therapy because it was poisoning my system. I knew there was a risk that I would not be able to get on to further medication but by now I was being rolled around in a wheelchair, no longer able to walk.

My sister again took me to the doctor who had first diagnosed me. He recommended me to a specialist physician in a private hospital. I refused, knowing that I could not afford a private hospital. My sister ignored me and took me anyway. Thank God she did or I would have died that day. I had developed a severe reaction to the medication called lactic acidosis that was poisoning my entire system. I was admitted to ICU immediately. My new doctor asked who he should call. I said Paul, my churchwardens and my bishop. Soon after that I aspirated and lost consciousness. I am told that the bishop was there and gave me the last rites. My sisters and father came to see me – Paul had let them know. Paul, with whom I had shared the last two and a half years of my life, was left outside – only close family were allowed into ICU.

I survived. A caring and informed doctor had managed to coax me back to life. I became only the third person in the world to have survived that level of lactic acidosis and the first without having had a full liver transplant. After painful weeks of strengthening I was back at work. The other great challenge became finding medication. I was put on a second-line regimen by my new doctor. The church medical aid rejected it as it was too expensive. Another drug combination was suggested and even then I was left with a substantial amount to top up. The church was going through the process of finding a new medical aid and the new provider they were looking at did not offer nearly as much cover, particularly for HIV treatment, as the current one. I went in to speak to the diocesan chancellor about this. His simple response was: 'Why should the rest of the clergy be penalised with higher membership costs because of something you have brought on yourself?' Thankfully, Paul was responding extremely well to his trial medication and continued to improve in health.

I went to see the bishop and indicated to him that I really felt that God was calling me to do something to assist the church in dealing with HIV. He was again very supportive. The church, however, did not have the money to support me in an initiative like this, so if I found the money to support myself I had his blessing. In the August of the following year a single event took place that would forever change my life.

In 2001 the Archbishop of Cape Town had been charged with drawing together 'An All-African Anglican Consultation on HIV and AIDS', which included a number of archbishops from around the continent. How does a simple parish priest from Mayfair in Johannesburg get invited to the biggest consultation of this kind to have happened in the Anglican communion? You bribe your way in! A dear friend who had been doing much of the spade work finally said: 'You don't sneak in – you keep your head down and pretend you are meant to be there.' At the opening service a young priest from Uganda addressed the assembled delegates: 'My name is Reverend Gideon Byamugisha. I am an Anglican priest and I am HIV positive.' For the first time I knew I was not alone. During the consultation I met and talked to Gideon. He shared with me a dream he had of holding a retreat for HIV positive clergy; a retreat to give support and help them to understand they were not alone.

By the following February the meeting was taking place in Nyanga Hills in eastern Zimbabwe. The challenge had been how to identify participants. A broad invitation had been made for clergy who were really interested in HIV in the hope that some who were really interested in HIV would be so because they were HIV positive. Eventually the meeting took place and 40 people attended. Eight of us were HIV positive, one having tested HIV positive at the mobile voluntary counselling and testing (VCT) site set up as part of the retreat. We believed that more needed to be done and a follow-up meeting was planned. By then Gideon had been made a canon within his diocese of Namarembe and the spade work for the meeting was done by a newly established group called the Friends of Canon Gideon Foundation (FOCAGIFO).

Again 40 clergy and lay people gathered. This time it was at the Collins Hotel in Mukono, Uganda and all the participants were either living with or personally affected by HIV. I had been asked to facilitate the meeting. We emerged with a newly formed network, ANERELA. We developed a vision, mission, goals and objectives. We were to be a support network that challenged stigma and discrimination around HIV and AIDS, and we were to help our respective faith communities engage more fully on HIV. The bold vision said it all: 'A world where HIV and AIDS related stigma, transmissions and deaths are eliminated.' Right from the start we acknowledged that the stigma and discrimination around HIV were not unique to the Christian church but were something faced by all faith communities. Henceforth, we would be an inter-faith network seeking to establish country-based networks that would mobilise members and empower them into positive living and stimulating congregational responses. A steering committee was elected and I was asked to co-ordinate the work of this new network.

There was no money and a co-ordinator who had no idea about writing funding proposals – it's not the sort of thing you are taught in a seminary. I started the work on this network in my parish office in Mayfair. News of the network slowly grew and within a relatively short period of time I was being invited to speaking engagements across Africa and later the world. On one such occasion, at the International Conference on AIDS and Sexually-Transmitted Illnesses in Africa (ICASA) held in Nairobi in September 2003, mere months after the network had begun, I sat with a friend who worked for USAID and he helped me to develop the first funding proposal. At the same conference I also met the international co-ordinator of the Global Network of People Living with HIV and AIDS (GNP+). We were immediately invited to come and launch this new network at their conference for people living with HIV, which was to take place the next month in Kampala. Space was created within the very busy Thirteenth International Conference for People Living with HIV. Never before had ordained members of faith communities been willing to publicly state their HIV status and identify in that way with people living with HIV. An evening launch of ANERELA was planned and very well attended. The network had consciously elected to identify strongly with people living with HIV by launching in this forum.

ANERELA started launching country networks. The first was Kenya, followed quickly by South Africa, Uganda and Malawi. We soon realised that if we were to overcome the stigma related to HIV, we would have to address the prevention messages being used. The popular message of the day (as it still is in many places) was ABC. The challenge with ABC was that it applied hierarchically and addressed sex only as a means of transmission. As one would typically say: 'Abstain; if you cannot abstain be faithful; and if you cannot be faithful use a condom.' There were, of course, many challenges with this. It meant that only sexually promiscuous people needed the condom, an opinion that led many faith communities to reject the condom as a means of HIV prevention. Then there was the issue of virgins getting married and as soon as they went to the clinic for their first pregnancy, they tested HIV positive. No one had spoken to them of the need to know both your own and your spouse's HIV status. This model did not address discordant couples; nor did it address different issues like prevention of mother-to-child transmission (PMTCT), people who use drugs (injecting drug use) and cultural scarification (particularly circumcision with a common spear). It also did not take into consideration social and environmental factors that increased vulnerability to HIV, thus placing the entire burden of HIV on an individual. Our response was to develop the SAVE prevention strategy (Safer practices, Available medical and nutritional interventions, Voluntary but regular counselling and testing, and Empowerment).

As 2004 arrived, the network was reaching ever more people and my health was again experiencing challenges. When it comes to cholesterol I have always been told the simple motto is 'strive for five'. The medication I was on (by this time a battery of protease inhibitors) was driving up my cholesterol. My doctor started panicking when my cholesterol reached 14.3 as I should have been having heart attacks or strokes. In addition, the last component of my anti-retroviral treatment (ART) regimen was a drug that fell into the thymidine category which, as can happen in some cases, started driving my lactic acid levels up again. It started with slight stiffness in my legs and was soon affecting my walking. Lactic acidosis had set in yet again. I was immediately admitted to hospital. This time I knew what lactic acidosis was. I had conducted a number of funerals for people who had died of lactic acidosis and now knew it was no joke. This time round I was really scared. I asked a friend to come and see me in hospital and she helped me draft my last will and testament. I know these sorts of things should always be in place but mine needed serious updating and I needed to make sure that both Paul and David were properly taken care of. They were to jointly benefit from my church pension. My sisters came in to see me. We cried together and tried to be strong together. Paul came to see me every day. We were all waiting for the worst and I was taken off all medication yet again. The problem is that it takes time for the body to clear toxic levels of lactic acid, mostly because the organs are themselves poisoned by high levels of lactic acid. Unbelievably, my levels began to drop and four days later I was back running the parish and ANERELA. I was taken off all medication. My doctor felt my body needed a break. We would keep off medication till my CD4 count indicated we should start again. It ended up being three years later.

Much has happened in the intervening years. My work at ANERELA grew to the point where I asked the Bishop of Johannesburg to release me from full-time parish work to become a self-supporting priest within the diocese. As a civil society speaker at the 2006 United Nations General Assembly review I was able to initiate the message, 'HIV is a virus, not a moral condition, not a moral issue'. Demand for the message and presence of ANERELA across the world led us to launch INERELA (International Network of Religious Leaders Living With or Personally Affected by HIV and AIDS) at the Seventeenth International AIDS Conference in Mexico City in 2008. ANERELA became INERELA Africa. As the years passed, through our own personal experience the message began to emerge: 'HIV is something you can live with, not something you have to die from.' With the knowledge we have today there is no reason why one more person needs to become infected with HIV; and certainly no reason why one more person needs to die of AIDS-related illnesses.

After being together for ten years, Paul and I finally got married on 26 April 2008. It was a very difficult decision. This had nothing to do with whether we loved each other or not – that much was obvious. It had to do with the response we would receive from the church. Having wrestled with it for many years, I came to understand that God created me the man I was with the sexuality I have. And just as it is with the rest of creation, when God created me God could look at me and say, 'It is good!' It was the church that had a problem with my sexuality, not God. I felt that I could no longer deny Paul the commitment and security the state now allowed us within the institution of marriage. The Anglican Church has to be true to its own statements, so I am no longer able to hold a licence as a priest within it. As painful as this has been, this has yet again led to an expanded vision and understanding of the call God has placed on my heart.

Again, through my own experience, I have come to understand that exclusion leads to vulnerability. Double the stigma will lead to double the discrimination. Double the discrimination will lead to double the vulnerability. As a result we see women, refugees, migrant labourers and sex workers; lesbian, gay, bisexual, transgender and inter-sex people (LGBTI); and disabled people all exposed to additional levels of vulnerability to HIV. It is not just about justice or human rights. If we as people of faith wish to respond fully to the love of God which is so generously extended to us, we are compelled to reduce each others' isolation and exclusion that leads to greater vulnerability to HIV. As I reflect on my journey over the past ten years of living positively and openly with HIV, I can see the remarkable healing touch of God on my life. I also see that God has chosen to use HIV as the lens through which we can observe communities of faith and through which God in infinite mercy chooses to bring healing to these communities. Through this process we are enabled to become more fully who God created us to be.

Contributors

NOKUTHULA BIYELA, co-ordinator of Siyaphila Community-Based Organisation for People Living with HIV and AIDS, is a community-based ARV treatment trainer and field worker for Ujamaa Centre for Theological Community Development and Research in the University of Kwa-Zulu Natal. Having lived with HIV for ten years, she is committed to fight for the protection of human rights for others living with HIV and to ensure there is greater involvement of HIV positive people in all policy decisions related to the epidemic.

GIDEON BYAMUGISHA is a goodwill ambassador on HIV and AIDS for Christian AID, United Kingdom and chair of the Friends of Canon Gideon Foundation, Uganda. He was the first HIV positive religious leader in Africa to publicly disclose his HIV status and is a passionate activist who seeks to fight stigma, shame, denial and discrimination associated with HIV and AIDS. He works extensively throughout Africa in promulgating comprehensive HIV prevention approaches.

EZRA CHITANDO is the theology consultant for the Ecumenical HIV and AIDS Initiative in Africa and associate professor of history and phenomonology of religion at the University of Zimbabwe. He has published widely on various aspects of religion in Africa and has recently been researching the area of masculinities and HIV and AIDS.

PAULA CLIFFORD is head of theology, Christian AID, United Kingdom. She has travelled extensively in Africa, South East Asia, the Caribbean, and central and South America. This has included working with Christian Aid partner organisations and church leaders on HIV and AIDS. She has published papers entitled 'Theology and the HIV/AIDS epidemic' and 'HIV in Asia: theological and cultural perspectives'.

STEVE DE GRUCHY was head of the School of Religion and Theology and professor of theology and development at the University of KwaZulu-Natal at the time of his death in February 2010. He was a senior researcher in the African Religious Health Assets Programme where he designed research tools and undertook research towards understanding the contribution of religion to public health in the HIV and AIDS context.

PHILIPPE DENIS is professor of history of Christianity at the School of Religion and Theology, University of KwaZulu-Natal. He is also director of the Sinomlando Centre for Oral History and Memory Work, which includes a programme of psycho-social support to orphans and vulnerable children in the context of HIV and AIDS. He is engaged in research on the history of HIV and AIDS in sub-Saharan Africa.

FARID ESACK is professor of the study of Islam and head of the Department of Religion Studies at the University of Johannesburg. He is a co-founder of Positive Muslims, a South African organisation working to support Muslims living with HIV. He has written extensively on the interface of Islam and HIV and with Sarah Chiddy has co-edited *Islam and AIDS: Between Scorn, Pity and Justice.*

MARTHA FREDERIKS is professor of missiology at the Faculty of Humanities of Utrecht University and director of the Centre for Intercultural Theology, Inter-Religious Dialogue, Missiology and Ecumenism. Her research focuses on inter-religious dialogue, particularly Christian-Muslim relations, and developments in African Christianity and theology. As part of the research into African theology, she co-ordinates a research programme on HIV, AIDS, religion and gender.

BEVERLEY HADDAD is director of the Theology and Development Programme and director of the Collaborative for HIV and AIDS, Religion and Theology at the School of Religion and Theology, University of KwaZulu-Natal. She is engaged in research in the field of gender and HIV, and the response of the Christian church to the epidemic.

UTE HEDRICH is an ordained pastor and head of the HIV and AIDS and Ecumenical Women's Affairs Departments in the Institute for Ecumenism, Mission and Global Responsibility of the Evangelical Church of Westphalia. She is also a board member and chair of the Committee on Ethics, Theology and HIV and AIDS of Action against AIDS, Germany, as well as a founding member of the German Church Network on HIV and AIDS Counselling.

GENEVIEVE JAMES is the project director of the Campaign for Learning at the University of South Africa. She is concerned with issues pertaining to violence against children and the consequent implications in the context of HIV and AIDS. She has prepared a story book and accompanying facilitator's guide for children in order to create awareness of rape and other forms of sexual abuse.

NYOKABI KAMAU is senior lecturer and director of the Institute of Life Long Learning, St Paul's University, Limuru in Kenya where she co-ordinates a Masters degree in Community Pastoral Care and HIV and AIDS. She has recently been appointed as the gender mentor for Oxfam in the Kenya and Tanzania pastoralist programmes. Her research interests include gender, sexuality, HIV and AIDS, culture, politics and education.

DOMOKA LUCINDA MANDA works for the College of Medicine, University of Malawi. Her research interests pay close attention to issues affecting women and women's health in Africa, especially in the context of HIV and AIDS. Her activist work involves addressing issues, including HIV and AIDS, that impact negatively on the education of girl children in Malawi.

GREG MANNING from Australia is a project officer in the Micah Network, an international network of evangelical Christian relief, development and justice organisations. He worked in India between 1993 and 2007 on the development and scaling-up of health care services designed by drug users and now applies these lessons about life, health, justice and respect to a range of issues emerging from the Micah Network's experiences of HIV and AIDS.

MONICA JYOTSNA MELANCHTHON is professor of Old Testament studies at Gurukul Lutheran Theological College, Chennai. She has researched and written in the area of gender and HIV and AIDS in India as well as the interpretation of biblical texts from the perspective of HIV and AIDS.

FAGHMEDA MILLER works for Positive Muslims, a non-governmental organisation operating in South Africa that focuses its programmes on Muslims living with HIV. She was the first Muslim woman in South Africa to publicly disclose her positive HIV status and works extensively in HIV and AIDS advocacy work through interviews on radio and television. She recently completed a documentary on her life story, *The Malawian Kiss*.

JOHANNES PETRUS MOKGETHI-HEATH is an ordained priest in the Anglican Church of Southern Africa. After publicly disclosing his HIV status, he assisted in establishing the African Network of Religious Leaders Infected or Affected by HIV or AIDS. He has since also established an international office of the organisation and is engaged in HIV and AIDS advocacy work globally.

ALISON MUNRO is director of the AIDS Office, Southern African Catholic Bishops Conference. She leads a programme providing education, home-based care, ARV treatment and support to children orphaned and made vulnerable by AIDS, and has a special interest in ongoing theological reflection on HIV and AIDS.

BENSON OKYERE-MANU from Ghana is the director of Newfrontier Aid Trust, a faith-based non-governmental organisation in South Africa. His doctoral research, which he completed at the School of Religion and Theology, University of KwaZulu-Natal, focused on the cultural underpinnings of stigma, discrimination and silence around HIV and AIDS.

JILL OLIVIER completed her Ph.D. at the University of Cape Town where she was also a research associate for the African Religious Health Assets Programme for which she has conducted research in several African countries on religion, health and development. She is currently a consultant with the World Bank-Development Dialogue on Values and Ethics in Washington, DC. Her main research focus is interdisciplinary research, multi-sectoral collaboration and non-state service delivery for HIV and AIDS, health and development.

GILLIAN PATERSON is an independent writer and researcher and a research fellow at Heythrop College, University of London. She has worked for many years with religious and other international organisations on health-related issues, especially in relation to HIV and AIDS. Her research interests focus on issues of stigma and the implications of the HIV epidemic for women and girls.

LILIAN SIWILA from Zambia lectures at Seth Mokitimi Methodist Seminary, Pietermaritzburg and completed her Ph.D. at the School of Religion and Theology, University of KwaZulu-Natal. Her research interest focuses on gendered religio-cultural practices and HIV and AIDS. She has worked extensively in churches in Zambia using theological resources to combat violence against women and children.

JAN BJARNE SØDAL is the project co-ordinator of the Nordic-FOCCISA One Body, a co-operation on HIV and AIDS between the national Christian councils in the southern African and Nordic European countries. His work engages North-South dialogue on the churches' perspectives and response to HIV, with particular reference to the issues of stigma, gender, sexuality, images of God, church, leadership and the involvement of people living with HIV.

ADRIAAN VAN KLINKEN is a Ph.D. fellow at the Centre for Intercultural Theology, Inter-Religious Dialogue, Missiology and Ecumenism in the Department of Religious Studies and Theology, Utrecht University. His doctoral study investigates the transformation of masculinities in the HIV era as envisioned and practised by African theologians and local churches in Zambia. His research interests include the study of religion and gender and the field of world Christianity.

EDWINA WARD is a research associate at the School of Religion and Theology, University of KwaZulu-Natal and director of the African Network of Higher Education and Research in Theology and HIV, which offers scholarships to Masters students studying in institutions throughout Africa on theology and HIV. She has worked extensively as a trainer for clinical pastoral education with special reference to counselling those who are HIV positive.

GERALD WEST is professor of Old Testament and biblical hermeneutics in the School of Religion and Theology at the University of KwaZulu-Natal and director of the Ujamaa Centre for Community Development and Research. He works with colleagues in the Ujamaa Centre to construct ways in which the Bible can be used for affirmation and life in the context of HIV.

BONGI ZENGELE is co-ordinator of the Solidarity Programme for People Living with HIV and AIDS in the Ujamaa Centre for Community Development and Research in the University of KwaZulu-Natal. She works extensively in communities throughout South Africa and in the rest of Africa with a special interest in forms of resilience in children, women and men impacted directly or indirectly by the HIV and AIDS epidemic.

PHUMZILE ZONDI-MABIZELA was for many years chief executive officer, KwaZulu-Natal Christian Council but has more recently worked as an independent consultant in the area of gender and HIV. She represents the faith-based sector on the KwaZulu-Natal Provincial Council on AIDS and is openly living with HIV. Her activism is concerned with ensuring that people living with HIV are meaningfully involved in the development and implementation of policies and positive theologies, as well as challenging religious organisations to speak out openly against HIV stigma, discrimination and denial.

Index

417

Professional
COM Applications
with ATL

Sing Li
Panos Economopoulos

Wrox Press Ltd. ®

Professional COM Applications
with ATL

Published by Wrox Press Ltd. 30 Lincoln Road, Olton, Birmingham, B27 6PA
Printed in USA
ISBN 1-861001-7-03

Trademark Acknowledgements

Wrox has endeavored to provide trademark information about all the companies and products mentioned in this book by the appropriate use of capitals. However, Wrox cannot guarantee the accuracy of this information.

Credits

Author
Sing Li
Panos Econopoulos

Editors
Tim Briggs
Victoria Hudgson
Chris Hindley
Daniel Maharry

Index
Seth Maislin

Copy Edit
Alex Zoro
Barnaby Zoro
George Briggs

Cover
Andrew Guillaume

Technical Reviewers
Tom Armstrong
David Gardner
Alex Homer
Claus Loud
Christian Nagel
Jonathan Pinnock
Will Powell
Michael O'Keefe
Marc Simkin
Michael Tracy
Byron Vargas

Design/Layout
Frances Olesch

About the Authors

Sing Li

First bitten by the computer bug in 1978, Sing has grown up with the microprocessor revolution. His first 'PC' was a $99 do-it-yourself Neutronics COSMIC ELF computer with 256 bytes of memory and a 1 bit LED display. Currently, Sing is an active author, speaker, consultant, instructor, and entrepreneur. He has participated in several Wrox projects, written for popular technical journals and is the creator of the 'Internet Global Phone', one of the very first Internet phones available. His wide-ranging consulting expertise spans multi-tiered Internet/intranet systems, distributed architectures, digital convergence technologies, computer integrated telephony, call center technology, multi-media messaging and embedded systems.

Sing works with the Willcam Group in developing and delivering intensive, advanced technical training. As the founder of Microwonders Inc, Sing is currently working on research for an end-to-end digital replacement for the conventional telephone. Other on-going research projects include various enabling 'infrastructural' technologies for the 'new millennium global citizen with no fixed physical address'. When back on earth, Sing is fascinated by the pragmatic technology offerings from Microsoft and is also a Java enthusiast.

Panos Economopoulos

Had Panos been born in an another era he would have certainly been an explorer. Luckily, the ever expanding frontiers of the digital age have been providing him with ample opportunity to do just that. He has been the architect, designer and leader of the development of a number of complex and successful distributed systems. He has extensive experience in a wide variety of areas including databases, multimedia, satellite and wireless communications. Currently, Panos is leading the development of an application in the area of interactive voice response systems and computer telephony integration. He is an active consultant to the industry and has developed and taught a wide range of courses at a number of universities as well as for professional developers. He has also carried out advanced research at the University of Toronto, the results of which have been published in several research journals.

Dedications

This book is dedicated to the guiding lights in my otherwise less than interesting life. To Kim, whose relentless brilliance and warmth has lit up all that is worth living for. To David and Meion Li, for the first breath of air and the first walking step. To Patrick and Alice Chow, whose Radio Shack transistor radio kit has launched a career. To Dr. Merv England, for my first 4-bit breadboard microprocessor, and for revealing that curiosity and creativity is a potent combination towards a fulfilling life. To Mr. Craig and Mrs. Murphy of Parkdale CI, for insisting that English is the ultimate computing language. To Scott Williams and Rob Price, for showing me that good learners can often make capable instructors. To John Franklin and David Maclean of Wrox, for convincing me that a keen reader makes an adequate writer. To Jon Erickson of DDJ, for taking a chance on a kid who wants to ramble on about using the Internet for phone calls. To Baris and Everlyn Dortok, for proving that determination and perseverance are the basic ingredients for any worthwhile achievement. To Allen Lee and Dr. Robert Lieberman, for lending me a light whenever my own flickers or threatens to extinguish. And last but not least, to the many other spot lights, flashing strobes, candles and blinking LEDs that continue to guide my way through this now fascinating life of endless possibilities. Shine on!

Sing Li

My gratitude goes to my wife-friend Marita, my children Nicolas and Aris and my parents Niko and Koula for their continuous and unwavering support.

Panos Economopoulos

Acknowledgements

Without our amazing editors at Wrox, Tim Briggs and Victoria Hudgson, the terse manuscript would not be read by anyone. Their dedication, encouragement and support were absolutely vital to the project's success. Thanks must go the John Franklin for his professional guidance. We are also grateful for the uncensored, hard-hitting, occasionally raw, but always accurate, honest and valuable comments from all our reviewers: Christian Nagel, Mark Simkin, Will Powell, Jonathan Pinnock, Michael O'Keefe, Claus Loud, David Gardner, Byron Vargas, Alex Homer, Tom Armstrong and Michael Tracy.

The absolute biggest 'thank you' goes to all the readers of the first edition, especially those who had taken the time to write to us. Each and every one of your comments, suggestions and criticism has contributed to improving the book this second time around.

Contact

Sing can be reached at **sing@willcam.com** or **singli@microwonders.com**. Panos can be reached at **epanos@interlog.com**.

Readers are encouraged to send any technical comments, suggestions and questions relating to this book to **feedback@wrox.com** for the fastest possible response and resolution.

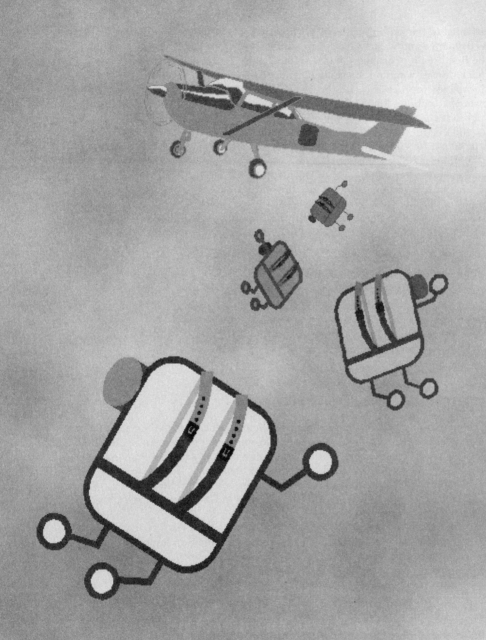

Table of Contents

Chapter 9: Microsoft Transaction Server and Distributed Objects with DCOM

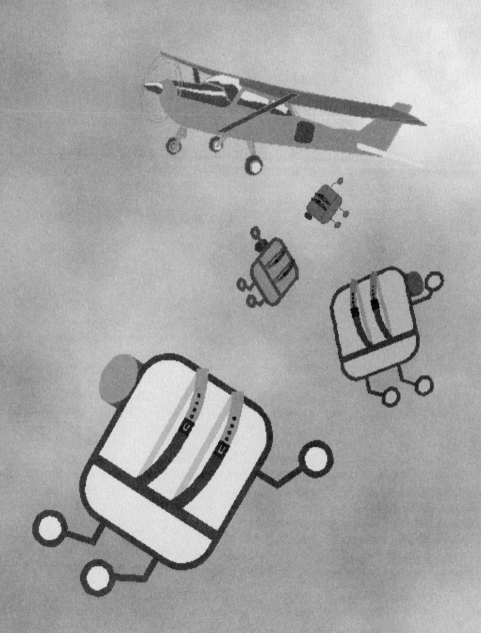

Introduction

Welcome to *Professional COM Applications with ATL*!

It has been one full year since the release of the first edition of this book, *Professional ActiveX/COM Control Programming*. In that book we explained our take on a stream of constantly evolving technology, so it came as no surprise when Wrox requested an updated second edition of the book.

What's new?

- ❑ Microsoft openly favors component-based development that spans three tiers, with the Distributed interNet Applications (DNA) architecture
- ❑ Visual C++ 6 and ATL 3 make COM development easier
- ❑ IE 4.01 is the first OC96-compliant container
- ❑ Development with MTS 2.0 has become irresistible, as it simplifies deployment of proxies and servers, security and makes transactions easy
- ❑ MSMQ is proving its worth and messaging as a concept is no longer alien
- ❑ OLE DB got easier, with provider and consumer templates, and standard providers
- ❑ Hybrid DHTML/Visual C++ components have the flexible UI of DHTML, and the event handling of C++
- ❑ UML is now a standard

So, what's changed in the book?

For those interested in the theory behind COM-based applications, we have greatly expanded our conceptual introduction to COM, with discussions covering threading models, marshaling, and security – the three subject areas that are most troubling to those beginning COM. In the advanced DNA sections, we cover the basic of transactions, MTS activities, just-in-time activation, the object-mapping layer, store-and-forward systems, asynchronous and disconnected systems, and much, much more. To facilitate understanding the concepts, we have increased the number of diagrams and charts, using the standard Unified Modeling Language (UML) notation wherever applicable. You will find more use case diagrams, more sequence diagrams, more collaboration diagrams, and three-tier component diagrams in this edition. For practitioners of object-oriented design patterns, we have also identified the use of design patterns within the COM infrastructure.

For those who have code flowing in their veins, we have included almost three times more code than the first edition. We will take you step-by-step through the construction of a non-trivial OC94-compatible calendaring ActiveX control, which uses native Win32 controls for its functionality, all the way to a fully-independent, OC96-compliant Windowless version with deferred activation. Along the way, we will implement:

- ❑ Middle-tier business objects
- ❑ MTS components
- ❑ Components using MSMQ
- ❑ Components that present a collection-based object model to automation clients
- ❑ Data access components that uses OLE DB templates
- ❑ A visual ActiveX control that uses Dynamic HTML for its user interface

We will use compiler COM support from Visual C++, and we will be getting our hands wet deploying many of the brand new features from Visual C++ 6 and ATL 3. The code included follows the latest ANSI C++ coding conventions. Any code-hungry developer will find plenty of ActiveX and DNA code in this book to sate their appetite. Plus, to save you any unnecessary frustration debugging DNA applications, we have even included a set of tips and caveats in the MTS and MSMQ sections, which document the pitfalls we have encountered in our own endeavors.

For the architects and system designers amongst us, this book documents the analysis, design, and implementation of an enterprise-wide, non-trivial, distributed calendaring system using the technologies that comprise Microsoft's DNA architecture. The use cases, design rationale, and implementation details for the system are presented end-to-end, from concept to deployment. We will see how we can create a component-based design approach to make ActiveX, DCOM, MTS, MSMQ, OLE DB and SQL Server work together in harmony to deliver a robust, scalable system for our desktop users, our departmental administrator, and even our disconnected administrators. For each technological area that we cover, we will look under the hood and see what makes it tick – and why it is designed that way. We will cover the design of COM, COM objects, DCOM, ActiveX controls, and the architecture of ATL, Universal Data Access (UDA) and OLE DB, MTS, and MSMQ. With each DNA technology, we analyze the capabilities it delivers today, and discuss the functionality promised in a future world of Windows NT 5 and COM+. In the chapter on security, we will discover that all DNA security is based on standard Windows NT security. We will see how DCOM security is built upon Windows NT security, how MTS simplifies the basic security model, and how MSMQ's security requirements are quite alien to 'regular' security requirements.

We believe that this book provides a technical, all-round and above-all practical introduction of COM, ActiveX and DNA.

What You Need to Use this Book

The basic requirement to use this book is Visual C++ 6, the latest version of Microsoft's best-selling C++ compiler and development environment. It runs on Windows 9x or NT 4, which means a 486 CPU or better and a minimum 16Mb of memory. For Visual C++, you'll need quite a lot of hard disk space – a typical installation is 170 Mb. You can do a minimal installation which takes up around 40 Mb, but this will mean longer compile times, as the CD will be utilized more often.

In the course of the book we'll test the calendar control with Visual Basic 6, FrontPage 98, Internet Explorer 4.01 and Visual J++ 6. And, to test the middle and backend tiers, you'll need at least one NT 4 server (with Service Pack 3), with SQL Server 6.5 (with Service Pack 4) and the NT 4 Option Pack for MSMQ and MTS.

> *You do not necessarily need a full install of SQL Server 6.5, either use the developer's edition that comes with the Enterprise edition of Visual Studio, or nick some database space from the MSMQ's (limited) installation of SQL server.*

Conventions Used

We use a number of different styles of text and layout in the book to help differentiate between different kinds of information. Here are some examples of the styles we use and an explanation of what they mean:

> **These boxes hold important, not-to-be forgotten, mission-critical details which are directly relevant to the surrounding text.**

Background information, asides and references appear in text like this.

- ❑ **Important Words** are in a bold font
- ❑ Words that appear on the screen, such as menu options, are in a similar font to the one used on screen, for example, the File menu
- ❑ Keys that you press on the keyboard, like *Ctrl* and *Enter*, are in italics
- ❑ All filenames are in this style: `Videos.mdb`
- ❑ Function names look like this: `sizeof()`

Code which is new, important, or relevant to the current discussion will be presented like this:

```
interface ICustomInterface : IUnknown
{
    HRESULT GetManagerName([out, retval] BSTR *lResult);
    HRESULT OkayToPublishInfo([in] long lyear, [in] long lmonth,
                             [out, retval] VARIANT_BOOL *bResult);
    HRESULT PeekCounters([out] long *lCount1, [out] long *lCount2);
}
```

However, code that you've seen before, or which has little to do with the matter at hand, looks like this:

```
interface ICustomInterface : IUnknown
{
    HRESULT GetManagerName([out, retval] BSTR *lResult);
    HRESULT OkayToPublishInfo([in] long lyear, [in] long lmonth,
                             [out, retval] VARIANT_BOOL *bResult);
    HRESULT PeekCounters([out] long *lCount1, [out] long *lCount2);
}
```

Support

The various Wrox Press web sites act as a focus for providing the following information and support to you, the reader:

❑ Title information
❑ Sample chapters
❑ Source code downloads
❑ Check/add errata
❑ Email newsletter
❑ Developer's Journal subscription
❑ Read articles and opinion on related topics

Check out the following sites:

http://www.wrox.com/
http://www.comdeveloper.com/
http://www.worldofatl.com/
http://rapid.wrox.co.uk/

Source Code

All the programs in the book are shown in full, or rather, the additions to the wizard-generated code are shown in full. However, for those who have better things to do than type it all in, the full source is available from the following URLs:

http://www.wrox.com/
ftp://ftp.wrox.com/
ftp://ftp.wrox.co.uk/

Tell Us What You Think

We've tried to make this book as accurate and enjoyable for you as possible, but what really matters is what the book actually does for you. Please let us know your views, whether positive or negative, either by returning the reply card in the back of the book or by contacting us at Wrox Press, either using email (feedback@wrox.com) or our website.

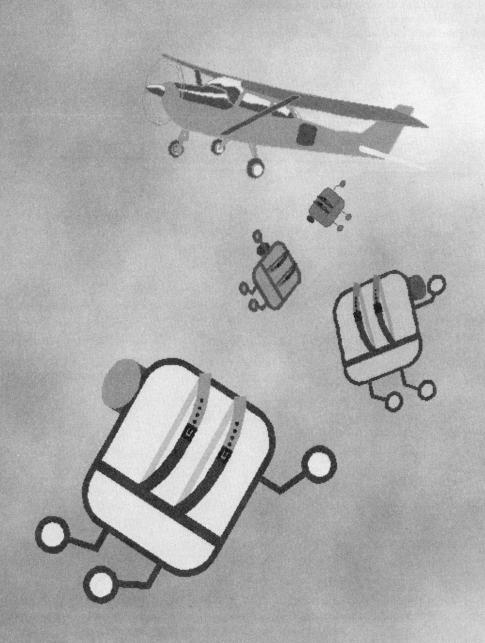

An Unusual Introduction to COM

It is most important to lay down a solid foundation before constructing a skyscraper. In this chapter and the next, we'll drive home the (thankfully simple) concepts underlying the Component Object Model, upon which an amazing, and increasing, number of skyscrapers are built (for example, Microsoft Transaction Server, Microsoft Message Queue, OLE DB and ActiveX to name just a few). It will be a fascinating journey behind the scenes of this utility 'object model', as we learn about the various types of COM objects. There'll be ground rules governing the interactions that these objects can have, and we'll take time to explain each one and why they are there.

Readers who are intimately familiar with basic COM principles should feel free to skip to Chapter 3, where we start designing and building an ActiveX control just using C++. For those who have no prior COM knowledge, who want to brush up on the basics, or who just want to explore an alternative view of what COM is all about, please read on.

On Win32-based systems, COM objects are built in very specific ways according to the COM Specifications – and we'll find out how. You can find a copy of the COM Specifications in the MSDN library distributed with Visual Studio 6. The COM support on Win32 systems provides many services and APIs, and we'll be taking a look at some of these. Appendix A contains a summary of how the system manages information concerning COM objects.

Throughout this chapter, and, indeed, the rest of the book, we'll be using plenty of UML (Unified Modeling Language) diagrams, references to well-known design patterns, and other illustrations to aid understanding of new ideas and concepts. As the saying goes, 'A picture is worth a thousand words' – you be the judge.

Don't worry though – you won't need an in depth knowledge of each design pattern to follow the discussions, but if you want to find out more about them, then you should consult (of course) Design Patterns, by Gamma, Helm, Johnson and Vlissides (a.k.a. Gang of Four). If you are unfamiliar with the UML notation, take a look at Appendix B, which contains a handy reference. If you need more detail than this, check out Instant UML, by Pierre-Alain Muller.

In these first two chapters, instead of adopting a practical programming approach (which we'll use in the rest of the book), we will look at how COM achieves some of its magic, and why it is designed in that particular way. Hopefully, this will help the concepts stick in your mind. There's nothing particularly difficult about COM, once you understand why it was developed in the first place. Be aware, though, that COM does impose a set of design restrictions. Our job, in this chapter, is to enumerate the rules behind these restrictions, and convince you that they are indeed reasonable.

When you've completed this journey, you'll be familiar with all the conceptual pieces that are required to really make sense of the material presented in the rest of the book. I hope you'll agree with me that the effort is well worthwhile.

The Premise of COM

COM, the **Component Object Model** as specified by Microsoft, is a binary object interoperability standard. COM tries to solve the problem of object reuse, on a large scale, allowing for the independent and uncoordinated evolution of the interacting objects.

The word **binary**, here, is especially significant because it represents the lowest possible level of information/data/code exchange on a particular platform. By specifying the COM standard on a binary level, one can attempt to arrive at a standard that's independent of the operating system, the transmission medium, and the computer language used for implementation. Extending this with a binary protocol standard, object inter-operation can be made hardware platform and location independent. A **use case** is a description of an interaction between a person (or another system) and the system one is building. Here is a use case view of that requirement:

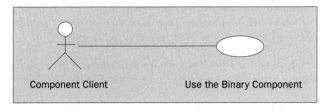

The actor (an actor is a UML element, approximately equal to 'client' or 'user') in this diagram is the 'component client'. Note that an actual 'component client' may also be a component itself. This means that it could provide certain functionality to others, while calling on other components for some of its own needs. In order to keep things simple, we are considering only one such 'client-to-component' relationship.

Constructing applications out of components has become highly fashionable lately. It is of no surprise, since it enables true code reuse, something that generic object-oriented design promised but did not deliver successfully. Fabricating applications out of highly configurable, pre-tested, pre-compiled components saves valuable development and testing time.

The component client in the diagram may have just created the component through a system API call, or may have located an existing instance of the component through some application specific means. To all intents and purposes, the component at this point is a simple **Binary Large OBject** (**BLOB**).

Binary Large Objects

A Binary Large Object, or BLOB, is simply a sequence of binary numbers stored in the memory and/or on disk. In this way, any piece of data, graphic or program can be viewed as a BLOB.

In the use case diagram, given a BLOB on a machine, which we know to be a software component (through some other mechanism, such as a 'component-blob-creation' system API), how can the actor (component client) make use of it? The answer to this question – the design of COM – will enable binary interoperability, as opposed to language-dependent or source-level interoperability.

To make things more concrete, let us look at an example. The following diagram depicts one such BLOB in memory, occupying memory addresses from $000000A0 to $00001FA0.

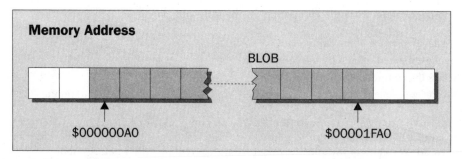

One design solution may be to jump to the first memory location ($000000A0) and start executing. This is a convention used frequently in operating systems for execution of programs and is similar to how dynamically linked libraries (DLLs) work. This design, however, is too simplistic, and adequate for only very restrictive 'execute once' type components.

The real-world problem is often more complicated. Most software components residing on a system don't simply 'execute', but provide many functions or services for other components or programs. They may also retain their internal state between calls to such functions. Therefore, it is also necessary for a calling program to find out what a BLOB can do, and find some way to execute these individual pieces of functionality accordingly. As an example, a refinement of our use case diagram below shows the typical things that a component client may want to do to the component:

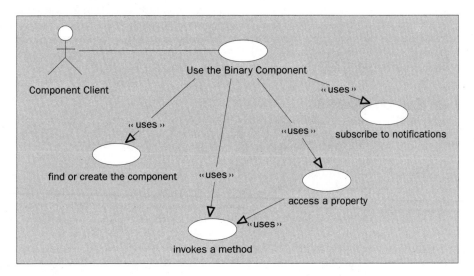

A component client should use the component in the following ways:

- ❑ Create an instance of the component
- ❑ Invoke a method offered by the component
- ❑ Access the component's properties
- ❑ Ask the component to notify the client whenever something exciting happens (to the client)

To greatly improve what we can do with the BLOB, we can mark a specific offset in the BLOB, and specify that it must be the entry point to a function. This function will tell the calling program what the BLOB can do. We can get the specific offset from the creation API when we obtain the BLOB, or it could be a convention that all BLOBs have the same special offset. The following diagram illustrates this:

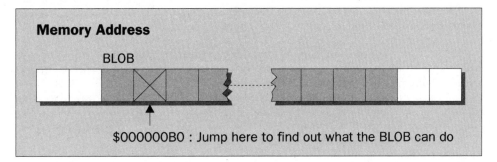

Now, the component client can take advantage of the services provided by the BLOB by calling the function at the specified offset to find out about its capabilities. Of course, the act of "calling the function" implies that a certain calling convention is followed (a specific usage of the stack for passing parameters and return values). Therefore, the designer of this solution must also specify the signature (the parameters and return values) and the calling convention associated with the function.

This design solution is all that we need to satisfy component clients on a simple operating system, like DOS, where there's only ever one executing program. However, in multitasking operating systems, it isn't uncommon for the BLOB components to be used by multiple calling programs/components within its lifetime. The 'clients' may also cause the BLOB to access shared resources at the same time. In order for the BLOB to properly handle these 'clients', maintain a consistent state for each one, and to determine its own lifetime, a convention has to be specified as to how the calling program can let the BLOB know that:

- ❏ It will be using the services of the BLOB
- ❏ It has finished using the services of the BLOB

To accomplish this, two more special offset locations in the BLOB can be marked. When a calling program/component calls into the function at offset #2, the BLOB will register that the component wants to use its services; if the function at offset #3 is called, the BLOB will assume the caller has finished using its services. Now, our 'marked' BLOB looks like this:

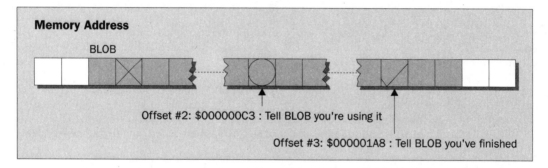

The X, O, and checkmark in the diagram above mark the three offsets. Since the three marked offsets (function entry points) on the BLOB are so very fundamental to the usability of the BLOB as a component on the system, one can group them together. By grouping together a set of pointers (function pointers) to these offsets, and specifying (dictating) that this group must be consecutively located within the BLOB, we have to specify only *one* single offset instead of three. For example, in our hypothetical case, simply specifying that memory $000000A6 is the offset is enough for the calling program:

Address	Meaning
$000000A6	Read the function pointer at this location and call the function there ($000000B0) to find out what the BLOB does.
$000000AA	Read the function pointer at this location and call the function there ($000000C3) to let the BLOB know that you're using it.
$000000AE	Read the function pointer at this location and call the function there ($000001A8) to let the BLOB know that you've finished using it.

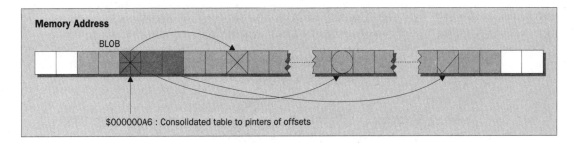

Memory Address

BLOB

$000000A6 : Consolidated table to pinters of offsets

What have we learnt

Notice that, up to this point, our discussion has been totally generic. We've specified a way of dealing with components that are represented by BLOBs that can be applicable to any computing machine with the Von-Neumann architecture (i.e. it stores program and data in memory locations during execution).

It may surprise you to find that what we've just covered represents a good portion of the fundamentals of COM. That is, the design we have described can be used to build a solution satisfying all the requirements of our use case.

Even though there's no Microsoft-specific jargon, no 'WINTEL' influences, no language specific constructs, it represents the heart and soul of a COM object. As a matter of fact, if you've created a BLOB according to the above specification, then you've officially created a COM object. This, hopefully, will strengthen your faith that this material can be applied generically to any new system that you may encounter.

Back to our discussion of the BLOB. It turns out that, despite repeated efforts by various groups of experts, it seems that the characteristics of a 'BLOB' representing a software component (a piece of self-contained, reusable software) can't be further agreed upon (in general) beyond the simple offset scheme illustrated above. Some historical component standards (such as DSOM and OpenDoc from IBM), tried to deal with component BLOBs on a higher level, and are now almost defunct. This is mainly because additions beyond the 'bare essentials' are often inapplicable in other problem domains, such as machine architecture or computing languages. Current component based technologies, such as CORBA or enterprise JavaBeans, tend to adopt the same minimalist approach when interoperating with foreign objects.

On the same machine, the binary interoperable nature of the above design enables a 'component client' written in COBOL to use a component written in C++, without re-compiling or linking the C++ code specifically for it. This is true provided both the 'component client' and the component itself have been compiled for the same machine architecture (for example, Intel x86 or Digital Alpha). Unlike enterprise JavaBeans, COM components are native executable images, and are dependent on the hardware platforms for which they are compiled. However, this is not necessarily a weakness, since the DCOM binary protocol extension, that we mentioned earlier, allows clients and COM components on different hardware platforms to inter-work with each other over a network. Having abstracted the problem of making component-based computing as universal as possible on a particular platform, let's look at how COM implements the three basic requirements of our BLOB.

Mapping what we know into Real COM

Let's translate our basic design into COM elements. First, it is customary to call member functions of components **methods**. We will switch our usage now:

- ❑ The 'function called to find out what the BLOB does' is named the `QueryInterface()` method, or `QI()` for short
- ❑ The 'function called to let the BLOB know you're going to be using it' is named the `AddRef()` method
- ❑ The 'function called to let the BLOB know you've finished using it' is named the `Release()` method

We'll look at the parameters of these methods in a moment. But first, let's think about what a **COM interface** means.

Going back to the BLOB design, we consolidated the pointers that pointed to these three functions in one place. There, they effectively form a table of function pointers. This table is the `IUnknown` interface.

Stepping back further, the client of the component holds a pointer to our table of pointers, in order to make its three basic calls. This translates to a pointer to an interface, or a pointer to a table of function pointers.

The important thing to note here is that the interface decouples the interaction of the client with the component's methods. The client can't directly call the methods of the IUnknown interface without more knowledge about the component than COM reveals, and without limiting the usefulness of the BLOB.

> **An interface is a table of function pointers.**

In other words, the `IUnknown` interface consists of the `QueryInterface()`, `AddRef()` and `Release()` methods. We'll describe them below in the 'official' format.

The IUnknown Interface

The most basic interface in COM is `IUnknown` and is called this because it defines an interface that all clients can talk to without having to know the exact workings of the component. The `IUnknown` interface contains three methods, and is the 'base' interface for *all* other COM interfaces.

Imagine that we want to do something useful in our component, so add a couple of methods to it, `MyMethod1()` and `MyMethod2()`. However, we must still implement the methods of the `IUnknown` interface as a subset of our new interface `IMyInterface`. We can say that `IMyInterface` inherits from `IUnknown`.

How is it possible to reuse the same implementation for both interfaces? Well, in C++, use of inheritance through a virtual base class automatically creates a virtual function table (vtable) that can be used to enforce the implementation of the `IUnknown` interface in all derived classes. Our inheritance hierarchy is shown in here:

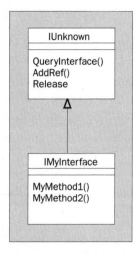

This also means that if you've obtained a pointer to any interface from an object, you can count on the methods of the `IUnknown` interface to be available from the interface pointer.

> **All COM interfaces are based on `IUnknown`. In other words, the first three methods of any COM interface are always `QueryInterface()`, `AddRef()`, and `Release()`.**

Except for the unfortunate name, which seems to tone down its importance, everything we've just seen emphasizes how important and how fundamental `IUnknown` really is. `IUnknown` is vital to even the most trivial operations using COM.

Back to the BLOB

We can now map the new COM terminology to our BLOB and the table of offsets. The existence of `IUnknown` within every interface implies that the first three offsets in any offset tables must point to the methods of the `IUnknown` interface:

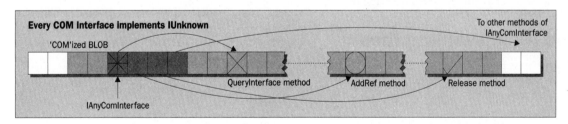

We can also map the representation of our BLOB into more concrete C++ constructs that we work with day to day. These tables of offsets (the darkly shaded memory regions in the above figure) are frequently called **vtables**. They are so named after a compiler-generated structure in the code image produced by the linker. More precisely, it is the way that Microsoft C++ compilers (and many others, although not all) create and handle tables of virtual functions for classes in C++. The original rationale for choosing this format probably has to do with making implementation of COM objects simple for C++ compiler users. This makes very good sense if you consider that:

❑ C++ is the most widespread object-oriented language to date
❑ At the time when COM was 'invented', the main development language for the Windows platforms was C/C++

It's important to understand, though, that this was just a convenient implementation choice. Indeed, the vtable format has taken on a life independent of C++. With appropriate programming, one can generate code images containing these vtable structures from almost any language from any vendor. In particular, there's ample coverage in popular programmer's magazines on how to create COM objects using C, Visual Basic, Visual J++, Delphi and even COBOL (Dr Dobb's Journal, Microsoft Developer's Journal, etc.).

Nevertheless, since this book is addressed to C++ developers and you'll use C++ to create and use COM interfaces and objects, we'll soon make the complete connection between COM and C++. In Chapter 3, where we actually create a COM object server using raw C++, you'll get a concrete idea of how to map C++ classes to COM interfaces and objects.

Let's take a more formal look at the members of the very important `IUnknown` interface. This is the format in which you will see most COM interfaces documented.

IUnknown::QueryInterface()

A client's call to `QueryInterface()` returns an interface pointer. As we discussed earlier, this is a pointer to the table of pointers that constitutes the interface, and these pointers themselves point to the component's methods.

Any calling program or component *must* interact with a component through its interfaces (obtained from `QueryInterface()`). For example, suppose I have a component that can check the validity of an employee ID and it exposes an interface called `IEmployeeIdentityCheck` (where the prefix `I` is used by convention). I can call `QueryInterface()` requesting that interface (quite how we do this will become clear very soon), and if this call succeeds, I can use the returned interface pointer to call the methods provided by the object through the `IEmployeeIdentityCheck` interface.

By carefully defining these interfaces, different capabilities of the component can be exposed to the component client.

Separating the interface specification from the actual implementation is very important for all component based technologies, and COM is no exception. So much so, that Microsoft uses an **interface definition language** (IDL) to define the attributes of the interface and the methods it contains. IDL also implements the COM interface inheritance scheme we saw earlier.

Here is the prototype for the QueryInterface() method:

```
HRESULT QueryInterface(REFIID iid, void** ppvObject);
```

Let's take a look at this in detail.

Parameters

Parameter	Description
iid	Identifier of the interface being requested. We'll be taking a look at where this identifier comes from in the section called *The Chicken and Egg Problem* later on.
ppvObject	This is the returned pointer to the requested interface. If the operation failed or the interface requested isn't supported by the component, this pointer will be set to point to NULL. If this is the case, use the HRESULT return value to determine why the call failed.

QueryInterface() Return Values

HRESULT Value	Description
S_OK	The requested interface is supported and a pointer is returned in the ppvObject argument.
E_NOINTERFACE	This object doesn't support the requested interface and NULL is returned in the ppvObject argument.

Comments

QueryInterface() is used to obtain any interface that a component may support, given an interface identifier specifying the interface required. Since we know that QueryInterface() is part of every COM interface, it follows that we can get any interface that a component provides, as long as we have a single interface pointer to the component. We'll examine the implications of QueryInterface() later on, in the section entitled *A Few Golden Rules*.

When an interface is returned by a call to QueryInterface(), it's assumed by the client that the component has already performed an AddRef() to the interface pointer before returning it, incrementing its reference count. The caller of QueryInterface() must remember to call Release() on the interface pointer when it has finished with it. Be very careful with this convention. Many of the most difficult-to-debug situations in COM stem from unmatched AddRef() and Release() calls. We'll have more to say about this later.

What's an HRESULT?

Error conditions in COM are indicated by a return code, instead of an exception mechanism. This is necessary for achieving programming language independence. An HRESULT is a 32-bit code that is a compromise between the ability to efficiently transfer error codes, while allowing for a reasonably large range that can be sub-divided for different uses. Let's take a quick look at how HRESULT accomplishes this.

The diagram shows how the bits in an HRESULT are partitioned:

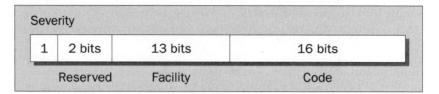

The severity field (1 bit) can be either 0 for SUCCESS or 1 for ERROR. This bit is used to determine if the method call has succeeded in performing its intended task. Note that we can actually differentiate between 'level of success' by combining this field with the rest of the HRESULT. What this means is that an operation can return from a call with more information than a simple Boolean SUCCESS/FAIL status. The reserved field (2 bits) must be zero, and not be used. The facility (13 bits) is pre-assigned to different 'groups' of related codes. Some common facilities are FACILITY_RPC for RPC related codes and FACILITY_DISPATCH for codes related to IDispatch (discussed in the next chapter). The only facility that's usable freely by user created components is FACILITY_ITF (ITF stands for the interface). This allows for the definition of code specific to any interface. In the code field (16 bits), COM will define its code within the range of 0x0000 to 0x01FF, leaving 0x2000 to 0xFFFF for the programmer. Two macros, SUCCEEDED() and FAILED() allow checking of the severity bit with all other bits masked. They should be used whenever you are concerned with only the success or failure outcome of a COM method call.

IUnknown::AddRef() and IUnknown::Release()

AddRef() and Release() are fundamental to the component's lifetime and resource management strategy. Typically, an internal counter holds the number of users referencing this component.

When the count reaches zero, it's okay for the object itself to free the interface/component and all its currently allocated resources from memory. Specific implementations of certain interfaces and objects, though, may not directly follow this convention. It's just a way to let the component/BLOB know that it's no longer wanted. However, what it wants to do with itself is up to the implementer of the object.

In some cases, this reference counting mechanism may be applied per interface (or set of interfaces) instead. This usually occurs in larger components that expose many interfaces. Distinct groups of interfaces may be responsible for their own resource allocation, depending on the component design.

The two functions are prototyped as:

```
ULONG AddRef();
ULONG Release();
```

Return Values

Usually returns a value between 1 and *x*, where *x* is the number of times that the interface has been referenced. However, program logic should never depend on the validity of this value. The COM specification doesn't require that the return value reflects the actual reference count, because COM optimizes the calls to AddRef() and Release().

Comments

Every interface pointer starts its life (on returning from `QueryInterface()`) with a reference count of 1. Every time the interface pointer is copied, the reference count should be incremented through calls to `AddRef()`. Every time a client finishes using it, or is about to wipe out its value, `Release()` should be called on it.

When the reference count of all interfaces on the object reaches zero, the component is expected to free itself from memory and free all the resources it owns. As previously mentioned, however, this isn't an absolute requirement. In system design scenarios where servers may be expected to 'stay around forever', the COM specification allows the forgoing of the reference counting convention.

Since the count maintained by `AddRef()` tracks the number of references to an interface pointer currently active, one must be very careful when making copies, passing interface pointers as arguments to functions or returning interface pointers from functions. All these actions essentially make an additional reference to the same interface, and the client must remember to call the `AddRef()` method on the interface. When the desired operation is finished, the holder of the interface pointer must remember to call the interface's `Release()` method.

Note that `AddRef()` *and* `Release()` *are the only standard COM interface methods that do not return an* `HRESULT`.

The Chicken and Egg Problem

We now know that there are special spots in the object (within our core memory) that make it usable as a component by other code or objects (via the COM `IUnknown` mechanism). But how does the object get into the computer memory in the first place?

That's a very good question. The idea is to bring alive a copy of an object that we want to use as a component. In object design or COM terms, this action is called **creating an instance** of the object, or **instantiating** the object. Why are we creating an 'instance'? Is there another running copy of the object (another instance) somewhere else?

Yes, the point is that there *could* already be another copy of the running object in the system. Since most modern operating systems are multitasking, it's possible that the object you want to use has already been instantiated by another running program. Furthermore, when getting an instance of the object, we don't know (and shouldn't care, if the object is designed properly) whether it's serving us alone, or if it's also being used by other clients.

While the concept of object instantiation or creation is generic, the actual implementation of this 'object creation process' is partially platform dependent. The platform dependent part of the system is called the **COM runtime**.

First, we definitely need a way to uniquely identify the type of object we want to 'instantiate'. Following object-oriented practice, the type of an object is called its **class** in COM. We need to be able to name our classes so that we (or our clients) can create instances of them at any time.

With you, me, my friend, his Aunt Martha and Aunt Martha's friends all defining COM classes, how do we cope with the assignment of names? If we give them text-based names, one can easily get into a situation where class names are duplicated. If two different objects with the same name are installed on the same system, one can imagine disastrous effects. One potential solution is to coordinate the assignment of names through some sort of centralized authority, in a scheme similar to the assignment of IP addresses for the Internet.

Microsoft's solution, and the solution in the industry in general, is to avoid these complex coordination issues. Instead, one can use an *almost* randomly generated, extremely large number. The algorithm used to generate such a number will ensure that the probability of generating the same number twice within several lifetimes is effectively nil. Wow! It turns out that one can generate a 16-byte (128-bit) number satisfying this property based on the current date and time, some ID (actually a network card's MAC address, which happens to be unique) on the machine generating the number and a random seed. The number created in this way is called a **Universally Unique Identifier** (UUID), or a **Globally Unique Identifier** (GUID), which is a slightly less ambitious name and used more often. There are two names for historical reasons – UUID was first used with DCE RPC to identify interfaces, and Microsoft adopted it and renamed it GUID under COM auspices. You've probably seen these beasts before, perhaps, without realizing what they were. A GUID typically looks like this:

```
{5CA735E0-2819-11D0-8DCF-000000000000}
```

Or this:

```
static const GUID myID = { 0x5ca735e0, 0x2819, 0x11d0, { 0x8d, 0xcf, 0x0, 0x0,
0x0, 0x0, 0x0, 0x0 } };
```

Now, armed with a way to absolutely and uniquely identify something, one may be tempted to start naming everything else (that needs a name) using the same mechanism. Well, Microsoft has done exactly that. As a matter of fact, UUIDs are currently used to name:

❑ COM classes – called class IDs or CLSIDs
❑ Interfaces – called interface IDs or IIDs
❑ Type information libraries – called library IDs or LIBIDs
❑ Categories of COM objects – called category IDs or CATIDs
❑ IDs for security configuration of DCOM objects – called APPIDs

We'll take a look at some of these other named items later on. One can easily extend this mechanism to name every fragment of code, every window instance and so on, since all these entities are unique in time. For now, it suffices to say that we can create an instance of an object provided we know its Class ID (CLSID). We just need to pass this to the COM runtime, and it will find and create the object we want. It's magic we'll explain further very soon, but first we need to elucidate the basic rules of COM interfaces.

A Few Golden Rules

Earlier, when we examined the COM BLOB, we ended up with a discussion of the `IUnknown` interface and its three methods. We've been dealing with these interface pointers, or 'pointers to a table of function pointers'. We can see that the services provided by the BLOB can be exercised purely through an `IUnknown` interface using a generic mechanism. Notice that at no time did we actually deal with a function pointer into the BLOB itself. This is not an oversight, but a fundamental feature/rule of COM itself. In fact, in DCOM, the actual BLOB may reside on another machine miles away.

> **The client of a COM object shall interact with the object only via its interfaces.**

As a matter of fact, even if we do have a pointer to the BLOB itself, there's very little we can do with it. For one thing, it may not be implemented in any language that we know or care about (remember that COM is language neutral). At least with an interface, we have a well-documented way of getting the BLOB to do something useful for us. This brings us to a second fundamental COM rule:

> **Each interface is a documented, binding contract between the COM object client and the object offering the interface. It is not subject to change, ever!**

The keywords here, as COM pundits proudly reiterate, are **contract** and **binding**. A contract, once specified, should never change. No minor revisions, no rethinking, no assorted excuses should ever change the terms of the contract. This means that the documentation to an interface is invaluable, and should be planned and worded very carefully. An interface is often said to be 'immutable'.

Notice, however, that while the rules say that the contract shall not change, they do not state that the ways in which we fulfill the contract can't change. This means that while the interface itself can't change (the number of methods, the parameters of the methods, what each method in an interface does, etc.), the implementation of the interface can change freely – as long as the contract is honored word for word.

This, in fact, is one of the powers of a COM interface. Once specified, it gives a true 'plug-in replaceable' fitting point for components. Imagine the following scenario, where our 'Banking Machine' object is using a Bank of America provided COM object through the `IGetBankUserInfo` interface. Since the `IGetBankUserInfo` interface is a well defined contract, the Banking Machine object could equally well connect to the `IGetBankUserInfo` interface of an object from the Wells Fargo Bank.

This may sound like something that standard subroutine libraries or DLLs can do, but upon deeper reflection, you'll see that the run time connection, language neutral, operating system neutral, and location neutral nature of COM object interactions goes far beyond the capabilities of conventional subroutine libraries.

Each and every interface provided by a COM object is given an interface ID (IID), and that ID is a GUID. For example, the only standard COM interface that we've covered so far, IUnknown, has an IID of:

```
{00000000-0000-0000-C000-000000000046}
```

All standard Microsoft defined COM and OLE interfaces have GUIDs that have been set aside and are of the following type:

```
{dw-w1-w2-C000-000000000046}
```

dw is a DWORD and w1, w2 are WORDs. However, the GUIDs that are generated for the objects that you and I create (we'll shortly see how) definitely look more random than that!

Since interfaces are done deals as soon as they're specified and published, how do we cope with the changing environments of real-world applications?

Like any other contractual situation, you draft up another one! Examining the COM and OLE documentation from Microsoft, you'll find many situations where this happens. For example, there exists an IClassFactory interface (which we'll cover later, so don't worry about what it does just yet), and an IClassFactory2 interface that is an enhancement of the original. It isn't uncommon, in in-house projects, to see an interface named Ixxxx, Ixxxx2, Ixxxx3, Ixxxx4,... in the specification of a COM object that has 'served its time'. The bottom line is that an interface, once specified and documented, must never change.

Recall our earlier discovery:

> **All COM interfaces are based on IUnknown. In other words, the first three methods of any COM interface are always QueryInterface(), AddRef(), and Release().**

A unique corollary to this rule is:

> **Given any interface pointer to an object instance, you can get the pointer to any other interface implemented by the object via the QueryInterface() method.**

This is vitally important – once you have any interface pointer to an object (including the guaranteed IUnknown), you can get the object to do anything that it is capable of doing!

At this point, it is appropriate to introduce another rule associated with `QueryInterface()`:

> **For any object instance, if `QueryInterface()` for an interface succeeds once, it must always succeed for the lifetime of the instance. Conversely, if the initial `QueryInterface()` fails for a requested interface, it must always fail.**

The rule ensures that the interfaces supported by an object instance do not dynamically change, and that functionality doesn't suddenly disappear.

Often in COM programming, we need to deal with multiple instances of an object. For example, later on in this book, we will be creating a corporate event calendar where each event in the calendar is an instance of the same COM class. Since we never have a pointer to an object itself (and we surmised that we really have no need for such a pointer), how do we determine if two interface pointers we hold refer to the same object? Enter another special property of the magical `IUnknown` interface:

> **A COM object must return the** *same* **`IUnknown` pointer whenever the `IUnknown` interface is explicitly requested from the object via the `QueryInterface()` method of any of the object's interfaces.**

This property is called the **identity** of the object, and is used exclusively to compare COM objects. There exists no other reliable way to determine whether or not two interface pointers are actually refering to the same instance.

Creating an Object Instance

Finally, we have all the background we need to create an instance of a particular class. We can do this by calling:

```
HRESULT CoCreateInstance(CLSID rclsid,
                         LPUNKNOWN pUnkOuter,
                         DWORD dwClsContext,
                         REFIID riid,
                         LPVOID* ppvObj);
```

The `CLSID` is the class ID of the object you're instantiating. We'll get to the other parameters in a moment.

Wait a minute, there seems to be something very non-COM about this `CoCreateInstance()` function. It isn't a method of an interface!

That's correct, it's an API function, provided by your friendly COM runtime residing in your local operating system. The `Co` prefix is quite common amongst COM runtime API functions. There is also a variation of this API, called `CoCreateInstanceEx()`, that can be used to explicitly create remote DCOM object instances.

The implementation of CoCreateInstance(), however, is *mostly* operating system, platform, or programming language independent (although the C++ language is used in the reference implementation). And, believe it or not, your object is instantiated by a method of an interface obtained from an object – that is, pure COM!

Curious? Well, here's a simple-minded implementation of the CoCreateInstance() call:

```
HRESULT CoCreateInstance(CLSID rclsid, LPUKNOWN pUnkOuter,
                    DWORD dwClsContext, REFIID riid, LPVIOD* ppvObj)
{
    HRESULT hresult;
    IClassFactory* pCF;

    CoGetClassObject(rclsid, dwClsContext, NULL,
                                IID_IClassFactory, &pCF);

    hresult = pCF->CreateInstance(pUnkOuter, riid, ppvObj)
    pCF->Release();

    return hresult;
}
```

The code introduces the standard IClassFactory interface, and the CoGetClassObject() API call, both of which need additional explanation.

Let's look first at the IClassFactory interface and the reasons for its design.

Class Factories

As the name implies, the IClassFactory interface has knowledge on how to *manufacture* objects of a particular class.

A class that implements the IClassFactory interface is called a **class factory**. The class factory object is itself a COM object, and can expose other interfaces, if necessary. Even though a particular class factory typically knows how to manufacture only one type of object, it can create as many of them as you want. Class factories are useful little BLOBs!

The code above shows the CoGetClassObject() call using the IID of IClassFactory and the CLSID of the class we want to instantiate. From this we get an interface pointer to a class factory which implements a CreateInstance() method to manufacture a COM object.

> *You may often see a class factory referred to a **class object**, as it is obtained via a call to* CoGetClassObject()*. Note that a class object is not always a class factory, however. There could be some situations where only one object of a class ever needs to exist, i.e. a **singleton**. In these cases, it is okay to return this singleton directly through the* CoGetClassObject() *call.*

So, why does COM use class factories to manufacture objects of a class? For the answer, let's look at our first design pattern.

Factory Method Design Pattern

You may wonder why we need an extra 'factory object' in order to create an object. Couldn't we just invoke a magic API function to directly instantiate our object based on the CLSID? The answer is evident when we realize that this is a textbook application of the well-known **Factory Method** design pattern.

> *Design patterns are observed recurring interactions between classes playing certain roles in very large object-oriented design projects. Many of these patterns are documented in the now classic book, 'Design Patterns: Elements of Reusable Object Oriented Software', by Gamma et al. There is currently great interest in this area from the software development community, and new patterns are found and documented quite frequently. Interested readers who are not familiar with the topic are encouraged to refer to the book above.*

The Factory Method pattern has two roles, a Creator and a Concrete Creator. The pattern is used when a class (the Creator) doesn't know beforehand all the object subclasses that it will create. Instead, each subclass (Concrete Creator) is left with the responsibility of creating the actual object instances. Here is the design pattern, with all the roles played by COM elements in the collaboration:

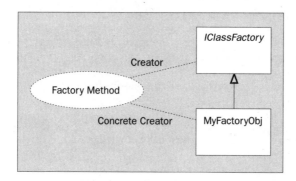

> *The UML diagrammatic convention above, using a parameterized collaboration to represent design patterns, is an approach documented in the book* UML Toolkit, *by Hans Erik and Magnes Penker (Wiley).*

In our scenario, the Creator is played by `IClassFactory`, while the Concrete Creator is played by our `MyFactoryObj`.

Thanks to the design pattern shorthand, we can now understand that COM uses a class factory to alleviate the need for the COM runtime to know about all the possible object types that might have to create ahead of time. Object creation may require acquisition of system resources, coordination among objects, etc. By introducing the `IClassFactory` interface, all details about the creation of a particular object can be hidden in a concrete derivation, manifested as a class factory. Now it's only the class factory that has to be explicitly created by the COM support system.

The COM specification also provides leeway for a class factory to implement its own class factory interface. This interface does not have to be derived from `IClassFactory`. Doing so, however, disqualifies the object from being created by COM helper APIs, such as `CoCreateInstance()` or `CoCreateInstanceEx()`. It also means that the component will not be compatible with some COM based DNA (Distributed interNet Achitechture) services, such as the Microsoft Transaction Server (MTS), which we will cover in detail in Chapter 9.

Let's now look at the complete `IClassFactory` interface.

The IClassFactory Interface

The `IClassFactory` interface is typically the only interface (besides `IUnknown`) exposed by a class factory. The class factory is typically a singleton and can be used to create multiple instances its corresponding class, through the `IClassFactory::CreateInstance()` method. A second method, `IClassFactory::LockServer()`, is provided for a client or the COM runtime system to maintain the class factory in memory if needed.

The COM runtime maintains the association of a CLSID with its object server, and the implementation specific manner of obtaining a class factory for that CLSID.

We already know that `CoCreateInstance()` uses `IClassFactory` internally to create the object. This suggests that, often, we could bypass using `IClassFactory` directly, and just let a helper function like `CoCreateInstance()` do the hard work. Other helper API functions include:

- ❑ `CoCreateInstanceEx()`
- ❑ `CoGetObjectEx()`
- ❑ `CoCreateInstanceFromFile()`

Interested readers are referred to the MSDN library included with Visual Studio 6 for more information on these APIs.

Since `IClassFactory` is a COM interface, it inherits from `IUnknown` and implements `QueryInterface()`, `AddRef()`, and `Release()`. The complete list of methods implemented by `IClassFactory` is:

Method Name	Base Interface	Description
`QueryInterface()`	`IUnknown`	Gets pointer to a supported interface and calls `AddRef()`
`AddRef()`	`IUnknown`	Increments reference count
`Release()`	`IUnknown`	Decrements reference count
`CreateInstance()`		Creates an uninitialized object
`LockServer()`		Locks or unlocks the class factory in memory. The locked state prevents the server from being unloaded

The two new methods are `IClassFactory::CreateInstance()` and
`IClassFactory::LockServer()`. Let's have a look at the definitions for these two methods.

IClassFactory::CreateInstance()

```
HRESULT CreateInstance(IUnknown* pUnkOuter,
                       REFIID riid,
                       void** ppvObject);
```

Parameters

Parameter	Description
PunkOuter	A pointer to an outer `IUnknown` (which, contrary to basic COM rules, is not `AddRef()`'ed) or `NULL`. An `IUnknown` is passed only if the client object wants to 'aggregate' the newly created object. The aggregation mechanism will be covered in the next chapter.
Riid	An Interface ID (IID) indicating the desired interface from the newly created object. Since we never hold any pointer to the object itself when working with COM, we always have to specify an IID in order to get hold of the new object. This parameter must be `IID_IUnknown` if aggregation is being performed. We will discuss the reason for this in our coverage of aggregation in the next chapter.
PpvObject	A pointer to the requested interface, if successful. Otherwise, it will be set to `NULL` upon return.

Return Values

Value	Description
S_OK	The method executed successfully
CLASS_E_NOAGGREGATION	The caller passed in a non-NULL outer `IUnknown`, indicating that aggregation was desired. The newly created object, however, doesn't support aggregation
E_NOINTERFACE	The newly created object doesn't support the interface requested
E_UNEXPECTED	An unexpected error has occurred
E_OUTOFMEMORY	The method ran out of memory during execution
E_INVALIDARG	The method has been called with invalid argument(s)

Comments

There are some legacy components (from 16 bit, Windows 3.1 heritage) which support `IClassFactory` on their class factory, but it can only create something called a 'single use' object. What this means is that the class factory may be used to create only one instance of the class at any time. If you should ever come across such a class factory and call `IClassFactory::CreateInstance()` after the object has already been created, then it is likely that you will get an `E_UNEXPECTED` error. Fortunately, there should be very few such components left around nowadays.

IClassFactory::LockServer()

If you need to create many instances of the same object, you can store away the `IClassFactory` interface pointer, and then lock the server module managing the class factory in memory to increase its object creation speed. To do this, we call the `IClassFactory::LockServer()` method:

```
HRESULT LockServer(BOOL fLock);
```

Parameter

Parameter	Description
fLock	TRUE indicates that you want to lock the server, and FALSE that you want to unlock it

Return Values

Value	Description
S_OK	The lock or unlock operation has been completed successfully
E_FAIL	The operation can't be performed
E_OUTOFMEMORY	The system was out of memory during the operation
E_UNEXPECTED	An unexpected error has occurred

Comments

Even though you hold a pointer to the `IClassFactory` interface (which you assumed would have been `AddRef()`'ed before it was given to you), you still need to call `IClassFactory::LockServer()`, if you want to be guaranteed the best possible performance in creating multiple instances under all circumstances. This is because the `AddRef()` on the `IClassFactory` interface will maintain the validity of the interface pointer itself, but doesn't semantically guarantee that the actual server module is going to remain 'in memory' all the time.

For COM objects implemented as EXE modules, the COM runtime will actually call `LockServer()` to keep the module loaded in memory.

Remember to match the number of `IClassFactory::LockServer(TRUE)` calls with `IClassFactory::LockServer(FALSE)` calls, to avoid stray servers hanging around. You should not invoke `IClassFactory::Release()` if you still have the server locked. Typical `IClassFactory` implementations will not free the class factory unless the object reference count and the lock count are both `0`.

CoGetClassObject()

If you look back at the `CoCreateInstance()` call that we saw earlier, `CoGetClassObject()` is called to somehow, from somewhere, obtain a pointer to an `IClassFactory` interface, indicated by `IID_IClassFactory`.

I am purposely being vague here because this is where generality stops. The implementation of `CoGetClassObject()` is absolutely platform and OS dependent. From a COM point of view, how it works is magic.

Have a look at the prototype for this function:

```
HRESULT CoGetClassObject(CLSID rclsid, DWORD dwClsContext,
                         COSERVERINFO* pServerInfo,
                         REFIID riid, LPVOID* ppv);
```

On Win32-based systems, the following is what actually happens.

Based on the CLSID passed in the `rclsid` parameter, the function goes to a system database and performs lookup operations. Typically residing in the system registry, the system database contains all the COM classes currently available for instantiation on the system (in the form of CLSIDs). Associated with each CLSID, there are many attributes. One of these attributes indicates the type of module in which the component actually resides. Such a module is called an **object server**. Under Win32, COM supports a 'DLL', an 'EXE', or an 'EXE'/'DLL' running on another machine. In more abstract COM terms, these are referred to an **in-process server**, a **local server**, and a **remote server** respectively. Remote DLL based servers are typically activated through the help of a 'surrogate' process. The sole purpose in life for a typical surrogate process is to support the activation of DLL servers.

The `dwClsContext` parameter specifies what type of server the client will accept. It can be any of the following values:

Value	Description
CLSCTX_INPROC_SERVER	Client accepts only in-process (often called 'in-proc') servers. Under Win32, the implementation is expected to reside in a DLL, and be executed in the same process as the client.
CLSCTX_LOCAL_SERVER	Client accepts only local servers. Under Win32, the implementation is expected to be in its own EXE file. The server will be running in a separate process from the client.

Value	Description
CLSCTX_REMOTE_SERVER	Client accepts only remote servers. Remote servers are enabled through Distributed COM (DCOM), an extension to basic COM. We'll look at DCOM in more detail in Chapter 9. The server providing the service resides on another machine in the network. The server and client are expected to be running on separate machines.
CLSCTX_SERVER	The client will accept service from this object from any of the above types of server.

There are two additional possible values, called CLSCTX_INPROC_HANDLER, and CLSCTX_ALL. We will not discuss them here, since they are typically used only by legacy OLE desktop applications.

If a match for the object and dwClsContext can be found in the database, the actual location (on disk) of where the object server resides will be noted. This information is stored as another attribute associated with the CLSID – the path name of the DLL or EXE, or Network Machine Name for a remote object server.

The CoGetClassObject() call will do different things depending on the dwClsContext value. The simplest and most interesting case for us right now is the case of an in-process server. For an in-process server, the system code implementing CoGetClassObject() loads the DLL and calls a function that all in-process servers *must* export on Win32 platforms – DllGetClassObject(). This 'magic' function creates a class factory and returns a pointer to the IClassFactory interface from the class factory.

> *Needless to say, implementations of DllGetClassObject() on other systems where DLLs aren't supported, say a UNIX variant, may be handled differently.*

If the object to be created is serviced by a local server (EXE), the EXE will be loaded and executed, if it isn't already running on the system. Following this, some magic code will be called to obtain an IClassFactory interface pointer from a class factory within the executable. We will defer discussion of the details of this code marshaling (an *abyss of complexity*) to the next chapter.

If the object to be created is serviced by a remote server, a rather complex sequence of events will occur, but again I'll defer discussion until Chapter 9, when we discuss DCOM.

In reality, an object may support the IClassFactory2 interface instead of IClassFactory. (Remember that an interface never changes? Well, Microsoft had to create a new one here.) IClassFactory2 supports licensing, which wasn't a concern addressed by the original IClassFactory interface. We won't be discussing licensing, since it generally doesn't apply to business objects development on intranets. The interested reader can consult the description of IClassFactory2 in the Platform SDK for more information, or look at *Professional ATL Programming* (Richard Grimes, Wrox Press). For our discussions, we'll assume that the in-proc object server which we're dealing with provides the IClassFactory interface for the class factory.

Singleton Pattern

The `DllGetClassObject()` function exported by the DLL server typically implements another design pattern; the **singleton**. This means that repeated calls to the DLL's `DllGetClassObject()` function – a well known access point – by different clients, or the same client, typically return the same instance of the class factory. Of course, this is not cast in stone, but it is a rarity *not* to use a singleton as a class factory.

A Word on Server Module Types

We've discovered that object servers come in three flavors:

- ❑   In-process
- ❑   Local
- ❑   Remote

In-process Servers

An in-process server provides objects that run in the same process as the client. On Win32 systems, they're usually created in the form of a DLL. A DLL, by definition, runs in the same process as its user.

Just to give you a feel of how pervasive in-process servers are, all the controls used in Visual Basic applications and the myriad of ActiveX controls used by Internet Explorer 4, and all MTS components are in-process servers.

Local Servers

A local server provides objects that run in an independent process. On Win32 systems, local servers are usually implemented in the form of an EXE. Depending on the nature of the application the server implements, one single EXE image may be able to manage multiple objects, or each object may correspond to a separate running EXE.

Proxy Design Pattern

The client of the local server communicates with the EXE through proxy code. The **proxy** is an in-process COM object running in the client process, exposing the same interface as the local server. This is an application of the Proxy design pattern.

Internally, the proxy implements the interface as Remote Procedure Calls (RPC) or alternative Inter-process Communications (IPC) mechanisms, communicating with the server in a separate address space (for another process). Most of the time, this activity is transparent to the client and the server; the client simply makes the interface call, and the server simply services the call.

The Façade Pattern

There's a significant difference between in-process and local servers, such that the local servers that exist today are typically implemented for the following reasons:

❑   The COM local server implements, or 'front ends', a more traditional server requiring efficient access to shared resources by multiple clients. This is an application of the façade design pattern. For example, a legacy, large, non-component based, or proprietary application wants to participate in a COM environment by offering its own subfunctions to external clients (a specific example may be the set of applications within the Microsoft Office 97 suite, such as Excel, Word, and PowerPoint). This provides customization and extension possibilities for an application without 'giving away the ship' by providing completely reusable components.

❑   As a means of providing fault isolation and access security to running COM objects.

❑   During development and testing, in order to decouple the client from the server until the server is stable enough to run within the client process.

❑   As a 'beta test' mechanism for DCOM-based remote objects before the DCOM software stabilizes and matures.

This last point is important because, for the client or object server developer, implementing a local server is almost identical to implementing a remote one. Code written to work with local servers will almost certainly run with very little change when moved to DCOM, since controlling an object and interacting with it across process boundaries is quite similar to interaction across machine boundaries. Therefore, with very little effort, the client/object server implementer can achieve location transparency with a common source base.

COM Diagram Conventions

Ladies and Gentleman, witness a COM object:

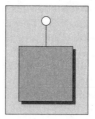

Don't ask me why, or whence it came. It seems that the notation for COM has descended from Microsoft's Ivory Tower and can now commonly be seen in contemporary trade publications, including many non-Microsoft ones. If you can't beat them, join them. The shaded block is an object, and the thing sticking out with a lollipop on top is an interface. When an interface is shown on top, it's usually IUnknown, while other, less privileged, interfaces stick out on the side, in whatever space they can find.

Actually, this isn't one of the more functional or particularly pretty schemes for diagramming objects and their interconnections, but it is the de facto standard for documenting COM interactions. For example, the earlier hypothetical banking example can be shown as:

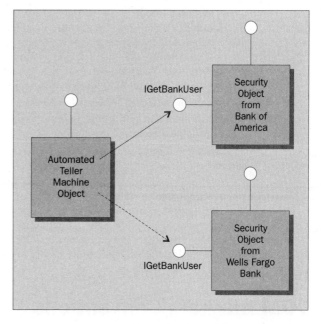

What these diagrams don't convey, however, is quite often the trickiest part of COM programming: the interactions between objects over time across multiple interfaces (or multiple methods in the same interface). This is especially true when the objects you write interact with objects which you didn't write. Typical documentation includes a static description of interface methods with some snippets of ad hoc scenarios of interactions with other objects. What isn't covered, we have to determine through trial and error. There is currently no tool or commonly accepted methodology to improve the situation. It is hoped that the highly integrated tools associated with the upcoming COM+ will address this problem.

Dynamic Modeling with Sequence Diagrams

Another diagramming scheme that we will use throughout this book is the UML sequence diagram. Such diagrams allow us to describe the dynamic interactions between components over time for a specific operation.

For example, the create object scenario described earlier for an in-process object server can be presented like this:

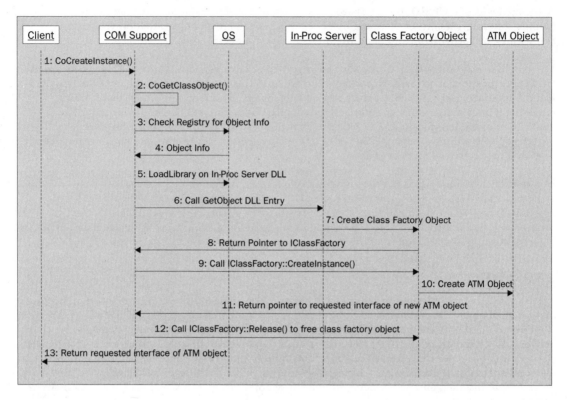

You can see how the client interacts with the COM runtime to find the class factory for the ATM object.

I hope you agree with me that the sequence diagram speaks volumes when you really want to know what's going on under the hood. Typically, the combination of the COM object/interface diagram, with the interface description, together with a set of sequence diagrams represents an acceptable set of programmer's documentation for individual components. Unfortunately, the subset of Rational Rose that Microsoft has licensed for the Microsoft Visual Modeler (a tool that comes with the Enterprise version of Visual Studio 6), does not include a facility for drawing sequence diagrams. You will need the full-blown Rose 98 (or another UML tool) for help in creating sequence diagrams.

Managing COM Classes

Obviously, to make good use of COM objects, there are other support services that are needed. One of the most important support services is the system database that we encountered earlier. This database provides information on every class of object that can be created and accessed on each machine.

Associated with the CLSID, the database keeps track of a 16-bit major and a 16-bit minor number to identify differing versions of the same object class. One can create objects that are 'backward compatible' by recognizing and handling these version numbers.

The database also stores IIDs. Interfaces, however, don't have version numbers. This is because in the COM specification, as we said earlier, an interface forms a contract between the interface provider and the interface user. This contract isn't subject to change. This is so important, that it bears repeating it once more. Once an interface is defined, it lives forever. The implementation or application of the interface may be changing on a case-by-case basis, but the actual 'contract' (interface) itself will never change. In order to modify the 'contract', a new one must be drawn up (that is, a new interface must be created).

Where is this database? This is a very interesting question. At the time of writing, the answer is the Windows 95 or Windows NT 4.0 registry. The COM support system manages the object location function. When you make a call to CoCreateInstance(), passing it a valid CLSID, the COM runtime will find information about the class factory from the database and will instantiate the COM object according to your request.

Class Store

This simple scheme, however, breaks down when one considers a network of computers all hosting thousands of object classes that need to be registered on each individual machine. With the arrival of Windows NT 5.0, this database will be migrating to the Active Directory service, managed by your network of NT servers. Called the 'Class Store', this database will be able to keep track of the COM classes available – per department, organizational unit or enterprise. Functionally, any classes that the component client needs, which may not be residing on the local machine, can now be downloaded, installed and instantiated, in one fell swoop if necessary. COM utopia will soon arrive with the Class Store.

Until the Class Store becomes a reality, you cannot create instances of classes that don't reside on your machine without first installing their server modules locally. If you are creating remote objects, you must ensure that the database entry for that object contains the network address of the machine on which the object is hosted. Either that, or you can undertake the even more undesirable task of hard-coding the address into your client code. Each and every network object must be 'wired' this way. MTS does provide some relief in this area for certain types of component – we'll be looking at MTS in Chapter 9.

Readers who are interested in the state of this database today are encouraged to go through Appendix A right now. Appendix A describes all the class attributes that are tracked in the registry based database by Windows 98 and Windows NT 4.0. It also describes the usage of a highly versatile COM utility called OLEVIEW.

Summary

In this chapter, the first of two introducing COM, we've introduced the basic concepts that we'll be building on throughout the book. The basic 'BLOB and OFFSETS' feature introduced at the start of this chapter is applicable in any operating system, using any programming language. Yet, with such a simple concept, real component-based software reuse is made possible.

In this chapter, we learned a number of things about the basics of COM, including:

- ❑ COM objects and the absolutely essential IUnknown interface, together with it's three methods – QueryInterface(), AddRef() and Release()
- ❑ Several 'golden rules' of COM programming
- ❑ How we can go about instantiating COM classes – the use of the Factory Method design pattern helped us to understand how we can use class factories for this purpose
- ❑ The IClassFactory interface supported by class factories
- ❑ The different flavors of server we can create – in-process, local and remote
- ❑ The various COM diagram conventions that we saw toward the end of the chapter facilitate documentation and understanding of COM objects and their interactions
- ❑ How the system keeps track of all the COM classes and where this is going in the future, with NT 5 and the Class Store

In the next chapter, we'll be taking a look at some of the more advanced features of COM, so stick around – it's going to be an interesting journey.

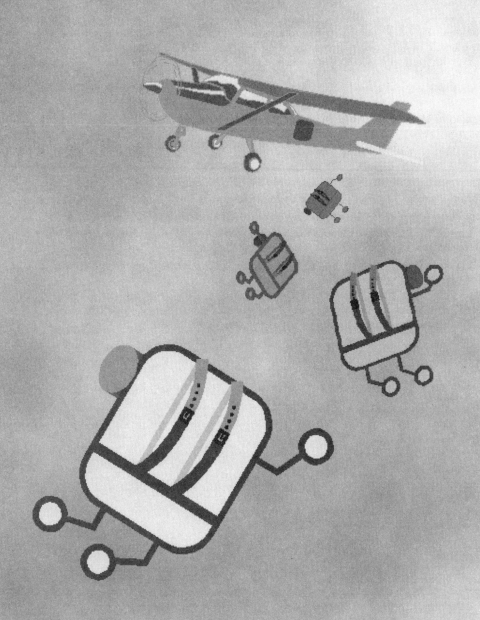

Just When You Thought It Was Safe...

In the first part of this chapter, we'll take a look at a several advanced COM concepts which enable 'component computing', another cornerstone of the Distributed interNet Applications (DNA) and the ActiveX movement. These concepts include:

❑ Automation
❑ Notification handling
❑ Containment
❑ Delegation
❑ Aggregation

Throughout our discussions, we will be very careful to avoid getting lost in the complexity that plagues many software designers when they first learn COM. This phenomenon accounts for a 'fuzzy period' of between three to six months of uncertainty about the technology, when developers feel that they can only follow rules blindly, without completely understanding them. Having spoken to many students of COM, we have come to realize that this complexity originates from *two* very specific, extremely complicated, yet fascinating technical areas:

❑ Marshaling
❑ Threading models

If one is careful when dealing with these issues (and resists the temptation of diving in head first), we believe that COM can be made readily understandable.

In this chapter, we will tread lightly upon these two 'complexity traps'. More detailed discussion of these areas will follow in later chapters, once you have become more comfortable working with the simpler facets of the technology.

Calling into the Object

In the last chapter, we learnt how to instantiate our component, obtain one of its interfaces, and now we're ready to party. So, how does the client out information about how to use the methods in the interface?

Of course, an interface is a contract, and therefore the methods in the interface must be documented somewhere. The user of the COM component, having read the documentation or contract, then makes the call according to the documentation.

However, we quickly realize that this is not always possible. More specifically, when we analyze our original 'component client/component' use case again, we found that the component client actor is actually two distinctly different subclasses of component clients. This is illustrated in the diagram:

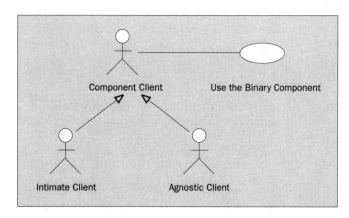

Here is a quick look at the two subclasses of component client.

Subclass Name	Description	Concrete Examples
Intimate Clients	These clients, in their compiled form, have built-in knowledge of the components that they will be making calls to. They are coded specifically to work with certain components only. This hard-code linkage results in high performance, but low flexibility.	C/C++ component clients. Compiled Visual Basic clients. Visual J++ clients. Clients of performance sensitive business objects for specific problems.

Subclass Name	Description	Concrete Examples
Agnostic Clients	These clients, in their compiled form, know nothing about components that they will be working with. Instead, they are interpreters. At runtime, driven by a script, they will discover the properties of the component that they work with. Scripting code is executed by these clients one line at a time. These clients will work with any components designed to be compatible with Automation (there is a section on this later in this chapter). For this extreme flexibility, these clients are willing to give up some runtime efficiency.	VBScript, JScript and JavaScript clients. Visual Basic for Applications. Certain Visual Basic and Visual J++ clients.

VTBL Binding

To satisfy the requirements of 'intimate clients' (especially C++ based ones) the actual binding between client and component must be established at compile time. To this end, the actual calls into methods of an interface are mapped onto vtable-based C++ method calls and compiled directly into the code. Calling methods, in this case, is extremely efficient, having the same overhead as calling a C++ virtual function, in the case of a loaded in-process server module. This approach of COM method invocation is known as **VTBL binding** (not to be confused with C++ virtual function binding terminology).

> *It's called a 'binding' because the user of a COM class essentially 'attaches' or 'binds' the client to an object at runtime.*

VTBL binding allows the compiler to calculate and prepare the most efficient way of 'attaching' to the component and make use of its services. Let's look once again at some code that we saw back in the last chapter:

```
HRESULT CoCreateInstance(CLSID rclsid, LPUKNOWN pUnkOuter,
                  DWORD dwClsContext, REFIID riid, LPVIOD* ppvObj)
{
    HRESULT hresult;
    IClassFactory* pCF;

    CoGetClassObject(rclsid, dwClsContext, NULL,
                  IID_IClassFactory, &pCF);

    hresult = pCF->CreateInstance(pUnkOuter, riid, ppvObj)
    pCF->Release();
    return hresult;
}
```

This code extract makes use of VTBL binding in its calls to IClassFactory::CreateInstance() and IClassFactory::Release().

Unlike conventional DLL or library calling, VTBL binding is not sensitive to COM class implementation changes, provided the new class exposes the same set of interfaces (that is, the vtable remains the same). This is, once again, a benefit of the *immutability* of an interface.

When We Cannot Perform VTBL Binds

For our 'agnostic clients', performance is important, but they are willing to sacrifice some runtime performance for the flexibility of rapid development. An example would be the interpretive mode of Visual Basic. These environments use interpretive techniques to allow rapid and easy development of applications by scripting pre-built components. Because of their interpretive nature, VTBL binding is not possible. VTBL binding demands that the client has an intimate knowledge of a component. In this case, however, an interpretive IDE, or a scripting engine, cannot possibly know all the COM components that it will ever work with and provide vtable linkage for them ahead of time.

Without the ability to perform VTBL binding early, what else can we do? Late binding, of course! Once again making use of the lifetime consistency inherent in an interface, the COM implementers have specified a special interface that can be used in this case. This interface is called IDispatch.

Through the IDispatch interface, it's possible for the client to discover, at runtime, what it can do with the COM object. Also through the IDispatch interface, the client can invoke methods supported by the component. So what we're actually saying is that the client would *VTBL bind* to the component's IDispatch interface, and then use it during runtime to discover and/or *late bind* to the component. Put another way, the 'agnostic clients, typically interpreters for scripting languages, know intimately about the vtable of the IDispatch interface, but they wouldn't have knowledge about the vtable of a custom user defined interface emanating from a custom component. Okay, this sounds feasible, but it still doesn't solve the semantics and interactions problem!

Automation

Let us take another quick look at the component client/compo- nent use case that we saw in the last chapter:

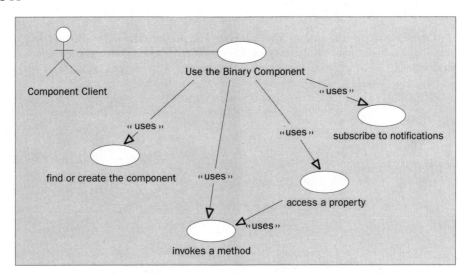

We are reminded here that once the component client has created the component, it uses it to:

- ❑ Invoke a method
- ❑ Access a property
- ❑ Subscribe to notifications

Accessing a property means the ability to read the value of a property or write to the property. This can actually be implemented using the 'invoking a method' use case. For example, in order to provide a `Modified` Boolean flag property for our component, we can define a pair of methods, `set_Modified()` and `get_Modified()`, in an interface of our component. All that we need now is some help from the COM support system to map these two methods semantically to the access of the `Modified` property. This help comes in the form of **Automation**.

Due to the overwhelming popularity of Microsoft's Office suite, its associated Visual Basic for Applications (VBA) language and Visual Basic itself, the late binding mechanism through `IDispatch` has been coined Automation. The term was chosen because the original motivation was the desire to enable the creation of macros (scripts) that could drive Microsoft Office applications to perform tedious or repetitive tasks using dialects of Visual Basic, without the presence of the end user (i.e. automatically or 'via automation').

A Taste of Automation

What follows is a fragment of Visual Basic code that illustrates how automation is used to access a COM object's property and methods.

Code written in scripting languages such as JavaScript, JScript or VBScript will be very similar.

The `Wrox.TipBlob1.1` object has one property and three methods:

- ❑ `InternalProperty`
- ❑ `GetManagerName()`
- ❑ `OkayToPublishInfo()`
- ❑ `PeekCounter()`

`Counter1`, `PropOut` and `Manager` in the code below are edit controls on a form of the Visual Basic application:

```
Private Sub Command2_Click()

    Dim flag As Boolean

    ' Late Binding Example
    Call CleanForm
    Dim AnObj As Object
    Set AnObj = CreateObject("Wrox.TipBlob1.1")
    AnObj.InternalProperty = 3333
```

```
        Manager.Text = AnObj.GetManagerName()
        flag = AnObj.OkayToPublishInfo(1990 + Int(Rnd * 100 + 1), _
                                       Int(Rnd * 12 + 1))
        If flag Then
           Okay.Text = "OKAY"
        Else
           Okay.Text = "NO WAY"
        End If
        Counter1.Text = Str$(AnObj.PeekCounter())
        PropOut.Text = Str$(AnObj.InternalProperty)
        Set AnObj = Nothing

     End Sub
```

Notice the natural syntax used to access the `InternalProperty` property. This maps to a method call, `set_InternalProperty(3333)`. A property is used as if it is a data member of a structure – we can use it on both sides of the assignment statement. The syntax for method invocation is also quite direct, as you can see from the above code.

The object is created with the following statements:

```
     Dim AnObj As Object
     Set AnObj = CreateObject("Wrox.TipBlob1.1")
```

The `AnObj` variable can be thought of as an interface holder. In fact, it will hold onto the `IDispatch` interface of the object. The `CreateObject()` call translates to a `CoCreateInstance()` call, with the string `"Wrox.TipBlob1.1"` translated to the CLSID required for `CoCreateInstance()`. This translation is again performed through the object class database that we are already familiar with. The `"Wrox.TipBlob1.1"` string is actually called a **ProgID**, and is essentially a human-friendly name for the CLSID. Typically, this is in the `<module>.<component>.<version>` form. We can see, though, that there could be problems with this, because ProgIDs may not be unique. Despite this, however, they are still extremely useful, as they eliminate those cryptic CLSIDs.

To summarize, COM objects that expose the `IDispatch` interface can implement a group of properties (semantically similar to C++ structure/class member variables) that we can `Get` and `Set`, through late binding to the underlying methods. They may also provide a set of methods (semantically similar to C++ structure/class member functions) that we can invoke through late binding.

Essentially, we're adding another layer of indirection to drive the object's actual functionality. What we pay for in terms of reduced performance, we gain in tremendous flexibility. Now, any application or development environment which implements the capability to drive a COM class through `IDispatch` can freely use any late binding COM classes *during runtime*. Any newly created class, as long as it implements late binding via `IDispatch`, can be immediately used by the existing application. This is quite powerful.

One remaining mystery is how the client discovers what methods or properties are available from the component. For example, in the code above, how would Visual Basic know that `InternalProperty` property for `AnObj` exists? How will it know what is the data type of the property? The only sure thing is that it *cannot* possibly know, or perform lookup, ahead of time. This is due to the fact that the argument to the `CreateObject()` call may not be determined until runtime. That is, the Visual Basic interpreter will not know what object to create until it actually interprets the line. The answer to this mystery lies again in the `IDispatch` interface.

Time to see how all this actually works.

The IDispatch Interface and Late Binding

For runtime 'dynamic' discovery of COM component functionality, the `IDispatch` interface has methods that facilitate retrieving information about the methods to be invoked, or properties to be retrieved or set. Here are the methods of the `IDispatch` inteface:

- ❑   `Invoke()`
- ❑   `GetIDsOfNames()`
- ❑   `GetTypeInfo()`
- ❑   `GetTypeInfoCount ()`

Let's look at these methods in more detail.

Firstly, we'll take a look at the all important `Invoke()` method.

IDispatch::Invoke()

This is the main method of the `IDispatch` interface. It invokes the requested method of the server interface.

```
HRESULT IDispatch::Invoke(DISPID dispidMember,
                          REFIID riid,
                          LCID lcid,
                          WORD wFlags,
                          DISPPARAMS FAR* pdispparams,
                          VARIANT FAR* pvarResult,
                          EXCEPINFO FAR* pexcepinfo,
                          unsigned int FAR* puArgErr );
```

Parameters

Parameter	Description
dispidMember	DISPID (see page 11) of the requested member. DISPIDs for arguments depend on their position in the method argument list, starting with 0 for the first one − we'll see more of these later. Most likely, it was obtained by using `GetIDsOfNames()`.
riid	Reserved. Must be IID_NULL.

Table Continued on Following Page

Parameter	Description
lcid	The locale context. May be necessary in order to interpret arguments. It's used by the GetIDsOfNames() function, and is passed to Invoke() to allow the object to interpret its arguments in a locale-specific way. Locale management is a topic in application internationalization, and is beyond the scope of this book. Interested readers are referred to their MSDN CD for more information.
wFlags	The flags help clarify how to interpret the requested member DISPID. See the table below for more information on these.
pdispparams	Pointer to a structure containing an array of arguments, an array of argument DISPIDs for named arguments, and counts for the number of elements in the arrays. The arguments are read-only except when the DISPATCH_PROPERTYPUTREF flag has been set.
pvarResult	Pointer to where the result is to be stored. Can be NULL (no return value). Notice that the VARIANT type is a union (in the C++ sense) of many different types of values or pointers.
pexcepinfo	Pointer to a structure containing exception information. This structure should be filled in if DISP_E_EXCEPTION is returned. Can be NULL (no exception information returned). In the context of IDispatch, an exception is really an error object.
puArgErr	The index of the first argument within pDispParams->rgvarg that has an error. It may have been set by the caller to indicate missing arguments. The object sets it when arguments of the wrong type have been passed into Invoke().

The wFlags parameter can be one of the following values:

Value	Description
DISPATCH_METHOD	The member is invoked as a method.
DISPATCH_PROPERTYGET	The member is retrieved as a property.
DISPATCH_PROPERTYPUT	The member is changed as a property.
DISPATCH_PROPERTYPUTREF	The member is changed via a reference assignment, rather than a value assignment. This flag is valid only when the property accepts a reference to an object. This is useful for clients implementing a scripting language that can assign objects by reference

Return Value

Here are some of the standard values, taken from the returned HRESULT:

Return value	Description
S_OK	Success.
DISP_E_BADPARAMCOUNT	Wrong number of arguments.
DISP_E_BADVARTYPE	Wrong variant argument type, puArgErr can be used to determine the offending argument.
DISP_E_EXCEPTION	An error occurred which should result in an exception. The error information has been filled in pexcepinfo.
DISP_E_MEMBERNOTFOUND	The requested member does not exist, or tried to set the value of a read-only property.
DISP_E_NONAMEDARGS	This implementation of IDispatch does not support named arguments.
DISP_E_OVERFLOW	One of the arguments in pDispParams->rgvarg could not be coerced to the specified type. Bear in mind that the arguments are passed as VARIANT types.
DISP_E_PARAMNOTFOUND	One of the parameter DISPIDs does not correspond to a parameter on the method. In this case puArgErr should be set to the first argument that contains the error.
DISP_E_TYPEMISMATCH	One or more of the arguments could not be coerced. The index of the first parameter within pDispParams->rgvarg that has the incorrect type is returned in the puArgErr parameter.
DISP_E_UNKNOWNINTERFACE	The IID passed in riid is not IID_NULL.
DISP_E_UNKNOWNLCID	Wrong locale information.
DISP_E_PARAMNOTOPTIONAL	A required parameter was omitted.

More errors, specific to the particular object, may be defined and returned.

IDispatch::GetTypeInfo()

This method retrieves a description of the object's programmable interface through a 'type information' interface (ITypeInfo). (Don't worry too much about this member now, we'll be covering it later in the section, *A Type Libraries Detour*.)

```
HRESULT IDispatch::GetTypeInfo(unsigned int itinfo,
                              LCID lcid,
                              ITypeInfo FAR* FAR* pptinfo );
```

Parameters

Parameter	Description
itinfo	The type information to return. Passing 0 asks for IDispatch type information.
lcid	The locale ID for the type information. An object may be able to return different type information for different languages (for example, localized member names). We can get the default by passing LOCALE_USER_DEFAULT.
pptinfo	Receives a pointer to the requested type information object.

Return Values

The return value obtained from the returned HRESULT is one of the following:

Return value	Description
S_OK	Success. The type information exists and was successfully retrieved
DISP_E_BADINDEX or TYPE_E_ELEMENTNOTFOUND	Failure. Asked for the wrong type info; itinfo argument was not 0

Comments

The retrieved type information interface can then be used to get specific information about the methods and properties we want to invoke, Get or Set.

Some clients, such as programming IDEs, may make use of the type information to display the component in a design-time palette for drag-and-drop deployment.

> *Readers who are familiar with Smalltalk, CORBA, or Java will recognize this 'type information' as meta-data or BeanInfo. The action of examining this information is sometimes called 'dynamic runtime discovery' or 'introspection'.*

IDispatch::GetTypeInfoCount()

The `IDispatch::GetTypeInfoCount()` function is very straightforward. It simply a count of type information interfaces via a pointer, `piTInfo`:

```
HRESULT GetTypeInfoCount(unsigned int FAR* piTInfo);
```

IDispatch::GetIDsOfNames()

Even though an Automation client may use user-readable names for the methods and properties of an Automation server (component), when it actually invokes them through `IDispatch::Invoke()`, an ID is used in order to signify exactly which property or method we want.

This layer of abstraction allows, for example, methods to have different names in different national languages – depending on the locality – but just one implementation. The type of the ID is a dispatch ID, or **DISPID** (it's really a `long` type). The purpose of `IDispatch::GetIDsOfNames()` is to return to the caller an array of DISPIDs, corresponding to an array of textual names that were passed in. The array contains either the name of a property, a method, or the name of a method followed by the names of its parameters. Thus, each invocation of `GetIDsOfNames()` refers to one property or one method only.

```
HRESULT IDispatch::GetIDsOfNames(REFIID riid,
                                 OLECHAR FAR* FAR* rgszNames,
                                 unsigned int cNames,
                                 LCID lcid,
                                 DISPID FAR* rgdispid );
```

Parameters

Parameters	Description
riid	Must be `IID_NULL`.
rgszNames	Array of names to be mapped.
cNames	Count of the names to be mapped.
lcid	The locale context in which to interpret the names.
rgdispid	Caller-allocated array, each element of which contains an ID corresponding to one of the names passed in the `rgszNames` array. If cNames is 1, the sole element of the `rgdispid` array corresponds to the method or property name passed in. Otherwise the first element represents the method name, while the subsequent elements represent each of the method's parameters. If any of the names aren't recognized, `DISPID_UNKNOWN` is stored in the corresponding position in the `rgdispid` array and `DISP_E_UNKNOWNNAME` is returned. Thus, the client (controller) knows which of the names weren't recognized. No specific ordering of names is required.

Return Value

The return value obtained from HRESULT is one of the following:

Return value	Description
S_OK	Success.
E_OUTOFMEMORY	Out of memory.
DISP_E_UNKNOWNNAME	One or more of the names were not known. The returned array of DISPIDs contains DISPID_UNKNOWN for each entry that corresponds to an unknown name
DISP_E_UNKNOWNLCID	The LCID wasn't recognized.

Comments

The member and parameter DISPIDs must remain static for repeated instantiation of the COM object. This allows a client to obtain the DISPIDs once and cache them for later use. A form of binding called ID-binding is used by some versions of Visual Basic (3 and 4) where the DISPIDs are obtained once and stored with the interpreted program.

DISPIDs are unique only within the same context (one interface). The same name may map to different DISPIDs, depending on context. For example, a name may have a DISPID when it's used as a member name with a particular interface, and a different DISPID for each time it appears as a parameter. It's worth noting in passing the kinds of values a DISPID may take:

DISPID Value	Description
DISPID_VALUE (0)	The default member of the IDispatch interface. In other words, if the object is invoked by name (let's say in a client's script), without further specifying a property or method, this member is going to be invoked.
Negative values	Standard DISPIDs, already reserved by Microsoft. For example, DISPID_UNKNOWN (-1) returned in the above API call signifies the name requested was not found. We will see many more examples when we work with 'stock properties' of ActiveX controls in Chapter 7.
Positive values	These are specified when the interface is defined. As we'll see later, when discussing the Interface Definition Language (IDL), there is a natural place where the DISPID for each method or property can be specified. The default member with DISPID DISPID_VALUE (0) is also specified when defining the interface.

Making Late Binding Work

To clear up any confusion, the sequence diagram is shown here, which illustrates how late binding is accomplished through the `IDispatch` interface. This scenario assumes the role of an interpretive macro language (for example VBScript). There is no need to 'discover' the capabilities of the component because the programmer who wrote the script being interpreted has already done so. However, if the script contains programming errors (for example, a property name of a component is misspelled), it will be caught during late binding at runtime.

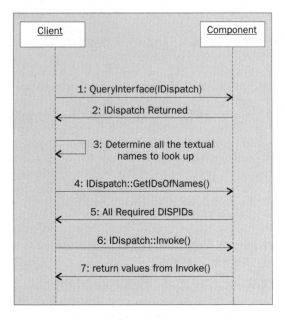

Basically, the client needs to first translate textual property, method and parameter names to DISPIDs, and then invoke the method indirectly through the `IDispatch::Invoke()` method. All arguments to the method are passed as `VARIANT` type, which is a wildcard C++ union that can represent most data types natively.

If our component supports the `IDispatch` interface, the `Invoke()` method can be quite complicated to implement from scratch. Fortunately, there is significant support in the form of standard Win32 API functions that take care of mundane, repetitive, but also very important tasks, such as parameter matching, parameter packaging, etc.. Look up the `CreateStdDispatch()`, `DispInvoke()`, `DispGetParam()` helper APIs on your MSDN CD if you are interested. However, this wouldn't be possible if standard ways of specifying the necessary type information were not available. This brings us right to the next section.

A Detour into Type Libraries

Compared to VTBL binding, late binding is extremely inefficient. Imagine having to use the `IDispatch` interface, each and every time, to obtain DISPIDs for a component's methods, and then for all the parameters for that method, and finally to invoke the method. Notice the number of function calls required between the client and the object in the sequence diagram above. It's quite bad, even when the server is running within the same process. Just imagine what it would be like if the server is a local server running in another process, requiring a context switch for every function call, or even across the network, requiring network transmission on every call. Definitely less than optimal performance!

A mechanism to find out quickly and easily what properties and methods are supported by an object would really improve things. If we know what the object can do ahead of time (although, still at runtime, not as far ahead as VTBL binding), then the only performance hit that we have to take is the unavoidable indirection through `IDispatch`. This will be the best thing that we can do with an `IDispatch` interface. Well, the COM folks have done it, and it's called a **type library**.

Type libraries have existed for a long time within the COM support system and the `IDispatch` interface. The `ITypeLib` interface (and its associated `ITypeInfo` interface) provides access to COM classes managing the type library information. What has been added more recently is an easy way for the developer of COM objects to create these type libraries. Instead of making a complicated series of calls into a type library object, one can simply use a text editor to describe the elements in a text file. Microsoft provides an enhanced version of the Interface Description Language (IDL) compiler **Midl.exe** that will read the text file (IDL file) and then call the appropriate API and interfaces on your behalf in order to create the library. We'll talk more about MIDL in Chapter 3.

Working directly with type libraries is of interest typically only to tools vendors or compiler writers, because of the libraries' very low level nature. For the rest of us, it will suffice to know that the Win32 API's `LoadTypeLib()` and `LoadTypeLibFromResource()` will load a type library file, create the necessary type library objects, and give the caller back an `ITypeLib` interface – ready for further manipulation and querying.

> *In due time, Microsoft will probably hide the complexity of type libraries from C++ COM programmers using something called 'attribute-based programming'. This will simplify COM programming significantly, and is a promised feature in their COM+ vision.*

A type library comprehensively describes almost everything contained and used by a particular object server. It can include definitions for:

- COM objects
- COM interfaces
- Custom interfaces (user defined)
- Dispatch interfaces
- Dual interfaces (that is, both custom and dispatch – see below)
- `IDispatch` properties
- `IDispatch` methods
- TYPE definitions
- STRUCTURE definitions

Once compiled, a type library becomes a binary resource. It can then be distributed in various forms:

- In its own `.tlb` file
- Bound into an EXE file as a resource
- Bound into a DLL file as a resource

The most convenient way of distributing a binary resource is to include it with the EXE or DLL file. For a COM server supporting `IDispatch` late binding, it's customary to register the type library information at the same time as the other class object attributes are being registered with the classes database.

Dual Interfaces

You like the efficiency of VTBL binding, and yet you like the flexibility offered by late binding. Since the code that implements the object's behavior has already been written, why not make it available to both VTBL and late binders?

This is especially important for interpretative development environments that can also compile to more efficient native or optimized runtime code. For example, Visual Basic version 4 uses late binding on properties and methods during application design and debug time, but will automatically take advantage of the higher performance VTBL binding if you 'make an EXE' using the compilation facility. Script languages such as VBScript, having no such compilation facility, continue to use late binding exclusively, while 'power' languages such as C++ work best with VTBL binding.

Applying a well-known design pattern called Command, one can define dual interfaces which exploit the best of both worlds.

To mark an interface as supporting both VTBL and late binding, it should be specified as `dual` when the type library is defined (we'll see how to do this in Chapter 4). Note that this is done only to let the client know that the interface or property is accessible both via VTBL and late bindings. It doesn't actually provide any code to implement `IDispatch` – you still need to do this.

A dual interface always derives from `IDispatch`, since all of the `IDispatch` methods must be implemented by a COM class supporting dual interfaces. A special restriction is imposed for dual interfaces that all member methods of the interface must return an `HRESULT` (**other than** `AddRef()` and `Release()`). Another less obvious restriction is that, since `IDispatch::Invoke()` only deals with method parameters of `VARIANT` compatible types, the vtable methods of a dual interface should only contain data types which are defined by the `VARIANT` union (more about this C++ union later).

The code to implement `IDispatch` support for the corresponding vtable methods is quite regular and tedious to code manually. A tool/library can assist with the implementation, and we'll see how the Active Template Library (ATL) makes dual interface support easy to implement in Chapter 4.

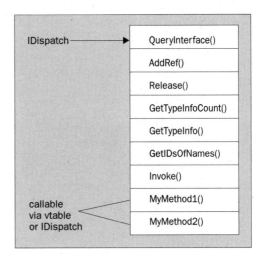

The [default] Interface

A COM component may expose one or more vtable interfaces, each providing a different set of capabilities. Each of these vtable interfaces can be accessed by the client through the QueryInterface() method. It is also possible that a number of these interfaces are implemented as dual interfaces. In this case, the object will have more than one IDispatch based interface. If a client does a QueryInterface() call for IDispatch, which one of these interfaces should be returned? To 'disambiguate' the situation, COM support allows you to specify one of these interfaces to be default in the type library. The methods and properties exposed on this interface will be used whenever an Automation client accesses the component through IDispatch without performing a QueryInterface() for a particular dual interface. Most development environments, such as Visual Basic and Visual J++, provide for working with multiple dual interfaces on a single component. Their scripting counterparts (VBScript, JavaScript), however, can only work with the default interface of a component.

Performing VTBL and Late Binding in C++

Recall that Automation clients expect the ability to access properties, while typical VTBL binding clients use the underlying direct method calls to the property access methods. This means that the methods specified for the default interface in a class supporting dual interfaces must be very carefully defined. For example, a method which sets a property called HeadCaption must follow the naming convention of put_HeadCaption(). In this way, the VTBL binding client can call put_HeadCaption() directly; meanwhile, the late binding client can set the HeadCaption property via the IDispatch::Invoke() call (or use ID binding as mentioned previously).

We will contrast how a VTBL binding client and a late binding client access a property. Both examples are written in C++ to emphasize the difference. In the following code snippet, pCustom is a valid pointer to our custom interface, obtained in the standard way that we have discussed:

```
HRESULT hResult;
BSTR newTitle = SysAllocString(_T("New Title"));
                        // allocate new string and copy value

if (newTitle)
   hResult = pCustom->put_HeadCaption(newTitle);

// check for errors
```

In the next chapter, we'll talk in more detail about the relevant data types (i.e. BSTR) and helper functions that (i.e. SysAllocString()).

For now, let's contrast the above code with the late binding case. Assume that we have somehow obtained a pointer to a dispatch interface (i.e. derived from IDispatch) called pDisp:

```
HRESULT hResult;
OLECHAR* szMember = _T("HeadCaption");
DISPID dispId;
DISPPARAMS dispParams;
VARIANTARG vargArgs[1];
hResult = pDisp->GetIDsOfNames(IID_NULL,
                        &szMember,    // name of the member
                        1,            // how many passed
```

```
                                        LOCALE_USER_DEFAULT, // default locale
                                        &dispId        // DISPID of the property
                                        );

// check for errors

// Strings should be passed in as BSTR. These are null-terminated
// strings that are prefixed by their length. No extra copy is
// required in order to pass them around across process boundaries.
dispParams.rgvarg = vargArgs;
dispParams.rgvarg[0].vt = VT_BSTR;

// allocate new string and copy value
dispParams.rgvarg[0].bstrVal = SysAllocString(_T("New Title"));

// because it is a property put
dispParams.rgdispidNamedArgs = DISPID_PROPERTYPUT;

dispParams.cArgs = 1;
dispParams.cNamedArgs = 1;

hResult = pDisp->Invoke(dispId,                // property DISPID
                        IID_NULL,              // fixed
                        LOCALE_USER_DEFAULT,   // default locale
                        DISPATCH_PROPERTYPUT,  // it is a property put
                        & dispParams,          // the value
                        NULL,                  // no result necessary
                        NULL,      // don't care about exceptions
                        NULL       // don't care about wrong arguments
                        );

// check for errors
```

Handling Notification

If you look back at the diagram we saw at the beginning of the chapter illustrating the component client/component use case diagram, you can see that, so far, we have covered how COM design satisfies three of the requirements:

- ❑ Finding or creating a component – using class factory objects
- ❑ Accessing a property – through IDispatch and late binding, or put_x()/get_x() methods and VTBL binding
- ❑ Invoking a method – via VTBL or late binding

The only requirement that we have not yet addressed is how to:

- ❑ Subscribe to notifications

In this case, the client wants the component to provide notification when something interesting happens. This ability to notify a client can be viewed as a characteristic of the component, as much as methods and properties. This means that it should be describable in the type library, and be discoverable at runtime with or without the type library. We can use an interface to implement this capability.

However, it is a very different interface to those we've seen previously. Instead of accepting incoming calls to methods and properties, the component agrees to make an outgoing call, back to the client, during notification. This also means that the client must be ready to implement the interface and accept the method call. What we are looking at is the COM component-based equivalent of a **common callback**.

An outgoing interface is marked in the type library as source to differentiate it from the common incoming interfaces.

Rather like Automation, script-based late binding clients cannot work with multiple outgoing interfaces from a component. Instead, they work with the outgoing interface that is marked as [default, source] in the type library. That is, the methods on this default interface are used exclusively for notification within the client.

The COM design solution takes the form of one of the following two mechanisms:

❏   Advise sinks
❏   Connection points

We will discuss each of these solutions in the following sections.

Observer (Publish/Subscribe) Pattern

Note that both advise sinks and connection points are implementations of the well-known Observer (or Publish/Subscribe) design pattern.

Advise Sinks

Advise sinks are the simpler of the two mechanisms, and solve the notification problem for our 'intimate' clients – that is, the client must have knowledge of the outgoing interface at compile time. An advise sink is basically an 'ear' in the client; it is listening out for notification of changes in the component. The actual COM advise sink mechanism is based on a single outgoing interface, IAdviseSink. The client must support this interface, and the component will only call methods defined in this interface. Unfortunately, advise sinks are not a generalized mechanism in COM, but rather, a protocol built upon COM by higher-level OLE layers to implement notifications.

Instead of describing the specific case used in OLE (see Mike Blazack's, "Professional MFC with Visual C++ 5" ISBN 1-86100 0146 for more information), we will look at advise sinks as a more general mechanism. We will not limit the notification interface to IAdviseSink, instead we will call our notification interface ICustomXAdviseSink to reflect an arbitrary notification interface. This interface can inherit from IAdviseSink, but has no need to. The X is a wildcard, indicating that the detail of the methods in the interface is agreed upon between the client and the component. As we will soon see, the IAdviseSink mechanism relies on a specific protocol between the client and component. Here are the objects and interfaces involved:

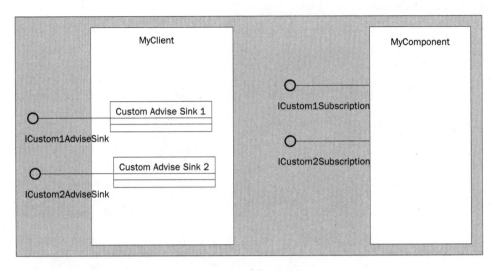

The client creates an instance of a custom advise sink object (that is, an object with an interface for callbacks) for each notification in which it is interested. Each instance of a custom advise sink object must support an ICustomXAdviseSink interface. The methods of the ICustomXAdviseSink interface(s) are used for callback from the component. So, one can choose to either use a single ICustomXAdviseSink interface with many notification methods – one for each notification – or many distinct ICustomXAdviseSink interfaces.

The client also provides a custom subscription interface, ICustomXSubscription, which the client will QueryInterface() for. The component indicates its support for a type of notification by implementing the corresponding custom subscription interfaces. Each ICustomXSubscription interface contains an Advise() and Unadvise() method, as well as other custom methods if necessary.

Once a client has obtained the ICustomXSubscription interface, it uses the Advise() method to pass the ICustomXAdviseSink interface from the corresponding custom advise sink object to the component. The component will return a 'session handle' value to indicate the accepted subscription. From now on, the component will call a notification method on the ICustomXAdviseSink interface whenever an event occurs. If the client wishes to terminate the subscription, it will call the ICustomXSubscription::Unadvise() with the 'session handle' to terminate the subscription. Internally, the component may manage an array of client-supplied advice sink objects. It will notify each of the clients holding a valid subscription.

Here is a sequence diagram showing what happens with advise sinks:

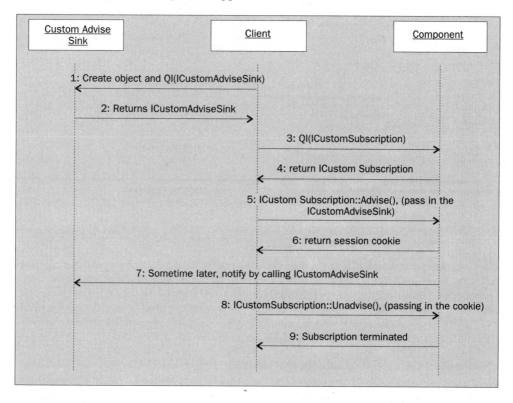

Observer Design Pattern

The Observer design pattern describes the relationship between a changing object (the subject) and an object that requires notification of such changes (the observer). The mapping of the advise sinks mechanism to the Observer design pattern is illustrated in the diagram below:

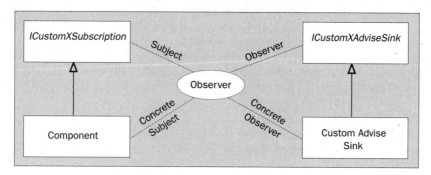

Here, the role of observer is played by the `ICustomXAdviseSink` interface, the Concrete Observer is the custom advise sink object inside the client, the subject is the `ICustomXSubscription` interface and the Concrete Subject is the component.

There are two disadvantages with this approach:

❑ Possible proliferation of interfaces: some implementations may require one subscription interface on the component, and an advice sink interface on the client for each type of notification
❑ It is not possible for agnostic clients to anticipate the type of component they may use and the incoming interfaces that they need to sink

Which leads us to...

Connection Points

Connection points are a significantly more generic mechanism for notifications. They are the notification mechanism of choice for ActiveX controls. If you need to support agnostic clients, it is necessary to use `IDispatch` and late binding in the notification mechanism. Connection points fit the bill and also overcome the need for defining a new interface for each new notification. The tradeoff is in the increased complexity of the connection points calling protocol.

Again, we should emphasize that connection points are a notification protocol/mechanism built on top of COM, and are by no means an intrinsic part of COM. However, they are used so frequently in late binding clients that they have become intimately associated with general COM component usage.

Here are the object classes and interfaces involved in the connection points mechanism:

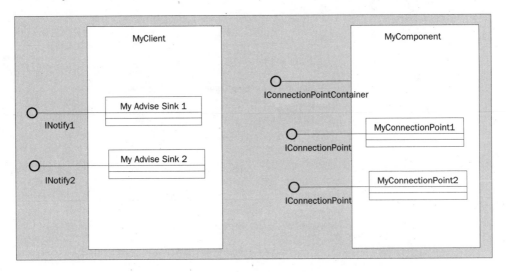

Instead of supplying specific interfaces for each notification supported, the component provides an `IConnectionPointContainer` interface to indicate that it supports at least one type of notification. Like the advise sinks situation, the client must be ready to sink events by creating custom advise sink objects. Similarly, each of these objects could sink an arbitrary advise interface. For supporting agnostic clients, this interface must be based on `IDispatch` (`INotifyX` in the diagram above).

Once the client has determined that the component supports notifications (that is, the
QueryInterface() for IConnectionPointContainer is successful), it can use the
IConnectionPointContainer::FindConnectionPoint() method to determine if the
component supports a specific type of notification, or it can use
IConnectionPointContainer::EnumConnectionPoints() to go through all the supported
notifications, one by one. In either case, the client will end up with the IConnectionPoint
interface of a connection point object within the component. This is the object that will fire the
notification to all subscribed clients, and IConnectionPoint is the generic subscription interface.
From this point on, the subscriber has located the subscription manager, and the mechanism is
identical to advise sinks. The client can use IConnectionPoint::Advise() to pass in the advise
interface of the corresponding sink object, receiving in turn a 'session handle'. The connection is now
established, and the component may call the methods in the advise interface to notify the client at
anytime. When the client wants to terminate the subscription, it will call
IConnectionPoint::Unadvise() and pass back the 'session handle' to terminate the
subscription with the component for that particular notification.

Here's a
sequence
diagram to
crystallize
the
concepts.

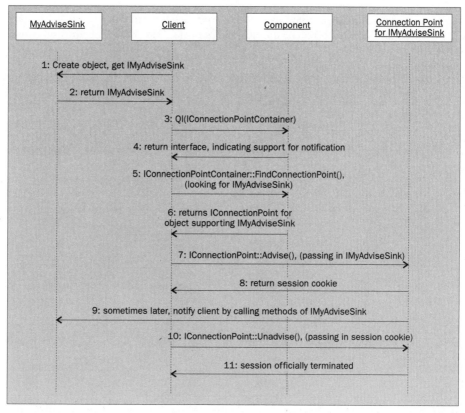

Notice that this design enables dynamic connection. The clients `QueryInterface()` for `IConnectionPointContainer` at *runtime*. For each connection point (type of notification) supported by the component, its outgoing interface can be obtained via `IConnectionPoint::GetConnectionInterface()`. Since this interface is based on `IDispatch`, the client can query its type library information and construct the appropriate sink object at *runtime* to mate and sink the corresponding notification. There needs to be no advance agreement between the client and the component, other than adherence to the connection points protocol, to enable notification subscription for agnostic clients.

Observer Design Pattern Again

The Observer design pattern reigns again. Here, the Observer is played by the `IDispatch` based notification interface, the Concrete Observer is the role of the corresponding sink object in the client, the Subject is the `IConnectionPoint` interface, and the Concrete Subject is the corresponding connection point object implemented by the component:

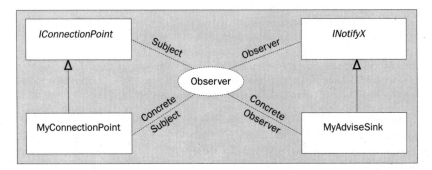

This concludes our discussion on how COM and its associated mechanism satisfies all the requirements of our "component client"/component use case analysis. Before moving on to a couple of code-reuse techniques, frequently used in the construction of COM components, we'll attempt to clarify a potential source of confusion.

Synchronous COM Calls vs Asynchronous Notification

At this time, all COM method invocations are synchronous. By synchronous, we mean that the client will stop execution when a method is invoked on a component, and will continue execution once the method returns. There is no exception to this rule with COM methods. This means that even method calls on the component's outgoing interface are synchronous. This behavior is exactly what we expect of a conventional callback. However, we sometimes see the description 'asynchronous notification'. Does this mean that some callbacks are asynchronous?

NO!

The 'asynchronous' in 'asynchronous notification' refers to the fact that there is no relationship between the time a notification subscription is made, and the time when the actual notification may occur. The actual method call used in the notification is still a synchronous call!

Real 'asynchronous COM calls' would mean 'call and forget – no return code', 'call and synchronize later – return code later', or 'call and get notification'. In each of these cases, two concurrent paths of execution exist once the call is made. Unfortunately, at the time of writing, COM does not support asynchronous calls. Microsoft has promised this ability with the COM+ vision. Today, similar behavior can be 'hard-coded' using MicroSoft Message Queue (we will examine MSMQ in Chapter 10).

Object Containment and Delegation

The most powerful thing about COM is the ability to use and reuse components dynamically in designing our systems. The idea of being able to encapsulate a concept, business rule, or a logical entity behind a component, and then use and reuse it in systems to solve practical problems is the grail of software design. Given this, it is entirely predictable that, in implementing our own COM classes, we may want to draw on the services of other predefined COM classes.

This delivers on one of the much vaunted benefits of object design, allowing us to use our software investment in any future project. How can we accomplish this using COM?

The most obvious way is to simply create other COM objects during our own operations and make them work for us. The COM specification allows this, and it's a great way of implementing COM classes, leveraging the code already encapsulated in other components.

When we create other COM objects during runtime, in order to use their services, this approach is known in COM as **containment**, since in fact, the main object we're creating is seen by the system as containing the worker object.

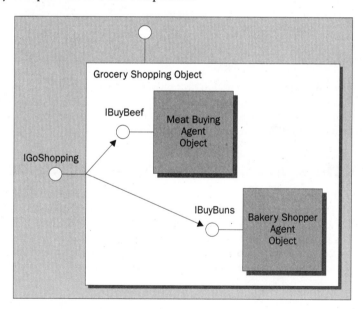

Containment is easy on the client because the client application, or object, doesn't even have to know about the existence of the contained object.

The action of calling a method in the worker object, in response to a method call on one of our own interfaces is called **delegation**. This is because we're delegating the work, or a piece of the work, to the worker object that we've created.

The simplistic example in the figure above shows containment and delegation in action. In this case, we're designing a grocery shopping object for client applications over the Internet. We provide an interface called `IGoShopping` that any client can call to get our COM class to do the shopping for them. In reality, we actually have two worker objects:

❑ A Meat Buying Agent object, which knows how to get the best quality and prices for all sorts of meat

❑ A Bakery Shopper Agent object, which knows about all the finer details of good baking.

Our Grocery Shopping object is said to **contain** both the Meat Buying Agent object and the Bakery Shopper Agent object. When our client calls our `IGoShopping::BuyForMeNow()` method, we immediately **delegate** the task to our two worker objects. To get the hard work done, the Grocery Shopping object calls the methods of the `IBuyMeat` interface from the Meat Buying Agent object, as well as the methods of the `IBuyBuns` interface from the Bakery Shopper Agent object. When the client retires our Grocery Shopping object after shopping concludes, we will, in turn, release our Meat Buying Agent and Bakery Shopper Agent objects.

Our Grocery Shopping object adds value to the client by constantly tracking and soliciting the services of the best possible meat and bakery buying agents in the entire info-universe. Any client object can reap the fruits of our labor simply by requesting the service of our Grocery Shopping object.

And that's all there is to it. To better visualize the interactions occurring in this particular case of containment and delegation, see the following sequence diagram:

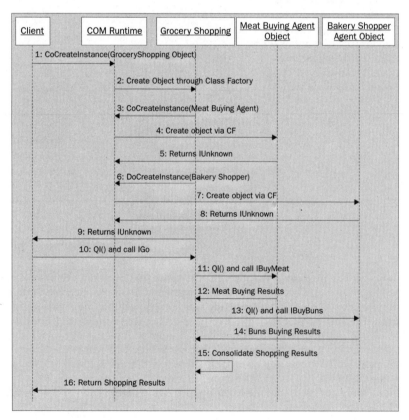

In our example, the worker objects are instantiated when our own object is instantiated, and destroyed when our own object is destroyed. There's nothing in the rule book that says one can't instantiate and destroy worker objects completely within one method call, or between invocation of different methods. However, significantly more attention must be paid in these cases to ensure that the design will have good performance (instantiating an object can be an expensive operation) and that it will be robust. It's difficult to enforce the calling pattern of methods. Consequently, it can be tricky to ensure that the worker objects are created and destroyed properly, if they last between multiple method invocations! Microsoft Transaction Server (MTS) offers a solution through just-in-time activation – we will see this in Chapter 9.

Object Aggregation

In our containment and delegation example, our Grocery Shopping object sits between our client and the actual shopping agent worker objects to provide added value. Frequently in COM programming, we'll find situations where the client of our object may be able to use the interface provided by our worker object directly. In these situations, if we were to use containment and delegation, our delegation code would become a simple wrapper that adds no specific value. The code will immediately call the corresponding method in the worker object.

To cater for these cases, COM provides a mechanism called **aggregation**, which allows our object (called the **aggregator**) to expose interfaces of our worker objects (called the **aggregates**) directly. Schematically, aggregation looks like this:

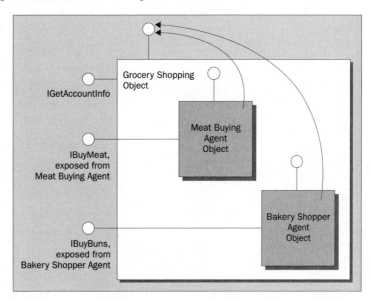

Let's start with our previous example. Now, suppose that owing to the increased volume of business that our shopping site is receiving, and the fragmentation of our customer's demographics, most customers are demanding that we provide specialized meat buying and bun buying services directly. To accomplish this, we've decided to expose the IBuyMeat interface from the Meat Buying Agent and the IBuyBuns interface from the Bakery Shopping Agent as our own interfaces. Meanwhile, we've implemented a new interface call IGetAccountInfo which the Grocery Shopping object implements itself. As far as any client of the Grocery Shopping object is concerned, the object implements all of the interfaces (IGetAccountInfo, IBuyMeat, and IBuyBuns). The client does not have to know, or care, that the Meat Buying Agent object and the Bakery Shopping Agent object are actually working behind the scenes.

In the figure, notice that there's a pointer from each of the aggregates to the outside IUnknown (top) lollipop of the aggregator. Why?

To understand the reason, let's imagine that a client has obtained a pointer to IBuyMeat. Now looking at the diagram, the client thinks that the interface belongs to the Grocery Shopping object and doesn't know about the existence of the Meat Buying Agent. In reality, it's the Meat Buying Agent's interface. What happens now if the client calls the IUnknown methods of IBuyMeat? What if the client calls IBuyMeat::QueryInterface() asking for interface IGetAccountInfo?

Of course, the IBuyMeat interface actually belongs to the Meat Buying Agent, and the Meat Buying Agent doesn't implement IGetAccountInfo, so in this case it would return E_NOINTERFACE. This is obviously not what we want, and it violates one of the golden rules of QueryInterface() – once QueryInterface() is successful for IGetAccountInfo, it must always be successful for the lifetime of the object.

Furthermore, consider the situation when a client holds a pointer to both IGetAccountInfo and IBuyMeat. Now if the client calls IGetAccountInfo::QueryInterface() asking for IUnknown, it would get a pointer to the IUnknown of the Grocery Shopping object. This is okay. However, if the client calls IBuyMeat::QueryInterface() asking for IUnknown, it would get a pointer to the IUnknown of the invisible Meat Buying Agent object. If the client compares the two pointers, they would be different! This breaks one of the golden rules of COM that we discussed in the last chapter – one of the properties of the IUnknown interface is 'identity'. I will repeat it here to refresh your memory:

> **A COM object must return the same IUnknown pointer every time the IUnknown interface is explicitly requested from the object via the QueryInterface() method of any interface.**

To fix these problems, COM takes a very straightforward approach. As revealed in the above figure, the aggregated object simply delegates the IUnknown methods of its interface to the outer object's IUnknown. Note that I did not say the aggregator's IUnknown, but rather the outer object's IUnknown. Let's try to absorb this.

Recall that every COM interface must implement the methods of IUnknown. Now, if a client calls QueryInterface(), AddRef() or Release() on any aggregated interface (except for the IUnknown interface), the corresponding methods of the IUnknown interface of the outer object will be called. It's important to realize that aggregation may be nested. In the nested situation, the innermost object's interface may be exposed by the outermost object as one of its interfaces (right 'through' all the intermediate objects in the nesting). In this case, the innermost object must obtain a pointer to the outermost object's IUnknown interface so that it may delegate its methods. The reason why we always want the outermost object's IUnknown is quite simple: it is **the only object** that is aware of the complete aggregation process, and it alone knows what interfaces it (the outermost object) is supposed to be exposing. Therefore, in our example, we would expect the IUnknown::QueryInterface() of the Grocery Shopping object to be implemented as:

```
// the following declaration assumes that the Grocery Shopping Ojbect
// implements its interfaces
// through multiple inheritance
// (more discussion in Chapter 5)

STDMETHODIMP GroceryShopper::QueryInterface(REFIID riid, LPVOID *ppv)
{
   if ( riid == IID_IUnknown )
      *ppv = (IUnknown *) this;
   else if ( riid == IID_IGetAccountInfo )
      *ppv = (IGetAccountInfo *) this;
   else if ( riid == IID_IBuyMeat )
      return m_pIUnknownMeatBuyer->QueryInterface( riid, ppv );
   else if ( riid == IID_IBuyBuns )
      return m_pIUnknownBakeryShopper->QueryInterface( riid, ppv );
   else
   {
   // notice that Grocery Shopper ONLY accepts IGetAccountInfo,
   // IBuyMeat and IbuyBuns, requests REGARDLESS of the total
   // capabilities of the inner objects — the Meat Buying Agent and
   // the Bakery Shopper Agent.  This is because it has to follow its
   // interface contracts with its own clients.  It exposes from the
   // aggregates only the functionality that it needs.
      *ppv = NULL
      return E_NOINTERFACE;
   }
   // AddRef the interface before returning it
   ( (IUnknown *) *ppv )->AddRef();

   return NOERROR;
}
```

Notice how it 'says yes' when asked if it's supporting either `IBuyMeat` or `IBuyBuns`. Also notice how it actually caches a pointer to the `IUnknown` of each of the aggregates. Without this 'real' `IUnknown` of the aggregate, it won't be able to obtain pointers to the implementations of the Meat Buying Agent and the Bakery Shopping Agent.

At this point, some of the earlier mysteries should start to clear up. Namely, when we examined `CoCreateInstance()`, there was a parameter called `pUnkOuter` that we said would be used only during aggregation: this is the outer unknown being passed into the aggregate. We also said that if `pUnkOuter` is non-NULL, then we must ask for `IUnknown`. This is clearly necessary, as that is the last chance to get the real `IUnknown` of the aggregate before the inner object delegates its `QueryInterface()` to the outer object.

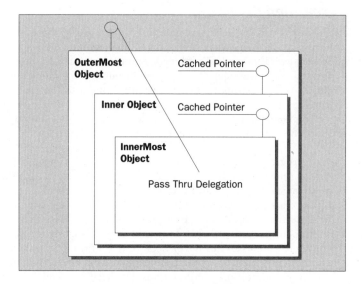

One can also deduce what the inner object should be doing with the pUnkOuter. The rules are general, and apply to any object we may want to make 'aggregatable'. In general, unless you have special reason not to, you should make any COM classes you write aggregatable. This enhances your component's potential usefulness to your users. The rules for the inner object are:

❑ Store the pUnkOuter in a variable within the class

❑ When QueryInterface(), AddRef() or Release() is called on any interface (except for IUnknown), delegate to pUnkOuter

❑ If this object aggregates any object, pass the pUnkOuter into the inner object as the pUnkOuter parameter

Conceptually, when nested aggregation occurs, the pUnkOuter is passed right through to the inner object, while the pointer to the actual IUnknown of each inner object is cached by its immediate aggregator.

Reference Counting

That's about as complicated as basic aggregation gets. However, reference counting in the above scenario is another can of worms entirely. Notice that when we pass the pUnkOuter into the aggregate, the pointer to IUnknown is not AddRef()'ed. This is the way it's done, and it's an allowed exception to the basic COM rule. In essence, the outer object and the inner objects are all part of one big happy family. The lifetime of the inner object is governed by the lifetime of the outer object (i.e. when the outer object dies, so does the inner one). Because of this, the interface pointers from the outer object, which an inner object may hold, must not be reference counted. This also avoids a cycle of references.

Inheritance vs Aggregation

There exists a school of thought that suggests aggregation is equivalent to the well-known object-oriented concept of inheritance. In many ways, this is true. One can imagine a situation involving a COM object that aggregates several other COM objects, and each, in turn, aggregating other COM objects. In this way, one particular interface can be passed through to the client without any of the intermediate objects actually implementing it. This is certainly similar to the concept of inheriting from a base class that provides an existing set of member functions. Our derived class gains the reuse of these methods with no implementation necessary. The analogy, however, falls apart when one considers overriding any of the base class's implementations of these methods.

In classical object-oriented programming, overriding the base class's method and member variables is allowed. It's even possible to selectively override certain members and methods, while inheriting others. As long as the new class is designed carefully, and has been fully tested, this is a very good way of reusing existing 'base class' code. Unfortunately, if a base class is used by more than one derived class (i.e. in any reuse situation), and the base class is changed (let's say a series of bug fixes were performed), it's possible for the derived class to break! This is because the combination of the new base class and the old derived classes has never been tested. Since the derived class has total freedom to override, or inherit, any element of the base class without restriction, thorough and complete testing of all the permutations and combinations of inheritance and override usually isn't feasible. This is frequently called the 'fragile base class' problem.

The real crux of the problem lies in the lack of clearly agreed responsibilities between the base class and the derived class. Inheritance and the capability to selectively override allow for this fuzziness. If this sounds like I'm leading on to something, you're absolutely correct. The interface contract! That's right, it's another use of COM's immutable interface.

With aggregation, as we've seen before, we can have interfaces passing through, from inner objects to the outer object, providing the benefits of inheritance. Since these interfaces are written to COM specifications, they are contracts with precise behavior. Essentially, they're contracts between the outer object and the inner object. Now, if the outer object decides to override the behavior of an interface, it *must* maintain the terms according to the contract. As a result, in the overriding situation, the onus is on the outer object to ensure that its implementation still conforms to the contract expressed by the interface. The COM object doesn't have the luxury of partial overrides: it must override one complete implementation of an interface at a time, and if it should decide to override, it must ensure that the overridden interface still conforms to the interface specification. Its because of this that COM provides a highly robust reuse mechanism.

Another thing that's worth noting about aggregation is that it's a purely runtime phenomenon. This means that there's no indication that a particular COM class uses aggregation to get its job done, until an object of that class is instantiated. For example, examining the type library or registry entry isn't going to give any clue as to whether aggregation is going to take place. Here, again, is a powerful feature in disguise. The implementation of a COM class can use (or not use) aggregation at will, with zero impact on its client or any other tools or utilities which work with the class or object of the class.

One major restriction of the aggregation technique is that it can only be used for in-process servers – DLL server modules only. The restriction is in place because the tricky reference counting semantics become unmanageable when servers are out of process.

As a result, even though aggregation can be a more efficient alternative for composing COM components, the simpler containment/delegation method is the preferred way of doing so. Composing components using containment/delegation will enable your resulting component to work under all COM server types. In the future, COM+ will make the containment/delegation style of object composition much easier to implement.

The Abyss of Complexity

Last, but definitely not least, we will take a brief look at the two aspects of COM that we have warned you about. Any casual diversion into these topics may cost you three to six months of puzzlement, research, and experimentation.

We will give you a taste of these topics here, and go on improve our understanding throughout the rest of the book. We cannot promise to cover all aspects by the end of the book, however, as one can easily write complete books on each of these topics. However, if you have understood everything we have covered so far, the following discussion should be sufficient to map these subject areas.

COM Threading Models

Let's start with a condensed history. In the beginning, man wrote monolithic single-threaded programs under Win32. Man was very happy. With COM, man was challenged to write 'component-based', multi-threaded programs... man became very troubled with COM threading models.

The key words here are *component-based*, and *multithreaded*. Component-based presumably means that the program makes good use of COM objects to simplify coding. Multithreaded means that somewhere within the program, more than one operating system thread has been created to improve the throughput of the system (hopefully).

Let us first take a step back in evolution, and examine a monolithic, multi-threaded application. Here's our representation of such a program.

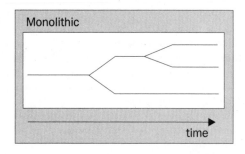

The fork-like structure represents the threads of execution, with time flowing to the right. The box represents the code of the monolithic program. The number of intersections with any vertical line on the graph will indicate the number of concurrent threads running at any moment in time.

Now, let us think about how we would write such a program. Some basic rules of thumb for multithreaded programming come to mind:

❏ **Protection of Shared Resources** – since each thread of execution runs inside the same address space, any variables or resources that may be accessed by more than one thread simultaneously must be protected

❏ **Thread Synchronization** – each thread of execution is independent of the others; if we need several of them to co-operate in accomplishing a task, some form of synchronization primitive must be used

Since this is a monolithic program, and we are writing the whole thing, these two rules are relatively straightforward to implement. Even though implementation may not be complex, testing is quite tricky, because we need to make sure we avoid:

❏ **Deadlocks** – two or more threads holding a resource that another thread wants, whilst waiting for another resource that someone else is holding, so that all the deadlocked threads end up waiting forever

❏ **Race conditions** – non-deterministic flow of execution due to timing dependencies (i.e. the program behaves differently with the same inputs)

Now imagine splitting up the same monolithic program into components.

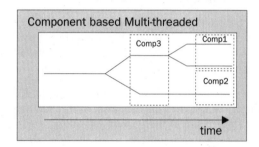

In this case, totally different people may write the code for the various components and the client. Since the program and its requirements did not change, all our concerns above (already quite complicated) are still valid, except now we need to make sure that the client and component together can still protect shared resources, provide thread synchronization, and avoid deadlocks and race conditions. This is precisely what makes the adherence to COM threading models important. It specifies a set of conventions and agreements between clients and components, which ensure that the resulting program will function correctly and in a robust manner.

Now, if you have constructed a component that doesn't protect the resources that it accesses, how can COM threading models help when the client using your component is multithreaded and may be using the component on multiple threads simultaneously?

However, if you have told both the client and the COM runtime system about this, together they can help you out. In this case, the COM runtime would intercept the client's calls, serialize them, and ensure that the client will never access your component on more than one thread simultaneously.

So, what COM threading models are available?

Here is a rundown.

The Simple 'Single Threaded' Model

Essentially, this is a legacy of the early days of COM, when it did not support more than one thread of execution. Even if the client is multithreaded, all COM usage under this model must be performed in the same thread; the one that called `CoInitialize()`. Only this single thread can use components that are created by the client.

`CoInitialize()`, `OleInitialize()`, or `CoInitializeEx()` are COM runtime APIs that must be called (any one of them) by a COM client before any other COM runtime APIs may be used.

A COM client that uses this model simply calls `CoInitialize()`. DLL based in-process COM components, which support this model, have a class database attribute entry "ThreadingModel", with value "None" (for in-process servers), or have no "ThreadingModel" entry at all. EXE-based COM components supporting the simple model inform the COM runtime by calling `CoInitialize()`.

COM components that support this model (including most legacy components) do not have to worry about protecting any variables or data access at all.

The Single Threaded Apartment (STA) Model

The old name for STA was the **Apartment model**. The term 'Apartment' will be defined shortly, once we have covered marshaling. You will find this naming in the configuration and calling flags. Essentially a 'transition' model for the legacy components, this model extends the single-threaded model to multiple threads.

Clients using this model must call `CoIntialize()` or `CoInitializeEx()` with the `COINIT_APARTMENTTHREADED` flag. Components supporting this model indicate via the value "Apartment" in the "ThreadingModel" class database entry (for in-process servers), or via `CoInitialize()`/`CoInitializeEx()` (for EXE servers).

The rules for the STA model say that multiple threads in a client can call `CoInitializeEx()` and create COM component instances. However, the components created on a particular thread can only be used on that very same thread. If it is absolutely necessary to use the COM component instance created on another thread, the client must enlist the help of the COM runtime and 'marshal' (see the next section) the COM interface across the threads, taking a performance hit (even for in-process servers) along the way. Let's consider an example: Say we have two threads, A and B. Thread A created, and is using, MyComponent. Now, thread B needs to call MyComponent, but must avoid conflicting with thread A's use of MyComponent. So thread B just asks thread A to make the call for it. Simple! The marshalling process coordinates the inter-thread communication – it receives the call request from thread B and passes it on to thread A.

The beauty of this model is that components supporting the model are still extremely easy to write. Most of the code, if you have any, from the single threaded component is preserved. Any shared variables used by the component logic do not have to be protected (since they're accessed only via one single thread anyway). However, any shared variables that are used outside of the component logic (variables used by the class factory object, global object counters, etc.) must be protected using Win32 synchronization primitives. Multiple threads from the client may access these variables simultaneously.

The Multithreaded Apartment (MTA) Model

This is frequently called the free-threaded model. It is the most flexible and high performance model when a multi-threaded client is used. Unfortunately, it is also the hardest one to code. Clients using this model should call CoInitializeEx() with the COINIT_MULTITHREADED flag. Components supporting the MTA threading model must have the registry key "ThreadingModel" with the "Free" string value (for in-process servers) or should call CoInitializeEx() (for EXE servers).

In the MTA model, the client may create as many threads as it wishes, create any component instance on any of the threads, and use the component instances on the same or other threads. A free-threaded model client always call methods of component instances directly, it never does any "marshaling". Because of this, it is the highest performance model, essentially indistinguishable from that of a monolithic program, when in-process (DLL) servers are used.

A component supporting the MTA model must protect *all* shared data. It cannot make any 'single thread access' assumption in any part of the code. These components must be written to be totally re-entrant (that is, being able to be executed by multiple threads at the same time). MTA components are very hard to code correctly.

One Last Variation: Both

In-process (DLL) components that are designed to support both STA and MTA clients may support all the models. This will allow the component writer to have the maximal compatibility and still maintain control over performance. A component supporting all the threading models has the class database entry "ThreadingModel" with the value "Both".

When coding such a component, as in the handling of the free-threaded model, protecting all shared data is still necessary. The component can be created safely in either an MTA by an MTA client, or in an STA by an STA client. COM runtime does not need to intervene during creation. Calls in MTA can be made from any thread without marshaling. Calls in an STA client from the creating STA can be made without marshaling, but calls from other STAs must still be marshaled.

The COM Runtime's Role

In our discussion of Threading Models thus far, we have concentrated on the agreement between client and component with regards to protecting shared resources. We have also said earlier that we must tell the COM runtime system about our threading models. Exactly what role does the COM runtime play in this case?

When a client supporting a particular threading model calls a method supplied by a component supporting the same model, everything is fine and dandy. Whenever the client's and the component's threading models don't match, the COM runtime steps in and does its job. In these cases, the COM runtime does whatever is necessary to make the client and component work together. This will free both the client and the component writers from worrying about a bewildering array of conditions. It turns out that the work that the COM runtime does in ensuring compatibility between client and component revolves around an activity called **marshaling**.

Marshaling

Marshaling is a term used frequently in RPC (remote procedure call) programming. Essentially, when a process makes an RPC call from one machine over the network to another machine, some code needs to be 'in the middle'. This code takes the call from the calling process, packages all the parameters, and sends them in some standard format across the network. Some other code then receives the data, unpackages the parameters, and makes the actual procedure call on the remote machine. Once this is complete, the remote code gathers the return value and ships this back to the calling machine. The code which sent the call then returns the value back to the process that made the call. This can all be done transparently to the calling process; that is, without letting it know that the call was made to a remote machine.

The bit of code on the calling process is called a **proxy**, and the bit of code taking the call on the remote machine is called a **stub**. Proxy and stub code is specific to a procedure, and is often generated by a programming tool. The act of packing and unpacking the parameters, and shipping them across the medium (network) is called **marshaling**. It looks something like this:

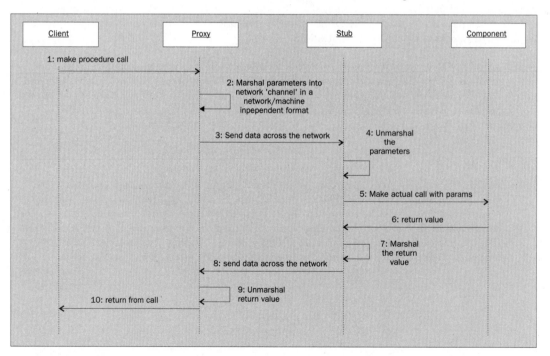

It comes as no surprise that the COM implementation is based on RPC. It uses the same terminology. In reality, COM provides an optimized object-oriented extension of the RPC mechanism.

- ❑ 'Optimized' because procedure calling between client and servers, on the same machine, uses alternative high performance mechanisms
- ❑ 'Extended' because the endpoints across which marshaling works are no longer machine or process address space boundaries; instead, marshaling is defined to be between apartments

In the case of a client invoking a method of a component in a remote server, the sequence of actions is identical to those of the standard RPC case. Even in the case of a client invoking a method of a component in a local server on the same machine, the action is very similar.

The real difference here from RPC, is that one can cross apartment boundaries even for calls within the same address space! That means that marshaling is required. To put it another way, even though you can load a DLL and obtain interfaces directly from a component, there are some cases where you *must* use marshaling code to make your calls into the DLL component, even if you have a pointer to the interface.

Apartments

What are apartments? We have avoiding defining an **apartment** in our threading model discussions so far. Now that we understand marshaling, we can define an apartment as *an end point for marshaling*. We can also conjecture that clients and components in the same apartment can call each other without marshaling i.e. directly.

Reading the above paragraph again and again, you will soon realize that all this apartment and marshaling business is about the classical thing that we need to watch out for in our monolithic, multithreaded program: thread synchronization!

Remember that a COM method call is synchronous. When a client in one apartment makes a call into a component in another apartment, what happens? Marshaling occurs *and* the caller is blocked until the call returns from the component's apartment. For a moment in time, we have synchronized the two threads of execution! We are getting serialization of work done from two potentially independent threads.

- ❑ *How does a thread get associated with an apartment?* When a client thread calls `CoInitializeEx()` or `CoInitialize()`, it marks the thread as entering an apartment.
- ❑ *How does a component get associated with an apartment?* A component is associated with the apartment in which it is created. This may not necessarily be the apartment associated with the client thread that creates the component, because the COM runtime may intervene and create the component in another apartment under certain circumstances. For example, if an MTA client attempts to create an STA component, the COM runtime will actually create a new STA (marshaling endpoint) for the component to execute in.

Now, let us revisit the apartment types again. For STAs, there can only be one physical OS thread associated with the apartment. Each STA thread must implement a message dispatch loop. This is not a strange requirement when we realize that Windows has its humble beginnings as a cooperative multitasking system (i.e. not pre-emptive). Under earlier incarnations, a message loop is the only way to implement logically separate threads of execution with a single 'real' thread. Furthermore, Windows today still makes use of the message loop mechanism to ensure that the user interface system is always responsive to the user. From this perspective, it should be clear that the only way to synchronize (from outside the thread) with the 'logical' threads of execution, or the user interface, is by putting a message in the message queue and wait for it to be processed. This is exactly what the stub code does during marshaling. Take the example of an object running in an STA on a local server (EXE). The diagram below shows what happens when an STA client makes a call into the object:

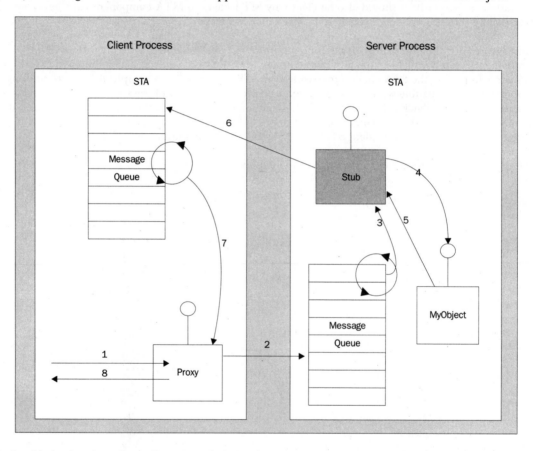

It should also be clear that calls within the STA can be made directly, without marshaling, since there can be no concurrency problem – the calling 'logical' thread has the physical thread all to itself at the moment. This is reminiscent of the action of the `SendMessage()` call in Windows 3.1.

For MTAs, there can be many threads in the apartment. However, there can only be one MTA per process. This is easy to understand when we realize that interface calls, by any thread, are safe at any time without marshaling. In this case, there is no need to differentiate between the threads that are in the apartment – they can call components running on any other threads at any time. Again, we can see that calls within the apartment do not require marshaling at all. If it sounds like difficult code, you are correct. Reusable and robust MTA components are notoriously difficult to write and test.

Now, let's look at the case of a client calling into an object running in an in-process server (DLL). It should be clear that STA client to STA component calls do not require marshalling. The component is created in the client's STA, so all calls into the object are made from the same thread on which it was created. If a client wants to use a component on another STA thread, it must manually marshal the interface. Similarly, it should also be clear why MTA client to MTA component calls never need marshalling – the component is created in the client's MTA.

An STA client calling into an MTA component, however, does require marshalling. If an MTA component is safely callable from any thread at any time, why do we need marshaling code? The answer is to protect the STA client. Once called, an MTA component is completely free to do things that may be incompatible with, or even disrupt, the proper operation of the STA client. Furthermore, in cases where a callback is involved, the MTA component will not guarantee that the call back will be made on the same thread. The component needs to be created in an MTA (created by COM if necessary) and calls from the client STA to the component MTA must be marshaled.

We will now ascend from the murky Abyss of Complexity!

Summary

Congratulations, together we've made it through the trenches! After everything we've seen and learned in these first two chapters, COM as a binary interoperability standard is no longer a stranger to us. In this chapter, we've been a tour of four advanced COM techniques – Automation, notification handling, containment and aggregation. All of these are powerful keys to the reusability and extensibility of COM based software components, yet relatively simple to grasp conceptually.

Adding icing to the cake, we finished up with a discussion of the two most complex topics in COM – threading models and marshaling. We studied all the currently available threading models, their client and component requirements, as well as *why* they are needed and designed that way. From the humble RPC origin of marshaling, we extended our discussion to COM's very own flavor of marshaling and saw how it dovetails nicely with the threading models.

It's amazing how much complexity (and flexibility) you can build on top of a simple 'BLOB and OFFSETS' binary code reuse scheme. In the next chapter, we'll apply these very principles to construct our first simple ActiveX control.

To hit the ground running, we will put into practice many concepts that we have covered in this chapter and build an ActiveX control completely from scratch.

For now, sit back and relax or go for a coffee, then come back and join us for an intensive coding session!

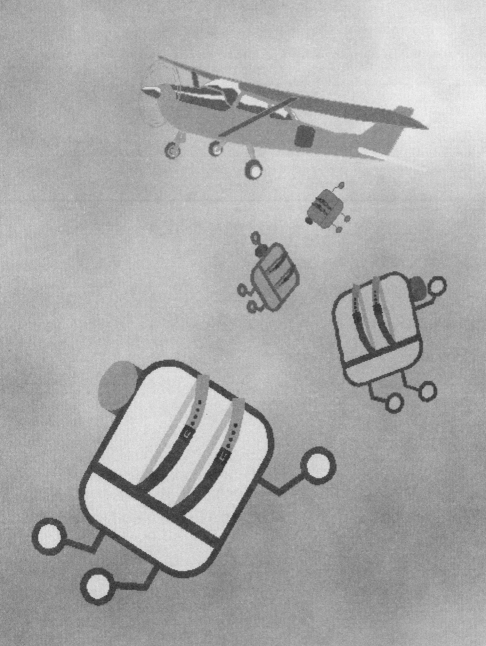

Writing An ActiveX Control From Scratch

Hopefully, after the last couple of chapters, COM is no longer a mystery to us. We can now proceed to write our first ActiveX control. To make sure that we really understand what was presented earlier, we'll forgo any assistance from wizards, and instead we'll create an ActiveX control from scratch. That's correct, we'll just use the trusty Visual C++ 6.0 compiler, without the help of the fancy Visual Studio 6.0 environment, the MFC or other class libraries. No doubt you'll find it refreshing to rediscover the command line interface to the compiler!

Granted, the ActiveX control that we create will be very minimal. It just passes as an ActiveX control, because it implements the IUnknown interface. However, in the process of creating this control, we'll gain an appreciation of what's involved, and how most of the tools do it 'under the hood'. It will give us more insight into how to take advantage of what the technology has to offer. As a bonus, it will make our next journey into building ActiveX controls using the Active Template Library 3.0 (ATL 3.0) much easier to follow.

We'll be constructing a hypothetical business rule ActiveX control for the Aberdeen & Wilshire intranet. The control is very simple, but its structure is a good example of how to construct business rule controls that have no user interface. Furthermore, it can be used to encapsulate existing legacy code, making it ActiveX-ready, and easy to use as a client control and/or server-side component. Our control can potentially be used by an event calendar control (which we'll build in Chapter 7) to determine the dynamic status of the department.

The control that we're going to construct has just one VTBL bound custom interface, which has three methods. The first one returns the current department manager's name, or the name of the person in charge at the time. In our implementation, we'll be hard-coding the name, but in real life, you would be more likely to consult other dynamic sources to provide the necessary information (for example, a shift schedule combined with a log from an attendance-tracking punch clock). The second method takes a year and a month, and determines what information should be published to the public for that month. Again, our implementation uses a trivial algorithm to determine if information should be published, but in a real-world situation, the actual business rule would be far more complex. The final method is more of a trace/debug method, providing a way to peek into the counters being maintained by the object.

In addition to creating and debugging our COM component, we'll also create a client program from scratch to understand how to code client programs. The client will be used to test our COM component. We'll go on to develop the client further, so that it really gives our COM component a thorough test. The final client program will allow the creation and testing of multiple instances of the COM object. It will enable experimentation with the COM threading model and marshaling, casting some much-needed light onto these deep dark topics.

We'll create an in-process server for our object, residing within a DLL. We'll also create the necessary interface description, type library, and registry update code to make it a good, well-behaved COM citizen. Trivial as this component may be, we will appreciate that it is 'Visual Basic 6 Ready' and may be deployed in a larger network of business objects immediately.

Describing the COM Component

First things first, we need to know what the class that we're creating looks like. Well, from the above description, we can tell that it's going to look something like this:

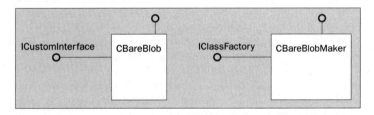

The server will implement two different types of object. CBareBlobMaker is the singleton class factory for the CBareBlob class. The CBareBlob class will implement a custom interface called ICustomInterface, which will provide the three methods:

- ❑ GetManagerName()
- ❑ OkayToPublishInfo()
- ❑ PeekCounters().

For each call to IClassFactory::CreateInstance(), a new instance of CBareBlob will be created on the heap by the CBareBlobMaker class object, using C++'s new operator.

The first step in creating this BLOB is to describe the object in an **IDL** file. IDL stands for **Interface Definition Language**, which is something of a misnomer for what it actually does. Historically speaking, objects, libraries, and interfaces were described in a text file called an ODL file (or Object Definition Language file). An ODL file can be used to generate a type library – the binary archive of metadata information describing the attributes of a component.

Originally, IDL files were used exclusively within the realm of RPC (Remote Procedure Call). RPC IDL files provide detailed descriptions of every remote procedure, covering in detail how each parameter of the procedure is to be marshaled across the network. The set of remote procedures in an RPC IDL file makes up its single "interface", thus the name "Interface Definition Language". One can turn the RPC IDL file into C++ proxy/stub code used for marshaling the procedure calls (and parameters, of course) by simply running it through a code generator called an IDL compiler. These generated files can then be used to implement the remote procedures transparently for any client programs that may need to use them.

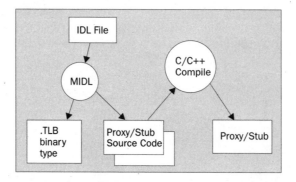

It is easy to see how COM calls across apartments are just an extension of this RPC mechanism. (We discussed apartments in the last chapter.) The most significant deviation being the fact that a COM component may expose multiple sets of remote procedures (methods), in the form of multiple interfaces. In earlier versions of Visual C++ (up to, and including, Release 4), you needed to create both an ODL and an IDL file for every COM component that was implemented (IDL files were necessary only for components requiring the generation of standard marshaling code). Since a typical interface and its methods needed to be described twice (once in each file), it wasn't long before developers (and competitors) started to complain loudly. Microsoft reacted and combined the two definition files into one, and enhanced its RPC IDL compiler – Midl.exe – to handle both type library generation, and marshaling proxy/stub code generation. The older type library generation tool, called Mktyplib.exe, quickly became a part of modern programming history. To this day, Midl.exe has maintained a compatibility option through its /mktyplib203 switch, as a tribute to the very last version of this well-used tool. This option can still be used to make old projects with ODL files.

Now, I think that it's about time we got down to some coding.

> *Remember that you can download all the code that accompanies this book from the Wrox Press web site at http://www.wrox.com. For the examples in this chapter, we're simply editing all the source code as text files – using Edit.exe or Notepad.exe – which we'll compile, using a makefile, later on.*

Our simple COM component is described in the following IDL file, which you can find in the source code in Ch3\baseblob\BareBlob.idl:

```
import "oaidl.idl";

[
    object,
    uuid(2740CBA0-274C-11d0-8DCF-000000000000),
]
interface ICustomInterface : IUnknown
{
    HRESULT GetManagerName([out, retval] BSTR *lResult);
    HRESULT OkayToPublishInfo([in] long lyear, [in] long lmonth,
                                            [out, retval] VARIANT_BOOL *bResult);
    HRESULT PeekCounters([out] long *lCount1, [out] long *lCount2);
}

[
    uuid(0B327BC0-274C-11d0-8DCF-006052008075),
    version(1.0),
]
library BareBlobLib
{
    importlib("stdole32.tlb") ;


    [
        uuid(048E11A0-2754-11d0-8DCF-000000000000)
    ]
    coclass CBareBlob
    {
        [default] interface ICustomInterface ;
    }
} ;
```

One thing that you should immediately notice is that even though we *are* implementing a class factory, its description is missing in the IDL description. As you may remember from our discussion in Chapter 1, the class factory is a special object. The COM runtime implementation takes care of the details of locating an instance of a class factory for any coclass defined in an IDL file, only the associated CLSID is required. How the COM runtime achieves this may be both OS and hardware platform dependent.

Don't worry if you don't understand everything that's going on in this file just yet. We'll be taking a detailed look at the IDL syntax shortly.

GUIDs Everywhere

Another thing you should notice are the various GUIDs, scattered throughout the file, which are used to identify the interface, the type library and the COM class. Each of these GUIDs is generated by the Uuidgen.exe utility, which ships with your Visual C++ compiler. They are 16 bytes, or 128 bits, long. You can try out this utility for yourself.

On your development machine, it's probably worthwhile setting up the default environment to contain all the binary and include paths and variables. This is automatically done with a Windows NT installation of Visual C++ 6. On Windows 95/98 systems, you can edit Autoexec.bat to include the variables that are found in the Vcvars32.bat file (you'll find this in the in the \Vc98\bin directory).

If you are running on a Windows 95 system, you must make sure the latest DCOM for Windows 95 (called DCOM98) update has been installed. This is already done for you if you have installed Internet Explorer 4.01 or above.

Open a command line prompt and type in uuidgen, and you will get a new GUID:

```
E:\vs8\VC98\Bin>uuidgen
5b723220-d375-11d1-a660-006052008075
```

Now try using the interface GUID generation option using the -i switch:

```
E:\vs8\VC98\Bin> uuidgen -i
[
uuid(93d1f560-d375-11d1-a660-006052008075),
version(1.0)
]
interface INTERFACENAME
{

}
```

This format is 'ready-to-go' for your IDL file, and is a handy feature for creating your own components. For example, uuidgen -i -n5 will create five GUIDs, in the above format, for your IDL file. You can ignore or delete the generated version(1.0) IDL statement. This statement is produced because Midl.exe and Uuidgen.exe also service pure RPC interfaces, which can be versioned. COM interfaces, however, cannot be versioned. Remember that a COM interface, once declared, cannot be changed.

If you should need to reference GUIDs directly within your C/C++ programs, you can also use the -s switch:

```
E:\vs8\VC98\Bin>uuidgen -s
INTERFACENAME = { /* 3a642ba0-d376-11d1-a660-006052008075 */
    0x3a642ba0,
    0xd376,
    0x11d1,
    {0xa6, 0x60, 0x00, 0x60, 0x52, 0x00, 0x80, 0x75}
};
```

A version of `Uuidgen.exe`, called `Guigen.exe`, has a GUI and works with windows clipboard, which makes it very useful to work with in the Visual Studio environment. To make `Guidgen.exe` available from the <u>T</u>ools menu of Visual Studio you need to:

1. Start Visual C++ 6 or Visual Studio 98.
2. From the <u>T</u>ools menu, select <u>C</u>ustomize... and go to the Tools tab. In the <u>M</u>enu contents: list you can see all the tools that are currently available to you through the <u>T</u>ools menu.
3. Go to the bottom of the <u>M</u>enu Contents listbox and double-click on the blank entry. Enter the description `Create a new &UUID`. Press return.
4. In the Command field, click on the ... button and locate your `Guidgen.exe` executable under the `\Vc98\Tools\bin` directory. Here, you can also add command line arguments to be passed to your new tool when invoked, and you can specify the initial directory in which to run.
5. Click on the Close button.
6. Now go to the <u>T</u>ools menu and verify that the tool is available there. Try it out!

BSTRs and VARIANT_BOOLs

Take a look at the IDL file that we've just created. In the definition of our business rule methods, `GetManagerName()` and `OkayToPublishInfo()`, we've deliberately used two COM/OLE specific data types, `BSTR` and `VARIANT_BOOL`. We could have easily used normal character arrays, such as `LPTSTR` and regular `BOOL`. However, doing so would be restricting the utility of the final business object. For automation COM clients (the ones we called "agnostic clients" back in Chapter 2), `BSTR` and `VARIANT_BOOL` are *the only ways* to pass string and Boolean data around. This is important because one of these clients is the scripting engine integral to Internet Explorer 4, which we'll be using as the primary client on our Intranet!

To avoid questions and headaches later, we've opted to introduce these data types at this point. But what are they? `VARIANT_BOOL`, if you look up the definition, is simply a short integer. The unique property of `VARIANT_BOOL` is that it will always be compatible with the `VARIANT` data type, which is heavily used in Automation (covered in Chapter 2). Being a fundamental type (`short`), `VARIANT_BOOL` needs no special handling.

`BSTR`, on the other hand, is a very interesting data type. It is **BASIC**ally a **STR**ing (terrible pun intended). Its origins lie in Visual Basic (the premiere Automation client across all of Microsoft's product line), and it's used to hold the value of a varying length string. With 32-bit COM support, `BSTR` always points to a UNICODE string. As a matter of fact, the entire OLE/COM runtime will deal with strings internally only as UNICODE. The unique thing about `BSTR` is that the length of the string is pre-calculated and stored in the word immediately *before* the storage of the actual character string (i.e. where `BSTR` actually points to). As with normal character strings, `BSTR` is NULL terminated. Having the string length traveling with the data all the time is extremely useful; repeated determination of string lengths, accomplished by scanning to the terminating NULL character, can waste a lot of computing cycles in a typical application. In the meantime, the convention of using NULL termination on a `BSTR` makes it compatible with all existing C/C++ string manipulation functions (though a `BSTR` may contain embedded `Null` characters which would cause the string to appear shorter than it is). Please note that the actual definition of a `BSTR` does not require the string to be `Null` terminated, although under most usage scenarios it is.

The design of BSTR turns out to be an excellent way to represent varying strings. So much so, in fact, that the MFC's CString class was 'revamped' to use a similar algorithm to represent strings in the library.

BSTRs are frequently used as parameters in Automation and other COM interface methods (such as our business object). Since a client and a server are involved in each parameter exchange, and may be in different processes or on different machines, there needs to be a convention specified, with respect to memory allocation for the BSTR. The convention is simple yet effective:

❑ For BSTRs passed by value (an input parameter), the caller has to allocate and free the BSTR data

❑ For BSTRs passed by reference, the caller allocates the BSTR data, but the party called has the option of returning the same data or newly allocated data (and freeing the old stuff); in either case, the caller must free the returned data

❑ For BSTRs passed by reference as an output parameter, the party called allocates the BSTR data, and the caller must free it

Closer examination of the above convention will reveal that it's designed for maximum flexibility, and yet it results in the minimal transference of data between the caller and the party called in a distributed network situation.

Memory allocation must always be made using a system supplied, guaranteed and sharable memory allocator (since the client and server could be implemented using different programming languages with different runtime libraries, etc.). The SysAllocString() and SysFreeString() family of functions in the Win32 API are designed to suit this purpose.

The Almighty MIDL

The MIDL compiler is a standard tool for anybody programming RPC and/or COM on Microsoft platforms. It reads an IDL file, prepared by the programmer, and generates the necessary proxy and stub source files for RPC operations. The C/C++ compiler can compile these source files. It will also generate a binary tokenized form of the IDL in a type library (.tbl file) for COM IDL files.

Midl.exe has a lot of command line options. The following table shows a brief description of those options that are most important in, and frequently used during, ActiveX development:

Option (case sensitive)	Usage
/I *directory list*	Specify one or more directories for the include path
/out *directory*	Specify the destination directory for output files
/syntax_check or /Zs	Check syntax only – do not generate output files
/D *name*[*=def*]	Pass #define name and an optional value to the preprocessor
/U *name*	Remove any previous definition (#undefine)

Table Continued on Following Page

Option (case sensitive)	Usage
`/error allocation`	Check for out of memory errors in generated stub code
`/align: {1|2|4|8}`	Designate the packing level of structures – default is 8, which is the natural alignment for most supported platforms.
`/Oicf`	Stub generation optimization switch for off-line, code-less, fully interpreted stubs – trade slightly slower marshaling for very small stub size
`/Os`	Stub generation optimization switch for in-line stubs – trade larger stub size for better marshaling performance.
@ *response_file*	Accept input from a response file
`/help` or `/?`	Display a list of MIDL compiler switches
`/o` *filename*	Redirects output from screen to a file

Proxy and Stub Generation

To create the type library, proxy and stub code for our COM component:

1. Open a command line prompt.

2. Make sure that your DOS environment variables are set up; if you're using Windows 95/98, you need to change directory to your `..\Vc98\Bin` directory and run a batch file called `Vcvars32.bat`.

3. Type `midl /Oicf BareBlob.idl`

If you get a message saying that certain include files can't be found, then most likely you haven't set the environment up correctly.

If you try compiling the `BareBlob.idl` file using `Midl.exe` as described above, then you will see that the process generates the following files:

File Name	Description
`BareBlob.tlb`	Binary type library file. The COM runtime can read the type library information directly from this file.
`BareBlob.h`	Part of the generated proxy/stub code includes a header file containing the actual definition of all the interfaces. This is a very handy include file for clients of the object server.

File Name	Description
BareBlob_i.c	Part of the generated proxy/stub code contains all of the interface IDs and class IDs in a C/C++ usable form. This is also a useful include file for clients of the object server.
BareBlob_p.c	Part of the generated proxy/stub code includes the actual marshaling code for the defined interfaces.
Dlldata.c	Part of the generated proxy/stub code, the DLL glue necessary to create a proxy/stub DLL.

Of these files, the two main ones that we'll be using are BareBlob.h and BareBlob_i.c. Both of these files need to be included into the source code of the BareBlob component. More specifically, we will include BareBlob.h in the control's header file and BareBlob_i.c in the implementation file, as you'll see when we come to write these files. BareBlob_p.c and Dlldata.c are generated files, which can be used to create proxy/stub codes. They're generated each time the IDL is compiled and should never be manually edited.

Notice that BareBlob.h is an MIDL generated file by default. This means that we can't name our program's header file by the same name. Instead, we'll be naming our actual source code BareBlob1.cpp and the header BareBlob1.h.

Notice also that, in our IDL description, we've defined the interface, ICustomInterface, and the COM object outside of the library definition. A library, in this case, refers to the type library (.TLB file) being generated as output of the compilation process. When you declare an interface in this way, MIDL will generate the required RPC proxy/stub code for marshaling the interface across machine or process boundaries. Another alternative is to declare the interface within the library description itself:

```
[
    uuid(0B327BC0-274C-11d0-8DCF-006052008075),
    version(1.0),
]
library BareBlobLib
{
    importlib("stdole32.tlb") ;
[   object,
    uuid(2740CBA0-274C-11d0-8DCF-000000000000),
]
interface ICustomInterface : IUnknown
{
        HRESULT GetManagerName([out, retval] BSTR *lResult);
        HRESULT OkayToPublishInfo([in] long lyear, [in] long lmonth,
                                        [out, retval] VARIANT_BOOL
*bResult);
        HRESULT PeekCounters([out] long *lCount1, [out] long *lCount2);
}
```

```
    [
        uuid(048E11A0-2754-11d0-8DCF-000000000000)
    ]
    coclass CBareBlob
    {
        [default] interface ICustomInterface ;
    }
} ;
```

Try it, and run MIDL on it in an empty directory (be aware that running MIDL again will not erase any previously generated files and so, if the directory isn't empty, mysterious mis-match problems can occur). You'll notice that no proxy/stub code will be generated, only the type library, `BareBlob.tlb`. An interface that's only used between the COM objects residing entirely within the same DLL or EXE doesn't need to be accessible outside, and so it doesn't require proxy/stub code to be generated. This style of interface specification is often used in defining 'in-process only' COM servers. However, if the interface needs to have any external visibility, proxy/stubs may be needed (see our discussion on COM threading models in Chapter 2 to determine when they are needed).

IDL Syntax

The combined syntax of the former ODL and IDL is a strange blend. While MIDL maintains compatibility with the old process of using an ODL/IDL combination, anyone creating new COM servers should really use the new combined IDL syntax that we've described above. After all, it does save you time and headaches by keeping all the definitions in one place. (If you work with sample programs or legacy code, you may still encounter the ODL and IDL combination once in a while.) Let's have a quick rundown of the new syntax. Instead of using the cryptic Backus Naur Form (BNF), or some parameterized notation, I'm just going to show you some general snippets of IDL declarations for a few things that ActiveX programmers frequently need to do.

Defining an Interface

This is the actual IDL for the `IClassfactory` interface that we talked about extensively in Chapter 1.

```
import "oaidl.idl";
[
    object,
    uuid(00000001-0000-0000-C000-000000000046),
]

interface IClassFactory : IUnknown
{
    typedef [unique] IClassFactory * LPCLASSFACTORY;

    [local]
    HRESULT CreateInstance([in, unique] IUnknown * pUnkOuter,
                           [in] REFIID riid,
                           [out, iid_is(riid)] void **ppvObject);

    [call_as(CreateInstance)]
    HRESULT RemoteCreateInstance([in] REFIID riid,
                                 [out, iid_is(riid)] IUnknown ** ppvObject);
```

```
    [local]
    HRESULT LockServer([in] BOOL fLock);

    [call_as(LockServer)]
    HRESULT __stdcall RemoteLockServer([in] BOOL fLock);
}
```

The `import` directive brings in definitions of standard types and interfaces used by COM, such as `IUnknown`, which our interface will use.

We tell the MIDL compiler that this isn't an RPC interface definition, but rather a COM interface definition, by using the `object` attribute. Remember that all COM interfaces derive from `IUnknown` and that interface inheritance is allowed only for COM interfaces. Inheritance in this sense means that the derived interface will implement all the methods of the base interface. Only single inheritance is supported.

The GUID following the `object` attribute is the **Interface ID (IID)** for this interface. Note that versioning of interfaces, common with RPC, isn't supported by the COM IDL. Each COM interface is immutable once defined, so the concept of versioning has no meaning here.

The rest of the code consists of the interface definition. There are also various parameter attributes:

- ❑ `[in]` for input parameters
- ❑ `[out]` for output parameters
- ❑ `[in, out]` for parameters which are both input and output
- ❑ `[out, retval]` to tag a return value to use in automation
- ❑ `[unique]` to indicate that pointers passed as parameters through a single method will never refer to each other indirectly
- ❑ `[call_as]` provides an alias for a method when it is invoked externally

Most of these attributes give MIDL some clues as to how to optimize the proxy and stub code generated, and owes its origin to RPC. For example, if a parameter is an `[in]` only parameter, the stub won't have to marshal its value back to the proxy. On the other hand, a parameter marked with `[in, out]` will always need to be marshaled both ways.

Defining A Type Library

Here is an IDL segment that defines a type library:

```
[
    uuid(6384D582-0FDB-11cf-8700-00AA0053006D),
    helpstring("Beeper 1.0 Type Library"),
    version(1.0)
]
library BeeperLib
{
    importlib("stdole32.tlb");
```

```
    //  Class information
    [ uuid(6384D586-0FDB-11cf-8700-00AA0053006D), helpstring("Beeper Object") ]
    coclass Beeper
    {
        [default] interface IBeeper;
    };
};
```

The code snippet starts with a GUID for the type library. We associate the string `"Beeper 1.0 Type Library"` with our library by using the `helpstring` attribute. This attribute can also be used to associate a string with a class, an interface or methods, and it means that the string will be available programmatically when a tool accesses the type library information. For example, the object viewer in Visual Basic 6 will display this `helpstring` to the user when they browse through the type library. The `version` attribute gives the type library a major (1) and minor (0) version number.

Within the definition of our type library, we use an `importlib` directive to make the standard definitions from the `Stdole32.tlb` type library available in this library. `Stdole32.tlb` includes the definition for some very common interfaces, including `IUnknown`. The `[default]` attribute is used typically by scripting engines to select the default interface to use – when there's more than one that may qualify to be a dispatch based automation interface (see coverage of default interface in Chapter 2).

Defining A COM Object

In the example code shown above, the `coclass` definition is the definition for a COM server object, bracketing the definition of all the interfaces that this object will support – simply `IBeeper` in this case. The UUID provided therein is the CLSID which identifies the class of the COM object. The exported interfaces are specified in the body with the keyword `interface`.

Defining A Type

Here is an IDL segment illustrating support for C++ type definitions:

```
typedef char * CHARPTR;

typedef interface IUnknown  *LPUNKNOWN;
```

You can use special keywords to specify the type that forms the base of the `typedef`. In this case, `LPUNKNOWN` is `typedef`'ed as a pointer to an interface. The `typedef` capability in MIDL is consistent with the standard C++ preprocessor conventions.

Defining A Structure

Here is how a structure is defined within IDL:

```
typedef struct tagCLIPDATA {
    ULONG cbSize;         // count that includes sizeof(ulClipFmt)
    long ulClipFmt;       // long to keep alignment
    [size_is(cbSize-4)]
    BYTE * pClipData;     // cbSize-sizeof(ULONG) bytes of data in clipboard format
} CLIPDATA;
```

Notice that the declaration is almost the same as you would write it in C++, except that IDL specifiers may appear before the types. The `size_is` attribute is useful for the marshaling proxy/stub. Without the `size_is`, when the structure of CLIPDATA is marshaled, there's no way for the proxy/stub code to figure out how many of the bytes pointed to by `pClipData` should be transferred 'across the wire'.

Making Interface Pointers

Defining the IDL file first forced us consider the interfaces provided by our ActiveX control up front. The output of the MIDL compiler provided us with a binary type library. What's more important, however, is that it also provided us with the `BareBlob.h` file. A lot of the 'dirty work' associated with assembling the required interface vtables (the table of function pointers within the BLOB) is automatically done for us. Let's take a moment to examine the generated `BareBlob.h` and see how our `ICustomInterface` interface is actually implemented.

A short way into the file `BareBlob.h`, we find the definition for our `ICustomInterface`:

```
MIDL_INTERFACE("2740CBA0-274C-11d0-8DCF-000000000000")
    ICustomInterface : public IUnknown
    {
public:
        virtual HRESULT STDMETHODCALLTYPE GetManagerName(
            /* [retval][out] */ BSTR __RPC_FAR *lResult) = 0;

        virtual HRESULT STDMETHODCALLTYPE OkayToPublishInfo(
            /* [in] */ long lyear,
            /* [in] */ long lmonth,
            /* [retval][out] */ VARIANT_BOOL __RPC_FAR *bResult) = 0;

        virtual HRESULT STDMETHODCALLTYPE PeekCounters(
            /* [out] */ long __RPC_FAR *lCount1,
            /* [out] */ long __RPC_FAR *lCount2) = 0;

    };
```

Notice that it's simply declared using a macro called `MIDL_INTERFACE(x)`. If we look up the definition of `MIDL_INTERFACE(x)` in `rpcndr.h` from the `\Vc98\Include` directory, we'll find that it's defined as:

```
/************************************************************************
 * Special things for VC5 Com support
 ***********************************************************************/

#if _MSC_VER >= 1100
#define DECLSPEC_UUID(x)      __declspec(uuid(x))
#define MIDL_INTERFACE(x)     struct __declspec(uuid(x)) __declspec(novtable)
#else
#define DECLSPEC_UUID(x)
#define MIDL_INTERFACE(x)     struct
#endif
```

It is essentially a `struct`. This isn't a problem at all, since a `struct` in C++ is exactly the same as a `class`, but with all methods and data members `public` by default rather than `private`. In our case, `ICustomInterface` is derived from `IUnknown`, another `struct`, which is defined in `\Vc98\Include\Unknwn.h` as:

```
MIDL_INTERFACE("00000000-0000-0000-C000-000000000046")
    IUnknown
    {
    public:
        BEGIN_INTERFACE
        virtual HRESULT STDMETHODCALLTYPE QueryInterface(
            /* [in] */ REFIID riid,
            /* [iid_is][out] */ void __RPC_FAR *__RPC_FAR *ppvObject) = 0;

        virtual ULONG STDMETHODCALLTYPE AddRef( void ) = 0;

        virtual ULONG STDMETHODCALLTYPE Release( void ) = 0;

    .....

        END_INTERFACE
    };
```

Under Win32 on Intel platforms, the `BEGIN_INTERFACE` and `END_INTERFACE` macros map to empty strings. What we're left with, essentially, is the pure virtual class definition for `QueryInterface()`, `AddRef()`, and `Release()`. Notice that the `Unknwn.h` was originally created by the MIDL compiler from the `Unknwn.idl` file.

You can create an instance of a pointer to `IUnknown` with the following syntax:

```
IUnknown *MyUnknown;
```

This allows `MyUnknown` to point to structures/classes which have the following in-memory footprint:

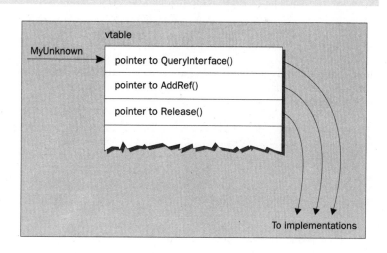

Since `ICustomInterface` derives from `IUnknown`, the pure virtual functions defined in `ICustomInterface` will be tagged on, right after the `IUnknown` entries, which means an `ICustomInterface` pointer is also good for the following vtable in

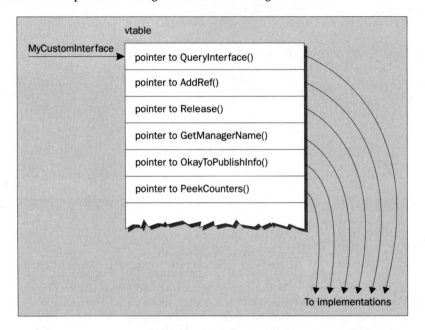

In the next section, we'll actually be creating and populating the vtable to which these 'interface pointers' can point. Basically, to assemble the vtables, you inherit from a base class or structure that has pure virtual functions defined – one for each method that the interface supports and in the order that the methods are defined.

So how do we go about implementing these methods? Well, it boils down to one of two alternative techniques using C++:

❑   Implement the interfaces via multiple inheritance
❑   Implement the interfaces via nested classes

Before we try coding this, however, let us take a quick refresher on the basic C++ syntax corresponding to these two techniques. This refresher will be helpful, because both implementation techniques use the more problematic features of C++ that programmers, striving for long term code maintainability, tend to avoid.

Multiple Inheritance

Consider the following code:

```
class base1
{
public:
    virtual int firstFunc(int i)=0;
    virtual int base1Func(int i)=0;
};

class base2
{
public:
    virtual int firstFunc(int i)=0;
    virtual int base2Func(int i)=0;
};

class derived: public base1, public base2
{
public:
    int firstFunc(int a) { return (a + 1); }
    int base1Func(int a) { return (a + 2); }
    int base2Func(int a) { return (a + 3); }
};
```

Here, the `derived` class inherits from both `base1` and `base2`. Both base classes are pure virtual, having two pure virtual member functions. The `base1` class has a vtable consisting of `firstFunc()` and `base1Func()`, while the `base2` class has a vtable consisting of `firstFunc()` and `base2Func()` entries. When `derived` inherits from these classes, it picks up the vtable from both base classes (in COM, it would have picked up two interface definitions). Both `base1` and `base2` have a virtual member called `firstFunc()`, but the `derived` class can only provide one implementation of this function. Therefore, the inherited vtables from both `base1` and `base2` would have their `firstFunc()` function pointing to `derived::firstFunc()`. This is the key to implementation through multiple inheritance. You could imagine `firstFunc()` implementing some interface methods which are common to all the interfaces inherited from, for instance, the `IUnknown` interface.

Multiple inheritance implementations are typically very concise and lean, maximizing code reuse, but are also relatively hard to maintain. Another obvious shortcoming of this implementation is its inability to handle those situations where the object implements two interfaces that have a method with the same name, but which require different implementations. This particular problem is easily solved if an implementation based on nested classes is used instead.

Nested Classes

The code extract below demonstrates the use of nested classes:

```
class base1
{
public:
    virtual int firstFunc(int i)=0;
    virtual int base1Func(int i)=0;
};
```

```
class base2
{
public:
    virtual int firstFunc(int i)=0;
    virtual int base2Func(int i)=0;
};

class derived
{
    class inner1: base1
    {
    public:
        int firstFunc(int a) { return(a+1); }
        int base1Func(int a) { return(a+2); }
    };

    class inner2: base2
    {
    public:
        int firstFunc(int a) {return(a+3); }
        int base2Func(int a) { return(a+4); }
    };

public:
    inner1 Abase1;
    inner2 Abase2;
};
```

The abstract base classes (base1 and base2) are exactly the same as in the multiple inheritance case, but in this example, however, the derived class does not derive from either of them. Instead, we have two nested class definitions, inner1 and inner2, which derive from base1 and base2 respectively. These nested classes also implement all the pure virtual functions of the inherited classes (equivalent to filling in the vtable for the two COM interfaces). inner1 and inner2 are locally scoped class definitions. We create an instance of each as a member of the wrapping derived class. These two instances are the Abase1 and Abase2 member variables of the derived class.

Note that, in this case, both inner1 and inner2 have an implementation of firstFunc(). Like the multiple inheritance case, the same vtable will be generated when the class is compiled. Unlike the multiple inheritance situation, we can have totally different implementations of the same function, firstFunc(), for each nested class. Translated, this means that we can have different implementations for methods with the same name across two interfaces. Obviously, if we *do* want the two implementations to be the same, we can create an implementation for firstFunc() in the derived class, make inner1 and inner2 C++ friends of the class, and then call this derived implementation from the inner classes. The multiple inheritance implementation is more suitable in this case.

In our case above, the syntax for calling the methods of the inner classes are:

```
derived a;
a.Abase1.firstFunc(1);
a.Abase2.firstFunc(1);
```

COM Interfaces: vtables in Other Environments

If you examine the source code of the include headers from our earlier MIDL experiment carefully, and follow through the #ifdef paths for the C language, you'll find that assembling vtables in C is somewhat more involved. Consequently, if you need to assemble these vtables on another platform (say, the Macintosh or UNIX), in another programming language (say, COBOL), or with another C/C++ compiler that doesn't handle vtables in this way (notably C/C++ compilers with heritage tracing back to the original AT&T CFront), then creating vtables/interfaces may require more sophisticated coding. The bottom line is that you need to know how code is generated, and you need to create the binary image in the object that represents an interface, as shown in the vtable diagrams earlier.

To date, there are very few computing languages that don't provide some means of access memory directly or that don't provide pointers of some type. Until the advent of Java, that is. The Java language itself doesn't support pointers, so one can't address the process's memory space, and it can run in a 'secure' interpretive environment. In this sort of scenario, creating vtables or implementing COM support within the language would not be possible without some sort of external intervention. There's no need to despair, however. Seeing that Java without COM can be a very lonely affair, Microsoft has provided just such an intervention. This extension is realized in their implementation of the Java interpreter (called a Virtual Machine, in Java lingo) which allows full bi-directional interoperation between Java and COM based objects. Using the Microsoft virtual machine, a Java class can be used as a COM object, and Java can use COM objects via class wrappers.

Assembling vtables: Implementing IUnknown

We have already seen that we can obtain a correctly formatted vtable by declaring the methods in IUnknown as pure virtual. Another advantage of declaring IUnknown in this way is that the end user of the interface is forced to implement its methods. Since you can't write a C++ program that leaves pure virtual functions in your class or subclass undefined, you're forced to implement the IUnknown methods of your interface – this is enforced by the compiler during the compilation phase. It's a kind of forced obedience to the terms of the contract. In this case, the side effect is highly desirable.

With no choice left for us, we implement IUnknown in BareBlob1.cpp (recall that the MIDL generates BareBlob.h, so we call our program and headers BareBlob1 instead). The code is shown below:

```
STDMETHODIMP    CBareBlob::QueryInterface(REFIID riid, void **ppv)
{
    *ppv = NULL ;

    if (riid == IID_IUnknown)
    {
        *ppv = this ;

    }
    if (riid == IID_ICustomInterface)
    {
        *ppv = &m_GutsOfBareBlob ;

    }

    if (*ppv == NULL)
    {
```

```
        return E_NOINTERFACE ;
    }
    (static_cast<IUnknown *>( *ppv))->AddRef() ;
    return NOERROR ;
}


STDMETHODIMP_(ULONG)    CBareBlob::AddRef(void)
{
    InterlockedIncrement( reinterpret_cast<LONG*>(&m_cRef) ) ;
    return m_cRef ;
}


STDMETHODIMP_(ULONG)    CBareBlob::Release(void)
{
    if (!InterlockedDecrement( reinterpret_cast<LONG*>(&m_cRef) ))
    {
        delete this ;
        return 0 ;
    }

    return m_cRef ;
}
```

The first thing you should notice is the use of macros in the definition of these functions. All implementations of the interface methods should use the STDMETHODIMP macro to declare the return type. By using the macro, it's guaranteed that the correct signature will be produced on all platforms. These macros essentially add HRESULT and __stdcall to the function. Taking a look at Winnt.h reveals how they're defined for Win32, C++ and Intel platforms:

```
#define STDMETHODIMP           HRESULT STDMETHODCALLTYPE
#define STDMETHODCALLTYPE      __stdcall
#define STDMETHODIMP_(type)    type STDMETHODCALLTYPE
```

__stdcall is a function-calling convention which is the 'standard' calling convention for 32-bit Windows on Intel platforms. Calling conventions affect how the compiler will generate code to implement a function and calls to functions. Under the __stdcall (some may recognize the similarity to the 16-bit PASCAL calling convention) convention, the called function is expected to clean up the stack before it returns from a call, and this convention is mandatory for the methods of the interfaces implemented by in-process COM servers. Clients such as Visual Basic 6, Internet Explorer, and Access 97 expect this when accessing an in-process COM object. By the nature of calling conventions, they are platform specific. There's a good chance that the standard calling convention for another OS or processor won't be the same as __stdcall.

HRESULT *must* be the return type of all interface methods. Only AddRef() and Release() may return any type other than HRESULT. The rest of the interface methods, including all the user defined ones, should always return HRESULT and must, therefore, be defined with STDMETHODIMP. One of the reasons for this uniform handling is the remoting case, when a COM server is accessed over a network. In this case, it's necessary for any method call to be able to return RPC or network failure information, which will come through as RPC_E_xxxx in the HRESULT value (which is acting as a network error reporter). This HRESULT handling also reflects the 'lowest common denominator' approach to method invocation, across all the programming languages that COM supports. For example, returning error information as structured exceptions isn't realistic, because few programming languages support such a mechanism, and anyway, implementations from different vendors are often non-uniform.

We should note that similar declaration macros exist for creating the .h file: STDMETHOD and STDMETHOD_(type). The methods are declared as virtual to ensure that the right (most derived) method is invoked in the case of class hierarchies. Look in the Objbase.h file and you will find:

```
#define STDMETHOD(method)        HRESULT (STDMETHODCALLTYPE * method)
#define STDMETHOD_(type,method)  type (STDMETHODCALLTYPE * method)
```

Notice the implementation of QueryInterface() in BareBlob1.cpp. Here, we simply:

❑ Check the requested IID for either IUnknown or ICustomInterface
❑ Return the interface pointer, after an AddRef() if it is one of the supported interfaces; otherwise return E_NOINTERFACE

With AddRef() and Release(), we play with a counter of type LONG, called m_cRef. To anticipate multiple simultaneous active users of our component (we'll make this happen later, with a multi-threaded client), we use the InterlockedIncrement() and InterlockedDecrement() Win32 API calls to manage our counter. These APIs ensure that the increment and decrement operation is totally atomic (i.e. complete, without the possibility of another processor or thread messing up the updating of the counter value). This gives our IUnknown implementation the robustness that it needs. In Release() we see how the object will be deallocated in the system, via:

```
if (!InterlockedDecrement( reinterpret_cast<LONG*>(&m_cRef) ))
{
    delete this ;
    return 0 ;
}
```

We saw in the last section how we can use either multiple inheritance or nested classes to assemble the vtable. If you take a look at available tools for building COM components originating from Microsoft, you'll find that MFC actually uses nested classes to implement the vtables, and that ATL took the multiple inheritance path. We will be using ATL 3, and hence the multiple inheritance method, almost exclusively throughout the rest of the book, but we will use nested classes here in order to contrast the implementations. To ensure that the generated binary code has the vtable, and exact ordering of functions, that we require, the CBareBlob class is defined as follows:

```
class CBareBlob : public IUnknown
{
    //   CGutsOfBareBlob
    ////////////////////////////////////////////
    // Nested class
    class CGutsOfBareBlob : public ICustomInterface
    {
        friend class CBareBlob ;

    public :
        // keep simple constructors or destructors in-line
        CGutsOfBareBlob():m_cRef(0),    m_outRef(0)
        {}


        ~CGutsOfBareBlob()
        {}

        //These are the methods of ICustomInterface
        STDMETHOD (QueryInterface)(REFIID riid, void **ppv);
        STDMETHOD_(ULONG, AddRef)(void);
        STDMETHOD_(ULONG, Release)(void);
        STDMETHOD(GetManagerName)(BSTR *bstrMgr);
        STDMETHOD(OkayToPublishInfo)(long lyear, long lmonth, VARIANT_BOOL *okay);
        STDMETHOD(PeekCounters)(long *lCount1, long *lCount2);

    private :
        ULONG      m_cRef ;          // ref count
        ULONG      m_outRef;         // spy on outer Ref
        IUnknown   *m_pUnkOuter ;    // controlling unknown
    }; // end of CGutsOfBareBlob nested class

public:
//an instance of our nested class
    CGutsOfBareBlob m_GutsOfBareBlob ;
    CBareBlob(IUnknown *punkOuter);
    ~CBareBlob();

    //These are the methods of IUnknown
    STDMETHOD(QueryInterface)     (REFIID riid, void **ppv);
    STDMETHOD_(ULONG, AddRef)     (void);
    STDMETHOD_(ULONG, Release)    (void);
private:

    ULONG      m_cRef ;           // ref count
    IUnknown   *m_pUnkOuter ;     // controlling unknown
};                               // end of CBareBlob class
```

Since CBareBlob derives from IUnknown, and we know the Microsoft C++ compiler stores the vtable to virtual functions at the very beginning of the object footprint, this makes the this pointer, of the instantiated CBareBlob object, the same as an IUnknown pointer to the object. CBareBlob also implements all the interfaces required by IUnknown (as we've seen earlier in this section), since they were specified to be pure virtual in the base class. The m_cRef in each class is used for interface reference counting.

Custom Interface Implemented as a Nested Class

Using the above idea, we can implement the ICustomInterface using a class that we've called CGutsOfBareBlob. We've nested the class definition to limit its scope (i.e. who it is visible to). It's possible to have many C++ classes within the same compilation unit, each implementing many interfaces. Limiting the scope of these definitions will avoid problems associated with namespace pollution (clashes of names).

The CBareBlob member, m_GutsOfBareBlob, is an instance of the CGutsOfBareBlob class, which inherits directly from ICustomInterface. CGutsOfBareBlob therefore implements the methods of ICustomInterface, and a pointer to the m_GutsOfBareBlob member is essentially an interface pointer. As expected, the CGutsOfBareBlob class populates the vtable entries with pointers to the actual method implementations. The inheritance hierachy at this point is:

IUnknown ← ICustomInterface ← CGutsOfBareBlob

In our case, having a member variable of type CGutsOfBareBlob called m_GutsOfBareBlob within our CBareBlob class, means that a CGutsOfBareBlob object is instantiated each and every time a CBareBlob object is instantiated. We've done this purely for simplicity and convenience. It is, of course, equally possible to simply have a member pointer to the CGutsOfBareBlob class:

```
CGutsOfBareBlob *m_pCGutsOfBareBlob;
```

In this case, you would dynamically create an object of the CGutsOfBareBlob class at runtime from the heap, when the CBareBlob object is instantiated:

```
m_pCGutsOfBareBlob = new CGutsOfBareBlob;
```

If ICustomInterface, implemented by CGutsOfBareBlob, is a very complicated and large interface, or if it is seldom required by clients, it may even be advantageous not to instantiate it until it's absolutely needed (i.e. when someone calls QueryInterface() for ICustomInterface). An interface that is implemented in this fashion is called a **tearoff interface**. This type of optimization technique works far better with the nested-classes implementation of COM interfaces. Under multiple inheritance implementation, interface methods aren't implemented independently on a per-interface basis, which makes the dynamic creation detailed above difficult.

The implementation of the CGutsOfBareBlob class can be found in BareBlob1.cpp. Recall that CGutsOfBareBlob actually implements the methods of the ICustomInterface. The first three methods are the obligatory IUnknown methods, and they're implemented, almost trivially, in BareBlob1.cpp:

```
STDMETHODIMP    CBareBlob::CGutsOfBareBlob::QueryInterface(REFIID riid, void **ppv)
{
    return m_pUnkOuter->QueryInterface(riid,ppv) ;
}

STDMETHODIMP_(ULONG)    CBareBlob::CGutsOfBareBlob::AddRef(void)
{
```

```
    return (m_outRef = m_pUnkOuter->AddRef()) ;
}

STDMETHODIMP_(ULONG)    CBareBlob::CGutsOfBareBlob::Release(void)
{
    return (m_outRef = m_pUnkOuter->Release()) ;
}
```

What we're doing here is being a good COM object and making sure we are aggregatable. Remember the aggregation discussion from Chapter 2; we must cater for a potential 'outer unknown' being passed in from some aggregator (that is, a pointer to the IUnknown interface from the outer object). The approach to follow is repeated here for convenience:

> When `QueryInterface()`, `AddRef()` or `Release()` is called on any interface (except for `IUnknown`), delegate to `pUnkOuter`.

Since `CGutsOfBareBlob` is providing the implementation of `ICustomInterface`, and not `IUnknown`, we must delegate the calls to `QueryInterface()`, `AddRef()`, and `Release()` to `pUnkOuter` as prescribed. Obviously, if the object isn't being aggregated, the outer unknown being passed in would be `NULL`. This case is handled in the constructor of the `CBareBlob` object itself (again found in the `BareBlob1.cpp` file):

```
CBareBlob::CBareBlob(IUnknown *punkOuter)
{
    ObjectCreated() ;
    m_cRef = 0 ;
    // if this is non-null, we're being aggregated
    if (punkOuter)
    {
        m_pUnkOuter = punkOuter ;
        m_GutsOfBareBlob.m_pUnkOuter = punkOuter ;
    }
    else
    {
        m_pUnkOuter = this ;
        m_GutsOfBareBlob.m_pUnkOuter = this ;
    }
}
```

If the object is not being aggregated during instantiation, `CBareBlob` will actually set the `m_pUnkOuter` variable to point to the `IUnknown` of the object itself (i.e. `this`). In this case, we're simply reusing the implementation for `QueryInterface()`, `AddRef()`, and `Release()`, which we already have in the `CBareBlob` class.

You'll notice that we call a function, `ObjectCreated()`, when a `CBareBlob` object is instantiated. This is simply a helper function that enables us to keep track of the total number of objects. There's another one of these, `ObjectDestroyed()`, which, unsurprisingly, we call from the object's destructor:

```
CBareBlob::~CBareBlob()
{
    ObjectDestroyed() ;
}
```

We declare a global value, `g_cObject`, in `BareBlob1.cpp` to keep a count of the total number of actual instances of `CBareBlob` objects that exist at any one time:

```
ULONG  g_cObject = 0 ;
```

This is quite different from the `m_outRef` reference counter, which is incremented and decremented by `AddRef()` and `Release()` respectively, and hence keeps track of the number of pointers to one particular instance of `CBareBlob`; it is *not* global. When `m_outRef` reaches zero, that instance of the `CBareBlob` class can be freed. When `g_cObject` reaches zero, there are no more instances of the `CBareBlob` class around in the system, and the entire server (DLL) can be freed. The two support functions that increment and decrement the global counter are shown below:

```
VOID ObjectCreated(VOID)
{
    InterlockedIncrement( reinterpret_cast<LONG*>(&g_cObject) ) ;
}

VOID ObjectDestroyed(VOID)
{
    InterlockedDecrement( reinterpret_cast<LONG*>(&g_cObject) ) ;
}
```

As you can see from the above code, these two functions are simply wrappers for the `InterlockedIncrement()` and `InterlockedDecrement()` APIs we've met before.

These global functions should be defined at the very top of the source file, or a forward declaration for the function must be made. These global functions and the global variable can be made static members of our class if only one COM server C++ class is involved in the DLL. Keeping them as globals, as we have done, is more flexible because it caters for multiple C++ COM server classes in the same DLL.

Getting back to our `CGutsOfBareBlob` class – this is where we must implement the 'real meat' methods of our COM component:

- ❑ `GetManagerName()`
- ❑ `OkayToPublishInfo()`
- ❑ `PeekCounters()`.

The following code extract from `BareBlob1.cpp` shows the implementations of these methods:

```
STDMETHODIMP CBareBlob::CGutsOfBareBlob::GetManagerName(BSTR * bstrMgrName)
{
    // the real business rule case should do whatever is
    // necessary
    *bstrMgrName = SysAllocString(L"J. Manzini");
    return S_OK;
}

STDMETHODIMP CBareBlob::CGutsOfBareBlob::OkayToPublishInfo(long year, long month,
VARIANT_BOOL *bResult)
{
    // again, do whatever is necessary to implement the business rule
    //
    if (((year + month) % 4) == 0)
        *bResult = VARIANT_FALSE;
    else
            *bResult = VARIANT_TRUE;
    return S_OK ;
}

STDMETHODIMP CBareBlob::CGutsOfBareBlob::PeekCounters(long *lRefCount, long
*lObjCount)
{
    *lRefCount = m_outRef;
    *lObjCount = g_cObject;
    return S_OK ;
}
```

`GetManagerName()` is a function which will return the name of the person in charge of the department, at the time the method is called. In an actual Intranet environment, the code may do whatever is necessary to determine the name (for example, check to see which manager has logged on to the system at that time). In our implementation, we've simply hard-coded the name of J. Manzini. Notice that we used `SysAllocString()` to create the `BSTR` variable. The caller must free this `BSTR` using `SysFreeString()`, just as we saw in the earlier `BSTR` discussion.

`OkayToPublishInfo()` determines, at the time of the call, whether it is okay to publish any event calendar information. This function can be used to stop external access to data while it's being updated, or to prevent viewing during a certain period of time. Again, the actual implementation can be more involved. Our method, however, takes the year and adds it to the month. If the resulting number is divisible by 4, then the method will return with a status code to prevent the viewing of events.

Finally, the `PeekCounters()` function acts as a kind of trace function by returning the value of the internal reference counter, `m_cRef`, as well as the 'number of objects' counter, `g_cObject`.

With both `CBareBlob` and `CGutsOfBareBlob` fully coded, we have now implemented both the `IUnknown` and the `ICustomInterface` required by the BareBlob, as specified in our IDL description. From the discussions we had in Chapter 1, you may remember the COM runtime needed a class factory in order to figure out how to create our `CBareBlob` object. In the next step, we must now define and create this class factory.

Implementing a Class Factory

Unlike `CBareBlob`, COM runtime creates a class factory in a system-specific way. This means that it isn't necessary to include the interface specifications of it in our IDL file, so that can stay the way it is for now.

The class factory exposes the `IClassFactory` interface. Thanks again to `\Vc98\Include\Objbase.h`, we don't have to assemble our own vtable structure for `IClassFactory`, we simply inherit from it.

> *A lesson can be learnt here. If you're rolling your own ActiveX control and you're implementing some interface already defined by Microsoft (or some other third party), it's a good bet that they'll have header files to make your vtable assembly job much easier. The way to find them is to use the Find in Files feature of Visual C++ 6. Look under the Edit menu for the Find in Files... selection. Point the In Folder field to* `\Vc98\include\`, *and type in the name of the interface you're looking for in the Find what field. Then you simply click the Find button and watch the output window.*

Our class factory is implemented by a C++ class named `CBareBlobMaker`. Its source code is found in the `BareBlob1.cpp` and `BareBlob1.h` files. The class definition for `CBareBlobMaker` is:

```
class CBareBlobMaker : public IClassFactory
{
public :

    CBareBlobMaker():m_cRef(0)
    {}

    STDMETHOD (CreateInstance)      (IUnknown *punkOuter, REFIID riid, void **ppv);
    STDMETHOD(QueryInterface)       (REFIID iid, void **ppv);
    STDMETHOD_(ULONG, AddRef)       (void);
    STDMETHOD_(ULONG, Release)      (void);
    STDMETHOD(LockServer)           (BOOL bLock);

private:

    ULONG   m_cRef ;        // refcount
} ;
```

As with all other COM interfaces, the `QueryInterface()`, `AddRef()`, and `Release()` methods must be implemented. In addition, the `IClassFactory` interface also has a `CreateInstance()` method, used here to create an instance of `CBareBlob`, as well as a `LockServer()` method which keeps the server in memory.

The `QueryInterface()` method of the class factory will only return pointers to `IUnknown` or `IClassFactory`. Any other interface request will get an `E_NOINTERFACE`:

```
STDMETHODIMP CBareBlobMaker::QueryInterface(REFIID iid, void **ppv)
{
    *ppv = NULL ;

    if (iid == IID_IUnknown || iid == IID_IClassFactory)
        *ppv = this ;
    else
        return E_NOINTERFACE ;

    AddRef() ;

    return S_OK ;
}
```

An interesting observation here is that the QueryInterface() call returns the same interface pointer for both IClassFactory and IUnknown! Why is this legal?

If we think about our binary vtable again, we can see that it's legal because the first three entries in the vtable are the same for IUnknown as well as IClassFactory. The golden rules of COM ensured that. So, passing a pointer to IClassFactory as an IUnknown pointer is totally legal. Conceptually, it's equivalent to a C++ dynamic_cast<> from the base class to a derived class. In essence, any COM interface pointer can be cast into an IUnknown pointer. So why didn't we also take this easy way out in our CBareBlob?

The answer lies in aggregation. If we can do exactly the same thing within the QueryInterface(), AddRef(), and Release() members, then we can do what our class factory does – make them the same. Unfortunately, for a COM class that supports aggregation, the handling of these members is required, by COM rules, to be different between normal interfaces and IUnknown. Because our CBareBlob was purposely designed to be aggregatable, we had to implement the IUnknown methods separately for each interface. Note that it's still possible – and quite common – for all the non-IUnknown interfaces to share an 'inner' set of these methods because, typically, they must all behave in the same general way. This reinforces our previous discussion on a multiple inheritance versus a nested class implementation of COM interfaces. A pure multiple inheritance implementation can't handle aggregation since all IUnknown methods *must* be implemented identically (by member functions of the derived class). However, an external class (outside the multiple inheritance hierarchy) can be created to remedy the situation. We will see this in action with ATL 3 in later chapters.

What I've been saying so far, then, indicates that the class factory isn't aggregatable. Well, we certainly created the class in a way that is incompatible with aggregation. While COM doesn't explicitly specify that a class factory is special and may not be aggregated, you're highly unlikely to meet a case where this would happen. In the Win32 implementation of COM, at least, you can rest peacefully knowing that you won't be aggregated during class factory instantiation by the COM runtime helper functions.

The `AddRef()` and `Release()` methods of `IClassFactory` (and `IUnknown`) for the class factory are implemented like this:

```
STDMETHODIMP_(ULONG) CBareBlobMaker::AddRef(void)
{
   return ++m_cRef ;
}

STDMETHODIMP_(ULONG)  CBareBlobMaker::Release(void)
{
   if (--m_cRef == 0)
   {
      delete this ;
      return 0 ;
   }

   return m_cRef ;
}
```

This is almost identical to the `CBareBlob` implementation.

Next, we'll look at the most interesting method from `IClassFactory`: the `CreateInstance()` method. Here it is:

```
STDMETHODIMP CBareBlobMaker::CreateInstance(IUnknown *punkOuter,
                                        REFIID riid, void **ppv)
{
   CBareBlob *cmg ;
   HRESULT hr ;

   *ppv = NULL ;

   if ((punkOuter) && (riid != IID_IUnknown))
   {
      return CLASS_E_NOAGGREGATION ;
   }

   cmg = new CBareBlob(punkOuter) ;

   hr = cmg->QueryInterface(riid, ppv) ;

   if (FAILED(hr))
   {
      delete cmg ;
      return hr ;
   }

   return S_OK ;
}
```

First, we perform a 'COM rule' consistency check to make sure that the client asks for IUnknown if it wants aggregation (punkOuter != NULL). Otherwise, we simply instantiate a CBareBlob object on the heap with the new operator, passing in the punkOuter controlling unknown. Next, we ask the newly instantiated object for the interface ID requested by the client. If the call is successful, we have the interface pointer, all is well, and we return S_OK. Otherwise, something is wrong, or the client really doesn't know what it's doing; we simply delete the object and return E_NOINTERFACE. Note that we're counting on the CBareBlob object to 'do the right thing' with the punkOuter passed in, and we also expect the CBareBlob to have AddRef()'ed any interface returning from a QueryInterface() call.

The last method to implement is LockServer(). From the client point of view, the aim of this call is to lock the server in memory, so as to improve object creation performance, thus avoiding the re-creation of the class factory each time the same COM server is instantiated. Wait a minute! Doesn't the class factory (providing the IClassFactory interface) have a reference count? And wouldn't that be enough to hold the class factory in memory? The answer turns out to be *no*! There is a quirk in COM's way of dealing with local servers (not in-process servers), which would cause deadlocks if we insist that the class object's reference count becomes zero before the server is unloaded. To overcome this, the LockServer() function must be used to hold the class factory and its server in memory. In our simple in-process server case, we'll just use the existing global 'object count' variable and increment it for lock, and decrement it for unlock. This is valid in our case, because the class factory actually lives in the very same DLL as the implementation of the object that it creates, and we aren't creating objects which require a lot of dynamically created resources.

```
STDMETHODIMP CBareBlobMaker::LockServer(BOOL bLock)
{
    if (bLock)
        ObjectCreated();
    else
        ObjectDestroyed() ;
    return S_OK ;
}
```

Hacking the System Attribute Database

That's about it. We've done everything that's required for a simple ActiveX control (or you can call it a COM object server). We have one task remaining – the creation of all the links required for the COM runtime to be able to find, and work with, our object. These are the links in the system attribute database. Until the Class Store (covered in Chapter 2) becomes available, the database is in the local machine's registry.

The registry entries that we want to add are:

```
\HKEY_CLASSES_ROOT\CLSID\{048E11A0-2754-11d0-8DCF-000000000000}\(default) = "CBareBlob"
\HKEY_CLASSES_ROOT\CLSID\{048E11A0-2754-11d0-8DCF-000000000000}\InProcServer32 =
                                                    "<path to
server>\BAREBLOB.DLL"
\HKEY_CLASSES_ROOT\CLSID\{048E11A0-2754-11d0-8DCF-000000000000}\ThreadingModel =
"Apartment"
\HKEY_CLASSES_ROOT\CBareBlob.1\(default) = "CBareBlob"
\HKEY_CLASSES_ROOT\CBareBlob.1\CLSID = {048E11A0-2754-11d0-8DCF-000000000000}
```

It's actually a requirement of ActiveX controls that they are self-registering (i.e. they're able to add the above registry entries into the registry itself). We'll implement this self-registration here. Under Win32, the requirements for an in-process server residing in a DLL are for the DLL to have the following entry point functions exported by name:

Function Name	Purpose
`STDAPI DllRegisterServer(VOID);`	An in-process server is expected to create its registry entries for all object classes it supports.
`STDAPI DllUnregisterServer(VOID);`	The in-process server should remove only those registry entries it created through `DllRegisterServer()`. It should leave alone any entries that currently exist for its object classes that it did not create. This is subtle since new attributes may be added by other programs after the component's registration.

`STDAPI DllGetClassObject(`
`REFCLSID rclsid,`
`REFIID riid,`
`LPVOID FAR *ppv);`
	This function is called by the COM runtime to get hold of the class object. Normally not invoked directly by client code, it is used to get an interface implemented by the class object, through which an instance of the requested object class can be created. `rclsid` is the requested object class id, `riid` is the REFID of the requested interface and `ppv` returns the interface pointer. Normally used to obtain `IClassFactory` interfaces.

`STDAPI DllCanUnloadNow(void);`	Determines whether the DLL that implements this function is in use. If not, the caller can safely unload the DLL from memory. Care should be taken if the DLL has loaded secondary DLLs on behalf of the client.

The `DllRegisterServer()` and `DllUnregisterServer()` entry points are typically used by a utility like `Regsvr32.exe` (which we'll explain and use shortly), while `DllGetClassObject()` and `DllCanUnloadNow()` are called directly by the COM runtime support. `CoGetClassObject()` will call the `DllGetClassObject()` for a DLL server, and `CoFreeUnusedLibraries()` will cause `DllCanUnloadNow()` to be called. In the next few sections, we'll be focussing on how to go about implementing these functions in our code.

In order to ensure that these functions are exported in the DLL, we'll create a `BareBlob.def` file. In the file, we explicitly export them by name:

```
DESCRIPTION    'a bare blob in a DLL'

EXPORTS        DllGetClassObject  PRIVATE
               DllRegisterServer  PRIVATE
               DllUnregisterServer PRIVATE
               DllCanUnloadNow PRIVATE
```

The PRIVATE keyword ensures that another client using the DLL couldn't accidentally import and call one of these functions when using the IMPLIB (or equivalent) tool. These entry points should only be called by the COM runtime explicitly.

We could have used the _declspec(dllexport) specifier in the declaration and definition of the functions to get them exported instead of using the BareBlob.def file. However, because of the way the COM macros such as STDAPI are defined, doing this will require some fairly ugly trickery. Instead, it's far cleaner to include a .DEF file. This also eliminates the chance of accidentally exporting mangled C++ function names.

Before we implement the exported functions, we need to have some global strings set up to make life a little easier. (Try typing in the CLSID several times without getting it wrong once!) We'll add these to the top of BareBlob1.cpp:

```
TCHAR tcSampleDesc[]       = _T("CBareBlob");
TCHAR tcInprocServer32[]   = _T("InprocServer32");
TCHAR tcSampleProgID[]     = _T("CBareBlob");
TCHAR tcProgID[]           = _T("BareBlobLib.CBareBlob1.1");
TCHAR tcThreadModel[]      = _T("ThreadingModel");
TCHAR tcFree[]             = _T("Apartment");
TCHAR tcCLSID[]            = _T("{048E11A0-2754-11d0-8DCF-000000000000}");
```

Note our use of the TCHAR type and the _T() macro. The _T() macro is the same as the TEXT() macro. These type and macro definitions originate from the Tchar.h header. They're extremely useful for keeping your application character set independent. Using these types and macros, you can write one set of source code for UNICODE, MBCS, or ANSI compilations. Basically, it will make internationalization of your application (adapting it for another country with another language) simpler in the future. Further discussion of internationalization is beyond the scope of this book, and the reader is encouraged to consult one of the many available books on the subject.

The DllRegisterServer Function

We now implement the DllRegisterServer() function for our server. It consists mainly of Win32 based registry manipulation calls.

```
STDAPI DllRegisterServer(VOID)
{
    HKEY     hKey  = NULL;
    HKEY     hKey2 = NULL;
    HKEY     hKey3 = NULL;
    DWORD    result;
    HRESULT hr = SELFREG_E_CLASS;
    TCHAR    cModulePathName[MAX_PATH];
```

```
// Create HKEY_CLASSES_ROOT\progid\CLSID
result = RegCreateKey(HKEY_CLASSES_ROOT, tcSampleProgID, &hKey);
if (result != ERROR_SUCCESS) goto lExit;

result = RegSetValue(hKey, NULL, REG_SZ, tcSampleDesc, _tcslen(tcSampleDesc));
if(result != ERROR_SUCCESS) goto lExit;

result = RegCreateKey(hKey, _T("CLSID"), &hKey2);
if (result != ERROR_SUCCESS) goto lExit;

result = RegSetValue(hKey2, NULL, REG_SZ, tcCLSID, _tcslen(tcCLSID));
if (result != ERROR_SUCCESS) goto lExit;

RegCloseKey(hKey);
RegCloseKey(hKey2);
hKey = NULL;
hKey2 = NULL;

// Create HKEY_CLASSES_ROOT\CLSID

// create CLSID key
result = RegCreateKey(HKEY_CLASSES_ROOT, _T("CLSID"), &hKey);
if (result != ERROR_SUCCESS) goto lExit ;

// create CLSID/GUID key
result = RegCreateKey(hKey, tcCLSID, &hKey2);
if (result != ERROR_SUCCESS) goto lExit ;

// put in sample description value into CLSID\GUID key
result = RegSetValue(hKey2, NULL, REG_SZ, tcSampleDesc, _tcslen(tcSampleDesc));
if (result != ERROR_SUCCESS) goto lExit ;

// get our path ..
 result = GetModuleFileName(static_cast<HINSTANCE>(g_hDllMain),
 cModulePathName, sizeof(cModulePathName) /sizeof(TCHAR));
if (result == 0) goto lExit ;

// create subkey under CLSID\GUID
result = RegCreateKey(hKey2, tcInprocServer32, &hKey3);
if (result != ERROR_SUCCESS) goto lExit ;

// set key value to the path obtained above
result = RegSetValue(hKey3, NULL, REG_SZ,
                        cModulePathName, _tcslen(cModulePathName));
if (result != ERROR_SUCCESS) goto lExit ;

// both
result = RegSetValueEx(hKey3, tcThreadModel, 0,
        REG_SZ, reinterpret_cast<BYTE*>(tcFree), sizeof(tcFree));
if (result != ERROR_SUCCESS) goto lExit;
RegCloseKey(hKey3);
hKey3 = NULL;

// PROGID
```

```
        result = RegCreateKey(hKey2, tcProgID, &hKey3);
        if (result != ERROR_SUCCESS) goto lExit;

        result = RegSetValue(hKey3, NULL, REG_SZ, tcSampleProgID,
                 _tcslen(tcSampleProgID));
        if (result != ERROR_SUCCESS) goto lExit;

        RegCloseKey(hKey3);
        hKey3 = NULL;


        hr = S_OK ;

lExit:

        // close up
        if (hKey) RegCloseKey(hKey);
        if (hKey2) RegCloseKey(hKey2);
        if (hKey3) RegCloseKey(hKey3);

        return hr;
}
```

If you perform a search (Tools\Find\Files or Folders...) into the header files under \vc98\include, you'll find that the STDAPI in front of DllRegisterServer() is defined to be equivalent to:

```
extern "C" HRESULT __stdcall
```

STDAPI takes care of making sure that DllRegisterServer() can be called by the client and that the name of the function won't be mangled by C++.

The implementation of DllRegisterServer() is quite straightforward, but one can see that this registry manipulation is quite tedious to write and test. The regular nature of it screams out for some sort of automatic generation. In the next chapter, we'll examine an automatic way of doing this based on a script language.

If you've read through the code carefully, then you may have noticed an undeclared identifier creeping in. It occurs when we set the path:

```
    // get our path ..
    result = GetModuleFileName(static_cast<HINSTANCE>(g_hDllMain), cModulePathName,
                              sizeof(cModulePathName) /sizeof(TCHAR));
    if (result == 0) goto lExit ;
```

The undeclared identifier is g_hDllMain, which is a global handle to the module instance itself (i.e. the DLL instance mapped into the current client EXE). We've stored this handle in a global variable, which needs to be added to the start of code, so that it's available. The following line should be at the top of the BareBlob1.cpp file.

```
HINSTANCE g_hDllMain;
```

However, we also have to initialize it. The best way of doing this is in the DLL entry point, namely `DllMain()`:

```
BOOL APIENTRY DllMain(HINSTANCE hDLLInst, DWORD fdwReason, LPVOID lpvReserved)
{
   switch (fdwReason)
   {
      case DLL_PROCESS_ATTACH :
         g_hDllMain = hDLLInst ;
   }
   return TRUE ;
}
```

The DllUnregisterServer Function

The `DllUnregisterServer()` function is almost a direct reversal of the `DllRegisterServer()` function. It's also rather uninteresting and screams out for some type of automatic generation.

```
STDAPI DllUnregisterServer(VOID)
{
    HKEY    hKey  = NULL;
    HKEY    hKey2 = NULL;
    DWORD   result;
    HRESULT hr = SELFREG_E_CLASS;

    result = RegOpenKey(HKEY_CLASSES_ROOT, tcSampleProgID, &hKey);
    if (result == ERROR_SUCCESS)
    {
        GuardedDeleteKey(hKey, _T("CLSID"));
        RegCloseKey(hKey);
        hKey = NULL;
        GuardedDeleteKey(HKEY_CLASSES_ROOT, tcSampleProgID);
    }

    result = RegOpenKey(HKEY_CLASSES_ROOT, _T("CLSID"), &hKey);
    result = RegOpenKey(hKey, tcCLSID, &hKey2);

    if (result == ERROR_SUCCESS)
    {
      GuardedDeleteKey(hKey2, tcInprocServer32);
      GuardedDeleteKey(hKey2, tcProgID);
      RegCloseKey(hKey2);
      hKey2 = NULL;
      GuardedDeleteKey(hKey, tcCLSID);
    }

    RegCloseKey(hKey);
    hKey = NULL;

    hr = S_OK;

    return hr;
}
```

There's one small but important issue we need to be aware of when working with registry entries during unregistration. If there are unexpected subkeys found under a key that we've created, we should not delete that key, since another object or utility may depend on the value of the key in order to perform properly.

> *You may have already noticed this behavior, when you've tried to uninstall a program and the uninstaller informs you that it can't remove all entries from the registry. It's reassuring to know that it follows standard procedures. Ironically, time has shown that acute registry bloating and crashes can be attributed to this "leave it alone if you don't know what to do with it" policy.*

In our implementation of `DllUnregisterServer()`, we have a function that makes this kind of check before allowing deletion. Shown below is the code for `GuardedDeleteKey()` function, which wraps the actual `RegDeleteKey()` Win32 API and allows it to be accessed 'safely'. Another very subtle reason for this function is the difference in implementation of `RegDeleteKey()` under Windows 98 versus Windows NT 4.0. `RegDeleteKey()` will recursively delete a tree of keys and subkeys under Windows 98, while the Windows NT version won't delete a key if it has any subkeys.

If you're following along and entering code, you need to make sure that this function is added at the beginning of the `BareBlob1.cpp` file:

```
LONG GuardedDeleteKey(HKEY hKey, LPCTSTR szSubKey)
{
    // check to see if the key to be deleted still has subkey,
    // if not delete it, otherwise fail this

    TCHAR cDumHolder[MAX_PATH+1];
    HKEY  hSubkey;

    if (ERROR_SUCCESS != RegOpenKey(hKey, szSubKey, &hSubkey))
       return REGDB_E_INVALIDVALUE;

    if (ERROR_SUCCESS == RegEnumKey(hSubkey, 0, cDumHolder,
                                    sizeof(cDumHolder)/sizeof(TCHAR)))
    {
       RegCloseKey(hSubkey);
       return REGDB_E_INVALIDVALUE;
    }

    RegCloseKey(hSubkey);
    return RegDeleteKey(hKey, szSubKey);
}
```

The DllGetClassObject Function

The `DllGetClassObject()` function provides an entry point for the COM runtime to get a hold of an instance of our class factory, and request its `IClassFactory` interface at the same time. The three parameters to this function are shown in the table below:

Parameter	Description
REFCLSID rclsid	The class ID (CLSID) for which you want a class object.
REFIID riid	The interface to request from the class factory – typically, either IClassFactory or IClassFactory2.
LPVOID FAR *ppv	(Output only.) Returns the interface requested, if successful; otherwise, it's set to NULL.

We implement DllGetClassObject() using the following code:

```
STDAPI DllGetClassObject(REFCLSID rclsid, REFIID riid, VOID **ppv)
{
    HRESULT  hr ;
    class CBareBlobMaker * pcf;

    *ppv = NULL ;

    if (rclsid != CLSID_CBareBlob)
    {
        return CLASS_E_CLASSNOTAVAILABLE;
    }

    pcf = new CBareBlobMaker() ;

    if (!pcf)
    {
        return CLASS_E_CLASSNOTAVAILABLE;    }

    hr = pcf->QueryInterface(riid, ppv) ;

    if (FAILED(hr))
    {
        delete pcf ;
        return hr ;
    }

    return S_OK ;
}
```

We first make a check to ensure that the caller (COM runtime) has requested a class factory able to create CBareBlobs (in this case rclsid == CLSID_CBareBlob). If not, we return an error since we don't have a class object for anything else in this server. If the client did indeed request a CBareBlob class object, we then instantiate a C++ CBareBlobMaker object. If this is successful, we then do a QueryInterface() on the new class factory instance for the IClassFactory interface. In this case, we're taking advantage of the fact that the CBareBlobMaker is actually a C++ class and, therefore, we make a call to its QueryInterface() member function directly. Note that for implementation simplicity, we have not implemented a singleton class object – we create a new instance of CbareBlobMaker, on the heap, for every call to DllGetClassObject().

The DllCanUnload Function

The last function we need to implement, `DllCanUnloadNow()`, is called by the COM runtime, from time to time, when it wants to determine whether or not a DLL server can be unloaded. This function is seldom called in the older 16-bit COM implementation, but is vital in the 32-bit implementation. A DLL can be unloaded if it isn't servicing any object and the server isn't locked, so the `DllCanUnloadNow()` function should work in conjunction with `LockServer()`. Since both the action of `LockServer()` and the creation of a new instance of `CBareBlob` will call `ObjectCreated()`, and hence increment the `g_cObject` counter, we can implement `DllCanUnloadNow()` by simply examining the object count. If the count hasn't reached zero, we return `S_FALSE`, which won't allow the server DLL to be unloaded:

```
STDAPI DllCanUnloadNow()
{
    return ( g_cObject == 0 ) ? S_OK : S_FALSE;
}
```

We have now implemented all the functionality required by our in-process COM server servicing `CBareBlob` objects, but before we proceed to the compilation and testing of the server, we have a few finishing touches to add. Our source code isn't quite complete yet, as there are the `#includes` required to make everything hang together.

Finishing up the Source Code

We'll start with the header file, `BareBlob1.h`. Up to now, the header file should contain just the class definitions of `CBareBlob`, `CGutsOfBareBlob` and `CBareBlobMaker`. As these classes are derived from interfaces (`IUnknown`, `ICustomInterface` and `IClassFactory` respectively), we need to tell Visual C++ about them. We do this by adding the following `#includes`:

```
#include <objbase.h>
#include "bareblob.h"       // this file generated by MIDL
```

The first of these, `objbase.h`, defines for us many COM types, prototypes of COM APIs, and standard interface vtables (pure virtual structures or classes), such as `IClassFactory` and `IUnknown`. The second, `BareBlob.h`, was generated by the MIDL when we compiled `BareBlob.idl` at the start of this chapter, and it contains a declaration for the custom interface `ICustomInterface` that we implemented in `BareBlob1.cpp`.

Moving on to `BareBlob1.cpp`, we find that we need to `#include` several headers – in particular, the `BareBlob_i.c` file generated for us by MIDL. This file contains all the UUIDs used in our IDL, including the library's UUID, the COM server's CLSID, and the interface's IID. We also need to `#include` the following:

- ❑ `Windows.h` to get a basic definition for the Win32 APIs that we call
- ❑ `Tchar.h` to get the `_T()` macro
- ❑ TCHAR type, as we've discussed earlier
- ❑ `Olectl.h` to get the Automation types like `BSTR` and `VARIANT_BOOL`, which we use as parameters for our business rule method implementation

```
#include <windows.h>
#include "bareblob1.h"
#include <tchar.h>
#include <olectl.h>
#include "bareblob_i.c"   // MIDL generated file,
                          // mainly for the UUID definitions
```

Compiling our Creation

Before we go on to compile the code, let's look at a quick summary of everything we've done so far. We have:

- ❑ Defined the appearance of our class in terms of the object and the interfaces it supports in an IDL file
- ❑ Run the IDL file through MIDL to generate proxy/stub code, as well as a binary type library
- ❑ Created source files for our project by including some useful output files from MIDL, which provide declarations for interfaces and definitions for IIDs and CLSIDs
- ❑ Coded and implemented the CBareBlob class by manually assembling the vtable, and using the nested class CGutsOfBareBlob
- ❑ Coded and implemented the CBareBlobMaker class which serves as a class object class for our CBareBlob class
- ❑ Created a module definition (.DEF) file for our COM server, exporting the routines required by the COM runtime
- ❑ Coded and implemented four in-process server support routines for registering and unregistering the server on the system

Now we're ready to compile our server.

From the feedback we have received for the first edition of this book, many readers would like to know about the actual compilation and link flags being used when creating an ActiveX control. The Visual C++ environment does a lot of wonderful things for us under the "push button" front-end, but when things don't quite work the way you expect, it is good to know what is actually happening under the hood. To this end, we have elected to use a rather 'raw' text Makefile to do the compilation and linkage for our BareBlob example. This will give you the confidence to "return to the command line" should Visual C++ 6 ever fail to follow your exact demands. After this chapter, though, we will revert back to the easy-as-pie Visual Studio 98 GUI interface, where everything *will* work as we expect.

Here is our Makefile for the BareBlob ActiveX Control. We'll take it one step at a time, and discuss what's happening at each stage.

```
TARGETOS=BOTH
APPVER=4.0
_WIN32_IE=0x0400

!include <win32.mak>
```

If you are curious, take a look at `win32.mak` in the `\vc98\include` directory. It has many macros defined which make writing `Makefile` easy. Here, the symbol `TARGETOS` specifies that we are building for both Win95/98 and Windows NT. The `APPVER` symbol specifies that Windows NT 4.0 or Windows 95/98 with DCOM is our target system, therefore some of the more advanced features of compilers and linkers should be enabled. Finally, the `_WIN32_IE` symbol indicates that we are building for an Internet Explorer 4.0 (rather than 3.0) target.

```
all:BareBlob.dll

cflags=$(cflags)
```

If you look up the `$(cflags)` definition in `win32.mak`, you will see that it specifies:

```
-c -W3 -DCRTAPI=_cdecl -DCRTAPI2=_cdecl -nologo -D_X86_=1  -D_WIN32_IE=0x0400 -
DWINVER=0x0400
```

Next, we define how to make a type library, given an IDL file:

```
BareBlob.tlb:BareBlob.idl
        midl /Oicf BareBlob.idl
```

Since the generated `BareBlob.h` file is vital for building the DLL, we also specify it as a dependency:

```
BareBlob.h:BareBlob.idl
        midl /Oicf BareBlob.idl
```

The next specification tells `nmake` how to create the object file:

```
BareBlob1.obj: BareBlob1.cpp BareBlob1.h BareBlob.h
    $(cc) $(cflags)  $(cdebug) $(cvarsmt) BareBlob1.cpp
```

The `$(cdebug)` macro will expand to a debug compile by default; a release build can be effected using `"NMAKE nodebug=1"`. We have elected to use the multi-threaded runtime library `$(cvarsmt)`, which maps to:

```
-Z7 -Od -DWIN32 -D_WIN32 -D_MT -DMT
```

Finally, we specify how to use the linker to build the DLL. Notice that the DEF file, which contains the exported entry points, is explicitly specified:

```
BareBlob.dll:  BareBlob1.obj BareBlob.def
    $(link) $(dlllflags) $(ldebug)
    -def:BareBlob.def -out:BareBlob.dll BareBlob1.obj $(olelibsmt)
```

$(ldebug) will link in debug information if necessary. Here, $(dlllflags) maps conveniently to:

```
/NODEFAULTLIB /INCREMENTAL:NO /PDB:NONE  /RELEASE /NOLOGO -
entry:_DllMainCRTStartup@12 -dll
```

And $(olelibsmt) maps to all the libraries that we will need:

- ❑   ole32.lib
- ❑   uuid.lib
- ❑   oleaut32.lib
- ❑   kernel32.lib
- ❑   libcmt.lib
- ❑   oldnames.lib
- ❑   ws2_32.lib
- ❑   mswsock.lib
- ❑   advapi32.lib

The last few lines in our Makefile help with cleanup when we perform an nmake clean:

```
clean:
    @del *.exe
    @del *.obj
    @del *.pdb
    @del *.ilk
    @del *.tlb
    @del BareBlob.h
    @del BareBlob_p.c
    @del BareBlob_i.c
    @del BareBlob.dll
    @del BareBlob.exp
    @del BareBlob.lib
    @del dlldata.c
```

That's all that we need for the makefile. To compile the BareBlob, simply type in NMAKE in a command prompt. When this is completed, you should see BareBlob.dll in your working directory.

Congratulations, you've just completed the creation of an ActiveX control from scratch!

Knowing this will probably be quite satisfying. However, seeing the object in action will be most gratifying. To do this, we must first register the server. How do we do this?

Registering The Server

In the \Vc98\Tools\bin directory, you should find a system utility called Regsvr32.exe. This is the utility that we'll use to register the server. On the command line, simply type:

```
REGSVR32 BAREBLOB.DLL
```

A message box will pop up shortly, announcing that the server has registered successfully:

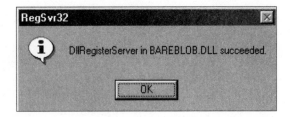

To unregister the server later, you may use:

REGSVR32 /u BAREBLOB.DLL

Again a message box will notify you of the status of the unregistration.

What happens inside Regsvr32.exe is actually quite simple. It calls LoadLibrary() on the DLL name that you've specified. If it is a register server request, it will make a call into the DllRegisterServer() entry point. If DllRegisterServer() returns a success code, it will report the success of registration; otherwise, the error message will be reported. If you've specified the unregister server operation, then it will call the DllUnregisterServer() entry point instead. You can see from this how useful these functions are for COM server self-registration.

Once you've successfully compiled and registered your server, you're ready to instantiate a CBareBlob – we can do this even without writing a client first. This is accomplished through the Oleview.exe utility (see Appendix A for an introduction if you have never used this tool).

Make sure you have Oleview.exe version 2.10.053 or later (check Help | About Oleviewer). If you have the Oleview.exe that comes with Visual C++ 6, then you're fine.

Start Oleview.exe on your system, and, on the left-hand pane, select the All Objects item (you'll have to make sure Expert Mode is turned on in the View menu). Look down the list of objects and find CBareBlob. It is there! You're being recognized by Oleview.exe!

Select the CBareBlob object on the left pane, and check out the attributes that Object Viewer knows about your class. As you can see, all of it came from the registry entry that you've added in the DllRegisterServer() function. Now, let's actually instantiate a copy of CBareBlob. You can do this by double-clicking on the CBareBlob entry of the left pane. After a brief pause, you can see a list of interfaces showing up. However, only IUnknown is shown; there is no sign of ICustomInterface. Believe it or not, you've actually instantiated a CBareBlob object.

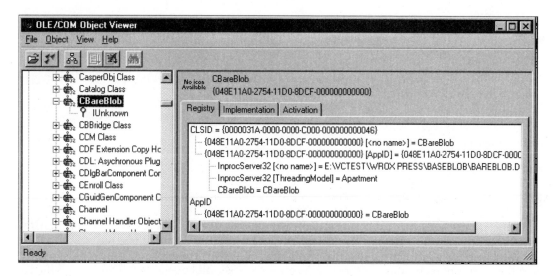

There's no outward sign that the object has been instantiated, however, because our object provides no user interface. Oleview.exe obtains the list of interfaces that you see by creating an instance of the COM class, obtaining a pointer to the IUnknown interface of the object, and finally going through a complete list of known interfaces and performing QueryInterface() on every one of them, noting which ones are supported.

In other words, not only has your poor object been instantiated, but it has also been interrogated by the system hundreds of times (looking for interfaces), while you're still trying to figure out if object creation actually worked.

Let's prove this. I suppose we could put an infinite loop inside the QueryInterface() method of CBareBlob and watch Object Viewer choke when it picks on your object, or we could meticulously rig up the debugger and do TRACE() inside the QueryInterface() implementation. Another, less offensive and easier, way to do this (which doesn't involve a recompile) is to manually define ICustomInterface() in the system registry. This will make the interface 'known' to the system (and hence Object Viewer), so that the next time your object is interrogated, this interface should be recognized. Sounds better? Let's do it.

Start Regedit.exe (or Regedt32.exe in Windows NT), expand HKEY_CLASSES_ROOT and go to the Interface key. Now manually add a key in this tree, and label it with the interface ID (IID) of ICustomInterface. Add a nameless (default) value of ICustomInterface. Finally, add a NumMethods subkey and set its default value to 6. A summary of keys to add is shown below:

```
\HKEY_CLASSES_ROOT\Interface\{2740CBA0-274C-11d0-8DCF-000000000000}\(default) =
"ICustomInterface"
\HKEY_CLASSES_ROOT\Interface\{2740CBA0-274C-11d0-8DCF-
000000000000}\NumMethods\(default) = "6"
```

Now you can go back to our friendly Object Viewer again, hit *F5* and then double-click on our CBareBlob once again to see its interfaces.

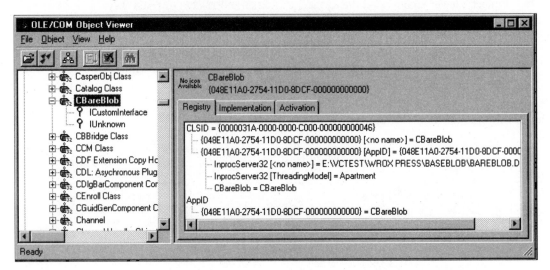

Ta-da! ICustomInterface is now recognized by the system! Our faithful object's QueryInterface() has returned and proudly announced to the world, 'Elementary, my dear Watson! I do support ICustomInterface.'

Before you start to curse me for making such a mountain out of a molehill, let me assure you that we'll spend a good part of the rest of this chapter building a far more sophisticated test harness for our BLOB object, and, indeed, for any future ActiveX control that we'll be designing.

But seriously, even in this seemingly trivial interaction, Object Viewer has already exercised over 80% of our code. Let's take a moment to look under the hood at what has been going on:

1. Object Viewer enumerated the \HKEY_CLASSES_ROOT\CLSID keys.

2. It then did a CoCreateInstance() on the CBareBlob CLSID when we double-clicked on CBareBlob, requesting IUnknown.

3. The COM runtime loaded our BareBlob.dll and made a call into DllGetClassObject() to get an IClassFactory interface from a class object.

4. Our implementation of the DllGetClassObject() instantiated a CBareBlobMaker object on the heap and returned a pointer to it to the COM runtime.

5. The COM runtime called IClassFactory::CreateInstance().

6. Our implementation of CBareBlobMaker::CreateInstance() created a CBareBlob object on the heap, QueryInterface()'d it for IUnknown and returned the pointer back to the COM runtime.

7. The COM runtime returned the `IUnknown` pointer to Object Viewer.

8. Object Viewer enumerated the `\HKEY_CLASSES_ROOT\Interface` keys.

9. For each IID entry enumerated, `IUnknown::QueryInterface()` of the `CBareBlob` was called to see if the interface is supported.

10. Object Viewer obtained the text representation of all the interfaces supported by `CBareBlob` from `\HKEY_CLASSES_ROOT\Interface` and displayed them.

The following interaction diagram illustrates what is going on here:

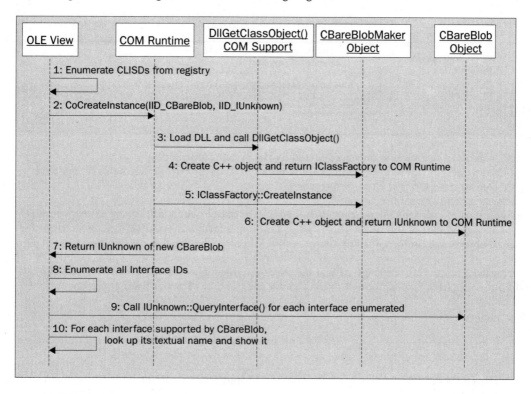

Testing our Object

Having finished writing a component that the system immediately recognizes is very exciting. Using Object Viewer to instantiate and 'test' our object is very easy, but also quite limited. For example, there's no way in Object Viewer to call our custom interfaces.

In order to further test our component (and prove to ourselves that our server is fully working), we now turn to writing a simple client. This client should instantiate an object of the `CBareBlob` class through COM, and then make calls into the methods of the `ICustomInterface`.

We'll be constructing the test harness client using straight C for simplicity of coding and ease of understanding. If you've followed along this far into the chapter, you're probably tired already, so I'll spare you the agony of going through any more complex code. Note that, if we wish, we could immediately use Visual Basic 6 to test our component, and this would work well for the two business rule methods on our custom interface. We cannot, however, use any scripting environment, such as Visual Basic for Applications or VBScript, in Internet Explorer 4. This is because we haven't implemented the IDispatch interface that's required for these clients.

Roughly speaking, we want our client code to implement the following steps:

1. Initialize COM subsystem.

2. Call CoGetClassObject() on CBareBlob's CLSID to get an IClassFactory interface and instantiate a class factory.

3. Call IClassFactory::CreateInstance() to create a CBareBlob object and get its IUnknown interface.

4. Release the IClassFactory interface.

5. Call IUnknown::QueryInterface() with the IID of ICustomInterface to get the object's ICustomInterface.

6. Release IUnknown

7. Call ICustomInterface::GetManagerName() and print the result.

8. Call ICustomInterface::OkayToPublishInfo() and print the result.

9. Call ICustomInterface::PeekCounters() and print the result.

10. Release ICustomInterface

11. Uninitialize the COM subsystem

Writing a Simple Client Test Harness

We've opted to create a very simple test-harness client as a console application. We really don't want to mess with GUI code; our focus is on the COM interactions. The following is our coding for the test harness. You will find this in the \Ch3\TestBlob directory, together with its own Makefile. The file, TestCont.cpp, is quite small; I'll annotate it as we examine it from the top:

```
#include "precomp.h"
#include "..\baseblob\bareblob.h"

#define IID_DEFINED
#include "..\baseblob\bareblob_i.c"
```

Notice how BareBlob.h and BareBlob_i.c come in handy again. Recall that they were MIDL generated files that include definitions for our custom interfaces, as well as definitions for the IIDs, CLSIDs, etc. These files are indispensable for clients of your COM class. Ensure that the #includes above (and INCDIR statements below) contain the correct path for your BareBlob.

Here is the content of `Precomp.h`:

```
#include <stdio.h>
#include <stdlib.h>
#include <time.h>

#define _WIN32_DCOM
#include <objbase.h>
#include <tchar.h>
#include <initguid.h>
```

We need to #include the `stdio.h` header file, so that we can use `printf()` to output information to the screen. Also #included are the headers `stdlib.h` and `time.h`, which, together, allow us to use the C runtime to generate a random number representing time. We need to define _WIN32_DCOM in order to get the definition of `CoCreateInstanceEx()` in our code to compile. The random numbers are used for the month and year inputs for testing the `OkayToPublishInfo()` function and to make the test more interesting. `objbase.h` was included again for the common COM type definitions.

```
int CRTAPI1 _tmain(int argc, TCHAR **argv, TCHAR **envp)
{

    IUnknown * pM;
    IClassFactory * pCF;
    ICustomInterface *pCI;
    long localRef, objCount;
    BSTR mgrName;

    srand( static_cast<unsigned>(time( NULL )) );
```

We declare pointers for the interfaces that we'll be getting from our blob and its class factory, and also two variables to hold the values from calls to our custom interface. The BSTR is for holding the manager's name that will be returned. We also take this chance to seed the random number generator of the C runtime, with the current time as a seed.

```
    HRESULT hRes = CoInitializeEx(NULL, COINIT_APARTMENTTHREADED);
```

The call to `CoInitializeEx()` is to make this the main thread in an STA based client.

```
    hRes = CoGetClassObject(CLSID_CBareBlob, CLSCTX_ALL, NULL,
        IID_IClassFactory,   reinterpret_cast<void **>( &pCF));

    if (SUCCEEDED(hRes))
    {
        printf("Got class factory!\n");
    }
    else
    {
        CoUninitialize();
        exit(1);
    }
```

Here, we try to obtain a class factory for `CBareBlob` by calling `CoGetClassObject()` and requesting a pointer to its `IClassFactory` interface. If we aren't successful, we uninitialize the COM subsystem and exit. Otherwise, we print a message out to the console.

```
    hRes = pCF->CreateInstance(NULL, IID_IUnknown,
        reinterpret_cast<void **>( &pM));
pCF->Release();
    if (pM != NULL)
    {
        printf("Made a bare blob!\n");
    }
    else
    {
        CoUninitialize();
        exit(1);
    }
```

With a call to `IClassFactory::CreateInstance()`, we create an instance of our `CBareBlob` object and ask for a pointer to its `IUnknown` interface. If successful, we print a message and notify the world. Otherwise, we clean up and exit gracefully. Once we've successfully created the `CBareBlob`, we can release the `IClassFactory` pointer and free the class factory, because we won't need it any more.

```
    // Get our custom interface!
    hRes = pM->QueryInterface( IID_ICustomInterface,
        reinterpret_cast<void **>( &pCI));
    pM->Release();
    if (pCI != NULL)
    {
        printf("Got its custom interface!\n");
    }
    else
    {
        CoUninitialize();
        exit(1);
    }
```

Using the `IUnknown` pointer, we `QueryInterface()` for `ICustomInterface`. Thanks to the definition in `BareBlob_i.c`, this is as easy as using the value `IID_ICustomInterface`. If we get the `ICustomInterface` pointer, we print a message. Otherwise, we exit gracefully after cleanup.

Now that we have a pointer to `ICustomInterface`, we're ready to call the 'real meat' of the `CBareBlob` object:

```
    hRes = pCI->GetManagerName(&mgrName);
#ifdef UNICODE
    _tprintf(_T("After calling GetManagerName : = %ls\n"); mgrName);
#else
    char * tp = new char[50];
    WideCharToMultiByte(CP_ACP,0, mgrName, -1, tp, 50, NULL, NULL);
    _tprintf(_T("After calling GetManagerName : = %s\n"),   tp);
    delete [] tp;
#endif
    SysFreeString(mgrName);
```

In this part of the code, we make a call into `ICustomInterface::GetManagerName()`, to get the manager name and print it out on the console. It turns out that this is not trivial, however. Recall that the `BSTR` type under Win32 is always in UNICODE. We need to print out the `BSTR` returned from `GetManagerName()`, but the way we do it will depend on whether the test client is compiled for UNICODE or not. The `Tchar.h` header is useless here, since it doesn't know about, or work with, `BSTR`s. Instead, we do our own checking and, if necessary, call the `WideCharToMultiByte()` function to convert the string before printing. The first parameter of this function is used to select the code-page for the multibyte character set, and setting this to `CP_ACP` gives us the ANSI character set.

> *The `WideCharToMultiByte()` function basically converts a UNICODE string to a multibyte character set string. The function has many parameters, and there are features catering for characters that can't be converted. We won't cover them at length here, but the Win32 API documentation explains it in detail.*

Notice that, according to `BSTR` usage conventions, we must call `SysFreeString()` to free the memory allocated. From our BSTR discussions earlier, you may recall that the caller must free the memory from an "output only" BSTR parameter.

```
long inYear, inMonth;
VARIANT_BOOL flag;
inYear = 1900 + rand() %100;
inMonth = rand() % 13 + 1;
hRes = pCI->OkayToPublishInfo(inYear, inMonth, &flag);

    _tprintf(_T("Checking for okay to publish info : year = %d, month = %d,
status = %s\n"), inYear, inMonth, (flag == VARIANT_TRUE) ? "OKAY": "NO WAY");
```

For testing the `ICustomInterface::OkayToPublishInfo()` function, we decided to use the `rand()` capability of the C runtime to make the test more interesting. The random number is used to enter random year and month values for the call. The returned value from the server is decoded, and either `OKAY` or `NO WAY` is output to the console.

```
hRes = pCI->PeekCounters(&localRef, &objCount);
_tprintf(_T
("After calling PeekCounters: we now have %d local references and
 %d object users.\n"),
localRef, objCount);
```

As you can see from the code above, the `ICustomInterface::PeekCounters()` testing is straightforward. For each call of `PeekCounters()`, we simply print out the values of the counters from the ActiveX control.

```
pCI->Release();
_tprintf(_T("Freeing the blob now!\n"));
CoUninitialize();
return 0;
}
```

Finally, we release interface pointers for `IUnknown` and `ICustomInteface`, and then call `CoUninitialize()` to uninitialize the COM subsystem. Now we are ready to compile and run the code.

The makefile is shown below:

```
# Nmake macros for building Windows 32-Bit apps
TARGETOS=BOTH
APPVER=4.0
_WIN32_IE=0x0400

!include <win32.mak>

INCDIR=..\baseblob

all:TestCont.exe


cflags=$(cflags)  -D_CONSOLE


TestCont.obj: TestCont.cpp $(INCDIR)\BareBlob.h $(INCDIR)\BareBlob_p.c
    $(cc) $(cflags) $(cdebug)  TestCont.cpp

TestCont.exe:  TestCont.obj
    $(link) $(conlflags)  -debug  -out:TestCont.exe TestCont.obj    $(conlibs)
$(olelibs)

clean:
    @del *.exe
    @del *.obj
    @del *.pdb
    @del *.ilk
```

The output you obtain should be similar to this:

```
Got class factory!
Made a bare blob!
Got its custom interface!
After calling GetManagerName : = J. Manzini
Checking for okay to publish info : year = 1927, month = 1, status = NOWAY
After calling PeekCounters: we now have 2 local references and 1 object users.
Freeing the blob now!
```

You may want to run `regsvr32 /u bareblob.dll` to unregister your server, and then try running the program again, just to see what happens.

If we add a loop around the custom interface calls, and run multiple copies of the program, each in its own command console, how come the counts from the `ICustomInterface::PeekCounters()` call stay constant? (Try it if you don't believe me.) This is actually a unique property of in-process servers. Since the server (DLL) runs inside the client's process, the copy running in each command console has a `CBareBlob` and its class factory all to itself. There's no sharing of any kind in this scenario between the instances.

Another good exercise would be to single-step through the program in debug mode and notice when the class object and the `CBareBlob` objects are actually allocated and freed.

The program we've just been looking at is a simple, yet effective test harness for ActiveX controls that implement only custom interfaces. There are, however, several aspects of an ActiveX object that aren't tested – the most notable one being the inability to create multiple, concurrent instances of `CBareBlob`s within the same process.

It turns out that one effective way to give our object a good workout is to write a client test harness which is multithreaded. In this way, each thread in the test harness process can create its own instance of `CBareBlob` and class factory. It can then test them simultaneously within the same process.

The following section introduces some of the basic concepts for those readers new to multithreaded programming. If you are familiar with this subject, then you should simply skip this section and move on to the next one, where we'll start coding up our multithreaded client.

An Aside on Threads and Synchronization Objects

Traditional Windows programs (Windows 3.1 and before) were all single-threaded programs. This was because the underlying operating system, DOS, could only execute one program at a time. A single-threaded program starts up, executes from beginning to end on the same CPU, and is never interrupted by the operating system. Non-preemptive multitasking, introduced by Windows 3.1, maps multiple logical threads to one single physical thread of execution; data is never accessed simultaneously, and no synchronization is necessary. With the advent of Windows 95 and Windows NT, application programs on Windows platforms not only gained the benefits of preemptive multitasking (many programs executing on the operating system simultaneously), but also multithreading.

A process under a Win32 based operating system can have many threads. The kernel, on Windows 95/98 and Windows NT, simply schedules threads. This means that each and every thread is conceptually executing simultaneously. In a system with multiple processors, this may actually be true. However, in most cases where the system only has one CPU, the scheduler uses 'time-slicing' to achieve the same effect. Each thread is given a slice of time to execute; it is then pre-empted, and another thread starts executing. Threads may also give up their right to execution if they're waiting for input/output or the availability of other resources. Since the scheduler works only with threads, a process must have at least one thread in order to be executed. Essentially, then, a process is, in this sense, a grouping of threads. It goes beyond this, however, since it is the process which gives the threads in its group the resources they need – for example, an address space (in virtual memory) in which to execute.

In many ways, a process can be viewed as the set of data structures tracking the utilization of system resources for a group of threads. Threads, on the other hand, can be viewed as a program counter location (the currently executing instruction) and a stack (for storage of temporary or automatic variables). On a system where only one process is running (but with multiple threads executing) the memory space of the process (group of threads) will never be swapped out, and other resources occupied by the process also need not be released. All that's happening in this situation is that each thread gets a chance at execution, with the operating system simply saving and restoring program counters and switching stacks. The registers, stack and other information, are called a context. When Windows NT or Windows 98 switches between threads it loads and unloads the thread's context.

When programming in a high level language such as C or C++, multithreaded programming is very similar to the multitasking programming of older operating systems (UNIX, for example), the only difference being the transparency of resource management. For example, when a UNIX process forks, it's assumed that there will be another execution context, but in order to get that other execution context to do something other than what the original process already does, we need to replace its instructions. With multithreaded programming, everything that a thread can do is defined in the 'thread function'. This thread function is given to a thread on its creation. In essence, the behavior of the thread is determined by the code in the thread function. We can create as many threads with as many thread functions (one per thread) as we want within an application, limited only by the system configuration. Even the 'main thread' of a process is simply the C runtime creating a thread using the operating system `CreateThread()` API, and giving it a thread function equivalent to your `WinMain()` routine. In this way, every thread within a process can be created equally, and the main thread in a process doesn't have any extra visibility or special privileges from the point of view of the operating system or scheduler.

Some aspects of multithreaded programming will take some time to get used to, if you come from the single-threaded programming world. The most important concept is the synchronization of shared resources. Since every thread is conceptually executing concurrently, any resource shared by more than one thread (for example, variables, graphic device contexts and disk files) can potentially get corrupted if some form of synchronization isn't implemented. Corruption occurs when two threads try to modify the same item at the same time, or if one thread holds some information about, or from, the shared resource, and assumes that it's the only one that has access to it.

Win32 offers many synchronization mechanisms for coordinating resource usage between threads and/or processes. The most lightweight and efficient of these is a critical section. Once created, any thread can 'enter' a critical section. If a thread tries to 'enter' the same critical section already being 'occupied' by another thread, the thread attempting to enter will be blocked, and will not continue execution until the thread in the critical section 'leaves' it. In this way, sections of code can be bracketed by 'enter' and 'leave' operations on a critical section object. These sections of code, then, are guaranteed to be executed by only one thread at a time. We'll use this technique later in our multithreaded client sample to protect the output to the console. Without this protection (you can try it if you like), the output from the threads may merge together, and become almost impossible to read.

While efficient, the critical section object has the special property that it can't be owned and it isn't visible outside of the process. Other synchronization objects, including mutexes, semaphores, and events, have different properties and some are accessible from other processes. Interested readers should consult the documentation of the Win32 SDK or other books on advanced Win32 programming (such as *Advanced Windows*, by Jeffrey Richter).

Another situation that frequently occurs in multithreaded programming is when a thread wants to wait for, and synchronize with, another thread. This may be necessary due to the differences in speed of execution or processing between the threads, or the situation may occur by design. In our multithreaded client, which we'll create in a moment, the main thread creates many threads with two seconds between each thread creation. After creating them, it has to wait for all of them to finish. Luckily, Win32 provides a way to do just that. The main thread can invoke the `WaitForMultipleObjects()` API call, and pass it an array of thread handles (obtained when the threads are created successfully). A thread is deemed 'signaled' if the thread has finished execution, or has terminated for other reasons. Therefore, when the main thread specifies in the `WaitForMultipleObjects()` call that it would like to wait for the entire array of threads to be signaled, it is essentially saying that it will wait for all threads to complete. `WaitForMultipleObjects()` is a very powerful call, allowing a thread to wait for a variety of conditions to be triggered before it continues execution. A variant of this is the function `MsgWaitForMultipleObjects()`, which allows the application to synchronize with objects such as threads, together with input events (like keyboard or mouse input) and is very useful for multithreaded COM programming.

Giving Our BLOB a Workout

Now it's time to get back to some coding. We're going to design a multithreaded client to test out our `BareBlob` object. In order to accomplish this, we'll start with the source code from the earlier client program as a base to work from. From this starting point, we'll make the following modifications:

1. Create a global critical section object to share the console, since each and every print statement should be executed by the reporting thread in an atomic fashion from beginning to end, otherwise the output would be impossible to read

2. Define `LOCK()` and `UNLOCK()` macros to make usage of the critical section easier within the code

3. Put the `LOCK()` and `UNLOCK()` macros before and after each and every `_tprintf()` statement

4. Put a loop around the custom interface calls to repeat them twenty times each

5. Move all the object creation and testing logic to a thread function

6. Create up to `MAX_THREAD` threads in the main program and store their handles in an array, allowing for some delay – say 2 seconds – between the creation of each thread

7. After the threads have been created, the main program should wait indefinitely for all the started threads to complete their work

8. After all threads have exited, the main thread should clean up by closing all thread handles and destroying the critical section object

Our main program is now called `MultiCont.cpp` and you can find the file in the `\Ch3\mtstblob` directory:

```
#include "precomp.h"
#include "..\baseblob\bareblob.h"
#define IID_DEFINED
#include "..\baseblob\bareblob_i.c"

#include <process.h>
#define MAX_THREAD          10
#define LOCK(x)             EnterCriticalSection(x);
#define UNLOCK(x)           LeaveCriticalSection(x);
CRITICAL_SECTION    g_Console;

unsigned _stdcall AThread(LPVOID lpParam);

int CRTAPI1 _tmain(int argc, TCHAR **argv, TCHAR **envp)
{
    HANDLE hThread[MAX_THREAD];
    long Params[MAX_THREAD];
    unsigned tpThreadID;
    long i,j;
    InitializeCriticalSection(&g_Console);
    CoInitializeEx(NULL, COINIT_APARTMENTTHREADED); // acts as main thread

    for (i=0; i<MAX_THREAD; i++)
    {
        Params[i] = i;
        hThread[i] = (HANDLE) _beginthreadex(NULL, 0, AThread,
        reinterpret_cast<void *>(&Params[i]),0, &tpThreadID);

        if ((reinterpret_cast<long>(hThread[i])) == 0)
        {
            LOCK(&g_Console);
            _tprintf(_T("Main: Thread creation failure!\n"));
            UNLOCK(&g_Console);
                break;
        }
        else
        {
            LOCK(&g_Console);
            _tprintf(_T("Main: Started thread %d!\n"),  i);
            UNLOCK(&g_Console);
        }
        Sleep(2000);    // 2 seconds between each thread
    }

    WaitForMultipleObjects(i, hThread, TRUE, INFINITE);
    for (j=0; j<i; j++)
    CloseHandle(hThread[j]);
    DeleteCriticalSection(&g_Console);
    CoUninitialize();

    return 0;
}
```

Before we enter `main()`, we declare the critical section and its associated macros, together with the declaration of the thread function, `AThread()`. If you look through the code for the main thread, you'll see that it follows the points listed above. The actual object creation and testing of the `ICustomInterface` takes place in the individual threads.

We have used an array of `long` values called `Params[]` to pass in a unique ID with which each thread can identify itself when printing messages to the console. Also, we're using the C runtime `_beginthreadex()` and `_endthreadex()` instead of the Win32 `CreateThread()` and `ExitThread()`. This is necessary for the C runtime resource management wrapper to do its job. Essentially, `_beginthreadex()` and `_endthreadex()` are wrapped calls to the underlying Win32 APIs. We needed to add `process.h` to the include list, so that we can use the thread related functions, such as `_beginthreadex()` and `_endthreadex()`. `_beginthreadex()` and `endthreadex()` are used instead of `_beginthread()` and `_endthread()` because we want the ability to explicitly close a thread handle (the latter pair will automatically close the handle when a thread terminates). Doing so allows us to avoid a potential race condition, since a thread may start and finish before we reach the `WaitForMultipleObjects()` call.

There's no endless loop or any hold/wait conditions in our thread function (which we'll look at in a moment), so all threads will eventually finish execution. The main thread will then be released from the blocking state and can continue on to the cleanup and shutdown activities.

In our `Makefile`, we must be careful to compile with multi-threaded flags, and link only with multi-threaded runtime libraries:

```
# Nmake macros for building Windows 32-Bit apps
TARGETOS=BOTH
APPVER=4.0
_WIN32_IE=0x0400

!include <win32.mak>

INCDIR=..\baseblob

all:MultiCont.exe

cflags=$(cflags)   -D_CONSOLE

MultiCont.obj: MultiCont.cpp $(INCDIR)\BareBlob.h $(INCDIR)\BareBlob_p.c
    $(cc) $(cflags)  $(cdebug) $(cvarsmt) MultiCont.cpp

MultiCont.exe:  MultiCont.obj
    $(link) $(conlflags)  $(ldebug)   -out:MultiCont.exe MultiCont.obj
$(conlibsmt) $(olelibsmt)

clean:
    @del *.exe
    @del *.obj
    @del *.pdb
    @del *.ilk
```

Remember that the former object creation and testing portion of the code has now been moved to the thread function. Each thread function does its own `CoInitializeEx()` at the beginning, and `CoUninitialize()` at the end. One's initial reaction is to use `CoInitializeEx()` and `CoUninitialize()` just once, on the main thread. But it turns out that these functions are designed for apartment model threading (the Single Threaded Apartment Model, mentioned in Chapter 2). This means that the COM runtime expects the same thread which calls `CoInitialize()` to call all the COM functions and the interface methods, so each thread must make a call to `CoInitialize()`. Our BareBlob component was marked as supporting the Apartment model (STA) when we set up our registry entries in `DllRegServer()`. However, having each thread call `CoInitializeEx()` and `CoUninitialize()` itself, works just fine for our purposes.

Here is the code for the thread function:

```
unsigned _stdcall AThread(LPVOID lpParam)
{
    long myNumber = *(reinterpret_cast<long *>(lpParam));
    IUnknown * pM;
    IClassFactory * pCF;
    ICustomInterface *pCI;
    HRESULT hRes;

    long localRef, objCount, inYear, inMonth;
    VARIANT_BOOL okFlag;
    BSTR mgrName;

    srand( static_cast<unsigned>(time( NULL )) );

    hRes = CoInitializeEx(NULL, COINIT_APARTMENTTHREADED);

    hRes = CoGetClassObject(CLSID_CBareBlob, CLSCTX_ALL, NULL,
    IID_IClassFactory,reinterpret_cast<void **>( &pCF));

    if (SUCCEEDED(hRes))
    {
        LOCK(&g_Console);
        _tprintf(_T("T%d: Got class factory!\n"), myNumber);
        UNLOCK(&g_Console);
    }
    else
    {
        CoUninitialize();
        _endthread();
    }
    hRes = pCF->CreateInstance(NULL, IID_IUnknown, reinterpret_cast<void **>(
&pM));
    // made one of those blobs, release the class factory
    pCF->Release();

    if (pM != NULL)
    {
        LOCK(&g_Console);
        _tprintf(_T("T%d: Made a bare blob!\n"), myNumber);
        UNLOCK(&g_Console);
    }
    else
    {
```

```
        CoUninitialize();
        _endthread();
    }

    // Get our custom interface!
    hRes = pM->QueryInterface( IID_ICustomInterface,
            reinterpret_cast<void **>( &pCI));
    pM->Release();

    if (pCI != NULL)
    {
        LOCK(&g_Console);
        _tprintf(_T("T%d: Got its custom interface!\n"), myNumber);
        UNLOCK(&g_Console);
    }
    else
    {
        LOCK(&g_Console);
        _tprintf(_T("T%d: Cannot get its custom interface!\n"), myNumber);
        UNLOCK(&g_Console);
        CoUninitialize();
        _endthread();
    }

    for (long i=0; i< 20; i++)
    {
        hRes = pCI->GetManagerName(&mgrName);

        inYear = 1900 + rand() %100;
                inMonth = rand() % 12 + 1;

        hRes = pCI->OkayToPublishInfo(inYear, inMonth, &okFlag);
        hRes = pCI->PeekCounters(&localRef, &objCount);

#ifdef UNICODE
        LOCK(&g_Console);
        _tprintf(_T("T%d: After calling GetManagerName : current manager is %ls\n"),
                                                    myNumber, mgrName );
        UNLOCK(&g_Console);
#else
        char * tp = new char[50];
        WideCharToMultiByte(CP_ACP,0, mgrName, -1, tp, 50, NULL, NULL);
        LOCK(&g_Console);
        _tprintf(_T("T%d: After calling GetManagerName : current manager is %s\n"),
                                                    myNumber, tp);
        UNLOCK(&g_Console);
        delete [] tp;
#endif
        SysFreeString(mgrName);

        LOCK(&g_Console);
        _tprintf(_T("T%d: After calling OkToPublishInfo : Year = %d,
                    Month = %d Status = %s\n"),myNumber, inYear, inMonth,
            (okFlag == TRUE) ? _T("OKAY"): _T("NO WAY"));
        UNLOCK(&g_Console);
```

```
            LOCK(&g_Console);
            _tprintf(_T("T%d: We now have %d local references and %d object users.\n"),
                                              myNumber, localRef, objCount);
            UNLOCK(&g_Console);

            Sleep(1000);  // sleep for about 1 second
        }

        pCI->Release();

        LOCK(&g_Console);
        _tprintf(_T("T%d: Freeing the blob now!\n"), myNumber);
        UNLOCK(&g_Console);

        CoUninitialize();

        _endthreadex(0);
        return 0;
    }
```

You'll notice very little difference between our previous _tmain() code and the AThread() thread function listed above. The most glaring difference being the LOCK() and UNLOCK() macros around the _tprintf()s, for synchronization, and the fact that a thread cannot simply exit() to terminate the program in case of error. Instead, a thread should use _endthreadex(), after cleaning up, in order to exit gracefully. Recall that the main thread, which starts all the test threads, will wait for the termination of every single thread before terminating itself.

We've used a pair of LOCK() and UNLOCK() macros around each and every _tprintf() statement (instead of one pair around the entire group) to give another thread a chance to 'sneak in' between the printing of every output line. This gives a somewhat finer-grained shuffle of the threads during execution.

Once you have the debug version compiled, you're ready to party. Execute it from a command console, and you should see an output similar to the following:

```
...
T0: After calling GetManagerName : current manager is J. Manzini
T0: After calling OkToPublishInfo : Year = 1928, Month = 11 Status = OKAY
T0: We now have 2 local references and 1 object users.
Main: Started thread 1!
T1: Got class factory!
T0: After calling GetManagerName : current manager is J. Manzini
T0: After calling OkToPublishInfo : Year = 1949, Month = 9 Status = OKAY
T1: Made a bare blob!
T1: Got its custom interface!
T1: After calling GetManagerName : current manager is J. Manzini
T0: We now have 2 local references and 1 object users.
T1: After calling OkToPublishInfo : Year = 1914, Month = 12 Status = OKAY
T1: We now have 2 local references and 2 object users.
T0: After calling GetManagerName : current manager is J. Manzini
T0: After calling OkToPublishInfo : Year = 1960, Month = 3 Status = OKAY
T0: We now have 2 local references and 2 object users.
T1: After calling GetManagerName : current manager is J. Manzini
```

```
T1: After calling OkToPublishInfo : Year = 1989, Month = 9 Status = OKAY
T1: We now have 2 local references and 2 object users.
T0: After calling GetManagerName : current manager is J. Manzini
T0: After calling OkToPublishInfo : Year = 1985, Month = 6 Status = OKAY
Main: Started thread 2!
T2: Got class factory!
T0: We now have 2 local references and 2 object users.
T1: After calling GetManagerName : current manager is J. Manzini
T1: After calling OkToPublishInfo : Year = 1979, Month = 2 Status = OKAY
...
```

Just before each thread completes, it releases the CBareBlob object – when you run this program, notice how the object users count goes up from 1 to 10 and then comes back down again, while the reference count is the same (2) for all cases. This is exactly what we'd expect. The user count reflects the total number of instances of CBareBlob that have been created within the client process, and it will increase as the main thread creates more and more threads. The reference count, on the other hand, is per instance. Because the calling sequence for all the interfaces remains the same across all instances (i.e. the same code is executing), the reference count is the same for all threads. You may find that the user count does not hit the maximum, if some threads start exiting before all of them have been created.

Next, try starting multiple command consoles, each running this code. Think about the relationships that you're observing. Recall that each in-process server (DLL) actually gets loaded into the process of the client; therefore each command console is running a separate copy of the executable and acts as a hard partition. Even though each program creates multiple instances of the CBareBlob object, the hard partitioning remains and each command console behaves independently from all others.

From an operating system point of view, though, the DLL (in-process server) is loaded only once in system memory – regardless of how many processes may be using it. It's interesting to imagine what sort of results we would see if CBareBlob were implemented via a local server (i.e. running in its own process) instead of in-process. Hold your curiosity for now; we'll be looking at this scenario in the next chapter.

Even though it's quite simple, the combination of BareBlob.dll and our test programs is a potent set of COM server/client utilities for experimenting with the various facets of COM or ActiveX programming. We'll be reusing the multithreaded version in later chapters, as we build more sophisticated, and complex, ActiveX components.

Now, for something interesting – bring up Oleview.exe and, on the Implementation tab, switch the ThreadingModel attribute of our BareBlob from Apartment to Free (from an STA supporter to an MTA supporter). Try running the Multicont.exe test harness again. What happens now? Your screen output should look something like this:

```
Main: Started thread 0!
T0: Got class factory!
T0: Made a bare blob!
T0: Cannot get its custom interface!
Main: Started thread 1!
T1: Got class factory!
T1: Made a bare blob!
T1: Cannot get its custom interface!
Main: Started thread 2!
```

```
T2: Got class factory!
T2: Made a bare blob!
T2: Cannot get its custom interface!
Main: Started thread 3!
T3: Got class factory!
T3: Made a bare blob!
T3: Cannot get its custom interface!
Main: Started thread 4!
T4: Got class factory!
T4: Made a bare blob!
T4: Cannot get its custom interface!
...
```

The threads are created, the class object located and new BareBlob instances created, but none of the interface method calls worked. This is very strange. We are calling from the same MultiCont.exe into the same BareBlob.dll using VTBL binding – which maps to a direct C++ virtual method call – all we have changed is an entry in the registry, and everything stopped working.

We had the same EXE to DLL linkage, and everything between client and component happens inside the same process, and yet COM has magically interfered. This might seem a little irritating at first. It appears to destroy our trust in the operations of Win32 DLLs and we would swear that Microsoft has somehow modified the OS or compiler. Just to make sure you're actually seeing it for real, switch the **ThreadingModel** attribute back to **Apartment** and check that MultiCont.exe works again. You should see that it does.

By this time, it should be crystal clear that COM is not simply a fancy way to dress up a Win32 DLL call! By using COM, we have somehow given up some 'to the metal' control. Big Brother is watching over us all the time, and can intercept and change calling behavior when necessary. Big Brother here is, of course, Microsoft's COM runtime.

This naturally leads us to revisit the complexity abyss that we ascended from at the end of Chapter 2. This time around, though, we have concrete code to show us what is involved, and the picture will become a little brighter.

Casting a Ray of Light into the Abyss

Yes, COM Threading Models and Marshaling again. If you recall our first encounter with this, back in Chapter 2, you may now have a clue as to why MultiCont.exe stopped working.

Examining the structure of MultiCont.exe from a threading model perspective, we can see that it is a pure STA client. This is the case because it creates multiple threads, and each thread calls the COM runtime with CoInitializeEx(NULL, COINIT_APARTMENTTHREADED), indicating to COM that the thread will support STA. In fact, after the CoInitializeEx(NULL, COINIT_APARTMENTTHREADED) call, the thread immediately enters the STA apartment. Since each thread creates an instance of CBareBlob, each instance lives happily in its own STA apartment.

When the BareBlob component is registered as supporting the Apartment model (STA), COM runtime decides that it is okay for the STA client to directly call the component's method. This was the case initially, and everything worked fine.

Next, we switched and told the COM runtime that `BareBlob` supported only Free Threaded model (MTA) clients directly. Then we ran `MultiCont.exe` (still an STA client) again, and the COM runtime knows that it must intercept and match the threading models. It does this by:

1. Creating an MTA in the process, since no MTA exists as yet

2. Creating the `BareBlob` (MTA supporting component) in the MTA

3. Marshaling an interface from the MTA back to the calling STA

4. Giving this interface to the calling `MultiCont.exe` thread

All this would have happened at the moment `CoCreateInstance()` is called by one of the threads in `MultiCont.exe`. Since marshaling is actually performed, the interface handed to the calling thread (in step 4) is actually a *proxy*, and not the object itself. Wait a minute... a *proxy*! Where did this come from? How does COM know how to create proxy for every custom interface, now and into the future? The answer is, of course, it doesn't know. Recall that `Midl.exe` created both a type library and generated proxy/stub code for `BareBlob`. The proxy/stub code from our project consisted of `BareBlob.h`, `BareBlob_p.c`, `BareBlob_i.c`, and `Dlldata.c`. But, we never compiled this, and this is why our code no longer works.

Essential Proxy and Stub

Without the proper proxy/stub supporting the `ICustomInterface`, the COM runtime does not know how to marshal the interface between the MTA, where the `BareBlob` is created, and the STA, where the `BareBlob`'s methods are invoked. Therefore, all we need to do is to go back and compile and register the proxy/stub objects.

In the `\Ch3\baseblob` directory, you will find the `BareBlobps.mak` file that we have created to compile the proxy/stub code. In fact, the proxy/stub itself is actually a bonafide COM object. The only difference for us is that we do not need to write any code for it – it is all generated by MIDL.

Here's the `BareBlobps.mak` file:

```
BareBlobps.dll: dlldata.obj BareBlob_p.obj BareBlob_i.obj
   link /dll /Zi /out:BareBlobps.dll /def:BareBlobps.def /entry:DllMain dlldata.obj
            BareBlob_p.obj BareBlob_i.obj kernel32.lib rpcndr.lib rpcns4.lib
            rpcrt4.lib uuid.lib oleaut32.lib
.c.obj:
   cl /D_DEBUG /DDEBUG /c /Ox /DWIN32 /D_WIN32_WINNT=0x0400 /DREGISTER_PROXY_DLL $<

clean:
        @del BareBlobps.dll
        @del BareBlobps.lib
        @del BareBlobps.exp
        @del dlldata.obj
        @del BareBlob_p.obj
        @del BareBlob_i.obj
```

If you look back, you'll see that this is almost identical to the way we compiled and linked BareBlob.dll. This is not too surprising, considering that they are both COM in-process servers. Look at BareBlobps.def:

```
LIBRARY         "BareBlobPS"

DESCRIPTION   'Proxy/Stub DLL'

EXPORTS
        DllGetClassObject       PRIVATE
        DllCanUnloadNow         PRIVATE
        GetProxyDllInfo         PRIVATE
        DllRegisterServer       PRIVATE
        DllUnregisterServer     PRIVATE
```

You can see the familiar DLL entry points exported, and there's another one here – GetProxyDllInfo(). This new function is implemented by the generated code. The important item to note in the Makefile is the /DREGISTER_PROXY_DLL switch. Without defining this symbol, the proxy/stub object created will not be able to self-register. Earlier versions of MIDL generated proxy/stub code that did not support this feature.

Now, we are ready to create the proxy/stub server:

nmake -f BareBlobps.mak

And of course, we need to register it:

regsvr32 BareBlobps.dll

Finally, we can go back and try running MultiCont.exe again. Everything works again, as expected – with the COM runtime assisting in the marshaling.

You may remember from our threading model discussion, in Chapter 2, that an STA client thread should dispatch messages. Our MultiCont.exe does not dispatch messages. In fact, an STA client only needs to dispatch messages if there is the possibility of a method call originating from another apartment, calling into objects created within the STA apartment. In our case, the logic flow of MultiCont.exe ensures that this would never happen.

Even More Threading Model Variations

The STA MultiCont.exe client now happily interoperates with both the Apartment model BareBlob or the Free Threaded BareBlob. The interested reader may want to attempt an MTA MultiCont.exe client. We'll look at such a client briefly in this section, and see what happens when we unregister BareBlobps.dll. We will also look at what is going on when BareBlob is marked with an Apartment, and then a Free, threading model.

You will find such a client in the \Ch3\mts2blob directory. It is a modified version of the original MultiCont.cpp. Instead of calling CoInitialize(NULL, COINIT_APARTMENTTHREADED), we now call CoInitializeEx(0, COINIT_MULTITHREADED) to cause all the threads to enter the MTA (recall that each process can only have one MTA).

```
void AThread(LPVOID lpParam)
{
    long myNumber = *(reinterpret_cast<long *>(lpParam));
    ......


        CoInitializeEx(0, COINIT_MULTITHREADED);
    hRes = CoGetClassObject(CLSID_CBareBlob, CLSCTX_ALL, NULL,
        IID_IClassFactory,(void **) &pCF);
```

Try out this new MultiCont.exe, first without the proxy/stub registered, against both Apartment and Free model versions of BareBlob. Next, try it with proxy/stub registered. This should help you to reinforce your understanding of threading models, the role of COM runtime, and marshaling in general. Notice specifically the improved throughput observed when both MultiCont.exe and BareBlob are MTA compatible. You may want to put some timing code in MultiCont.exe to actually measure the difference.

Now we ascend from the abyss once again!

There Must be a Better Way

Working through `BareBlob` and its drivers has given us a good feel for what raw COM programming is like, and what it involves. While tedious, raw COM programming is actually not as difficult as it may seem at first. However, in our commercial world, any tool that will allow us to do the job faster, more effectively, or more efficiently, will undoubtedly improve our competitiveness. To this end, as much as we may like to program every ActiveX control from scratch, the fact that there are tools and libraries out there that make the activity much easier certainly demands our attention.

For the rest of this book, we won't be returning to raw COM programming. There are several choices of tools and libraries that make ActiveX control programming significantly easier, and to maintain the competitive edge, you really should be using them. Besides, these tools allow you to focus more on the actual problem that the ActiveX control solves, instead of the idiosyncrasies of COM programming or interactions. However, just like COM and DCOM, many of these tools and libraries are in rapid evolution, and may be quite fragile. Whenever something doesn't work quite correctly, or if there are things that the tool or library doesn't handle, raw COM once again becomes the only game in town.

Should it ever be necessary to wing-it from scratch in your programming endeavors, you'll be glad that you spent the time reading the last three chapters. In addition, we hope that the focus of COM as a platform and operating system independent technology will instill in you a sense of the unlimited possibilities that component technology and distributed computing can offer. We hope that the ActiveX components you design will solve your urgent problems of today, and be part of the solution for those (as yet) unknown problems of tomorrow. This, at least, should be the goal of every software-component design.

The next chapter covers a library that makes building COM servers substantially easier. We will reconstruct our `BareBlob` object server in record time, and even add features to it – with almost no work. The new and improved `BareBlob` component that we'll create will be compatible with a larger variety of clients, including Visual Basic, Java, and even an automation scripting client like Internet Explorer 4!

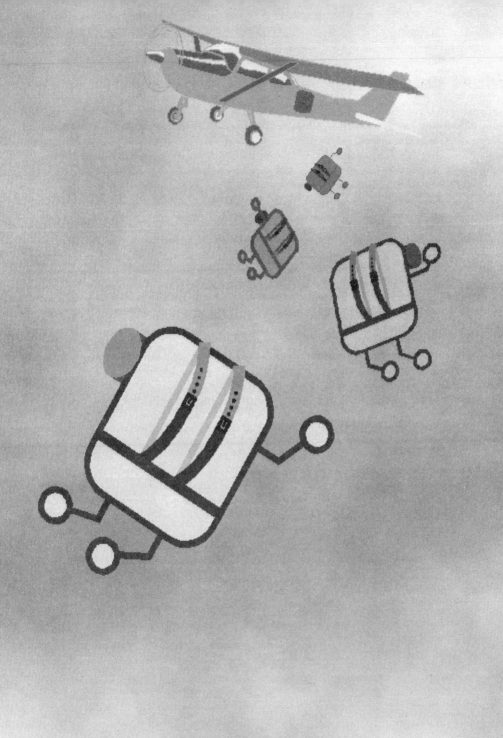

4

ActiveX Controls The Easy Way: ATL 3

There are many ways to create ActiveX Controls and COM business objects, and some are easier than others. When we are using C++, our primary choice from Microsoft is either the Microsoft Foundation Class (MFC) or Active Template Library (ATL). While MFC provides convenient features for building ActiveX controls, the generated code tends toward a large binary image footprint. Also, because of its heritage and comprehensive coverage, MFC is starting to show signs of becoming legacy-ware, potentially unable to keep up with the rapid pace of evolution. This really leaves ATL as the only choice for moving forward.

ATL is only a couple of years old. It is so new, that not long ago, the only way you could get a hold of it was to download it from the Internet. As we speak, its functionality is still being integrated into the base Visual C++ 6 product (in terms of proper wizard support for all its classes). If you aren't familiar with what a template is, don't despair. Take a look at Appendix C, which is a quick refresher on using templates in C++, to enable you to understand the ATL code. In this chapter, we'll introduce the ATL assuming only that you know C++.

We'll start this chapter with a look at how ATL has been designed to satisfy all the requirements of a template library that enables the user to create COM components. Our aim here is to provide you with enough background, design rationale and description of special techniques to make your own continued study of ATL more straightforward. Only time and patience studying and writing ATL source code will give you a comprehensive understanding of how to implement it, so our coverage here is design and usage based.

Of course, we will implement some code to give you a flavor for it. Later, we'll recreate both our `BareBlob` server (from the last chapter) using ATL so that it supports late binding and also our multithreaded `BareBlob` tester using the COM support from Visual C++ 6 that makes everything easier. We'll look at some programs to utilize our `BareBlob` business object in the following environments:

- ❑ Visual Basic 6
- ❑ Internet Explorer 4
- ❑ Visual J++6

You can be sure that it's going to be another intense journey. Along the way, we'll discover how the ATL 3 really simplifies the creation of highly functional ActiveX controls.

It's a logical next step to what we've done in the last chapter. Our business rule ActiveX control now 'grows up' and all sorts of new clients can use it. The ease of programming provided by ATL 3 will allow us to cover much more ground in this chapter; the hard work we endured in the last chapter will help us to understand how ATL 3 carries out its magic, and to customize or maintain the resulting generated code.

This is another chapter where we'll be investigating the foundation ActiveX technology, upon which flexible, multi-component, distributed applications can be built. Just in case you're wondering where all the more practical applications are, be assured that after this chapter on the fundamentals, we'll be on a rocket ride to building an actual distributed application for the DNA architecture.

By the end of this chapter, you'll be able to build your own reusable nonvisual ActiveX software components to implement any business rules, using Visual C++ 6 and ATL 3. These components can be used through Visual C++, Visual Basic, VBScript or JavaScript in Internet Explorer, Visual J++, or any other platform that supports ActiveX controls.

Discovering The Active Template Library

ATL used to be a small library, but that's history. ATL 3, included with Visual Studio 6 or Visual C++ 6, is anything but small. However, it is still not as hoggish as its MFC cousin, which, quite frankly, is way beyond a manageable size.

For those fortunate enough to grow up with ATL through versions 1.0, 1.1, 2.0, 2.1, etc, the additions and improvements in ATL 3 continue to make sense and be consistent with its original noble design and implementation styles. For the rest of us, getting to know ATL and knowing where to start just got a bit more difficult with ATL 3.

ATL 3 has added support for the following new types of components:

- ❑ Dynamic HTML based web control
- ❑ OLE DB Consumer Objects
- ❑ OLE DB Provider Objects
- ❑ Microsoft Management Console Snapin Objects

It has also improved support for OC96 compliant controls, and support for:

- ❑ Lite Controls
- ❑ Full Controls
- ❑ Dialog based Controls
- ❑ ASP Components
- ❑ Visual Studio Add-ins
- ❑ MTS compatible business objects

The inclusion of wizards for creating these controls in Visual Studio 6 makes life easier for the developer. We will see how to build many of these controls with ATL in later chapters.

There's no better way to learn about ATL than to see how its designers realized its core implementation in response to their original design goals. If we can understand how their ends justify their means, so to speak, understanding the rest of ATL 3 will be relatively simple – the extensions to the ATL 3 core have simply been created to address new problem areas that have arisen in COM programming.

Hopefully, you will soon agree with us that ATL 3 is an elegant and practical solution to an almost impossible problem – that of making C++ COM programming easy now and into the future – instead of a hopelessly complex library with notations cryptic enough to satisfy the geek supremo.

The Composition of ATL 3

As of the time of printing, ATL 3 includes the following files, which you can find under the `\Microsoft Visual Studio\vc98\atl\include` directory:

File Name	Size	Description
Atlbase.h	137k	Base level fundamental type and class definitions
Atlcom.h	136k	Most of the COM object handling
Atlconv.h	13k	String conversion utility classes from UNICODE and back
Atlctl.h	95k	ActiveX control support
Atldb.h	196k	OLE DB provider support
Atldbcli.h	104k	OLE DB consumer/client support
Atldbsch.h	38k	OLE DB schema classes
Atldef.h	4k	Macro definitions for ATL
Atlhost.h	73k	Dynamic HTML Hosting support
Atliface.h	76k	MIDL generated from `Atliface.idl` below.
Atlsnap.h	42k	Microsoft Management Console Snapin Support

Table Continued on Following Page

File Name	Size	Description
Atlwin.h	82k	Basic Windows support
Statreg.h	28k	Support file for static linking of registry update code
Atlconv.cpp	1k	String conversion implementation
Atlimpl.cpp	5k	Implementation of pieces that won't fit inline
Atlwin.cpp	1k	Implementation of windows support
Atlctl.cpp	1k	Implementation of ActiveX control support
Statreg.cpp	1k	Implementation for static linking of registry update code
Atliface.idl	12k	Interface description for IRegistrar for component registrar support

This is quite a collection of source code, and represents the distribution of ATL 3.

If you have ever had the pleasure of looking at the directory \Microsoft Visual Studio\Vc98\Mfc\Src (and include), which is another library which could help you write ActiveX controls, the reason should be clear why ATL is the inevitable alternative. The MFC source code collection looks like it is the encoding of the entire New York City white pages in the C++ language! Of course, it does carry with it legacy support for much more than ActiveX controls.

An optional DLL called Atl.dll (68k) is also supplied which, if installed will reside in your \WinNT\System32 directory. The previous version of Visual Studio saw this distributed in two forms – one for Windows 95 and the other for Windows NT – though thankfully Studio 6 contains only one version which works on all platforms. If you compile your ATL code with the project set as a Release MinSize build, your COM component will depend on this DLL for proper operation, but if your project is set as a Release MinDependency build, then your COM component will not have this dependency.

Template Libraries vs Binary Class Libraries/Frameworks

Let's take the chance here to review the differences between a class library and a template library. This is best illustrated with a diagram:

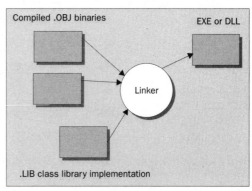

A class library is typically included at link time as a .lib file, providing more functions for the object that the user has created in addition to those in the compiler created .obj files. It is possible that the .lib file simply points to an external DLL to do this, but in general, most class libraries are written such that more code is linked into the final executable file than is actually needed.

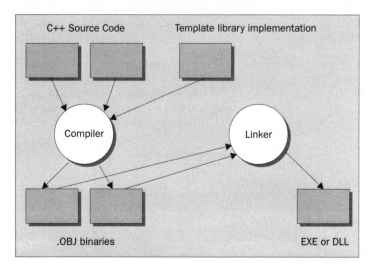

With a template library, the code is generated 'to spec' during compilation time. Essentially, a template library is a highly configurable code generator. A properly designed and written template library ensures that just enough code is generated for each application. Of course, this desirable feature can only be true if the library is used in the correct way.

The major difference between a conventional class library or framework and a template library can be summarized in the following sentence:

> **A binary class library or framework works at link time by combining static compiled code with new user code, whereas a template library works at compile time to configure and control code generation and its merging with the code of the user.**

Just because typical template library files are small, it doesn't mean that they do nothing. The code generation effect, if abused or misused, can potentially create a gigantic, unbounded final footprint size.

Template libraries are typically very concise. Because of this, their source code tends to be more difficult to understand than the code based on application frameworks. Due to their relatively recent rise in popularity and their code generation nature, the corresponding compile time error and debugging support are often difficult to understand today. This may completely change in the near future as the C++ compilers and debugger technology supporting templates mature.

A Brief Account of ATL's Brief History

The predecessor of ActiveX controls – OLE controls – were notoriously complex to implement. Much of the code involved in the implementation of such controls was repetitious between each implementation, yet didn't factor out easily, so that it could be isolated and re-used.

MFC, Microsoft's flagship development class framework, quickly rose to the challenge by patching its Document/View model to handle OLE controls. This worked, but was by no means an optimal solution. Each patch required a new patch to solve new problems and soon MFC development was reduced to a vicious loop creating new patches rather than optimizing the library to incorporate them. The end result of that legacy today is that the MFC runtime is frequently over 1Mb in size, MFC-based ActiveX controls are similarly bulky, adding a feature to the MFC itself requires a low level knowledge of its bloated framework and its adopted programmer base is significantly less than it was.

Meanwhile, as the Microsofties put it... "The Internet happened to Bill".

Downloading an ActiveX control through predominantly slow connections (then 14.4 to 28.8 Kbps) further aggravated the MFC control fabrication community. There needed to be a leaner and meaner alternative for creating ActiveX controls.

Enter the Active Template Library!

The Early Years in "ATL Time"

The early days of ATL – some tens of months ago – were fraught with perils. Junior programmers with bright fresh-from-college ideas were struggling with a well established, proven effective cabinet of senior architects. Templates were regarded as "impure" and too complex, while the legacy framework (MFC) was still enjoying the triumph from much historical industry recognition and a huge user base. In fact, the first few attempts at template implementation within the Microsoft C++ compiler itself were full of crippling bugs.

Then the customer base spoke out, and they were louder than ever... "We need a lightweight alternative to MFC, and we need it yesterday."

Microsoft responded by merging the ATL development team with the MFC development team, further "accelerating the synergistic growth between the two technology bases". Clearly a "let them battle out their differences fast" in typical, noncommittal, middle management speak.

That was then, and this is now. Visual Studio 6 and Visual C++ 6 represent the first fruits of the labor of this new "high synergy" team. It comes complete with co-existence "wizards" that allow you to merge ATL and MFC code together in one harmonious binary (formerly the domain of MFC hackers), so you can judge for yourself the merit of ATL against or in combination with MFC.

ATL User Requirements

The secret of successful ATL programming lies in understanding why the library is designed the way it is. To get a grip on this, one must go back to the beginning and examine the original problem domain that ATL addresses: the original ATL User Requirements. Here's a cut at a use case diagram for ATL.

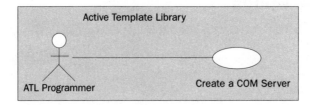

Examining the use case further, it is clear that a user needs to:

- Create modules containing COM servers in various forms – a local server (EXE module), in-proc server (DLL module), or NT Service (specialized EXE module)
- Manage multiple COM servers in the same EXE or DLL module
- Implement a class object for each COM server class, and support different strategies when creating /locating instances of the COM server
- Implement COM servers that can be used via vtable or `IDispatch`, by C++, Automation, or scripting clients
- Implement custom behaviors in Microsoft defined interfaces
- Implement custom behaviors in user defined interfaces
- Implement `IUnknown` and support aggregation semantics if necessary
- Write COM server code which fits a specific threading model – STA or MTA
- Create COM components of a particular category, supporting a well defined set of interfaces and its associated protocol
- Manage individual COM server lifetimes, based on a variety of strategies depending on the application
- Optimize the implementation of interfaces if necessary

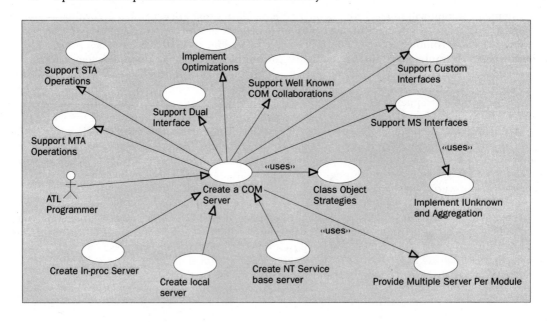

The ATL Way of Things

So how does ATL, a relatively small template library (at the core), satisfy all these requirements?

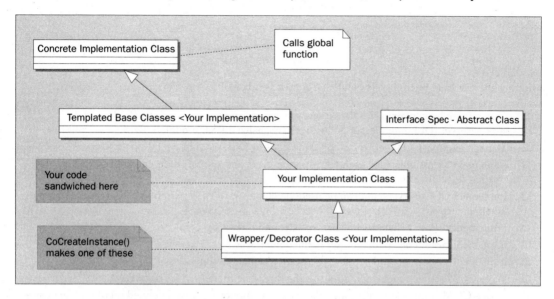

At the core of this magic is your COM object implementation class – a C++ class. In fact, your implementation is in the middle, sandwiched between a top layer (below you in the hierarchy) of ATL generated code, and a bottom layer (above you in the hierarchy) of ATL generated/implemented code.

Your implementation will inherit from templated base classes that are generated according to your custom specifications – a number of macros and flags which control the template instantiation and its runtime behavior. Another set of ATL 'wrapper classes' will be generated as a top layer that will inherit from your implementation. You will also control much of their behavior through macros.

CoCreateInstance() and other COM runtime helper functions create only instances of wrapper classes. Since these wrapper classes inherit from your implementation, they gain all the functionality provided by your coding. However, they also have the option to alter the behavior of the entire server and/or override methods you provide if necessary. These wrapper classes can elect to take first hit on any interface methods of the object it wants. In fact, the wrapper classes can work in conjunction with the templated base classes that your implementation inherit from to perform work for you. It can pass requests right through your implementation to the bottom layer transparently. This is a very powerful mechanism.

The templated base classes provide the code for complex interfaces like IDispatch, meaning you need only worry about the implementation of interfaces which inherit from them. Your own interface can inherit from as many of them as you need to implement as many interfaces as you need. Those interfaces for which ATL does not provide implementations (hopefully few), you need to inherit from the interface specification abstract class and implement all the methods yourself.

In the templated base classes, the concrete implementation of a method is done in the top-most global concrete classes or global functions whenever possible to produce the highest call and execution performance – i.e. no virtual table lookup, total freedom on resource/memory allocation, etc.

The main function of the wrapper classes in ATL is to provide `IUnknown` handling, aggregation support, threading models, and object lifetime support. The implementation of this support code requires library (ATL) code intervention before your specific implementation code is executed. The fact that object factory instantiation, and module initialization are all performed by this top layer of code provides the developer with flexible configuration options without requiring tedious detailed coding.

Design Patterns At Work

In terms of design patterns, the conceptual design of ATL 3 is the application of a combination of the Template Method design pattern together with a variation of the Decorator design pattern – with your own implementation class sandwiched in between. The bonus here is that the design structure is incredibly easy to remember, and applying it in practice becomes very 'natural'.

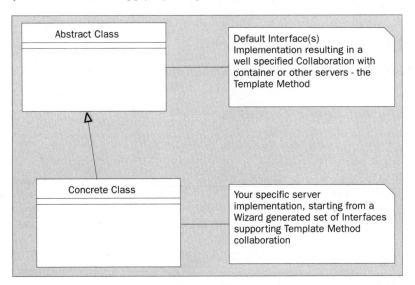

ATL provides a set of wizard-generated default interface implementations, whose behavior follows some well-specified interaction semantics. The implementation of these interfaces uses the Template Method design pattern. The default collaboration between the wizard-generated object and its container (or other components) is the conceptual template method. Your specific implementation will modify the behavior of the interfaces, without changing the collaborative behavior.

In ATL, the default implementation of the `IUnknown` interface and its support for aggregation are handled via a variation of the Decorator design pattern. Your implementation is being "decorated" by a `CComObject<>` or `CComAggObject<>` class which adds features transparently to your class. Both implement `IUnknown` and transparently provide support for aggregation according to your chosen threading model and exposed interfaces.

Role of Human Developer in the ATL 3 Loop

Ultimately, the main role of a human programmer within the "ATL 3 loop" can be summarized as:

> **Configure the code generating ATL 3 to generate the code that you need, and add your own code at the right place to do the required work.**

To make the entire 'code with ATL' process even easier, you can and should let the Wizards in the Visual Studio 6 IDE automatically generate the bulk of ATL configuration code for you. Then you can modify the code generated by the wizard to better meet your own requirements. This whole process is actually equivalent to a meta-code generator: a parameterizing wizard generates code for ATL, which in turns parameterizes code for the actual COM control.

At any time during this discussion, if you would like to see some of the concepts discussed in action, feel free to skip directly to the section entitled 'Examining the Code' and go as far as you need to. Once you become more comfortable after seeing the code, you may resume this exploration.

Fulfilling The User Requirements

Now for some specifics. Let us take a look at the design mechanism solving each of the use cases one at a time.

Supporting Different Server Contexts

In order to support the creation of COM objects as local servers, in-proc servers or specialized NT services, ATL provides the CComModule class.

CComModule is an implementation class, not a template. You typically create an instance of this class in a DLL based server, or derive from it for an EXE based server. If you use the ATL COM AppWizard to create your project, then this is automatically done for you. For example, if you create a DLL with this wizard, then you'll find the following statement in StdAfx.h:

```
extern CComModule _Module;
```

In this section, we'll be looking at how CComModule helps ATL to provide default, configurable implementations for all server context and threading model permutations typically found in COM servers. By using these default implementations, you can save valuable time in coding and debugging.

For DLL in-proc servers, the ATL 3 object wizards allow you to select a threading model, and they automatically generate all the required code for the object to support the model. In addition, the CComModule class also implements methods that assist in the implementation of the four required entry points:

In-proc Server DLL Entry Point	Corresponding CComModule Method
DllGetClassObject()	GetClassObject()
DllCanUnloadNow()	GetLockCount() in conjunction with Lock() and Unlock() to keep the global object count.
DllRegisterServer()	RegisterServer()
DllUnregisterServer()	UnregisterServer()

These methods are automatically implemented for you in the main .cpp file of your project:

```
/////////////////////////////////////////////////////////////////////////////
// Used to determine whether the DLL can be unloaded by OLE

STDAPI DllCanUnloadNow(void)
{
    return (_Module.GetLockCount()==0) ? S_OK : S_FALSE;
}


/////////////////////////////////////////////////////////////////////////////
// Returns a class factory to create an object of the requested type

STDAPI DllGetClassObject(REFCLSID rclsid, REFIID riid, LPVOID* ppv)
{
    return _Module.GetClassObject(rclsid, riid, ppv);
}


/////////////////////////////////////////////////////////////////////////////
// DllRegisterServer - Adds entries to the system registry

STDAPI DllRegisterServer(void)
{
    // registers object, typelib and all interfaces in typelib
    return _Module.RegisterServer(TRUE);
}


/////////////////////////////////////////////////////////////////////////////
// DllUnregisterServer - Removes entries from the system registry

STDAPI DllUnregisterServer(void)
{
    return _Module.UnregisterServer(TRUE);
}
```

Remember the work we had to do to implement these functions without the aid of ATL in the last chapter?

CComModule also knows how to register and revoke COM component class objects for EXE based local servers (via the RegisterClassObjects() and RevokeClassObjects() methods).

For EXE based servers, the call from the COM runtime is made through a stub and performed directly in the context of the invoking RPC thread. The default-generated code derives a `CExeModule` class from `CComModule`. You can see this in `StdAfx.h`:

```
class CExeModule : public CComModule
{
public:
      LONG Unlock();
      DWORD dwThreadID;
      HANDLE hEventShutdown;
      void MonitorShutdown();
      bool StartMonitor();
      bool bActivity;
};
extern CExeModule _Module;
```

If Apartment threading is selected and you do not change any generated code, then your object instances will be created on the EXE server's only STA thread. This means that many instances of all the classes that the EXE local server support may be running on this single thread. To get a higher degree of concurrency (more worker threads) using STAs, you will need to use a variation of `CComModule` called `CComAutoThreadModule`. With this module type, you can change the default server into a MTA server by defining the `_ATL_FREE_THREADED` symbol (in `StdAfx.h`) and deriving your COM server from `CComObjectRootEx<CComMultiThreadModel>`.

`CComAutoThreadModule` is a replacement for `CComModule`, used for EXE based local servers (or Windows NT services). If you derive your `CExeModule` from a `CComAutoThreadModule`, and use the `DECLARE_CLASSFACTORY_AUTO_THREAD()` macro in your C++ server implementation.

```
      // module class definition
class CMyServerModule : public CComAutoThreadModule
{
public:
      HRESULT RegisterServer(BOOL bRegTypeLib, BOOL bService);
      HRESULT UnregisterServer();
      void Init(_ATL_OBJMAP_ENTRY* p, HINSTANCE h, UINT nServiceNameID, const
GUID* plibid = NULL);
      void Start();
      void ServiceMain(DWORD dwArgc, LPTSTR* lpszArgv);
      void Handler(DWORD dwOpcode);
.....
      // COM server class definition

class ATL_NO_VTABLE CIntCnv:

public CComObjectRootEx<CComMultiThreadModel>,
      public CComCoClass<CIntCnv, &CLSID_IntCnv>,
      public IDispatchImpl<IIntCnv, &IID_IIntCnv, &LIBID_TYPECNVRTLib>
      {
public:
      CIntCnv()
      {
      }
      DECLARE_CLASSFACTORY_AUTO_THREAD()
.........
```

The resulting EXE server will be using a thread pool to create COM server objects. The default server will have a pool of threads equal to four times (overridable) the number of actual SMP processors, and will be using a round robin thread selector to schedule work for server objects. CComAutoThreadModule is invaluable when you are creating your own components based scalable servers that can run on SMP machines. In Chapter 9, we will try to convince you that you don't want to do this (most of the time), and should let MTS do all the hard work for you.

The following table summarizes ATL's ability to support different server contexts:

If You Want To Build...	Be Aware Of This...	Do This...
DLL/ in-proc (single threaded)	Runs only in the "main thread" STA of client. All access to data are already serialized.	Specify Single during wizard code generation.
DLL/ in-proc (apartment threaded)	Runs in the same STA where it is created. Access to global data needs to be serialized.	Specify Apartment during wizard code generation.
DLL/ in-proc (free threaded)	Runs on any thread, nothing is serialized. Must protect anything shared.	Specify Free threaded during wizard code generation.
DLL/ in-proc (both threaded)	Supports either STA or MTA clients without marshaling. Must protect anything shared.	Specify Both during wizard code generation.
EXE/ local or NT Service (Single STA)	All object instances run on the single main STA thread of the server.	Default generated code with CExeModule deriving from CComModule.
EXE/ local or NT Service (Multiple STAs)	Server object instances distributed over multiple STA threads, using default round-robin allocator.	Modify CExeModule to derive from CComAutoThreadModule, and use DECLARE_CLASSFACTORY_ AUTO_THREAD() macro.

Table Continued on Following Page

If You Want To Build...	Be Aware Of This...	Do This...
EXE/ local or NT Service (MTA)	Server object instances are invoked by whichever thread COM runtime happens to be in (RPC thread context).	Define _ATL_FREE_THREADED symbol and derive object from CComObjectRootEx<CComMulti ThreadModel>
EXE or DLL in-proc, local, or NT Service (Custom Threading Model)	ATL places no restrictions on what you can do when custom coding your threading behavior.	You can roll your own threading by creating your own threads and using the DECLARE_CLASSFACTORY_EX() macro.

Managing Multiple COM Servers in Same Module

This is achieved in ATL using an **object map**. The object map is an array of _ATL_OBJMAP_ENTRY structures. This map is specified by you (typically through a wizard), and read by the CComModule (or a derived class) in managing and creating the class object associated with your COM server. Specifically, this happens when the CComModule::init() method is invoked (either from the main() routine of an EXE or from DllMain() in a DLL). The object map looks something like this:

```
BEGIN_OBJECT_MAP(ObjectMap)
OBJECT_ENTRY(CLSID_YourComServer, CYourComServer)
OBJECT_ENTRY(CLSID_AnotherComServer, CAnotherComServer)
END_OBJECT_MAP()
```

A CComModule based module can provide services for as many COM servers as you wish. Each of these "externally creatable" objects *must* have an entry in the object map. Exactly how instances of objects are created by the class object depends on your parameterization of the CComCoClass<>, which we'll look at in the next section.

Implementing Class Factory Objects With Different Strategies

For the implementation of a class factory object for each COM server, ATL provides various DECLARE_CLASSFACTORY_XXX() configuration macros:

- ❏ DECLARE_CLASSFACTORY()
- ❏ DECLARE_CLASSFACTORY2()
- ❏ DECLARE_CLASSFACTORY_AUTO_THREAD()
- ❏ DECLARE_CLASSFACTORY_SINGLETON()
- ❏ DECLARE_CLASSFACTORY_EX()

ATL 3 provides configurable default implementations for the different strategies you may want to use when implementing instance creation within the class factory object. In fact, you do not typically have to implement your own class object explicitly (as we had to with our BareBlob in the last chapter) unless ATL's default implementation fails to address your needs.

Let's take a look at some of the different strategies you might want to use, and at the implementations ATL provides for such strategies:

❑ DECLARE_CLASSFACTORY()
The default class factory object implementation provided by ATL creates new instances of your server on the heap. This is done with the DECLARE_CLASSFACTORY() macro, which you inherit from the CComCoClass<>, so you do not have to explicitly specify this macro in your code. It uses the CComClassFactory<> template class to do the work.

❑ DECLARE_CLASSFACTORY2(*class_name*)
To provide default licensing aware class object implementation, and have new instance of your server created on the heap, use DECLARE_CLASSFACTORY2(). This macro uses the CComClassFactory2<> template class, which implements the IClassFactory2 interface, an extension of IClassFactory. It takes one argument, a class that implements VerifyLicenseKey, GetLicenseKey, and IsLicenseValid.

❑ DECLARE_CLASSFACTORY_SINGLETON(*class_name*)
To implement a Singleton (where the only object instance is statically defined and all calls are directed to the single instance of the object), then you should use DECLARE_CLASSFACTORY_SINGLETON(). This macro uses the CComClassFactorySingleton<> template class to be the class factory and takes the name of your class as an argument.

❑ DECLARE_CLASSFACTORY_AUTO_THREAD()
To implement a heap based instance creation that caters for a multi-threaded STA local server (discussed in the *Supporting Different Server Contexts* section), use: DECLARE_CLASSFACTORY_AUTO_THREAD(). This macro uses the CComClassFactoryAutoThread<> template class as the class factory. In this case you would need to use the CComAutoThreadModule class rather than CComModule.

❑ DECLARE_CLASSFACTORY_EX(*class_factory*)
Finally, if none of the above default implementations provided by ATL suits your needs, then you can provide a custom class factory implementation (for example, a heap based singleton), using DECLARE_CLASSFACTORY_EX() and implement your own class object logic. This macro takes the name of your custom built class factory class, which must derive from CComClassFactory, as its one argument.

The coverage is quite complete, given that the last macro is an escape into your own code. Normally, the default implementations suffice, and, in most cases, you'll not have to write any class object implementation code when you are using ATL 3.

These macros should be used within your class definition .h file. Here is an example:

```
class ATL_NO_VTABLE CLeftDeco :
    public CComObjectRootEx<CComSingleThreadModel>,
    public CComCoClass<CLeftDeco, &CLSID_LeftDeco>,
    public ILeftDeco
{
public:
    CLeftDeco()
    {
    }
DECLARE_REGISTRY_RESOURCEID(IDR_LEFTDECO)
DECLARE_CLASSFACTORY_SINGLETON(CLeftDeco)
......
```

Supporting vtable Or IDispatch Based Interfaces

As we discussed in Chapter 2, a COM server needs to support the IDispatch interface in order to allow clients to use early or late binding. ATL provides a default implementation of this interface with the IDispatchImpl<> template class. This is parameterized by your interface, its IID, and the type library's CLSID.

The IDispatchImpl<> class takes care of all the details of implementing the complex methods of IDispatch, namely:

- ❏ Invoke()
- ❏ GetTypeInfo()
- ❏ GetIDsOfNames()
- ❏ GetTypeInfoCount()

You only have to implement the relevant methods of your interface once – in the vtable interface. The ATL IDispatch implementation will call the corresponding vtable interface method. This is a tremendous time saver. You only have to inherit from an instantiation of IDispatchImpl<> to get this for free. Note that this is done automatically for you if you use the ATL Object Wizard and specify that you want a dual interface.

Supporting Microsoft Specified Interfaces

Many of the standard interfaces specified by Microsoft have a default implementation in ATL 3. These default implementations are handled by the set of template classes of the form, IXXXImpl<>. In fact, these classes account for the bulk of the library. If you want to implement a standard interface, simply look for a corresponding IXXXImpl<> template class, parameterize it with your own interface and inherit from an instantiation of it – as in the previous section. You can always override any implementation if the default behavior does not suit your exact purposes.

Note that many interfaces work in conjunction with each other, according to some published protocol/collaboration specification. This is especially true in the case of ActiveX controls with visual elements. For example, the ActiveX control specification (see your MSDN Library CD) details a set of interfaces and protocols between an ActiveX control and its container which we'll look at in Chapter 5. The default behavior of such interfaces also takes this "typical" collaboration into consideration, making the coding of the interaction easier. Later on, the section *Supporting The Rapid Creation of Component with Interface Grouping* provides some well-known examples of such interface groupings, and describes how ATL 3 assist in the implementation of such groupings.

For Microsoft specified interfaces that ATL 3 does not provide a default implementation for (the ATL team hope these interfaces are in the minority), you can simply inherit from the interface itself and implement its methods within your own C++ implementation. We will see how this is done later in our coding.

Supporting User Specified Custom Interfaces

The Visual C++ 6 IDE makes the creation of user specified custom interfaces very simple indeed. We'll see this shortly, when we go on to a full working example later in the chapter. It is possible to select an interface and define its associated methods directly using the ClassView window. The IDE will then take care of:

- ❑ updating the IDL file
- ❑ updating the .h header file
- ❑ creating a function skeleton in the .cpp source file for the implementation of the interface method

The only requirement for this to be operational is that you have compiled your IDL file and have a type library available. The interface specification in this IDL file need not contain any method declaration.

Implementing IUnknown and Aggregation Semantics

Implementation and control for IUnknown behavior and aggregation support is distributed between several ATL classes to allow for maximal flexibility. These classes are:

- ❑ CComObjectRootEx<>
- ❑ CComCoClass<>
- ❑ CComObject<>
- ❑ CComContainedObject<>
- ❑ CComAggObject<>

The way in which these ATL library classes will work together for you is configured by your C++ implementation class. The class hierarchy is illustrated in the diagram below:

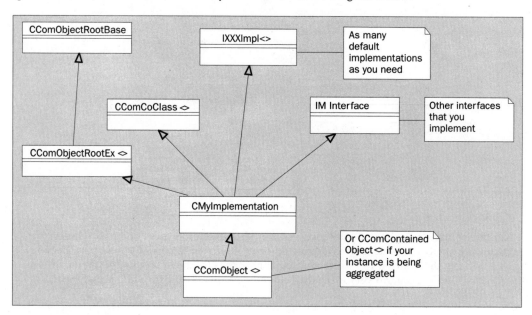

The implementation of the IUnknown interface involves two major concepts:

- ❑ Dynamic discovery through QueryInterface()
- ❑ Reference counting through AddRef() and Release()

The way that IUnknown is implemented for an in-proc server will depend on whether or not it can support aggregation. The reasons for this were discussed in some detail in Chapter 2.

The CComObject<> class is used by ATL to create instances of your implementation and it is always the most derived. From the diagram above, you can see that it inherits from your C++ implementation class. Its main purpose in life is two-fold.

Firstly, it provides a means of creating a non-aggregating COM object, which is based on your C++ class implementation. This object is created on the heap using C++ new operator, calling the appropriate ATL FinalConstruct() during the process. This method is provided as an initialization hook for the server object so it is not subjected to the C++ constructor limitations – i.e. virtual functions can be called safely.

Secondly, CComObject<> implements IUnknown for you transparently. It does this by redirecting reference counting calls right through your C++ class implementation to its partnering CComObjectRootEx<> class – one of your base classes. This implementation in turn calls the appropriate threading model version of AddRef() and Release() for the server (see the later section *Supporting STA and MTA Model for COM Servers*). This is a powerful mechanism that is totally transparent to your code. To the developer, IUnknown implementation is taken care of automatically by ATL once you've configured its behavior using the DECLARE_XXX_AGGREGATABLE() macros (see next section).

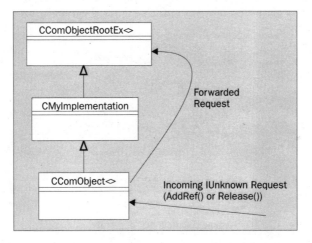

When an object instance is created under aggregation, the situation is more complex. Under aggregation, we need to be able to provide two different implementations of IUnknown. Back in Chapter 2, we saw the drawback of using multiple inheritance to implement COM interfaces – it makes just this kind of scenario very difficult. To overcome the difficulties, ATL uses an instance containment approach.

During aggregation, ATL uses the template class `CComAggObject<>` to provide the implementation of the explicit `IUnknown` methods for your object to the aggregator object. Unlike `CComObject<>`, `CComAggObject<>` doesn't derive from your implementation but `CComContainedObject<>` which provides the second implementation of `IUnknown`, does. This second implementation is actually the `m_contained` member of the `CComAggObject<>` implementation, with its `Addref()`, `Release()` and `QueryInterface()` methods delegating to `OuterAddRef()`, `OuterRelease()` and `OuterQueryInterface()` functions provided by `CComObjectRootBase`, as shown.

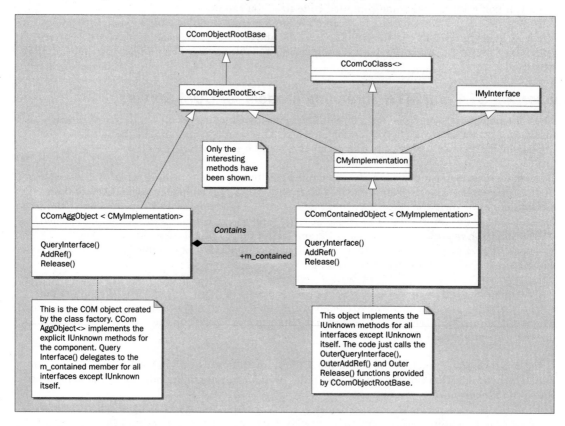

From a developer's perspective, one only need to make sure that the C++ implementation derives from `CComObjectRootEx<>` and `CComCoClass<>`. The `CComCoClass<>` class provides the default aggregation behavior through the macro, `DECLARE_AGGREGATABLE()`. This macro is already defined in the `CComCoClass<>` definition, and you need not explicitly specify it. You can find the declaration in `\vc98\atl\include\atlcom.h`:

```
template <class T, const CLSID* pclsid = &CLSID_NULL>
class CComCoClass
{
public:
    DECLARE_CLASSFACTORY()
    DECLARE_AGGREGATABLE(T)
    typedef T _CoClass;
.......
```

If you are implementing components for an EXE based server, then you know your components will never be aggregated. In this situation, you should override this behavior by defining the DECLARE_NOT_AGGREGATABLE() macro in your implementation.

If the server you create should only be used under aggregation (proxy/stub objects are good example of this), then define the DECLARE_ONLY_AGGREGATABLE() macro.

Finally, if you want to save some compiled code size, you can use the DECLARE_POLY_AGGREGATABLE() macro for implementing aggregatable servers. Instead of using either CComObject<> or CComAggObject<>, the above macro uses a single class CComPolyObject<> to handle both cases, providing vtable saving. The tradeoff is a slight runtime penalty.

Supporting STA and MTA Threading Models for COM Servers

The C++ object that you create in ATL to implement the COM server always derives from an instance of CComObjectRootEx<> template class. This template class, unlike the interface implementation classes, takes only one parameter – and it is not your C++ class.

Instead, the parameter it takes is a class to implement the required threading model, for example, the CComSingleThreadModel or CComMultiThreadModel non-template classes. Each of these classes defines its own Increment() and Decrement() methods, as well as providing typedefs for AutoCriticalSection, CriticalSection, and ThreadModelNoCS. Essentially, when CComSingleThreadModel is passed as parameter, all these symbols, together with the Increment()/Decrement() methods, are all mapped to the fastest possible implementation code, without the use of synchronization primitives.

On the other hand, if CComMultiThreadModel is passed to CComObjectRootEx<>, then the symbols, and the Increment()/Decrement() methods are all mapped to use implementation code which utilizes a critical section for synchronization (see Atlbase.h in the \vc98\Atl\include directory for more details).

Using this technique, much of the rest of the ATL simply proceeds with bracketing protecting code around synchronization sensitive areas, and relies on the compiler to optimize away the definitions should no synchronization be necessary.

For STA (Apartment model) servers, we can safely use CComSingleThreadModel, since the COM server will only be used by one thread at a time. The client guarantees that direct calls into the object instance will only be made from the thread that created the object instance. On the other hand, with MTA (Free threaded) servers, we must use CComMultiThreadedModel and its associated critical section to ensure integrity.

Wait a moment! That might not always work... as some of you will find. What about counters used at the class factory level, or on the module level? What protects them? In fact, for STA in-proc servers, the global object counter (and any other global, non-per instance variables) maintained by the class object must be synchronized. ATL provides for this by internally using a finer granularity of distinction, through the CComObjectThreadModel and CComGlobalThreadModel type definitions. Here is how they are defined depending on the actual threading model supported:

Threading Model	CComObjectThreadModel	CComGlobalThreadModel
Single	CComSingleThreadModel	CComSingleThreadModel
Apartment	CComSingleThreadModel	CComMultiThreadedModel
Free	CComMultiThreadedModel	CComMultiThreadedModel
Both	CComMultiThreadedModel	CComMultiThreadedModel

From the above mapping, it is clear that synchronization can be ensured if ATL simply use the CComObjectThreadModel and CComGlobalThreadModel classes to manipulate per-instance and global variables respectively. In fact, you as an end user can also use these classes to maintain a threading model independent implementation!

This is how ATL makes the implementation of COM servers for the various threading models easy. The ATL object wizards supplied with Visual C++ 6 will generate this code for you when you select the threading model. Here is an example, we have selected the Apartment threaded model:

```
class ATL_NO_VTABLE CIdealCase :
public CComObjectRootEx<CComSingleThreadModel>,
    public CComCoClass<CIdealCase, &CLSID_IdealCase>,
    public IDispatchImpl<IIdealCase, &IID_IIdealCase, &LIBID_EXESERVERLib>
{
public:
    CIdealCase()
    {
    }
DECLARE_REGISTRY_RESOURCEID(IDR_IDEALCASE)
......
```

In fact, if you use the Visual C++ 6 wizards to create a DLL based in-proc server, the wizard will even generate an automated script code that updates the threading model attributes registry key to your specified threading model!

Supporting The Rapid Creation of Components with Interface Grouping

Interfaces are typically not defined in isolation. Instead, families of interfaces are defined for a specific problem domain, and components implementing these interfaces collaborate with each other in carrying out the actual work. Some recognizable families of interfaces include:

- ❑ MAPI (messaging API)
- ❑ OCX specifications (OLE control interfaces)
- ❑ OC'96 specifications (OCX Internet extension and ActiveX control)
- ❑ OLE DB specifications

You will become intimately familiar with many of these families by the end of this book.

ATL 3 enables rapid creation of COM servers supporting these families of interfaces through extensive use of object wizards. These wizards are essentially miniature applications, whose main purpose in life is to accept user customization input, and then generate custom ATL and related code. With Visual C++ 6, there are ATL wizards to create the following categories of COM servers (implementing the associated family of interfaces):

COM Component Target	Description
Simple Object	Simple ActiveX control, only IUnknown and registration support
Add-in Object	Add-in component to enhance the functionality of the Visual Studio 98 IDE
Internet Explorer Object	Simple, non-visual, Internet Explorer 4 compatible ActiveX control
MS Transaction Server Component	Component compatible with Microsoft Transaction Server (MTS) and the required header files
Component Registrar	Component that can be used to programmatically modify the component attributes database (registry)
MMC SnapIn	Component that can be used to add functionality to the Microsoft Management Console (MMC)
Property Page	Property page COM component
Full Control	Visual ActiveX control which can be used in all containers and supporting the full OC'96 specification
Lite Control	Visual ActiveX control which can be used in Internet Explorer 4, only supporting the required interfaces
HTML Control	Visual ActiveX control which uses a Dynamic HTML page as its user interface
Composite Control	Visual ActiveX control which is composed of other visual ActiveX controls and uses them to achieve its own functionality
Lite HTML, Lite Composite controls	Same as their full counterparts, but only support enough interfaces for using Internet Explorer 4 as a container
Dialog	COM component which displays a dialog
DB Provider	COM component which can act as an OLE DB provider
DB Consumer	COM server which can act as an OLE DB consumer/client

Each of the above components has a family of associated COM interfaces, and ATL provides basic implementations for all them. The wizard will provide customization assistance during the initial generation of ATL code. We will be examining the full control (Chapter 7), the MTS object (Chapters 9, 10), the HTML control (Chapter 10), and the DB consumer (Chapter 8, 9) in details.

Managing Server Lifetime

Internally, ATL has to create COM servers with differing lifetime management requirements. Many of the classes used by ATL for this purpose can also be utilized by the end user in achieving certain server lifetime management goals. The table below includes some of the available template classes for creating COM servers with different reference counting characteristics.

In actual usage, these classes are always the most derived (they inherit from your C++ implementation class). In addition, most of them also assume that you derive your implementation from the usual `CComObjectRootEx<>` and `CComCoClass<>`.

Class Name	Type Of Object	When to Use
CComObject<>	A regular heap based object. Reference counting is supported automatically. The last Release() will delete object from heap.	Used when a normal heap based independent object is required. ATL uses it to create instances of your server implementation when an object instance is not being aggregated.
CComObjectGlobal<>	An object whose lifetime depends on the lifetime of the module containing it. For example, an object in an EXE server that stays around until the EXE exits.	Typically used in a class object that is implemented as a singleton. All instance requests and calls go to the same object instance in this case.
CComObjectNoLock<>	An object whose reference count is independent of the lock count of the module containing it.	ATL uses this class for class objects in EXE based modules, and it implements reference counting semantics. These objects are created and registered when the EXE starts up, and stays around until the EXE explicitly revokes them.

Table Continued on Following Page

Class Name	Type Of Object	When to Use
CComObjectStack<>	A function scoped object instance. This object is created on the stack and disappears when it exits the function scope.	Use this when you need a function scoped, temporary COM object. It *will* call your FinalConstruct() method in its constructor, and FinalRelease() in the destructor. The IUnknown implementation is a benign one. The object will not exist past the scope of one method call, no reference counting is necessary.
CComObjectCached<>	An object that stays around once created. Reference count will always be at least 1.	When you need repeated fast access to an object. ATL uses this internally for the class object of a DLL in-proc server.

Optimize Server Size and Performance

The ATL designers and coders went to great length to meet the objective of optimization. Doing so required an enumeration of the possible usage scenarios, and then examining each one to see where optimization could be performed.

The space we have here does not allow for an in depth analysis of all the possible optimization techniques used or usable within ATL. Instead, we'll point out several common examples of such optimization techniques.

Size Optimization: ATL_NO_VTABLE

Since one cannot reasonably guess what an ATL user may be using ATL to build, it is necessary to adopt an ultra-conservative approach to space optimization.

Simply put, every extra byte that is not needed is one byte too many. One area of routinely wasted space (and time) during the instantiation of a C++ object is the vtable building scan process, down a class hierarchy with many pure virtual classes. Imagine, for example, the following class hierarchy:

```
class A
{
  virtual int func_a(int val) = 0;
}
class B: public A
{
int func_b(int val)  { return val+5; }
}
class C: public B
{
int func_a(int val) { return val+3; }
}
```

Since class B does not implement the func_a() virtual function, it also is a pure virtual class, like A. When an object instance of class C is created, a vtable is still built for the base class A and B during the scanning process down the hierarchy.

In this situation, class A and class B are pure virtual and can never be instantiated, and we know for a fact that they will never implement func_a(), so the actual allocation of vtables for them is a waste of time and memory.

This is the purpose of the ATL_NO_VTABLE macro used in ATL generated code for your C++ implementation. This macro is defined as the Visual C++ supported __declspec(novtable) directive. It specifies that, while a vtable pointer should be allocated for such class, it should not be initialized. Specifically, this directive can be used in the definition of pure virtual classes (which can never be instantiated), and should only be used for those classes which do not call virtual functions in their constructor. Our ATL COM server implementation class fits this category. It is a pure virtual class (some virtual functions defined by the base class is not implemented; i.e. IUnknown support) and an instance of it is never created directly by ATL, an instance of the CComObject<> class derived from the implementation is. Secondly, all initialization involving virtual functions should be performed in the FinalConstruct() initialization hook method, therefore no virtual method call needs to be in the constructor.

By using ATL_NO_VTABLE, the vtable allocation for the abstract class is not performed during the vtable scan process, which occurs when an instance of an object from a concrete derived class is instantiated. The directive also provides for some linker optimization. It saves on both space and time.

Size Optimization: Applying Template Specialization

Often, a member variable of a template class is only required when the template is instantiated with a specific type. For example, for the CComObjectRootEx<> template class, the member variable containing a critical section handle (m_critsec) is not required if the parameterization is CComSingleThreadModel. ATL 3 uses a template specialization to ensure that the extra 4 bytes are not taking up valuable space in the final executable and during runtime (see vc98\atl\include\atlcom.h).Here is the regular template code:

```
template <class ThreadModel>
class CComObjectRootEx : public CComObjectRootBase
{
public:
  .......
private:
    _CritSec m_critsec;
};
```

And the specialization without the critical section member variable:

```
template <>
class CComObjectRootEx<CComSingleThreadModel> : public CComObjectRootBase
{
public:
    ......
};
```

Performance Optimization: IUnknown Implementation

For a busy COM server, the `AddRef()` and `Release()` code in the `IUnknown` implementation can be executed quite frequently. Performance optimization here can benefit many library users across all applications. In this vein, ATL makes sure that the more performance expensive `InterlockIncrement()` and `InterlockDecrement()` calls are used only if the server absolutely needs it. This leaves most servers with the simple and fast `var++` and `var--` for reference counting.

Using the mechanisms that we have described so far, ATL can be extended to support the default implementation of (hypothetically) a million interfaces. If you only need to support three interfaces, you can easily inherit from ATL's implementation, and override any the methods that you need. Unlike non-template, binary class libraries, the other 999,997 interfaces don't enter the picture. They are not part of the class hierarchy, their implementation does not consume valuable vtable space, and you do not have to wade through their source code to customize what you're interested in.

That is all we need to know to apply ATL 3 when building COM components. Let us now give our itchy fingers a chance at the bare metal: that of using ATL 3 to re-construct our beloved `BareBlob` object from the last chapter.

Before moving on, I will assume that you have Visual C++ 6 or Visual Studio 6 fully installed with ATL 3. If you have an earlier version of the C++ compiler or ATL, you may not be able to follow along.

Modernizing Our BareBlob with ATL

I hope you haven't forgotten about our `BareBlob` yet. We are now going to recreate it with ATL 3. During the process, you'll see how similar it is to the raw COM coding that we've already done. In contrast, you'll discover how much easier it is with ATL. The background material presented earlier will assist you in quickly understanding the code generated by the various ATL wizards.

As usual, the first step in the process is to define our object in an IDL file. ATL is so helpful that it automatically creates a "starter IDL file" for us. And that's not all, it will create all of the required C++ and header files as well. You'll be glad that you've gone through the process of creating an ActiveX control from scratch because these files will be fully recognizable.

Let's recreate our `BareBlob` in ATL. You should be pleasantly surprised by how quick this will be. Start Visual C++ 6 and select **New...** from the **File** menu, and make sure you have the **Project** tab selected. The **New Project** dialog will now pop up:

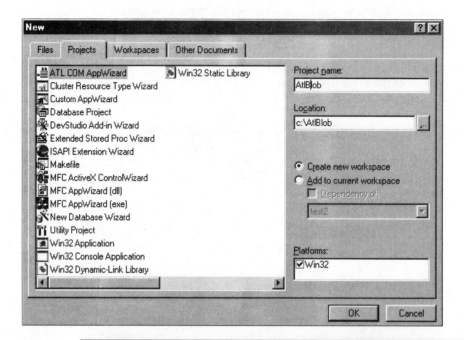

From the selection of project wizards, select the **ATL COM AppWizard**. Give the project a name; use `AtlBlob` for this project. Make sure the **Create new workspace** radio button is checked and press the **OK** button. Next, the wizard will startup and prompt you with its one and only screen:

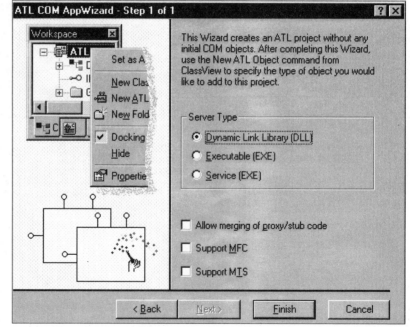

We're creating an in-proc server, so we select the **Dynamic Link Library** server type. Note that we have an option to merge the proxy/stub code into the DLL – this will put the proxy and stub objects into the same module, thus cutting down the number of files required for distribution. We won't need this in our case, however, since we already know how to compile and register proxy/stubs when they are needed. The **Support MFC** option will include the appropriate headers if selected. This will allow you to use some of the MFC data classes (CString, for example). The downside of this is that your server will require the MFC runtime DLL, increasing the effective distribution size.

Now click <u>F</u>inish and the wizard will summarize its activities:

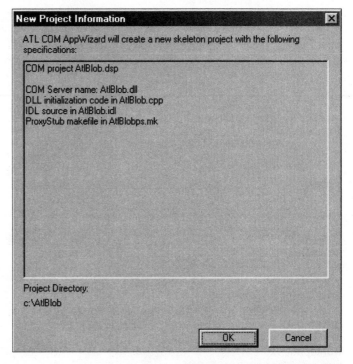

Notice how it offers to write both the IDL and the DLL initialization code for us (recall the four required export functions for COM DLL servers). Click **OK** to have the code generated, then check the **FileView** tab of the project to see the files generated.

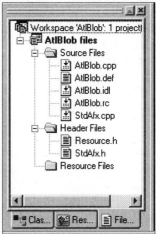

This is the complete skeleton ATL project. However, it doesn't yet contain or support any COM object. To add object support, select Insert | New ATL Object.... The ATL Object Wizard will pop up and offer you a large choice of target objects (see earlier *Supporting Rapid Creation of Components with Interface Grouping* section).

To implement our `BareBlob`, we need only the Simple Object:

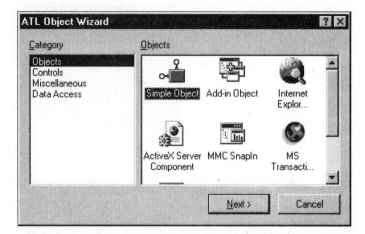

Click Next> to start the wizard on its way. We'll now be prompted with more questions to configure (and generate ATL code for) our object:

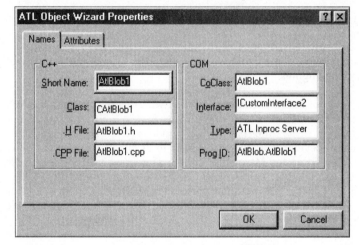

Fill in the object information as shown above, to approximately match our initial `BareBlob` project. We need to change the name of the interface to `ICustomInterface2` and give it a new interface ID because we'll be adding more methods to the interface and also modifying one of them. Recall from Chapter 2 that a COM interface, once specified, can't be changed – this means we must create a new name for our interface.

Note that the name we entered in the CoClass field above will appear in the generated IDL file, the Type field (which we have changed to ATL Inproc Server) will actually be inserted into the registry when the generated type library (`.tlb` file) is registered, and the Prog ID will be a string representation of the CLSID, which can be used in a client's call to create an object.

Now select the **Attributes** tab to continue the configuration:

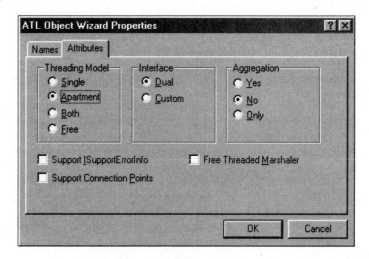

Here, we can select the threading model of our object. Like our original `BareBlob`, we'll support the Apartment threading model.

For the type of interface, we'll select **Dual**. Remember that the interface that we've implemented for `BareBlob` was vtable only. Selecting **Dual** here gets ATL to help us with implementing an `IDispatch` based interface (by inheriting from `IDispatchImpl<>`). This makes our component more popular in the COM world, as it will be able to talk to many more potential clients, including scripting engines.

We will not be supporting aggregation with this simple `BareBlob`. This will cause the wizard to generate a `DECLARE_NOT_AGGREGATABLE()` in order to override the default. The `ISupportError` interface (which provides rich error and context reporting) and connection points (for firing events from the object back to its client) will also not be supported, neither will we check the **Free Threaded Marshaller** option. The Free Threaded Marshaller (FTM) is typically used only by COM servers that support "both" in the threading models (see Chapter 2). The FTM allows the server to ensure that cross-apartment calls made by an STA client will not be marshaled. We will not be covering this specialized advanced scenario in this book. Interested readers should check out Richard Grimes' *Professional ATL Programming* (ISBN 1-861001-40-1).

Finally, press the **OK** button to have the wizard generate the code according to your specifications. After code generation (it may take a little while), you'll find that two extra files have been added to your project:

- ❑ `AtlBlob1.cpp`
- ❑ `AtlBlob1.h`

This is beginning to look very much like the 'from scratch' project we did in the last chapter. The only discernible differences are:

- ❑ An RC file, which is used for storing system strings, and registry update information for the ATL library
- ❑ Our `Precomp.h` is replaced by the `StdAfx.h` in ATL

❏ An `Atlblob1.rgs` file holding a script for automated attributes database updates via the **registrar** (see the *Automated Registry Manipulation* section later in this chapter)

Other files you'll recognize from the `BareBlob` project:

❏ `Atlblob.idl` is an input for the MIDL compiler
❏ `Atlblob.h` and `Atlblob_i.c` (not part of the project) are generated by MIDL when it is run on `Atlblob.idl`
❏ `Atlblob.def` lists all the exported routines from the DLL for server registration
❏ `Atlblob1.h` contains the declaration of the actual `CAtlblob1` class – unlike our `CBareBlob` class, though, it has quite a few ATL macros in there

You'll also recognize the `Atlblob.cpp` file once you open it. Inside you'll find the implementation of the `DllMain()`, `DllRegisterServer()`, `DllUnregisterServer()`, `DllCanUnloadNow()` and `DLLGetClassObject()` functions. We saw how these were implemented earlier in the chapter using the methods of the `CComModule` class.

The `Atlblob1.cpp` file is like our `Bareblob1.cpp` file, where we'll be implementing the methods of `ICustomInterface2`.

The `.rgs` and the `.rc` files didn't exist in the old project. You'll also not be able to find registry modification and update routines like the ones we had to code in the `CBareBlob` case. It turns out that the `.rgs` and the `.rc` files contain the required information regarding the registry keys to be added and deleted during the registration/de-registration process. ATL will handle this for us, so we don't need to do any tedious, explicit coding or painful testing.

That accounts for every file that ATL has generated for us, and we can see that there's really nothing very mysterious about ATL. It's following very much the same pattern as we did in our raw COM coding example.

To get a different perspective on the same code, click on the **ClassView** tab, and see which classes have been generated for us:

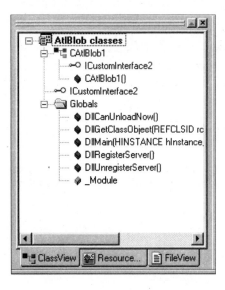

Note that the five required entry point functions, DllCanUnloadNow(), DllGetClassObject(), DllMain(), DllRegisterServer(), and DllUnregisterServer() are already in place. So is the declaration of the CAtlblob1 class in the C++ source file and the header file. That wasn't so bad for a few mouse clicks, was it?

Spoon Feeding a COM Interface

The little 'spoon like' thing next to ICustomInterface2 is the 'visual COM interface' feature of Visual C++ 6. We can use this spoon to define our methods and properties for the interface from this view. The system will actually update all the relevant files for us! Thank Microsoft for the spoon.

Now, let's define the methods and properties of this new interface. Recall our discussion from Chapter 2 about the IDispatch interface and its ability to provide Automation properties which a client such as VBScript can easily access and configure. We'll add one such property here in our ICustomInterface2, called ThreadID. This property will be read-only, and will give the operating system the thread ID of the thread on which the component is executing. In addition to being an example of how to implement an Automation compatible property, it will also help us to understand threading models better. Lastly, we'll carry forward our GetManagerName() and OkayToPublishInfo() business rule implementations from the last chapter. For PeekCounters(), we change it to PeekCounter() and return only one counter value (the count of the total number of instances of our object) since the other one was less than interesting.

To summarize, we have:

Methods and Properties	Description
HRESULT GetManagerName([out, retval] BSTR* pbstrMgrName);	Obtain the name of the current manager in charge of the department.
HRESULT OkayToPublishInfo([in] long lYear, [in] long lMonth, [out, retval] VARIANT_BOOL* bOkayFlag);	Determine if it's okay to publish Events Calendar information for a particular month in a particular year.
HRESULT PeekCounter([out, retval] long* lCounter);	Show the number of current objects being served (and class factory server locks) by the server.
long ThreadID;	A read-only property supporting Get() to demonstrate the implementation of an Automation property using ATL 3.

To add these definitions to the project, simply highlight the ICustomInterface2 spoon, and press the right mouse button. Select **Add Method**, and enter the specification for GetManagerName():

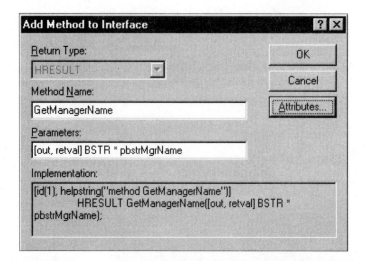

Repeat the above procedure to add `OkayToPublishInfo()` and `PeekCounter()`. Finally, select the spoon again, right click, and select **Add Property**, to add the `ThreadID` property:

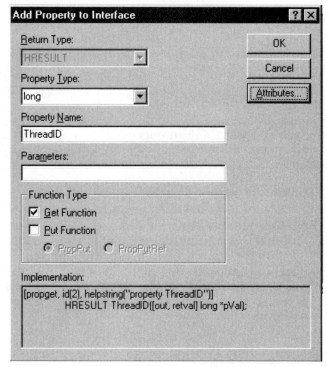

The `ThreadID` property, which supports only the `Get` (not `Put`) operation, ends up being implemented by an interface method, the `get_ThreadID()` member function in the `CAtlblob1` class.

It's a good time to take a look at the ClassView pane again, to see that indeed these new methods and properties have been added to the ICustomInterface2 definition. Notice also that the CAtlblob1 class also has skeleton member functions ready for your implementation.

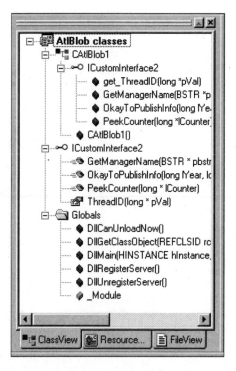

Just in case you may have made some mistakes in data entry while following along, you will appreciate that Visual C++6 provides for deletion of interface methods. Simply highlight the method in question, right click and select **Delete**. Clearly, this is a complex process involving the following steps:

❑ Delete its definition from the .idl file.
❑ Delete the member function(s) declaration in the .h header file.
❑ Delete the implementation of the member function(s) in the .cpp source file. (Visual C++ 6 will actually comment the code out instead of deleting it, just in case you change your mind).

Notice that in the above diagram, the ICustomInterface2 instance under the CAtlBlob1 class is an internal implementation instance, while the one outside by itself is an external instance. The external instance displays Automation methods and properties while the internal instance shows only the raw implementation methods.

Examining the Code

Now, let's see exactly what ATL 3 did to handle the ICustomInterface2. First, as in CBareBlob, we can open and examine the .idl file that ATL has generated for us.

The IDL File

The IDL is called Atlblob.idl. Notice where the interface is defined — outside the library definition. This ensures that MIDL will generate the proxy/stub code that we require

```
// Atipblob.idl : IDL source for Atipblob.dll
import "oaidl.idl";
import "ocidl.idl";
    [
        object,
        uuid(7882E1CD-D8A2-11D1-A660-006052008075),
        dual,
        helpstring("ICustomInterface2 Interface"),
        pointer_default(unique)
    ]
    interface ICustomInterface2 : IDispatch
    {
        [id(1), helpstring("method GetManagerName")]
            HRESULT GetManagerName([out, retval] BSTR* pbstrMgrName);
        [id(2), helpstring("method OkayToPublishInfo")]
            HRESULT OkayToPublishInfo([in] long lYear,
            [in] long lMonth, [out, retval] VARIANT_BOOL* bOkayFlag);
        [id(3), helpstring("method PeekCounter")]
            HRESULT PeekCounter([out, retval] long* lCounter);
        [propget, id(4), helpstring("property ThreadID")]
            HRESULT ThreadID([out, retval] long *pVal);
    };
[
    uuid(7882E1C1-D8A2-11D1-A660-006052008075),
    version(1.0),
    helpstring("Atlblob 1.0 Type Library")
]
library ATLBLOBLib
{
    importlib("stdole32.tlb");
    importlib("stdole2.tlb");

    [
        uuid(04476DFC-D784-11D1-A660-006052008075),
        helpstring("ATL Inproc Server")
    ]
    coclass Atlblob1
    {
        [default] interface ICustomInterface2;
    };
};
```

One important point to notice is the specification of the interface as dual. This is saying that we'll also support the late binding of our methods in ICustomInterface2. Indeed, we can see that ICustomInterface2 inherits from IDispatch instead of IUnknown. Recall our discussion in Chapter 2 on late binding. Late binding requires the server to support the IDispatch interface. The IDispatch interface contains several complex methods to obtain type library information, invoke methods by and translate symbolic information to dispatch IDs. The IDispatchImpl<> class in ATL makes our work trivial. Supporting IDispatch opens up a whole new world of clients to our object. As a rule of thumb, one should, if possible, always consider making a COM class' interfaces dual, to maximize reuse potentials by the large number of Automation compatible clients.

When supporting `IDispatch`, one has to be careful about the format and data types of arguments for our methods. Only certain 'Automation compatible' data types may be used, which rules out any custom structures, etc. Thankfully, we've coded our sample from the beginning to use only Automation compatible data types. (A list of such data types is included later on in this chapter.) In our discussion on late binding, we learned that the `IDispatch::Invoke()` model supports the setting and getting of properties, as well as the invocation of methods. We can see in the IDL that ATL has assigned dispatch IDs to all of our methods and properties (from `id(1)` to `id(4)`).

The Class Definition

Let's take a look now at the methods and the new property that ATL has generated for us. First, we examine the class definition in the `AtlBlob1.h` file:

```
///////////////////////////////////////////////////////////////
// CAtlBlob1
class ATL_NO_VTABLE CAtlBlob1 :
    public CComObjectRootEx<CComSingleThreadModel>,
    public CComCoClass<CAtlBlob1, &CLSID_AtlBlob1>,
    public IDispatchImpl<ICustomInterface2, &IID_ICustomInterface2,
                                            &LIBID_ATLBLOBLib>
{
public:
    CAtlBlob1()
    {
    }

DECLARE_REGISTRY_RESOURCEID(IDR_ATLBLOB1)
DECLARE_NOT_AGGREGATABLE(CAtlBlob1)

DECLARE_PROTECT_FINAL_CONSTRUCT()

BEGIN_COM_MAP(CAtlBlob1)
    COM_INTERFACE_ENTRY(ICustomInterface2)
    COM_INTERFACE_ENTRY(IDispatch)
END_COM_MAP()

// ICustomInterface2
public:
    STDMETHOD(get_ThreadID)(/*[out, retval]*/ long *pVal);
    STDMETHOD(PeekCounter)(/*[out, retval]*/ long* lCounter);
    STDMETHOD(OkayToPublishInfo)(/*[in]*/ long lYear, /*[in]*/
        long lMonth, /*[out, retval]*/ VARIANT_BOOL* bOkayFlag);
    STDMETHOD(GetManagerName)(/*[out, retval]*/ BSTR* pbstrMgrName);
};
```

Note the commented out IDL attributes with the method declarations. These are in to save you a potential trip to the IDL file while editing code.

You can see here that the ATL wizard has already created our class, `CAtlBlob1`, for us, and added declarations for all the methods of `ICustomInterface2`. At the top of the file, we can see that the `ATL_NO_VTABLE` optimization being applied. Take a look at the classes from which `CAtlBlob` derives:

- ❏   CComObjectRootEx<>
- ❏   CComCoClass<>
- ❏   IDispatchImpl<>

CComObjectRootEx<> implements the IUnknown reference counting for us in a manner appropriate for our threading model. In this case, it has the parameter CComSingleThreadModel, because we specified that we wanted apartment threading when we were generating the code with the ATL Object Wizard. Our QueryInterface() calls will be processed through the **COM interface map**, which is described below.

CAtlblob1 also inherits from CComCoClass<> to obtain the default definition for class factory and aggregation mode – all externally creatable COM objects in ATL inherit from this class.

Finally, CAtlblob1 inherits from IDispatchImpl<> to get the free IDispatch implementation.

ATL COM Interface Map

Inside the class definition, we can also see the COM map:

```
BEGIN_COM_MAP(CAtlBlob1)
    COM_INTERFACE_ENTRY(ICustomInterface2)
    COM_INTERFACE_ENTRY(IDispatch)
END_COM_MAP()
```

This contains two COM_INTERFACE_ENTRY() macros, one with ICustomInterface2 in it and the other with IDispatch. The COM interface map gives ATL the proper information it needs to perform its QueryInterface(). It is an internal ATL-managed table, which maps out all the interface IDs supported by the COM server. We see here, in our interface map, that the object is claiming to support IDispatch, which is true since ICustomInterface2 is derived from IDispatch *and can be used as* IDispatch.

Method Declarations

The method declarations in Atlblob1.h are almost identical to the CBareBlob case from the last chapter. If you look at our good old Objbase.h file, you'll find the definition of STDMETHOD() macro. Look at the declaration of GetManagerName() in atlblob1.h:

```
STDMETHOD(GetManagerName)(BSTR* pbstrMgrName);
```

This translates as:

```
    virtual HRESULT __stdcall GetManagerName(BSTR* pbstrMgrName);
```

The DECLARE_REGISTRY_RESOURCEID() macro is used by ATL to find the compiled script, when it has to update the registry during server registration and unregistration. The .rgs source file is actually packed into the .rc file as a custom resource, which is loaded by ATL using this macro.

The Class Implementation

The class definition is now completed. We'll now proceed to implement the logic for methods and properties of our object. To do this, we'll work on the `Atlblob1.cpp` file generated by ATL. The following listing highlights the additions that we key in:

```cpp
// AtlBlob1.cpp : Implementation of CAtlBlob1
#include "stdafx.h"
#include "AtlBlob.h"
#include "AtlBlob1.h"

/////////////////////////////////////////////////////////////////
// CAtlBlob1

STDMETHODIMP CAtlBlob1::GetManagerName(BSTR *pbstrMgrName)
{
    *pbstrMgrName = SysAllocString(L"J. Manzini");
    return S_OK;
}

STDMETHODIMP CAtlBlob1::OkayToPublishInfo(long lYear, long lMonth, VARIANT_BOOL
*bOkayFlag)
{
    if (((lYear * lMonth) % 4)==0)
        *bOkayFlag = VARIANT_FALSE;
    else
        *bOkayFlag = VARIANT_TRUE;
    return S_OK;
}

STDMETHODIMP CAtlBlob1::PeekCounter(long *lCounter)
{
    *lCounter = _Module.GetLockCount();
    return S_OK;
}

STDMETHODIMP CAtlBlob1::get_ThreadID(long *pVal)
{
    *pVal = GetCurrentThreadId();
    return S_OK;
}
```

If you look at the implementation for `GetManagerName()` and `OkayToPublishInfo()`, you can see that these have not been changed from the last chapter. `PeekCounter()`, however, needs modification to work in `CAtlblob1`. The counter we want to keep track of is in the `CComObjectRootEx<>` class, which implements global module reference counting, and was instantiated in `AtlBlob.cpp`:

```cpp
CComModule _Module;
```

Notice the use of the Win32 `GetCurrentThreadID()` function call to implement our `get_ThreadID()` method, which in turn implements the `ThreadID` property. The function used to get the property's value must be of the form:

```cpp
get_<PropertyName>()
```

This is enforced so that any Automation compatible handling code (from our 'agnostic' clients) will know, without you having to define more tables, which function to call when the Get operation is invoked on a property, via the IDispatch::Invoke() method.

Compiling

So far, we have:

- ❏ Used the ATL COM AppWizard to create a skeleton ATL project called Atlblob
- ❏ Used the **Insert ATL Object...** option to activate the ATL Object Wizard to insert a **Simple Object** into the ATL project, specifying that it implements the ICustomInterface2 COM interface and that the interface should be implemented as dual
- ❏ Added methods to ICustomInterface2, and at the same time added skeletal code in the CAtlblob1 class to implement the interface
- ❏ Added a new read-only property to ICustomInterface2, called ThreadID
- ❏ Added our implementation to all the methods of the CAtlblob1 class, modeling it on our earlier BareBlob implementation

What else remains to be done for our ActiveX control? Would you believe... nothing!

Try building the project now. Notice how Atlblob.dll is created and the server registered with the system automatically. If you look back in ClassView, you will see that type library for Atlblob has also been created and stored in the file Atlblob.tlb. More on that later.

Now, run the OLE/COM Object Viewer utility and examine the new ActiveX control that you've just created. Click on the **All Objects** folder on the left pane. Look for an **ATL InProc Server** entry. Click on it and notice all the registry entries (on the right-hand pane) that ATL has registered for you without any work. Double-click on the **ATL InProc Server** entry, this will actually instantiate a CAtlblob1 object, and notice the interfaces that it supports. It should look like this:

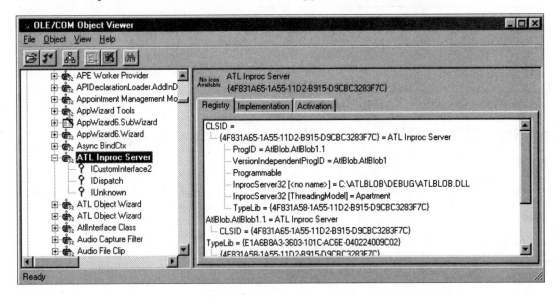

Unlike our old `CBareBlob` class, our ATL Inproc Server claims support for the `IDispatch` interface, as well as the `ICustomInterface2` that we've just defined. Double click on the `IDispatch` interface, and an `IDispatch` viewer will now pop up. If you now click on the View Type Info button, you'll notice that our methods and properties of `ICustomInterface2` show up:

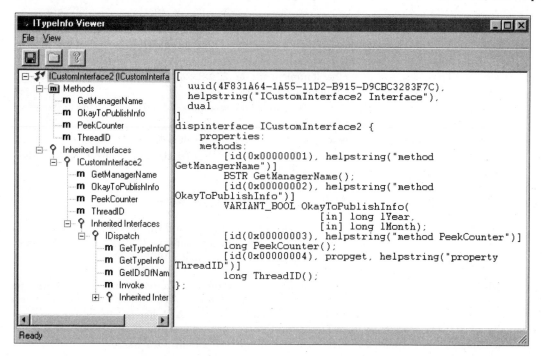

Recall that we've defined `ICustomInterface2` to be `dual` in the IDL file. Furthermore, `ICustomInterface2` actually derives from `IDispatch` rather than `IUnknown`, which was the case with `ICustomInterface` in `CBareBlob`. What the `IDispatch` viewer actually does is to find out what methods the object supports directly, using `IDispatch::GetTypeInfo()` and `IDispatch::GetIDsOfNames()` to get the information about the dispatch interface (in our case `ICustomInterface2`). This simple test has confirmed that ATL has implemented the methods of `IDispatch` for us in our COM server painlessly.

Creating COM Clients with Visual C++ 6 Native Support

Now, since the interface is dual – supporting both `IDispatch::Invoke()` and vtable calls – we should still be able to call it using VTBL binding from C/C++. Let's prove it with our multithreaded tester client. Since we've 'modernized' our `BareBlob` object, we're going to modernize our test client, too.

To do this, we'll draw on some cool built-in features of Visual C++ 6 and its native support for COM client programming.

Testing VTBL Binding

We saw in the last chapter how to program a vtable binding test client for the object. Looking back through the code from that chapter, you'll discover that this was a fairly complicated process.

In our .cpp file, we had a dependence on a myriad of header files, especially those that defined the required CLSID and interface definitions for CBareBlob. For example, our former multithreaded test client had to include:

```
#include "..\baseblob\bareblob.h"
#define IID_DEFINED
#include "..\baseblob\bareblob_i.c"
```

We also went through a multistep process to obtain an interface pointer to ICustomInterface. This involved obtaining a class factory, creating the BareBlob object and then querying for ICustomInterface. Here is an excerpt from our previous client showing what was necessary:

```
    hRes = CoGetClassObject(CLSID_CBareBlob, CLSCTX_ALL, NULL,
    IID_IClassFactory, reinterpret_cast<void **>( &pCF));
....
    hRes = pCF->CreateInstance(NULL, IID_IUnknown,
                                  reinterpret_cast<void **>( &pM));
....
    hRes = pM->QueryInterface( IID_ICustomInterface,
                                  reinterpret_cast<void **>( &pCI));
```

Error handling code was dispersed throughout. Just examine the source code from our previous test client and you'll see that almost half of the code deals with error conditions and handling. Finally, we had to take careful consideration during design to ensure that reference counting rules for all instantiated objects were observed.

Now, what if:

- ❑ We can create a COM client without having to deal with multiple include files
- ❑ We create the interface that we need simply by instantiating a single C++ object
- ❑ We can handle all errors in a centralized location in the source file
- ❑ We don't have to worry about reference counting at all during coding

Seasoned COM programmers will say that we're in dreamland, and newcomers to COM client programming probably will never program any other way (and swear that COM is dead simple). Welcome to the wonderful new world of Visual C++ 6 "native" COM support!

The core code of our new test client will be reduced to **4** simple lines:

```
ICustomInterface2Ptr pCI(__uuidof(Atlblob1));
mgrName = pCI->GetManagerName();
okFlag = pCI->OkayToPublishInfo(inYear, inMonth);
objCount = pCI->PeekCounter();
```

181

What are the new elements that make all this possible? Are we not still working within a C++ language? Let's take a look at this now.

Native COM Client Support Features of Visual C++ 6

Indeed, we're still working within the confines of the C++ language. Behind the smoke and mirrors, it's all done with:

- ❑ Several new compiler/preprocessor specific directives
- ❑ A set of utility wrapper classes
- ❑ Smart pointer wrapper classes for COM interfaces

We'll look at each of these pieces in turn, and at the same time examine our revamped multithreaded tester to illustrate the points.

New Compiler Directives

Let's take a look at the most important new preprocessor directive, called the #import directive. In one sentence:

> #import **reads a type library and generates all the wrapper classes you need for easy COM programming.**

This is precisely what this new directive does. Let's look at it in action with our test harness client program.

You can find the source code in the \Ch4\Atlmtst\AtlMulti.cpp *file which downloadable from the Wrox Press Ltd. site at* http:\\www.wrox.com

Right at the very top of the file AtlMulti.cpp, you'll see the #import directive for Atlblob.tlb, the type library file we created as a result of compiling our Atlblob project.

```
#include "stdafx.h"
#import "..\atlblob\Atlblob.tlb" no_namespace
```

You will find the same set of #includes as our earlier BLOB testing program in stdafx.h:

```
#include <stdio.h>
#include <stdlib.h>
#include <time.h>
#include <tchar.h>
#define _WIN32_DCOM
#include <objbase.h>
#include <comdef.h>
#include <initguid.h>
#include <process.h>
```

There is one additional include file here, `Comdef.h`. This file contains a definition of basic smart pointer support, and the `BSTR` and `VARIANT` wrappers which are necessary for everything to work properly (we'll cover these in the next section).

Note that we no longer have to include files containing CLSIDs, interface descriptions, etc. The preprocessor, upon seeing the `#import` directive, will reverse-engineer a binary type library, and generate all the headers required! Hurrah! This also means that the type library can be embedded anywhere: in a binary TLB file, as a resource within an EXE or a DLL, etc.

The `no_namespace` attribute (and its variations) can be used to isolate the symbolic information from the reverse engineering process in its own C++ namespace. Specifically, in dissecting very large type libraries, it's possible for the type library to introduce symbols that are already defined in your main source code, or its include files. By isolating the symbols in their own C++ namespace, the `#import` directive can proceed without any name conflicts. It's also possible to selectively rename certain symbols from the `#import` process. Since our `AtlBlob` type library is tiny, we use the `no_namespace` attribute to avoid creating any namespace. Otherwise, a namespace of ATLBLOBLib (from the 'library' statement of our IDL file) will be generated by default.

Another very useful attribute to note in passing is the `raw_dispinterfaces` attribute. If you specify this then the code generated will be using `IDispatch::Invoke()` to access the properties and methods of the COM object, essentially acting as an Automation controller. Without this attribute, the `#import` directive will create code which accesses the COM object via direct vtable interface calls. We want to access the object via VTBL binding, so we will not specify the `raw_dispinterfaces` attribute here.

See the Visual C++ 6 documentation for other attributes for the `#import` directive.

On compiling our `Atlmtst` project, the `#import` directive will generate two files:

- ❑ `AtlBlob.tlh` – Type Library Headers
- ❑ `AtlBlob.tli` – Type Library Includes

We'll see this in action later, when we put together out multithreaded test program and compile it, but let's take a look now at the files that are generated from our `AtlBlob` type library using the `#import` directive.

The .tlh File

The `AtlBlob.tlh` file is logically included with the definition (header) files, while the `AtlBlob.tli` file is logically included with the source code. Here's our `AtlBlob.tlh` file:

```
// Created by Microsoft (R)
// C/C++ Compiler Version 12.00.8047.2 (4d2fdae6).
//
// c:\atlmtst\AtlBlob.tlh
//
// C++ source equivalent of Win32 type
// library ..\atlblob\AtlBlob.tlb
// compiler-generated file created 04/21/98
// at 07:40:46 - DO NOT EDIT!
```

```
#pragma once
#pragma pack(push, 8)

#include <comdef.h>

//
// Forward references and typedefs
//

struct /* coclass */ Atlblob1;
struct __declspec(uuid("7882e1cd-d8a2-11d1-a660-006052008075"))
/* dual interface */ ICustomInterface2;

//
// Smart pointer typedef declarations
//

_COM_SMARTPTR_TYPEDEF(ICustomInterface2, __uuidof(ICustomInterface2));

//
// Type library items
//

struct __declspec(uuid("04476dfc-d784-11d1-a660-006052008075"))
Atlblob1;
    // [ default ] interface ICustomInterface2

struct __declspec(uuid("7882e1cd-d8a2-11d1-a660-006052008075"))
ICustomInterface2 : IDispatch
{
    //
    // Property data
    //

    __declspec(property(get=GetThreadID))
    long ThreadID;

    //
    // Wrapper methods for error-handling
    //

    _bstr_t GetManagerName ( );
    VARIANT_BOOL OkayToPublishInfo (
        long lYear,
        long lMonth );
    long PeekCounter ( );
    long GetThreadID ( );

    //
    // Raw methods provided by interface
    //
```

```
        virtual HRESULT __stdcall raw_GetManagerName (
            BSTR * pbstrMgrName ) = 0;
        virtual HRESULT __stdcall raw_OkayToPublishInfo (
            long lYear,
            long lMonth,
            VARIANT_BOOL * bOkayFlag ) = 0;
        virtual HRESULT __stdcall raw_PeekCounter (
            long * lCounter ) = 0;
        virtual HRESULT __stdcall get_ThreadID (
            long * pVal ) = 0; };

//
// Wrapper method implementations
//

#include "e:\atlmtst\AtlBlob.tli"

#pragma pack(pop)
```

Other than the few new types that we'll cover in a moment, this code is completely understandable. You can see the type library disassembly process here. Notice how our ICustomInterface2 has been reverse-engineered and its member methods reassembled under a new C++ pure virtual structure.

However, you will also notice that the actual calling syntax of the methods has been modified from the interface implementation to reflect the retval specification. For example, GetManagerName() is declared with a _bstr_t return type. Note that there's a set of virtual methods with the raw_ prefix that matches our interface definition, method for method. The reason for these virtual members is that they provide the vtable through which the smart interface pointer will call the methods of the actual object.This will become evident when we take a look at the .tli file later. For now, let's look at another couple of new compiler keywords that cropped up in this file:

❑ __declspec()
❑ __uuidof()

__declspec(uuid())

The __declspec(uuid()) declaration specifier will associate a GUID with a structure or class, and keep this association for later retrieval. For example, our CAtipblob1 class is associated with its CLSID (decoded by the preprocessor) in the statement:

```
struct __declspec(uuid("04476dfc-d784-11d1-a660-006052008075"))
Atlblob1;
```

__uuidof()

Retrieval of the associated GUID can be performed by using the __uuidof() keyword on the type. The compiler's symbol table component will handle the storage. For example, the GUID from ICustomInterface2, was retrieved with:

```
__uuidof(ICustomInterface2)
```

In practice, the __uuidof() keyword is typically used in conjunction with smart pointer features to handle GUIDs transparently (see the *Smart Pointers Save the Day* section later in this chapter).

__declspec(property())

The __declspec(property()) construction provides compiler shorthand for calling the 'virtual data members' of a class. These data members are virtual because they do not actually exist, but their Set and Get behaviors map to member functions of the class.

For example, in the code above, we saw the following declaration:

```
__declspec(property(get=GetThreadID))
long ThreadID;
```

Now, if the compiler were to encounter the following code:

```
long a;
a = obj.ThreadID;
```

Then, provided that obj is an instance of a class derived from the ICustomInterface2 type, the actual code generated will be:

```
long a;
a = obj.GetThreadID();
```

Most of these declaration specifiers make use of the compiler's symbol table to carry out their task.

The .tli File

The code from the AtlBlob.tli file that is generated from our AtlBlob type library is shown below. Here, we can see how the actual functions are implemented:

```
// Created by Microsoft (R)
// C/C++ Compiler Version 12.00.8047.2 (4d2fdae6).
//
// c:\atlmtst\AtlBlob.tli
//
// Wrapper implementations for Win32
// type library ..\atlblob\Atlblob.tlb
// compiler-generated file created 04/21/98
// at 07:40:46 - DO NOT EDIT!

#pragma once

//
// interface ICustomInterface2 wrapper method implementations
//

inline _bstr_t ICustomInterface2::GetManagerName ( ) {
    BSTR _result;
    HRESULT _hr = raw_GetManagerName(&_result);
    if (FAILED(_hr)) _com_issue_errorex(_hr, this, __uuidof(this));
    return _bstr_t(_result, false);
}
```

```
inline VARIANT_BOOL ICustomInterface2::OkayToPublishInfo ( long lYear,
                                                           long lMonth ) {
    VARIANT_BOOL _result;
    HRESULT _hr = raw_OkayToPublishInfo(lYear, lMonth, &_result);
    if (FAILED(_hr)) _com_issue_errorex(_hr, this, __uuidof(this));
    return _result;
}

inline long ICustomInterface2::PeekCounter ( ) {
    long _result;
    HRESULT _hr = raw_PeekCounter(&_result);
    if (FAILED(_hr)) _com_issue_errorex(_hr, this, __uuidof(this));
    return _result;
}

inline long ICustomInterface2::GetThreadID ( ) {
    long _result;
    HRESULT _hr = get_ThreadID(&_result);
    if (FAILED(_hr)) _com_issue_errorex(_hr, this, __uuidof(this));
    return _result;
}

}
```

We can see above that the member functions actually wrap around the raw_ series of direct COM interfaces calls and will raise an exception via a _com_issue_errorex() call to throw an exception with a _com_error object. The catcher of the exception can use this object's various member functions to obtain extended information about the error. If the COM object issuing the error supports IErrorInfo (which we've elected not to do to keep the code readable), then the object itself can return extended error information, accessible through members of the _com_error class. This effectively translates the HRESULT based error handling to C++ exception handling. The caller to these functions can thus use a try/catch block to put all the error handling code in one location.

COM Wrapper Classes for Data Types

There are a couple of utility classes provided by Visual C++ runtime that ease the handling of certain data types frequently used in COM. These include _bstr_t to wrap BSTR and _variant_t to wrap VARIANT. Using these wrapper types will save you a lot of unnecessary coding when working with these data types.

_bstr_t

You can use the _bstr_t class to create new BSTR objects. More useful, however, is the capability to attach an existing BSTR to a new _bstr_t object. For example, if you were passed a BSTR variable called bstrInput, the following statement will create a _bstr_t object called newBstr, and attach an existing BSTR variable to it:

```
_bstr_t  newBstr(bstrInput);
```

This is just one of many ways to construct a _bstr_t object. You can also use a UNICODE or ANSI string to create a BSTR compatible _bstr_t object, or you can construct a BSTR type variable from a VARIANT variable holding a BSTR (a sort of logical casting).

In general, using _bstr_t instead of BSTR will make handling and conversion simpler, and eliminates the frequent calls to the SysAllocString() family of functions, because the _bstr_t implementation handles all of this for us.

_bstr_t also has a number of other useful features:

- Supports concatenation, through the + operator
- Supports comparison, through the <, >, and == operators
- Implements a copy constructor
- Supports automatic reference counting, so the internal allocation for the actual string data will be freed automatically

We will see how it really simplifies the handling of our BSTR variable for the manager's name a little later.

In fact, the code generated by the #import directive will use the _bstr_t to represent BSTR variables exclusively. For the convenience it offers you, you should consider doing this in your code as well. See the Visual C++ 6 documentation on _bstr_t for more details on the member functions and operators that this class supports.

_variant_t

Like the _bstr_t class, the _variant_t class makes handling of VARIANT variables considerably easier. You can create new _variant_t variables, or create one based on an existing VARIANT variable using the constructor:

```
_variant_t newVar(inVariant);
```

An alternative is to use the Attach() member function:

```
_variant_t newVar;
newVar.Attach(inVariant);
```

A Detach() member also exists to recover the VARIANT variable controlled by a _variant_t object. The underlying data in the _variant_t object can be extracted using a variety of extraction operators. The type can be converted (if a conversion exists) using the ChangeType() member function, and a Clear() member function is provided to clear out the _variant_t object. There is also a SetString() member function, which allows the setting of a BSTR _variant_t object when only an MBCS string is passed in.

The encapsulation provided by _variant_t ensures that the VARIANT variable being represented is always in a consistent state.

The code generated by the #import directive will use the _variant_t to represent VARIANT variables exclusively. See the Visual C++ 6 documentation on _variant_t for the various members and operators possible with this class.

Smart Pointers

Smart pointers are pointer objects that perform automatic lifetime management by encapsulating the operation of reference counting. Essentially, the smart COM object pointer will perform the AddRef() and Release() for you, so you do not have to worry about coding it yourself.

Sounds too good to be true? Well, it is true. Smart COM object pointers work as advertised, *as long as all access to the underlying objects is performed through the same pointer* (i.e. you or the runtime you deal with does not 'steal' the actual interface pointer from you and do its own thing for a while). In certain COM programming exercises, our multithreaded testing client, for example, maintaining full control of the pointer is totally acceptable and is all that will be needed. In other scenarios, especially when you have to pass the underlying pointer to a third party (component or COM runtime), maintaining full control of the pointer may not be possible.

_com_ptr_t Class

The _com_ptr_t class encapsulates the functionality of the smart COM pointer. The IUnknown methods (QueryInterface(), AddRef() and Release()) are all called automatically by the implementation. This gives the programmer an apparent 'instantiate and use' flexibility.

You create a smart pointer class using the COM_SMARTPTR_TYPEDEF() macro. This will actually create an instantiation of the _com_ptr_t class for the COM object you specify as a parameter. The two parameters taken by this macro are:

- ❑ The interface of the object that this pointer refers to.
- ❑ The IID of the interface.

For example, in AtlBlob.tlh, the #import preprocessor has created a smart pointer for our ICustomInterface2 interface using:

```
_COM_SMARTPTR_TYPEDEF(ICustomInterface2,
                      __uuidof(ICustomInterface2));
```

Here, we see the use the __uuidof() keyword in conjunction with smart pointers to retrieve the IID associated with the ICustomInterface2 class/structure. After the execution of this macro, there will be a type called ICustomInterface2Ptr (note the Ptr postfix; this will always be the case with this macro). When instantiated with the appropriate object's CLSID, ICustomInterface2Ptr will create the smart pointer and QueryInterface() in one simple step.

A typedef of a template will not actually generate any code until the new type is actually used in a declaration. See Appendix C if you want more details.

Take, for example, the following single line of code:

```
ICustomInterface2Ptr pCI(__uuidof(Atlblob1));
```

This will actually perform the following steps:

1. Call `CoGetClassObject()` on the CLSID of `AtlBlob1` object to obtain a class factory

2. Call `CreateInstance()` of the class factory to create an `AtlBlob1` object

3. Call `IUnknown::QueryInterface()` of the `AtlBlob1` object to obtain an interface to `ICustomInterface2`

4. Create a `__com_ptr_t` smart pointer object around this pointer

5. Throw an exception with a self-describing `__com_error` object if anything should go wrong with the above

The code 'surface area' (actual lines of code in programmer-maintained source files) decreases substantially between the conventional way of using C++ or C based COM programming and the use of smart pointers. Since the complexity of code design and maintenance is directly proportional to the number of lines of code, smart pointer COM programming does indeed simplify COM programming for everyone. We will see a rapid progression of this technology as Microsoft heads towards "attributes based" programming in COM+ (see http://www.microsoft.com/COM/ or http://www.comdeveloper.com for more details).

Multithreaded Test Client Using Smart Pointers

We now have enough background to take a look at the new multithreaded tester. You can find the listing in the \ch4\atlmtst\atlmtst.cpp file from the source code you can download from http://www.wrox.com. We've already seen the #import and #include directives at the start of the file:

```
#include "stdafx.h"
#import "..\atlblob\Atlblob.tlb" no_namespace
```

We then have a routine that will decipher (print to the console) a _com_error object, which is thrown during a COM exception. Since our object doesn't actually support IErrorInfo, this will only decode error information originating from other portions of COM.

```
void dump_com_error(_com_error &e)
{
  _tprintf (_T("Ooops - hit an error!\n"));
  _tprintf(_T("\a\tCode = %08lx\n"), e.Error());
  _tprintf(_T("\a\tMessage = %s\n"),e.ErrorMessage());
}
```

The next portion of the code contains declarations and the main() function implementation. Nothing here has changed from the original multithreaded client of the last chapter, so it is not repeated it in its entirety here:

```
#define MAX_THREAD        10
#define LOCK(x)           EnterCriticalSection(x)
#define UNLOCK(x)         LeaveCriticalSection(x)
CRITICAL_SECTION          g_Console;
```

```
unsigned _stdcall AThread(LPVOID lpParam);
int CRTAPI1 _tmain(int argc, TCHAR ** argv, TCHAR **envp)
{
    .
    .
    .
}
```

Finally, we arrive at the thread function, where the smart pointer usage really simplifies things:

```
unsigned _stdcall AThread(LPVOID lpParam)
{
    long myNumber = *(reinterpret_cast<long *>(lpParam));
    HRESULT hRes;
    long objCount, inYear, inMonth;
    VARIANT_BOOL okFlag;
    _bstr_t mgrName;
```

Here, we have used the `__bstr_t` type for our `mgrName`, in order to simplify our code.

```
srand( static_cast<unsigned>(time( NULL )) );
hRes = CoInitializeEx(NULL, COINIT_APARTMENTTHREADED);

    try
    {
        ICustomInterface2Ptr pCI(__uuidof(Atlblob1));
```

This is it. After this statement, `pCI` will be pointing to `ICustomInterface2` in a newly created `AtlBlob1` object. If this isn't the case, then an exception would have occurred and the thread terminated (you can see what happens in such a situation in code at the end of the thread function).

```
        LOCK(&g_Console);
            _tprintf(_T("T%d: Made a bare blob!\n"), myNumber);
        UNLOCK(&g_Console);
```

We bracket each `_tprintf()` with `LOCK()` and `UNLOCK()` to enable finer granularity of interleaving when multiple threads are all printing.

```
        LOCK(&g_Console);
            _tprintf(_T("T%d: Got its custom interface!\n"),myNumber);
        UNLOCK(&g_Console);

            for (long i=0; i< 20; i++)
            {
            mgrName = pCI->GetManagerName();  // note usage
```

The smart pointer allows us to use the simpler `[retval]` syntax to call a method. Note how easy the assignment of the `BSTR` variable is when done with the `mgrName` `_bstr_t` variable.

```
        LOCK(&g_Console);
        _tprintf(_T("T%d: After calling GetManagerName : current manager
                is %s\n"), myNumber, (TCHAR *) mgrName );
        UNLOCK(&g_Console);
```

Here again, the use of _bstr_t has eliminated the former, more convoluted, #ifdef UNICODE and call to WideCharToMultiByte(). We also no longer have to call SysFreeString(), since the _bstr_t reference counting will do this for us automatically.

```
inYear = 1900 + rand() %100;
inMonth = rand() % 12 + 1;
okFlag = pCI->OkayToPublishInfo(inYear, inMonth);
LOCK(&g_Console);
_tprintf(_T("T%d: After calling OkToPublishInfo : Year = %d,
        Month = %d Status = %s\n"),myNumber, inYear, inMonth,
        (okFlag == VARIANT_TRUE) ? _T("OKAY"): _T("NO WAY"));
UNLOCK(&g_Console);

objCount = pCI->PeekCounter();
LOCK(&g_Console);
_tprintf(_T("T%d: We now have %d object users.\n"),
        myNumber, objCount);
UNLOCK(&g_Console);
long tid = pCI->ThreadID;
```

Notice in the last line here, the very "natural" syntax for accessing the property.

```
LOCK(&g_Console);
_tprintf(_T("T%d: Running on thread ID %lx\n"), myNumber, tid);
UNLOCK(&g_Console);
 Sleep(1000);  // sleep for about 1 second
    }
```

The method calling and printing logic remains largely the same.

```
LOCK(&g_Console);
_tprintf(_T("T%d, Freeing the blob now!\n"), myNumber);
UNLOCK(&g_Console);
    }
```

This is the end of the try block, also the place where our smart pointer goes out of scope, releasing the AtlBlob1 object instance.

Finally, we implement the exception handling by dumping out to the console a (hopefully) deciphered error message, uninitializing COM, then terminating the thread.

```
catch (_com_error &e)
    {
        dump_com_error(e);
        CoUninitialize();
        _endthreadex(0);
    }
    CoUninitialize();
    _endthreadex(0);
    return 0;
    }
```

And that's it for the code.

As I've mentioned before, you can find the source and project files in the \ch4\atlmtst directory of the source code download from http://www.wrox.com . Try building the test client now and executing it. Notice how the client works exactly as our older implementation without smart pointers. Notice also how the new ATL ActiveX control behaves just like our 'from scratch' BareBlob object showing that non-IDispatch VTBL binding is still working. Through the newly implemented ThreadID property, you can also see that the thread ID for each loop iteration remains constant. This reassures us that COM runtime did not intervene since both our client and component conform to STA/Apartment threading model.

Typical output from this program is shown below:

```
...
T8: We now have 3 object users.
T8: Running on thread ID ffc201a3
T9: After calling GetManagerName : current manager is J. Manzini
T9: After calling OkayToPublishInfo : Year = 1999, Month = 5 Status = OKAY
T9: We now have 3 object users.
T9: Running on thread ID ffc201a3
T7: Freeing the blob now!
T8: After calling GetManagerName : current manager is J. Manzini
T8: After calling OkayToPublishInfo : Year = 1940, Month = 5 Status = NOWAY
T8: We now have 2 object users.
T8: Running on thread ID ffc201a3
T9: After calling GetManagerName : current manager is J. Manzini
...
```

Automated Registry Manipulations

In our eagerness to test our ATL control and explore the benefits of Visual C++ 6 native COM support, we've neglected an important topic. The topic is the handling of registry updates through ATL.

An implementation of a **Registrar** component is supplied. Using the Registrar, one can describe all the operations to be performed during the component registration and de-registration process in a text based **script** file. The benefit of this approach is clear. Instead of the raw coding using the registry APIs, we have the ability to quickly change the actions performed in the script, without having to write and test tedious code again and again.

The Registrar works on a .rgs file. The entire file is actually compiled into a custom resource. The Registrar component will interpret this resource during runtime (i.e. when DllRegisterServer() or DllUnregisterServer() is called) and call the appropriate registry API function to modify the registry.

In our `AtlBlob1.h` file, the ATL generated line within the `CAtlBlob1` class definition handles the mapping:

```
class ATL_NO_VTABLE CAtlblob1 :
    public CComObjectRootEx<CComSingleThreadModel>,
    public CComCoClass<CAtlblob1, &CLSID_Atlblob1>,
    public IDispatchImpl<ICustomInterface2, &IID_ICustomInterface2,
&LIBID_ATLBLOBLib>
{
public:
    CAtlblob1()
    {
    }
DECLARE_REGISTRY_RESOURCEID(IDR_ATLBLOB1)
```

The `DECLARE_REGISTRY_RESOURCEID()` macro translates to a static function declaration, which is found in the `Atlcom.h` file:

```
#define DECLARE_REGISTRY_RESOURCEID(x)\
    static HRESULT WINAPI UpdateRegistry(BOOL bRegister)\
    {\
        return _Module.UpdateRegistryFromResource(x, bRegister);\
    }
```

This function is called indirectly (through another function and a mapping of the `OBJECT_ENTRY` map) through the `DllRegisterServer()` and `DllUnregisterServer()` implementations.

The `.rgs` file for our `AtlBlob` project is listed here:

```
HKCR
{
    AtlBlob.AtlBlob1.1 = s 'ATL Inproc Server'
    {
        CLSID = s '{4F831A65-1A55-11D2-B915-D9CBC3283F7C}'
    }
    AtlBlob.AtlBlob1 = s 'ATL Inproc Server'
    {
        CLSID = s '{4F831A65-1A55-11D2-B915-D9CBC3283F7C}'
        CurVer = s 'AtlBlob.AtlBlob1.1'
    }
    NoRemove CLSID
    {
        ForceRemove {4F831A65-1A55-11D2-B915-D9CBC3283F7C}
                = s 'ATL Inproc Server'
        {
            ProgID = s 'AtlBlob.AtlBlob1.1'
            VersionIndependentProgID = s 'AtlBlob.AtlBlob1'
            ForceRemove 'Programmable'
            InprocServer32 = s '%MODULE%'
            {
                val ThreadingModel = s 'Apartment'
            }
            'TypeLib' = s '{4F831A58-1A55-11D2-B915-D9CBC3283F7C}'
        }
    }
}
```

The syntax is actually readable and very easy to understand. Each successive level of curly braces indicates another level of subkeys. From the very top, we have HKCR, which is shorthand for HKEY_CLASSES_ROOT.

Right underneath this root, we create the second subkey which is AtlBlob.AtlBlob1 and it has a default string value of "ATL Inproc Server". Underneath this subkey, we have a named value called CLSID that has a string value of '{4F831A65-1A55-11D2-B915-D9CBC3283F7C}', and a named value called CurVer (this is the version dependent ProgID), with string value of AtlBlob.AtlBlob1.1.

The rest of the file follows the same pattern. Just compare this with all the code we had to write in the previous chapter, and imagine having to maintain that code!

There are a number of items worth mentioning here. All the keys specified in the .rgs file will be deleted during the unregister server phase. The deletion of a key by default is done during the unregistration process, but to prevent a subkey from being deleted at this time, you can use the NoRemove attribute before the subkey (for an example, see the CLSID subkey above). You don't have to mark the root key with NoRemove, since the registrar will not remove a root key. If you want to force the recursive deletion of a subkey prior to creation (at registration time), you can use the Force Remove attribute before the subkey. ATL has done this for us with the CLSID entry. It's also possible to precede a key name with the Delete attribute and have the key deleted during registration time.

The %MODULE% macro will be replaced by the actual qualified path of the executable or DLL during execution. A value can be preceded by an s, for a string value, or d, for a numeric DWORD value in decimal; there's no provision for hex entries, simply convert to decimal. You can also create a named value, instead of a subkey and a default value, using the val prefix.

Back to Our Object: Sing Along with Visual Basic

We've been saying for a long time that our object is an ActiveX control, yet we haven't seen any solid proof of this. An ActiveX control, thanks to the Internet extensions of the OC96 specification from Microsoft, is any in-process COM class that implements the IUnknown interface and can perform self registration/de-registration. Since AtlBlob is definitely an in-process COM class, we know that it implements the IUnknown interface, and we have see how ATL has provided self registration capabilities, we can safely say that it is an ActiveX control. Case closed!

To make you a full believer, we can investigate what more we need to do to get AtlBlob to work with Visual Basic 6 (assuming you have VB6 installed). It turns out, at least on the machine where you've been developing the ActiveX control, that there is nothing more you need to do! The control is ready to go. To enable your control in Visual Basic 6, all you need to do is add your type library to the list of project references. Select the References... option from the Project menu and look for the Atlblob 1.0 Type Library reference. Select it, then click OK:

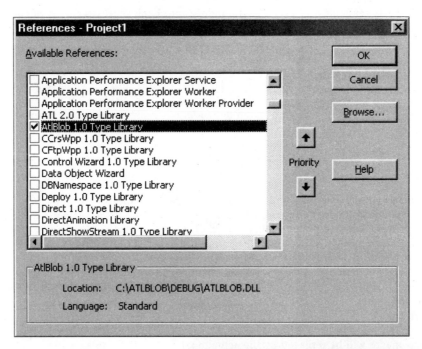

Visual Basic 6 can actually read and decipher the binary metadata inside the type library, and then can custom manufacture code to call your control. To see this for yourself, open the object browser (you can do this from the View menu or by hitting *F2*) and double click on the AtlBlob1 in the left hand window. You can then select the ATLBLOBLib entry to see the methods and the ThreadID property that we've created. Visual Basic is now ready to use the object!

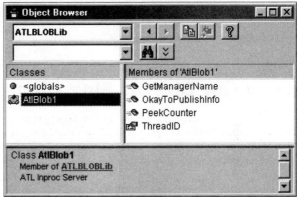

We'll create a very simple program now that tests out the ActiveX control. This program can be found in the \Ch4\atlmVB6 directory of the source distribution. It consists of a sample form with three buttons and four text fields on it. Whenever a button is pressed, an object instance of AtlBlob1 is created, its methods are called and the property values are set first, then read back. The instance is immediately released. A new instance of AtlBlob1 is created for each button press.

The form we'll use is shown below:

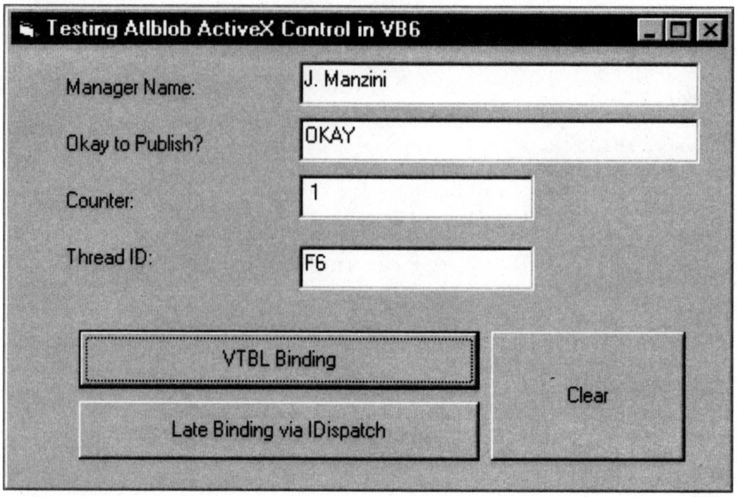

If you press the **Late Binding via IDispatch** button, late binding will be used. The following code will be executed:

```
Private Sub butLate_Click()

    Call butClear_Click
    Dim AnObj As Object
    Set AnObj = CreateObject("Atlblob.Atlblob1")

    txtManager.Text = AnObj.GetManagerName()
    flag = AnObj.OkayToPublishInfo(1990 + Int(Rnd * 100 + 1),
                                    Int(Rnd * 12 + 1))

    If flag Then
        txtOkay.Text = "OKAY"
    Else
        txtOkay.Text = "NO WAY"
    End If

    txtCounter.Text = Str$(AnObj.PeekCounter())
    txtThread.Text = Hex$(AnObj.ThreadID)
    Set AnObj = Nothing

End Sub
```

In this case, the `AnObj` variable is dimensioned as an `Object`. Visual Basic doesn't know anything about the object until one of its methods is called or the property is accessed. At that time, the `IDispatch::GetIDsOfNames()` method will be called, to get the ID of the method or property, and then `IDispatch::Invoke()` will be called, in order to manipulate the property or invoke the method. Nothing in this code took advantage of Visual Basic's ability to read the type library information.

If you press the **VTBL Binding** button, another routine with very similar code will be called. There are only two lines in this routine that are different:

```
Private Sub butEarly_Click()

    Call butClear_Click

    Dim AnObj As AtlBlob1
    Set AnObj = New AtlBlob1

    txtManager.Text = AnObj.GetManagerName()
    flag = AnObj.OkayToPublishInfo(1990 + Int(Rnd * 100 + 1),
                                    Int(Rnd * 12 + 1))

    If flag Then
        txtOkay.Text = "OKAY"
    Else
        txtOkay.Text = "NO WAY"
    End If

    txtCounter.Text = Str$(AnObj.PeekCounter())
    txtThread.Text = Hex$(AnObj.ThreadID)
    Set AnObj = Nothing

End Sub
```

The Clear button simply clears all the text boxes. It is shown here for completeness:

```
Private Sub butClear_Click()

    txtManager.Text = ""
    txtOkay.Text = ""
    txtCounter.Text = ""
    txtThread.Text = ""

End Sub
```

If you key this code in by hand, you will notice that Visual Basic 6 will use auto-completion to guide you everytime you're entering a method or property of AnObj.

In the early binding case, we have specifically pointed out to Visual Basic that AnObj will contain an object of the AtlBlob1 variety. Since Visual Basic has already read and understood the type library information of the Atlblob1 class, it knows the methods that the ICustomInterface2 interface supports, the arguments and the type of the arguments that the functions will require, their return values, and even the vtable order of the functions, given a pointer. In this case, Visual Basic can elect to either call into IDispatch::Invoke() using the information, or call into the vtable entries directly. This has tremendous benefit in terms of improving performance (typically doubling or more), since each and every call doesn't have to go through IDispatch::GetIDsOfNames() anymore. Visual Basic 6 can now take advantage of vtable binding. One can imagine the possibilities of combining the best of what Visual Basic and the native C++ language has to offer in a complex application. As a bonus with the ActiveX component approach, the same component is reusable by others within any other compatible programming language or programming environment.

Let's now revisit one key statement that was made earlier. We basically said (no pun intended) that Visual Basic was able to find our ActiveX control only on the machine where the control was compiled and built. Why? It turns out that Visual Basic was able to find information regarding our control because its type library was registered with the system. Recall that a type library contains the information (in a binary form) that we've placed into the IDL file (the interfaces, methods, properties, IIDs, object descriptions, etc.). By default, the ATL generated registration routine will register the type library and interfaces of the COM server with the system. This is done in the implementation of the DllRegisterServer() function inside the AtlBlob.cpp file:

```
STDAPI DllRegisterServer(void)
{
    // registers object, typelib and all interfaces in typelib
    return _Module.RegisterServer(TRUE);
}
```

If you don't want to register the type library information, you can pass FALSE as a parameter into the _Module.RegisterServer() call. Since the build file that ATL creates for you will automatically load your DLL and execute the DllRegisterServer() call, the type library and interface information was entered into the registry. If you were to move the COM server (DLL) to another machine, you must remember to run REGSVR32 ATLBLOB.DLL to get this information into the registry before Visual Basic will be happy. You can do this within your Setup utility if you're distributing more than a few copies.

Deploying Our ActiveX Control on a Web Page

Next, we'll try to operate our ActiveX control from a web page viewed from Internet Explorer 4. Later, in our Intranet programming, this will be performed frequently. We'll assume that we're using a WYSIWYG tool to create the web page. In our case, we'll use FrontPage 98, which supports the laying out of ActiveX controls.

The sample web page can be found in the \Ch4\atlmFP98 directory of the source code download. Unlike Visual Basic, FrontPage 98 doesn't read the type libraries registered with the attributes database to come up with its list of ActiveX controls. Instead, it depends on an extra subkey under the HKEY_CLASSES_ROOT\CLSID\{---} entry to determine if a specific COM object is a control. Appropriately enough, the key is named Control. Be aware, though, that this is the 'old' way of identifying COM objects as ActiveX controls. Microsoft is recommending a new standard based on UUIDs, called components categories, in the OC96 specifications. We'll give a synopsis of the OC96 specification in Chapter 5. In the (hopefully near) future, more and more containers will implement this new standard. For now, though, just adding the Control subkey to our .rgs file and rebuilding the project will suffice.

The new .rgs file now looks like this:

```
HKCR
{
...

    NoRemove CLSID
    {
```

```
ForceRemove {04476DFC-D784-11D1-A660-006052008075}
                = s 'ATL Inproc Server'
    {
        ....
        'TypeLib' = s '{7882E1C1-D8A2-11D1-A660-006052008075}'
        'Control' = s ' '
    }
  }
}
```

Now, we should be ready to start up the FrontPage 98 editor. Click on the Insert menu, select the Advanced... selection, and then choose ActiveX Control.... We'll see the ATL Inproc Server as a selection. Give it a name: myAtlBlob, and then click the OK button:

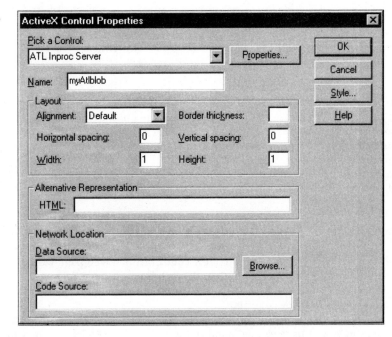

At this point, the control automatically is embedded into the page, and you're ready to call its methods and set its property from the scripting language. The actual HTML involved in embedding the ActiveX control is shown here:

```
<object ID="myAtlblob" WIDTH="1" HEIGHT="1"
    CLASSID="CLSID:04476DFC-D784-11D1-A660-006052008075"></object>
```

Since our target browser is Internet Explorer 4, we have a choice of using either VBScript or JScript for scripting. For illustration purposes, we'll be using VBScript. We'll set up a web page with various HTML form controls which looks and acts very similar to our Visual Basic example. Using FrontPage 98 you can lay out a page as follows (you can use Notepad or Visual Interdev instead if you find it more comfortable):

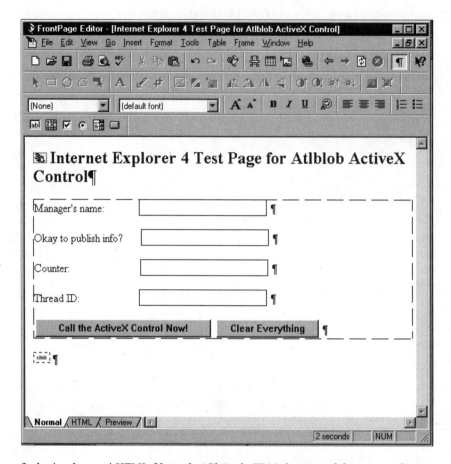

You can find a 'ready-to-go' HTML file in the \Ch4\atlmFP98 directory of the source code distribution. However, you'll need to change the CLSID of the control if you created the control yourself.

The four input fields and the two buttons are HTML form elements. We used standard HTML form controls instead of the ActiveX equivalent from FrontPage 98, so that the actual HTML page was kept simple. You can see a **FrontPage bot** (this is a markup bot which allows me to add raw HTML into the code generated) right at the top – within this bot, we have defined a VBScript procedure. A FrontPage bot is a runtime agent that performs a specific function when the web page is accessed. The ActiveX control is embedded in the lower left-hand corner (appearing as a gray square, since we don't do any UI). We call the methods and the property of the AtlBlob ActiveX control in the ONCLICK event of the button labeled Call the ActiveX Control Now!

If you're following along using Notepad as an HTML editor, the following is the required HTML file:

```
<html>

<head>
<title>Internet Explorer 4 Test Page for AtlBlob
ActiveX Control</title>
</head>

<body>
<script LANGUAGE="VBScript">
<!--
Sub ClearForm()
Document.MyForm.txtOkay.value = ""
Document.MyForm.txtManager.value = ""
Document.MyForm.txtCounter.value = ""
Document.MyForm.txtThread.value = ""
end sub
-->
</script>

<p><strong>
<big><big>Internet Explorer 4 Test Page
for AtlBlob ActiveX Control </big> </big> </strong></p>

<form ACTION="--WEBBOT-SELF--" METHOD="POST" NAME="MyForm">

<p>Manager's name:
<input TYPE="text" SIZE="20" NAME="txtManager">
</p>

<p>Okay to publish info?
<input TYPE="text" SIZE="20" NAME="txtOkay"> </p>
<p>Counter:
<input TYPE="text" SIZE="20" NAME="txtCounter"> </p>

<p>Thread ID:
<input TYPE="text" SIZE="20" NAME="txtThread"> </p>

<p><input LANGUAGE="VBScript" TYPE="button" VALUE="Call the
ActiveX Control Now!"
   ONCLICK="Document.MyForm.txtManager.value =
                              myAtlBlob.GetManagerName()
randomize

inYear = rnd() * 100 + 1900
inMonth = rnd() * 12 + 1

Flag = myAtlBlob.OkayToPublishInfo(inYear, inMonth)
if Flag then
 Document.MyForm.txtOkay.value = &quot;OKAY&quot;
else
 Document.MyForm.txtOkay.value = &quot;NOWAY&quot;
end if

Document.MyForm.txtCounter.value = myAtlBlob.PeekCounter()
```

```
Document.MyForm.txtThread.value = Hex(myAtlBlob.ThreadID)"
  NAME="CallBut"> <input TYPE="reset" VALUE="Clear Everything" NAME="ClearBut">
</p>
</form>

<p>
<object ID="myAtlBlob" WIDTH="1" HEIGHT="1" align=" "
CLASSID="CLSID:04476DFC-D784-11D1-A660-006052008075">
</object>
</p>
</body>
</html>
```

Notice the code in the ONCLICK handler of the CallBut button. The syntax here is quite similar between VBScript and Visual Basic. However, there isn't any Dim or Set statement for object manipulation, because the model of operation is quite different. With Visual Basic applications, we have the flexibility to instantiate and free the ActiveX control/COM server whenever we want programmatically. Under Internet Explorer, the lifetime of an ActiveX control on a page is the same as the lifetime of the page. When it is in view and active, the ActiveX control is initialized and ready for action. As soon as the user moves to another page, the object instance is released and the functionality is no longer available, so there's no way that you can manage object lifetime programmatically using VBScript.

Since you can't use the Dim or Set statements, you can't control the binding method that's used. VBScript in IE 4 will always use the lower performance late binding. This is plainly evident during debugging, since the script engine will not detect a method that belongs to the object until the method is actually invoked. You can use the VBScript debugger that comes with Visual Studio 98 to debug your VBScript programs. Every variable in VBScript is a variant. The variant type is a monstrous union of almost all the frequently used data types, and a few of the quainter ones.

Here are some of the most common data types. The VARTYPE value (enumerated value) is used to signify the type of the variant. Special functions exist (and their use is strongly encouraged) that convert between variant types:

VARTYPE values	Description
VT_EMPTY	No value specified
VT_U1	Unsigned 1-byte char
VT_I2	2-byte integer
VT_U2	Unsigned 2-byte integer
VT_I4	4-byte integer
VT_U4	Unsigned 4-byte integer
VT_R4	4-byte real value
VT_CY	8-byte currency number

Table Continued on Following Page

VARTYPE values	Description
VT_BSTR	A string in a <length, data> format
VT_NULL	Null value
VT_ERROR	An error information structure
VT_BOOL	A Boolean value (0 or 0xFFFF)
VT_DATE	Date represented as a double-precision number
VT_DISPATCH	Pointer to an object implementing IDispatch
VT_UNKNOWN	Pointer to an object implementing IUnknown
VT_ARRAY	Array of data of any kind

Using VARIANTs make script programming substantially easier – the engine will always try to convert types to fit whatever the programmer is doing, freeing him or her from ever worrying about type conversions. In practice, we know from experience that there are many problems associated with a 'one type fits all' system. These systems frequently end up making us understand and memorize a complex set of often inconsistent type conversion situations and rules.

Finally, we can test our ActiveX control on a web page. Try it out by loading the page that you've created using Internet Explorer 4, press the button. Depending on your security settings, you should be greeted by a security alert dialog when you try to call the control:

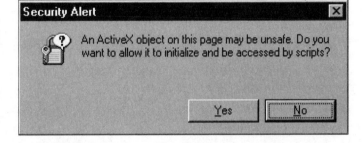

The default security level of IE 4 (medium) will warn about ActiveX controls being used by a script that is not marked "Safe for Scripting". If you select Yes, then the page will work normally. While FrontPage 98 does *not* support the Component Categories specification in OC96, Internet Explorer 4 does. Therefore, it is anticipating a CATID key in the attributes database, which indicates that the control is safe for scripting. We can add this to our .rgs file and recompile the AtlBlob project.

```
HKCR
{
...

    NoRemove CLSID
    {
        ForceRemove {04476DFC-D784-11D1-A660-006052008075}
                            = s 'ATL Inproc Server'
        {
            ....
            'TypeLib' =
                    s '{7882E1C1-D8A2-11D1-A660-006052008075}'
```

```
            'Control' = s' '
           'Implemented Categories'
           {
               '{7DD95801-9882-11CF-9FA9-00AA006C42C4}'
               '{7DD95802-9882-11CF-9FA9-00AA006C42C4}'
           }
       }
    }
}
```

The GUIDs above are the required CATIDs. "Safe for Scripting" simply means that the control cannot harm the computer client even by malicious scripts. An ActiveX control is likely to be safe provided it doesn't allow a script to specify (through any methods) the source or target of any file and/or registry operations.

If you try the HTML page again, everything should work fine without the security alert. The page should look like this:

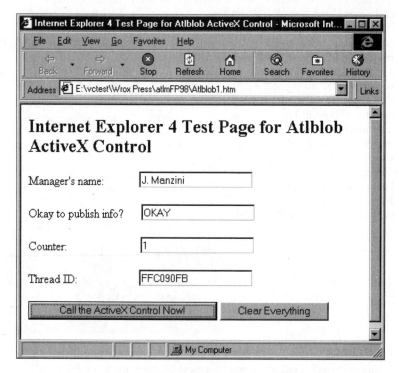

Now, try selecting File|New|Window, press the call button again, notice that the user count is now 2 and that the thread ID is now different! This reveals how Internet Explorer 4 handles threading – one new STA thread per Internet Explorer 4 window. ActiveX controls supporting Apartment threading works great inside IE 4. We can easily use IE 4 as a replacement multithread test tool for our AtlBlob!

Deploying Our ActiveX Control within Visual J++ Applications

Being able to use our AtlBlob business object from C++, Visual Basic and Internet Explorer has assured us of the programming language neutrality of COM components. As a final example, we will take a look at the very popular language for the Internet: Java. Specifically, we will see how to make use of the same object within a Visual J++ 6 application. We will be using the Visual J++ 6 IDE and the Windows Foundation Classes (WFC) components to create our user interface.

Open your Visual J++ IDE and create a new Windows Application target project. Name this project atlmJAVA. You can also find the related source code in the \Ch4\atlmJAVA directory of the source code download from the Wrox Press website.

Next, you need to create a Java code wrapper for the AtlBlob. Visual J++ is superior to FrontPage 98 in this aspect since it, too, reads registered type library information to make our life easier. The Java code wrapper can be generated automatically from the type library information by selecting **Add Com Wrapper...** from the **Project** menu:

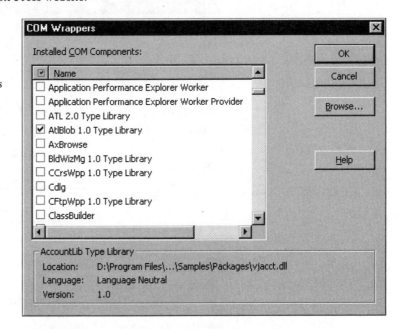

Select the AtlBlob type library as shown above, and Visual J++ will generate the appropriate wrapper classes – enabling you to access its methods directly.

Next, layout the form using the Form Designer and the WFC components to look like this. We name the edit boxes (from top to bottom) txtManager, txtOkay, txtCounter and txtThread. The two buttons we'll call butCall and butClear:

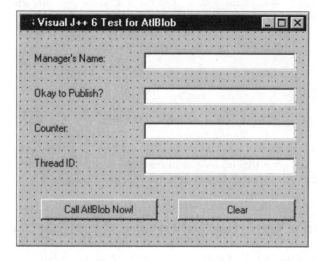

Add the following lines to the header portion of the code generated by Visual J++ 6:

```
import com.ms.wfc.app.*;
import com.ms.wfc.core.*;
import com.ms.wfc.ui.*;
import atlblob.*;
import java.util.*;
```

The import atlblob.* brings the COM wrapper classes into the namespace, and the java.util.* is used for random number generation and float to integer conversion. Finally, we add the onclick event handler for both buttons.

```
private void butCall_click(Object source, Event e)
{
    Random myRand = new Random();
    Atlblob1 myBlob = new Atlblob1();
    txtManager.setText(myBlob.GetManagerName());
    int iYear = Math.round(myRand.nextFloat() * 100) + 1900;
    int iMonth = Math.round(myRand.nextFloat() * 12);

    if (myBlob.OkayToPublishInfo(iYear,iMonth))
        txtOkay.setText("OKAY");
    else
        txtOkay.setText("NOWAY");

    txtCounter.setText(Integer.toString(myBlob.PeekCounter()));
    txtThread.setText(Integer.toHexString(myBlob.getThreadID()));
}
```

This code is amazingly similar to the Visual Basic vtable binding example, you don't even have to know Java to appreciate it. The click handler for `cmdClear` is trivial:

```
private void cmdClear_click(Object sender, Event e)
{
    txtManager.setText("");
    txtOkay.setText("");
    txtCounter.setText("");
    txtThread.setText("");
}
```

That's it. All you need to do now is build the application and run it. It works as expected, re-assuring us once again that a piece of business logic built as an ActiveX control can be used and re-used by applications written in any language.

Ready for the Intranet Challenge

ATL 3, while still young in its age, is becoming a robust, mean-and-lean library for building high performance, just-big-enough software components. Visual C++ 6's support for integrating MFC with ATL provides the best of both worlds for application developers – the ability to use a mature, robust directory for maintaining legacy code, and leveraging all of ATL's features at the same time. In this chapter, we have examined the design objective and rationale behind ATL. We browsed inside and studied the architecture of ATL and saw what makes it tick.

The powerful simplicity of ATL 3 has allowed us to cover a lot of ground in this chapter. The native COM support of Visual C++ 6 really simplifies COM programming, and reduces the amount of code we have to write to build great COM clients. We completed the construction of our business rule ActiveX control using ATL 3 with great ease, and implemented our interface as a dual interface, allowing it to be used by scripting languages and Internet Explorer 4 immediately. We tested the control with C++, Visual Basic, and VBScript, J++, and it worked equivalently well on every platform.

Now, armed with a solid understanding of COM fundamentals and a powerful tool collection like Visual C++ 6 and ATL 3, we're ready to tackle more Intranet programming problems with an eye towards component based solutions. Along the way, we'll be covering a few more advanced COM topics, and showing how ATL and other tools can really help in constructing highly functional Distributed interNet Applications.

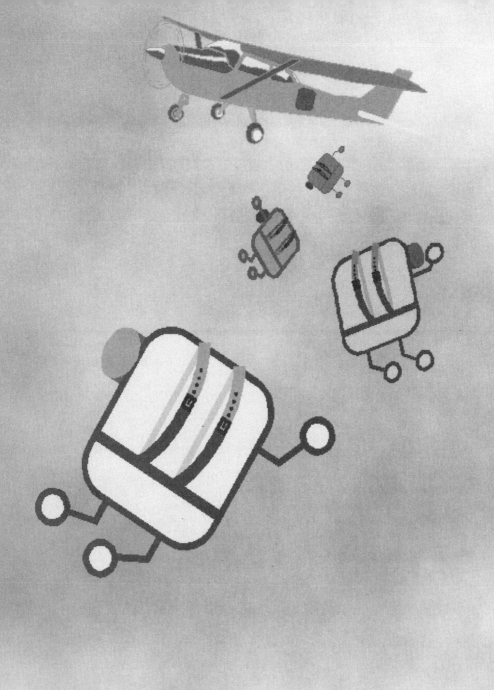

5

All About Controls

In this chapter, we start by examining what constitutes a full control, and how these relate to the simple ActiveX controls that we have been building in the last two chapters. We'll go on to take a detailed look at the OC94 and OC96 specifications for ActiveX controls and at the way controls need to implement interfaces to support these standards. There are several performance optimization techniques in this specification that are supported by modern containers (such as Internet Explorer 4.01 and later) that we will be examining.

Along the way, we'll see what help we can get from ATL 3 in the implementation of these interfaces, and how Visual C++ and ATL really simplify the construction of visual components conforming to optimizations in the newer OC96 specifications. In Chapter 7, we'll get a chance to put some of this theory into practice when we create a visual calendar control.

By the end of Chapter 7, you will be comfortable with both the OC94 and OC96 specifications, understand the requirements and implications of building visual ActiveX controls, and be able to build them quickly using ATL 3 and Visual C++ 6. This topic alone used to consume entire books, but the 'power-tool' nature of ATL 3 and Visual C++ 6 allow us to cover the same material in the space of two intensive chapters.

Sources of Confusion

Before we begin, let's clear up a likely source of confusion. It's important to realize that Microsoft's marketing department is pushing a multiyear, multimillion dollar effort in establishing a brand identity for **Distributed interNet Application** (DNA) architecture. Everything and anything coming out of Microsoft that's associated with multi-tiered, Internet or intranet-based applications will be labeled under the DNA technology umbrella. Unfortunately, this can be confusing because many of the newly labeled pieces already have well-established, accepted industry names.

A good example is an ActiveX control. When an ActiveX control is used in the middle-tier (on a server attached to the client), it is now called a **DNA business object**. To further mix metaphors, the set of DNA (intranet applications) within the enterprise is also branded as the 'Digital Nervous System' of the enterprise.

In order to clarify things, let's define some terms we're using throughout this book:

❑ **COM component** – Implements IUnknown

❑ **ActiveX control** – A COM component that is self-registering

❑ **Full control** – An ActiveX control that implements the OC94 and/or OC96 specifications

❑ **Business object** – A design / architectural term, referring to an ActiveX control that performs a specific function, and forms a part of a 'black box' component

There are some legacy terms that we will avoid:

❑ OLE control – The ideas are subsumed into ActiveX and full controls

❑ OCX – This is a full control, and the interfaces supported by a control are more important than the file extension

❑ Lite control – A term from the Insert ATL Object wizard; such controls support the OC96 specification, but they aren't really that 'lite' compared to the 'full' controls (13 as opposed to 19 interfaces)

Any control that has elements applicable to Internet/intranet use should be labeled as ActiveX. We will sub-classify non-visual controls that work in the three-tier server space as middle-tier DNA business objects and data-tier objects, depending on their role.

However, in our coverage of the specifications (i.e. OC96), we'll attempt to use the terminology adopted by the particular specification being examined.

Advance Warning for Avid Readers

If you're the type of reader who likes to read chapters in a book in sequential order, please pay close attention. It's now a good time to power off your development station, and get a pot of coffee ready. In this chapter, we'll condense several complex specifications from Microsoft, and nail down numerous advanced concepts. All this is in preparation for the equally intense coding chapters to follow.

We have adopted this style of presentation to deliver the maximum amount of practical technology information within the confines of this book. If you find going through this chapter rather rough on first reading, don't worry – many of the concepts will be reinforced by actual code in later chapters. Overall, this chapter lends itself to a 'quick read' the first time through, and then serves as a reference point for later explorations.

Introduction to ActiveX Controls

We'll start with an introduction to visual ActiveX controls. In this section, we'll also examine in some detail the evolution of the *de facto* standards and new specifications that Microsoft is pushing. At the same time, we'll note the subtle ways in which this evolution has been influenced by the Internet and intranet.

Creating a Product Family

Visual Basic 3.X created a rapidly growing component market that surprised many pundits. By using code to arrange and orchestrate its self-contained user interface made up of 'visual components', the Visual Basic programmer can rapidly create sophisticated applications from well-tested, industrial strength components. The entire process is simple, and most construction steps are highly visual. This simplicity in application construction has attracted over three million programmers to the tool in its five short years of existence.

The VBX components used in Visual Basic 3.X were fundamentally flawed, since they took advantage of many specific 16-bit Windows/Intel platform features. Microsoft's answer was the OLE Control (or OCX). By the time Visual Basic 4.0 was released, most of the VBX vendors had migrated to the new OCX architecture for their bread-and-butter components. The OCX architecture was designed so that Visual Basic was no longer the sole 'hosting' application.

In addition, Microsoft has taken great pains to expand the tools with which one can create full ActiveX controls.

Anatomy of a Full Control

In this section, we'll take a brief look at some of the ideas and terminology involved with full ActiveX controls, including:

- ❏ Methods and properties
- ❏ Ambient and extended properties
- ❏ Event sourcing
- ❏ Interactions between the control and the container
- ❏ Persistence

Methods and Properties

Methods are functions that the users of a control may invoke; this is identical in action to the interface methods that we created for our COM components in the early chapters. **Properties** are attributes of the component that the component user can change, although some may be read-only and/or hidden. In actual implementation, properties too are functions. Each read/write property corresponds to two functions, one to 'get' the value of a property, and one to 'set' its value. This is direct application of automation properties, which we discussed in Chapter 2.

Ambient Properties

Optionally, the container or hosting application may also provide something called **ambient properties**. Visual Basic as a host provides a comprehensive set of ambient properties. Ambient properties are properties through which the hosting environment can indicate 'preferences' or 'hints' to all the child components that it contains. Essentially, these are suggestions that the control should follow if it doesn't want to appear alien to the end user. For example, one ambient property may contain the suggested font for the object to use, while another one may contain the suggested background color. In this way, the component can blend in with the host application.

Extended Properties

In addition to ambient properties, if the container is a programming tool, it may optionally provide a set of **extended properties** with each embedded control. To the programmer using the control, these extended properties look no different from those implemented by the control. However, they are actually implemented by the programming tool container (support provided at runtime by the programming tool's runtime library) and are made available to the programmer together with all the properties provided by the control. Some typical extended properties include the Top, Left, Width, and Height properties of a control in Visual Basic. Since the container implements these properties for every control, they save the control implementer a significant amount of work.

A property may also be classified in other ways:

❑   As persistent (saved with the container) or transient (not saved, and valid only while the object is instantiated)

❑   As available at runtime only, at both runtime and design time, or design time only

Events

Another powerful mechanism that the full control provides, and that ActiveX controls in general can use, is **event sourcing**. Event sourcing allows the control to trigger actions in the container. For example, a method in the container (or say, a Visual Basic procedure managed by the container) can be called whenever a user clicks on the visual representation of the full ActiveX control. This sort of 'reverse calling' action is implemented through the versatile **connection points** mechanism that we discussed in Chapter 2.

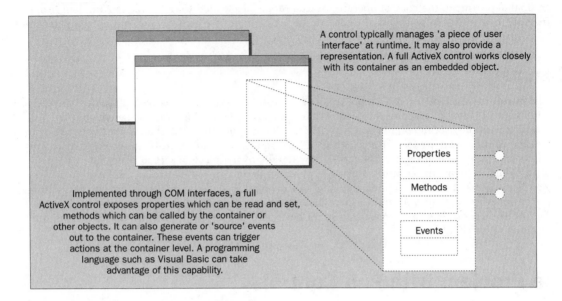

A control typically manages 'a piece of user interface' at runtime. It may also provide a representation. A full ActiveX control works closely with its container as an embedded object.

Implemented through COM interfaces, a full ActiveX control exposes properties which can be read and set, methods which can be called by the container or other objects. It can also generate or 'source' events out to the container. These events can trigger actions at the container level. A programming language such as Visual Basic can take advantage of this capability.

Properties

Methods

Events

Interactions with Container

Interactions between a hosting container and a control are performed through a well-defined set of COM interfaces – that is, the container uses a well known contract (interface) to access the component. These interfaces are issued by Microsoft, so that components can be written independently of containers, and the application put together at runtime, if necessary.

Support for Persistence

Properties of a full ActiveX control can be set or changed visually within visual programming environments, such as Visual Basic. Either the design time host (e.g. Visual Basic) or the control itself may provide a set of property sheets for modifying the value of the properties. These property values can be set at design time, and then **persisted**, or saved as blobs into the container's image, which will be compiled into a part of the final executable. When the program is executed by the end user, these persisted properties are restored and the control will initialize as it was configured.

Run (User) Mode vs Design Mode

For development environment such as Visual Basic 6 and FrontPage 98, it is often important for a full ActiveX control to determine whether it is being manipulated during the development process, or whether it is being actually deployed in the final application. Take, for example, a control that displays different graphics when not under actual deployment. When our calendar control (which we'll create in Chapter 7) is being configured, it displays a fake grid without connecting to the backend database. When a developer is working with the control in the development environment, the control is operating in **Design Mode**.

In final deployment, the control operates in **Run Mode** (also called **User Mode**). An ambient property from the container can be accessed to determine which mode the control is in, but unfortunately, not all containers support these modes, so you must be careful to check for this.

Summary

The main difference between a simple ActiveX control (like the one we coded in the last chapter) and a full control is that a full control typically manages certain visual user interface elements, and interacts with the user in conjunction with its containing application. All interactions between control and the container are performed through COM interfaces, so a full control implements many more COM interfaces. The full ActiveX control may literally own a piece of screen real estate within a form (which contains the control). During application design time, a control is displayed in a 'What You See Is What You Get' manner, showing how it would look in the final application. This allows the designer to tweak its appearance incrementally without having to recompile and test each time. The ActiveX controls we've constructed so far have no user interface elements, and implement only a minimal set of COM interfaces.

The Problem with Full Controls

There is only one problem with building full controls – it's notoriously hard to do! In order to build a full control that can be hosted in a variety of containers, one has to create code which implements a very large set of complex COM interfaces. This assumes that the builder is completely familiar with COM, the OLE Control interface specifications, as well as the style of COM support provided by the development tool or code library.

Let's look at a typical full control, the 'Microsoft Forms 2.0 CommandButton' from Visual Basic 6, and see what COM interfaces it implements. Here's what you'll see when you look at it through Oleview.exe:

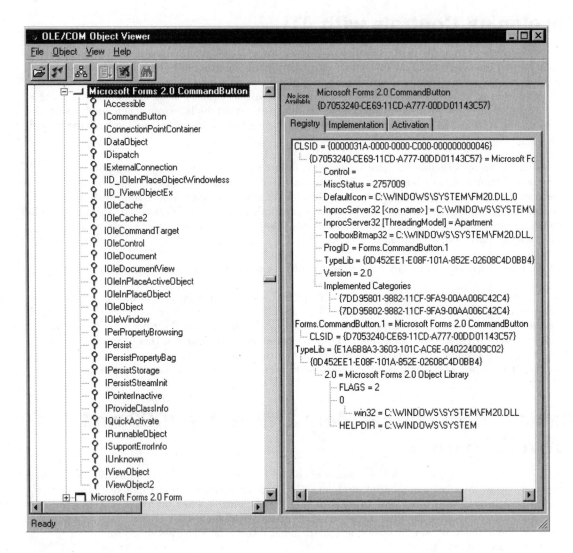

Interface Overload

Besides the `IUnknown`, `IDispatch`, and a custom `ICommandButton` interface, the full control shown in the above screenshot implements a long list of other complex, yet essential interfaces. Remember that all this particular control does for a hosting application is to provide a button that the end user can click on!

Contrast its almost trivial function with the amount of work required above and beyond a simple `CreateWindow()` call, and you'll see what we mean by hard work.

Developing Controls with ATL

Even though we can apply the techniques that we've covered in the COM and ATL chapters to construct all the required COM interfaces, significant time and effort still needs to be spent on implementing and testing all the interfaces and methods. Even just to walk you through the code necessary to implement the above button control alone would require a book of a similar size to this one! Most of this monumental work needs to be done just so that the full control can coexist with the hosting application. We haven't even thought about coding the actual processing logic for the control yet.

A tool to make constructing full controls easier is an obvious necessity. The 'configurable code generating' nature of C++ templates, which we discussed in Chapter 4, is perfect for creating lean controls that contain just enough code to implement the required functionality and satisfy the OLE control specifications. What's more, ATL is ideal for implementing the COM based interfaces of a full control, as it makes use of C++'s ability to multiply inherit from default implementations and override ones that require custom implementation.

At the time of writing, ATL is by far the most popular way of creating ActiveX controls in C++.

Highly competitive development by Sun Microsystems with Java and JavaBeans has forced Microsoft into providing easier and easier way of building ActiveX controls. To this end, Microsoft has poured tremendous resources into ensuring that Visual Basic 6, Visual J++ 6, and scripting languages like VBScript and/or JavaScript can be used to quickly create ActiveX controls. However, due to the heavy runtime support and (typically) interpreted nature of these programming languages/environments, there is some loss of performance, flexibility, and code compactness.

Making OLE Controls More Efficient – OC96 and ActiveX Controls

ATL provides us with a more efficient means of coding controls, but the fact remains that the controls require support for a large number of interfaces. Component software vendors had just barely finished migrating their 16-bit VBX to the new 32 bit OLE controls when the Internet frenzy hit. In an effort to accommodate the then current controls and allow them to coexist peacefully in a world soon to be populated by newer, leaner, and more generic controls, Microsoft opted for a subclassification hierarchy.

This was done through the **OLE Control 96** (or **OC96**) specification, and a subsequent addendum known as the 'ActiveX Control/COM Objects for the Internet'. The earlier specification for OLE controls is now called **OC94**, a term we'll use from now on to differentiate the two specifications.

Optimization of control size and performance is the prevailing theme in OC96. New interfaces replace older, bulkier interfaces and perform various optimizations. The dependency on a Windows handle, the very last remaining link between controls and the underlying Windows operating system, is now made optional. The OC96 controls are not only smaller and run faster, but may also be adapted to operate on a variety of operating systems or hardware platforms. Since many of the optimizations in the OC96 specification require the developer to re-design and re-code both the container and control, the migration to the new standard is proceeding rather slowly. In fact, Internet Explorer 4.01 arriving in mid 1997, is the first stable and widely available OC96 container in the world. Visual Studio 98 is the first Microsoft development suite providing hosting containers (in Visual Basic 6, Visual C++ 6, and Visual J++ 6 applications) supporting the OC96 specification.

In order to qualify as an ActiveX control in OC96, a COM object is required only to implement the IUnknown interface and support self-registration. As we've learnt in previous chapters, this makes almost any COM object technically an ActiveX control compliant with OC96. Such controls, although not full controls, can implement business rules or provide support for hosted full controls.

In this chapter, we'll study in detail many of the new optimizations introduced by OC96, and how ATL 3 simplifies the implementation of these.

Server-side ActiveX Controls – DNA Business Objects

Having successfully fueled the flame of excitement for component-based design for desktop applications, Microsoft moved to the more formidable task of component-based software construction on the server side. In theory, it is as simple as moving non-visual ActiveX controls from the desktop client to the back-end server. In reality, the picture is considerably more complex. First and foremost, Microsoft does not yet own the server market!

The server-side market is currently dominated by a mix of mid-range, high-availability UNIX servers and low to high end mainframe machines, all running software untouched by Microsoft. The MIS business world, even today – two decades after the proclaimed death of the mainframe – is still full of plush and elegant multi-million dollar 'human networking' executive pow-wows, followed by renewal of equally high valued hardware upgrade plans, software rental and/or maintenance contracts. Microsoft's way of doing business appears guerilla in comparison.

Microsoft's Windows NT operating system is gaining momentum and making in-roads into departmental and (some) enterprise servers of medium to large size businesses. At the same time, the BackOffice servers are growing steadily to handle the varying requirements of business clients. Notwithstanding earlier versions of the stable SQL Server (which originally was a spin-off from early collaboration-turned-competition effort with Sybase), most of the servers in the BackOffice suite are brand-new code. This is not a feature to tout when you ask corporations to bet their business on your server operating system. However, a Windows NT based enterprise solution, despite all the risks associated with it, has one big advantage over its competition – it is an order of magnitude lower in cost!

Two decades of unchanged existence should convince anybody that a revolution in the server computing world is unlikely, and that a grassroots evolution is the only sane route to take. As part of this, a clear division of labor has to be laid out between Microsoft and their developers while they work to change the way that medium and small businesses do their computing. The 'component strategy' is a good strategy, since it has proven its worthiness on the desktop.

An ActiveX control can use the services of the Windows NT operating system. These services are enhanced by the variety of BackOffice servers available for Windows NT 4 Server. Here is just a partial list:

- SQL Server – for relational database management
- Transaction Server – for deploying distributed applications and managing distributed transactions
- Message Queue Server – for providing transaction compatible 'store and forward' capability
- Internet Information Server – for Web based services and applications
- System Management Server – for enterprise wide hardware and software configuration and management
- Exchange Server – for messaging (text based email, or eventually multimedia voice and video)
- Certificate Server – for implementing public-key based security
- SNA Server – for interoperability with legacy mainframe systems

With these generic services in place, Microsoft can safely convince developers that most of their hard work has already been done for them – for the measly cost of the servers themselves. Taking a page from the mainframe software development book, Microsoft is working towards alleviating some core server application development difficulties:

- Working efficiently for multiple concurrent user requests
- Handling resource contention in a high-concurrency environment
- Scaling the application from small to large to giant systems
- Maximizing computing resources when more than one processor and/or server machine is available
- Maintaining system integrity and surviving hardware failures

It is true that if you use all the tools and OS facilities available on Windows NT, you can implement solutions that achieve some of the above benefits – at great cost and effort. On the other hand, as long as you're willing to create ActiveX controls which conform to certain requirements laid down by Microsoft, you can enjoy all the above mentioned benefits without tackling any of the above issues yourself. By fitting into this framework, a server-side ActiveX control can be written as if it is servicing only a single user on a single thread. By virtue of being (deep) inside the framework, Microsoft will ensure that the work performed by the control can take advantage of all the items above.

ActiveX controls written in this fashion are typically quite simple, and encapsulate a single piece of domain specific business logic. For this reason, these controls are frequently called **DNA business objects**. The logic they implement – the business rules – typically reflects how an organization conducts business. Thus, one frequently reads this buzzword-filled reference: *DNA business objects encapsulate business rules in the middle tier*. Since they have no need to manage any user interface or to access any low-level system resources, Visual Basic 6 and Visual J++ 6 are frequently used to create DNA business objects. Such objects typically maintain their state in a database server and orchestrate other actions through the services of the BackOffice servers, so the minor performance penalty imposed by the interpretive environment is easily justified by their ease of use and prototyping.

In later chapters, we will be constructing our own set of DNA business objects using ATL 3 for our calendaring system.

ActiveX Controls Genealogy

With DNA business objects and OC96 containers in full force, combined with the component vendor's slow conversion to full OC96 compliance, the ActiveX control landscape is more confusing than ever. The following diagram attempts to summarize the variety of controls you're likely to find on your systems (and in the market place):

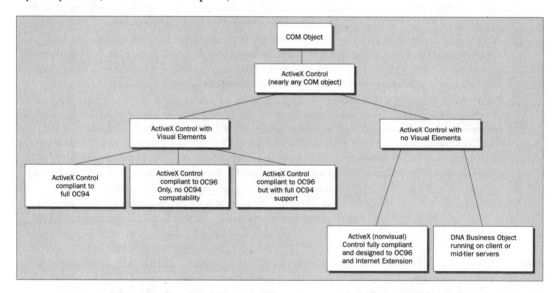

❑ **ActiveX Control** – This refers to nearly any COM object by Microsoft's definition. Any object that implements IUnknown and is self-registering is qualified as an ActiveX control.

❑ **Visual ActiveX Control** – These are closer to what we typically considered to be a 'control'. They usually have a visible appearance, such as a button, list box, combo box or a text box. Besides managing the actual data processing or manipulation, these controls also handle their own user interface interactions. They co-operate extensively with the container in managing the user interface.

- ❏ **Non-visual ActiveX Controls** – These are frequently called hidden or invisible controls. Typically, they don't handle any user interface interactions. Instead, they may handle data conversion, data processing, validation or business rule implementations. Not having to deal with the complex and tricky user interface handling, non-visual ActiveX controls allow the developer to concentrate on the data processing problem, without introducing unnecessary complexity. Such controls split task responsibility and can feed many visual controls.

- ❏ **Visual Control (Compliant with OC94 only)** – Most existing controls fall into this category. These are typically large controls that implement all the required OC94 interfaces. They are marked as a 'control' in the registry under the HROOT\CLASSES\<CLSID> subkey. These controls work well with all currently available containers including Visual Basic 6, Visual C++ 6, Internet Explorer 4 and FrontPage 98. They also work with the previous generation of containers including Visual Studio 97 and Internet Explorer 3.

- ❏ **Visual Control (Compliant with OC96 only)** – Sometimes also called **lite controls**, these are newer lightweight controls built to the optimizations specified in the OC96 specification (of which we'll see more very soon). These sort of controls have been unpopular so far, *not* due to complexity in implementation, but mainly due to lack of commercial containers which support the full OC96 specifications. This has changed with the arrival of Internet Explorer 4.01 and Visual Studio 6.

- ❏ **Visual Control (Compliant with OC96 and OC94)** – Also called **full controls**, this type is for control developers or vendors who are committed to supporting both standards fully, either for the widest market share or for backward compatibility. These controls are typically registered under \HKEY\CLASSES\ROOT, as well as listed under the component categories key.

- ❏ **Non-visual Control (Fully Compliant with OC96)** – Although they are non-visual, these controls assist the container in handling and rendering the control to the end user. They do so by providing an icon and one or more component categories to allow the container to determine whether the control is one that it would like or is allowed to host.

- ❏ **Non-visual Control (DNA Business Objects)** – These non-visual ActiveX controls may run on the client desktop, or any server in a multi-tiered distributed system. Each control encapsulates the implementation of a business rule or some business objects. These controls perform their data manipulation through services provided by the BackOffice family of servers. Instead of being compliant with OC96 standards, these controls are typically compliant to the requirements of the BackOffice servers, whose services they may use (MTS, for example, has specific requirements).

- ❏ A bonus is that OC96 strongly recommends that any new containers should be prepared to accommodate any ActiveX controls, although the control only has to implement one interface, IUnknown. Most new OC96 compliant containers should be able to host these minimal COM controls.

Internet Explorer 4 has legitimized the creation of OC96 compliant controls. All visual ActiveX projects starting today should be built to this standard to 'future proof' them. The Visual Studio 6 suite of development tools makes creating these controls straightforward. With the increasing focus on Dynamic HTML to create all Windows user interfaces, including traditional dialog boxes and forms, OC96 compliance will become a 'must have' for any component-based product.

Visual Controls vs Non-visual Controls

Having worked with visual controls, it may be difficult to imagine why anyone would want to create controls that are non-visual. With visual programming tools, it is tempting to tightly couple together the data, application logic and user interface into a monolithic component which handles all aspects related to a set of data objects. This is certainly consistent with classical object-oriented encapsulation (an object should know how to show itself, modify itself and manage its own data). It turns out, however, that this 'pure' form of encapsulation doesn't scale well. That is, as the number of users or the size of the data collection increases, the resources required for the design to work grows explosively.

The distributed model of computing is based on inter-operating components and takes the best from object-oriented and client-server computing, applying this in a pragmatic way to solve large and complex system design problems. Much of this activity is spurred on by the popularity of the Internet, which is causing the industry to redefine the term 'scaling to a very large user base or data collection size'. The former maximum user limit has grown from hundreds and thousands to millions, and the data collection size has grown from megabytes to terabytes.

Within the currently favored distributed model, the business rules are separated from the user interface and from the data management tasks. Each task is managed and encapsulated in a component (business object running on a server), and the interoperating network of components together forms an 'n-tier' client-server network that solves the problem. Careful design of solutions using this architecture will ensure scalability to very large user base or data collection size.

In fact, we'll be designing and implementing several business objects in our intranet implementation. As you'll soon see, they are invaluable for encapsulating business rules within software components that can be reused in a location and even context independent manner.

Meanwhile, we need to fully understand the interfaces that the OC94 and OC96 specifications require, and what help ATL provides for control development. In fact, ATL Wizards can often generate 'ready to compile' code for us for many of these interfaces.

Fundamental OC94 Interfaces and ATL 3

Our discussion will stay on the high level, but we'll go into enough detail to ensure that the places where customization may be performed are evident. Our approach will be COM interface-centric; we'll cover the ActiveX control interfaces (actually older OC94 interfaces) one by one and point out the way in which they are implemented and handled by ATL. To gain a better understanding of the required interfaces, and appreciate their richness and complexity, we will be going through the interface groups by functional areas and describing the corresponding OC94 specification requirements. Along the way, we'll learn about the traditional OLE controls in general.

Sharing User Interface with the Container

Sharing the user interface between a control and a container involves working with legacy interfaces that span more than two generations of COM-based embedding technology.

Before controls, monolithic applications such as Microsoft Word and Microsoft Excel allowed portions of their document to be embedded inside other applications that supported Object Linking and Embedding (**OLE**). In OLE 1.0, this was the extent to which one could have a **compound document**. When the user double clicked on the embedded document, the application that worked with the embedded document started up in a separate window, allowing the user to edit what has originally been embedded. The interfaces defined for OLE 1.0, between the embedded document and the container are the **object linking and embedding interfaces**.

In the next generation, OLE 2.0, the compound document user interface became more complex. Instead of starting a new application for each type of embedded object, **in-place activation** was introduced. With in-place activation, double clicking on an embedded object no longer starts the associated application in a separate window. Instead, the application is started as an invisible 'server'. In fact, the hosting application 'rests' without shutting down its own user interface, and the newly activated, in-place application takes over user interaction. The in-place nature of this switch means that no new windows will popup; instead, the embedded application actually takes over a portion of the hosting application's screen real estate during its interaction with the end user. Furthermore, the hosting application can share the menus, toolbar and keyboard accelerators (shortcut keys) with the in-place application.

From our discussion of full ActiveX controls, it should be obvious that a control requires some features from both sets of OLE interfaces. Conversely, it should also be obvious that many of the features from the OLE and compound documents are not immediately applicable to ActiveX controls.

However, in the interests of using the existing OLE containers to host controls, Microsoft reused all the defined OLE 1 and 2 interfaces, even if those interfaces were only marginally reusable. The impact of this conservative reuse is felt even today; all visual ActiveX controls have to carry around massive legacy OLE interfaces even when they only use one or two methods.

This is a classic example of the tension between:

- ❑ Visionary interface factoring – if they had known about the eventual popularity of controls when they designed OLE, the interfaces would have been factored differently
- ❑ Compatibility – making sure the first controls could be embedded in existing OLE containers
- ❑ Reuse – trying to avoid interface proliferation by reusing existing interfaces

While the design decision made may not please everyone, you've got to accept that this way, the design doesn't break existing containers with new controls, and new containers with existing controls.

Let's take a moment to recap. In order to share a user interface between a control and its container, controls make use of most legacy interfaces originating from OLE, which can be tracked by their respective technology generation:

- ❑ OLE 1– interfaces supporting object embedding
- ❑ OLE 2 – interfaces supporting in-place activation

Legacy compatibility with OLE compound documents dictates that a control with a visual user interface is also an embeddable OLE in-process server, which can be in-place activated. That is, the control will have to implement a whole slew of interfaces defined for object embedding within the OLE compound document architecture. We saw this earlier in our examination of the 3D button control from Visual Basic and its many interfaces.

Let's take a look at why we need some of these interfaces.

Interfaces Supporting Object Embedding

We can easily appreciate that a hosting application/container can have more than one embedded control. The control, once embedded in the container, can obtain the ownership of a portion of the container's display area. Communications between the container and the control are carried out solely using COM-based interfaces. The container must provide one **site** object for each embedded control. These sites are analogous to 'chip sockets' in the hardware world; they provide the location on the container's display and the COM-based connections for the 'control chip' to communicate with the container application.

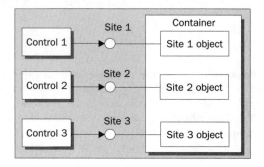

The communications protocol between the control and the container can be broken up into two general categories:

- Services provided by the container to the embedded object
- Control interfaces provided by the embedded object to the container

The split between interfaces is shown in the this diagram:

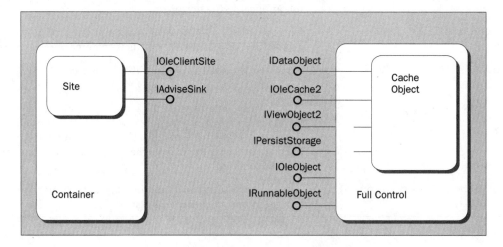

Note that the IPersistStorage *and* IViewObject2 *interfaces are purposely drawn disconnected.* IDataObject *and* IOleCache2 *are typically implemented directly by a Cache Object, and the* IViewObject2 *and* IPersistStorage *are implemented usually by the control, with assistance from the Cache Object. This is typically true for compound document controls, but not necessarily for ActiveX controls. We will have more to say about the Cache Object in a later section, when we describe the Data Management interfaces.*

Services provided by the Container to Embedded Object

In the first category, the container provides two service interfaces for this purpose:

- ❑   IOleClientSite
- ❑   IAdviseSink

One set of these interfaces is provided for each embedded control. They provide services to the embedded object, allowing the object to get information from the container, or make requests or supply notification information to the container. Most of the COM interfaces described below aren't defined specifically for control operations, but are also usable for legacy OLE compound document interactions. As a result, you'll frequently find that some methods of an interface may not be used by a control. Let's take a quick look at these interfaces and their methods:

The IOleClientSite Interface

Methods	Description
SaveObject()	Requests that the object be saved in the container's persistent storage synchronously — typically used in handling of the Close verb for an embedded application. Usually not applicable to controls.
GetMoniker()	Used in object linking to get a moniker (an object that acts as a locator for another object) corresponding to the container or the object relative to the container. Usually not applicable to controls.
GetContainer()	Can be called by the control to get a pointer to the IOleContainer interface of the container object.
ShowObject()	A request from the control for it to be shown in the container.
OnShowWindow()	Notifies the container that the object is changing from visible to invisible or vice versa when the object opens a separate window to display itself. This will allow the hosting container to display a hatched area where the object is embedded.
RequestNewObjectLayout()	Lets the container know that the object wants more or less room on the container's display.

ATL Implementation

ATL handles most of the required calls through IOleClientSite for you automatically. The client site object is also available as a data member of CComControlBase (from which all ActiveX controls in ATL are derived) in case you need to call these methods directly. ATL stores an interface pointer to the client site object inside the m_spClientSite smart pointer member.

The IAdviseSink Interface

Methods	Description
OnDataChange()	Notifies the container that the data in the object has changed. Used by data objects in uniform data transfer, typically not used by controls.
OnViewChange()	Lets the container know that the view has changed.
OnRename()	Notifies the container that the name of the object has changed. Used for linked objects, typically not by controls.
OnSave()	Lets the container know that the object has been saved to disk. Typically not used by controls.
OnClose()	Lets the container know that the object has been closed. Typically not used by controls.

ATL Implementation

IAdviseSink is a classic application of the advise sink mechanism, which was covered in Chapter 2. It allows an object to send notifications to the container asynchronously whenever the object wishes. As such, it's used under various circumstances in OLE, but not all the methods apply to controls.

Again, the CComControlBase class shields most of the notification calls to IAdviseSink::OnViewChange() wherever possible.

In fact, the control redraw action is typically a direct consequence of the usage of the IAdviseSink interface. In this case, when ATL detects that the display needs to be refreshed, it invokes CComControlBase::FireViewChange() on the container. Later, at a time convenient to the container, the container will invoke the control's IViewObject2::Draw() method. The CComControlBase class will in turn call the method, CComControlBase::OnDrawAdvanced(). This method will normalize the device coordinates and then call CComControlBase::OnDraw(). Most of the time, simply overriding CComControlBase::OnDraw() is all that is necessary when creating controls with ATL.

The diagram below shows this action:

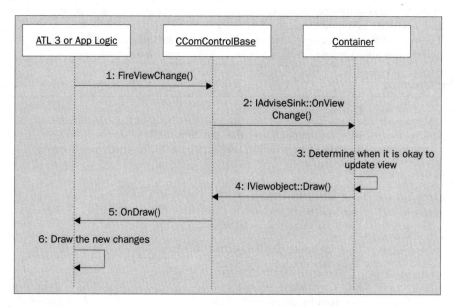

The actual firing of the `IAdviseSink::OnViewChange()` notification is through an inline member function called `SendOnViewChange()`, also in the `CComControlBase` class.

As with `IOleClientSite`, ATL 3 maintains a `CComControlBase` data member smart pointer to the advise sink. This smart pointer member can be accessed if necessary as `m_spAdviseSink`. However, direct use of this smart pointer is strongly discouraged – the `CComControlBase::FireViewChange()` method should be used instead in almost all cases.

This first set of interfaces deals with the protocols between the containing application and the control, when sharing the user interface.

Control Interfaces provided by the Control to the Container

In the second category of interfaces supporting object embedding, the interfaces are implemented by the control, and used by the container. These OLE interfaces are monstrosities and reveal their age. In fact, the set of interfaces dealing with cache handling is quickly dropping out of use – as the OC96 optimizations have made them obsolete. However, since an interface cannot be changed once it is defined, their reign of terror continues.

The IOleObject Interface

First, the unwieldy, yet mandatory, interface that *must* be implemented by a full control is the `IOleObject` interface. Be aware that some of the terminology used in describing these methods is a legacy from age of OLE/document centric computing.

The methods of the `IOleObject` interface are shown in the table below:

Methods	Description
Advise()	Establishes an advise link between the container and the embedded object. The caller gets back an advise token. It will be notified should the OLE object be renamed, saved or closed.
Close()	Called when an executing object should be closed or should revert back to the loaded but not running state.
DoVerb()	Called when a specific **verb** is to be performed by the object due to client request. Verbs are user-level requests (for example, Open, Edit, Show, Hide, etc.) This is typically called during a complex handshake between the container and the embedded object when the user interacts with the user interface.
EnumAdvise()	Called to obtain an enumeration object enumerating all the advise connections active. Used by the container to release connections prior to Close().
EnumVerbs()	Used to obtain an enumeration object enumerating all the supported verbs; it can also provide the necessary content to display a drop-down menu with the supported verbs.
GetClientSite()	Called to obtain the client site associated with the embedded object. This client site object is supplied by the container and manages the area of the container occupied by the embedded object's UI.
GetClipboardData()	Called to get an IDataObject representing the object itself. The caller can create a new object with the same data as the original using the IDataObject interface. This can be used in drag and drop implementations across applications via the clipboard.
GetExtent()	A container calls this as part of the size negotiation during initialization. The object being called must be running for this to work. The returned rectangle should be the control application's preferred size.
GetMiscStatus()	Returns the miscellaneous status bitmap used to indicate particular characteristics of the control; this is the same as the MiscStatus key value in the registry for the control.
GetMoniker()	Called in object linking scenarios, this should return a moniker (like a system name) for the object.
GetUserClassID()	Returns the CLSID of the object.

Table Continued on Following Page

Methods	Description
GetUserType()	Returns the OLE string representation (AppID) of the object.
InitFromData()	This method is called when initializing a newly created data object from a data object, typically from the container or clipboard.
IsUpToDate()	Called to determine if all linked objects are up-to-date, or if the Update() method needs to be called.
SetClientSite()	Called by the container during initialization handshaking to supply the object with a client site that will manage the screen real estate (on the container display surface). This method is essential to control operations. Most controls will insist that this is called by the container even before the common IPersist* methods are called, this supplies the control with ambient properties values. Unfortunately many containers don't follow this convention.
SetColorScheme()	Sends a recommended palette for the object to use during graphics drawing operations.
SetExtent()	Called by the container to 'dictate' a size for the embedded object to fit into. Can only be called for a running, active object.
SetHostNames()	Provides the application name and compound document name for the embedded object.
SetMoniker()	Called to provide the object with either a full moniker or the container's moniker, used in object linking situations.
Unadvise()	Breaks an active advisory link. The input parameter is the management token.
Update()	Used only for linked objects to update any linked representation.

IOleObject is a monster-interface, carrying with it all the methods supporting an embedded (or linked) object that aren't specified anywhere else.

> *Older 'OLE object' specifications require the implementation of IOleObject, IDataObject and IPersistStorage as the minimal set of interfaces to qualify a blob as an OLE object. Once you've gone through this interface, you'll appreciate the big step Microsoft took in OC96 in allowing an ActiveX Control to have only one required interface*

ATL 3 Implementation

You should be pleased to know that ATL 3 has code to implement all of the relevant methods in this complex IOleObject interface for you. Many of these methods have standard implementations by now. They are typically used by legacy OLE 1 and OLE 2 containers and are not very likely to change. All you need to do is to multiply inherit from the IOleObjectImpl<> template class, supplying your own class as the parameter.

Again, almost all of the work is done inside the `CComControlBase` to which almost all the `IOleObjectImpl<>` methods delegate:

Method Called	`IOleObjectImpl<>` or `CComControlBase` **Member Function Handling it**	Description
`Advise()`	`Advise()` delegating to `CComControlBase::IOleObject _Advise()` member	Delegates to the system call `CreateOleAdviseHolder()` to manage multiple advise sinks. The system call returns an instance of a default advise holder object, which is accessible through the smart pointer member `m_spOleAdviseHolder`. There is very little reason to override this in general.
`Close()`	`Close()` delegating to `CComControlBase::IOleObject _Close()` member	In-place deactivate (if necessary), save data (if necessary), release reference on client site, and restore control back to loaded state. You may want to override this if there is more to do for your control that is semantically equivalent to a close operation.
`DoVerb()`	`DoVerb()` delegating to a series of `CComControlBase::DoVerbXXX()` methods which in turn perform the required work.	Although unlikely, you may want to override the `OnPreVerbXXX()` and `OnPostVerbXXX()` methods, should you need them for hooking in pre-activation and post-activation work.
`EnumAdvise()`	`EnumAdvise()`	Delegate to the helper advise holder object, `m_spOleAdviseHolder`, see `Unadvise()` and `Advise()`.

Table Continued on Following Page

Method Called	`IOleObjectImpl<>` or `CComControlBase` **Member Function Handling it**	Description
EnumVerbs()	EnumVerbs()	Unlikely to ever require overriding, ATL 3 implements the following verbs: PRIMARY, OPEN, SHOW, HIDE, INPLACEACTIVATE, UIACTIVATE, DISCARDUNDOSTATE, PROPERTIES
GetClientSite()	GetClientSite() **delegating to** CComControlBase::IOleObject_GetClientSite()	Fetch the site interface from smart pointer member, m_spClientSite, if available. With controls, this site interface is used to query for other interfaces offered by the site object.
GetClipboardData()	GetClipboardData()	Stubbed only
GetExtent()	GetExtent()	Return the value of m_sizeExtent member
GetMiscStatus()	GetMiscStatus()	Make system call to OleRegGetMiscStatus(). If necessary, you may want to override and modify the flag from the registry stored value.
GetMoniker()	GetMoniker()	Stubbed only
GetUserClassID()	GetUserClassID()	Return CLSID
GetUserType()	GetUserType()	Make system call to OleRegGetUserType
InitFromData()	InitFromData()	Stubbed only
IsUpToDate()	IsUpToDate()	Stubbed only
SetClientSite()	SetClientSite() **delegating to** IOleObject_SetClientSite()	Saves client site interface to smart pointer member, m_spClientSite, queries the site for its ambient dispatch, and saves it to smart pointer member m_spAmbientDispatch

Method Called	IOleObjectImpl<> or CComControlBase **Member Function Handling it**	Description
SetColorScheme()	SetColorScheme()	Stubbed only
SetExtent()	SetExtent() delegating to CComControlBase::IOle Object_SetExtent()	Older containers just dictate the control's size to it. Newer containers implement the size negotiation protocol, as we'll see later in the section *Control Sizing and IViewObjectEx Enhancements.*
SetHostNames()	SetHostNames()	Stubbed only
SetMoniker()	SetMoniker()	Stubbed only
Unadvise()	Unadvise()	Delegate to the helper advise holder object, m_spOleAdviseHolder, see Advise() and EnumAdvise().
Update()	Update()	Stubbed only

It is important to note that one major legacy affecting control implementers is the fact that activation, in-place activation, and UI activation are all done through the DoVerb() methods of this interface. While the COM interface itself didn't change, its semantics has expanded significantly with the addition of new control states. Yes, folks, it has achieved its goals of not breaking new code, but it isn't pretty.

Isn't it great to have ATL do all the work? For a typical visual control, there is no need to override any of these methods. However, it is good to know what ATL is doing under the hood, and where it is squirreling away the client site interface, the ambient dispatch, and the advise holder – just in case you need to tweak something.

The IRunnableObject Interface

The IRunnableObject interface is another required legacy interface. It is used to control the transition of state from loaded to running and to manage the object's running state. In OLE 1.0, when IRunnableObject was created, these were the only two states that a control could be in.

With in-place active support, a full control can have more states:

❑ Passive (on disk)
❑ Loaded but not activated
❑ In-place activated (has window, usually)
❑ UI activated (has focus)

When a control is loaded, its persistent representation is accessible but it is still not visible. The control may be activated with its user interface showing either in a separate window (**activated**), or in a window of its own inside the container window (**in-place activated**). A container may have many in-place activated controls, but at any point in time only one may have the focus and interact with the user. The control with the focus is in a **UI activated** state. A control can be changed between UI activated and in-place activated, as the focus is shifted to and from the control by the container. In general, for efficiency purposes, it is desirable to deactivate controls as soon as possible when they're not being used.

`IRunnableObject` was intended to provide methods for getting the CLSID of the running object (which may be different from the originally requested CLSID – see description of handlers in the next section), to lock a running object, or to deal with local server extensions. Most modern containers no longer use this interface, and it is completely stubbed out by ATL 3 in the `IRunnableObjectImpl<>` template class. If you inherit from this template class, you save yourself from having to create your own stubs.

Data Cache Management Interfaces

In the days of OLE, monolithic applications such as Microsoft Word, had to run out-of-process when servicing an activated embedded object. In order to avoid the penalty of calling out-of-process for each and every user interface change, a type of OLE server known as a **handler** was very popular. The handler runs in-process to the container, providing most of the UI handling in this high speed environment, and delegates any data manipulation to the out-of-process application. The `IRunnableObject` interface and the data cache management interfaces described below are essential for the proper operation of these handlers.

With the arrival of OC94 and OC96, however, all such controls are deemed in-process, and there no longer exists any need for these elaborate interfaces. Unfortunately, legacy containers that check for, or depend on, some of these interfaces are still in wide circulation. As a result, it is still good to know what they do and what ATL 3 does with them.

The data cache management interfaces involved in object embedding are typically implemented using a default **cache object** provided by the OLE runtime support libraries. This means that an ActiveX control can either use containment or delegation to implement these interfaces through the default cache object. The object can be created using the `CreateDataCache()` Win32 helper function. The interfaces implemented by the default cache object include:

- ❑   `IOleCache2`
- ❑   `IDataObject`
- ❑   `IPersistStorage`
- ❑   `IViewObject2`

What do these interfaces do and why does the container require them? In short, these interfaces provide the container with a way of displaying the embedded document without activating it. OLE 1 and 2 containers, which can host many foreign document objects, usually prefer not to do the work of activating each associated monolithic application unless it's necessary. That is, if the end user isn't going to interact with a particular application, why spend the computing time required to load and run the associated application? Imagine opening an MS Word document with an embedded Excel spreadsheet, Powerpoint picture, and Visio drawing, and having to open *all* the applications!

The cache object provides the container with a mechanism for saving an image (usually in a metafile representation) of the embedded document, as it was last activated. The next time the document is loaded, this saved image can be retrieved and drawn in the container's display area, without having to run the monolithic application. The container will only need to activate the application when the user actually starts interacting with it (e.g. by double clicking on it). This way it is also possible to send, for example, a Word document with an embedded Excel object to a user who doesn't have Excel installed. The user receiving the document can now see the resulting metafile-output of the Excel object! There's just no possibility to activate the embedded object.

As you will soon see, delayed activation is precisely the goal of the optimizations provided in OC96. However, there is no point in providing redundant implementation. As most modern day containers designed for controls do not make use of these data cache interfaces at all, they have been unofficially deprecated.

In fact, ATL 3 creates controls that do not implement the IOleCache2 interface at all, and only implement the other interfaces to the extent that popular containers use them.

ATL 3 Implementation of Legacy Cache Object Interfaces

The following table describes what ATL 3 does to handle each interface used in this context:

Interfaces supplied by Cache Object	ATL Implementation
IDataObject	Formerly used to store and read back data or metafile rendering of the control from the cache object. This worked in conjunction with IOleCache2. Most modern ActiveX controls do not implement IOleCache2. However, a container may still create its own cache and may require a metafile rendering from IDataObject.
	With IDataObjectImpl<>, ATL 3 implements only the GetData() method and stubs out the rest. GetData() actually delegates to CComControlBase::IDataObject_GetData(), where ATL checks for metafile rendering request, and then asks the control to render the metafile.
	This interface is included only if you specifiy a Full Control as target when using the ATL wizards
IPersistStorage	Allows the container to tell the object to 'persist in' or 'persist out' its internal state to a storage supplied by the container.
	See the section *Saving the Control's Internal State* later on. for more details.
	Original OLE specifications made this interface mandatory when IOleCache2 is implemented, mainly for embedded compound documents. Modern ActiveX controls typically implement IPersistStreamInit instead of this interface.
	This interface is included by ATL 3 only if you specify a Full Control as target when using the ATL wizards. See the later section on OC96.

Table Continued on Following Page

Interfaces supplied by Cache Object	ATL Implementation
IViewObject2	Allows the container to tell the object to render its representation to a specific device. Can also be used by a container to get the set of colors used in rendering the object, to cause the object to freeze further updates to the view or to request the size of the object. This is also the interface used in passing a pointer to the container's IAdviseSink interface to the object. ATL 3 implements IViewObjectEx, which is a descendent of IViewObject2 and IViewObject. The implementation is in IViewObjectExImpl<>, all other IViewObject2 methods are stubbed out except for Draw(), GetExtent(), QueryHitPoint(), QueryHitRect() and the advise management methods. GetExtent() simply returns the **value of** m_sizeExtent member, as it did in IOleObject::GetExtent().
IOleCache2	Allows the container to control caching of the object's view or data. With OCXs, this interface was formerly only used to turn view caching on and off. It is unofficially deprecated.

Interfaces Supporting In-place Activation

OLE 2 introduced the concept of in-place activation, and, along with it, yet another formidable set of new interfaces.

The container supports three new interfaces for in-place activation:

❑ IOleInPlaceSite is an additional interface that is supported by the container-supplied client site object to support in-place activation.

❑ IOleInPlaceFrame is implemented to enable embedded documents to negotiate sharing of menus and toolbars with the MDI frame. This is usually unnecessary with controls.

❑ IOleInPlaceUIWindow allows even finer granularity of negotiation, but is seldom implemented by containers.

As a minimum requirement, in-place activation demands two other interfaces from the control:

❑ IOleInPlaceActiveObject
❑ IOleInPlaceObject

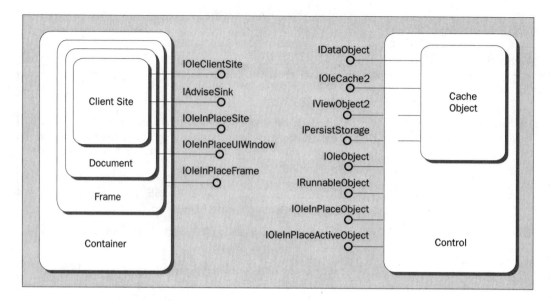

Let us see what surprises the new control-supported interfaces bring, and how ATL help us to handle them.

The IOleInPlaceObject Interface

The `IOleInPlaceObject` interface is the state-transition interface for any embedded object which needs to be in-place active (in other words, all visual controls). It derives from `IOleWindow` interface, and thus contains the `GetWindow()` and `ContextSensitiveHelp()` methods from the classic interface. Typically, the caller to these methods is the immediate container of the control. Here you can find methods that complement the `IOleObject` monster interface.

This interface also has methods controlling the extent to which the control should be visible when activated. Note that a control can be UI deactivated, and plain deactivated. The difference is that transition between UI deactivation and UI activation should be inexpensive; nothing needs to be cleaned up by the control. Deactivation, however, should be handled with a complete UI cleanup by the control. In any case, final control cleanup should really be deferred to either the `IOleObject::Close()` call, or until reference count for the control goes to zero. The lack of corresponding 'activate' method should not be a surprise if you recall our earlier discussion of `IOleObject::DoVerb()`.

The methods of the IOleInPlaceObject interface are outlined in the following table:

Methods	Description
GetWindow()	Obtains the window handle associated with the object, if any.
ContextSensitiveHelp()	Signals to the embedded object to enter or exit the context sensitive help mode of operation. Containers that support this mode will change the cursor to a pointer with a question mark.
InPlaceDeactivate()	Called by the container when the object is deactivated, and its undo state should be cleared.
ReactivateAndUndo()	Called to reactivate a deactivated object and to restore it to a previously saved state.
SetObjectRects()	Notifies the object about how much of its rectangle is visible.
UIDeactivate()	Called when a UIActive object is being deselected. UIActive is a state where the object currently has the focus and handles the user interactions directly.

ATL Implementation of IOleInPlaceObject

ATL 3 implements the methods of the IOleInPlaceObject interface through the class IOleInPlaceObjectWindowlessImpl<>. The IOleInPlaceObjectWindowless interface is an OC96 specified extension of IOleInPlaceObject.

This implementation stubs out the ContextSensitiveHelp() method and the ReactiveateAndUndo() method. The InPlaceDeactiveate() method delegates to CComObjectBase::IOleInPlaceObject_InPlaceDeactivate(), and the SetObjectRects() and UIDeactivate() methods are implemented similarly. These methods are essential to the proper behavior of the ATL full control within a container. Shown below is an interaction diagram, which shows how these interfaces work to transition the state of the control:

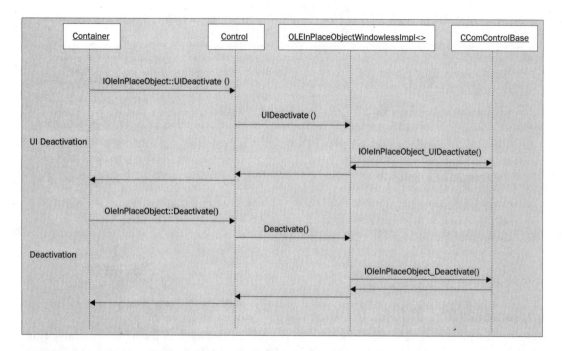

The IOleInPlaceActiveObject Interface

The `IOleInPlaceActiveObject` interface provides the user interface sharing portion of the in-place active operation. An MDI model of application construction is assumed. Three parties are involved:

- ❑ The object itself
- ❑ The document window in which the object is embedded
- ❑ The outermost frame window of the application

Here are the methods of the `IOleInPlaceActiveObject` interface.

Methods	Description
`EnableModeless()`	Used to disable an object's modeless dialog display while the container displays modal dialog boxes.
`OnDocWindowActivate()`	Called when the document window is activated or deactivated.
`OnFrameWindowActivate()`	Called when the application frame window is activated or deactivated.

Table Continued on Following Page

Methods	Description
ResizeBorder()	Notifies an object that it needs to adjust its border space, which may be due to the resizing of the document or frame window. The object should resize its border and adornments (hash lines, drag handles, etc.).
TranslateAccelerator()	Passes down the menu acceleration keys to the in-process object for translation.

The main function of this interface are for the container to:

❑ Notify the control when the frame and various document windows of the container are activated
❑ Let the activated control process menu accelerator keys
❑ Let the control know if it needs to resize itself.

The IOleInPlaceActiveObject interface also derives from IOleWindow and has the GetWindow() and ContextSensitiveHelp() methods.

ATL Implementation of IOleInPlaceActiveObject

You need to inherit from IOleInPlaceActiveObjectImpl<> to get ATL's implementation. This is automatically done for you if you use the Lite Control or Full Control options in the ATL Object wizard.

ATL implements the IOleWindow methods in exactly the same way as for IOleInPlaceObject. ATL's OnDocWindowActivate() implementation checks for deactivation, and calls IOleInPlaceObject_UIDeactivate() if necessary. The implementations of OnFrameWindowActivate(), ResizeBorder(), and EnableModeless() are stubbed, since the handling of MDI applications has gone (unofficially) out of fashion. It is unlikely that you will need to override these methods.

TranslateAccelerator() is handled by ATL by coordinating the keyboard accelerator translation protocol between the control and the container – see the section *Keyboard Hotkeys and Shortcut Handling* later in this chapter.

Beyond OLE 2: Interfaces Supporting Control-Specific UI Functionality

Finally, we get to a third generation interface designed not for OLE, but specifically for OC94. What better name to call it than IOleControl!

The IOleControl Interface

In IOleControl, we will find all those methods that are necessary for controls, but not found in IOleObject, IOleInPlaceObject, or IOleInPlaceActiveObject.

Methods	Description
GetControlInfo()	Called by the container to obtain accelerator information from the control.
OnMnemonic()	When a corresponding mnemonic key sequence is detected by the container, this call is made to the control with the key information.
OnAmbientPropertyChange()	Called by the container when an ambient property of the container has changed. The IDispatch DISPID of the property is passed in.
FreezeEvents()	A call to this method with a TRUE value indicates that the container will ignore any events sent by the control until it is called again with FALSE.

ATL Implementation of IOleControl

IOleControl is called by the container to notify the control of ambient property changes, get control information, handle mnemonics, or tell the control to stop sending events for a while. As usual, ATL implements it with a templated IOleControlImpl<> class.

The default implementations of all the interface methods are stubbed, except for FreezeEvents(), where a member counter m_nFreezeEvents is incremented or decremented depending on the request.

When you are creating controls, you will frequently find it necessary to override these methods and provide your own. If the state or appearance of your control depends upon ambient properties (and it should), you will need to override the OnAmbientPropertyChange() method in order to reflect the change in your control. If your control fires events to the container, it should check to make sure the m_nFreezeEvents is zero before firing the event.

If your control uses keyboard shortcuts, you will want to override GetControlInfo() and/or OnMnemonic().

Now would be a good time to breakaway from ATL implementation discussion, so we can take a look at the protocol used between the control and container to manage keyboard shortcuts and hotkeys.

Managing Keyboard Hotkeys and Shortcuts

Keyboard hotkeys and shortcuts are also called accelerators and mnemonics in the Win32 programming world. The handling of these keystrokes is trivial in monolithic applications, because the application always has complete control of the keystroke flow.

With OLE 1 object embedding, there was no problem, since any activated object always ran independently in its own window. Each monolithic application still continued to process keystrokes in the normal way, and could therefore filter and handle any shortcut keys.

With the OLE 2 introduction of in-place activation, the problem becomes a little more difficult. In this case, the UI active embedded object has the focus, and gets all the keystroke input. If a container has multiple embedded objects, the keystrokes flow will be transferred as the focus is changed from one object to another. At the same time, the user shouldn't be aware that they are dealing with multiple applications.

In order to give this 'single application' feeling to the end user, a container with multiple controls shares their keystroke input and hotkey information via a well-defined protocol. First, a control may have certain hotkeys or shortcuts which are applicable only while it is in focus, let us call these its **accelerators**. Other hotkeys or shortcut keys are more global, and we want the container to make sure that it will pass them to the control when it gets them – regardless of who is in focus, we call these global hotkeys a control's **mnemonics**.

Once we have established this terminology, we can proceed to give the container ultimate responsibility for keeping track of all the mnemonics from all the controls. This is reasonable, since the container will always be around while controls may come and go. This means that the container must have some way of getting the mnemonics from the control to build its **accelerator table**, and it does: through `IOleControl::GetControlInfo()`. Together with mnemonic information, `GetControlInfo()` will also indicate to the container whether the control will consume the *Enter* and *Escape* key during keyboard processing. Now, if the container determines that one of the control's registered mnemonics has been pressed by the user, while the control is in-place active, the container can call `IOleControl::OnMnemonic()` to let the control perform the associated action.

This is all fine, but we must remember that the container doesn't directly get the keyboard input stream – only the currently UI active control will. Therefore, it is the responsibility of a UI active control to give the container 'first dip' on any keyboard input encountered. This is done through `IOleControlSite::TranslateAccelerator()`. If this method returns and the container has not processed the accelerator, the control can then check its own set of accelerators for a match. We will cover the `IOleControlSite` interface in the next section.

There are two other important points to consider here. First, if a control ever changes its set of associated mnemonics, it should call `IOleControlSite::OnControlInfoChanged()` to notify the container of the change. Second, the container depends on each control to tell it when the focus (UI active or not) changes from one to another, this can be done by the control through `IOleControlSite::OnFocus()`.

When these rules are followed, the container can manage a dynamic set of controls, each with a dynamic set of mnemonics and still give the end user the same keyboard accelerator 'feel' of a conventional monolithic application. The interaction is illustrated in the following sequence diagram:

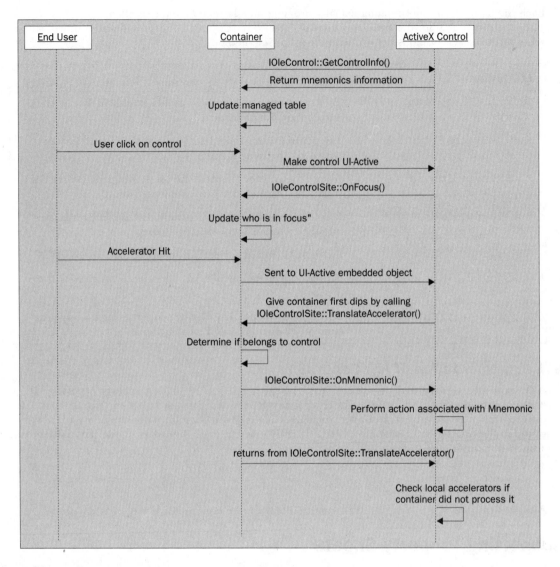

IOleControlSite Interface from Container

By now, it should be no surprise that the container-supplied `IOleClientSite` and `IOleInPlaceSite` interfaces are insufficient for all control needs. These older interfaces were designed without regards to control. `IOleClientSite` provides the control with information about the container, as well as allowing it to ask the container to ensure the control's visual representation is visible. `IOleInPlaceSite` encapsulates the requests and notifications an in-place control can send to its container.

Each site object from the container actually provides an additional interface called IOleControlSite for the associated control. The IOleControlSite provides the control with a set of further services and is defined with the following methods:

Methods	Description
OnControlInfoChanged()	Tells the container that the control's mnemonics information has changed.
LockInPlaceActivate()	The control wants to be kept in-place active until further notice via the same method.
GetExtendedControl()	Allows the control to access the properties provided by the container's extended control implementation.
TransformCoords()	Provides a service for the control to transform coordinates into the container's coordinate system.
TranslateAccelerator()	Provides keyboard accelerator mapping for this control.
OnFocus()	Notifies the container site that the control has gained or lost focus.
ShowPropertyFrame()	Called by the control to display property pages to give the container a chance to add its own pages.

ATL Implementation of IOleControlSite

ATL implemented control code will use the IOleControlSite methods whenever necessary. It does not provide any specific means for control developers to access the IOleControlSite interface from the site object. However, since the client site interface from the same object is always stored in the smart pointer member CComControlBase::m_spClientSite, one can easily obtain a smart pointer to the IOleControlSite interface via:

```
CComQIPtr<IOleControlSite, &IID_IOleControlSite> spControlSite(m_spClientSite);
```

After this call, the m_spControlSite smart pointer can be used to access any of the methods.

Supporting Property Sheets

IDEs like Visual Basic 6 and Visual J++ 6 that are control-friendly have their own panels for editing properties, where the properties value of a control can be readily modified by the end user. For environments where an editor like this is not available (for example, FrontPage 98), the control may still want to present a user interface for modifying its properties. This is the main reason for property sheets.

Occasionally, property sheets may also be used to supplement the properties editor provided by the IDE. If you have a control with complex properties that the regular editors do not handle well, you may need to create your own property editor for it.

Here is an example of a set of property sheets from Microsoft's slider control:

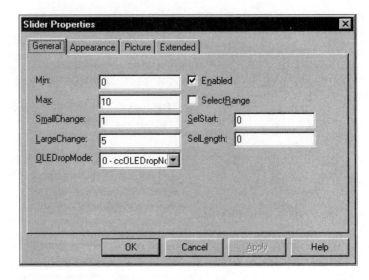

The interfaces required for property sheets support are:

- ❏ ISpecifyPropertyPages
- ❏ IPerPropertyBrowsing
- ❏ IPropertyPage
- ❏ IPropertyPage2

ISpecifyPropertyPages

ISpecifyPropertyPages allows the container to enumerate the CLSIDs of the property page objects supported by the control. This implies that each and every property page (shown as an independent tab on the top) should be implemented as a separate COM object.

This is a very simple interface with only one method, GetPages(), which returns an array of CLSIDs for the property pages of the control.

IPerPropertyBrowsing

The IPerPropertyBrowsing interface provides the container with metadata information of the properties.

Methods	Description
GetDisplayString()	GetDisplayString() gives a textual descriptive name of a property, given a DISPID.
GetPredefinedStrings()	For a specific DISPID, provides a selection of textual options for the value of the DISPID. Each textual option also has an associated DWORD token.

Table Continued on Following Page

Methods	Description
GetPredefinedValue()	Retrieves the VARIANT value associated with the DWORD token corresponding to a predefined string returned by the GetPredefinedStrings() method.
MapPropertyToPage()	Returns the CLSID of the property sheet associated with a specified DISPID.

Note that this interface does not give access to the actual properties themselves. This is not a limitation, since we already know that properties and methods of any ActiveX control can be accessed via their default IDispatch interface.

IPropertyPage and IPropertyPage2

These interfaces are not directly exposed by the control, but each property page object must support one of them. They also have access to an interface, IPropertyPageSite, provided by the property sheets container. One can view the relationship between a property sheet and its container as a specialized case of embedding. Instead of dealing with the mega-interfaces of conventional containers and controls, however, the Microsoft engineers have provided a customized lean set of specialized interaction interfaces. We will not go in-depth here into the methods of these interfaces, but the interested reader can read the COM documentation and easily understand the semantics, since they provide effectively a specialized subset of the control functionality.

One interesting point to note is that since property pages are independent COM objects, it is totally possible for a (property sheet) container to be working with only the property sheet without the actual control being displayed or active. Also, one property page object can be used by different controls. Stock property pages are such objects.

ATL Implementation of Property Sheet Interfaces

Again, ATL makes supporting property sheets a drag-and-drop affair. First off, since each property page is a separate COM object, the ATL Object wizard has a property page target. Using this target, you can visually paint the appearance of your property page using the dialog editor.

If you use the ATL wizard to create your property sheets, it will also edit the #include file of your control to add a set of property map macros. Here's an example of the macros:

```
BEGIN_PROP_MAP(CCalendar)
PROP_PAGE(CLSID_DateInitPage)
PROP_ENTRY("Start Date", 1, CLSID_DateInitPage)
PROP_ENTRY("Stop Date", 2, CLSID_DateInitPage)
END_PROP_MAP()
```

Note that the BEGIN_PROPERTY_MAP *macros used in ATL 2.x have been deprecated*

If you check under the hood, this set of macros builds a global (static) array of information associating each property with the property page.

ATL 3's implementation of `ISpecifyPropertyPages`, all done within the `ISpecifyPropertyPagesImpl<>` templated class, will walk the global property map array for information when necessary. You only have to:

- ❑ Define your property map
- ❑ Design your property pages visually
- ❑ Write code to support your property page object
- ❑ Inherit from `ISpecifyPropertyPagesImpl<>` to get the functionality

Similarly, you can inherit from `IPerPropertyBrowsingImpl<>` will to get the free implementation which gets its data from your property map.

Since each property page is a separate ATL-implemented COM object, they are pre-generated by the wizard to inherit from `IPropertyPage2Impl<>` to support `IPropertyPage` and `IPropertyPage2`. You are simply left with the actual implementation of the dialog/property sheets interaction.

When a property is defined within the ATL 3 property map, it will automatically be used in supporting state persistence. The next section has more details on this.

Other Interfaces not Related to UI Handling

Not all interfaces supported by a control deal with manipulating the user interface. In this section, we'll cover other important control interfaces that are not directly related to UI handling.

Saving the Control's Internal State

Visual development environments, such as Visual Basic 6, allow a developer to design applications visually using a control, setting its properties to certain values, and then 'freezing' the control in that state by saving the project or creating an executable. When the project is reloaded, or the executable ran, the control involved is expected to start up with the saved values in its properties. To make this possible, the Visual Basic 6 container must be able to ask the control to save itself into a storage medium. This medium may be a file itself (seldom), a storage within a compound file (infrequent), a stream in a compound file (frequent), or memory (frequent). **Persisting** is so called because, once the state is saved, it is assumed to be permanent, although `IPersistMemory` may be considered an oxymoron in this context.

Hence, there are a series of `IPersistXXX` interfaces for persisting the control's properties to and from storage mediums. All controls with persistent properties should implement some of these. The following are four such interfaces:

- ❑ `IPersistStreamInit` – persists to a stream
- ❑ `IPersistStorage` – persists to a storage object in a compound file
- ❑ `IPersistPropertyBag` – persist to ASCII file
- ❑ `IPersistMemory` – persist to memory

Of these four interfaces, IPersistStreamInit is by far the most frequently requested by typical containers, thanks in part to the popularity of MFC to construct application containers. For scripting development environments and/or Visual Basic, you should also implement IPersistPropertyBag. Otherwise, IPersistStorage and IPersistMemory should be implemented if the container you design requires them.

The methods of these interfaces are very similar, so let us take a quick look at them here:

IPersist

All the IPersistXXX interfaces derive from IPersist. Its only method, GetClassID(), returns the CLSID of the object which can be persisted.

IPersistMemory

The IPersistMemory interface is a new optimization interface implemented by more recent controls. It allows an object to persist itself to and from fixed-size memory blocks. It also allows for initialization the first time the object is restored from the memory block. The behavior of this interface is identical to that of IPersistStreamInit.

Methods	Description
GetSizeMax()	Returns the size of the memory block required to persist the object.
InitNew()	Used to initialize the object to a default state. If this method is called, the Load() method should not be called. For full controls, this is typically called the first time a control instance is created.
IsDirty()	This method indicates whether the persistent properties of the object have changed and therefore need to be written to the storage medium.
Load()	Initializes the object from previously persisted properties. For full controls, this can be called many times as the form containers come and go.
Save()	Saves the object's persistent properties into the memory block supplied.

IPersistStorage

The IPersistStorage interface allows an object to be persisted into a compound document, within its own storage.

Methods	Description
HandsOffStorage()	Called when the container wants the object to release all storage.
InitNew()	Passes in an IStorage interface for a newly created object.
IsDirty()	Same as IPersistMemory.

Methods	Description
Load()	Loads the persistent properties/data from a specified storage.
Save()	Saves the persistent properties/data to a specified storage.
SaveCompleted()	Notifies the object that the IStorage may be used again if necessary after a HandsOffStorage() method call.

IPersistStreamInit

The interface behaves identically to the IPersistMemory interface covered earlier, except the object can persist to or from a stream storage provided by the host, rather than memory.

Methods	Description
GetSizeMax()	Same as in IPersistMemory
InitNew()	Same as in IPersistMemory
IsDirty()	Same as in IPersistMemory
Load()	Same as in IPersistMemory, except that it works with a generalized IStream
Save()	Same as in IPersistMemory, except that it works with a generalized IStream

IPersistPropertyBag

We'll describe part of this interface below, and later in the OC96 coverage.

ATL Implementation of IPersistXXX Interfaces

ATL provides implementations for IPersistStreamInit, IPersistStorage, and IPersistPropertyBag with the IPersistStreamInitImpl<>, IPersistStorageImpl<> and IPersistPropertyBagImpl<> templated classes respectively.

The only state of a control that you will be persisting to and from the storage medium corresponds to the values of properties, and ATL has taken advantage of this situation and made support for the IPersistXXX interfaces very easy. In fact, all you need to do is declare the persistent properties in a property map (discussed earlier in *ATL Implementation of Property Sheet Interfaces*), and their persistence is taken care of automatically.

Source code for IPersistStreamInitImpl<>, IPersistStorageImpl<>, and IPersistPropertyBagImpl<> can be found in Atlcom.h file, instead of the usual Atlctrl.h. The implementation of IPersistStorageImpl<> actually calls on IPersistStreamInitImpl<> to do the work.

In fact, all it does is call:

```
pStorage->OpenStream(OLESTR("Contents"),....);
```

This creates a stream in the storage with name `"Contents"`, and then calls on
`IPersistStreamInitImpl<>` to do the persisting. This delegates to
`IPersistStreamInitImpl<>::IPersistStreamInit_Save()`, which in turn ends up calling
a global function `AtlIPersistStreamInit_Save()` to do the actual work. The `Load()` method
follows the same delegation pattern. A Boolean member called `m_bRequiresSave` is used in
`IsDirty()` to determine the properties which need saving.

`IPersistPropertyBagImpl<>` follows a similar pattern, first delegating to
`IPersistPropertyBagImpl<>::IPersistPropertyBag_Save()` and then to a global
function called `AtlIPersistPropertyBag_Save()` to do the actual work with the property map.

Of course, one can probably come up with contrived cases where there is a need to persist more than
property value. Remember, however, that a typical control which works with non-UI related data
always has a 'natural' place to store that data already — in a database or file, and so on. Storing
additional domain-specific data in the container's control 'state' persist stream is not a good design
choice. Therefore, there is seldom any need to override any of the `IPersistXXX` interface methods
yourself. The only potential exceptions to this statement that come to mind are:

❑ If you need to do something the very first time an instance of the control is created, override
   `IPersistStreamInitImpl<>::InitNew()`
❑ To optimize for speed, by taking advantage of a situation-specific condition.
❑ You are persisting properties with complex automation-compatible data types that the default
   implementation does not implement

Providing Metadata to Development Tools

In our study of the `IDispatch` interface back in Chapter 2, we looked at the descriptive power of
the binary type library. Much of the information regarding the interfaces, the methods, and the
properties supported by any ActiveX control can be interpreted from the type library. This is what is
commonly referred to as **metadata**. Metadata is essential to development tools. It also allows such
tools to work with any new control that it didn't know about at the time the tool itself was compiled.
It allows the tool to provide property viewing and editing capability to the end user for any control
which provides this type information.

There are two interfaces, typically supported by a control, that can provide metadata information:

❑ `IProvideClassInfo`
❑ `IProvideClassInfo2`

IProvideClassInfo

This interface is used in obtaining type library information.

The solitary `GetClassInfo()` method returns an `ITypeInfo` interface for the caller to access the
type library information for the object.

IProvideClassInfo2

This interface is based on IProvideClassInfo and extends it to cover events, providing an additional method, GetGUID().

The caller to GetGUID() can specify the type of GUID to obtain. Currently, it's used to obtain the default event set interface ID from the control.

ATL Implementation of Metadata Interfaces

To implement the above interfaces, you need to inherit from IProvideClassInfoImpl<> and/or IProvideClassInfo2Impl<>. The operation of these interfaces is direct and simple. They locate the type library and pass the information to the caller. Since the ATL environment creates and maintains your type library for you, it knows how to get at it. You almost never need override these methods.

Spilling a Can of Metadata Worms

It is true that IDispatch itself provides much of the metadata information required for method invocation and property access, and that the type library information associated with a control can be fetched directly from the registry. In fact, the actual binary type library information may be attached to the control, independent in its own file, or attached to some other module, thus providing flexibility.

Conceptually, however, a control should be self-describing. The two interfaces above give a container the illusion that the control is self-describing. Unfortunately, the actual location of the type library may vary greatly. This is irritating to developers who may need to track versions and evolution. Microsoft is well aware of this, and will centralize type library information once and for all in the upcoming COM+ offering.

Giving Meaningful Rich Error Messages

Recall that almost all COM interface methods return an HRESULT. This uniformity allows COM to operate in any environment, OS, and programming language that supports simple function calls, but does not allow for passing of meaningful exceptions or error information between the caller and called. To solve this problem, the additional information can be **tunneled** through the limited mechanism. The ability to supply rich error reporting information is set on a per-interface basis.

A COM interface is specifically designed for this purpose:

❑   ISupportErrorInfo

The interface has one single method called InterfaceSupportsErrorInfo(). When passed an interface ID, this function will return S_OK if the interface supports rich error reporting.

ATL Implementation of Rich Error Messages

When you create your control using the ATL Object Wizard, you can check a checkbox marked Support ISupportErrorInfo. If you do this, the wizard will generate code to implement the InterfaceSupportsErrorInfo() method. You can look in the <project>.cpp file to see this code. Your C++ class will also inherit from the ISupportErrorInfo interface. The code generated maintains a global (static) array of the interface IDs that support rich error reporting, to which you should add the ID of any new interface into this array if it also supports rich error reporting.

ATL also provides a default implementation called ISupportErrorInfoImpl<>. You should use this implementation if your object has only one interface and it supports rich error reporting.

This is all that is required from the control. When an error occurs, the code within the interface must fill in the details on an error object and pass it back to the caller. Thankfully, ATL 3 has six member functions in CComCoClass called Error() to do this all for you. Each Error() function has a different parameterization. Check out the source file Atlcom.h to see the variety of information you can pass back with the error. All the Error() functions end up calling the globally scoped AtlReportError() functions to do their work.

To retrieve this rich error information, the caller first checks to make sure that the interface supports rich error reporting by querying the object's ISupportErrorInfo interface. Next, if one of the interface methods returns a return code other than S_OK, the caller can use the global Win32 function, GetErrorInfo(), to retrieve the rich error information. If the client is multi-threaded, each thread has its own rich error support object and can perform this query independently.

Major Features and Optimizations in OC96

Thus far, we have only been talking about the COM interfaces which affect all visual controls. Now we turn our attention to OC96 compliant controls. Thanks to the new optimizations specified, these controls show their true colors when working with new containers. Let's take a look now at some of these features and how ATL 3 helps us to implement them. They include:

- ❑ Deferred Activation Optimization
- ❑ Optimized Drawing
- ❑ Flicker-free Activation and Deactivation
- ❑ Quick Activation
- ❑ Windowless Control Support
- ❑ Improved Undo Model
- ❑ Negotiated Control Sizing

Deferred Activation Optimization

When a container plays host to many controls, activating all of them when the container starts and deactivating them when it closes can become a very expensive proposition. The simple action of creating a Window is both a time and resource intensive operation, particularly when there are many windows to create – one for each contained control. To compound the problem, the original OC94 specification provided an OLEMISC_ACTIVATEWHENVISIBLE flag, which was used by almost all controls in their implementation of IOleObject::GetMiscStatus() (called by the container) because it greatly simplified coding. When this flag is specified by the control, the container is obliged to activate the control upon initialization. The control stays in this 'in-place active' state and processes its own mouse messages to detect UI Activation.

In many cases, a control embedded in a container may not actually be used by the end user (if, for example, only some other control hosted in the same container is required), but must be activated simply to get the control to draw itself for the container.

By decoupling the drawing process from the activation of the control, it can be activated 'just-in-time', as and when the end user actually needs to use it.

A control which has been loaded in by the container and has an appearance on the container's surface, but has not yet been activated is called an **inactive object** – an object in the 'inactive' state. This is a pseudo-state introduced by OC96, which specifies an interface, IpointerInactive, for containers to support these new controls.

The IPointerInactive Interface

The IPointerInactive interface, as discussed above, contains three methods:

Methods	Description
GetPointerActivationPolicy()	Obtains the instantaneous activation policy of the control. Called by the container when the mouse enters the inactive control display area.
OnInactiveSetCursor()	Used by the container to ask or command the object to set the mouse cursor.
OnInactiveMouseMove()	Used by the container to forward mouse move messages to the inactive object while the mouse is over the object's display area.

ATL Implementation of IPointerInactive

ATL provides a skeleton IPointerInactiveImpl<> class which stubs out all of the methods. If you would like to implement inactive object behavior, you must inherit from IPointerInactiveImpl<> (or alternatively IPointerInActive) and then override (implement) the methods to provide your own behavior.

Inactive Object Support

A protocol is established between the container and the control. Under the inactive object protocol, the mouse and drag-and-drop detection is performed by the container, and the control will be activated 'just-in-time' to handle the core interactions. In this way, controls that aren't used by the user may never need to be activated even though their container is displayed.

A portion of this 'windowless exchange' of messages is similar to the support for new OC96 windowless objects that we will cover later.

Controls which support inactive object operation should support the IPointerInactive interface, and also use the new flag OLEMISC_IGNOREACTIVATEWHENVISIBLE to signal to the container that it should not be activated as a matter of course upon initialization. This flag indicates to a container that the control supports inactive object activation. (Obviously, the container also needs to support this.) Note that the OLEMISC_ACTIVATEWHENVISIBLE flag still needs to be set for containers that may not know about inactive object activation.

Let's summarize this, since it is entirely anti-intuitive:

> **You need to remember to set both** OLEMISC_ACTIVATEWHENVISIBLE **and** OLEMISC_IGNOREACTIVATEWHENVISIBLE **flags in your implementation of** GetMiscStatus().

For an example, look in viscal1.5\viscal.cpp.

This effectively decouples the control behavior from the requirement for the control to actually have an active Window, essentially using a non-visual control in a visual way. There can be a large performance gain as it is no longer necessary to activate and negotiate painting with every control on a form. Since the unmarshalable IViewObject isn't involved, nor is any windows handle, it opens up the possibility of DCOM enablement in the future when high speed links are available.

The Deferred Activation Support Protocol

An inactive object is initially displayed by the container when the object is called to render its metafile representation – or by the container from a previously cached version of the metafile. After container initialization, the container will start the protocol to pass mouse messages to the control, without activating it. The container will call IPointerInactive::GetActivationPolicy() upon every WM_SETCURSOR or WM_MOUSEMOVE message, when the mouse is over the area occupied by the inactive object.

The control can return the activation policy dynamically, and may return a combination of POINTERINACTIVE_ACTIVATEONENTRY and POINTER_DEACTIVATEONLEAVE flags. If the POINTERINACTIVE_ACTIVATEONENTRY is specified, the container will immediately in-place activate the control and pass the same message to it once again for processing. The control can then process mouse messages within its own window – the old fashioned OC94 way. If the POINTER_DEACTIVATEONLEAVE is set as well, the object will be deactivated the moment the cursor leaves the control's display area. We can show this in a sequence diagram:

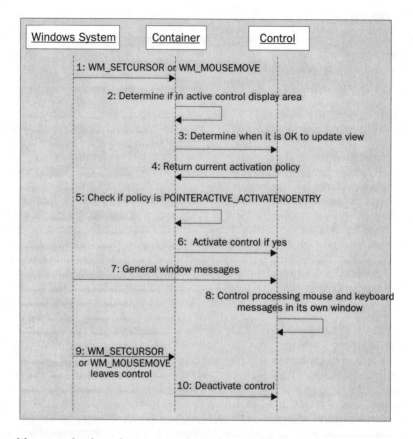

Note that, unlike a windowless object, an inactive object can't draw, or capture the mouse. It's restricted to giving feedback by changing the mouse cursor. If a control needs to provide user feedback beyond this, it must return POINTERINACTIVE_ACTIVATEONENTRY as part of its activation policy, and become activated in order to draw into its window or capture the mouse.

Since the activation policy is generated dynamically by the control, it can indicate that it doesn't want to be in-place activated. In this case, the container will continue to forward WM_MOUSEMOVE messages by calling OnInactiveMouseMove(), and forward WM_SETCURSOR messages by calling OnInactiveSetCursor() to the inactive control. The control can use these messages to fire events without ever having to be in-place activated.

While inactive, the control can wake up 'just in time' to handle drag and drop if necessary. Without a supporting window, the inactive control can't register directly to be a drop target. The container determines whether an inactive control supports drop targets by checking to see if the control supports the IPointerInactive interface. If it does, it assumes it is a potential drop target. An inactive control can act as a drop target by having the container activate it as soon as something is dragged over the display area. In this case, the control should return POINTERINACTIVE_ACTIVATEONDRAG for the activation policy.

Optimized Drawing

The old protocol of control drawing required the control to select and deselect the GDI resources (such as font, brush or pen) into and out of the container supplied device context, each time `IViewObject::Draw()` was called. Since many controls on the same form may use the same set of font, brush and pen, this creates some undue inefficiencies.

OC96 specifies a protocol where the `pvAspect` parameter of the `IViewObject::Draw()` method, previously always NULL, can point to a `DVASPECTINFO` structure specifying the optimization.

Not all containers cater for optimized drawing, so a control must check for the case where optimized drawing isn't supported (the `pvAspect` parameter for `Draw()` will be NULL). Objects that participate in optimized drawing may leave GDI objects selected into the device context, allowing the next object to use them without having to reselect them. The container is responsible for ensuring that the GDI objects are deselected from the device context at the end of container drawing. Participating objects are responsible for deleting the GDI objects that they select into the device context (on an as-needed basis or based on the Least Recently Used algorithm).

This optimization speeds up rendering in a container with many controls, since each object no longer needs to select and deselect the required GDI resources when the container repaints. The actual cleanup may be a little harder to implement, but the significant performance gain is well worth the redesign.

ATL Implementation of Optimized Drawing

ATL supports optimized drawing by checking for the container support in `IViewObject2::OnDraw()` using `IViewObjectExImpl<>` or the `OnDraw()` methods in the `CComControlBase` class. It then sets the `bOptimize` member of an `ATL_DRAWINFO` structure accordingly. This structure is passed through `OnDrawAdvanced()` to `OnDraw()`. When you override the `OnDraw()` method of `CComControlBase`, you can check this flag on the `ATL_DRAWINFO` structure passed in, and perform the optimized GDI resource handling as necessary.

Flicker-Free Activation and Deactivation

Before the enhancement of flicker-free activation and deactivation, an OCX had to repaint itself every time it was activated and have the container repaint it when deactivated. This, combined with the need for an object to be activated in order to handle mouse interaction, often causes a flickering display as objects are activated and deactivated on a form – since most UI repaint involves clearing the display area and redrawing.

With this enhancement, the container will provide the `IOleInPlaceSiteEx` interface to coordinate redraw as necessary during activation and deactivation. If a particular control's display is the same whether it is activated or not, this enhancement will eliminate the additional unnecessary update. This new interface, derived from `IOleInPlaceSite`, provides specific clues to the validity of a control's visual presentation.

ATL Implementation of Flicker-Free Activation

During in-place activation, ATL will query the container's site object for support of `IOleInPlaceSiteEx`. If the container supports this interface, a Boolean member called `m_bInPlaceSiteEx` is set to true, and the smart pointer member `m_spInPlaceSite` will hold an `IOleInPlaceSiteEx` interface.

ATL will make use of the `IOleInPlaceSiteEx`, if available, to coordinate activation redraw. You can use the `IOleInPlaceSiteEx` interface directly to tell the container not to redraw when deactivating if you like, but that would require a complete override of the `CComControlBase::IOleInPlaceObject_InPlaceDeactivate()` method.

Quick Activation

Any control supporting `IQuickActivate` can be loaded and initialized by the container in one single COM method call. This contrasts with the complex handshake required for conventional controls. Essentially, the `IQuickActivate` allows for a 'batching exchange' of all information (including status information and interface pointers) between container and control, doing it all in one shot prior to control initialization.

Containers supporting quick activation will first query a control for the new `IQuickActivate` interface. If found, this will be the preferred interface used for in-place activation. If either the control or the container does not support quick activation, the regular in-place activation mechanism through `IOleObject::DoVerb()` will be used instead.

ATL Implementation of Quick Activation

ATL provides a complete implementation for quick activation in the `IQuickActivateImpl<>` template class. If you inherit from this class, your COM object will provide support for quick activation automatically.

ATL implements this interface by delegating to either `IOleObjectImpl<>` for the methods dealing with extends, or an inline global function called `IQuickActivate_QuickActivate()` for the actual interface exchanges. You can find the details of this function in `Atlctl.h`. It implements all that is required for quick activation according to OC96 specification, so there should be little reason to change this.

Windowless Control Support

We are so used to a control having its own window, that there appears to be something ironic about a visual windowless control. Yet, this is one of the greatest inventions since the original VBX. Many of the OC96 optimizations above revolve around minimizing the number of windows created by the container. In the limit, the container should only create its own window. The legacy of the VBX, where a control is essentially a sub-classed or super-classed Window with attached data, is the only thing that binds us into thinking that a visual control must have a window.

In fact, the study of inactive object support should convince us that a control need not have a window if it is not activated. It can even handle drag and drop and mouse messages (to a certain extent) without activating or creating a window. This actually takes us halfway to complete windowless control support. The only missing part is to simulate the activation process without creating a window for the control. This turns out to be relatively easy. OC96 specifies two new interfaces:

- ❑ `IOleInPlaceObjectWindowless` (supplied by the control)
- ❑ `IOleInPlaceSiteWindowless` (supplied by the container through a site object)

These interfaces inherit from and add several methods to the `IOleInPlaceObject` and `IOleInPlaceSiteEx` interfaces respectively.

A bonus of not having a window associated with a control is that the control no longer has to be rectangular! That is, it can be a circle, a star, or any arbitrary shape. The container still allocates a rectangular bounding area where the control draws itself, but the control can now do the appropriate 'hit-testing' to determine whether a mouse click within the bounding area actually hit the control. A new interface, IViewObjectEx, inheriting from IViewObject, is defined by OC96 to provide this support for nonrectangular hit-testing.

With windowless control support, you can create completely windowless visual objects. Essentially, the normal window message queue handling is replaced by interaction between container and object via COM interfaces. Not only is efficiency greatly improved, but it is now also possible for a container to contain hundreds or even thousands of controls without bogging down the system or running out of resources. Imagine a spreadsheet where every cell is a control, or a drawing program where every line is a control; seemingly outrageous implementations, but it is all possible now because of OC96. Let me leave you with another two "blue-sky" uses for windowless controls:

❑ Taking advantage of non-rectangular hit-test support to provide 3D interactive controls (for example, a rotating cube with six 'clickable' sides).

❑ Scaling the user interface with Symmetric MultiProcessing (SMP). Traditionally, the user interface can only run as fast as the fastest CPU available; it isn't intrinsically scaleable. With windowless objects, even the user interface can potentially scale in terms of performance when more processor resources are added.

The IOleInPlaceObjectWindowless Interface

The following table shows the additional methods provided by the control's IOleInPlaceObjectWindowless interface:

Methods	Description
OnWindowMessage()	Tunneling mechanism for the container to pass window messages for processing by the in-place active windowless control (see following text).
GetDropTarget()	Called by the container to let a windowless control participate in drag-and-drop.

A typical scenario starts with the control being in-place activated. The control then queries the site object for the IOleInPlaceSiteWindowless interface. Once the interface is successfully obtained, its CanWindowlessActivate() is invoked to determine if it is OK to activate them in a windowless state. On the other hand, if IOleInPlaceSiteWindowless isn't supported, the control must proceed with creating a window in the normal way.

The container, by supporting IOleInPlaceSiteWindowless, is specially designed to activate controls in a windowless state. It relies on IOleInPlaceObject::GetWindow() to determine when, and if, the control actually has a window at any time. To complete the activation protocol, the windowless control must also call OnInPlaceActivateEx() with the ACTIVE_WINDOWLESS flag bit instead of the standard OnInPlaceActivate() call.

Windows messages are dispatched from the container, and tunneled through to the activated control, without the use of a window, via the method `IOleInPlaceObjectWindowless::OnWindowMessage()`. The `IOleInPlaceSiteWindowless` interface even provides an `OnDefWindowMessage()` method to serve the same function during message processing as the Win32 `DefWindowProc()` API. In essence, the entire Windows message processing has been mapped to an inter-component communications protocol between the container and the windowless control. Now, the container is given the duty of logically managing a message queue for each embedded control.

The drawing of an in-place active windowless object is still performed through `IViewObject2::Draw()`. However, the input `lprcBounds` rectangle parameter is now `NULL` to indicate that the control is being drawn windowless. The aspect and device context properties are also handled differently. Despite this, even for a windowless control, a container may sometimes call `IViewObject2::Draw()` with a non-null `lprcBounds`, to do drawing into a separate device context for display or printing.

Windowless controls can even support drag and drop. This is done by implementing an `IDropTarget` interface and passing it to the container when the container invokes the `IOleInPlaceObjectWindowless::GetDropTarget()` method. The container will then coordinate the passing through of the `IDropTarget::DragOver()` and `IDropTarget::DragEnter()` methods.

The IOleInPlaceSiteWindowless Interface

The container supporting windowless activation provides a comprehensive set of services to assist in the windowless control presentation through `IOleInPlaceSiteWindowless`. The following table shows these methods:

Methods	Description
CanWindowlessActivate()	Asks the container if it can support windowless activation
SetCapture()	Provides mouse capture for the windowless control
GetCapture()	Called to determine if the control still has mouse capture
SetFocus()	Sets focus to the windowless control
GetFocus()	Determines if the windowless control has focus
OnDefWindowMessage()	Provides default message processing for any tunneled message from the container
GetDC()	Gets a handle to a device context from the container
ReleaseDC()	Releases the device context obtained from `GetDC()`
InvalidateRect()	Specify that a portion of the windowless control visual needs updating

Table Continued on Following Page

Methods	Description
InvalidateRgn()	Specifies that a region of the windowless control visual needs updating
ScrollRect()	Scrolls a portion of the windowless control's visual representation. It is invoked by the object to give the container a chance for optimized scrolling.
AdjustRect()	Adjust clipping for caret display

There is almost a one-to-one mapping between these methods and the standard Win32 functions for managing a window display. This completeness in service will ensure that windowless controls can enjoy the same expressiveness as their less-efficient windowed cousins.

ATL Implementation for Windowless Controls

ATL provides implementation of IOleInPlaceObjectWindowless through its IOleInPlaceObjectWindowlessImpl<> templated class. You can create a windowless control by inheriting from this interface. In order to trigger the proper activation sequence, you must also set the member flag m_bWindowed to FALSE.

To make implementation of windowless control as painless as possible, ATL's implementation of IOleInPlaceObjectWindowless actually routes the window messages tunneled from the container through an ATL control's message map. Since this is the exact same message map that a windowed control uses for display management, most existing code for windowed controls can be reused immediately.

With ATL's support for windowless controls, it is easy to write to the new windowless standard. Furthermore, we have code remaining compatible with containers that require windowed controls. This is because ATL will transparently provide a window if necessary. Getting your control to work without a window actually requires significantly more discipline in coding than doing conventional windowed controls. So, you may not even realize the dependencies of your control on its window until you've tried coding windowless controls.

Unfortunately, there was a period of time where every control programming book and manuals preached the virtues of sub-classing or super-classing standard window controls or other windowed controls when constructing your own control. This was all done in the name of simplicity and code-reuse. Ironically, while it was the 'fad of the year' to build controls out of existing controls for the programming public, almost all commercial control vendors, including Microsoft, built most of their own controls from scratch. Now, with the transition to windowless controls, these commercial vendors have a solid code base from which to convert, while those who had been using standard window controls found themselves caught between a rock and a hard place.

The lesson here is simple. If you are building new visual controls, definitely build them to be OC96 compliant and support windowless operations. There's no going back now. If you already have visual controls that don't use standard window controls or other controls internally, migrate them to windowless operation as soon as possible. This will require some work and re-thinking, but it should not be impossible. If you already have visual controls that use standard window controls or other controls, you must weigh the (typically very significant) effort to rewrite the control for windowless operations, or leave it the way it is and rely on the backward compatibility of most containers. As of the time of writing, there is no known OC96 compliant containers that would break legacy compatibility – yet.

Other Advanced OC96 Features

The OC96 standard also covers various features that apply to more specialized control projects. This section contains a quick summary of some of these other features. We will make note of ATL 3 support where applicable.

New IViewObjectEx and IAdviseSinkEx Interfaces

This extension of the `IViewObject` interface provides more efficient and flicker-free drawing capabilities for non-rectangular objects and objects with transparent areas. It does so by providing for a choice of drawing algorithms without dictating a policy.

New here is a 'two-pass' drawing scheme where objects are drawn front-to-back in the first pass and back-to-front in the second pass. The intention is to have the object do most of its drawing during the first front-to-back pass, avoiding flickering by relying on (hopefully) speedy clipping computations. The frequently used double buffering, off-screen drawing technique is still supported.

Since this is a behavior applicable to very specific controls, ATL 3 allows you to implement the behavior, but does not provide any default implementations.

An Improved Undo Model

Another new feature of OC96 is an extensible model for handling `Undo` in a component based application. This improvement is significant in cases where you are building a document centric application completely from components following the compound document model.

OC96 specifies the following new interfaces:

- ❏ `IOleUndoUnit`
- ❏ `IOleParentUndoUnit`
- ❏ `IServiceProvider`
- ❏ `IOleUndoManager`

It also introduces a centralized `Undo` manager service for tracking an application-wide undo stack across all inter-operating components within the application. Individual components are responsible for creating 'undo unit' objects and submitting them to the `Undo` manager. Undo units can be nested, reflecting the nested network of inter-operating components with undo states. Components or objects that have changed state, and can't be undone, can choose to clear the undo stack of the manager when it is their turn to submit an undo object.

In the two years since the completion of OC96, the popularity of compound document based applications has dwindled significantly. It appears that other than the office automation applications in which Microsoft has dominance (word processing, spreadsheets, presentation graphics and so on), there are few other applications that fit this model well. The Internet revolution has placed the 'view only' browser, instead of the editable document, as the centerpiece of the user experience.

ATL provides minimal assistance in the form of `IServiceProviderImpl<>` and a set of service map macros. Fortunately, the probability that you would ever have to worry about working with centralized Undo Manager when creating controls is very slim.

Control Sizing and IViewObjectEx Enhancements

One of the trickier parts to code for any control is the negotiation for the size of screen real-estate between the container and the control – and maintaining/adjusting the size throughout the life of the control. One element of complexity originates from conversions between mapping modes and associated coordinates space. 32-bit OLE promises to cure this with standardization on the `HIMETRC` mapping mode. More complexity originates from compromising the various sizing requirements of containers and controls, and working with the protocol required between the two to fulfill these requirements. We will take a look at the evolution of this protocol for controls.

Historically, the problem was solved quite simply. The first two generations of OLE assume that the container has absolute say on the control display size. Some containers simply call `IOleObject::SetExtent()` to dictate a size for the running embedded object.

To be more sensitive to the control's desire and preferences, the OLE guidelines request that container calls `IOleObject::GetExtent()` from the control (or `IViewObject2::GetExtent()` for inactive or non-running objects). This allows the control to specify a preferred size. The container can then account for this preference when it comes to decide on how much screen real-estate to give to the control (when it calls `IViewObject::Draw()`). In any case, the parameter passed in during `IViewObject::Draw()` indicates the final rectangle allocated for the control within the container's client area, in which the control should draw itself.

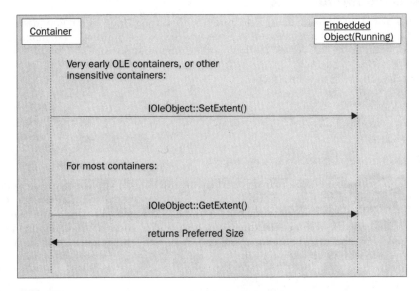

The introduction of OC96 extends this simplistic size negotiation protocol to a more flexible one. An 'autosizing' protocol is defined where the control, if possible, is given the responsibility to determine and change its own size. In an actual application, this is typically due to some action on the control by the user – for example, changing the label text for a label control in Visual Basic 6. In this case, the protocol for size determination becomes:

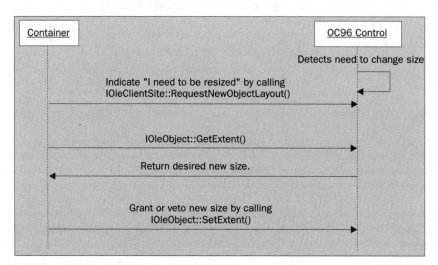

The above picture is slightly different if the control is inactive or windowless. In this case, the control would call `IOleInPlaceSite::OnPosRectChange()` to initiate resizing while the container responds with `IOleInPlaceObject::SetObjectRects()`.

OC96 also concretely specifies two ways to perform container-based control sizing:

- ❑ Content sizing
- ❑ Integral sizing

Both of these sizing protocols are supported by the `GetNaturalExtent()` method of the `IViewObjectEx` interface.

Content sizing is very similar to the OLE embedded object-sizing protocol. The container calls `IViewObjectEx::GetNaturalExtent()` specifying `DVEXTENT_CONTENT`, and the control returns a `SIZEL` structure containing the preferred size.

Integral sizing allows for a very specific action: user initiated rubber-banding in design mode. During this action, the user changes the size of a 'rubber-band' box displayed by the container, and the size of the control changes accordingly. The container calls `IViewObjectEx::GetNaturalExtent()` with `DVEXENT_INTEGRAL` and a `SIZEL` structure containing the proposed new size (of the current rubber-band box) within a `DVEXTENTINFO` structure. The control should examine the extent and determine the next 'integral' size that it wants to resize to – typically by adjusting the height based on the current width of the rubber-band box – and return it in the `SIZEL` structure parameter.

ATL supports the traditional mode of embedded object sizing, as well as all the new flavors of control sizing (with the exception of the specialized integral sizing). ATL has default implementation for all the interface methods associated with these control-sizing protocols. You can customize its behavior by changing a set of member Boolean flags (covered below) at any time. During control drawing, or when implementing complex protocols such as integral sizing, the current size information is available via several member variables in the CComContolBase class:

- ❑ m_sizeNatural – contains the 'natural' size that the control wants to be
- ❑ m_sizeExtent – contains the size in which the container has told the control to draw
- ❑ m_rcPos – an additional RECT structure, containing the current position of the control in pixels; a handy variable for use inside the normalized OnDraw() implementation

The first two member variables are in HIMETRIC units, consistent with OLE 32 conventions.

There exists a set of Boolean flag member variables that can be set to influence how ATL handles the resize protocols. m_bAutoResize can be set to indicate that this control is an autosizing control and should be the one to initiate the resizing protocols as detailed earlier. In this case, the ATL control will always use m_sizeNatural as the size that it 'wants' to be.

You can cause your control to adjust its 'natural' size based on a container's call to SetExtent() by setting the m_bResizeNatural member variable to TRUE. This can be useful when handling archaic containers or if the control is willing to scale to any size.

Setting the m_bDrawFromNatural flag will cause your control to draw to the natural extent, rather than the extent specified by the container. This may be useful in some cases when you want to preserve the natural size of the control in lieu of having appeared to be clipped with the container.

Another flag is worth mentioning here, although it is not directly related to sizing. The m_bRecomposeOnResize, together with a control flag called OLEMISC_RECOMPOSEONRESIZE, supports controls that require more than simple scaling and clipping handling when resized. In this case, the control's SetExtent() implementation will make sure that the control becomes activated and is completely repainted. An example of such control is one that displays flowing raw-text or renders HTML; in these cases, the graphical appearance of the control depends on its width and height.

IPersistPropertyBag for Persisting to ASCII Files

IPersistPropertyBag is now formally documented for persisting an object out to a text file. This interface allows a control to persist its properties in or out in textual format to a **property bag**, provided by the container. This is done through the container's IPropertyBag interface. A property bag is a logical collection that holds named values where the name is typically in textual form. When persisted out, it can take a human-readable ASCII form, for example:

```
Property Name 1 = 0x10000
Property Name 2 ="A Textual Property"
```

The sequence of interactions between the container and the control is very similar to the other interfaces in the IPersistXXX series of interfaces.

As we saw earlier, ATL supports the `IPersistXXX` interfaces, including `IPersistPropertyBag`, through the property map mechanism. At the time of writing, though, this support is not yet complete, so properties of certain data types cannot be persisted through the `IPersistPropertyBag` interface without user-supplied support routines.

Interested readers can find more information on this in Beginning ATL Programming, from Wrox Press.

Component Categories

Many newcomers to the COM scene ask the question, 'Is it possible to find all the COM objects that support a particular interface on a system?' While common sense and a keen belief in Microsoft's marketing propaganda would lead you to conclude that this would allow best-of-breed selection for performing any task – you may be surprised by the answer you get from COM gurus and architects alike.

'Why would you want to do this?'... 'You don't want to do this.'...

It turns out that, while the marketing team was trumpeting virtues of component technologies and the ability to work with best-of-breed applications, the business and design teams seldom had this goal at the top of their list. After all, why would you go out of your way to let another vendor's application or component displace your own value-added functionality? It just simply doesn't make any business sense. Simply put, Microsoft component interfaces were largely designed to work well with Microsoft applications.

Microsoft's OC94 partial solution was to introduce a value in the registry to find all controls that belong to a particular ad hoc category. For example, you will see the value 'control' below the CLSID of the object for a lot of components. How does an Office-container find out about all controls that can be inserted in a Microsoft Word document? Microsoft introduced a different keyword, 'insertable', and when Word is started, the Office Application scans all 'insertable' entries in the registry. When the user asks for Insert |Object, it displays a list of insertable controls. A problem arises here in that more and more clients are being built which need specific interfaces in servers, and the naming of these categories is not guaranteed unique.

Notice that I never said that 'best-of-breed' or 'interchangability' operations are impossible, it simply wasn't a priority in design or implementation. This explains the variety of answers you get when you ask the infamous question.

Times change and you just can't keep on answering the question vaguely forever. With the proliferation of ActiveX controls on a typical system, thanks to the Internet revolution, a solution is required to address the problem. A draft for a specification called 'ActiveX Control and Control Container Guideline' arrived at about OC96 timeframe and provided the answer to these sort of questions through a specification for something called **Component Categories**. Since then, the specification has been merged with the Platform SDK, and the component categories section has quietly migrated to become part of the core COM specifications.

Component categories attempt to address a more generic problem than the one we have staged. They allow COM components to be classified as either implementing certain features, or requiring certain features from the container. 'All components that implement `IMyInterface`' can certainly fit this scenario, but 'Components that can be safely scripted by a scripting language' or 'Components that require the Microsoft Java VM for operation' can also fit the model.

Component categories are implemented via the new `ICatInformation` and `ICatRegister` interfaces. Controls use the `ICatRegister` interface to register with the system the component categories that they support. A user can query this information with the `ICatInformation` interface, before deciding on which component to use. These interfaces are typically provided by a COM runtime object, called the **component manager**. The container specification provides a 'starter set' of definitions for standard component categories, but is wide open for definition of custom categories.

Because they're an afterthought, component categories were not supported in Windows environments prior to Windows 98 (and Windows NT 5). Instead, a separate COM support redistributable DLL called `comcat.dll` must be installed on the target system. This makes dependable, general, usage of the component categories technology impossible prior to Windows 98 (or Windows NT 5).

Component Categories are identified by UUIDs, just as interfaces or classes are, and these UUIDs are called CATIDs. They are typically kept in the system registry, and have a local specific 'human-friendly' text description associated with each one. The nature of CATIDs requires them to be definable by anyone and be applicable universally. To realize this, it is recommended that a CATID be treated in the same way as an interface – once defined and advertised, do not change it. You need to create new CATIDs as needed for evolution and backward compatibility.

The Microsoft rationale for component categories is for ActiveX controls to be able to state explicitly the interface(s) or semantic interactions that they support, as well as the minimal level of service that they demand from the container. On the flip side, a container can also find out the requirements of a control, and what the control may expect – this can allow a smart container to decide not to host controls which it cannot handle. In fact, a mechanism has been specified to provide a 'default class' to be associated with a category, using the 'TreatAs' registry key on the CATID. This allows for creation of adaptive containers that can use 'better implementations' of certain functionality, if the associated ActiveX control is available, but still provide 'minimal implementation' of the functionality if no value-added component is available. Our original best-of-breed intentions are finally fulfilled if and when these containers arrive.

ATL 3 provides flexible support for component categories through **category maps**. Similar to other maps, you simply define your categories via ATL macros, and a global (static) table will be built for you automatically. The generated ActiveX control registration code will automatically register the categories for you by walking the global table and using `ICatRegister` from the component manager to register your component. If a component manager is not available at the target system, ATL will simply skip the process.

Here is a typical segment of code illustrating the ATL category map:

```
BEGIN_CATEGORY_MAP(CCalendar)
IMPLEMENTED_CATEGORY(CATID_Insertable)
REQUIRED_CATEGORY(CATID_PersistToStreamInit)
END_CATEGORY_MAP()
```

The proliferation of ActiveX controls in a typical system is phenomenal. As more and more ActiveX controls take advantage of Component Categories, management of these categories can become a nightmare.

Fear not, thanks to the 'just-in-time' arrival of the enterprise-wide Active Directory service from Windows NT 5. Component Categories extend and work naturally within the class store provided by Active Directory. The same component category registration and search/location facility will be available on a departmental or enterprise wide basis through the **class store**. The centralized class store will ease the installation, dependency management, and version tracking problems associated with ActiveX control proliferation.

Summary

We started this chapter by looking at exactly what is meant by the terms COM component, ActiveX control and full control. In order for a control to be a full control, it needs to implement the OC94 and/or OC96 specifications, so we also spent a good deal of time looking at what these specifications require.

We also examined how Visual C++ 6 and ATL 3 help us to implement the multitude of interfaces that are laid down by the OC94 and OC96 specifications.

For the OC94 specification, we looked in particular at the interfaces associated with:

- ❑   Object linking and embedding
- ❑   In-place activation
- ❑   Control specific UI functionality
- ❑   Support for property sheets

Finally, we turned our attention to the new features of OC96, and saw how we could implement:

- ❑   Deferred activation
- ❑   Optimized drawing
- ❑   Quick activation
- ❑   Flicker-free activation and deactivation
- ❑   Support for windowless controls

This concludes our examination of what makes a visual ActiveX control click. Now is a good time to put the theory into practice. First, however, we'll take a little time out to examine the requirements and the design of the case study that we'll be coding up in the chapters to come.

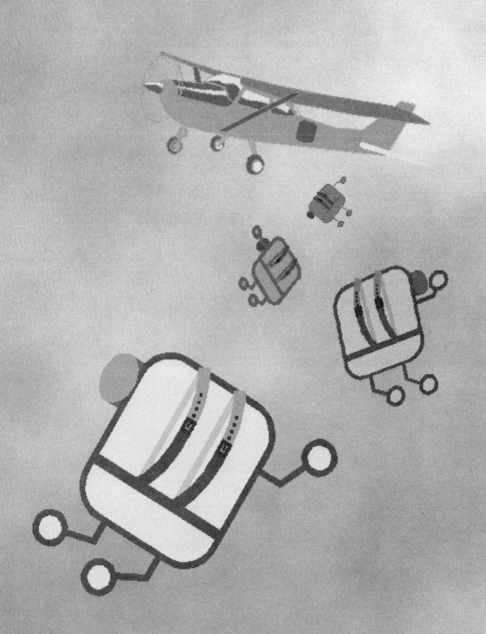

Designing a Distributed Calendar System

Armed with our knowledge of basic COM principles, our experience of creating an ActiveX control from scratch, using the Active Template Library, and what we learnt about controls in the last chapter, we're ready to apply our knowledge to a more complex problem. Instead of some concept demonstration, this will be a 'near production quality' application designed to solve a real-world problem.

In this chapter, we'll lay the foundations for the case study whose construction will occupy the following four chapters. We'll go through:

- ❑ Requirements analysis
- ❑ Use case analysis
- ❑ Architectural considerations
- ❑ Partitioning your application
- ❑ Initial class design

Overview

We're a consultant team and have been asked to evaluate the applicability of an intranet for a fictitious company called Aberdeen & Wilshire International.

Aberdeen & Wilshire is a San Francisco-based company with branches in Dallas, New York, Washington D.C., Vancouver, Toronto, and London. The headquarters is in San Francisco, with a sales office in every other location, though assembly and manufacturing is mostly done in Dallas. The company employs around 900 people.

The Requirement Analysis

In the first consultation session, we met with the Chief Information Officer, and representatives from the Human Resources, Sales, Logistics, and Manufacturing departments. During our meeting, we distilled the following requirements for the system:

❑   Want to take a 'least risk' approach to 'phase-in' an intranet. Ideally, the system should be implemented for the headquarters' and sales staff first.

❑   Want to get the intranet up and running within three months and need to obtain immediate results to allay the anxieties expressed by the CEO and Board of Directors. The longer term strategic value of such a system must be clearly visible after the first phase of implementation.

❑   Must be able to set metrics to measure success.

❑   Staging must ensure that full-scale corporate-wide deployment is possible.

❑   Need to minimize expenditure, especially capital expenditure, since the budget is particularly tight this financial year.

Existing Network Topology

The CIO has explained that the company has achieved its 'PC on every desk goal' throughout the corporate offices (except for manufacturing). However, the hardware configurations are not uniform: some of the offices PCs are 486s while those in the corporate headquarters are at least Pentium 200s. Furthermore, the variety of OSes they're using is mind blowing:

❑   There are 200 PCs in San Francisco, and about 50 Macintoshes. Most of the PCs are running Windows 95 or Windows NT Workstation as the desktop environment.

❑   There are about 20 PCs in Toronto running a mixture of OS/2 Warp and Merlin.

❑   15 workstations in Dallas are UNIX based.

❑   In Washington DC, Vancouver, and London, there are approximately 50 networked computers at each site consisting of 45% PCs running Windows 3.11 and Windows 95 – the rest being Macintoshes.

Every PC is networked within the department via Ethernet. Most departments operate on Novell 2.x or 3.x file servers, with an occasional Microsoft based peer-to-peer workgroup LAN. All departments are inter-networked through routers and leased lines. Servicing the backbone are a set of HP UNIX Servers – acting mainly as the conduit for email, ftp, telnet, networked FAX, and remote printing services. San Francisco, New York, and Toronto have their own Windows NT departmental servers running the Microsoft BackOffice suite. All access to the corporate backbone is via TCP/IP based clients or utilities.

Identified Problematic Areas

After explaining the value of an intranet and what it can do for Aberdeen & Wilshire, the group as a whole has identified the following areas which lend themselves to almost immediate intranet application:

The A&W personnel directory

It is currently being administered at the San Francisco headquarters. The cost of maintenance is high. A full-time staff member is responsible for the coordination, update, production, planning, layout, and distribution of the directory. Unfortunately, with the high turnover experienced within recent years, it has become increasingly difficult to keep the information up-to-date. The directory is published twice a year, and, often, the printed copies aren't completely distributed before the information is outdated.

Distribution of Memos regarding Corporate and Departmental Events

Their current paper circulation of event notification is expensive, wasteful, and inefficient, especially when using couriers to the Canadian and UK offices. An attempt has been made to use email for these notifications. Unfortunately, higher level management and directors (who are invited to many of the departmental events) often missed them because they received a mailbox full of such announcements. People working across departments or disciplines are often bombarded with a barrage of 'junk announcements'. Maintenance and update of mailing lists for distribution of event notices is also a significant chore.

This is the area we'll be looking at during the course of the book.

Automation in Human Resources

The Human Resources department is swamped with forms. Company policies and government regulations have forced the department into keeping both current and historical employee records. With the recent resource cuts, the department is under heavy pressure to provide improved services with significantly fewer personnel. Given this situation, the head of Human Resources is looking to Automation in order to alleviate the most voluminous and common Human Resource interactions. The two most common areas requiring human interactions or paper form processing are:

- ❑ Inquiries about policies, procedures, and processes
- ❑ Change of personal employee information

Our Proposal

While the above company and situation is hypothetical, you're likely to find similar (if not identical) requirements and situations in most modern corporations. It serves as a good basis for the rationale of introducing an intranet, which can address many of these requirements almost immediately.

In order to guide Aberdeen & Wilshire to an intranet-based system that they can operate and maintain in the long term, we realize that the project must be implemented in a phased approach. Many of the staff members that will be responsible for the upkeep of the intranet lack the necessary skills and will require extensive training. However, the team's unusually high enthusiasm for this intranet effort should mean that the smoothing out of the rough spots is an easy process.

Also, to address the CIO's comment on risk and immediate results, we must make the first phase of the project simple, quick, and effective. To this end, we've planned the project in two phases:

Phase I: Proof of Concept

In the first phase, we'll implement the Aberdeen & Wilshire Events calendar, which will announce corporate-wide and departmental events. The major architectural parts of the intranet will be put in place in this phase. Initially, they will be used solely to provide the data to the calendar, but it's the plan that extending the intranet won't involve major changes to the underlying architecture, just the addition of new business logic and database tables.

Phase II: Extending the Intranet's Functionality

The intranet we'll design will cover the following additional areas:

- ❑ The Employee Directory; maintaining an up-to-date directory for employee names, departments, email addresses, and phone numbers.
- ❑ Human Resources will pilot the replacement of forms for changing of employee's personal information including address and phone numbers. It will also require that the system can be administered *securely* over the intranet.

One week after presenting this proposal to the Aberdeen & Wilshire intranet team, the proposal received the team's unanimous approval. Our consultancy was asked to assist in the planning, design, and coordination during the two phases of the project. Within two weeks, higher-level management commitment was obtained and funding was available for beginning the project.

Getting Started

Our target system, the one we'll be developing over the next few chapters, is the distributed system handling the Aberdeen & Wilshire corporate calendar of events.

The design is one where computation and event data will be distributed over multiple machines via an intranet. Each department hosting events can keep track of their own data using their own database and departmental servers, on whatever hardware platform they choose to host such data. As long as they all agree to provide a well-specified component interface into the system, the components making up the system can be changed or upgraded independently with no effect on others. This will illustrate how COM technology can be used to 'wrap' dissimilar systems in a distributed intranet.

This calendaring system will be a complete end-to-end corporate application, frequently called an 'intranet application'. And because of its use of ActiveX and Internet technology, it's also a **Distributed interNet Architecture** (DNA) application.

To give you a map for the project, we will be covering the following topics in order:

- ❑ System requirements and architecture
- ❑ The visual ActiveX control calendar component
- ❑ The non-visual Visual Basic compatible components

❑ The middle-tier Business Object components
❑ Handling the data tier with ATL 3 OLE DB Templates
❑ Integrating Microsoft Transaction Server 2.0 for application deployment and distributed transactions
❑ Creating an administrative component user interface using ATL 3 Dynamic HTML support
❑ Enabling remote operation through Microsoft Message Queue Server

In this chapter, we will examine the objective of our project, and perform the necessary analysis and high-level design for our system. Through UML diagrams and design descriptions, we will formulate the solution for the Aberdeen and Wilshire problem, and define the various components within the system and their associated roles.

At the core of this process is the design of the visual calendar control, which is the client of the completed, distributed Calendar system. It's a miniature application that will be used on the web pages within our intranet. As such it has two roles:

❑ It will provide the user interface and handle all the required user interactions
❑ It will allow the Aberdeen & Wilshire corporate calendar of events to be viewed at any time from any employee's desktop, with live data

We'll go on to code and test this control in the next chapter.

The A&W Calendaring System Requirements

The following is the first attempt at a use case diagram for the A&W Calendar system.

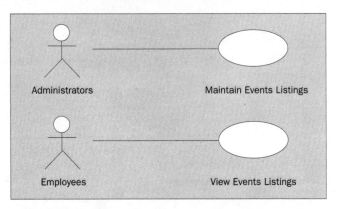

This first level use case is overly simplistic, but does establish the basic consumer-producer relationship. The administrator creates and deletes the event listings, and the employees view the event listings at their leisure. Here, we can also establish the read/write nature of the administrator's access to the event data, as well as the read-only nature of the employee's access.

Analysis

The system depicted in this first level use case is not necessarily a distributed one. In our case, however, we actually have multiple departmental administrators responsible for the maintenance of event information for their own department; while employees across all departments may well be interested in event information from other departments.

Other than the fact that multiple departmental administrators are involved, we have also discovered that some administrators work off-line. These administrators may be creating new event information while they are on the road. To accommodate these users, the administration client software must be functional when executed from a notebook computer in a disconnected mode.

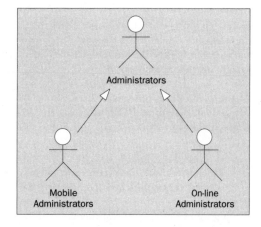

The final, more complex use case diagram summarizes what we've been saying. It fully specifies the different type of actors and use cases involved in the distributed system.

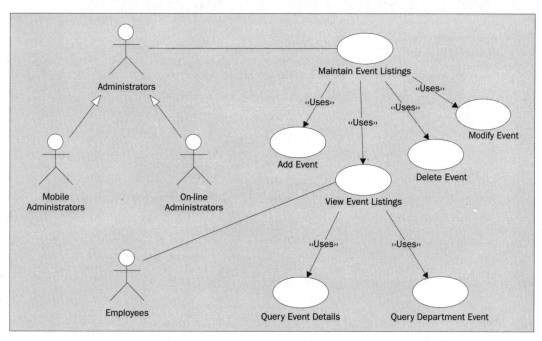

Actor: Employees

All employees of A&W who have access to their PC. All have IE 4 installed.

Actor: On-line Administrators

These are departmental administrators whose PCs are directly connected to the intranet. Each administrator is responsible for keeping the list of events available on his/her department's database server.

Actor: Mobile Administrators

These are departmental administrators who are working in a disconnected environment using notebook computers. Each administrator is responsible for keeping the list of events available on his/her department's database server, which is always connected to the intranet.

Use Case: View Events

See a count of all the events that are available for a particular day across all the departments – in a month-at-a-glance format.

Use Case: Query Department Events

See the headers of all the events available for a particular day, for a particular department.

Use Case: Query Event Detail

See the details for a particular event.

Use Case: Add Event

Add an event to the departmental event list maintained at the departmental data server.

Use Case: Delete Event

Remove an event from the departmental event list maintained at the departmental data server.

Use Case: Modify Event

Change the details of an event already existing in the event list maintained at the departmental data server.

> *We will not implement the Modify Event use case in order to avoid repetition. The actual design and implementation can be easily deduced from the way we implement the Delete Event and Add Event use cases.*

Data Access Profile

We have also learnt from the A&W MIS team that there are a total of 15 departments in the corporation, and close to 900 employees in total. A typical employee would view the calendar over the intranet an average of three times a day. We have established, through a study over the last three months that there are an average of five events per department per month across all the departments. The probability of event cancellation or information change once listed is 5% according to our study. We also found that 65% of all events are announced less than one day prior to the event occurrence and 20% of them are announced less than one week but more than one day prior. This allows us to characterize our data access requirement as:

- ❑ Frequently read
- ❑ Infrequently written/modified
- ❑ Requires immediate update after modification

For the design of any distributed system, it is very important to understand in advance the data access profile and requirement of the target system. Ideally, the profile should be broken down by users (use case actors), dataset type (if many sets of data are involved), access type (read, read/write, write) and access frequency (frequency scaled 1 to 10). This is vital because, due to the limitation of distributed technology today, the actual data access profile/pattern will heavily influence the design and implementation of the final system.

High-Level Design

Our analysis of the system leads us naturally to the following high-level design. We decompose the problem into the now-classic three-tier architecture. Within each tier, we will be using ActiveX controls and DNA business objects to accomplish the task required.

Here is a high-level view of this structure.

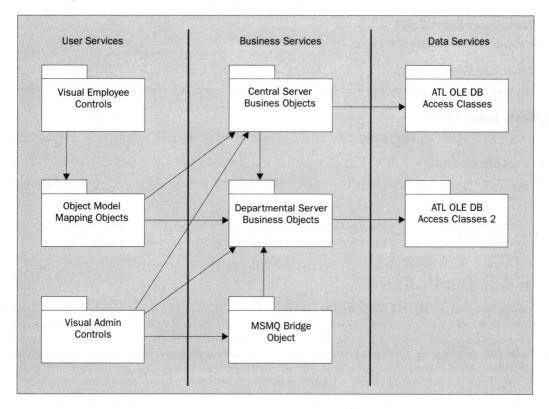

In the first tier, where the user interface is presented to the actors, we have one of three visual controls:

- ❏ A month-at-a-glance visual calendar ActiveX control – Used by employees
- ❏ A Dynamic HTML-based visual administration control for on-line usage – Used by on-line administrators
- ❏ A Dynamic HTML-based visual administration control for off-line usage – Used by mobile administrators

Together with this first tier of user-interface presentation, we have a series of components that present the Automation compatible object model. It is through these components that the calendar control will access the event data. These components, the **object model mapping objects**, in turn use the services of the middle-tier DNA business objects to retrieve event information.

On a conceptual level, this series of Automation compatible components represents a layer which performs the relational-to-object mapping. While the business objects in the middle tier enforce certain business rules during data access, they do not provide the mapping required for easy access from the visual ActiveX control. We selected this approach also to demonstrate potential reuse of the object model by ActiveX controls written using Visual Basic, Visual J++, or any supported scripting languages. This opens up the event data for use by any new client applications.

The visual administration controls, however, talk directly with the second-tier business objects. This linkage is not necessarily Automation compatible, but is typically more efficient. Of course, it is also possible to introduce an additional layer of Automation compatible relational-to-object mapping components in this case; however, we will forego this option to avoid repetitive coverage.

If we look into the details of the DNA business objects in the second tier, we will discover that they serve two vital functions:

- ❏ Managing a local **caching data server** to provide for frequent client access *without* contacting departmental servers
- ❏ Enforcing certain **data access rules** (so called business rules) across distributed database updates

Finally, the business objects themselves make use of objects in the third tier. Residing in the third tier are data access objects created to work with OLE DB. Specifically, we will be using ATL 3's new OLE DB data consumer templates to quickly create these third tier data objects.

A DNA Solution

Our problem is not easily solvable without DNA technologies. Here are some of the issues that must be addressed:

- ❏ Information on some events will be viewed frequently, but it should not cause network traffic directly to the responsible departmental database. This implies some form of information caching.
- ❏ When event administrators add or delete events, the new events (or deleted event) should be reflected immediately on the system.

❑ The mobile administrators should use exactly the same user interface to add/delete an event as their on-line counterparts.

❑ Addition or removal of departmental servers to the system should be handled dynamically, without 'taking down' the system.

❑ The distributed system should have minimal downtime.

To deal with some of these issues, let us take a look at the various use cases in action.

Use Case 1: View Events

This is what the Employee actor would be faced with:

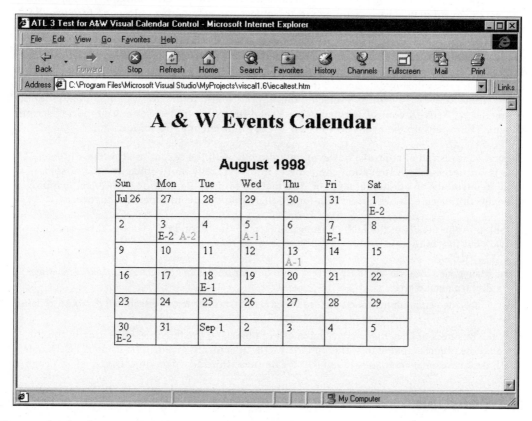

The visual calendar control displays events in a month-at-a-glance view. It only displays the following information for each day in a particular month being viewed:

❑ Departments with events, where A stands for Accounting and E stands for Engineering

❑ The number of events for the department

Use Case 2: Query Department Events

When the Employee actor clicks on one of the date cells in the calendar, the following dialog will pop up:

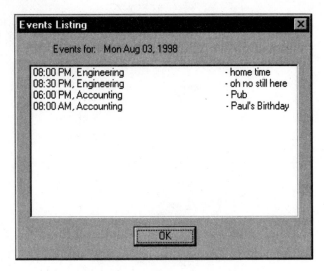

Use Case 3: Query Events Details

This provides further header information into the events available from the department. If the actor is interested in a particular event, he/she can click on the event to get the complete details:

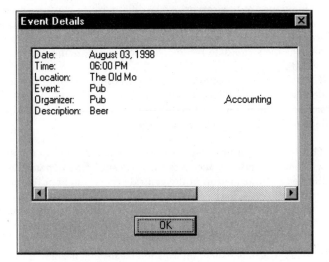

Network Topology Analysis

We are now going to take a look at a simplified view of the network serving the A&W enterprise. Network and server availability and connectivity as well as administrative issues will provide us with further information that will aid our continuing analysis and will restrict the space of acceptable design alternatives.

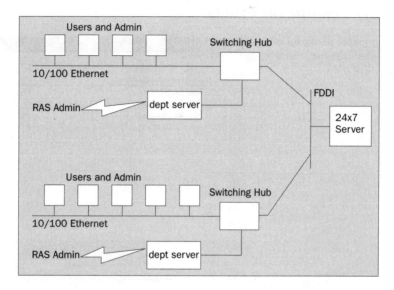

Notice the 24x7 server available as the central data server. It is the single server enjoying the widest connectivity from most part of the intranet. However, due to the high cost of administration and maintenance of this server, A&W don't wish to consider a completely centralized calendaring solution. This situation is further complicated by politics (as are most real world administration scenarios). Each departmental administrator wishes to have complete control over their own event data, as the same data is often simultaneously being used in other contexts.

To divert most of the event viewing traffic away from the slower portion of the intranet, we have decided to cache the departmental and event count (not headers) information on the centralized 24x7 server. Although we will maintain the cache, we have decided not to use it for our first release but leave using it for future optimization.

This implies that use case 1 will require access only to the centralized server, and use case 2 and 3 will require network access to the corresponding departmental server. We have decided not to cache the header information in the central server (i.e. handling use case 2) for the following reasons:

❑ Caching only the count (handling use case 1) may already be sufficient and the implementation is significantly simpler. We can always modify the strategy in a subsequent release – once we get the basic architecture working

❑ Caching header information means that header information would be stored in both the centralized server and the departmental server redundantly, which significantly complicates system recovery planning and may affect stability

❑ If both header and count are available from centralized server, and only details are stored in departmental servers – we are in a borderline 'centralized update' and 'replicate' situation

This design sufficiently addresses the first issue from the section *A DNA Solution*.

Enhancing Perceived System Uptime

Since the Calendar control only depends on use case 1 to become active, the system is also 'up' as long as the 24x7 centralized server is up. While one can argue that every other departmental server, or portion of the Intranet could be down, the DNA application embedding the calendar control would still appear to be 'up' and can effectively work with any connected departmental server that is still 'up'. This is an excellent example of how a distributed system can take advantage of the 'greatest common factor' uptime, instead of reflecting the more common and depressing 'least common denominator' uptime. Since we can enjoy 24x7 uptime as long as our connection to the centralized server, and the server itself stays up, the requirement for minimal downtime is sufficiently addressed by this design.

More Use Cases

Administrator actors have very different requirements, their responsibilities are reflected in the other use cases:

Use Case 4: Add Event

Administrators, whether on-line or mobile, uses a visual ActiveX control to add events to the system.

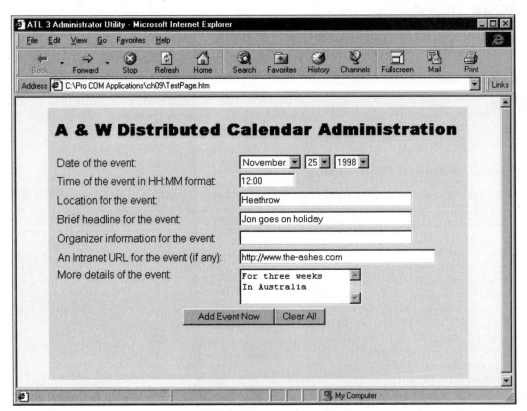

The event is added to the system once the Administrator presses the 'Add Event' button. It is expected that the event information will be updated shortly after, and every Employee actor in the system will have access to that data.

In the case of a mobile Administrator, the actual event information submission will be deferred until the next time the notebook computer is connected to the intranet, either directly through the office docking station or over the Internet via virtual private network connection.

Use Case 5: Modify Event

This use case is not implemented to avoid redundant coverage.

Use Case 6: Delete Event

Administrators, on-line or mobile, use the following visual ActiveX control to delete an event from the system.

The event deleted is to be reflected in the system shortly after the Administrator presses the 'Delete Event' button. Every Employee actor accessing the system at this time should not see the deleted event.

Yet More Use Cases

Finally, to ensure the dynamic addition and removal of departmental servers doesn't necessitate service interruption, it is important to add two more use cases to our analysis.

Use Case 7: Add Department

Adds information relating to a department to the central server's database. This information includes the department number, the name of the department, and its network connection information. Typically, this is used by a departmental server during its startup, in order to let the central server know that it is ready for event requests.

Use Case 8: Remove Department

Deletes a particular department's record from the central server's database. This is typically used by a sentinel process on the central server. The sentinel process occasionally checks for connectivity with departmental servers, and removes any departmental servers which are unreachable.

These additional use cases are associated with a sub-analysis where we treat the departmental servers as actors against the database server residing on the centralized server. In this analysis, which we will not go into in-depth for brevity's sake, we want the departmental servers to add themselves to the central server's database whenever they come up. We also want a way to detect that a departmental server is down, and remove the department information from the central server's database.

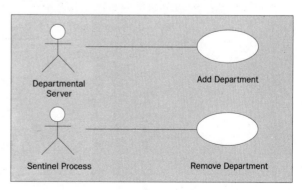

In the next chapter, we will commence our detailed design by examining in more detail the specific components in each layer that makes up our DNA application.

Proceeding with the Visual Calendar Control Design

Before commencing with the code of the calendar control, the subject of the next chapter, we should take a look at the design details.

Detailed Design

In our design, the software will consist of three main classes:

- ❏ CViscal – A user control module
- ❏ CCellMgr – Calendar cells manager
- ❏ CDataMgr – Back-end data manager

The classes interact in the following manner:

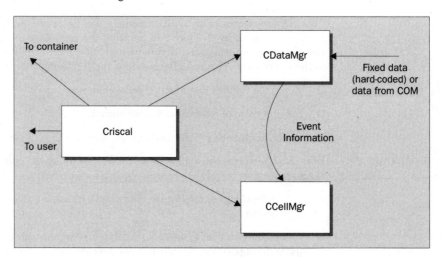

The CViscal is the core of the control that handles the display of the user interface, and input from the user. It's also the coordinator of activities between the instance of the CDataMgr class and an instance of the CCellMgr class.

Here's a high-level design description of the code modules:

Module Name	Description
CViscal	This is the core ActiveX control, its functions include: ❑ Coordinating the action of its m_DataMgr (an instance of CDataMgr) and m_CellMgr (an instance of CCellMgr) ❑ Interacting with the ATL support environment for visual ActiveX control operations ❑ Drawing and managing the presentation display to the user ❑ Handling user interactions and displaying the required form or data ❑ Exposing and implementing custom properties and interfaces for the ActiveX control user
CCellMgr	This class manages an array of calendar cells. Each cell contains coordinate information used by Cviscal in painting the presentation display, as well as specific event information obtained from CDataMgr's routine for direct access to the event data. This module provides the following functions: ❑ Reads the value of calendar cell array elements ❑ Sets the value of calendar cell array elements ❑ Performs hit testing to determine if the user clicked on a cell
CDataMgr	This class performs the actual data access, and hides the complexity of data access from the rest of the control. The class provides: ❑ A high-level logical interface to data access, hiding the actual data access mechanism ❑ Calendar event data to the CViscal class, either through hard-coded data or through support from middle-tier business objects

One conscious design decision we've made is to use an array of data structures to represent the calendar cells instead of using an array of actual controls. In our design, the Calendar control paints and manages the entire canvas area. This is done mainly for efficiency. In an alternative design, one may create 42 Windows controls in a control array to represent the calendar cells. However, creating 42 Windows controls on the Calendar control would require the creation of at least another 42 windows during runtime. While the alternative design may simplify some of the coding and hit testing required, the runtime resource consumption and performance would make it an undesirable choice.

Testing Environment

We'll be testing the function of this ActiveX control inside the Visual Studio 98 ActiveX control test container, Internet Explorer 4, and Visual Basic 6.

As a completely self-contained intranet mini-application, the Calendar control really doesn't need too many externally configurable parameters. This allows easy deployment of the control, and simpler overall support. While it's possible to create extremely configurable controls for more generic use using Visual C++, we'll focus on applying it to our hypothetical Aberdeen & Wilshire intranet.

The Calendar control will have the following properties and methods exposed to the user:

Property Name	Type	Description
TitleFontName	String (Default = "Arial")	The typeface described by this name will be used to draw the 'Month' title of the calendar.
TitleFontSize	Integer (Default = 10)	This font size in points specified by this value will be used to draw the 'Month' title of the calendar.
TitleFontBold	Boolean (Default = TRUE)	When set to TRUE, the typeface of the 'Month' title will be set to bold. When set to FALSE, the title typeface will be set to normal.
ButtonVisible	Boolean (Default = TRUE)	When set to FALSE, the two arrow buttons for advancing the month will not be drawn.

Method Prototype	Description
void AdvanceMonth(Long I);	Call this method to advance the month displayed on the calendar. The number passed indicates the number of months to advance the calendar by, and can be either positive or negative.

Our calendar ActiveX control will not generate any ActiveX events for the container.

Initially, in order to test our control, the CDataMgr access routines will be coded to access back-end COM server objects to obtain data. In the next chapter, we'll use these back-end components without going into them in any depth. In the chapter after that, we'll examine the construction of these components using some advanced ATL techniques. In addition, we'll hook up the components across a network to obtain live event data available from the individual departments using DCOM-based technology. In all cases, though, we'll be artificially setting the data into the back-end components upon initialization. This frees us from having to set up real data sources for testing and demonstration purposes.

Let's take a detailed look at the two core classes that make up our Aberdeen & Wilshire calendar control.

The CDataMgr Class

CDataMgr manages access to back-end event data. It provides a set of member functions that allow the calendar logic to be independent of where the data may be stored. Many of the data structures used in processing of event data are defined by this class. For sample purposes, our implementation of the event system is limited to handling up to ten events each day from up to three departments. These limits can easily be changed and are defined in CalDefs.h:

```
const kMaxEvents = 10;
const kMaxDepts = 3;
```

The structure of an event for the calendar cells is defined in CEvents.h

```
struct CCalEvent
{
    CDateTime DateTime;
    tstring Location;
    tstring Heading;
    tstring Organizer;
    tstring OrgDept;
    tstring Details;
    tstring Hlink;
};
```

This structure matches the calendar event detail information that we may obtain from the back-end data components. The types CDateTime and tstring encapsulate what their names intuitively suggest and will be examined in more detail in the next chapter.

Before drawing the calendar with information, the control needs to find out all the participating departments that may have events. The details of the department, including the initial character used and the color to draw the information in is kept in the following structure:

```
struct CCalDept
{
    tstring DeptName;
    tstring DeptNumber;
    bool CanRead;
    bool CanPostNew;
    tstring Symbol;
    OLE_COLOR Color;
};
```

Another data structure defined in CEvents.h is CDeptEvents, which maintains a collection of the dates on which a particular department may have events.

```
struct CDeptEvents
{
    CCalDept Dept;
    CDatesList OnDates;

    ULONG GetNumEventsOnDate(const CDateTime& inDate) const;
};
```

`CDatesList` is declared as follows:

```
class CDatesList : public vector<CDateTime>
{
};
```

By inheriting from `vector<>`, rather than using `vector<>` directly, we allow potential future changes of the implementation method of the `CDateTime` collection without affecting the rest of the code.

The `CDataMgr` class provides several high-level functions for obtaining data. The actual details of data retrieval are encapsulated completely within the `CDataMgr` class. This allows us, initially, to hard-code the data, and eventually obtain the data through the middle-tier business objects.

The CCellMgr Class

The cell manager class manages the 'data' associated with the displayed calendar cells. It does not directly do any drawing of the data for the calendar. All the drawing is done by the `CViscal` class. However, the cell manager class does manage all required data for drawing. The `OnDraw()` member of `CViscal` class works closely with the cell manager to display calendar information.

The work is done by managing a private array of cell structures, one associated with each cell displayed on the calendar. Each cell corresponds to a day. A cell structure is defined as:

```
class CCalCell
{
public:
    CCalCell();
    ~CCalCell();

    void ClearContent();

    CDateTime date;
    tstring dayNumber;
    bool hasEvent;
    tstring label;
    CRect rect;
    CellAttachment attach[kMaxCellAttachments];
};
```

Note that besides the values used to paint the representation of the cell, it also contains optional attachments (which aren't used in our example) – the actual date represented, a string label for the day, and the location information of the cell on the ActiveX control's client area. (The `CRect` class will be examined in the next chapter). The location information is used by the control when the user clicks on the control. At this time, the control will check all the cells that have events, to determine if the user has clicked on one of the cells.

Ready to Code!

In this chapter, we've laid out the framework for a hypothetical intranet consultancy assignment. While consulting for Aberdeen & Wilshire, we met with the executives and developers to discuss the major business objectives and
formulated an agreed approach to launch an intranet. We've also laid the foundations of our design.

In the next chapter will show the steps taken in creating the control, and analysis of the code involved in the implementation of the control. Our coding will make extensive use of ATL's support for many of the OC94 and OC96 interfaces we looked at in Chapter 5.

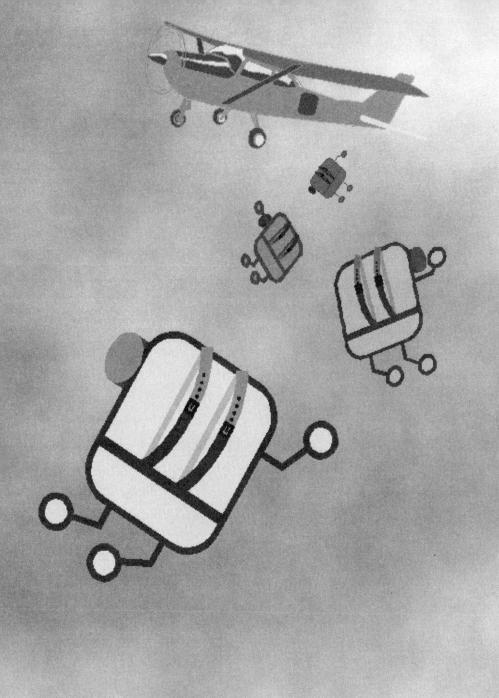

Building an ActiveX Calendar Control

In this chapter, we'll be coding a visual calendar control using ATL 3 and Visual C++ 6, putting to work all those complex interfaces that we covered in Chapter 5. We'll also be looking at various ways to test the control in different real-world containers.

The control is not very interesting by itself, so we'll provide some calendar event data for it to display. To obtain this data, we'll take a look at the design of middle-tier business objects that can supply the calendar control with vital real-time event data for display to the user. Our analysis will cover the object model presented by these components. The same model can easily be incorporated into other COM-based clients, including Visual Basic and Visual J++ based applications. In other words, these middle-tier objects can be easily reused by front-end applications, supporting a variety of methods of presentation to the end user.

> **Because we will be going through several iterations of the code and we don't want the chapter to dominate the book, we haven't shown every line of code. There'll be listings of the support classes in Appendix E, but we still advise you to use the downloaded source code when looking at this chapter.**

In the next chapter, we'll go on to examine the business objects in the middle tier, and see how business rules are enforced. We'll also discuss relational-to-object mapping. Visual C++ 6 will again be used in building these components. Finally, in later chapters, we'll test the entire system, including the calendar control, business objects, and database access objects – all communicating through COM in a distributed three-tier combination.

Creating the Calendar Control with Visual C++ 6

Throughout this chapter, you'll see how Visual C++ 6, together with the ATL 3 wizards, eases the task of coding complex visual ActiveX controls in C++. We will be going through a total of six separate iterations in the construction of our visual calendar control. With each iteration, we will add a significant new feature to our visual control. The six iterations are:

1. Creating a basic ActiveX control project using AppWizard and ATL 3, implementing ambient properties which will include a system-managed font resource

2. Adding child windows as contained windows, using an alternate message map, resizing contained windows and adding drawing code

3. Adding a method for the ActiveX control, hooking up buttons to behaviors, drawing calendar cells, and adding date calculation and display logic

4. Adding a custom property for the ActiveX control, working with font resources, adding backend logic, and interfacing with middle-tier objects, performing a hit test, and implementing and managing popup dialogs using ATL

5. Implementing OC96 deferred activation

6. Implementing an OC96 windowless control while maintaining compatibility with legacy containers

Iteration 1: The Basic Control

In this iteration, we will be creating the skeleton of a complete control, and implementing support for ambient properties, including a system-managed font resource.

Creating an ActiveX Control Project Using AppWizard

The steps in generating the skeletal code to support a visual ActiveX control are similar to the creation of any ATL project. Remember the simple `ATLBlob` project we created back in Chapter 4? First, we must create a new ATL COM project using the AppWizard, and we call the project `viscal1`. In general, you must choose the name of your project carefully, since this will be the name of the target DLL or executable.

> *You can find all the code for this in the* `\Ch06\viscal1` *directory of the source download for this book from* http://www.wrox.com.

Since this is a visual ActiveX control, and we will later make it OC96 compliant, it will always be in-process. The detailed reason for this is that the necessary `IViewObject` interface is unmarshalable, as we explained in Chapter 5.

We will leave the proxy-stub code in its own DLL, to keep the generated code straightforward. As we do not require any help from the MFC library, we'll also leave the Support MFC option unchecked. Also, we will not use any MTS features in the creation of this control, so you can leave the final option unchecked.

Later on in the book, in Chapter 9, we will be creating business objects with MTS (Microsoft Transaction Server) support, and the visual control we're creating here will make use of these middle-tier objects during its operation.

All you need to do now is press the Finish button, and then click OK when the AppWizard shows a summary of the code to be generated.

This completes the generation of the skeleton code. Now let's add an ATL object using the ATL Object Wizard. (Remember that you can do this by selecting New ATL Object from the Insert menu.) Instead of the Simple Object that we looked at in Chapter 5, we will now create a Full Control. Select Controls from the Category listbox, and Full Control from the Objects pane:

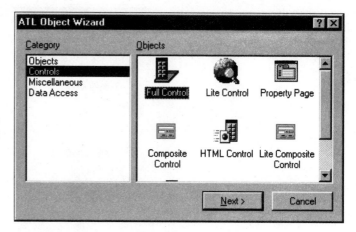

The difference between Full and Lite versions lies in the interfaces that they support. Lite versions of controls should live happily in Internet Explorer 4 and newer OC96-compliant containers. Full versions of control may be necessary if you need to maintain compatibility with existing and legacy containers.

There are quite a few properties to look at here, so let's take this form one tab at a time.

Names

First, we need to name our control and its associated C++ class and COM libraries. Enter viscal in the C++ Short Name field, and adjust the ProgID to reflect the `<library>.<component>` syntax. The library name is the same as the name of the target module, while the component name is the short name we entered above.

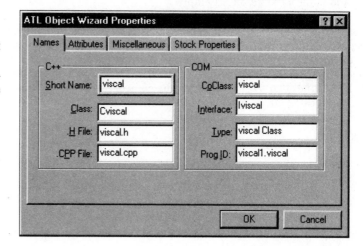

Attributes

Now switch to the Attributes tab. Our in-process server will support the higher performance apartment threading model and flexible dual interfaces. We decide to support aggregation since many IDEs, such as Visual Basic 6, use aggregation to present additional extended properties to end users. We will also implement support for rich error reporting by checking the Support ISupportErrorInfo checkbox.

This control will not support generic connection points (for firing custom events back to the container), nor will it aggregate the Free Threaded Marshaler:

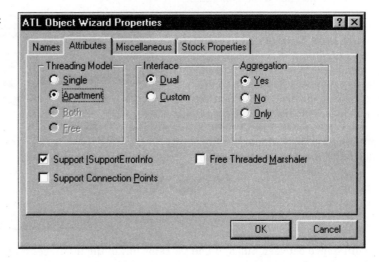

Miscellaneous

Move to the Miscellaneous tab, and take a look at the options there. The screen area that we manage within the ActiveX control will have an opaque and solid background. If we leave these boxes checked, then this will prevent containers that care about transparency from worrying about whether the control has a transparent visual representation. We are not sub-classing standard Win32 controls, so we'll leave the Add control based on list empty.

The Misc Status group indicates that the requested flags should be set under the MiscStatus key in the registry. The first one, Invisible at runtime, is for controls that should be visible at design time (so that, for example, their properties can be set) but should be invisible at runtime (examples would be a timer control, a control that monitors a device, or one that receives notifications from an application server etc.) The other two flags specify that the control has some specific behavior. None of these flags apply to our visual calendar, so we'll leave them alone.

In the Other group box, we leave the Normalize DC box checked, so that ATL will generate code to normalize the device context (setting the mapping mode to MM_TEXT, and the window and viewport origin to (0, 0)). It does this by implementing a CComControlBase::OnDrawAdvanced() method, which will eventually call OnDraw() with the normalized context. This makes our painting code significantly simpler.

We also check the Windowed Only option, since this first iteration will not support OC96 windowless operation. Finally, we check the Insertable option, for the control to be registered with Insertable key in the registry. This is important because many OLE heritage containers will depend on this key to determine which COM object can be embedded. We will see the effect of all these selections later, when we take a look at the generated code.

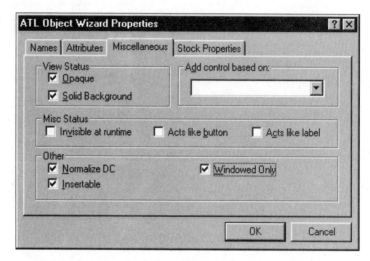

Stock Properties

Finally, we move on to the Stock Properties tab. To illustrate how one would handle and manage complex ambient properties, we will implement two stock properties: Background Color, and Font. Font handling, due to the complex resource structures involved, will be especially interesting. Other stock properties could easily be added using the same techniques that we will demonstrate in this chapter.

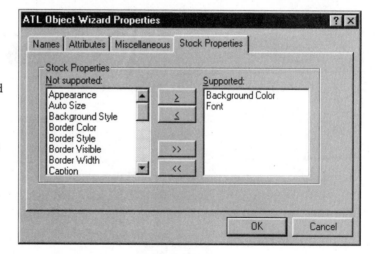

If you click OK at this point, the Object Wizard will proceed to generate the support code for our visual control. After code generation, you can examine the ClassView pane to see all the classes and code that you do not have to write:

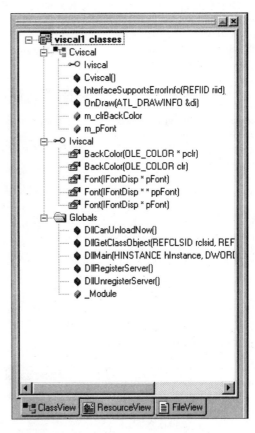

We can see from this that the ATL Object Wizard has carried out the following tasks for us:

1. Defined the default dual interface (Iviscal), together with the access routines for the two stock properties (these are also implemented, if you look at the code)

2. Implemented an InterfaceSupportsErrorInfo() method

3. Defined two member variables to hold the value of the background color and font stock properties

4. Put in all the usual ActiveX control support code (self-registration, IUnknown support, etc.)

5. Generated an OnDraw() member for our implementation of the drawing code

Let's take a look now at the actual code generated. If you examine viscal.h, you can see all the interfaces that the object wizard decided to implement, based on our input:

```
class ATL_NO_VTABLE Cviscal :
    public CComObjectRootEx<CComSingleThreadModel>,
    public CStockPropImpl<Cviscal, Iviscal, &IID_Iviscal, &LIBID_VISCAL1Lib>,
```

```
      public CComControl<Cviscal>,
      public IPersistStreamInitImpl<Cviscal>,
      public IOleControlImpl<Cviscal>,
      public IOleObjectImpl<Cviscal>,
      public IOleInPlaceActiveObjectImpl<Cviscal>,
      public IViewObjectExImpl<Cviscal>,
      public IOleInPlaceObjectWindowlessImpl<Cviscal>,
      public ISupportErrorInfo,
      public IPersistStorageImpl<Cviscal>,
      public ISpecifyPropertyPagesImpl<Cviscal>,
      public IQuickActivateImpl<Cviscal>,
      public IDataObjectImpl<Cviscal>,
      public IProvideClassInfo2Impl<&CLSID_viscal, NULL, &LIBID_VISCAL1Lib>,
      public CComCoClass<Cviscal, &CLSID_viscal>
```

Since we have indicated that the control should always be activated with its own window, ATL has configured the IOleInPlaceObject handling of ATL 3 by setting the m_bWindowOnly flag to TRUE in the constructor:

```
public:
    Cviscal()
    {
        m_bWindowOnly = TRUE;
    }
```

As we have saw in Chapter 4, the COM_MAP configures ATL to handle QueryInterface() calls. The code generated in viscal.h shows the mapping, but we will make one minor modification here, which is shown by the highlighted line below:

```
BEGIN_COM_MAP(Cviscal)
    COM_INTERFACE_ENTRY(Iviscal)
    COM_INTERFACE_ENTRY(IDispatch)
    COM_INTERFACE_ENTRY(IViewObjectEx)
    COM_INTERFACE_ENTRY(IViewObject2)
    COM_INTERFACE_ENTRY(IViewObject)
//    COM_INTERFACE_ENTRY(IOleInPlaceObjectWindowless)
    COM_INTERFACE_ENTRY(IOleInPlaceObject)
    COM_INTERFACE_ENTRY2(IOleWindow, IOleInPlaceObjectWindowless)
    COM_INTERFACE_ENTRY(IOleInPlaceActiveObject)
    COM_INTERFACE_ENTRY(IOleControl)
    COM_INTERFACE_ENTRY(IOleObject)
    COM_INTERFACE_ENTRY(IPersistStreamInit)
    COM_INTERFACE_ENTRY2(IPersist, IPersistStreamInit)
    COM_INTERFACE_ENTRY(ISupportErrorInfo)
    COM_INTERFACE_ENTRY(ISpecifyPropertyPages)
    COM_INTERFACE_ENTRY(IQuickActivate)
    COM_INTERFACE_ENTRY(IPersistStorage)
    COM_INTERFACE_ENTRY(IDataObject)
    COM_INTERFACE_ENTRY(IProvideClassInfo)
    COM_INTERFACE_ENTRY(IProvideClassInfo2)
END_COM_MAP()
```

We comment out the `IOleInPlaceObjectWindowless` entry in the COM map, so that a call to `QueryInterface()` requesting the `IOleInPlaceObjectWindowless` interface will fail. We do not support windowless operation in this version. (We will, however, be coming back to this later in the chapter.) Regardless of our indicated support (or lack, thereof) of the `IOleInPlaceObjectWindowless` interface, we are still inheriting from the `IOleInPlaceObjectWindowlessImpl<>` implementation class since it provides the implementation for `IOleInPlaceObject` methods.

We learnt in Chapter 5 that property persistence is done through the `PROP_MAP` macros. The generated code shows how the two stock properties (`BackColor` and `Font`) are persisted, together with the x and y co-ordinates of the control. To this property map, we will add two stock pages for editing the stock properties. ATL 3 will provide the support of `IPersistStreamInit` based on these declarations:

```
BEGIN_PROP_MAP(Cviscal)
    PROP_PAGE(CLSID_StockColorPage)
    PROP_PAGE(CLSID_StockFontPage)
    PROP_DATA_ENTRY("_cx", m_sizeExtent.cx, VT_UI4)
    PROP_DATA_ENTRY("_cy", m_sizeExtent.cy, VT_UI4)
    PROP_ENTRY("BackColor", DISPID_BACKCOLOR, CLSID_StockColorPage)
    PROP_ENTRY("Font", DISPID_FONT, CLSID_StockFontPage)
END_PROP_MAP()
```

If you go to the end of the file, you'll see that the two stock properties are declared as public member variables of our `Cviscal` control class:

```
OLE_COLOR m_clrBackColor;
CComPtr<IFontDisp> m_pFont;
```

Mediator Pattern Applied: Font Resource Management

Before OC96 and the new ActiveX control support, controls had to act like normal Windows applications. They had to allocate, manage, and destroy their own font resources. The font resource, which is essentially a shared data structure between the Windows application and the GUI system, is quite large and complex. Because of this, and the relatively scarce availability of the system heap, each control would have to create the font, select it into the device context, use it, select it out, and then delete it – each and every time it repaints. If a container has many active controls, and each one is doing this repeatedly on every repaint, one can imagine the computing resources devoted to this tedious and inefficient task.

Not only is this very expensive in term of computation time and memory consumption, but the code to make this happen is also tremendously verbose and therefore extremely error-prone. To solve this problem, a solution was proposed where, essentially, the COM/OLE runtime system becomes the *mediator* between the ActiveX control and the Win32 GUI system. This solution is the mediator design pattern. You can find more coverage of this design pattern in the *Design Patterns* book.

The COM/OLE runtime assists by maintaining ownership of the font resources. It can decide to maintain a reusable pool of these resources on an application or system-wide basis, without affecting the application and/or the Win32 GUI system. As a matter of fact, the current runtime implementation improves overall application performance when accessing font resources by strategically 'caching' frequently-used fonts.

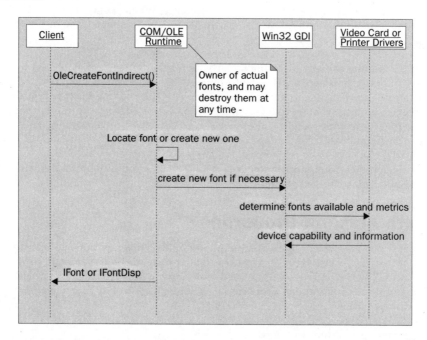

This functionality is accessible through the `OleCreateFontIndirect()` call, which triggers the caching mechanism as shown in the above diagram. For anyone who struggled with control font resources the hard way, this improvement makes a day-and-night difference in programming. The new interaction to obtain a font resource now becomes:

```
OleCreateFontIndirect(&DefaultFontDesc, IID_IFontDisp,
                    reinterpret_cast<void**>(&m_pFontDisp));
```

Or:

```
OleCreateFontIndirect(&DefaultFontDesc, IID_IFont,
                    reinterpret_cast<void**>(&m_pFont));
```

`DefaultFontDesc` is a `FONTDESC` structure, defined in `olectl.h`, which contains font information, such as typeface, point size, and weight. We define this in the `public` part of our `viscal` header file after the declaration of `m_pFont`:

```
static FONTDESC DefaultFontDesc;
```

The use of these functions and types will be explained in detail in the next section.

There are two interfaces you use to access the created font:

❑   IFont – A vtable interface
❑   IFontDisp – A dispatch interface

While easier to use, IFontDisp is more limited in functionality. When programming in C/C++, IFont is typically used for maximum flexibility. One can easily obtain one interface from another using standard QueryInterface().

Since the COM/OLE runtime actually owns the underlying font resources, it may choose to free or release them at any time it deems appropriate. Unfortunately, a user may also have selected the actual font in a device context. In order to communicate to the COM/OLE runtime that the font should not be destroyed, a reference counting scheme, like that of IUnknown, is used. The control or application wishing to hold the font for a while should call IFont::AddRefHfont() to the font, and when the font is no longer needed, it should call IFont::ReleaseHfont().

This solution is so elegant that other large system resources, such as graphics bitmaps in picture resources, are also managed in the same fashion.

Working with Ambient Properties

Recall from Chapter 5 that ambient properties are supplied by the container and can be accessed through the IOleClientSite interface. Our visual calendar depends on the ambient properties BackColor and Font. These properties will be used to determine how the calendar should display itself. This is the main purpose of ambient properties – enabling a control to 'blend' well into the container when it displays itself.

To support these ambient properties, we must:

❑   Initialize them
❑   Be notified when they change and reacquire their new value

The most convenient way to initialize ambient properties is by implementing the IOleObject::SetClientSite() method. This is the method called by the container to enable the control to get the site interface pointer from the container. Given this site pointer, we can then access the ambient properties. ATL 3 provides a default implementation for most of this functionality. First, we'll add a declaration for this method in our header file just beneath the message map declaration:

```
// IOleObjectImpl
   STDMETHOD(SetClientSite)(IOleClientSite* pClientSite);
```

Now, add the following method to the Cviscal class, located in the viscal.cpp file:

```
STDMETHODIMP Cviscal::SetClientSite(IOleClientSite* pClientSite)
{
    IOleObjectImpl<Cviscal>::SetClientSite(pClientSite);
```

```
        // initialize ambient properties
        if ( FAILED(GetAmbientBackColor(m_clrBackColor)) )
            m_clrBackColor = RGB( 255, 255, 255);

        // in case set client site called twice -- for some containers
        if (m_pFont)
            m_pFont.Release();

        if (FAILED(GetAmbientFontDisp(static_cast<IFontDisp**>(&m_pFont))))
        {
            OleCreateFontIndirect(&DefaultFontDesc,
                                  IID_IFontDisp,
                                  reinterpret_cast<void**>(&m_pFont));
        }

        return S_OK;
    }
```

In this method, we start by calling ATL 3's implementation of
`IOleObjectImpl<>::SetClientSite()`, which does most of the hard work for us. As covered in
Chapter 5, the ATL implementation stores the site pointer from the container in a smart pointer, and
provides a series of `CComControlBase` methods to access the ambient properties. We use the
`CComControlBase::GetAmbientBackColor()` and
`CComControlBase::GetAmbientFontDisp()` methods to simplify coding. Note the use of a static
constant `DefaultFontDesc` to specify a default system font resource. This default descriptor is defined
at the top of `viscal.cpp` as:

```
FONTDESC Cviscal::DefaultFontDesc =
{
    sizeof(Cviscal::DefaultFontDesc),
    OLESTR("Arial"),
    FONTSIZE(12),
    FW_BOLD,            // weight
    DEFAULT_CHARSET,   // char set
    FALSE,              // italic
    FALSE,              // underline
    FALSE               // strike-through
};
```

You also need to add the member to `viscal.h`:

```
    static FONTDESC DefaultFontDesc;
```

This basically specifies an Arial bold 12-point font as our default. This font exists on almost all current
Win32 systems. We use the `FONTSIZE()` macro and constants such as `FW_BOLD` and
`DEFAULT_CHARSET`, found in `wingdi.h`, in filling out this `FONTDESC` structure. They greatly ease the
construction of default descriptors. (We will defer the more difficult task of filling out non-default font
descriptors to a later section.)

Another characteristic of ambient properties is that they may be changed at any time (typically by the user, during design mode). The container that is managing the ambient properties will notify each control of the change through the IOleControl::OnAmbientPropertyChange() method. We need to implement this method, catch the new ambient property values, and reflect them on the visual display. The implementation is in our OnAmbientPropertyChange() method. Again, we need to declare this first in the header file:

```
// IOleControl
   STDMETHOD(OnAmbientPropertyChange)(DISPID dispid);
```

And this is what our implementation looks like:

```
STDMETHODIMP Cviscal::OnAmbientPropertyChange(DISPID dispid)
{
   switch(dispid)
   {
   case DISPID_AMBIENT_BACKCOLOR:
      if ( FAILED(GetAmbientBackColor(m_clrBackColor)) )
      {
         m_clrBackColor = RGB( 255, 255, 255);
      }
      FireViewChange();
      break;
```

The FireViewChange() call of the CComControlBase method ensures that the visual control will be updated properly at the next available opportunity.

```
   case DISPID_AMBIENT_FONT:
      if (m_pFont)
         m_pFont.Release();

      if (FAILED(GetAmbientFontDisp(static_cast<IFontDisp**>(&m_pFont))))
      {
         OleCreateFontIndirect(&DefaultFontDesc,
                         IID_IFontDisp,
                         reinterpret_cast<void **>(&m_pFont));
      }
      FireViewChange();
      break;
   }

   return S_OK;
}
```

If your control requires getting more than just a few ambient properties, you may consider creating a handler function for getting each one. You could invoke these handlers either through a long switch statement, similar to the one above, or by implementing a function dispatch array mapping each DISPID to the corresponding handler.

Implementing IViewObject2::Draw()

We learnt in Chapter 5 that ATL 3 will call our OnDraw() member whenever the visual display of the control needs to be redrawn. This is true whether the rendering is to go to an actual window, to a portion of the container's client area directly, or to a metafile. In fact, IOleObject::GetData() and IViewObject2::Draw() both call the OnDraw() routine.

When the rendering is to either the container's client area or to a metafile, one cannot depend on the device context being a screen device context from an actual Win32 window. In order to minimize the conditional code within OnDraw(), ATL passes in two device contexts. One device context can dependably be used to get information about the device to be rendered to in all cases. The other context is the actual context to render into. If your OnDraw() code follows this convention, it is possible to code one routine to render for all these different destinations.

The signature of OnDraw() is:

```
HRESULT Cviscal::OnDraw(ATL_DRAWINFO& di)
```

The drawing DC (device context) can be accessed at:

```
di.hdcDraw
```

And the information DC can be accessed at:

```
di.hicTargetDev  // hic is Handle to Information Context
```

Let us take a closer look at ATL_DRAWINFO declared in atlctl.h

```
struct ATL_DRAWINFO
{
    UINT cbSize;
    DWORD dwDrawAspect;
    LONG lindex;
    DVTARGETDEVICE* ptd;
    HDC hicTargetDev;
    HDC hdcDraw;
    LPCRECTL prcBounds;
    LPCRECTL prcWBounds;
    BOOL bOptimize;
    BOOL bZoomed;
    BOOL bRectInHimetric;
    SIZEL ZoomNum;
    SIZEL ZoomDen;
};
```

Here is a brief explanation of each ATL_DRAWINFO member:

Member	Description
cbSize	Size of the struct.
dwDrawAspect	Specifies how is the object going to be drawn. DVASPECT_CONTENT is the most common value and signifies the visual representation of the control.
lindex	Specifies part of the control to be drawn. Depends on the view aspect (dwDrawAspect).
ptd	If NULL, then we are drawing to the default target device (typically the screen). If not NULL, then ptd provides information about the drawing device, in conjunction with hicTargetDev.
hicTargetDev	Information context for the target device in ptd from which the control can find the device metrics and capabilities. Valid only if ptd is not NULL. .
hdcDraw	Device context on which to draw.
prcBounds	The rectangle on hdcDraw in which the control should be drawn.
prcWBounds	If hdcDraw is a metafile, prcWBounds specifies the bounding rectangle of the metafile. prcBounds is contained within prcWBounds. The RECTL contains the window origin and extent of the bounding rectangle.
bOptimize	Set to true by the ATL implementation if it has saved the current DC. Since ATL can restore it before returning to the container, we can do whatever we want with hdcDraw.
bZoomed	Set to true if the control has been zoomed, that is its extent on the screen is different from its natural extent.
bRectInHimetric	If true, rectangle coordinates are in HIMETRIC.
ZoomNum	Zoom numerator (width and height of bounding rectangle) .
ZoomDen	Zoom denominator (width and height of the natural size of the object).

Despite this mapping, it is still occasionally necessary for the ActiveX control to know whether rendering is done to a window or a metafile. Our code in OnDraw() determines this by examining the hdcDraw member of the structure directly:

```
bool inMetafileContext = (GetDeviceCaps(di.hdcDraw, TECHNOLOGY) == DT_METAFILE);
```

Also, in `OnDraw()`, we only draw the control if asked to do so for the visual representation of the control embedded in a container. This is so if `di.dwDrawAspect` is equal to `DVASPECT_CONTENT`.

```
if ( di.dwDrawAspect != DVASPECT_CONTENT )
    return S_OK;
```

Using IFontDisp Font Resources for Drawing

The `IFontDisp` interface, which we use to access the font, is implemented by a font object managed by the COM runtime, and we hold onto this interface through the `m_pFont` smart pointer. Other clients of the COM runtime may also use the very same GDI font, and the runtime needs a way of finding out when a particular client has finished using it. On the flip side, a client having a font selected into a device context will not want it to be destroyed suddenly by the COM runtime. This means that we must lock it in place while we have it selected for drawing in a device context.

The 'locking' is done by first querying the font dispatch interface, `IFontDisp`, for an `IFont` interface. We call `IFont::get_hFont()` to get a handle to the actual font, and then we increment the reference count (not to be confused with a COM reference count) using `IFont::AddRefHfont()`. The font handle can then be used as we please. Finally, after the drawing, the `hFont` handle is released back to the system pool via `IFont::ReleaseHfont()`. The code that does this is in the `OnDraw()` method, which we'll put in `viscal.cpp` in place of the generated version in `viscal.h`:

```
HRESULT Cviscal::OnDraw(ATL_DRAWINFO& di)
{
    RECT&      rc = *(LPRECT)di.prcBounds;
    HDC        hdc = di.hdcDraw;
    COLORREF   backClr;
    HBRUSH     hOldBrush, hBrush;
    bool       inMetafileContext = (GetDeviceCaps(di.hdcDraw, TECHNOLOGY) ==
                  DT_METAFILE);

    // we can only draw content not an icon or a thumbnail yet
    if ( di.dwDrawAspect != DVASPECT_CONTENT )
        return S_OK;

    // translate the stock property from OLECOLOR to a COLORREF type
    OleTranslateColor( m_clrBackColor, NULL, &backClr );
    COLORREF oldBkColor = SetBkColor(hdc, backClr);
    hBrush = CreateSolidBrush( backClr );
    hOldBrush = (HBRUSH) SelectObject( hdc, hBrush );

    COLORREF cForeColor = RGB( 0, 0, 0 );

    HPEN hPen = CreatePen( PS_SOLID, 0, cForeColor );
    HPEN hOldPen = (HPEN) SelectObject( hdc, hPen );

    FillRect( hdc, &rc, hBrush );
    CComPtr<IFont> pIFont;
    m_pFont->QueryInterface(IID_IFont, (void**) &pIFont);

    HDC    attrDC = ( di.ptd != NULL ) ? di.hicTargetDev : ::GetDC(m_hWnd);
    HFONT  curFont;
```

```
        pIFont->get_hFont(&curFont);
        pIFont->AddRefHfont(curFont);
        HFONT hOldFont = (HFONT) SelectObject( hdc, curFont );
        HFONT hOldAttrFont = (HFONT) SelectObject( attrDC, curFont );

        PaintGrid(hdc, attrDC, rc, inMetafileContext);

        SelectObject( hdc, hOldFont );
        SelectObject( attrDC, hOldAttrFont );
        pIFont->ReleaseHfont(curFont);
        SelectObject( hdc, hOldPen );
        DeleteObject( hPen );
        // deselect brush from DC in order to delete it
        SelectObject( hdc, hOldBrush );
        DeleteObject( hBrush );

        SetBkColor(hdc,oldBkColor);
        return S_OK;
    }
```

Note the line,

```
    HDC   attrDC = ( di.ptd != NULL ) ? di.hicTargetDev : ::GetDC(m_hWnd);
```

where we make sure we have an information device context. If we are drawing to a non-default device, we are guaranteed to be passed one in the ATL_DRAWINFO structure. Otherwise, we must acquire it. The actual drawing is done inside the PaintGrid() method. We declare this as a protected member in viscal.h:

```
    protected:
        void PaintGrid(HDC hdc, HDC attrDC, const CRectangle& rect,
                       bool inMetafileContext);
```

We will evolve this PaintGrid() method substantially throughout the code iterations. In this first iteration, though, we will simply be drawing the grid and title. Note that CRectangle is a utility class that encapsulates a RECT and will be covered shortly:

```
    void Cviscal::PaintGrid(HDC hdc, HDC attrDC, const CRectangle& rect,
                            bool inMetafileContext)
    {
        // do intermediate calculations in float to eliminate
        // round-off errors when scaling
        float x1, x2, y1, y2;
        float cellWidth, halfCellWidth;
        float cellHeight, halfCellHeight;
        float topMargin, leftMargin;
        float xPad = 2, yPad = 2;
        ULONG numRows, numCols;
        ULONG offsetY;
        ULONG i;
```

First, we calculate the margins around the cell grid. We allow space for one more cell width and 2 cell heights around the grid:

```
numRows = kRowsDisplayed + 2;
numCols = kDaysInWeek + 1;
cellWidth = rect.Width() * 1.0f / numCols;
cellHeight = rect.Height() * 1.0f / numRows;
halfCellWidth = cellWidth / 2;
halfCellHeight = cellHeight / 2;
topMargin = halfCellHeight;
leftMargin = halfCellWidth;
offsetY = ULONG( cellHeight * 1.8 );
```

Note the kRowsDisplayed *and* kDaysInWeek *constants. You'll find these defined in* CalDefs.h, *in Appendix E.*

Calculate and draw the vertical lines:

```
for ( i = 0; i < numCols; i++ )
{
    // top point
    x1 = leftMargin + i * cellWidth;
    y1 = offsetY;
    // bottom point
    x2 = x1;
    y2 = y1 + kRowsDisplayed * cellHeight;
    // draw line
    MoveToEx( hdc, x1, y1, NULL );
    LineTo( hdc, x2, y2 );
}
```

Calculate and draw horizontal lines:

```
for ( i = 0; i < kRowsDisplayed + 1; i++ )
{
    // left point
    x1 = leftMargin;
    y1 = offsetY + i * cellHeight;
    // right point
    x2 = rect.Width() - x1;
    y2 = y1;
    // draw line
    MoveToEx( hdc, x1, y1, NULL );
    LineTo( hdc, x2, y2 );
};
```

Now, we draw the title line:

```
TEXTMETRIC tm;
SIZE tex;
LPCTSTR psTitle = _T("A&W Calendar");
::GetTextMetrics(attrDC, &tm);
::GetTextExtentPoint32(attrDC, psTitle, lstrlen(psTitle), &tex);
::SetTextAlign(hdc, TA_LEFT | TA_TOP);
::ExtTextOut(hdc, (rect.Width() - tex.cx)/2, (rect.Top() + 5),
    ETO_CLIPPED, (RECT *) &rect, psTitle, lstrlen(psTitle), NULL);
}
```

Note that the font used to draw the title line is specified by the ambient property Font. This font has been selected into the device context in the OnDraw() method prior to the call to PaintGrid().

Rectangles and Strings

We need some utility classes that will take shape with the development of our main classes. You can find them in CalUtils.h and CalUtils.cpp. Here we'll take a look at the kind of strings we use and the way we encapsulated rectangles. We'll describe the date/time related utility classes in a subsequent section.

It is well known that many developers have been using MFC, even for simple non-visual applications, just so they can use the extremely powerful CString class. Admittedly, strings (null-terminated character arrays) are a necessity and good string handling is not to be given up lightly. In the world of ATL, the Standard Template Library (part of the standard C++ library) provides the solution in the form of an extremely flexible basic_string<> template class. Its power partly stems from the fact that it does not rely on a char type as the type of a character but rather it accepts any type as character as long as its properties are accessible through another template class – char_traits<>. Strings of the fundamental character types char and wchar_t are easily available since they have been typedef'd as follows:

```
typedef basic_string<char> string;
typedef basic_string<wchar_t> wstring;
```

In our case, we want to be able to use either of the above types. Windows already provides us with the macro TCHAR which compiles either as a simple or as a wide character (in order to support Unicode). In STL it is easy to accommodate TCHAR's through the following type definition,

```
typedef basic_string<TCHAR> tstring;
```

which you will find in CalDefs.h. Some examples of its use include,

```
tstring t = _T("Hello");
tstring s = t.append(_T(" ") ).append( _T("world"));
```

printing into a buffer,

```
TCHAR buf[BUFSIZ];
wsprintf(buf, _T("%"), s.c_str() );
```

and getting a sub-string:

```
tstring(t, 0, 5);
```

The CRectangle class allows for easy construction and operations on a rectangle. The actual dimensions are stored in the data member r of type RECT. Since CRectangle is not much more than a RECT, and to allow easy access to its dimensions, we decided to make it a struct. The class provides for coordinate conversion, hit testing and conversions to/from RECT.

```
struct CRectangle
{
    CRectangle() { SetRectEmpty(); }
    CRectangle(ULONG left, ULONG top, ULONG right, ULONG bottom)
                { SetRect(&r, left, top, right, bottom); }
    CRectangle(const CRectangle& other)
                { r = (RECT)other; }
    CRectangle(const RECT& rc)
                { r = rc; }
    CRectangle(const POINT* points)
                { r.left = points[0].x; r.top = points[0].y;
                  r.right = points[1].x; r.bottom = points[1].y; }
    CRectangle(const SIZE& s)
                { r.left = r.top = 0; r.right = s.cx;
                  r.bottom = s.cy; }
    ~CRectangle() {}

    CRectangle& SetRectEmpty(void)
                { ::SetRectEmpty( &r ); return *this; }
                operator RECT&() { return r; }
                operator const RECT&() const { return r; }
    bool operator==(const CRectangle& o) const
                { return EqualRect( &this->r, &o.r ) == TRUE; }
    bool operator!=(const CRectangle& o) const
                { return EqualRect( &this->r, &o.r ) == FALSE; }
    CRectangle LPtoDP(HDC hdc) const;
    CRectangle DPtoLP(HDC hdc) const;

    LONG  Left() const    { return r.left; }
    LONG  Top() const     { return r.top; }
    LONG  Right() const   { return r.right; }
    LONG  Bottom() const  { return r.bottom; }

    LONG  Width() const   { return abs(r.right - r.left); }
    LONG  Height() const  { return abs(r.bottom - r.top); }

    CRectangle Center(const SIZE& size);
    bool PtInRect(const POINT& pt) const;

    RECT r;
};
```

Compiling and Linking the Control

You can find the complete source code for Iteration 1 in the directory Ch06\viscal1.1. It is configured for a debug target on Windows 9x or NT.

A note on including the necessary STL header files in the project. Since STL is used throughout, the most appropriate place is stdafx.h. Also, bear in mind that STL provides its own implementation of the C++ stream classes which cannot coexist with the older header files. Here is the right sequence of includes:

```
#include <string>
#include <iostream>
#include <fstream>
#include <iomanip>
#include <vector>
#include <functional>
#include <algorithm>
```

In order not to have to apend the std namespace identifier to the STL classes (for example, std::string, or std::vector etc.) we declare that we will be using the std namespace

```
using namespace std;
```

And last, but not least, we need to change the name of the control. Go to the viscal.rgs and change all the instances of 'viscal Class' to 'A&W viscal Class'. You'll see the effect of this in the next section.

Once you have built the project successfully, it is time to get a feel for the control by testing it. Let's turn our attention to that now.

Testing in the ActiveX Control Test Container

One of the most flexible test containers for ActiveX controls is the ActiveX Control Test Container application (Tstcon32.exe) supplied as part of Visual Studio 6.0 or Visual C++ 6. This test container supports dynamic configuration of container capability, and tests all major interfaces and features of a control. If you have used the previous version of this container, in Visual C++ 5.0, you will be quite at home when you browse through its menus and dialogs. In this new release, it has provision to test all OC96 container and control features, and also has macro scripting capability, using any Active Scripting engine, to perform regression tests on visual ActiveX controls.

Though the simplicity and flexibility of the container makes it a great tool, thorough testing still requires careful planning. In fact, casual testing with this container frequently gives a false sense of confidence for many control writers. I warn you now, and again later in this book, that the ActiveX control test container is not a sufficient tool to be the sole test tool in a production environment. To this end, it is vital that an ActiveX control be tested in all the containers that it intends to be used in – and not just in this reference container.

To try out our skeletal control in the ActiveX control test container, start it and click on the New Control button:

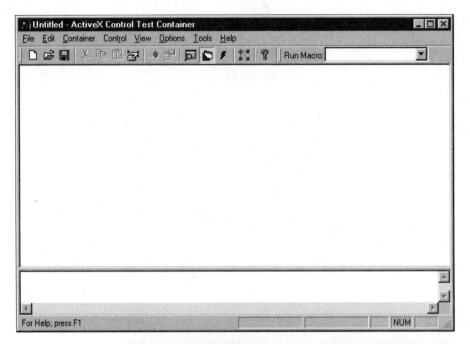

Select from the list box the entry called **A&W viscal Class**:

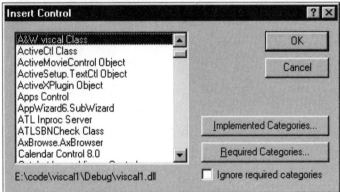

This will insert an instance of the control in the client area of the test container. You can use the various facilities of the test container to test the control. For our calendar control, you can try changing the Font and BackColor ambient properties that we have just implemented.

> *Note that there is a minor problem with the beta version of the test container which will hopefully be gone in the final release. The second and subsequent times you attempt to change the* BackColor *or* ForeColor *property, the* **Ambient Properties** *dialog does not set the* **Property Type** *to* VT_COLOR *but rather to* VT_UI4. *You must set the type manually to* **VT_COLOR** *so that the* **Choose Color...** *button appears allowing access to the standard* **Color** *dialog.*

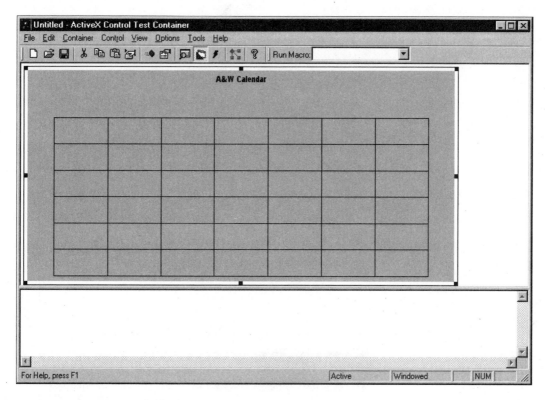

Testing in Visual Basic

We have provided a Visual Basic 6 project to test the control. The project can be found under the Ch06\VBTest source directory, or you could also easily create your own.

To add our visual calendar control to Visual Basic's control palette, right click on the palette and select Components...

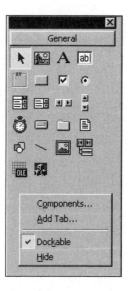

Look through the list and select the viscal1 1.0 Type Library entry from the Controls tab.

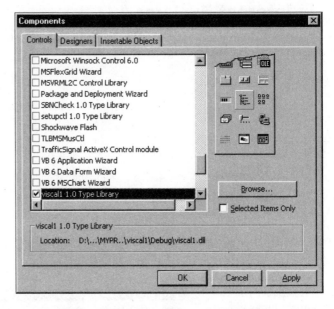

After adding the control to the palette, you can use it in any Visual Basic 6 project, just as you would use any of the other controls provided there. In this example, we have modified the two ambient properties. Try this out for yourself!

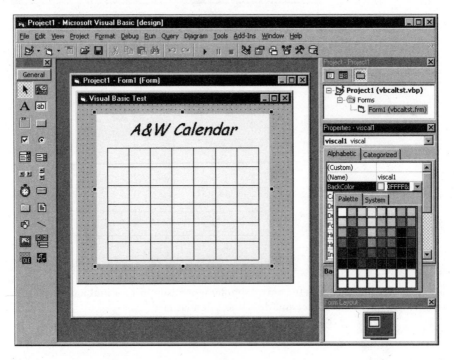

You can easily add functionality by using other ActiveX control and new logic using Visual Basic 6.

Testing in Internet Explorer 4

To test under Internet Explorer 4.x, you can use our provided page in the Ch06\IETest directory, or create your own Dynamic HTML test page:

```
<html>
<head>
<title>ATL 3 Test for A&W Visual Calendar Control</title>
</head>

<body bgcolor="#f0f3f8">
<center><h1>A & W Events Calendar</h1>
<object id="calendar"
   classid="CLSID:B59F7C1B-F96B-11D1-A660-006052008075"
   align="baseline" border="0"
   width="500" height="300">
</object>
</p>
<center>
</body>
</html>
```

If you open up this page, you can see what our control looks like in Internet Explorer:

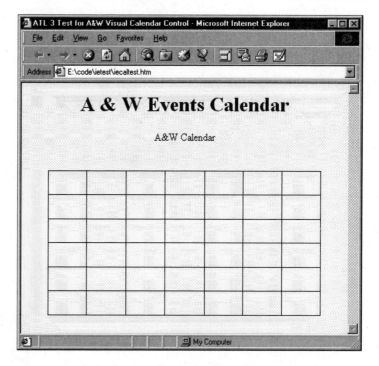

In this first iteration, we created a complete control, implemented support for ambient properties, including a system-managed font resource, and drew the calendar grid.

Iteration 2: Adding Child Controls and Drawing Code

So far, we have successfully implemented and tested some code to draw our calendar and handle the ambient properties. Now is a good time to implement more required code into our control.

In this section, we will add two child button controls, hook them up to some function, and make sure that they resize with the control. Once the basics are out of the way at the end of this iteration, we'll pick up some speed. All the code we use in this iteration can be found in the Ch06/viscal1.2 directory of the source code download for this book available at http://www.wrox.com.

Working with ATL 3 Contained Windows

Our visual calendar needs two buttons, for moving the month displayed forwards and backwards. The easiest way to do this is simply to create two Win32 buttons as child windows to the control's window and let them handle the user interface. This can be easily done using the CContainedWindow class provided by ATL 3.

We add two protected member variables in the Cviscal class to hold these contained controls:

```
protected:
    void PaintGrid( HDC hdc, HDC attrDC, const CRectangle & rect,
                    bool inMetafileContext );

    CContainedWindow m_ctlButBack;
    CContainedWindow m_ctlButFore;
```

The constructor of CContainedWindow does not actually create the contained window, but it does initialize the type of control (the Win32 window class), the class containing an alternate message map, and the alternate message map number. A good place for us to carry out this initialization is in our own in-line constructor:

```
Cviscal() : m_ctlButBack(_T("Button"),this,1),
                              m_ctlButFore(_T("Button"),this,2)
{
    m_bWindowOnly = TRUE;
}
```

The numbers 1 and 2 that we pass to the CContainedWindow constructor refer to the number of the alternate message map in our Cviscal class. This will route the button's window messages to our Cviscal class for processing. The message we are interested in is the button click message.

Using Alternate Message Maps

In a classic application of the Chains of Command pattern, the Windows message queue is augmented by the ATL implemented message map. In effect, our use of alternate message maps allows us to redirect window messages originally destined for the contained windows, and process them ourselves. The contained windows are initialized with a pointer to the parent object (so that they can access its message map) and an alternate message map number.

The message map of the parent object contains ALT_MSG_MAP(n) macros which precede message handlers for messages originally destined for the contained window, which have now been redirected to the message map of the parent (by the CContainedWindow implementation).

To map the messages from the two buttons' alternate maps, we need to add the following entries to the generated message map, which you'll find in the Cviscal header file:

```
BEGIN_MSG_MAP(Cviscal)
    CHAIN_MSG_MAP(CComControl<Cviscal>)
    DEFAULT_REFLECTION_HANDLER()
ALT_MSG_MAP(1)
    MESSAGE_HANDLER(WM_LBUTTONDOWN, OnBackButton)
ALT_MSG_MAP(2)
    MESSAGE_HANDLER(WM_LBUTTONDOWN, OnForwardButton)
END_MSG_MAP()
```

The CHAIN_MSG_MAP(CComControl<Cviscal>) macro performs the default message processing by passing the message to the message map of the base class CComControl<Cviscal>. Our own message handlers must precede this macro. Similarly, the DEFAULT_REFLECTION_HANDLER() provides a default handler for notifications reflected back to the control. It should be obvious that this mechanism is very similar to the MFC message maps.

This message map will map the left mouse button down event from the first button to an event handler function called Cviscal::OnBackButton(), and from the second button to Cviscal::OnForwardButton().

We must also declare the two message handling functions in the protected block of viscal.h:

```
LRESULT OnBackButton(UINT uMsg, WPARAM wParam, LPARAM lParam, BOOL& bHandled);
LRESULT OnForwardButton(UINT uMsg, WPARAM wParam, LPARAM lParam,
                                                  BOOL& bHandled);
```

Since the constructor does not create the actual buttons, we need to do this ourselves as soon as possible after the control window is created.

Creating Win32 Windows for CContainedWindow Operation

At what point should we create the child window buttons?

The best time to create the button windows is not as part of the container-to-control protocol. Instead, we should create them when the actual window for our calendar control is created (and we know that a window will be created because we set m_WindowOnly to TRUE as a result of choosing the Windowed Only wizard option during control creation). Therefore, we need to process the WM_CREATE window message.

You can add a new window message handler by right-clicking on `Cviscal` in Class View and selecting **Add Windows Message Handler....** From the list of messages, select `WM_CREATE`, and click on the **Add and Edit** button:

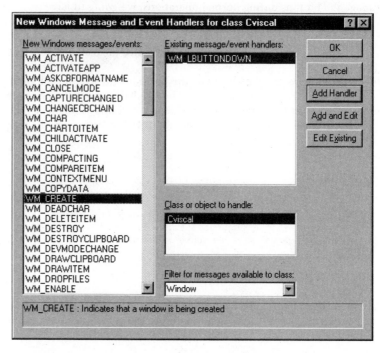

This is a convenience feature of Visual C++, but you can also add the handler manually. A new skeleton implementation for an `OnCreate()` method will be added for you in `viscal.h`. Just change this to a function declaration – we'll see how to implement this in the `.cpp` file in the next section.

```
LRESULT OnCreate(UINT uMsg, WPARAM wParam, LPARAM lParam, BOOL& bHandled);
```

If you now take a look at the message map, you'll see that a new entry has been added:

```
BEGIN_MSG_MAP(Cviscal)
    MESSAGE_HANDLER(WM_CREATE, OnCreate)
    CHAIN_MSG_MAP(CComControl<Cviscal>)
    DEFAULT_REFLECTION_HANDLER()
ALT_MSG_MAP(1)
    MESSAGE_HANDLER(WM_LBUTTONDOWN, OnBackButton)
ALT_MSG_MAP(2)
    MESSAGE_HANDLER(WM_LBUTTONDOWN, OnForwardButton)
END_MSG_MAP()
```

You may find that the wizard has added the entry for the message handler at the bottom of the message map. You must be sure to move it to the top, otherwise it becomes part of the second alternate message map, and your `OnCreate()` *method will not be called on the creation of the control.*

To manage the buttons during normal operations, we going to have to:

- ❑ Create the buttons at a default position and size
- ❑ Reposition and resize the button every time the control is resized

In order to do this, we need to calculate the position and size of each button, given the current size of the control window. Since this calculation will be needed in more than one place, we'll write a helper function to factor out the common code. You can add this as member function by right-clicking on `Cviscal` in **ClassView** and selecting **Add Member Function** from the drop-down menu.

```
void Cviscal::ButRectHelper(LPCRECT inrectWin, LPRECT rectBack, LPRECT rectFore)
{
    CRectangle rectWin(*inrectWin);
    long cmdHeight = rectWin.Height()/6;
    rectBack->left = 2;
    rectBack->right = rectBack->left + cmdHeight;
    rectBack->top = rectFore->top = 5;
    rectBack->bottom = rectFore->bottom = rectBack->top + cmdHeight;
    rectFore->left = rectWin.Width() - 2 - cmdHeight;
    rectFore->right = rectFore->left + cmdHeight;
}
```

The two buttons are calculated to be equal size squares, with each size one sixth the height of the control. They are positioned at five units from the top of the control window and two units from the left and right side respectively.

Implementing WM_CREATE Handling

Now that we the code to calculate the size and position of buttons in place, we can code up the `OnCreate()` handler like this:

```
LRESULT Cviscal::OnCreate(UINT uMsg, WPARAM wParam, LPARAM lParam, BOOL& bHandled)
{
    RECT rectWin, rectBack, rectFore;
    GetWindowRect(&rectWin);
    ButRectHelper(&rectWin, &rectBack, &rectFore);
    m_ctlButBack.Create(m_hWnd, rectBack, _T("<<"),
                        WS_CHILD | WS_VISIBLE | WS_BORDER);
    m_ctlButFore.Create(m_hWnd, rectFore, _T(">>"),
                        WS_CHILD | WS_VISIBLE | WS_BORDER);

    return 0;
}
```

`GetWindowRect()` is a method of `CWindow` and `Create()` is a method of `CContainedWindow` that creates the underlying Win32 window.

Resizing Contained Windows with the Control

Now it's time to write the code that will reposition and resize the buttons when the control is resized. We can do this by implementing the `IOleObject::SetExtent()` function, and adjusting the button size and position after calling the default ATL implementation.

`::SetWindowPos()` allows us to specify the left and top position, width and height to which the window corresponding to its first handle argument should be set. This is a rich function, accepting a variety of sizing and positioning flags, which, however, are not relevant to our button windows. Also, notice that the control engages in button size and position calculations only if it is asked to draw itself as an embedded object in the container (dwDrawAspect == DVASPECT_CONTENT):

```
STDMETHODIMP Cviscal::SetExtent(DWORD dwDrawAspect, SIZEL* psizel)
{
    HRESULT hr = IOleObjectImpl<Cviscal>::SetExtent(dwDrawAspect, psizel);
    if ((dwDrawAspect == DVASPECT_CONTENT) && (psizel != NULL))
    {
        RECT rectBack, rectFore;
        ButRectHelper(&m_rcPos, &rectBack, &rectFore);
        ::SetWindowPos(m_ctlButBack.m_hWnd,
                       NULL,
                       rectBack.left,
                       rectBack.top,
                       rectBack.right - rectBack.left,
                       rectBack.bottom - rectBack.top,
                       0);
        ::SetWindowPos(m_ctlButFore.m_hWnd,
                       NULL, rectFore.left,
                       rectFore.top,
                       rectFore.right - rectFore.left,
                       rectFore.bottom - rectFore.top,
                       0);
    }
    return hr;
}
```

Recall from our discussion in the Chapter 5 that `SetExtent()` plays an essential role in the negotiation between a container and the control about the control size and position. Its lineage extends back to the days of OLE 1, so you can guarantee that containers from all generations will support the protocol, calling this method whenever the visible size of the ActiveX control changes.

Handling Contained Button Clicks

Finally, we need to hook up the mouse click with actual function, which we can do by implementing the mouse button handlers:

```
LRESULT Cviscal::OnBackButton(UINT uMsg, WPARAM wParam, LPARAM lParam,
                              BOOL& bHandled)
{
    ATLTRACE( _T("***Cviscal::OnBackButton\n") );
    bHandled = FALSE;
    return 0;
}
LRESULT Cviscal::OnForwardButton(UINT uMsg, WPARAM wParam, LPARAM lParam,
                                 BOOL& bHandled)
{
    ATLTRACE( _T("***Cviscal::OnForwardButton\n") );
    bHandled = FALSE;
    return 0;
}
```

These two handlers will simply print out trace messages for now, but later we'll use them to change the month displayed, once we have the date calculation routines in place.

Note that you must explicitly set bHandled to FALSE. If you don't do this, then it will default to TRUE and will prevent the button from doing its own user-interface rendering. This behavior clearly indicates that we are getting the window message *before* the actual ContainedWindow instance gets a chance to process it, and therefore are actually superclassing rather than subclassing the window.

> *Both **subclassing** and **superclassing** refer to the ability of an application to intercept and process messages destined to a particular window before the window has a chance to process them. This is done by diverting the messages to a new window procedure which has a chance to process the message first. It may then choose to send the message to the original window procedure, unaltered or not. The difference is that, while in subclassing, we modify the window class by substituting its window procedure with our new one, in superclassing we create a totally new window class (to which the messages are diverted). The superclass uses the original class as a base class to which it may divert messages.*

Testing Iteration 2

The project up to this stage can be found in the directory Ch06\viscall.2 of the source code distribution. If you compile the project now and try it out in the containers, it will look like this:

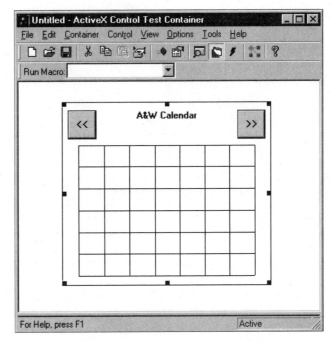

If you click one of the buttons, it will provide its default 'push-in/pop-out' UI, and a message will be output to the debug window (if you run the control under debug mode). It is not too interesting if you are not running under debug mode.

> *In order to run the control in debug mode, you need to go to the* Debug *tab on* Project | Settings, *and make sure that the* Executable for debug session *is pointing to the location of* Tstcon32.exe.

It's about time we hooked up the buttons for more action. We'll this do in Iteration 3.

Iteration 3: Bringing Life to The Calendar

The work we have done so far has set up the container – now would be a good time to add some real functionality to the calendar itself. We'll add some code to display the days of the month on the calendar, and also to hook up the buttons for changing these values.

First, however, we need to add a method to the `Iviscal` interface. Back in Chapter 4, we saw how we can do this by right-clicking on the name of the interface in **ClassView**, and selecting **Add Method**. When we add a method in this way, the interface wizard will add code automatically for us at three different locations:

- ❏ `viscal1.idl`
- ❏ `viscal.h`
- ❏ `viscal.cpp`

The details of the method that we will be adding to our `Iviscal` interface are shown in the following table:

Return Type	Method Name	Parameters	Description
HRESULT	AdvanceMonth	[in] long inc	Will be used in moving the displayed month forward or backward

Hooking up the Buttons to Change the Month Displayed

With the `AdvanceMonth()` method in place (we will provide the actual implementation shortly), we can now hook the buttons up to call it. The button on the right will advance the calendar by one month and the button on the left will move it back by one. In the last iteration these button event handlers did nothing useful, so let's add the real implementation here:

```
LRESULT Cviscal::OnBackButton(UINT uMsg, WPARAM wParam, LPARAM lParam, BOOL&
bHandled)
{
    AdvanceMonth(-1);
    bHandled = FALSE;
    return 0;
}
LRESULT Cviscal::OnForwardButton(UINT uMsg, WPARAM wParam, LPARAM lParam, BOOL&
bHandled)
{
    AdvanceMonth(1);
    bHandled = FALSE;
    return 0;
}
```

As you can see, this is very straightforward. Notice how we set the bHandled flag to be FALSE – this causes the message map mechanism to call the default handler for the mouse click events. As mentioned earlier, this essentially means that the child windows themselves (Win32 buttons) will have a chance to complete their UI display by handling the message.

You may be wondering why we added the AdvanceMonth() method to the Iviscal interface, since we are calling it directly. Please take a moment to realize that by exposing the method we allow users of the control to change the displayed month programmatically, either by calling the method directly or through Automation (e.g. through VBScript).

Managing the Cells: The CCellMgr Class

Each square within the calendar grid is a cell. Leaving viscal.cpp and viscal.h for a while, we'll start work on the cells. At the moment, our draw routine only paints a grid of cells. Each cell, however, can contain various pieces of information:

❏ The date of the month to which it corresponds
❏ The actual location of the cell with respect to the control's client area
❏ Event information associated with the day of the month

This information is a natural candidate for encapsulation in a C++ class. We are now entering into the territory of a Controller in a Model-View-Controller (MVC) design pattern. We model the cell-specific information in a class called CCalCell which you can find in CCellMgr.h.

```
class CCalCell
{
public:
    CCalCell();
    ~CCalCell();

    void ClearContent();              // clear cell content
    CDateTime date;                   // day the cell represents
    tstring dayNumber;                // text number of the date
    bool hasEvent;                    // does it have events?
    tstring label;                    // optional label associated with cell
    CRectangle rect;                  // where the cell is in the client area
    CellAttachment attach[ kMaxCellAttachments ]; // optional attachment
};
```

Each cell in the currently displayed grid will have an instance of this CCalCell class associated with it. Since this class does not utilize any system resources (windows, device contexts, etc.), allocating and working with an array of instances is exactly the same as a regular array of C/C++ structures, and is therefore quite efficient. We have a second class to encapsulate this grid of cells, which is called CCellMgr, and represents the Controller role in the design pattern.

Here are the details of the CCellMgr class in CCellMgr.h:

```
class CCellMgr
{
public:
   CCellMgr();
   ~CCellMgr();
   void ClearCellContents();
   ULONG GetNumCells(void) const;
   void SetDate(const CDateTime& d );

   void SetMonthYearLabel(const CDateTime& d);
   const tstring& GetMonthYearLabel(void) const;

   const tstring& GetCellLabel(int i) const;
   const tstring& GetCellDayNumber(int i) const;
   const CDateTime& GetCellDate(int idx) const;

   bool GetCellHasEvent(int idx) const;
   void SetCellHasEvent(int idx, bool hasEvent);

   void SetCellCoords(int i, const CRectangle& rect);

   bool CellHitTest(const POINT& pt, int* pi) const;
   bool CellHitTestWithEvents(const POINT& pt, int* pi) const;

   void OnLMouseButtonDown(const POINT& pt);
   bool OnLMouseButtonUp(const POINT& pt, int* pCellIndex);

   bool CellCoordsHaveBeenSet(void) const;
private:
   CCalCell m_Cells [ kRowsDisplayed * kDaysInWeek ];
   ULONG    m_NumCells;
   tstring  m_MonthYearLabel;
   int m_CellPressed;      // index of cell pressed
};
```

Here is a brief explanation of each of the class' methods:

Method Name	Description
ClearCellContents()	Clears the contents of all the cells in the grid
GetNumCells()	Returns the number of cells in the grid
SetDate()	Sets the current month being displayed by the grid
SetMonthYearLabel()	Sets the title text for the calendar
GetMonthYearLabel()	Gets the title text for the calendar
GetCellLabel()	Gets the label text for a cell
GetCellDayNumber()	Gets the day number represented by the cell
GetCellDate()	Gets the date represented by the cell

Table Continued on Following Page

Method Name	Description
GetCellHasEvent()	Indicates whether any events occur on the date represented by the cell.
SetCellHasEvent()	Sets an indicator if at least one event occurs on the date represented by the cell.
SetCellCoords()	Sets the rectangle occupied by each of the cells in the grid. This is necessary before we can perform hit tests.
CellHitTest()	Determines if one of the cells within the grid has been clicked.
CellHitTestWithEvents()	Performs a hit test – if a cell has been clicked, indicates if the date represented by the cell holds an event.
OnLMouseButtonDown()	Handles a left mouse button down event by performing a hit-test on all cells with events. Makes a note of the cell that has been hit.
OnLMouseButtonUp()	Handles a left mouse button up event by performing a hit-test on all cells with events, and compares to the cell that has potentially been hit on the mouse-down event .
CellCoordsHaveBeenSet()	Indicates if a valid SetCellCoords() has been called since creation or the last call to ClearCellContents() – basically checking whether the data in the CCellMgr instance is valid.

Here is the SetCellCoords() method:

```
void CCellMgr::SetCellCoords(int i, const CRectangle& rect)
{
    _ASSERTE( i>=0 && i <= m_NumCells );
    m_Cells[i].rect = rect;
}
```

Cviscal::SetCellCoords() performs similar calculations to those in PaintGrid() in order to find the rectangle corresponding to each cell. It then invokes CCellMgr::SetCellCoords() to actually set the cell coordinates:

```
void Cviscal::SetCellCoords(const CRectangle& rect)
{
    TCHAR buf[BUFSIZ];
    wsprintf(buf, "      x [ %3d %3d ]   y [ %3d %3d ]\n",
             rect.Left(), rect.Right(), rect.Top(), rect.Bottom());
    ATLTRACE(buf);

    float curX, curY;
    float cellWidth, cellHeight;
    float leftMargin;
    ULONG numRows, numCols;
```

```
    ULONG offsetX, offsetY;
    ULONG counter;
    ULONG i, j;

    // calculate margins and spacing. Allow space for one more
    // cell width and 2 cell heights around the grid
    numRows = kRowsDisplayed + 2;
    numCols = kDaysInWeek + 1;
    cellWidth = rect.Width() * 1.0f / numCols;
    cellHeight = rect.Height() * 1.0f /numRows;
    leftMargin = cellWidth / 2;

    // if we have a window, client coordinates passed to us,
    // e.g. for mouse messages, start at (0, 0)
    offsetX = 0;
    offsetY = ULONG( cellHeight * 1.8 );
    counter = 0;
    for (i = 0; i < kRowsDisplayed; i++)
    {
        curY = offsetY + i * cellHeight;
        for (j = 0; j < kDaysInWeek; j++)
        {
            curX = offsetX + leftMargin + j * cellWidth;
            // set cell coordinates
            m_CellMgr.SetCellCoords( counter,
                        CRectangle( curX, curY,
                                    curX + cellWidth, curY + cellHeight ));
            counter++;
        } // for i
    } //for j
}
```

You can find the rest of the implementation of this class in the file CCellMgr.cpp (in Appendix E). These member functions shed some light on how the class manages the set of CCalCell instances, which represent the cells within the grid. We can also observe that a flag is used within each cell to indicate whether or not a particular day has an event.

The actual data elements of the event are not contained in CCellMgr class, however, but in the CDataMgr class. This is the Model part of the Model-View-Controller pattern.

Our main concern in this section is the mechanics of displaying the month, and we will look at the data management class in the next section.

Integrating the Cell Manager

Let's put the CCellMgr class to work. First, we need to add a protected member to the Cviscal class, in the viscal.h file:

```
    CCellMgr m_CellMgr;
```

Next, we initialize the cell manager in our override of the `CComObjectRootEx::FinalConstruct()` method in the `viscal.cpp` file. We'll have more to say about the use of `FinalConstruct()` a little bit later.

```
STDMETHODIMP Cviscal::FinalConstruct(void)
{
    m_CurrentDate = CDateTime::CurrentTime();
    m_CellMgr.SetDate(m_CurrentDate);
    return S_OK;
}
```

Of course, we need to add the declaration for this method to the header as well:

```
// CComObjectRootEx<> overrides
   STDMETHOD(FinalConstruct)(void);
   void FinalRelease(void);
```

This will ensure that the current month will be shown when the ActiveX control is first instantiated. Next, we can fill in the implementation of the `AdvanceMonth()` method, which we created earlier:

```
STDMETHODIMP Cviscal::AdvanceMonth(long inc)
{
    m_CurrentDate = m_CurrentDate + CDateTimeDiff(0, inc, 0, 0, 0, 0);
    m_CellMgr.SetDate(m_CurrentDate);
    FireViewChange();
    return S_OK;
}
```

Once we have calculated the new date by adding `inc` months to it, we call the `CCellMgr` member to recalculate the contents of all cells using its `SetDate()` method. Finally, we inform the container that a repaint of the control is necessary by calling `FireViewChange()`.

Here, we're using two extremely versatile utility classes we have developed: `CDateTime` encapsulates dates and times and `CDateTimeDiff` encapsulates time differences. The `m_CurrentDate` member is added to the `Cviscal` class and is used as a state variable reflecting the month being shown on the calendar.

```
    CDateTime m_CurrentDate;
```

That is all that we have to do to wire up the buttons.

The Versatile CDateTime Utility Class

Throughout our ActiveX control implementation, we have used the features of our `CDateTime` utility class extensively. This is an extremely versatile class when dealing with information associated with date or time. We developed it in the absence of anything better provided by ATL and drew inspiration from the MFC `COleDateTime` class.

```
class CDateTime
{
public:
   CDateTime();
   CDateTime(int year, int month = 1, int day = 1, int hour = 0,
                                      int minute = 0, int second = 0 );
   CDateTime(const CDateTime& other );
   CDateTime(const time_t other );
   CDateTime(const SYSTEMTIME& sysTime );
   CDateTime(const FILETIME& fileTime );
   CDateTime(const DATE date );
   ~CDateTime();

   CDateTime& operator=( const CDateTime& other );
   CDateTime& operator=( time_t other );
   CDateTime  operator+( const CDateTimeDiff diff ) const;

   int GetYear() const;        // 1970 - 2036
   int GetMonth() const;       // 1- 12
   int GetDay() const;         // 1 - 31
   int GetHours() const;       // 0 - 23
   int GetMinutes() const;     // 0 - 59
   int GetSeconds() const;     // 0 - 59
   int GetDayOfWeek() const;   // 0 == Sunday, 1 == Monday ...
   int GetDayOfYear() const;   // 0 == Jan 1, to 365

   operator time_t() const;   // convert to time_t
   operator tstring() const;  // convert to tstring

   tstring Format( LPCTSTR fmt ) const; // pass format string as per strftime()

   DATE ConvertToDATE() const;

   CDateTime& Clear(void);

   // class static
   static CDateTime CurrentTime(void);

private:
   time_t t;
   TCHAR m_buf[BUFSIZ];    // for debugging
};
```

Internally, the CDateTime class maintains a date/time value in C runtime format, time_t. Externally, the class provides a DATE based access to the value, as well as:

❑ String-based access to a formatted date/time representation
❑ Conversion to and from time_t type
❑ Direct access into the month, year, and day component of the date/time value

All this is done to facilitate the kind of access typically required for a date/time value. Finally, a static member method, CurrentTime(), is provided in the CDateTime class for working with the current time, which is obtained through C runtime calls.

CDateTime provides for conversions from and to the DATE data type which, as a member of VARIANT, is used to pass dates within Automation. DATE encapsulates a date/time combination in an 8-byte floating-point number. We used this extensively in the routines setting the days. One example is the SetDate() member function of the CCellMgr class:

```
void CCellMgr::SetDate( const CDateTime& d )
{
   // clear the cells
   ClearCellContents();

   int i, offset;

   // first day of current month
   CDateTime currDate( d.GetYear(), d.GetMonth() );

   // weekday of first day of current month
   int weekDay = currDate.GetDayOfWeek();

   // set the cell labels for days of past month, if any,
   // that should appear in the calendar.  Note that the day
   // of the first cell is 'firstWeekDay' days before 'firstDay'.
   CDateTime pastMonthDate((time_t)((time_t)currDate - weekDay * kSecondsInADay));

   int   pastMonthDay = pastMonthDate.GetDay();
   for ( i = 0; i < weekDay; i++, pastMonthDay++ )
   {
      m_Cells[i].dayNumber = Int2TString( pastMonthDay );
      m_Cells[i].date = pastMonthDate + CDateTimeDiff( 0, 0, i, 0, 0, 1 );
   }

   // add label for past month, if any
   if ( weekDay > 0 )
      m_Cells[0].label = CMonthInfo().GetMonthShortName( pastMonthDate );

   // set the cell labels and date for current month
   // cells corresponding to current month are 'firstWeekDay'
   // offset into m_Cells
   offset = weekDay;
   for ( i = 0; i < CMonthInfo().GetDaysInMonth( currDate ); i++ )
   {
      m_Cells[i + offset].dayNumber = Int2TString( i + 1 );
      m_Cells[i + offset].date = currDate + CDateTimeDiff(0, 0, i, 0, 0, 1);
   }
   // set the cell labels for next month, if any
   CDateTime nextMonthDate( (time_t)( (time_t)currDate +
         CMonthInfo().GetDaysInMonth( currDate ) * kSecondsInADay) );

   // offset into m_Cells of cells corresponding to next month
   offset += CMonthInfo().GetDaysInMonth( currDate );
   for( i = 0; i < m_NumCells - offset; i++ )
   {
      m_Cells[i + offset].dayNumber = Int2TString( i + 1 );
      m_Cells[i + offset].date = nextMonthDate + CDateTimeDiff(0,0,i,0,0,1);
   }

   // add label for next month, if any
   if ( offset < m_NumCells )
      m_Cells[offset].label = CMonthInfo().GetMonthShortName(nextMonthDate);
```

```
        // set the control label
        SetMonthYearLabel( currDate );
}
```

Another very useful capability of the CDateTime class is the set of the date-based arithmetic operations, which are performed in conjunction with the CDateTimeDiff class. A CDateTimeDiff variable can represent time intervals as days, hours, minutes, or seconds. It can represent either a positive interval into the future or a negative interval back through the past. You'll find CDateTimeDiff defined in CalUtils.h:

```
class CDateTimeDiff
{
public:
    CDateTimeDiff(int year, int month = 0, int day = 0, int hour = 0,
                  int minute = 0, int second = 0 );
    operator time_t() const;

private:
    struct tm tm_t;
    // we could provide accessor but this way is easier
    friend class CDateTime;
};
```

Internally, CDateTimeDiff wraps a tm_t C runtime structure representing a time interval. The sole purpose of this class is to provide for the addition of a time interval to a CDateTime value which will yield another CDateTime value. The CDateTime class has a specific + operator defined to work with CDateTimeDiff. This operator provides for adjusting a CDateTime value by any arbitrary time interval.

Please refer to CalUtils.cpp if you are curious as to how any of the CDateTime or CDateTimeDiff members are implemented. Using the CDateTime and CDateTimeDiff class has significantly reduced the overall coding burden of our control.

That little diversion over, we now need to add code to the paint handler in order to put the correct labeling on the cells.

Drawing the Calendar Labels

To draw the calendar cell labels, the OnDraw() method must be enhanced to query the CCellMgr member for the appropriate label to draw. In our case, the OnDraw() method actually calls the PaintGrid() method to do the drawing. Here is what the PaintGrid() method will look like:

```
void Cviscal::PaintGrid(HDC hdc, HDC attrDC, const CRectangle& rect,
                                            bool inMetafileContext )
{
    // do intermediate calculations in float to eliminate
    // round-off errors when scaling
    float x1, x2, y1, y2;
    float curX, curY;
```

```
float cellWidth, halfCellWidth;
float cellHeight, halfCellHeight;
float topMargin, leftMargin;
float xPad = 2, yPad = 2;
ULONG numRows, numCols;
ULONG offsetY;
ULONG counter;
ULONG i;
ULONG j, k;
...
```

The new variables required have been highlighted in the above code. The first part of this method simply calculates spacing and draws the horizontal and vertical lines that form the grid. We have seen this already, so that part of the code will not be repeated here.

The next part of the method iterates through the cells, one by one, and calls the CCellMgr member to get the cell label. The highlighted code segment shows this interaction between view and controller.

```
::SetTextAlign(hdc, TA_LEFT | TA_TOP);
// draw data in each cell
counter = 0;

for (i = 0; i < kRowsDisplayed; i++)
{
    curY = offsetY + i * cellHeight;

    for (j = 0; j < kDaysInWeek; j++)
    {
        curX = leftMargin + j * cellWidth;

        // draw cell(i,j)
        tstring text = tstring( m_CellMgr.GetCellLabel( counter ) )
                        .append( _T(" ") )
                        .append( m_CellMgr.GetCellDayNumber( counter ) );

        // clip inside cell rectangle
        CRectangle clipRect ( int( curX + xPad ),
                              int( curY + yPad ),
                              int( curX + cellWidth - xPad ),
                              int( curY + cellHeight - yPad ) );
        ::ExtTextOut( hdc, clipRect.Left(), clipRect.Top(),
                    ETO_CLIPPED, &((RECT)clipRect)
                  , text.c_str(), text.size(), NULL );
        counter++;
    } //for j
} //for i
```

The title containing the month and year is obtained from the CCellMgr and printed:

```
// center and draw the control label
const tstring&   label = m_CellMgr.GetMonthYearLabel();

SIZE  labelSize;
::GetTextExtentPoint32( attrDC, label.c_str(), label.size(), &labelSize ) ;
CRectangle labelRect = CRectangle(labelSize);
```

```
      // determine the bounding rectangle for the label
      int    labelOffset = 6;
      CRectangle labelBoundingRect(
              max( kCalLeftMargin + m_CurButtonSize + labelOffset,
                   (rect.Width() - labelRect.Width())/2 ),    // left
              max( labelOffset,
                   (kCalTopMargin + m_CurButtonSize - labelRect.Height())),
              min( rect.Width() - kCalLeftMargin - m_CurButtonSize - labelOffset,
                   (rect.Width() + labelRect.Width())/2 ),    // right
              kCalTopMargin + m_CurButtonSize               // bottom
        );

      // draw label
      ::ExtTextOut(hdc, labelBoundingRect.Left(), labelBoundingRect.Top(),
                               ETO_CLIPPED, &((RECT)labelBoundingRect),
                               label.c_str(), label.size(), NULL);
```

Finally, we print the column headings containing the days of the week labels. This is done through a static class named CMonthInfo().

```
      // draw the names of the days of the week
      for ( i = 0; i < kDaysInWeek; i++ ) {
          TEXTMETRIC    tm;
          GetTextMetrics( attrDC, &tm );    // use attribute DC
          curX = leftMargin + i * cellWidth;
          curY = offsetY - 1.1f * tm.tmHeight;
          CRectangle clipRect( curX, curY, curX + cellWidth, curY + cellHeight );
          const tstring&    name = CMonthInfo().GetDayOfWeekName(i);
          ::ExtTextOut(hdc, clipRect.Left(), clipRect.Top(), ETO_CLIPPED,
                               &(RECT)clipRect, name.c_str(), name.size(), NULL);
      }
  } // Cviscal::PaintGrid()
```

The use of CMonthInfo() class here provides a kind of global constant, without cluttering up CCellMgr with something that is not directly related. You can find the definition of this class in the CalUtils.h file:

```
class CMonthInfo
{
public:
    tstring       monthName;
    UINT          daysInMonth;

    CMonthInfo() : daysInMonth(0) {}
    CMonthInfo(const tstring name, const UINT num)
        : monthName(name), daysInMonth(num) {}

    const tstring GetMonthLongName  (const CDateTime& d) const;    // 1 - 12
    const tstring GetMonthShortName (const CDateTime& d) const;    // 1 - 12
    int           GetDaysInMonth    (const CDateTime& d) const;    // 1 - 12
    const tstring GetDayOfWeekName  (const int i) const;           // 0 == Sun
private:
    // class statics -- declaration
    static CMonthInfo months[];
    static tstring dayNames[];
};
```

The actual initialization of the static class is contained in `CalUtils.cpp`. Here we see the months,

```
CMonthInfo   CMonthInfo::months[] =
{
    CMonthInfo( _T("January"),   31 ),
    CMonthInfo( _T("February"), 28 ),
    CMonthInfo( _T("March"),     31 ),
    CMonthInfo( _T("April"),     30 ),
    CMonthInfo( _T("May"),       31 ),
    CMonthInfo( _T("June"),      30 ),
    CMonthInfo( _T("July"),      31 ),
    CMonthInfo( _T("August"),    31 ),
    CMonthInfo( _T("September"),30 ),
    CMonthInfo( _T("October"),   31 ),
    CMonthInfo( _T("November"), 30 ),
    CMonthInfo( _T("December"), 31 )
};
```

and here the names of the weekdays:

```
tstring CMonthInfo::dayNames[] = {
    _T("Sunday"),
    _T("Monday"),
    _T("Tuesday"),
    _T("Wednesday"),
    _T("Thursday"),
    _T("Friday"),
    _T("Saturday") };
```

The other data access members of this class are quite straightforward, so they will not be repeated here to save some space. Refer to `CalUtils.cpp` in Appendix E, if you are interested.

Trying out the Monthly Display

This concludes our task of displaying the month/day information and hooking up the two buttons for changing the date.

The visual calendar control is now 60% functional; the only task remaining is to hook up the actual event data to be displayed. You can find the code up to this stage in the `Ch06\viscal1.3` directory of the source distribution. You will notice some additional changes to the code from the previous iteration which we haven't covered in detail. These include:

- Adding new constants in `CalDefs.h` – for example `kMaxCellAttachments` and `kCalLeftMargin`
- Implmentation of `CCellMgr` and `CCalCell`
- Including `CCellMgr.h` in the source files
- Changes to `Cviscal` (adding `m_CurButtonSize` and modifying the methods `OnCreate()` and `ButRectHelper()`).

Using Visual Basic 6, you can deploy the calendar control, and try out its basic month-changing functions. A test program is available under the `Ch06\VBTest` directory of the source distribution:

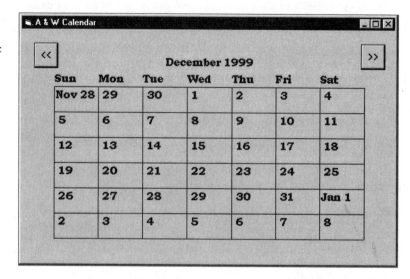

Iteration 4: Adding Custom Properties and Middle Tier Data

Were going to pick up the pace a bit now, and add everything else that is necessary to make our control fully functional. First, we'll start with some custom properties.

Adding Custom Properties to the Control

Let's just start with a brief rundown of what we have achieved thus far. We have:

- ❑ Created our basic control skeleton using ATL 3
- ❑ Added some visual behavior to it
- ❑ Enabled it to handle ambient and extended properties
- ❑ Added our own method and implemented it
- ❑ Attached the 'controller' (our cell manager) from a MVC pattern.

The stock properties supplied by ATL 3 allow us to easily implement the most common properties that a visual control requires by default. For our specific functionality, we'll also need to define some new custom properties. In this case, the onus is on us to ensure that the custom properties get initialized, and persisted properly when the control is persisted.

For our visual ActiveX calendar control, we need separate control over the font used in printing the month and year across the top of the calendar display. Instead of having the same size and weight as the font used to label the cells, we typically want a larger and heavier weight font for the title. Unfortunately, the stock properties only provide for one font setting, and we are already using this for the default-labeling font. It is therefore necessary for us to create some custom properties that will facilitate control of the title font.

To add a custom property to the control, we add get/set methods to its default dispatch (in this case, dual) interface. From the **ClassView**, right-click on the `Iviscal` interface and select **Add Property**.

> *You'll be able to see from this dialog that we can create a read-only or write-only property by defining only a* Get *method or* Put *method.* PropPut *will set the property with a value, while* PropPutRef *allows the object to be set by reference.*

Add the following properties to the `Iviscal` interface:

Property Type	Property Name	Parameters	Function Type
BOOL	TitleFontBold	empty	Get, Put, PropPut
long	TitleFontSize	empty	Get, Put, PropPut
BSTR	TitleFontName	empty	Get, Put, PropPut

Once you have added these, take a look at the code the property wizard has generated.

We need to make the following changes to the generated IDL code:

```
enum {DISPID_TITLEFONTNAME = 2, DISPID_TITLEFONTSIZE = 3,
                                DISPID_TITLEFONTBOLD = 4};

    interface Iviscal : IDispatch
    {
        ...
        [id(1), helpstring("method AdvanceMonth")] HRESULT AdvanceMonth(
                                                [in] long inc);
        [propget, id(DISPID_TITLEFONTNAME), helpstring("property TitleFontName")]
            HRESULT TitleFontName([out, retval] BSTR *pVal);
        [propput, id(DISPID_TITLEFONTNAME), helpstring("property TitleFontName")]
            HRESULT TitleFontName([in] BSTR newVal);
        [propget, id(DISPID_TITLEFONTSIZE), helpstring("property TitleFontSize")]
            HRESULT TitleFontSize([out, retval] long *pVal);
        [propput, id(DISPID_TITLEFONTSIZE), helpstring("property TitleFontSize")]
            HRESULT TitleFontSize([in] long newVal);
        [propget, id(DISPID_TITLEFONTBOLD), helpstring("property TitleFontBold")]
            HRESULT TitleFontBold([out, retval] BOOL *pVal);
        [propput, id(DISPID_TITLEFONTBOLD), helpstring("property TitleFontBold")]
            HRESULT TitleFontBold([in] BOOL newVal);
```

The header file, `viscal.h`, contains the definitions for the get/set methods:

```
public:
    STDMETHOD(get_TitleFontBold)(/*[out, retval]*/ BOOL *pVal);
    STDMETHOD(put_TitleFontBold)(/*[in]*/ BOOL newVal);
    STDMETHOD(get_TitleFontSize)(/*[out, retval]*/ long *pVal);
    STDMETHOD(put_TitleFontSize)(/*[in]*/ long newVal);
    STDMETHOD(get_TitleFontName)(/*[out, retval]*/ BSTR *pVal);
    STDMETHOD(put_TitleFontName)(/*[in]*/ BSTR newVal);
    ...
```

You can see how the Property Wizard has created three new properties for us. The above example illustrates how to create and handle custom properties of different types (BOOL, long, and BSTR, for example). These font-related properties allow a user of the calendar control to change attributes of the title font, one at a time, without calling any font functions.

We will now discover how we can internally manage a system font resource that is not exposed directly as a property.

First, we must declare additional members in the Cviscal class to hold the state of these new properties:

```
        CComPtr<IFontDisp> m_pFont;
        static FONTDESC DefaultFontDesc;

protected:
        CComBSTR          m_TitleFontName;
        long              m_TitleFontSize;
        BOOL              m_TitleFontBold;;
        CComPtr<IFont> m_pTitleFont;
        BOOL              m_bInitDone;
```

The font's textual name is held in m_TitleFontName, using the versatile CComBSTR class; the font's size and weight are held in m_TitleFontSize and m_TitleFontBold respectively. The actual font used will be a system-managed font to which we keep a reference using the m_pTitleFont smart pointer (as we did with the Font stock property).

The CComBSTR Class

Of particular interest here is the use of an ATL-defined class, CComBSTR, to handle the BSTR data type. This is especially convenient and saves on code, as all of the construction, copying, conversion, and release coding is performed automatically by the CComBSTR class.

Briefly, the ATL CComBSTR class includes these members:

CComBSTR Member	Type	Description
Attach()	method	Attaches an existing BSTR to the object to use its method and operators
CComBSTR()	method	Constructor uses a UNICODE string or an ANSI string. A copy constructor is also supplied as well as a default constructor
Copy()	method	Creates and returns another copy of the represented BSTR
Detach()	method	Detaches a BSTR from the object after performing operations
Empty()	method	Frees the associated BSTR
Operator BSTR	operator	Casts a CComBSTR object to a BSTR, allowing direct reference

Table Continued on Following Page

CComBSTR Member	Type	Description
Operator =	operator	Allows assignment from UNICODE, ANSI, or another CComBSTR
Operator &	operator	Returns a pointer to the represented BSTR
Operator +=	operator	Concatenates another BSTR to the end
Operator !	operator	Returns TRUE if the represented BSTR is NULL, returns FALSE otherwise (for example, if (!m_strAString) abort();)
Operator ==	operator	Returns TRUE if the two BSTR are equal
m_str	member variable	The member variable containing the actual BSTR

Implementing the Font Control Properties

We need to hook up the get/set methods in Cviscal to get and set the appropriate member variable implementing each property. First, let's look at the string name of the title font:

```
STDMETHODIMP Cviscal::get_TitleFontName(BSTR* pVal)
{
    return m_TitleFontName.CopyTo(pVal);
}
```

Here, we use the CopyTo() method of the CComBSTR class, which is new to ATL 3.

```
STDMETHODIMP Cviscal::put_TitleFontName(BSTR newVal)
{
    if (!newVal)
        return S_OK;

    if (m_TitleFontName != newVal)
    {
        m_TitleFontName = newVal;
        SetDirty(TRUE);
        RefreshTitleFont();
        FireViewChange();
    }
    return S_OK;
}
```

In this method, we first check to make sure that the string is not empty, then we check to make sure it is not the same as the currently used font. Only when the font name is different, we assign it into the m_TitleFontName member. The remaining lines call the refresh routines to update the appearance of the title font on the control.

Next, the size of the font is checked and set in a similar way, as illustrated in the following code fragments.

```
STDMETHODIMP Cviscal::get_TitleFontSize(long* pVal)
{
    *pVal = m_TitleFontSize;
    return S_OK;
}

STDMETHODIMP Cviscal::put_TitleFontSize(long newVal)
{
    if (m_TitleFontSize != newVal)
    {
        m_TitleFontSize = newVal;
        SetDirty(TRUE);
        RefreshTitleFont();
        FireViewChange();
    }
    return S_OK;
}
```

Finally, the weight of the title font is got and set in the same way:

```
STDMETHODIMP Cviscal::get_TitleFontBold(BOOL* pVal)
{
    *pVal = m_TitleFontBold;
    return S_OK;
}

STDMETHODIMP Cviscal::put_TitleFontBold(BOOL newVal)
{
    if (m_TitleFontBold != newVal)
    {
        m_TitleFontBold = newVal;
        SetDirty(TRUE);
        RefreshTitleFont();
        FireViewChange();
    }
    return S_OK;
}
```

These methods take care of transferring the property values into and out of the Cviscal member variables, but we still haven't touched the actual system font (the m_pTitleFont smart pointer). In fact, we only need to work with this extra font when we paint the title of the calendar. Our strategy here is to delay and isolate the code that deals with the extra font inside.

The PaintGrid() method (called by OnDraw()), and two extra helper methods, RefreshTitleFont() and SetTitleFont(), are declared as follows:

```
protected:
    void RefreshTitleFont();
    void SetTitleFont();
```

Here is the first of the two helper methods, implemented in `viscal.cpp`:

```
void Cviscal::RefreshTitleFont()
{
    if (m_pTitleFont)
        m_pTitleFont.Release();
    SetTitleFont();
}
```

This method first tests whether or not `m_pTitleFont` is currently assigned, and if so, it releases the old font. We then simply reassign the font using a call to `SetTitleFont()`, which works with the `FONTDESC` structure that we saw earlier in the working with stock properties section.

The `FONTDESC` structure is one of the most badly documented system structures in the Microsoft platform SDK. Note that font size is specified as a 64-bit `LONGLONG` value in the form of a `CY` (Currency) structure. `CY` itself is defined as either a double precision floating point number or a `struct` consisting of a 'low' long value and a 'high' long value. The font size must be in the lower long value portion and must be 10000 times the actual point value.

```
void Cviscal::SetTitleFont()
{
    FONTDESC tmpFontDesc = DefaultFontDesc;
    if (m_TitleFontName)
        tmpFontDesc.lpstrName = (LPOLESTR) m_TitleFontName ;
    CY tpCy = {m_TitleFontSize * 10000, 0};
    tmpFontDesc.cySize = tpCy;
    tmpFontDesc.sWeight = m_TitleFontBold ? FW_BOLD: FW_NORMAL;
    OleCreateFontIndirect(&tmpFontDesc, IID_IFont, (void **) &m_pTitleFont);
}
```

Here again, `OleCreateFontIndirect()` is used to request the system to locate or create the font that we wish to use, saving us the agony of working with complicated font APIs or managing its allocation.

We can be sure that the right font is created and ready for use by the drawing routine, because each of the get/set methods for the font properties will call `RefreshTitleFont()` whenever a property is changed.

Drawing the Title in a Different Font

We now need to make some minor modification to the `PaintGrid()` method when painting the title with the user-specified font. The additional code used, both to select the font into the device context before label printing, and the de-selection after, is shown below. This is identical to the way we have used our stock font property.

```
    . . .

    // work out the current font for title
    if (!m_pTitleFont)
    {
        SetTitleFont();
    }
    HFONT tmpFont;
```

```
m_pTitleFont->get_hFont(&tmpFont);
m_pTitleFont->AddRefHfont(tmpFont);
HFONT hOldFont = (HFONT) SelectObject( hdc, tmpFont );
HFONT hOldAttrFont = (HFONT) SelectObject( attrDC, tmpFont );

// center and draw the control label
const tstring& label = m_CellMgr.GetMonthYearLabel();

SIZE labelSize;
::GetTextExtentPoint32( attrDC, label.c_str(), label.size(), &labelSize ) ;
CRectangle labelRect = CRectangle(labelSize);

// determine the bounding rectangle for the label
int labelOffset = 6;
CRectangle labelBoundingRect(
                    max(kCalLeftMargin + m_CurButtonSize + labelOffset,
                        (rect.Width() - labelRect.Width())/2 ),    // left
                    max(labelOffset, kCalTopMargin + m_CurButtonSize -
                        labelRect.Height()) ),                     // top
                    min(rect.Width() - kCalLeftMargin -
                        m_CurButtonSize - labelOffset,
                        (rect.Width() + labelRect.Width())/2 ),    // right
                    kCalTopMargin + m_CurButtonSize                // bottom
                    );

// draw label
::ExtTextOut( hdc, labelBoundingRect.Left(), labelBoundingRect.Top(),
                            ETO_CLIPPED, &((RECT)labelBoundingRect),
                            label.c_str(), label.size(), NULL );

SelectObject(hdc, hOldFont);
SelectObject(hdc, hOldAttrFont);
m_pTitleFont->ReleaseHfont(tmpFont);

// draw the names of the days of the week
for (i = 0; i < kDaysInWeek; i++)
{
    TEXTMETRIC tm;
    GetTextMetrics(attrDC, &tm);    // use attribute DC
    curX = leftMargin + i * cellWidth;
    curY = offsetY - 1.1f * tm.tmHeight;
    CRectangle clipRect(curX, curY, curX + cellWidth, curY + cellHeight);
    const tstring& name = CMonthInfo().GetDayOfWeekName(i);
    ::ExtTextOut(hdc, clipRect.Left(), clipRect.Top(), ETO_CLIPPED,
                        &(RECT)clipRect, name.c_str(), name.size(), NULL);
}
}
```

Persistence Support for Custom Properties

The user can now manipulate the font properties, and the control will visibly respond to the change of setting. We should now ensure that the states of these member variables (properties) are consistent at all times, and that they can be persisted in and out with the rest of the (stock) properties properly.

To make sure that the properties are persisted properly, all we need to do is add them to the property map macro in the `viscal.h` file. Although the ATL Wizard automatically adds entries for the stock properties to the property map, it doesn't do the same for the custom properties.

```
BEGIN_PROP_MAP(Cviscal)
    PROP_PAGE(CLSID_StockColorPage)
    PROP_PAGE(CLSID_StockFontPage)
    ...
    PROP_ENTRY("TitleFontName", DISPID_TITLEFONTNAME, CLSID_NULL)
    PROP_ENTRY("TitleFontSize", DISPID_TITLEFONTSIZE, CLSID_NULL)
    PROP_ENTRY("TitleFontBold", DISPID_TITLEFONTBOLD, CLSID_NULL)
END_PROP_MAP()
```

These are the DISPIDs we defined earlier in `viscal1.idl`.

To ensure that each member variable contains a reasonable default value when the C++ object is created, we initialize them in the `Cviscal` constructor:

```
Cviscal():m_ctlButBack(_T("Button"),this,1),
          m_ctlButFore(_T("Button"),this,2),
          m_CurButtonSize(10),
          m_clrBackColor(0xffffff),
          m_TitleFontBold(FALSE),
          m_ButtonVisible(TRUE),
          m_TitleFontSize(16),
          m_bInitDone(FALSE)
{
    m_bWindowOnly = TRUE;
}
```

Depending on the container, a persisted ActiveX control may be initialized via either the `IPersistStreamInit` or `IPersistStream` interface. If `IPersistStreamInit` is used, the container is interested in explicitly initializing the newly created control to a well defined default state, and will call the `InitNew()` method. Here is our code for `InitNew()`, resetting all the member variables back to their default:

```
STDMETHODIMP Cviscal::InitNew()
{
    if (m_bInitDone)
        return E_UNEXPECTED;

    m_TitleFontName = "Arial";
    m_TitleFontSize = 16;
    m_TitleFontBold = TRUE;
    SetDirty(TRUE);
    RefreshTitleFont();
    m_bInitDone = TRUE;

    return S_OK;
}
```

Most modern containers should support IPersistStreamInit, and would distinguish between initializing the control for the very first time after instance creation (by calling InitNew()) or initializing a control from a persisted stream (by calling IPersistStreamInit::Load()). If the container only supports IPersistStream for controls, only the IPersistStream::Load() member should be called.

```
STDMETHODIMP Cviscal::Load(LPSTREAM pStream)
{
    if (m_bInitDone)
        return E_UNEXPECTED;
    m_bInitDone = TRUE;
    return IPersistStreamInitImpl<Cviscal>::Load(pStream);
}
```

The Load() member calls IPersistStreamInitImpl<>::Load(), which will in turn restore the persisted property values from the stream automatically. The m_bInitDone flag, added as a data member to Cviscal, is used to ensure that a misbehaving container doesn't end up initializing the ActiveX control twice.

C++ Constructor, FinalConstruct() versus InitNew()

It is appropriate here to note the different initialization points available in an ActiveX control. Here is a summary:

Point of Initialization	Description	Comment
C++ class constructor	C++ object may not be completely constructed.	Can be used to set object members to reasonable default values – avoiding potential coding errors, but has no significant COM semantics; cannot safely call virtual members.
FinalConstruct()	ATL-based 'post constructor' hook, guarantees that C++ object has been completely created when called. It is a code library (ATL) adjunct to compensate for C++'s weakness.	Can be used to initialize state of C++ object which depends on the constructor having completed successfully; for example, it can call virtual C++ members. Still has no significant COM semantics.

Table Continued on Following Page

Point of Initialization	Description	Comment
`InitNew()` or `Load()`	COM/OLE specified initializer, after a new instance of a COM object has been completely constructed.	Typically used to initialize the state of the COM object after an instance of the COM object is completely created; note that this has *no* C++ relevant semantics. As a matter of fact, the implementation of this member may not even be in the same object with the C++ source.

When you have initialization work to perform for an ActiveX control, the above table will help you to decide where you should place such code. Inappropriate use of these functions is often a source of great confusion, and of annoying bugs. This is because they can frequently be substituted for each other.

This wraps up the required code for implementing the title font properties. Now we move on to implementing a stub backend for our control, so that we can actually complete the visual user interface for viewing event data.

The Event Data Backend

The backend calendar data in our system is accessed through a three-tier DNA scheme. Within our calendar control, all the dirty data-access work is hidden away from the View and Controller in the MVC pattern. As a matter of fact, the `CDataMgr` class, which plays the role of the Model in the MVC pattern, is the only class that is 'data aware'. Its idea of the data follows an object model presented by a system of middle tier objects. The object model abstraction facilitates easy access to the data through Automation, by using any compatible languages and/or environments (for example, Visual Basic 6 or Visual J++ 6).

> *The containment and interaction relationship of objects within, or 'behind', a component is sometimes called its **object model**. The object model gives the user of a component a mental image of how things work behind the scenes. It serves as a visualization tool for providing documentation of how to use the set of COM interfaces exposed by a component. This may sound more complex than it actually is, but never fear, we'll be looking at a concrete example of this through our project.*

In our example, the client for these middle tier objects is the `CDataMgr` class. The client can manipulate objects through the object model, and obtain event data. The fact that this COM component uses one or more other COM components to do its job is transparent to the View and Controller portion of the control. Let's examine the object model for the calendar control.

The Object Model and the CDataMgr Class

You can find the source code for the `CDataMgr` class in `CDataMgr.cpp` and `CDataMgr.h` (see Appendix E for a full listing).

For the calendar control to work, we want the control to go out over the network and 'pull' the event data 'live' from all the departments providing event information. This contrasts with the need for departments to publish event data to a centralized server. In Chapter 5 we discussed the ramifications of these requirements.

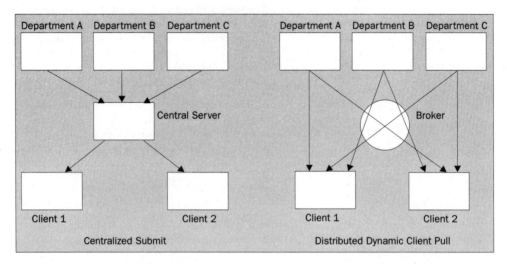

To enable this architecture, an 'event finder' business object works with individual 'departments with events' objects to complete the object model. In order to keep the sample simple, and so that it can work initially on just Windows 9x machines, we've implemented these objects without actually giving them real data access capabilities.

Diagrammatically, the object model looks like this:

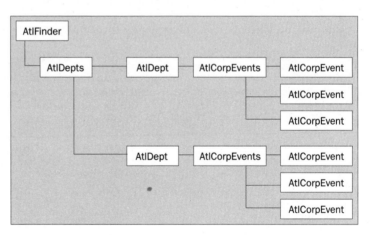

The above diagram says that the event finder object, ATLFinder, has a property with a value of type ATLDepts. An ATLDepts object is a collection of individual ATLDept objects. In turn, each ATLDept object has a property with a value of type ATLCorpEvents, and an ATLCorpEvents object is a collection of individual ATLCorpEvent objects. The ATLCorpEvent objects contain the details of a specific event. The following is a more detailed and specific description of the objects making up the model.

Class name	Object Represented	Description
ATLFinder	Finder for departments with events.	The broker object locating all the departments with event information given a date. It keeps the collection of departments with events in an EventfulDept property holding a collection of department objects. This property is an instance of the ATLDepts class.
ATLDepts	A collection of departments.	A generic collection of departments. We have added a 'secret' (that is, non-publicized) Add() function to add departments for testing purposes without having to set up data sources.
ATLDept	A single department.	Department containing name, symbol, and color information; also holds an instance of a KnownEvents property holding a collection of events.
ATLCorpEvents	Collection of events.	A generic collection of events.
ATLCorpEvent	A single event.	An event contains description, header, organizer, and detail information.

The above classes will be explained in the next chapter in greater detail.

Typically, a user of this object model (one example of which is our calendar control) will do the following:

Please note that the arrows to the left denote that we have an interface pointer to an object, while the arrows pointing to the right denote invoking a method on the object at the tip of the arrow.

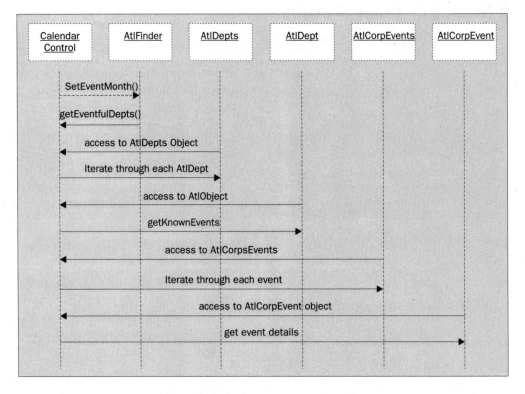

1. Call `ATLFinder.SetEventMonth()` to set the date of the month of interest for the component

2. Access the `ATLFinder.EventfulDept` properties to get a list of all the departments with events to post during the month

3. Obtain access to an `ATLDepts` object through its `IATLDepts` COM interface

4. Iterate through the list of departments, and for each department, perform steps 5 to 10

5. Obtain access to an `ATLDept` object through its `IATLDept` COM interface

6. Access the `KnownEvents` member of the department to get a list of all the events available

7. Obtain access to an `ATLCorpEvents` collection object through its `IATLCorpEvents` COM interface

8. Iterate through the list of events performing steps 9 and 10 for each one

9. Obtain access to an `ATLCorpEvent` object through its `IATLCorpEvent` COM interface

10. Get the event details

The diagram above shows how the entire series of interactions boils down to property access and method invocations across different objects/components. It's this simple object interaction scheme, supported by COM and Automation, which will allow other developers to easily extend our application.

Data Manager Class Details

The CDataMgr class is defined in CDataMgr.h as:

```
class CDataMgr
{
public:
   CDataMgr();
   virtual ~CDataMgr();

   bool CreateFinder();
   void ReleaseFinder();

   const CCalDept& GetDept(ULONG idx) const;
   ULONG GetDeptCount() const;

   ULONG GetNumDeptEventsInMonth(ULONG inDept) const;

   void GetNumEventsOnDate(const CDateTime& inDate,
                              vector<ULONG>& eventCount) const;

   void GetDeptEventsOnDate(const ULONG inDept, const CDateTime& inDate,
                              CCalEventList& events) const;

   void GetAnEvent(const CDateTime & inDate, ULONG inDept, ULONG idx,
                              CCalEvent & anEvent) const;

   void GrabActiveDepts();
   bool InfoAvail();
   void ResetState();

   void SetEventMonth(const CDateTime & inMonth);

protected:
   Finder::IATLFinder1Ptr* m_MyFinder;
   bool m_InfoAvail;
   CDeptEventList m_DeptEventList;
};
```

We can see that CDataMgr actually wraps a COM object with an IATLFinder interface (via m_MyFinder), and an instance of a C++ class called CDeptEventList (via m_DeptEventList). Before we look at this C++ class, here is a tabulation of the CDataMgr methods and a brief description what each one does:

Method	Description
CreateFinder()	Using compiler COM support, creates an instance of the ATLFinder COM server, so that departments and events will be obtained through this broker
ReleaseFinder()	Releases the interface on the ATLFinder COM server
GetDept()	Get a CCalDept instance with details on the department

Method	Description
GetDeptCount()	Gets the number of departments
GetNumDeptEventsInMonth()	Gets the number events for a department in a particular month
GetNumEventsOnDate()	Gets the number of events on a particular date
GetDeptEventsOnDate()	Gets the total number of events on a particular date for a particular department
GetAnEvent()	Gets a CCalEvent instance with details on the event. See the following text for the CCalEvent structure definition
GrabActiveDepts()	Obtains all the departments that participate in the event calendar, from the ATLFinder broker
InfoAvail()	Indicates that the data manager has been filled at least once with department information since the last ResetState() call
ResetState()	Clears the data manager, enabling it to query for a new department and event data
SetEventMonth()	Sets the month for which to fetch data (this is where we 'stuff' our backend component with test data)

Most methods defined for the CDataMgr class (the model in the Model-View-Controller pattern) are custom tailored to the requirements of the CCellMgr (Controller) class and Cviscal (View) class.

The files CEvents.cpp and CEvents.h contain helper classes encapsulating events for the data manager. The CDeptEventList class, which is used by CDataMgr, is defined in CEvents.h, simply as a vector of CDeptEvents:

```
class CDeptEventList : public vector<CDeptEvents> {};
```

CDeptEvents, in turn, is defined as:

```
class CDeptEvents
{
    CCalDept Dept;
    CDatesList OnDates;

    ULONG GetNumEventsOnDate( const CDateTime& inDate ) const ;
};
```

The structure used to hold information about each department, CCalDept, as shown here:

```
struct CCalDept
{
    tstring   DeptName;
    tstring   DeptNumber;
    bool      CanRead;
    bool      CanPostNew;
    tstring   Symbol;      // single character symbol
    OLE_COLOR Color;
};
```

The Symbol and Color members are used to display the number of events for each department within each calendar cell.

CCalEvent, the structure used to hold information about each event, has the following members:

```
struct CCalEvent
{
    CDateTime DateTime;    // day and time of event
    tstring   Location;
    tstring   Heading;     // one line title of event
    tstring   Organizer;
    tstring   OrgDept;     // department resp
    tstring   Details;     // detail description
    tstring   Hlink;       // web link to event info
};
```

Creating and Maintaining a Backend COM Server

In our code, we must create the ATLFinder object at the appropriate time. Since network operation is relatively expensive, we should do this only when it is absolutely necessary. In the viscal.cpp file, we wrap the creation of the ATLFinder object in the InitializeBackend() method declared as:

```
void InitializeBackend();
```

and defined as:

```
void Cviscal::InitializeBackend()
{
    if(InAmbientUserMode() && !m_DataMgr.InfoAvail())
    {
        m_DataMgr.CreateFinder();
        m_DataMgr.SetEventMonth( m_CurrentDate );
        m_DataMgr.GrabActiveDepts();
        FireViewChange();
    }
}
```

The InAmbientUserMode() method deserves a few words of explanation:

```
bool Cviscal::InAmbientUserMode()
{
    BOOL bUserMode = FALSE;
    return ( SUCCEEDED( GetAmbientUserMode( bUserMode) ) && bUserMode );
}
```

If the container does not support ambient dispatch, `CComControlBase::GetAmbientUserMode()` will fail. If it does, it will set `bUserMode` to `TRUE` if we are indeed in user mode.

Back in `InitializeBackend()`, the `!mDataMgr.InfoAvail()` expression will evaluate to `TRUE` only if the `CDataMgr` instance does not yet contain retrieved data. In this case, the `ATLFinder` object is created, the current month of interest is set, and the data manager is asked to grab a list of departments with events in the month. The `FireViewChange()` call ensures that the calendar display will be updated with the appropriate event information.

We'll need to free the `ATLFinder` backend COM server with a call to `ReleaseFinder()`. The only applicable spot, where we are guaranteed we don't need it any more, is during the destruction of the ActiveX control – in the `FinalRelease()` member:

```
void Cviscal::FinalRelease(void)
{
    m_DataMgr.ReleaseFinder();
}
```

This is enough code to create the `ATLFinder` backend server when we first need it, and release it when we no longer need it. The `InitializeBackend()` method will cause the `CDataMgr` class to fetch data for the calendar display, but what we have not yet discussed is when and where this `InitializeBackend()` member should be called. As it turns out, determining when to initialize the backend is a non-trivial analysis, due to compatibility concerns.

Hooking Backend Action to UI Activation Protocol

If the visual control design exercise appears thus far to be the black art of 'determining where to hook in logic', then you have grasped the essence of the toughest part of visual ActiveX control programming. We have spent significant time in covering all the OLE 1, OLE 2, OC94, and OC96 specifications, and shown ATL implementations of them in Chapter 5 – hopefully enabling you to readily determine the best and most appropriate place to place these 'hooks' for your specific application.

It is indeed an art, because the precision of it depends on the container's implementation of these specifications. If you will only target one or two specific 'fixed version' containers, your job should be quite straightforward – you simply need to understand how much of the specifications these containers have implemented. However, if you need to write ActiveX controls for *all* containers, you will have a tougher job – and potentially have a lot to learning to do along the way.

The most common and sensible approach to writing controls for executing in all containers is to *make no assumption about the container(s) and perform thorough testing with each supported container.* Take a conservative approach and code against all potential points of failure. It's better not working fully with a container's enhanced feature, than to crash the entire application.

In our case, we want to activate the backend and fetch all the event count information essential for displaying the calendar via a call to `InitializeBackend()`. We need to determine where to add hooks. If we can articulate our requirements clearly, the solution should be staring us in the face. A first attempt to articulate our requirement may be:

❑ Whenever we need to draw the calendar grid

Upon further reflection, we really don't want the backend activated and network data fetch performed, if we are in design mode within an IDE. Therefore, we can refine our requirement to be:

❑ Whenever we need to draw the calendar grid and we are in user mode (not design mode)

Now, we need to refine the definition of 'we need to draw the calendar grid'. What this means specifically is that 'the ActiveX control is in-place active'. The action of initializing the backend should be flexible, so that repeated calls to the routine will not cause inefficient multiple initialization. That is, it must keep an internal state that indicates whether or not the backend has already being initialized. Our final refined specification is:

❑ Initialize the backend once when the control first goes in-place active and we are in user mode (not design mode)

The above line of thought reflects what you would do frequently with each piece of logic attached to the visual control. In our case, the definition of 'control first goes in-place active' would be an ideal candidate for an `OnInPlaceActivate()` method of one of the OLE interfaces. But, having visited all the interfaces in Chapter 5, we realize that legacy OLE compatibility dictates that activation is done through OLE Verbs. In the ATL implementation, it is also hard to find one clear point where we can hook in to capture all activation scenarios. Instead, we must hook into each of the following three places:

1. In `IOleObjectImpl<>::PreVerbInPlaceActivate()` where we have the following code:

```
HRESULT Cviscal::OnPreVerbInPlaceActivate()
{
    InitializeBackend();
    return S_OK;
}
```

This method is invoked by the ATL implementation before the invocation of `CComControlBase::InPlaceActivate()` which brings the control to the in-place activated state.

2. In IOleObjectImpl<>::PreVerbUIActivate() where we have:

```
HRESULT Cviscal::OnPreVerbUIActivate()
{
    InitializeBackend();
    return S_OK;
}
```

When the control acquires the focus it is transitioning to the UI activated state. This method is invoked by the ATL implementation before the invocation of `CComControlBase::InPlaceActivate()` (with different arguments than before) which brings the control to the UI-activated state.

3. In `IQuickActivate::QuickActivate()` for OC96 containers (as we will see shortly):

```
STDMETHODIMP Cviscal::QuickActivate(QACONTAINER* pCont, QACONTROL* pCtrl)
{
    HRESULT hres = IQuickActivateImpl<Cviscal>::QuickActivate(pCont, pCtrl);
    InitializeBackend();
    return hres;
}
```

Depending on the container, any one (or more than one) of these hooks can be called during the first in-place activation, so our implementation of `InitializeBackend()` must be repeatedly callable with no ill effects. Recall that our implementation checks the `mDataMgr.InfoAvail()` member before initializing, making the call safe for repeated use.

Displaying 'Live' Middle-tier Data

After `InitializeBackend()` has created `ATLFinder` and retrieved the data for the `CDataMgr` object, it calls `FireViewChange()`, which in turn causes the container to ask the ActiveX control to repaint. As we are familiar by now, the repaint procedure calls `PaintGrid()` to do much of its work. It is the `PaintGrid()` method to which we must add the display logic for the event data, as obtained from the `CDataMgr` class. The additional code to display cell events is highlighted below:

```
for (i = 0; i < kRowsDisplayed; i++)
{
    curY = offsetY + i * cellHeight;

    for (j = 0; j < kDaysInWeek; j++)
    {
        curX = leftMargin + j * cellWidth;
        // draw cell(i,j)
        tstring text = tstring( m_CellMgr.GetCellLabel( counter ) )
                    .append( _T(" ") )
                    .append( m_CellMgr.GetCellDayNumber( counter ) );

        // clip inside cell rectangle
        CRectangle clipRect ( int( curX + xPad ),
                            int( curY + yPad ),
                            int( curX + cellWidth - xPad ),
                            int( curY + cellHeight - yPad ) );
        ::ExtTextOut( hdc, clipRect.Left(), clipRect.Top(),
                    ETO_CLIPPED, &((RECT)clipRect)
                    , text.c_str(), text.size(), NULL );

        // Display cell data
        if ( InAmbientUserMode() && m_DataMgr.InfoAvail())
        {
            // paint in event indications
            float cellX = curX + cellWidth / 20;
            float cellY = curY + cellHeight / 2;
```

```
                   // get the number of events for each department on this day
                   vector<ULONG>  evCount;
                   m_DataMgr.GetNumEventsOnDate(
                           m_CellMgr.GetCellDate( counter ), evCount );

                   // proceed only if there is at least one department with events
                   // on the date corresponding to the current cell

                   if ( evCount.size() != 0
                           && find_if( evCount.begin(), evCount.end(),
                           bind2nd( not_equal_to<ULONG>(), 0 ) ) != evCount.end()
                      )
                   {
                     m_CellMgr.SetCellHasEvent( counter, true );

                     // output dept symbol and number of events
                     // for the departments that do have events
                     for ( k = 0; k < evCount.size(); k++ )
                     {
                       if ( evCount[k] != 0 )
                       {
                         tstring deptStr = tstring( m_DataMgr.GetDept(k).Symbol )
                                   .append( _T("-") )
                                   .append( Int2TString( evCount[k] ) )
                                   .append( _T(" ") );

                         COLORREF hOldColor = ::SetTextColor( hdc,
                               m_DataMgr.GetDept(k).Color );
                         clipRect = CRectangle( curX, curY, curX + cellWidth,
                               curY+ cellWidth);
                         ::ExtTextOut( hdc, cellX, cellY,
                                   ETO_CLIPPED, &((RECT)clipRect),
                                   deptStr.c_str(), deptStr.size(), NULL );
                         ::SetTextColor( hdc, hOldColor );

                         // move current position over for the next dept
                         SIZE deptStrExtent;
                         ::GetTextExtentPoint32( attrDC, deptStr.c_str(),
                               deptStr.size(), &deptStrExtent);

                         cellX += deptStrExtent.cx + cellWidth/20;
                       } // if evCount[k]
                     } // for k
                   } // if evCount.size
                } // if ( InAmbientUserMode() && m_DataMgr.InfoAvail())
             counter++;
          } //for j
       } //for i
```

The code above directly obtains data from `m_DataMgr`, and for each department that has an event for a particular day, it draws the department's symbol (from `CCalDept`) and the number of events in the department's selected color (again from `CCalDept`).

Interacting with User: Performing Hit Testing

As it stands, our code will allow users to do the following:

❏ Move the month displayed backwards and forwards through time
❏ Display the events available for the currently displayed month

Now, we need to add some code which will detect a mouse click within a cell representing a day, and then pop up more information on the events for that day. Simply put, we need to handle a mouse click that occurs within any cell that has events.

To this end, we will be handling the mouse down and mouse up events from the ActiveX control's window. This is what we want the message map to end up looking like (don't write this in just yet):

```
BEGIN_MSG_MAP(Cviscal)
    MESSAGE_HANDLER(WM_CREATE, OnCreate)
    MESSAGE_HANDLER(WM_LBUTTONDOWN, OnLeftMouseButtonDown)
    MESSAGE_HANDLER(WM_LBUTTONUP, OnLeftMouseButtonUp)
    CHAIN_MSG_MAP(CComControl<Cviscal>)
    REFLECT_NOTIFICATIONS()
ALT_MSG_MAP(1)
    MESSAGE_HANDLER(OCM__BASE + WM_COMMAND, OnBackButton)
ALT_MSG_MAP(2)
    MESSAGE_HANDLER(OCM__BASE + WM_COMMAND, OnForwardButton)
END_MSG_MAP()
```

Notice that we have slightly changed our previous message handlers (in preparation for future iterations). The WM_LBUTTONDOWN message and its companion are now handled by the main message map for hits on the cell grid, while the reflection macro REFLECT_NOTIFICATIONS() allows us to handle the reflected WM_COMMAND message in the alternate message map used by the contained button.

Having altered the alternate message maps, we can use Visual C++ 6 to add the two Windows event handlers for OnLeftMouseButtonDown and OnLeftMouseButtonUp – just click the drop-down list next to the magic wand icon and select **A**dd Window Message Handler. Define a handler for WM_LBUTTONDOWN, and one for WM_LBUTTONUP in the wizard dialog box (we saw how to do this earlier in the chapter). The wizard will update the message map in viscal.h automatically. You'll need to change the skeleton methods to method declarations and then alter them to point to the message handler implementations in viscal.cpp that we're about to create.

For the stub function in viscal.cpp, we need to add the following code:

```
LRESULT Cviscal::OnLeftMouseButtonDown(UINT msg, WPARAM wParam, LPARAM lParam,
                                       BOOL &bHandled)
{
    if (InAmbientUserMode())
    {
        POINT pt = {LOWORD(lParam), HIWORD(lParam) };
        m_CellMgr.OnLMouseButtonDown(pt);

        bHandled = TRUE;
    }
    return 0;
}
```

First we check that the ActiveX control is in user mode, or there's no need to display any data. The
`CCellMgr` controller object is given a chance to handle the mouse click via the call to
`m_CellMgr.OnLMouseButtonDown()`:

```
LRESULT Cviscal::OnLeftMouseButtonUp(UINT uMsg, WPARAM wParam,
                                      LPARAM lParam, BOOL &bHandled)
{
    int cellIndex;
    if (InAmbientUserMode())
    {
        POINT pt = {LOWORD(lParam), HIWORD(lParam)};

        if (m_CellMgr.OnLMouseButtonUp(pt, &cellIndex))
        {
            CEventListDlg dlg;
            dlg.SetParent(*this );
            dlg.SetDateToShow( m_CellMgr.GetCellDate(cellIndex));
            dlg.DoModal();
            bHandled = TRUE;
        }
    }
    return 0;
}
```

When the mouse button up is detected, `m_CellMgr.OnLMouseButtonUp()` will be called. This
essentially does a hit test for any cell, and returns `TRUE` if the mouse click was in one of the 'eventful'
cells. In this case, the cell index number is returned. We then show a popup dialog box displaying all the
departments with events on this day.

Implementing Popup Dialog Boxes Using ATL 3

In this section, we'll look at creating two dialog boxes: one for listing many events and the other for
showing the details of a particular event.

The dialog resource itself can be defined in Visual Studio
6 by right-clicking on the root node viscal1 resources in
Resource View, and then selecting Insert:

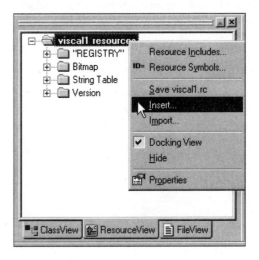

Form the Insert Resource popup, select Dialog and then click the New button to create a new dialog box:

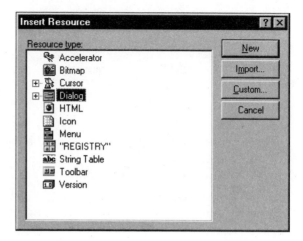

Using the dialog editor with Visual Studio 6, create one dialog called IDD_EVENTLISTDLG for the event list dialog. The layout of this dialog box is shown below:

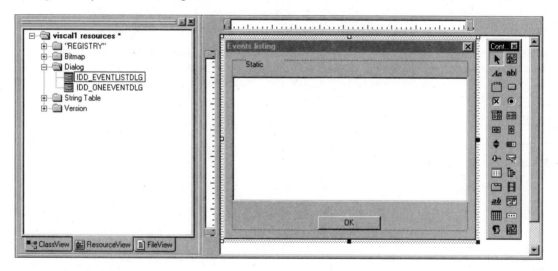

Note above that there is a static label above the list box on the dialog, where we will show the date of the events displayed in the listbox below it. The listbox is called IDC_EVENTLIST, the label IDC_EVENTLISTDATE.

We can implement this dialog box using our CEventListDlg class. The definition of this class can be found in EventListDlg.h file:

```
class CEventListDlg : public CDialogImpl<CEventListDlg>
{
public:
    CEventListDlg();
    ~CEventListDlg();
```

```
        enum { IDD = IDD_EVENTLISTDLG };

BEGIN_MSG_MAP(CEventListDlg)
    MESSAGE_HANDLER(WM_INITDIALOG, OnInitDialog)
    COMMAND_ID_HANDLER(IDOK, OnOK)
    COMMAND_ID_HANDLER(IDCANCEL, OnCancel)
    COMMAND_HANDLER(IDC_EVENTLIST, LBN_DBLCLK, OnDblClickList) \
END_MSG_MAP()

    LRESULT OnInitDialog(UINT uMsg, WPARAM wParam, LPARAM lParam, BOOL& bHandled);
    LRESULT OnOK(WORD wNotifyCode, WORD wID, HWND hWndCtl, BOOL& bHandled);
    LRESULT OnCancel(WORD wNotifyCode, WORD wID, HWND hWndCtl, BOOL& bHandled);
    LRESULT OnDblClickList(WORD wNotifyCode, WORD wID, HWND hWndCtl, BOOL&
            bHandled);

    void SetDateToShow( const CDateTime& d );
    void SetParent( const Cviscal & ctl );
    void FillEvents( const CDateTime& d );

private:
    CDateTime          m_DateToShow;   // dialog shows events on that date
    CDeptEventInfoList m_Events;       // list of events to show
    const Cviscal *    m_pCalCtl;      // parent control.
};
```

This class takes advantage of `CDialogImpl<>` implementation in ATL, which handles the display of a dialog box based on a predefined Win32 dialog resource. If you use the ATL 3 Wizard to add a dialog class, the Wizard creates a dialog resource with an **OK** and **Cancel** buttons and adds the `OnOK()`, `OnCancel()`, and `OnInitDialog()` methods and handlers.

Here's a description of each of our class' methods and what functions they serve:

Method	Description
OnInitDialog()	Initializes the dialog listbox display by calling `FillEvents()`
OnOK()	Terminates the dialog
OnCancel()	Terminates the dialog
OnDblClickList()	Shows the selected event's detail in its own instance of `COneEventDlg`
SetDateToShow()	Sets the date to display events for
SetParent()	Sets a pointer back to the `Cviscal` control parent
FillEvents()	Fills up the listbox with department and event information

You may want to refer to the source code in `EventListDlg.cpp` to see how these methods are implemented.

Next, create another dialog resource, called `IDD_ONEEVENTDLG`, which is used only to display one single event, as follows:

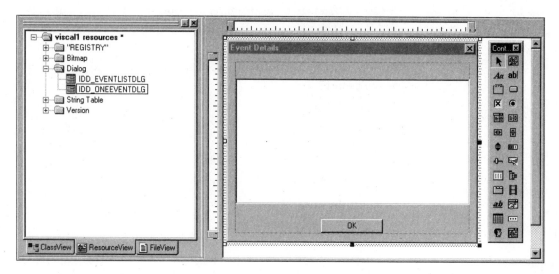

The list box here is called IDC_EVENTDETAILS.

The class for this second dialog is defined in OneEventDlg.h, which is somewhat simpler than its CEventListDlg cousin:

```
class COneEventDlg :
    public CDialogImpl<COneEventDlg>
{
public:
    COneEventDlg();
    ~COneEventDlg();

    enum { IDD = IDD_ONEEVENTDLG };

BEGIN_MSG_MAP(COneEventDlg)
    MESSAGE_HANDLER(WM_INITDIALOG, OnInitDialog)
    COMMAND_ID_HANDLER(IDOK, OnOK)
    COMMAND_ID_HANDLER(IDCANCEL, OnCancel)
END_MSG_MAP()

    LRESULT OnInitDialog(UINT uMsg, WPARAM wParam, LPARAM lParam, BOOL& bHandled);
    LRESULT OnOK(WORD wNotifyCode, WORD wID, HWND hWndCtl, BOOL& bHandled);
    LRESULT OnCancel(WORD wNotifyCode, WORD wID, HWND hWndCtl, BOOL& bHandled);

    COneEventDlg& SetCalEvent( const CCalEvent& ev );
    void FillDetails(void);
private:

    void InitListbox( void );
    void AddLine( const tstring& s );

    CCalEvent m_Event;
};
```

Here is a list of the methods of `COneEventDlg` together with a brief description of what each one does:

Method	Description
OnInitDialog()	Initializes the dialog by filling up the list box with the details of the event to be displayed
OnOK()	Terminates the dialog
OnCancel()	Terminates the dialog
SetCalEvent()	Sets the event to be displayed
FillDetails()	Fills in the listbox with event details, called by OnInitDialog()
InitListBox()	Sets the attributes of the listbox control
AddLine()	Adds a line to the listbox for display

If we now revisit the `Cviscal::OnLeftMouseButtonUp()` handling, we can better understand the code fragment:

```
LRESULT Cviscal::OnLeftMouseButtonUp(UINT uMsg, WPARAM wParam,
                                           LPARAM lParam, BOOL &bHandled)
{
    ATLTRACE( _T("CCalCtl::OnLeftMouseButtonUp\n") );

    int cellIndex;
    if (InAmbientUserMode()) {
        POINT pt = { LOWORD(lParam), HIWORD(lParam) };

        if (m_CellMgr.OnLMouseButtonUp(pt, &cellIndex) && InAmbientUserMode())
        {
            CEventListDlg    dlg;
            dlg.SetParent(*this );
            dlg.SetDateToShow(m_CellMgr.GetCellDate( cellIndex ) );
            dlg.DoModal();
            bHandled = TRUE;
        }
    }
    return 0;
}
```

This code does the following:

1. Performs a hit test to see whether a cell with event is clicked, and, if so, stores the index of the cell in `cellIndex`
2. If a cell with event is clicked, creates an Event List Dialog and sets its parent to the control window
3. Prepares the dialog by setting the date for which to show the event list
4. Displays the dialog as a modal dialog

This results in a popup dialog display like this:

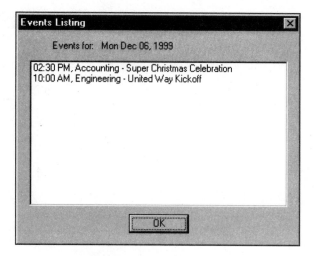

Once the list of events is displayed by the Events Listing Dialog, further interaction at this point is handled directly by the dialog. If the user double clicks on one of events in the list, `CEventListDlg::OnDblClickList()` will be called. This method is implemented like this:

```
LRESULT CEventListDlg::OnDblClickList(WORD wNotifyCode, WORD wID,
                                      HWND hWndCtl, BOOL& bHandled)
{
    // get the current selection
    int idx = CWindow(GetDlgItem(IDC_EVENTLIST)).SendMessage( LB_GETCURSEL, 0, 0);

    // find out the corresponding event.
    for ( int di = 0; di < m_Events.size(); di++ )
    {
        int numOfDeptEvents = m_Events[ di ].Events.size();
        if ( idx < numOfDeptEvents )
            break;
        else
            idx -= numOfDeptEvents;
    }

    // the event we clicked on is  m_Events[ di ].Events[ idx ]

    COneEventDlg dlg;
    dlg.SetCalEvent(m_Events[ di ].Events[ idx ]);
    dlg.DoModal();
    return 0;
}
```

Basically, the above code performs the following steps:

❑ Gets the index of the selected item (just double clicked) from the listbox
❑ Translates the index into an actual event. Note that the i-th entry in the m_Events container is the count of events for the i-th department on the selected day, and that the listbox presents all events for all departments on the selected day.
❑ Sets the details of the event into the COneEventDlg() and displays the dialog as modal

This will display a second-level modal popup dialog, showing the details of the selected event:

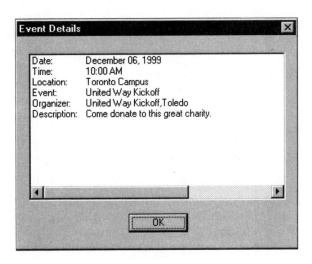

Testing the Visual Control with Backend Model

We just need to document some additional changes to the code from the previous iteration, which we have not been covered so far. They include the introduction of a new `Cviscal` method,

```
const CDataMgr & Cviscal::GetDataMgr() const
{
    return (m_DataMgr);
}
```

with its declaration in `viscal.h`:

```
const CDataMgr & GetDataMgr() const;
...
protected:
...
CDataMgr m_DataMgr
```

There are also modifications to

- ❏ `OnAmbientPropertyChange()` – adding a handler for `DISPID_AMBIENT_USERMODE`
- ❏ `OnCreate()`
- ❏ `SetExtent()`
- ❏ `AdvanceMonth()`

This completes all the code we need for the visual calendar control. We can now test the new custom properties implemented for the control, together with their persistence behavior, and try out the control with properly displayed backend and event information data.

Since this sample uses the backend objects, please make sure that `ATLFinder.exe` and `ATLDept.dll` have been compiled and registered. Without these backend components, the calendar will not compile. Alternatively, you can register the `ATLDept.dll` under the `ATLDept` build subdirectory by invoking `regsvr32 ATLDept.dll` and `ATLFinder.exe` under the `ATLFinder` build subdirectory by invoking it with the argument `/register`.

The completed control with all the code up to this point is found in the `Ch06\viscal1.4` directory of the source distribution. You should try it out in the ActiveX Control Test Container, Visual Basic 6, and Internet Explorer 4.x.

> *Note that in order to see the data from the ActiveX Control Test Container, you'll need to turn off* Design Mode *from the* Options *menu.*

Here is what our test under Internet Explorer 4.x looks like:

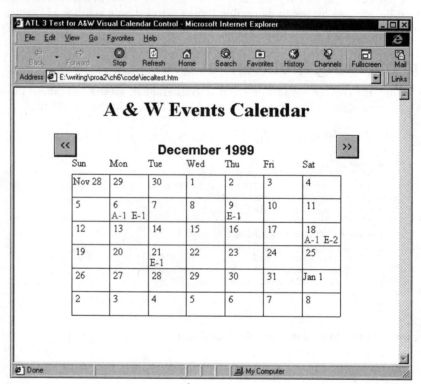

You can find the HTML page used for this test in the `Ch06\IETest` directory.

Iteration 5: Adding OC96 Deferred Activation Behavior

In line with our desire to initialize the backend as late as possible, thus avoiding the performance hit due to slow network activity, OC96 specifies a way of delaying the activation of the ActiveX control itself as late as possible. We have covered how this mechanism works in Chapter 5, and we will now implement this deferred activation.

The net effect of this deferred action is that the control will not in-place activate or UI-activate until the user moves the mouse over the calendar grid, indicating his or her desire to use the control. This scenario seems very sensible if one imagines an application composed of the calendar plus other visual controls on the same form. There could be a situation where the user brings up the form to use one of the other controls, but not the calendar. In such a situation, there would be no point at all in activating the control or initializing the backend.

Deferring Calendar Activation to as Late as Possible

Implementing deferred activation requires us to co-operate with the container in processing mouse messages. A protocol is established whereby the container will pass all mouse messages to us whenever the user passes the cursor over the client area where the visual of our ActiveX control is being displayed. We then do our own hit test to determine if the control should activate and return the appropriate value. In our case, if the mouse is over the ActiveX control but outside the grid, we will not activate the control.

Implementing IPointerInactive

Let's modify the code to support deferred activation. First, we need to inherit the interface definition from `IPointerInactiveImpl<>` provided by ATL 3. Add this to `viscal.h`:

```
////////////////////////////////////////////////////////////////////////////
// Cviscal
class ATL_NO_VTABLE Cviscal :
    public CComObjectRootEx<CComSingleThreadModel>,
    public CStockPropImpl<Cviscal, Iviscal, &IID_Iviscal, &LIBID_VISCAL1Lib>,
    public CComControl<Cviscal>,
    public IPersistStreamInitImpl<Cviscal>,
    ...
    public IQuickActivateImpl<Cviscal>,
    public IDataObjectImpl<Cviscal>,
    public IProvideClassInfo2Impl<&CLSID_viscal, NULL, &LIBID_VISCAL1Lib>,
    public IPointerInactiveImpl<Cviscal>,
    public CComCoClass<Cviscal, &CLSID_viscal>
{
public:
```

Also, we need to add an entry into the COM map:

```
BEGIN_COM_MAP(Cviscal)
    COM_INTERFACE_ENTRY(Iviscal)
    COM_INTERFACE_ENTRY(IDispatch)
    COM_INTERFACE_ENTRY(IViewObjectEx)
    ...
    COM_INTERFACE_ENTRY(IProvideClassInfo)
    COM_INTERFACE_ENTRY(IProvideClassInfo2)
    COM_INTERFACE_ENTRY(IPointerInactive)
END_COM_MAP()
```

Next, we add a new Boolean member variable, `m_bWantActivation`, to our `Cviscal` class, which indicates that the control wants to be activated (and wants to stay activated):

```
    protected:
        BOOL m_bWantActivation;
        void RefreshTitleFont();
    ...
```

We will be using this variable to hook the activation. Once the user has activated the control and the backend data has been retrieved from the network, we want the control to act just like a control that does not support `IPointerInactive()`.

While this is the behavior that we want, bear in mind that it may not be typical of the use of `IPointerInactive()`. In other uses of `IPointerInactive()`, you may want the control actually to deactivate each and every time the cursor moves out of the display of the ActiveX control. One example of this is to achieve a 'mouse-over' effect, changing the display of the ActiveX control depending on whether the mouse is over the control or not.

Indicating Support of Deferred Activation to the Container

Recall from Chapter 5 that we had an `OLEMISC` value in the registry for our control, which indicates to a supporting container that we want activation when we are visible (`OLEMISC_ACTIVATEWHENVISIBLE`). The value is entered in the registry during the registration of the control. This is very bad for our control, because, as we discussed above, we don't want the control to be activated every time it is visible. The `OLEMISC` value is accessed by the container through a call to `IOleObject::GetMiscStatus()`, so we can override this function to provide the appropriate behavior.

Here is where the `m_bWantActivation` flag comes in handy. Essentially, we want the container to ignore the `OLEMISC_ACTIVATEWHENVISIBLE` attribute *before* the deferred activation takes place. Once the control is activated, however, we want the container to honor the `OLEMISC_ACTIVATEWHENVISIBLE` attribute again. The following code in `viscal.cpp` accomplishes this:

```
STDMETHODIMP Cviscal::GetMiscStatus(DWORD dwAspect, DWORD *pdwStatus)
{
    ATLTRACE( _T("Cviscal::GetMiscStatus\n") );

    // get the standard flags for this control, set in the registry
    // by default by the wizard.  Instruct the container to ignore
    // ACTIVATEWHENVISIBLE to give us more control over when to let
    // the container activate the control.
    HRESULT hr = IOleObjectImpl<Cviscal>::GetMiscStatus( dwAspect, pdwStatus );
    if ( SUCCEEDED(hr) )
    {
        if (!m_bWantActivation)  // once activated, stay that way
            *pdwStatus |= OLEMISC_IGNOREACTIVATEWHENVISIBLE;
    }

    return hr;
}
```

The Subtle Meaning of Activation

In the last few sections, we have been looking at what is meant by **deferred activation**, and how we go about implementing it for our control. Our control also supports **quick activation**, and you should bear in mind that the meaning of the word *activation* in these two phrases is subtly different. Quick activation was covered in Chapter 5.

Our `Cviscal` class is derived from the `IQuickActivateImpl<>` class, so we inherit ATL's default implementation of the `IQuickActivate` interface. We need to modify the `QuickActivate()` method, because quick activation is done independently of `IPointerInactive`-deferred activation.

The result of this is that quick activation no longer really 'activates' anything. However, the quick activation call is still performed by a supporting container, because it speeds up the exchange of interface pointers between the control and the container, but semantically it is no longer a real activation. In our case, we definitely do not want to call `InitializeBackend()` at this time. We should comment out the call in `viscal.cpp`:

```
STDMETHODIMP Cviscal::QuickActivate(QACONTAINER* pCont, QACONTROL* pCtrl)
{
    HRESULT hres = IQuickActivateImpl<Cviscal>::QuickActivate(pCont, pCtrl);
//  InitializeBackend();
    return hres;
}
```

Working with the Container to Process Mouse Messages

A container supporting deferred activation tunnels its mouse messages through `IPointerInactive::OnInactiveMouseMove()` to the ActiveX control. In our implementation of this method, we perform a hit-test against the grid. You can find this method in the `viscal.cpp` file. Let's look at it a one step at a time:

```
STDMETHODIMP Cviscal::OnInactiveMouseMove(LPCRECT pRectBounds,
                                          long x, long y, DWORD dwMouseMsg)
{
    ATLTRACE(_T("Cviscal::OnInactiveMouseMove\n"));

    if(CRectangle(*pRectBounds) != CRectangle(m_rcPos))
    {
        if(!m_CellMgr.CellCoordsHaveBeenSet())
            SetCellCoords( *pRectBounds );
    }
```

Here, we determine if our cell manager is ready to do a hit-test first. It may not be ready if the size of the control has recently changed, or if the container calls `OnInactiveMouseMove()` before any `OnDraw()` after a resize. In these cases, we must do our own call to `SetCellCoords()` in order to calculate the hit test co-ordinates.

```
    POINT pt = {x - pRectBounds->left, y - pRectBounds->top};
```

This translation makes sure that the mouse co-ordinate is relative to the top-left corner of our ActiveX control, instead of the container's client area.

```
        if (m_CellMgr.CellHitTest(pt, NULL))
            m_bWantActivation = TRUE;

    return S_OK;
}
```

Finally, we perform the hit-test on the grid by calling the `CellHitTest()` method on the `CCellMgr` class – this returns TRUE if a cell in the grid has been clicked. If this is the case, it is time to start the activation process, so we set the m_bWantActivation flag to TRUE.

Telling the Container to Activate NOW!

Following OC96 specifications, the container will call `IPointerInactive()::GetActivationPolicy()` on every mouse message, and the control should return POINTERINACTIVE_ACTIVATEONENTRY when it wants to be activated. In other words, the container will continuously poll the control for its preferred activation policy. We implement this method by taking into account the latching effect of m_bWantActivation flag. That is, we want to return 0 to the container, until a hit test within the grid has been confirmed. Once it is confirmed, we want to always return POINTERINACTIVE_ACTIVATEONENTRY to the container. Since we know that in-place activation should proceed shortly, we will also call `InitializeBackend()` at this point:

```
STDMETHODIMP Cviscal::GetActivationPolicy(DWORD *pdwPolicy)
{
    if ( m_bWantActivation )
    {
        InitializeBackend();
        *pdwPolicy = (POINTERINACTIVE_ACTIVATEONENTRY );
    }
    return S_OK;
}
```

Deferred Activation is not always Windowless

It is important to keep in mind that OC96 deferred activation and OC96 windowless control support are two different things. Even though the initial 'painting' of a deferred activation control is done on a windowless basis, the control is often windowed once it is activated. This is indeed the case for our control. Take a look at the constructor for `Cviscal`:

```
Cviscal():m_ctlButBack(_T("Button"),this,1),
          m_ctlButFore(_T("Button"),this,2),
          m_CurButtonSize(10),
          m_clrBackColor(0xffffff),
          m_TitleFontBold(FALSE),
          m_ButtonVisible(TRUE),
          m_TitleFontSize(16),
          m_bInitDone(FALSE),
          m_bWantActivation(FALSE)
{
    m_bWindowOnly = TRUE;
}
```

We can see that this is a full-fledged windowed ActiveX control, because the m_bWindowOnly flag is set to TRUE. Note that we have added a new initializer here to set m_bWantActivation flag to FALSE.

The initial painting of the control *is* performed before its window is created. In this case, the PaintGrid() routine is called (when the container calls the IViewObject2::Draw() method) to draw directly into its own client area. We need to modify the PaintGrid() routine slightly, making sure that it will not paint event information before it is activated:

```
      . . .
         // Display cell data
         // if the backend is not initialized yet,
         // we will wait for the next draw request
         if ( m_bInPlaceActive && InAmbientUserMode() && m_DataMgr.InfoAvail())
         {
            // paint in event indications
            float    cellX = curX + cellWidth / 20;
            float    cellY = curY + cellHeight / 2;
      . . .
```

Testing the Visual Control with Deferred Activation

In this iteration, we have seen everything you need to do to convert a visual control to support deferred activation. Some other minor changes are also required in:

- ❑ SetExtent()
- ❑ InitializeBackend()

Summarizing the steps:

- ❑ Be careful not to execute logic that you shouldn't unless the control has already been activated
- ❑ Decide when you want to activate and let the container know about it by implementing the IPointerInactive interface. Ensure you perform accurate hit testing by ensuring you have the latest size information available.

Please refer to the code for the details. Although in a couple of places the technique we use is not immediately obvious, the work overall was quite painless. Furthermore, the optimized behavior we gain definitely justifies the effort.

The completed control supporting deferred activation may be found in the Ch06\viscal1.5 directory of the source distribution. The control may be tested in ActiveX Control testing container, Visual Basic 6, or Internet Explorer 4.x. Try it out and notice how the events and buttons only appear only after you have moved the mouse over the dormant grid.

Iteration 6: Retrofitting for OC96 Windowless Control Support

OC96 containers like IE4.x are crying out for the higher performance windowless compliant control. We saw in Chapter 5 why windowless controls are 'higher performance' – creating windows is an expensive proposition. Unfortunately, our control has been designed exclusively to work only when a window is created and available.

We will really need to go through our code with a fine toothcomb to make it windowless compliant. In doing so, we must be careful to ensure that the ActiveX control remains compatible with older non-OC96 containers. Even though, theoretically, a windowless control can work directly within a legacy container just by having ATL create a host window for it (which ATL 3 will do automatically), this is not as straightforward in practice as it sounds.

Hey, ATL 3! We're Going Windowless!

First things first, we need to inherit from ATL 3's `IOleInPlaceObjectWindowlessImpl<>` in `Cviscal`. This is already in place:

```
class ATL_NO_VTABLE Cviscal :
    public CComObjectRootEx<CComSingleThreadModel>,
    ...
    public IOleInPlaceActiveObjectImpl<Cviscal>,
    public IViewObjectExImpl<Cviscal>,
    public IOleInPlaceObjectWindowlessImpl<Cviscal>,
    public ISupportErrorInfo,
    public IPersistStorageImpl<Cviscal>,
    public ISpecifyPropertyPagesImpl<Cviscal>,
    ...
    public CComCoClass<Cviscal, &CLSID_viscal>
{
public:
```

Next, we uncomment the entry to the COM map to facilitate operations of `QueryInterface()` from the container specifying `IOleInPlaceObjectWindowlessImpl`:

```
BEGIN_COM_MAP(Cviscal)
    COM_INTERFACE_ENTRY(Iviscal)
    ...
    COM_INTERFACE_ENTRY(IViewObject)
    COM_INTERFACE_ENTRY(IOleInPlaceObjectWindowless)

    COM_INTERFACE_ENTRY(IOleInPlaceObject)
    ...
    COM_INTERFACE_ENTRY(IProvideClassInfo2)
    COM_INTERFACE_ENTRY_IMPL(IPointerInactive)
END_COM_MAP()
```

We now remove the m_bWindowOnly flag in the constructor of Cviscal to let ATL 3 know that we are now a windowless control:

```
Cviscal():m_ctlButBackW(_T("Button"),this,1),
          m_ctlButForeW(_T("Button"),this,2),
          m_CurButtonSize(10),m_clrBackColor(0xffffff),
          m_TitleFontBold(FALSE),
          m_ButtonVisible(TRUE),
          m_TitleFontSize(16),
          m_bInitDone(FALSE),
          m_bWantActivation(FALSE),
          m_ctlButBack(1),
          m_ctlButFore(2)
     {
//        m_bWindowOnly = TRUE;
     }
```

Notice the strange m_ctlButBackW() and m_ctlButForeW() in the initializer list – we will see why they are necessary in the next section. There are more than a few gotchas to watch for when changing a windowed control to be windowless compliant. Let us examine two of the most prominent ones here and see how we can deal with them. In a windowless control:

❑ We can't use ATL's CContainedWindow implementation for our buttons
❑ We can't assume a paint origin at (0,0) when drawing our control

Windowed ATL 3 ContainedWindows Clash

It is unfortunate but true that the two handy Win32 buttons, which made use of the CContainedWindow class, are inadequate for the windowless control. What started out to be a simplification in implementation in an earlier iteration has resulted in significant effort when moving to windowless control here. Since we can no longer count on the control having a window of its own, we cannot simply use the ATL 3 contained window implementation to create our buttons (which assumes a Win32 parent/child window relationship). Hopefully, in a future version of ATL, we may see a more adaptive CContainedWindow class – freeing us from the agony of re-creation from scratch.

At this time, the best that we can do though is to create our own buttons from scratch to:

❑ Draw the visual representation of the buttons
❑ Handle mouse click behavior of the buttons

The code for our very own button is contained in CCalButton.h:

```
class CCalButton
{
public:
   CCalButton(long ID);
   ~CCalButton();

   void        ResetSize( const CRectangle& winRect );
   void        ResetHitTestSize(const CRectangle & hitRect);
   void        Show(BOOL visible);
```

```
    const          CRectangle& GetRect( void ) const {return m_rect;}
    BOOL           IsClicked(void) const {return m_bClicked;}
    void           DrawClicked(HDC hdc);
    void           DrawFlash(HDC hdc);
    void           DrawNormal(HDC hdc);
    void           DrawClear(HDC hdc);
    void           ReDraw(HDC hdc);
    bool           HitTest(const POINT & pt) const;

private:
    long           m_ID;
    BOOL           m_bClicked;
    CRectangle     m_rect;
    CRectangle     m_hitrect;
    BOOL           m_bVisible;
};
```

We can tell from the private members that this class encapsulates the states of a button. Here is a list of the methods and what each one does:

Method	Description
ResetSize()	Resets the button size based on an input CRectangle instance
ResetHitTestSize()	Resets both the size and location of the button based on an input CRectangle instance for hit-test purposes only – not for paint
Show()	Controls the visibility of the button (not currently used)
GetRect()	Gets the rectangle where the button is currently displayed
IsClicked()	Determines if the button is in a 'clicked' state
DrawClicked()	Draws the button in a clicked state
DrawFlash()	Draws the button with a flash (not currently used)
DrawNormal()	Draw the button in a non-clicked state
DrawClear()	Erase the button, not currently used
ReDraw()	Repaint the button, reflect the clicked state in drawing
HitTest()	Determine if mouse click is within button display area

For the two windowless buttons, we create two new member instances of CCalButton in our Cviscal class:

```
protected:
//    CContainedWindow m_ctlButBack;
//    CContainedWindow m_ctlButFore;
```

```
CContainedWindow m_ctlButBackW;
CContainedWindow m_ctlButForeW;
CCalButton m_ctlButBack;
CCalButton m_ctlButFore;
```

You'll need to #include CalButton.h *for these new member variables.*

Note how we have renamed the windowed button with a W at the end. One thought that comes to mind is to derive CCalButton from CContainedWindow and implement a 'dual mode' button class that can 'do the right thing', depending on whether the control is windowed or windowless. We thought we'd spare you from examining even more code, though – and leave the ATL 4 team with something to work on for Visual Studio 2000!

Creating Windowless Child Buttons

We saw earlier that the windowed buttons were created when we receive the WM_CREATE message, whenever our control is activated with a window. Now, what about the *windowless* buttons?

Well, we don't have to create them, because they are already a part of the Cviscal class – as member variables. Their visible appearance in the calendar, however, is brought about by some additional code in the PaintGrid() method:

```
// draw the windowless buttons
if(!inMetafileContext && m_bInPlaceActive && m_bWndLess)
{
    RECT rectBack, rectFore;
    ButRectHelper(&(rect.r), &rectBack, &rectFore);

    m_ctlButBack.ResetSize(rectBack);
    m_ctlButFore.ResetSize(rectFore);
    m_ctlButBack.ReDraw(hdc);
    m_ctlButFore.ReDraw(hdc);
}
```

This combination of coding will ensure that the windowed buttons are created when we have a window, and the windowless buttons are drawn for supporting OC96 containers.

Handling Mouse Clicks from Windowless Child Buttons

Now, it's time for a bit more complexity. ATL 3, as we learnt in Chapter 5, will route mouse messages destined for the ActiveX control through the message map, regardless of whether or not the control is windowed. This means that we must modify the OnLeftMouseButtonDown() and OnLeftMouseButtonUp() methods to handle both cases appropriately.

If ATL 3 provided a windowless model and did a complete mapping, we would not need to do any new work here. Unfortunately, ATL 3 does not, so our code becomes quite involved in this area.

Here is how we handle the left button down message:

```
LRESULT Cviscal::OnLeftMouseButtonDown(UINT msg, WPARAM wParam,
                                        LPARAM lParam, BOOL &bHandled)
{
    POINT pt = {LOWORD(lParam), HIWORD(lParam)};
```

The above extracts the *x* and *y* mouse coordinates from the DWORD parameter.

```
    if (m_ctlButBack.HitTest(pt))
    {
```

Here, we test to see if the left button is hit.

```
        if (m_spInPlaceSite && m_bWndLess)
        {
```

We also need to verify that we have the container's site, and that we are indeed windowless.

```
            HDC tpDC;
            if (SUCCEEDED(m_spInPlaceSite->GetDC(NULL, 0, &tpDC)))
            {
                m_ctlButBack.DrawClicked(tpDC);

                m_spInPlaceSite->ReleaseDC(tpDC);
                m_spInPlaceSite->InvalidateRect(&(m_ctlButBack.GetRect().r),TRUE);
                m_spInPlaceSite->SetCapture(TRUE);
                bHandled = TRUE;
            }
```

Shown above is the implementation for the interaction of the button with the mouse. We use the prescribed way of interacting with the container by requesting its device context through its IOleInPlaceSite interface, and then draw the button in the container's client area, invalidate *only* the button area, and then set the mouse capture.

```
        }
    }
    else
    {
        if (m_ctlButFore.HitTest(pt))
        {
            if (m_spInPlaceSite && m_bWndLess)
            {
```

If, on the other hand, it is the right button that has been clicked, we do the same thing with the right button:

```
                HDC tpDC;
                if (SUCCEEDED(m_spInPlaceSite->GetDC(NULL, 0, &tpDC)))
                {
                    m_ctlButFore.DrawClicked(tpDC);
```

```
                          m_spInPlaceSite->ReleaseDC(tpDC);
                          m_spInPlaceSite->InvalidateRect(&(m_ctlButFore.GetRect().r),TRUE);
                          m_spInPlaceSite->SetCapture(TRUE);
                          bHandled = TRUE;
                      } // of SUCCEEDED
                  } //of m_spInPlaceSite
              } // of HitTest
```

If neither of the two buttons have been clicked, we check for click inside one of the event cells in the grid – this was the former body of the message handler before we added the windowless handling.

```
              else
              {
                  if (InAmbientUserMode())
                  {
                      m_CellMgr.OnLMouseButtonDown( pt );

                      bHandled = TRUE;
                  }
              } // of HitTest
          }
      return 0;
  }
```

We haven't finished yet, though. For the left mouse button up, we must implement the other half of the windowless button behavior:

```
LRESULT Cviscal::OnLeftMouseButtonUp(UINT uMsg, WPARAM wParam,
                                     LPARAM lParam, BOOL &bHandled)
{
    POINT pt = {LOWORD(lParam), HIWORD(lParam)};
    int cellIndex;
```

Here, we extract the mouse coordinates as before, and create a local variable, cellIndex, for storing the cell that is being clicked on.

```
    if (m_ctlButBack.IsClicked())
    {
        if (m_spInPlaceSite && m_bWndLess)
        {
```

We have to make sure that left button is in a clicked state, and also that this is the windowless control.

```
            m_spInPlaceSite->SetCapture(FALSE);
            HDC tpDC;
            if (SUCCEEDED(m_spInPlaceSite->GetDC(NULL, 0, &tpDC)))
            {
                m_ctlButBack.DrawNormal(tpDC);

                m_spInPlaceSite->ReleaseDC(tpDC);
                m_spInPlaceSite->InvalidateRect(&(m_ctlButBack.GetRect().r),TRUE);
                bHandled = TRUE;
            }
```

In the code above, we release the mouse capture and get the container's device context from the container's `IOleInPlacesite` interface. We then paint the normal button appearance and invalidate just the button area. This completes our 'emulation' of the button behavior, and we can finally perform the actual action of the button.

Here, we simply call the windowed button handling routine directly:

```
            if (m_ctlButBack.HitTest(pt))
            {
                // AdvanceMonth here
                OnBackButton(uMsg, wParam, lParam, bHandled);
            }
        }
    }
```

The next code fragment is identical to the above, but checks only for the right button.

```
    else
    {
        if (m_ctlButFore.IsClicked())
        {
            if (m_spInPlaceSite && m_bWndLess)
            {
                m_spInPlaceSite->SetCapture(FALSE);
                HDC tpDC;
                if (SUCCEEDED(m_spInPlaceSite->GetDC(NULL, 0, &tpDC)))
                {
                    m_ctlButFore.DrawNormal(tpDC);

                    m_spInPlaceSite->ReleaseDC(tpDC);
                    m_spInPlaceSite->InvalidateRect(&(m_ctlButFore.GetRect().r),TRUE);
                    bHandled = TRUE;
                }
                if (m_ctlButFore.HitTest(pt))
                {
                    // AdvanceMonth here
                    OnForwardButton(uMsg, wParam, lParam, bHandled);
                }
            }
        }
    }
```

We merge the former message handling code here for hit testing a cell click, and displaying event information:

```
    else
    {
        if (InAmbientUserMode())
        {
            POINT pt = {LOWORD(lParam), HIWORD(lParam)};

            if(m_CellMgr.OnLMouseButtonUp(pt, &cellIndex) && InAmbientUserMode())
            {
                CEventListDlg  dlg;
                dlg.SetParent( *this );
                dlg.SetDateToShow( m_CellMgr.GetCellDate( cellIndex ) );
```

```
                    dlg.DoModal();
                    bHandled = TRUE;
            }
        } //of if InAmbientUserMode()
    } // of else
} // of outter else
return 0;
}
```

This is the all the additional code that we need to support the windowless child buttons. Note that the button click from the two contained windows, if they are ever created, will be routed to `OnBackButton()` and `OnForwardButton()` 'manually'. This eliminates the need to modify these tested methods. Now, let us examine another 'gotcha'.

Not Assuming Paint Origin at (0,0)

We have heard about this warning over and over again whenever we implement ActiveX controls. However, it turns out that, as long as we are creating a windowed ActiveX control, it is still possible to have many implicit dependencies within our code for the paint origin to be (0,0). This assumption, along with several other drawing problems surfaced for us when we went windowless.

Let us take a look at the code change that is necessary within the `PaintGrid()` method in order to prevent our control from drawing inappropriately.

```
    ...
    cellWidth = rect.Width() * 1.0f / numCols;
    cellHeight = rect.Height() * 1.0f / numRows;
    halfCellWidth = cellWidth / 2;
    halfCellHeight = cellHeight / 2;
    topMargin = halfCellHeight;
    leftMargin = halfCellWidth;
    offsetY = cellHeight * 1.8 ;
```

This line used to be:

```
    offsetY = ULONG( cellHeight * 1.8 );
```

This looks extremely innocent, since an offset should always be positive, analogous to a padding value...NOT! The `rect` structure passed in to the `PaintGrid()` method may not have origin at (0,0)! As a matter of fact, the `rect` may not even have positive co-ordinates. If one of the origin co-ordinates is negative, we must keep the correct sign on the offset. Otherwise, a strange and intermittent problem happens. It is very unfortunate that the Visual Studio 6 ActiveX Control Test Container always passes in a `rect` with origin (0,0), rendering it useless to test for this problem. Note how indirect and subtle this dependency on the origin really is.

Printing Labels under Deferred Action

Another part of the `PaintGrid()` method that we need to be extremely careful about is the code that deals with where the year and month labels of the calendar are painted. The old code depends on the button height being already calculated, which would be true if the buttons have been displayed at least once. Since we cannot rely on the buttons being drawn when we paint the calendar year and month label, we must do our own calculations.

Here are the changes to the `PaintGrid()` method:

```
void Cviscal::PaintGrid(HDC hdc, HDC attrDC, const CRectangle& rect,
                                          bool inMetafileContext)
{
    ...
    float xPad = 2, yPad = 2;
    // use long instead of ULONG...
    // intermediate results may be made unsign (yuk) making life difficult to debug
    long numRows, numCols;
    long offsetY;
    long counter;
    long i, j, k;

    ...

    offsetY = cellHeight * 1.8;

    for ( i = 0; i < numCols; i++ )
    {
        ...
        // draw line
        MoveToEx( hdc, rect.Left() + x1, rect.Top() + y1, NULL );
        LineTo( hdc, rect.Left() + x2, rect.Top() + y2 );
    }

    for ( i = 0; i < kRowsDisplayed + 1; i++ )
    {
        ...
        // draw line
        MoveToEx( hdc, rect.Left() + x1, rect.Top() + y1, NULL );
        LineTo( hdc, rect.Left() + x2,rect.Top() + y2 );
    }

    ...

    for (i = 0; i < kRowsDisplayed; i++)
    {
        curY = rect.Top() + offsetY + i * cellHeight;

        for (j = 0; j < kDaysInWeek; j++)
        {
            curX = rect.Left() + leftMargin + j * cellWidth;

            ...
            // Display cell data

        } //for j
    } //for i

    // draw the windowless buttons

    // center and draw the control label

    // work out the current font for title

    ...
```

```
    // determine the bounding rectangle for the label
    int supposedButtonSize = rect.Height() / kButSizeToHeightRatio;
    int    labelOffset = 6;
    CRectangle labelBoundingRect;
    labelBoundingRect = CRectangle(
        rect.Left() + max( kCalLeftMargin + supposedButtonSize + labelOffset,
                    (rect.Width() - labelRect.Width())/2 ),   // left
        rect.Top() + max( labelOffset, (kCalTopMargin + supposedButtonSize
                    - labelRect.Height()) ), // top
        rect.Left() + min(rect.Width() - kCalLeftMargin
                                    - supposedButtonSize - labelOffset,
                    (rect.Width() + labelRect.Width())/2 ),   // right
        rect.Top() + kCalTopMargin + supposedButtonSize          // bottom
        );


    ...

    // draw the names of the days of the week
    for ( i = 0; i < kDaysInWeek; i++ )
    {
        TEXTMETRIC    tm;
        GetTextMetrics( attrDC, &tm );    // use attribute DC
        curX = rect.Left() + leftMargin + i * cellWidth;
        curY = rect.Top() + offsetY - 1.1f * tm.tmHeight;


        ...
    }
} // Cviscal::PaintGrid()
```

Note the painstaking care in the highlighted code to ensure that we do not depend on origin equaling (0,0)!

Yet another location where we need to be careful (and explicitly so) of the origin assumption is the management of the hit-test co-ordinates of the individual cells. Our design stores these coordinates in a CCellMgr instance. Unfortunately, the coordinates must reflect the windowed or windowless mode of operation. This is because the position of each cell is measured in the coordinate system of the container in the windowless case, but with respect to the (0,0) origin of the control's own window in the windowed mode of operation.

Here is the new version of SetCellCoords() that can work with the windowless version of our control. The modified code is highlighted:

```
void Cviscal::SetCellCoords(const CRectangle &rect)
{
    float    curX, curY;
    float    cellWidth,   cellHeight;
    float    leftMargin;
    ULONG    numRows, numCols;
    ULONG    offsetX, offsetY;
    ULONG    counter;
    ULONG    i, j;

    numRows = kRowsDisplayed + 2;
    numCols = kDaysInWeek + 1;
    cellWidth = rect.Width() / numCols * 1.0f;
```

```
      cellHeight = rect.Height() / numRows * 1.0f;
      leftMargin = cellWidth / 2;
      if (m_bWndLess)
      {
         offsetX = rect.Left();
         offsetY = rect.Top() + ULONG( cellHeight * 1.8 );
      }
      else
      {
         offsetX = 0;
         offsetY = ULONG( cellHeight * 1.8 );
      }

      counter = 0;
      for (i = 0; i < kRowsDisplayed; i++)
      {
         curY = offsetY + i * cellHeight;
         for (j = 0; j < kDaysInWeek; j++)
         {
            curX = offsetX + leftMargin + j * cellWidth;
            // set cell coordinates
            m_CellMgr.SetCellCoords(counter, CRectangle(curX, curY,
                                              curX + cellWidth, curY +
cellHeight));
            counter++;
         }
      }
   }
```

One final necessary modification involves code to reposition the windowed buttons. This used to happen whenever resize was detected for our control. In the SetExtent() method, we should now only reposition the windowed buttons if the control is operating in the windowed mode:

```
STDMETHODIMP Cviscal::SetExtent(DWORD dwDrawAspect, SIZEL *psizel)
{
    HRESULT hr = IOleObjectImpl<Cviscal>::SetExtent(dwDrawAspect, psizel);

    if (!m_bWndLess)
    {
       if ((dwDrawAspect == DVASPECT_CONTENT) && (psizel != NULL))
       {
          RECT rectBack, rectFore;
          if (m_hWnd)  // only if we've activated
          {
             ButRectHelper(&m_rcPos, &rectBack, &rectFore);
             ::SetWindowPos(m_ctlButBackW.m_hWnd,
                         NULL,
                         rectBack.left,
                         rectBack.top,
                         rectBack.right - rectBack.left,
                         rectBack.bottom - rectBack.top,
                         0);

             ::SetWindowPos(m_ctlButForeW.m_hWnd,
                         NULL, rectFore.left,
                         rectFore.top,
                         rectFore.right - rectFore.left,
```

```
                              rectFore.bottom - rectFore.top,
                              0);
                }
        }
        // define hit-test co-ordinates
        SetCellCoords(m_rcPos);
    }
    return hr;
}
```

Combining OC96 Deferred Activation with OC96 Windowless Controls

With our implementation of OC96 deferred activation, there is nothing special we need to do to make it co-exist with windowless support. It just works.

Retain Code which Maintains Compatibility with Legacy Containers

Our implementation of the OC96 windowless compatibility has been more complex than most sample programs. This is a result of our goal to maintain backward compatibility with the legacy containers that earlier versions of the control worked with. Indeed, this is what almost all production ActiveX controls need to achieve.

Testing the Windowless Deferred Activation Control

We made some additional changes to the code that we haven't discussed. In particular, we:

- Modified the `OnCreate()` message handler due to the name change of the windowed buttons
- Modified `ButRectHelper()` in order to deal with the problem of not having origin at (0,0)
- Modified `AdvanceMonth()` and `InActiveMouseMove()`
- Overrode the default `SetObjectsRects()` implementation with the following code:

```
STDMETHODIMP Cviscal::SetObjectRects(LPCRECT prcPos,LPCRECT prcClip )
{
   HRESULT hr =  IOleInPlaceObjectWindowlessImpl<Cviscal>::SetObjectRects(
              prcPos, prcClip);
   RECT rcIXect;
   BOOL b = IntersectRect(&rcIXect, prcPos, prcClip);
   RECT rectBack, rectFore;

   if (m_bWndLess)
   {
       // this is done redundantly... IE 4 may or maynot call this
       // before painting the screen... if it doesn't, the calculation
       // is done in the draw again
       // appears to be some mapping mode bug in current IE 4 version

       ButRectHelper(&m_rcPos, &rectBack, &rectFore);
       m_ctlButBack.ResetHitTestSize(rectBack);
       m_ctlButFore.ResetHitTestSize(rectFore);
```

```
        // define hit-test co-ordinates
        SetCellCoords(m_rcPos);
    }
    return hr;
}
```

You can try out the final control, the source code can be found in `Ch06\viscal1.6` directory.

Try it out in the test container. If you go to the Container menu and select Options, you can see what happens when you switch on and off the support for windowless activation. Try it under Visual Basic 6, and Internet Explorer 4.x. IE 4.x is a fully compliant OC96 host for windowless control, you can test the control's compatibility there.

Lessons We Have Learnt

Through the six iterations involved in developing this visual control, we can conclude that:

- ❑ Visual ActiveX controls can be written to multiple levels of container support and expectations
- ❑ Half of the battle in designing and coding a visual ActiveX control is figuring out where to 'hook in' specific non-visual control logic
- ❑ The Visual Studio 6 ActiveX Control Test Container is not a sufficient container for production level testing of ActiveX controls
- ❑ Test every production control in each of its intended containers thoroughly, this is *the only reliable way* to ensure compatibility – relying on the preciseness of the OLE specification or its interpretation is futile
- ❑ Upgrading former windowed standard ActiveX controls to the OC96 delayed activation and windowless operation is non-trivial if the control is a non-trivial control
- ❑ An OC96 windowless control, created using ATL 3, cannot easily be used in legacy containers, which can only deal with windowed controls, unless you design very carefully up front – you must take into account specific requirements of the container and interactions of the container with the control

ATL 3 helps in the implementation of many OC96 control features, but does not necessarily provide coherent models or complete feature sets. It is therefore important to be familiar with its limitations before embarking on a project.

Now that we have a fully OC96 windowless compliant, visual calendar control, we can focus our efforts on the design and coding of the middle-tier and data access components, within the A & W Corporate Events Calendaring system. It is to these components that we will turn our attention in the next chapter.

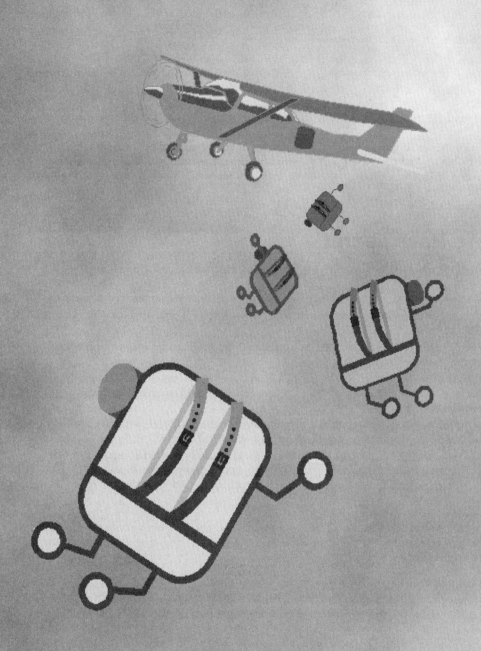

Data Management with OLE DB

8

In this chapter, we'll first focus on the design and implementation of two core business objects that can be accessed by presentation components (such as our Visual Calendar control). These objects provide a simple object model that is Automation compatible. We will take a look at some advanced ATL issues as we apply them to the coding of these components. These include:

- ❑ Manipulating the IDL code
- ❑ Using smart pointers and COM compiler support
- ❑ Working with enumerations

In the second half of the chapter, we'll turn our attention to OLE DB – our chosen data access technology. We introduce OLE DB concepts and show how ATL 3 makes it easy to create OLE DB consumers. Finally, we show how our business objects can use these OLE DB consumers for their operation. We will cover:

- ❑ OLE DB as a universal access layer
- ❑ Typical data access situations and what OLE DB objects fit
- ❑ Building an OLE DB consumer using ATL 3
- ❑ Parameterized queries
- ❑ Creating Accessor objects

Then, in the next chapter, we'll tie the middle-tier and data-tier components together using MTS and get the application working.

Implementing Automation Compatible Mid-tier Components

If you recall the architecture diagram of Chapter 6, we need two business object servers to provide the event data for the calendar control:

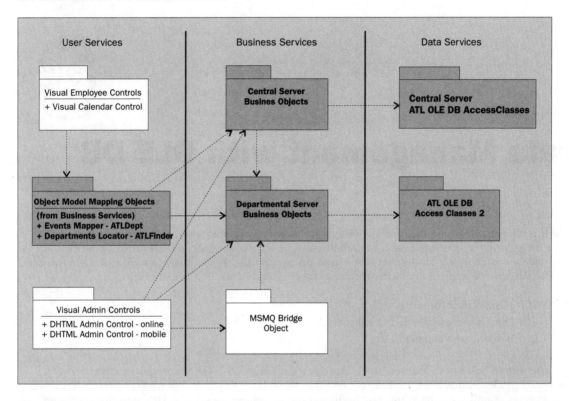

We discussed the employee and calendar controls in Chapter 6. The items in the highlighted area of the diagram will be covered in this chapter and the next. The business objects are implemented by two COM servers – `Atlfinder.exe` and `Atldept.dll`. These components will provide a simple object model to the end user (including scripting engines, Visual Basic and Visual J++). We examined this model in the first two chapters.

Construction of both servers is very similar, since they both contain collections of other objects (`ATLFinder` has `m_spEventfulDepts`–a list of departments with events occuring within a specified month, and `ATLDept` has `m_spKnownEvents`–the list of events for the department occuring within a specified month). However, `Atldept.dll` is slightly more involved because it maintains data for both the 'department' objects that it represents, as well as the 'departmental event' objects. We'll look, therefore, at the construction of `Atldept.dll` first.

The ATLDept In-process COM Server

For `ATLDept.dll`, we'll need to implement the following objects:

- `ATLDept1` – The department object
- `ATLCorpEvents1` – The events collection
- `ATLCorpEvent1` – An event object

Examining this list of objects, we see that the client will only ever need to create instances of the `ATLDept1` class externally, since the `ATLCorpEvents1` and `ATLCorpEvent1` objects will be created by `ATLDept1`. Consequently, we should not give external clients the ability to create instances of the `ATLCorpEvents1` and `ATLCorpEvent1` classes – something we can accomplish by making the appropriate modification to the `ATLDept.idl` file. We'll only provide a `coclass` definition for the `ATLDept1` class. This will be shown in the *Defining COM Interfaces in IDL* section below.

Since we've worked through several complete ATL projects already, we'll breeze through this portion to keep you from getting bored!

To create a project for the `ATLDept.dll` server:

- Create an ATL project in Visual Studio, call it `ATLDept` and select the in-process server checkbox
- Add three simple ATL objects using the wizard, each with dual interfaces and name them `ATLDept1`, `ATLCorpEvents1`, and `ATLCorpEvent1` respectively; make them all non-aggregatable

Defining COM Interfaces in IDL

We now have to specify the properties and methods for our COM interfaces in our `IDL` file. Let's start with those of the `ATLDept1` class.

Property	Property Type	Function Type
Name	BSTR	put/get
Number	BSTR	put/get
CanRead	BOOL	put/get
CanPostNew	BOOL	put/get
Symbol	BSTR	put/get
Color	BOOL	put/get
KnownEvents	VARIANT	get
Date	DATE	put/get
Host	BSTR	put/get

You can use the ClassView, or edit the IDL file directly, to add the properties above. The resulting IDL file looks like:

```
[
        object,
        uuid(8C80B86E-93C9-11D0-891C-004095E279DD),
        dual,
        helpstring("IATLDept1 Interface"),
        pointer_default(unique)
]
interface IATLDept1 : IDispatch
{
        // Name
        [propget, id(1), helpstring("property Name")] HRESULT
                                        Name([out, retval] BSTR *pVal);
        [propput, id(1), helpstring("property Name")] HRESULT
                                        Name([in] BSTR newVal);
        // Number
        [propget, id(2), helpstring("property Number")] HRESULT
                                        Number([out, retval] BSTR *pVal);
        [propput, id(2), helpstring("property Number")] HRESULT
                                        Number([in] BSTR newVal);
        // CanRead
        [propget, id(3), helpstring("property CanRead")] HRESULT
                        CanRead([out, retval] VARIANT_BOOL *pVal);
        [propput, id(3), helpstring("property CanRead")] HRESULT
                                CanRead([in] VARIANT_BOOL newVal);
        // CanPostNew
        [propget, id(4), helpstring("property CanPostNew")] HRESULT
                        CanPostNew([out, retval] VARIANT_BOOL *pVal);
        [propput, id(4), helpstring("property CanPostNew")] HRESULT
                                CanPostNew([in] VARIANT_BOOL newVal);
        // Symbol
        [propget, id(5), helpstring("property Symbol")] HRESULT
                                Symbol([out, retval] BSTR *pVal);
        [propput, id(5), helpstring("property Symbol")] HRESULT
                                        Symbol([in] BSTR newVal);
        // Color
        [propget, id(6), helpstring("property Color")] HRESULT
                                Color([out, retval] OLE_COLOR *pVal);
        [propput, id(6), helpstring("property Color")] HRESULT
                                        Color([in] OLE_COLOR newVal);
        // KnownEvents
        [propget, id(7), helpstring("property KnownEvents")] HRESULT
                        KnownEvents([out, retval] VARIANT *pVal);
        [propget, id(8), helpstring("property Date")] HRESULT
                                        Date([out, retval] DATE *pVal);
        [propput, id(8), helpstring("property Date")] HRESULT
                                        Date([in] DATE newVal);
        [propget, id(9), helpstring("property Host")] HRESULT
                                        Host([out, retval] BSTR *pVal);
        [propput, id(9), helpstring("property Host")] HRESULT
                                        Host([in] BSTR newVal);

};
```

The only tricky looking thing is the KnownEvents property – KnownEvents is a collection of event objects. It is handled through the ATLCorpEvents1 interface. Since ATLCorpEvents1 is a dual interface, it inherits from IDispatch, and can be accessed directly by script languages. This also allows us to pass the collection back (as an object reference) via a VARIANT type, to any client (since a VARIANT can contain an IDispatch and IDispatch can be used to access the object).

Notice the straightforward mapping of an Automation property to a propget or propput method:

- ❑   The string type used is a Visual Basic compatible BSTR type
- ❑   The Visual Basic Color type maps to an OLE_COLOR value

The IATLDept1 interface above is also a dual interface derived from IDispatch. It will be specified as the default interface for the ATLDept1 object, as we'll see in the declaration of the CATLDept1 class later on. This coding pattern can be applied, in general, to Automation interfaces that are compatible with scripting languages – the default interface for an object should contain all the required methods and properties that are to be exposed to the Automation client. The object, of course, may expose additional interfaces, which are needed by non-Automation clients.

For access to the ATLCorpEvents1 class, we have defined an IATLCorpEvents1 interface. Use the ClassView to add these properties for the interface:

Property	Property Type	Function Type	HelpString
Count	long	get	Returns number of items in the collection
_NewEnum	LPUNKNOWN	get	Returns an enumerator for the collection
Item	long	put/get	Given an index, returns an item in the collection

And the methods on this interface:

Method	Parameters	Return Type
Add()	[in] DATE DateTime, [in] BSTR bstrLocation, [in] BSTR bstrHeading, [in] BSTR bstrOrganizer, [in] BSTR bstrOrgDept, [in] BSTR bstrDetails, [in] BSTR bstrHlink	HRESULT
DeleteFirst()		HRESULT

You can also edit the IDL file by hand, instead of with the ClassView, to add the properties and methods. The IDL file should finally look like:

```
[
        object,
        uuid(8C80B871-93C9-11D0-891C-004095E279DD),
        dual,
        helpstring("IATLCorpEvents1 Interface"),
        pointer_default(unique)
]
interface IATLCorpEvents1 : IDispatch
{
        [propget, id(1),
                helpstring("Returns number of items in collection.")]
                HRESULT Count([out, retval] long *pVal);
        [id(2)] HRESULT Add([in] DATE DateTime, [in] BSTR bstrLocation,
                [in]BSTR bstrHeading, [in]BSTR bstrOrganizer,
                [in] BSTR bstrOrgDept, [in]BSTR bstrDetails,
                [in] BSTR bstrHlink);
        [id(3)] HRESULT DeleteFirst();
        [propget, id(DISPID_NEWENUM),
            helpstring("Returns an enumerator for the collection."),
            restricted] HRESULT _NewEnum([out, retval] LPUNKNOWN *pVal);
        [propget, id(DISPID_VALUE), helpstring
            ("Given an index, returns an item in the collection.")]
            HRESULT Item(long Index, [out, retval] VARIANT *pVal);

};
```

The `ATLCorpEvents1` class is an Automation collection class. It has a method called `_NewEnum()`, which has a `DISPID` value of `DISPID_NEWENUM` (=-4), and has a `restricted` attribute.

> *When adding this property with the class viewer, you have to change the* `DISPID` *later in the IDL file. The class viewer doesn't support the adding of negative* `DISPID`s.

The method is provided to enable the `For Each...Next` syntax of Visual Basic and scripting languages. We'll have more details on implementing enumerations in the *Working with Enumerations in ATL* section of this chapter.

We set the `Item` property to be the default property by setting its `DISPID` to `DISPID_VALUE`. The `Item` property is frequently designated as the default property of a collection. This allows a Visual Basic program to simply name the collection to index one of its members. For example:

```
MyDept.KnownEvents(6)
```

is equivalent to:

```
MyDept.KnownEvents.Item(6)
```

When the Item property is accessed, scripting languages like VBScript will expect an object reference to be returned, such as an ATLCorpEvent1 object reference. As stated earlier, a VARIANT can be used to pass the IDispatch based interface, representing an object reference (to an ATLCorpEvent1 object in this case), back to the client.

Here are the specifications of the IATLCorpEvent1 interface. Use the ClassView to add the properties:

Property	Property Type	Function Type
DateTime	DATE	put/get
Location	BSTR	put/get
Heading	BSTR	put/get
Organizer	BSTR	put/get
Details	BSTR	put/get
Hlink	BSTR	put/get
OrgDept	BSTR	put/get

This generates the following IDL:

```
[
        object,
        uuid(8C80B873-93C9-11D0-891C-004095E279DD),
        dual,
        helpstring("IATLCorpEvent1 Interface"),
        pointer_default(unique)
]
interface IATLCorpEvent1 : IDispatch
{
        // DateTime
        [propget, id(1), helpstring("property DateTime")]
                        HRESULT DateTime([out, retval] DATE *pVal);
        [propput, id(1), helpstring("property DateTime")]
                        HRESULT DateTime([in] DATE newVal);
        // Location
        [propget, id(2), helpstring("property Location")]
                        HRESULT Location([out, retval] BSTR *pVal);
        [propput, id(2), helpstring("property Location")]
                        HRESULT Location([in] BSTR newVal);
        // Heading
        [propget, id(3), helpstring("property Heading")]
                        HRESULT Heading([out, retval] BSTR *pVal);
        [propput, id(3), helpstring("property Heading")]
                        HRESULT Heading([in] BSTR newVal);
        // Organizer
        [propget, id(4), helpstring("property Organizer")]
                        HRESULT Organizer([out, retval] BSTR *pVal);
        [propput, id(4), helpstring("property Organizer")]
                        HRESULT Organizer([in] BSTR newVal);
```

```
                // Details
                [propget, id(5), helpstring("property Details")]
                              HRESULT Details([out, retval] BSTR *pVal);
                [propput, id(5), helpstring("property Details")]
                              HRESULT Details([in] BSTR newVal);
                // Hlink
                [propget, id(6), helpstring("property Hlink")]
                              HRESULT Hlink([out, retval] BSTR *pVal);
                [propput, id(6), helpstring("property Hlink")]
                              HRESULT Hlink([in] BSTR newVal);
                // orgDept
                [propget, id(7), helpstring("property orgDept")]
                              HRESULT OrgDept([out, retval] BSTR *pVal);
                [propput, id(7), helpstring("property orgDept")]
                              HRESULT OrgDept([in] BSTR newVal);
        };
```

The final `coclass` definition for the IDL file is quite interesting.

```
        library ATLDEPTLib
        {
             importlib("stdole32.tlb");
             importlib("stdole2.tlb");

             [
                  uuid(8C80B86F-93C9-11D0-891C-004095E279DD),
                  helpstring("ATLDept1 Class")
             ]
             coclass ATLDept1
             {
                  interface IATLCorpEvents1;
                  interface IATLCorpEvent1;
                  [default] interface IATLDept1;
             };
        };
```

> *Note that if you used the* **ATL COM AppWizard** *to create the* `ATLCorpEvents1` *and*
> `ATLCorpEvent1` *classes, it will have created* `coclass` *definitions in the IDL file. You need
> to edit these out.*

Here, we see that the type library consists of the definition of the three interfaces and one `coclass`.
Only the `CATLDept1 coclass` is defined, and we specified `IATLDept1` as its default interface
(Automation compatible objects are allowed only one default incoming `IDispatch` interface). What
happened to the `CATLCorpEvents1` and `CATLCorpEvent1` classes?

Actually, we'll provide full implementation of these classes within our code. However, since instances
of these classes are never created externally by clients, we will not register them through the type
library. When the time comes to create them, we will not use `CoCreateInstance()`, but create
directly using the `CoComObject<>` class from ATL. This technique provides effective encapsulation
and protection for dependent objects within an object model. When ATL's object wizard creates code
for us, however, it has already generated the required class factory support for all our objects. It is
therefore necessary to manually remove this code from our project.

Removing ATL Class Factory Support for Non-Externally Creatable COM Objects

You must take three additional steps to remove the ATL-generated class factory support code.

1. First, you must remove the line of code in your class declarations for CATLCorpEvents1 and CATLCorpEvent1 where they inherit from the CComCoClass template. Also comment out the relevant DECLARE_REGISTRY_RESOURCEID(). These lines are found in ATLCorpEvents1.h and ATLCorpEvent1.h respectively.

```
class ATL_NO_VTABLE CATLCorpEvents1 :
    public CComObjectRootEx<CComSingleThreadModel>,
//    public CComCoClass<CATLCorpEvents1, &CLSID_ATLCorpEvents1>,
    public IDispatchImpl<IATLCorpEvents1, &IID_IATLCorpEvents1,
                                          &LIBID_ATLDEPTLib>
{
....

//DECLARE_REGISTRY_RESOURCEID(IDR_ATLCORPEVENTS1)
....
};


class ATL_NO_VTABLE CATLCorpEvent1 :
    public CComObjectRootEx<CComSingleThreadModel>,
//    public CComCoClass<CATLCorpEvent1, &CLSID_ATLCorpEvent1>,
    public IDispatchImpl<IATLCorpEvent1, &IID_IATLCorpEvent1,
                                         &LIBID_ATLDEPTLib>
{
....

//DECLARE_REGISTRY_RESOURCEID(IDR_ATLCORPEVENT1)
....
};
```

2. Then, you must remove the corresponding entries in the application Object Map.

```
// ATLDept.cpp : Implementation of DLL Exports.

...

BEGIN_OBJECT_MAP(ObjectMap)
OBJECT_ENTRY(CLSID_ATLDept1, CATLDept1)
//OBJECT_ENTRY(CLSID_ATLCorpEvent1, CATLCorpEvent1)
//OBJECT_ENTRY(CLSID_ATLCorpEvents1, CATLCorpEvents1)
END_OBJECT_MAP()

...
```

3. Lastly, you need to remove the two RGS files from the project to stop them from being registered as separate objects.

This completes all the steps involved in making `ATLCorpEvents1` and `ATLCorpEvent1` creatable only from `ATLDept1`. Note that unlike regular C++ classes, instances of `CATLCorpEvents1` and `CATLCorpEvent1` classes are bona-fide Automation compatible COM objects. Even though they are not externally creatable, they *are* externally accessible – just like any other COM object – by Automation clients, once a reference is obtained.

Implementation of the IATLDept1 Interface

With the IDL description out of the way and the class factory code removed, we're ready to code the actual methods of the interfaces.

Let's first take a look at the ATL COM map entries. For the `CATLDept1` object, `IATLDept1` is the default `IDispatch` interface. Here is the generated source code in `ATLDept1.h`.

```
class ATL_NO_VTABLE CATLDept1 :
    public CComObjectRootEx<CComSingleThreadModel>,
    public CComCoClass<CATLDept1, &CLSID_ATLDept1>,
    public IDispatchImpl<IATLDept1, &IID_IATLDept1, &LIBID_ATLDEPTLib>
{
public:
    CATLDept1()
    {
    }

DECLARE_REGISTRY_RESOURCEID(IDR_ATLDEPT1)
DECLARE_NOT_AGGREGATABLE(CATLDept1)
DECLARE_PROTECT_FINAL_CONSTRUCT()

BEGIN_COM_MAP(CATLDept1)
    COM_INTERFACE_ENTRY(IATLDept1)
    COM_INTERFACE_ENTRY(IDispatch)
END_COM_MAP()

    . . .
```

To maintain the property values in our object, we need to add a set of member variables which keep the value of the properties of the object, as well as the property access methods themselves.

```
    . . .

// IATLDept1
public:
    STDMETHOD(get_Host)(/*[out, retval]*/ BSTR *pVal);
    STDMETHOD(put_Host)(/*[in]*/ BSTR newVal);
    STDMETHOD(get_Date)(/*[out, retval]*/ DATE *pVal);
    STDMETHOD(put_Date)(/*[in]*/ DATE newVal);
    STDMETHOD(get_KnownEvents)(/*[out, retval]*/ VARIANT *pVal);
    STDMETHOD(get_Color)(/*[out, retval]*/ OLE_COLOR *pVal);
    STDMETHOD(put_Color)(/*[in]*/ OLE_COLOR newVal);
    STDMETHOD(get_Symbol)(/*[out, retval]*/ BSTR *pVal);
    STDMETHOD(put_Symbol)(/*[in]*/ BSTR newVal);
    STDMETHOD(get_CanPostNew)(/*[out, retval]*/ VARIANT_BOOL *pVal);
```

```
        STDMETHOD(put_CanPostNew)(/*[in]*/ VARIANT_BOOL newVal);
        STDMETHOD(get_CanRead)(/*[out, retval]*/ VARIANT_BOOL *pVal);
        STDMETHOD(put_CanRead)(/*[in]*/ VARIANT_BOOL newVal);
        STDMETHOD(get_Number)(/*[out, retval]*/ BSTR *pVal);
        STDMETHOD(put_Number)(/*[in]*/ BSTR newVal);
        STDMETHOD(get_Name)(/*[out, retval]*/ BSTR *pVal);
        STDMETHOD(put_Name)(/*[in]*/ BSTR newVal);
        HRESULT FinalConstruct();
protected:
        CComBSTR      m_bstrName;
        CComBSTR      m_bstrNumber;
        VARIANT_BOOL m_bCanPostNew;
        VARIANT_BOOL m_bCanRead;
        CComBSTR      m_bstrSymbol;
        OLE_COLOR     m_Color;
        CComPtr<IATLCorpEvents1>  m_spKnownEvents;

        CComBSTR m_bstrHost;
        DATE m_CurDate;
};
```

Note how each `propget` *and* `propput` *attribute in the* IDL *has become a* `get_` *or* `put_` *member function of the class.*

Data Types

The `VARIANT_BOOL` data type, while looking especially threatening because of the word `VARIANT`, is actually currently defined to be a `short` value. It can thus be handled as an elementary data type.

We declare the `m_spKnownEvents` collection member variable as a smart pointer, again freeing us from tracking `AddRef()` and `Release()` on the object.

```
    CComPtr<IATLCorpEvents> m_spKnownEvents;
```

Finally...

ATLCorpEvents1 is not externally creatable, but it is externally accessible via VTBL binding, or Automation, as long as a reference (interface) to the object is available. From this perspective, the ATLDept1 object acts as a kind of custom class factory for ATLCorpEvents1 objects.

Unlike a non-COM C++ object, instances of `ATLCorpEvents1` are reference counted. This means that in order to keep an embedded COM object (the `m_spKnownEvents` property) within our `CATLDept1` object, we must always keep the COM object's reference count greater than zero until `CATLDept1` itself is destroyed. We will rely on the `CComPtr<>` smart pointer class to do this for us, as it will do the final release when the variable goes out of scope (that is, when `CATLDept1` is destroyed).

When a COM object of the class `CATLDept1` is created, we need to create its associated `KnownEvents` COM object. The embedded object must be created by the time that construction of the parent COM object is completed, so that it can be referenced immediately. To accomplish this, we need to construct a `CATLCorpEvents1` object immediately after the construction of the `CATLDept1` object. An ATL COM object derived from the `CComObjectRoot` ATL class can override the `FinalConstruct()` and `FinalRelease()` functions for this purpose. In our case, the `CATLDept1::FinalConstruct()` function creates the `KnownEvents` object and 'ransoms' it by holding an `IUnknown` pointer to the object for its entire lifetime.

```
HRESULT CATLDept1::FinalConstruct()
{
    CComObject<CATLCorpEvents1>  * tpPtr;
    HRESULT hTmp = CComObject<CATLCorpEvents1>::CreateInstance(&tpPtr);
    _ASSERTE(SUCCEEDED(hTmp));
    // hold this object with smart pointer as long as we live
    tpPtr->QueryInterface(IID_IATLCorpEvents1,
                          reinterpret_cast<void **>(&m_spKnownEvents));

    return S_OK;
}
```

Note how the `CComObject<>` template class allows us to create an instance of a COM class internally, without calling `CoCreateInstance()`. `CoCreateInstance()` would not have worked anyway, in our case, because the `CATLCorpEvents1` has no class factory implementation (we removed it earlier).

Here is the code from `\Vc98\Atl\Include\atlcom.h` for `CComObject<>::CreateInstance()`:

```
template <class Base>
HRESULT WINAPI CComObject<Base>::CreateInstance(CComObject<Base>** pp)
{
    ATLASSERT(pp != NULL);
    HRESULT hRes = E_OUTOFMEMORY;
    CComObject<Base>* p = NULL;
    ATLTRY(p = new CComObject<Base>())
    if (p != NULL)
    {
        p->SetVoid(NULL);
        p->InternalFinalConstructAddRef();
        hRes = p->FinalConstruct();
        p->InternalFinalConstructRelease();
        if (hRes != S_OK)
        {
            delete p;
            p = NULL;
        }
    }
    *pp = p;
    return hRes;
}
```

The important lines are highlighted above, we can see that the COM object is created on the heap, its associated `FinalConstruct()` is always called, and the newly created object reference is left at zero.

When our `CATLDept1` object terminates, there is no need to do anything. The smart pointer will free the attached object for us.

Whenever a client accesses the `KnownEvents` property of an `ATLDept1` object, we need to return the interface pointer to the events collection object. This is done by setting a `VARIANT` type variable with the `ATLCorpEvents` (derived from `IDispatch`) interface from the collection object:

```
STDMETHODIMP CATLDept1::get_KnownEvents(VARIANT * pVal)
{
    // get the IDispatch of the embedded collection and return it
    VariantInit(pVal);
    IDispatch* pDisp;
    if (m_spKnownEvents)
    {
        m_spKnownEvents->QueryInterface(IID_IDispatch,
                                reinterpret_cast<void**>(&pDisp));
        pVal->vt = VT_DISPATCH;
        pVal->pdispVal = pDisp;
        return S_OK;
    }
    else return E_FAIL;
}
```

`VariantInit()` is worth mentioning. It's used to initialize variables of type `VARIANT` by setting their tag field to `VT_EMPTY`.

The Rest of the Implementation

The rest of the implementation follows. It consists of pretty straightforward `put`/`get` methods for the remaining properties of `ATLDept1`.

```
STDMETHODIMP CATLDept1::get_Name(BSTR * pVal)
{
    if (pVal == NULL)
        return E_POINTER;
    *pVal = m_bstrName.Copy();
    return S_OK;
}

STDMETHODIMP CATLDept1::put_Name(BSTR newVal)
{
    m_bstrName = newVal;
    return S_OK;
}

STDMETHODIMP CATLDept1::get_Number(BSTR * pVal)
{
```

```
     if (pVal == NULL)
     return E_POINTER;
     *pVal = m_bstrNumber.Copy();
     return S_OK;
}

STDMETHODIMP CATLDept1::put_Number(BSTR newVal)
{
     m_bstrNumber = newVal;
     return S_OK;
}

STDMETHODIMP CATLDept1::get_CanRead(VARIANT_BOOL * pVal)
{
     *pVal = m_bCanRead;
     return S_OK;
}

STDMETHODIMP CATLDept1::put_CanRead(VARIANT_BOOL newVal)
{
     m_bCanRead = newVal;
     return S_OK;
}

STDMETHODIMP CATLDept1::get_CanPostNew(VARIANT_BOOL * pVal)
{
     *pVal = m_bCanPostNew;
     return S_OK;
}

STDMETHODIMP CATLDept1::put_CanPostNew(VARIANT_BOOL newVal)
{
     m_bCanPostNew = newVal;
     return S_OK;
}

STDMETHODIMP CATLDept1::get_Symbol(BSTR * pVal)
{
     if (pVal == NULL)
     return E_POINTER;
     *pVal = m_bstrSymbol.Copy();
     return S_OK;
}

STDMETHODIMP CATLDept1::put_Symbol(BSTR newVal)
{
     m_bstrSymbol = newVal;
     return S_OK;
}

STDMETHODIMP CATLDept1::get_Color(OLE_COLOR * pVal)
{
     *pVal = m_Color;
     return S_OK;
}
```

```
STDMETHODIMP CATLDept1::put_Color(OLE_COLOR newVal)
{
    m_Color = newVal;
    return S_OK;
}
STDMETHODIMP CATLDept1::get_Date(DATE *pVal)
{
    *pVal = m_CurDate;
    return S_OK;
}

STDMETHODIMP CATLDept1::put_Date(DATE inDate)
{
    m_CurDate = inDate;
    return S_OK;
}

STDMETHODIMP CATLDept1::get_Host(BSTR *pVal)
{
    if (pVal == NULL)
    return E_POINTER;
    *pVal = m_bstrHost.Copy();
    return S_OK;
}

STDMETHODIMP CATLDept1::put_Host(BSTR newVal)
{
    m_bstrHost = newVal;
    return S_OK;
}
```

Working with Enumerations in ATL

The CATLCorpEvents1 class is an Automation collection class; that is, it contains a collection of CATLCorpEvent1 objects. In this section, we'll see how an Automation collection class can be implemented using ATL. During the description of the IDL, we've already seen how the Item property can be assigned the DISPID_VALUE which makes it the default method, and how assigning the DISPID_ENUM to the _NewEnum() method makes it the method for obtaining an IEnum interface to a new enumerator object. The _NewEnum() method was also given the attribute of restricted to keep it hidden in most object browsers.

Besides serving as a For Each...Next mechanism for Automation clients with scripting or macro language capabilities, enumerators are frequently used in COM programming to iterate through a collection of objects in a consistent manner.

The CComEnum<> templated class takes the following arguments:

```
CComEnum<Base Interface Name,
        Pointer to IID of Interface,
        Object to Enumerate,
        Class for deep Copy of Object>
```

Now, let's look at how the CATLCorpEvents1 class itself is defined and how CComEnum<> is used.

The Implementation of the CATLCorpEvents1 Class

We can see that, unlike CATLDept1, this class isn't subclassed from CComCoClass. This isn't required since the class isn't externally creatable. We have, however, defined the IDispatch interface to be the same as the IATLCorpEvents1 interface, enabling the Automation client to get at the properties and methods.

```
class ATL_NO_VTABLE CATLCorpEvents1 :
    public CComObjectRootEx<CComSingleThreadModel>,
    public IDispatchImpl<IATLCorpEvents1, &IID_IATLCorpEvents1,
                                          &LIBID_ATLDEPTLib>
{
public:
    CATLCorpEvents1() {}

DECLARE_NOT_AGGREGATABLE(CATLCorpEvents1)
DECLARE_PROTECT_FINAL_CONSTRUCT()

BEGIN_COM_MAP(CATLCorpEvents1)
    COM_INTERFACE_ENTRY(IATLCorpEvents1)
    COM_INTERFACE_ENTRY(IDispatch)
END_COM_MAP()

. . .
```

The Count, Item, and _NewEnum properties are read-only, and they are declared in the class definition as:

```
. . .

STDMETHOD(get__NewEnum)(/*[out, retval]*/ LPUNKNOWN *pVal);
STDMETHOD(get_Item)(long Index, /*[out, retval]*/ VARIANT *pVal);
STDMETHOD(get_Count)(/*[out, retval]*/ long *pVal);

. . .
```

We need two overloaded Add() functions:

❑ One is the 'back-door' Add() – part of the interface – that we used in the control to initialize the department with specific values from the client during initial testing
❑ The other one is an actual Add() for adding a new member to the collection.

Let's add the second one here:

```
. . .

STDMETHOD(Add)(DATE DateTime, BSTR bstrLocation,
               BSTR bstrHeading, BSTR bstrOrganizer,
               BSTR bstrOrgDept, BSTR bstrDetails, BSTR bstrHlink);
void Add(CComVariant& var) { m_VarVect.insert(m_VarVect.end(), var); }
. . .
```

We restricted the delete function to delete only the very first member of the collection, and named it `DeleteFirst()`.

```
...

STDMETHOD(DeleteFirst)();

...
```

Internal to the class, the actual collection is implemented via a template-based vector class. This class is taken from the Standard Template Library (STL), which is completely integrated into Visual C++ 6's library support. The STL provides an extremely handy templated implementation of classical data structures (for example, lists, vectors, hash tables, etc.). It allows for rapid creation of type-safe and efficient data structure classes with minimal coding.

Lastly, we have an `Init()` method (for testing), and a vector for the `DeleteFirst()` method implementation:

```
    ...

    void Init(ULONG n);
protected:
    vector<CComVariant, allocator<CComVariant> > m_VarVect;

};
```

Two more steps are necessary in order to use the STL vector class. First, the necessary include file needs to be added to the `stdafx.h` file

```
#include <vector>
#if _MSC_VER>1020
using namespace std;
#endif
```

Second, since integration between ATL and STL isn't yet totally seamless, we must define two comparison operators that work on `CComVariant` types. These operators are not defined by `CComVariant`, but are required by STL vectors. Here, we will be providing only a dummy stub for the operators – the operators will not be used in our case. Add the following to `ATLCorpEvents1.cpp`,

```
bool operator< (const CComVariant l, const CComVariant r)
{
    _ASSERTE(false);
    return true;
}

bool operator==(const CComVariant l, const CComVariant r)
{
    _ASSERTE(false);
    return true;
}
```

and the corresponding declarations to the top of the ATLCorpEvents1.h file, outside the class declaration:

```
bool operator<(const CComVariant l, const CComVariant r);
bool operator==(const CComVariant l, const CComVariant r);
```

Because STL makes use of C++ exception handlers, the default project settings must be changed to support exceptions. You can do this by selecting the **Project** menu, then **Settings...**, click the **C/C++** tab, select **C++ Language** from the category list, and click the **Enable exception handling** checkbox.

By defining the following for CATLCorpEvents1, we've created an Automation compatible collection:

❑   A Count property
❑   An Item property
❑   A _NewEnum property returning an enumerator object

Taking a look at how each of these properties is implemented in ATLCorpEvents1.cpp, we see:

```
STDMETHODIMP CATLCorpEvents1::get_Count(long* pVal)
{
    if (pVal == NULL)
        return E_POINTER;
    *pVal = m_VarVect.size();
    return S_OK;
}
```

The Count property is delegated to the size() member function of the STL vector class.

```
STDMETHODIMP CATLCorpEvents1::get_Item(long Index, VARIANT* pVal)
{
    if (pVal == NULL)
        return E_POINTER;
    VariantInit(pVal);
    pVal->vt = VT_UNKNOWN;
    pVal->punkVal = NULL;
    // use 1-based index, VB like
    if ((static_cast<unsigned long>(Index) < 1) ||
               (static_cast<unsigned long>(Index) > (m_VarVect.size())))
        return E_INVALIDARG;
    VariantCopy(pVal, &m_VarVect[Index-1]);
    return S_OK;
}
```

The Item property is implemented via an extraction from the vector, as long as the index required isn't out of range of the vector. Remember, assigned into the vector is actually an IDispatch pointer within a VARIANT pointing to a CATLCorpEvent1 object.

The _NewEnum property is most interesting: it somehow has to create a new enumerator object which provides an IEnumVariant interface. We need to return an IEnumVariant object to allow the client to enumerate through the event collection, while internally we have an STL vector of events. Thanks to ATL, we have a very easy way of performing this mapping.

```
STDMETHODIMP CATLCorpEvents1::get__NewEnum(LPUNKNOWN* pVal)
{
    if (pVal == NULL)
        return E_POINTER;

    *pVal = NULL;
    typedef CComObject<CComEnum<IEnumVARIANT, &IID_IEnumVARIANT, VARIANT,
                                        _Copy<VARIANT> > > enumvar;
    enumvar* pEnumVar = new enumvar;
    _ASSERTE(pEnumVar);
    HRESULT hRes = pEnumVar->Init(m_VarVect.begin(), m_VarVect.end(), NULL,
                                                    AtlFlagCopy);

    if (SUCCEEDED(hRes))
        hRes = pEnumVar->QueryInterface(IID_IEnumVARIANT,
                                    reinterpret_cast<void**>(pVal));

    if (FAILED(hRes))
        delete pEnumVar;

    return hRes;
}
```

Notice that we have parameterized the CComEnum<> template with:

```
typedef CComObject<CComEnum<IEnumVARIANT, &IID_IEnumVARIANT, VARIANT,
                                    _Copy<VARIANT> > > enumvar;
```

The IEnumVARIANT is our base interface, with an IID pointer of &IID_IEnumVARIANT, and we want the enumeration object to enumerate VARIANT objects. The copy class is _Copy<VARIANT> as predefined by ATL. Other predefined copy classes in ATL include:

- ❑ _Copy<LPOLESTR>
- ❑ _Copy<OLEVERB>
- ❑ _Copy<CONNECTDATA>
- ❑ _CopyInterface<>

Once an instance of the COM object represented by our enumerator class (which we have named pEnumVar) is created, we take advantage of the guaranteed consecutive storage property of the vector<> STL class, and initialize the enumerator with our vector of VARIANT IDispatch pointers.

```
HRESULT hRes = pEnumVar->Init(m_VarVect.begin(),
                            m_VarVect.end(), NULL, AtlFlagCopy);
```

The construction of the enumerator object is now complete and we can return the IEnumVARIANT interface pointer to the calling Automation client. The following statement sets the value of the incoming IUnknown pointer to the IEnumVARIANT interface of the newly created enumerator object.

```
hRes = pEnumVar->QueryInterface(IID_IEnumVARIANT,
                              reinterpret_cast<void**>(pVal));
```

Using the above technique, one can quickly implement Automation collections or fulfil other IEnum requirements as they surface during COM programming.

> Besides the IEnumVARIANT *interface commonly found when dealing with Automation clients,* *there are other* IEnum *interfaces that you may encounter during COM programming. They* *include* IEnumUnknown, IEnumMoniker, IEnumString, IEnumFORMATETC, IEnumSTATSTG, IEnumSTATDATA, *and* IEnumOLEVERB.

The remainder of the class implementation is:

```
STDMETHODIMP CATLCorpEvents1::DeleteFirst()
{
    VARIANT firstNode;

    get_Item(1, &firstNode);

    if ( firstNode.punkVal != NULL)
    {
        // free the COM object before the C++ one!
      (static_cast<IUnknown *>(firstNode.punkVal))->Release();
    }

    m_VarVect.erase(m_VarVect.begin());

    return S_OK;
}
```

And finally a test method capable of creating n instances of ATLCorpEvent1 objects during testing. It makes use of the fact that a CATLCorpEvent1 class will be a C++ friend of the CATLCorpEvents1 class. There is more coverage in the next section.

```
void CATLCorpEvents1::Init(ULONG n)
{
    for (int i=0; i<n; i++)
    {
        CComObject<CATLCorpEvent1> * pAnEvent;
        HRESULT hTmp = CComObject<CATLCorpEvent1>
                                        ::CreateInstance(&pAnEvent);
        _ASSERTE(SUCCEEDED(hTmp));

        // take advantage of the friendship to do some direct
        // manipulation
        pAnEvent->m_dDateTime = 0;
        pAnEvent->m_bstrLocation = "A Location";
```

```
        pAnEvent->m_bstrHeading = "My Heading";
        pAnEvent->m_bstrOrganizer = "I'm an Organizer";
        pAnEvent->m_bstrDetails = "Some Details";
        pAnEvent->m_bstrHlink = "What Link";
        pAnEvent->m_bstrOrgDept = "Super Dept";

        // get IDispatch pointer
        LPDISPATCH lpDisp = NULL;
        pAnEvent->QueryInterface(IID_IDispatch,
                              reinterpret_cast<void**>(&lpDisp));
        _ASSERTE(lpDisp);

        // create a variant and add it to the collection
        CComVariant var;
        var.vt = VT_DISPATCH;
        var.pdispVal = lpDisp;
        Add(var);
    }
}
```

The remaining 'backdoor' Add() function will be presented in the next section.

Implementing the CATLCorpEvent Class

Having gone through the implementation of the CATLDept1 class, which included an attached COM object represented by the m_spKnownEvents property, and seen how the CATLCorpEvents1 class implements an Automation collection, the CATLCorpEvent class may seem relatively uninteresting. The class definition is shown here:

```
class ATL_NO_VTABLE CATLCorpEvent1 :
    public CComObjectRootEx<CComSingleThreadModel>,
    public IDispatchImpl<IATLCorpEvent1, &IID_IATLCorpEvent1,
                                        &LIBID_ATLDEPTLib>
{
public:
    CATLCorpEvent1()    {}

DECLARE_NOT_AGGREGATABLE(CATLCorpEvent1)
DECLARE_PROTECT_FINAL_CONSTRUCT()

BEGIN_COM_MAP(CATLCorpEvent1)
    COM_INTERFACE_ENTRY(IATLCorpEvent1)
    COM_INTERFACE_ENTRY(IDispatch)
END_COM_MAP()

// IATLCorpEvent1
public:
    STDMETHOD(get_OrgDept)(/*[out, retval]*/ BSTR *pVal);
    STDMETHOD(put_OrgDept)(/*[in]*/ BSTR newVal);
    STDMETHOD(get_Hlink)(/*[out, retval]*/ BSTR *pVal);
    STDMETHOD(put_Hlink)(/*[in]*/ BSTR newVal);
    STDMETHOD(get_Details)(/*[out, retval]*/ BSTR *pVal);
    STDMETHOD(put_Details)(/*[in]*/ BSTR newVal);
```

```
        STDMETHOD(get_Organizer)(/*[out, retval]*/ BSTR *pVal);
        STDMETHOD(put_Organizer)(/*[in]*/ BSTR newVal);
        STDMETHOD(get_Heading)(/*[out, retval]*/ BSTR *pVal);
        STDMETHOD(put_Heading)(/*[in]*/ BSTR newVal);
        STDMETHOD(get_Location)(/*[out, retval]*/ BSTR *pVal);
        STDMETHOD(put_Location)(/*[in]*/ BSTR newVal);
        STDMETHOD(get_DateTime)(/*[out, retval]*/ DATE *pVal);
        STDMETHOD(put_DateTime)(/*[in]*/ DATE newVal);
protected:
        DATE m_dDateTime;
        CComBSTR m_bstrLocation;
        CComBSTR m_bstrHeading;
        CComBSTR m_bstrOrganizer;
        CComBSTR m_bstrDetails;
        CComBSTR m_bstrHlink;
        CComBSTR m_bstrOrgDept;
        friend class CATLCorpEvents1;
};
```

Being a leaf node in the class tree of the object model, the main purpose of this class is to contain data. All of that data is stored in the protected members. Notice that the CATLCorpEvents1 class is made a friend of this class. This was done mainly for performance reasons. The CATLCorpEvents1::Add() backdoor function actually sets these variables directly:

```
STDMETHODIMP CATLCorpEvents1::Add(DATE DateTime, BSTR bstrLocation,
                 BSTR bstrHeading, BSTR bstrOrganizer, BSTR bstrOrgDept,
                 BSTR bstrDetails, BSTR bstrHlink)
{
    CComObject<CATLCorpEvent1> * pAnEvent;
    HRESULT hTmp = CComObject<CATLCorpEvent1>::CreateInstance(&pAnEvent);
    _ASSERTE(SUCCEEDED(hTmp));

    // take advantage of the friendship to do some direct manipulation
    pAnEvent->m_dDateTime = DateTime;
    pAnEvent->m_bstrLocation = bstrLocation;
    pAnEvent->m_bstrHeading = bstrHeading;
    pAnEvent->m_bstrOrganizer = bstrOrganizer;
    pAnEvent->m_bstrDetails = bstrDetails;
    pAnEvent->m_bstrHlink = bstrHlink;
    pAnEvent->m_bstrOrgDept = bstrOrgDept;

    // get IDispatch pointer
    LPDISPATCH lpDisp = NULL;
    PAnEvent->QueryInterface(IID_IDispatch,
                                       reinterpret_cast<void**>(&lpDisp));
    _ASSERTE(lpDisp);

    // create a variant and add it to the collection
    CComVariant var;
    var.vt = VT_DISPATCH;
    var.pdispVal = lpDisp;
    Add(var);
    return S_OK;
}
```

Without the `friend` statement, one would have to call the `CATLCorpEvent1::set_` methods for each of the properties to set. Some extra computing time would have been wasted in moving string data back and forth between memory locations. The `CATLCorpEvents` class takes advantage of this tightly coupled C++ relationship to optimize its operations. External COM clients accessing the event object must use the `CATLCorpEvent1::get_` methods through vtable or Automation instead.

As an aside, note again that the `IDispatch` pointer of the `CATLCorpEvent1` object is the actual item stuffed into the `VARIANT` array. This is the most direct way to provide the Automation client with something to immediately access the properties and methods of the object. It is what Visual Basic will expect when accessing an Automation collection.

For completion, here is the implementation of the rest of the `CATLCorpEvent1` methods in `ATLCorpEvent1.cpp`. They are pretty trivial `get`/`put` property functions:

```
STDMETHODIMP CATLCorpEvent1::get_DateTime(DATE * pVal)
{
    *pVal = m_dDateTime;
    return S_OK;
}

STDMETHODIMP CATLCorpEvent1::put_DateTime(DATE newVal)
{
    m_dDateTime = newVal;
    return S_OK;
}

STDMETHODIMP CATLCorpEvent1::get_Location(BSTR * pVal)
{
    if (pVal == NULL)
        return E_POINTER;
    *pVal = m_bstrLocation.Copy();
    return S_OK;
}

STDMETHODIMP CATLCorpEvent1::put_Location(BSTR newVal)
{
    m_bstrLocation = newVal;
    return S_OK;
}

STDMETHODIMP CATLCorpEvent1::get_Heading(BSTR * pVal)
{
    if (pVal == NULL)
        return E_POINTER;
    *pVal = m_bstrHeading.Copy();
    return S_OK;
}

STDMETHODIMP CATLCorpEvent1::put_Heading(BSTR newVal)
{
    m_bstrHeading = newVal;
    return S_OK;
}
```

```
STDMETHODIMP CATLCorpEvent1::get_Organizer(BSTR * pVal)
{
     if (pVal == NULL)
          return E_POINTER;
     *pVal = m_bstrOrganizer.Copy();
     return S_OK;
}

STDMETHODIMP CATLCorpEvent1::put_Organizer(BSTR newVal)
{
     m_bstrOrganizer = newVal;
     return S_OK;
}

STDMETHODIMP CATLCorpEvent1::get_Details(BSTR * pVal)
{
     if (pVal == NULL)
          return E_POINTER;
     *pVal = m_bstrDetails.Copy();
     return S_OK;
}

STDMETHODIMP CATLCorpEvent1::put_Details(BSTR newVal)
{
     m_bstrDetails = newVal;
     return S_OK;
}

STDMETHODIMP CATLCorpEvent1::get_Hlink(BSTR * pVal)
{
     if (pVal == NULL)
          return E_POINTER;
     *pVal = m_bstrHlink.Copy();
     return S_OK;
}

STDMETHODIMP CATLCorpEvent1::put_Hlink(BSTR newVal)
{
     m_bstrHlink = newVal;
     return S_OK;
}

STDMETHODIMP CATLCorpEvent1::get_OrgDept(BSTR * pVal)
{
     if (pVal == NULL)
          return E_POINTER;
     *pVal = m_bstrOrgDept.Copy();
     return S_OK;
}

STDMETHODIMP CATLCorpEvent1::put_OrgDept(BSTR newVal)
{
     m_bstrOrgDept = newVal;
     return S_OK;
}
```

Lastly, you need to #include the header files for CATLCorpEvents1 in CATLDept, and those for CATLCorpEvent1 in CATLCorpEvents1. In ATLDept1.cpp you should have:

```
#include "stdafx.h"
#include "ATLDept.h"
#include "ATLCorpEvents1.h"
#include "ATLDept1.h"
```

and in ATLCorpEvents1.cpp:

```
#include "stdafx.h"
#include "ATLDept.h"
#include "ATLCorpEvents1.h"
#include "ATLCorpEvent1.h"
```

Compiling and Testing the DLL Server

You can now compile the DLL server by building ATLDept.dll in Visual Studio. Thanks to the ATL AppWizard, the DLL will also automatically be registered in the registry via a custom build step.

Remember, however, that in order to install this DLL COM server on another system, you must perform the following:

- ❏ Copy ATLDept.dll to the target machine.
- ❏ Run regsvr32 ATLDept.dll on the target machine.

Forgetting to do step two can easily lead to hours of frustrated debugging.

Finally, to perform a quick test of the newly created COM object server, we can use the Oleview.exe Viewer utility.

We can try to create an instance of the ATLDept1 object (and thus an invisible embedded CATLCorpEvents1 object) by double-clicking on the ATLDept1 entry under either All Objects or Automation Objects:

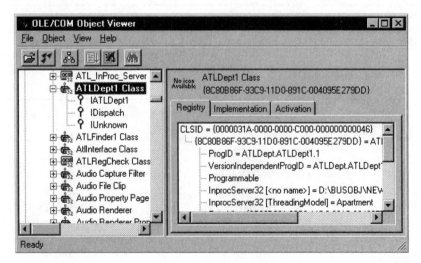

We can see the `IATLDept1` interface being supported. If we double-click on the `IDispatch` interface, the `IDispatch` decoder can also be used to view the Automation accessible methods and properties of this interface.

The ATLFinder Local COM Server

We are now going to repeat the entire process again in creating the new `ATLFinder` server. Unlike `ATLDept`, which is DLL based and in-process, `ATLFinder` is an EXE based local server. Earlier in the chapter, in the high level design description, we discovered that the `ATLFinder` is a business object that allows us to locate all the departments within the enterprise that have events posted for any specified month. It will return a collection of `ATLDept` objects. We can then drill down into each of the `ATLDept` objects and obtain each one's collection of available events.

Please hang on! We are going to move rapidly in order to make the coding process less tedious.

To implement the `ATLFinder` we start by creating an ATL COM AppWizard project for a local (EXE) server. We then insert two ATL 'simple objects' for the `ATLFinder1` and `ATLDepts1` classes.

Going through the same steps as with the `ATLDept1` project, we need to restrict the `ATLDepts1` object by:

- Modifying the IDL file so that it does not contain a `coclass` for `CATLDepts1`
- Removing inheritance from `CComCoClass<>`
- Removing the `DECLARE_REGISTRY_RESOURCEID()` from the class declaration
- Removing the corresponding entry from the application Object Map
- Removing `ATLDepts1.rgs` from the project

The properties and methods can be added through the ClassView. For the `IATLFinder1` interface, they're:

Property	Property Type	Function Type
EventfulDepts	VARIANT	get

and for its single method:

Method	Parameters	Return Type
SetFindDate()	[in] DATE inDate	HRESULT

While for the `IATLDept1` interface they're:

Property	Property Type	Function Type
Count	VARIANT	get
Index	VARIANT	get
_NewEnum	LPUNKNOWN	get

And for its two methods:

Method	Parameters	Return Type
Add	[in] BSTR bstrName, [in] BSTR bstrNumber, [in] VARIANT_BOOL bCanRead, [in] VARIANT_BOOL bCanPostNew, [in] BSTR bstrSymbol, [in] long lColor, [in] BSTR bstrHost, [in] DATE inDate	HRESULT
DeleteFirst		HRESULT

The resulting IDL should be (or you can modify it by hand if you are not using the ClassView):

```
import "oaidl.idl";
import "ocidl.idl";
    [
        object,
        uuid(BEF0D4CE-9490-11D0-891C-004095E279DD),
        dual,
        helpstring("IATLFinder1 Interface"),
        pointer_default(unique)
    ]
    interface IATLFinder1 : IDispatch
    {
        [propget, id(1), helpstring("property EventfulDepts")]
        HRESULT EventfulDepts([out, retval] VARIANT *pVal);
        [id(2), helpstring("method SetFindDate")]
        HRESULT SetFindDate([in] DATE inDate);
    };
    [
        object,
        uuid(BEF0D4D0-9490-11D0-891C-004095E279DD),
        dual,
        helpstring("IATLDepts1 Interface"),
        pointer_default(unique)
    ]
    interface IATLDepts1 : IDispatch
    {
        [propget, id(1),
            helpstring("Returns number of items in collection.")]
            HRESULT Count([out, retval] long *pVal);
        [propget, id(DISPID_VALUE), helpstring
            ("Given an index, returns an item in the collection.")]
            HRESULT Item([in] long Index, [out, retval] VARIANT *pVal);
        [propget, id(DISPID_NEWENUM),
            helpstring("Returns an enumerator for the collection.")]
            HRESULT _NewEnum([out, retval] LPUNKNOWN *pVal);
        [id(4)] HRESULT Add([in] BSTR bstrName, [in] BSTR bstrNumber,
            [in] VARIANT_BOOL bCanRead, [in] VARIANT_BOOL bCanPostNew,
            [in] BSTR bstrSymbol, [in] long lColor, [in] BSTR bstrHost,
```

```
                        [in] DATE inDate);
            [id(5)] HRESULT DeleteFirst();

    };


[
    uuid(BEF0D4C1-9490-11D0-891C-004095E279DD),
    version(1.0),
    helpstring("ATLFinder 1.0 Type Library")
]
library ATLFINDERLib
{
    importlib("stdole32.tlb");
    importlib("stdole2.tlb");
    interface IATLFinder1;
    interface IATLDepts1;

    [
        uuid(BEF0D4CF-9490-11D0-891C-004095E279DD),
        helpstring("ATLFinder1 Class")
    ]
    coclass ATLFinder1
    {
        [default] interface IATLFinder1;
    };
};
```

Implementing ATLFinder

Here's the class declaration of the `ATLFinder1` object, found in `ATLFinder1.h`,

```
class ATL_NO_VTABLE CATLFinder1 :
    public CComObjectRootEx<CComSingleThreadModel>,
    public CComCoClass<CATLFinder1, &CLSID_ATLFinder1>,
    public IDispatchImpl<IATLFinder1, &IID_IATLFinder1, &LIBID_ATLFINDERLib>
{
public:
    CATLFinder1() {}
DECLARE_REGISTRY_RESOURCEID(IDR_ATLFINDER1)
DECLARE_NOT_AGGREGATABLE(CATLFinder1)
DECLARE_PROTECT_FINAL_CONSTRUCT()
BEGIN_COM_MAP(CATLFinder1)
    COM_INTERFACE_ENTRY(IATLFinder1)
    COM_INTERFACE_ENTRY(IDispatch)
END_COM_MAP()

// IATLFinder1
public:
    STDMETHOD(SetFindDate)(/*[in]*/ DATE inDate);
    STDMETHOD(get_EventfulDepts)(/*[out, retval]*/ VARIANT *pVal);
    HRESULT FinalConstruct();
private:
    CComPtr<IATLDepts1> m_spEventfulDepts;
    DATE m_dCurStartDate;
};
```

and the corresponding implementation in `ATLFinder1.cpp`:

```
STDMETHODIMP CATLFinder1::get_EventfulDepts(VARIANT * pVal)
{
     // get the IDispatch of the embedded collection and return it
     VariantInit(pVal);
     IDispatch* pDisp;
     m_spEventfulDepts->QueryInterface(IID_IDispatch,
                                 reinterpret_cast<void**>(&pDisp));
     pVal->vt = VT_DISPATCH;
     pVal->pdispVal = pDisp;
     return S_OK;

}

STDMETHODIMP CATLFinder1::SetFindDate(DATE inDate)
{
     m_dCurStartDate = inDate;
     return S_OK;
}

HRESULT CATLFinder1::FinalConstruct()
{
     CComObject<CATLDepts1> * tpPtr;
     // Create and hold ransom our contained object
     HRESULT hTmp = CComObject<CATLDepts1>::CreateInstance(&tpPtr);
     _ASSERTE(SUCCEEDED(hTmp));
     // hand control over smartpointer
     tpPtr->QueryInterface(IID_IATLDepts1,
                           reinterpret_cast<void **>(&m_spEventfulDepts));
     return S_OK;
}
```

Here is the class declaration for `ATLDepts1` in `ATLDepts1.h`:

```
class ATL_NO_VTABLE CATLDepts1 :
     public CComObjectRootEx<CComSingleThreadModel>,
public IDispatchImpl<IATLDepts1, &IID_IATLDepts1, &LIBID_ATLFINDERLib>
{
public:
     CATLDepts1() {}
DECLARE_NOT_AGGREGATABLE(CATLDepts1)
DECLARE_PROTECT_FINAL_CONSTRUCT()

BEGIN_COM_MAP(CATLDepts1)
     COM_INTERFACE_ENTRY(IATLDepts1)
     COM_INTERFACE_ENTRY(IDispatch)
END_COM_MAP()

// IATLDepts1
public:
     STDMETHOD(DeleteFirst)();
     STDMETHOD(Add)(/*[in]*/ BSTR bstrName,  /*[in]*/ BSTR bstrNumber,
                    /*[in]*/ VARIANT_BOOL bCanRead,
                    /*[in]*/ VARIANT_BOOL bCanPostNew,
```

```
                        /*[in]*/ BSTR bstrSymbol, /*[in]*/ long lColor,
                        /*[in]*/ BSTR bstrHost, /* [in] */ DATE inDate);
        STDMETHOD(get__NewEnum)(/*[out, retval]*/ LPUNKNOWN *pVal);
        STDMETHOD(get_Item)(/*[in]*/ long Index,
                            /*[out, retval]*/ VARIANT *pVal);
        STDMETHOD(get_Count)(/*[out, retval]*/ long *pVal);
        void Add(CComVariant& var);
protected:
// internal data
        vector<CComVariant, allocator<CComVariant> > m_VarVect;
};
```

And here's the implementation from `ATLDepts1.cpp`. Notice the similarity with the `CATLCorpEvents1` method implementation:

```
STDMETHODIMP CATLDepts1::get_Count(long * pVal)
{
        if (pVal == NULL)
            return E_POINTER;
        *pVal = m_VarVect.size();
        return S_OK;
}

STDMETHODIMP CATLDepts1::get_Item(long Index, VARIANT * pVal)
{
        if (pVal == NULL)
            return E_POINTER;
        VariantInit(pVal);
        pVal->vt = VT_UNKNOWN;
        pVal->punkVal = NULL;
        // use 1-based index, VB like
            if ((static_cast<unsigned long>(Index) < 1) ||
                (static_cast<unsigned long>(Index) > (m_VarVect.size())))
            return E_INVALIDARG;
        VariantCopy(pVal, &m_VarVect[Index-1]);
        return S_OK;
}

STDMETHODIMP CATLDepts1::get__NewEnum(LPUNKNOWN * pVal)
{
        if (pVal == NULL)
            return E_POINTER;
        *pVal = NULL;
        typedef CComObject<CComEnum<IEnumVARIANT, &IID_IEnumVARIANT, VARIANT,
                                    _Copy<VARIANT> > > enumvar;
        enumvar* p = new enumvar;
        _ASSERTE(p);
        HRESULT hRes = p->Init(m_VarVect.begin(), m_VarVect.end(), NULL,
                                                        AtlFlagCopy);
        if (SUCCEEDED(hRes))
            hRes = p->QueryInterface(IID_IEnumVARIANT,
                                        reinterpret_cast<void**>(pVal));
        if (FAILED(hRes))
            delete p;
        return hRes;
}
```

```
STDMETHODIMP CATLDepts1::Add(BSTR bstrName, BSTR bstrNumber, VARIANT_BOOL
bCanRead, VARIANT_BOOL bCanPostNew, BSTR bstrSymbol, long lColor, BSTR bstrHost,
DATE inDate)
{
        // we need to create a Dept COM object here,
        // no more luxury of it being a local C/C++
        // object
        IATLDept1 * pITmpDept;

        HRESULT hTmp = CoCreateInstance(CLSID_ATLDept1, NULL, CLSCTX_INPROC,
                        IID_IATLDept1, reinterpret_cast<void**>(&pITmpDept));
        _ASSERTE(SUCCEEDED(hTmp));

        // make use of the dual interface ability to
        // set the data using C++ preferred VTBL binding
        pITmpDept->put_Name(bstrName);
        pITmpDept->put_Number(bstrNumber);
        pITmpDept->put_CanRead(bCanRead);
        pITmpDept->put_CanPostNew(bCanPostNew);
        pITmpDept->put_Symbol(bstrSymbol);
        pITmpDept->put_Color(lColor);
        pITmpDept->put_Host(bstrHost);
        pITmpDept->put_Date(inDate);

        // get IDispatch pointer
        LPDISPATCH lpDisp;
        lpDisp = NULL;
        pITmpDept->QueryInterface(IID_IDispatch,
                                  reinterpret_cast<void**>(&lpDisp));
        _ASSERTE(lpDisp);

        pITmpDept->Release();

        // create a variant and add it to the collection
        CComVariant var;
        var.vt = VT_DISPATCH;
        var.pdispVal = lpDisp;
        Add(var);
        return S_OK;
}

STDMETHODIMP CATLDepts1::DeleteFirst()
{
        VARIANT firstNode;
        get_Item(1, &firstNode);
        if ( firstNode.punkVal != NULL)
        {
                // free the COM object before the C++ one!
                (static_cast<IUnknown *> (firstNode.punkVal))->Release();
        }
        m_VarVect.erase(m_VarVect.begin());
        return S_OK;
}
```

```
}

void CATLDepts1::Add(CComVariant& var)
{
    m_VarVect.insert(m_VarVect.end(), var);
}
```

Note that we need to add the necessary includes for STL vector to Stdafx.h:

```
#include <vector>
#if _MSC_VER>1020
using namespace std;
#endif
#define IID_DEFINED
```

We should also provide declarations and definitions (in the ATLDepts1.h and ATLDepts1.cpp files, respectively) for the missing operators from CComVariant<> since the STL vector definition will require them to compile. As before, we will be stubbing them out:

```
bool operator<(const CComVariant l, const CComVariant r);
bool operator==(const CComVariant l, const CComVariant r);
bool operator<(const CComVariant l, const CComVariant r)
{
    _ASSERTE(false);
    return true;
}

bool operator==(const CComVariant l, const CComVariant r)
{
    _ASSERTE(false);
    return true;
}
```

We also need the CLSIDs for ATLDept1, so, in the ATLDepts1.cpp, include the MIDL-generated ATLDept.h and the ATLDept_i.c file that contains them:

```
#include "..\ATLDept\ATLDept.h"
#include "..\ATLDept\ATLDept_i.c"
```

That is all the code in the two middle-tier object model presenters. At this time, we have coded them for easy testing with the Visual Calendar Control that we completed in the last chapter. Later on, we will retrofit them to use other mid-tier objects.

Time to move on again. The next section looks at another tier of business objects that actually works with data residing in multiple relational databases. Ultimately, these objects supply actual data to be used by ATLFinder.exe and ATLDept.dll.

Accessing Databases

In the remainder of the chapter, we'll cover an important up-and-coming data access technology from Microsoft called OLE DB, part of Microsoft's Universal Data Access strategy. Before we begin, though, we need to recap on some basic concepts.

Hierarchical Multi-user to Relational Client/Server

Back in pre-history, databases were almost all hierarchical. A hierarchical database can be thought of as a persistent version of a C structure. Essentially, the relationship between the data elements stored in the database (defined by its schema, or blueprint) is static and fixed. It's therefore vital to analyze the data storage and access problem thoroughly before committing to a specific schema. All the potential ways of adding, modifying, and querying data must be considered. Properly designed schema enable very fast access to the underlying data, since the physical data layout is optimized for access. The problem with this approach is that it is not conducive to change. Modification of the schema typically requires considerable analysis and manual labor in migrating the existing data.

But, as is the way of things, a new breed of database, using relational technology, arrived and has made large inroads on client-server systems. **Relational DataBase Management Systems** (RDBMSes) allow dynamic definition of data schema, and promise flexible, yet quick, access to the data. This fits in perfectly with organizations' desire to evolve their data access capabilities with minimal effort. This works very well in the era of client/server computing, where high-speed connections between client and server enable new levels of interactivity for database applications.

Meanwhile, a decade old 'revolution' in object-oriented database systems is still taking place; giving the RDBMS stronghold companies a chance to fortify their defenses – adding OO-like 'extensions' to their predominately relational database engines. OO database technology has to fight an up-hill battle against the relational model, not unlike the one that RDBMSes fought, and won, over hierarchical systems. Ironically, the current differentiating factor for OO database vendors is the tremendous access speed advantage they have, over RDBMSes, when working with certain highly-interrelated data pieces (which is, of course, in no way reminiscent of the very strength of its archaic hierarchical forefather…).

What's a Programmer to Do?

Given the options here, and that's before we include flat-file data, what's an application's programmer to do? Microsoft's idea is simple:

> **Universal Data Access (UDA) – Use the same access methods (mostly relational friendly at the moment) to access data of any arbitrary type in its native format – in an object-like manner**

Speed is not of the essence here – and you will not find it mentioned anywhere in the literature. Rather, it is the ability to access, manage, and perform *ad-hoc* queries against an arbitrary data set that forms the underlying appeal.

Before we look at the set of technological components that make up **Universal Data Access** in their glorious technical detail, let's take a quick refresher on the fundamentals.

Quick Relational Database Basics

Instead of providing a formal introduction to relational databases (which you can find many references and textbooks on, a classic being *An Introduction to Database Programming* by Chris Date), we will try to breeze through some basics.

Data is stored as records in **rows** of a **table** within a RDBMS. A table is used to store information about entities, whether tangible (i.e. customer, company, product, etc.) or intangible (i.e. a training course, a hotel booking). Here is a picture of two such tables:

	Vacations		
Teacher	Start	End
3	8/12/99	8/26/99
1	7/1/99	7/7/99
2	5/16/99	6/3/99

Teachers

ID	First Name	Last Name
1	Joe	Cook
2	Joan	Willis
3	Jack	Morgan

Each cell of a row is sometimes called a **field**, and is used to store one specific attribute with respect to the table (i.e. the first name of a customer, the model number of a product). Some **columns** in a table may contain data that is duplicated in columns in another table. These columns are used to 'link' the two tables together – this is the basis of the ad-hoc query capability.

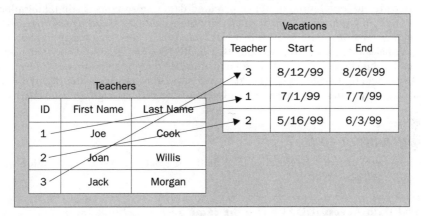

For fast retrieval of records, a table is typically **indexed** based on certain fields. This involves the allocation of extra 'indexing storage' to store the index information. The most frequently used index on a table is known as its **primary key**, and is the ordering system used by default.

For performance reasons, 'links' between two tables are always performed through fields which have been indexed. A field, which has been linked to another table's primary key, is called a **foreign key** of the table. By definition, foreign keys are also indexed.

An operation in relational theory, called **normalization**, allows one to systematically arrive at an optimally linked set of tables, given any initial configuration. This will always work. In practice, however, specific knowledge about the data access patterns will always override this 'schoolbook' normalization to arrive at a reasonably workable set of linked tables. The trade-off (often called the **denormalization** process) made after the normalization process involves trading duplication of data (more tables with fewer fields of duplicated data) against anticipated access patterns (grouping frequently retrieved fields together, anticipating deletion of records or key modifications, etc.).

To manipulate relational data, a standard language called **Structured Query Language** (SQL) is used. ANSI-standard SQL levels are available – most vendors implement the standard and add many proprietary extensions. The SQL syntax uses textual commands, and can be divided roughly into two categories:

- ❑ **Data Definition Language** (DDL) – You can use DDL to create and maintain tables, indexes, views (pre-defined joins), etc.
- ❑ **Data Manipulation Language** (DML) – You use DML to actually perform ad-hoc queries against the data stored in the database

The ODBC Way of Looking at Databases

Microsoft has a phenomenally successful standard for database access with its **Open DataBase Connectivity** (ODBC) initiative. The premise was quite simple: create a 'standard' middleware layer that all database clients will be written to, and then have database vendors provide individual drivers for their own database product to plug into this middleware layer.

Here is a simplified diagram of how ODBC fits into the picture:

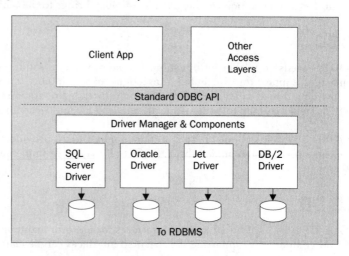

After half a dozen iterations of the ODBC specification, now standing at version 3.51, ODBC is a mature form of cross-vendor data access. It is well understood that some performance has to be sacrificed for flexibility, but specially tuned ODBC drivers, such as the ODBC driver for SQL Server from Microsoft, make the performance sacrifice extremely small.

Today, ODBC is extensively used in data applications that obtain and consolidate data from many heterogeneous data sources (for example, in decision-support applications). When portability or heterogeneous vendor support is not an important agenda, most projects revert back to the more tightly coupled, and higher efficiency, vendor-specific client access technology.

Microsoft takes Ownership of the Client

The success of ODBC and Windows has allowed Microsoft to take ownership of a 'Universal Desktop Client'. Essentially:

Microsoft Windows Operating system + ODBC Support = Universal Desktop Client

Microsoft Universal Data Access (UDA) Technologies

This is a group of existing, and evolving, data access technologies that together enable the n-tier client server computing vision of DNA. Currently, this group includes:

- ODBC
- OLE DB
- ADO
- RDS

Microsoft is unmistakably leaning towards the COM-based OLE DB, ADO and RDS in the long-term. Let us take a look at what each technology brings to the table.

ODBC

ODBC needs no further introduction. The latest version features a functional client-side cursor manager, support for distributed transactions (of which more in the next chapter), connection-pooling capability, thread safety for server-side multi-threaded operations, and many other improvements. ODBC will continue to be the de-facto standard for multi-vendor data access for a long time to come.

ODBC 3.51 delivers one of the first functional OLE DB providers for ODBC. In due course, as OLE DB matures, it is anticipated that ODBC itself may be re-implemented, on top of OLE DB, to reverse the picture.

OLE DB

OLE DB is a COM-based layer of interfaces for uniform manipulation of arbitrary data types. The COM components supporting the specified interfaces can be classified as:

- **Providers** – exposes OLE DB interfaces (and typically manages physical persistence data)
- **Consumers** – make use of OLE DB interfaces
- **Service components** – these are both consumers and providers These service components aggregate the rudimentary interfaces provided by simple providers, and expose a superset of the interfaces (their added value) to the consumer

The current OLE DB specification is closely tied to relational data through the **rowset** access model (a rowset is a set of rows, each row containing columns of data). However, OLE DB, in general, does not restrict the data being manipulated to relational data.

OLE DB interfaces are factored and designed with flexibility and efficiency as goals, and so they are not generally Automation compatible – making C/C++ the natural programming languages for leveraging their power.

We will have much more to say about OLE DB in the next section.

ADO

The generality of OLE DB means it has a monster set of interfaces (as we will see in the next section). Not only is coding OLE DB a tedious and involved exercise, the fact that it is based on custom COM interfaces makes it totally unsuitable for direct access using scripting languages, Visual Basic or Visual J++.

To cater for these development platforms, ActiveX Data Object (ADO) was introduced to provide an Automation compatible access to OLE DB. The object model provided by ADO is similar to the OLE DB component factoring, but not identical. In many ways, the ADO model is much simpler and easier to understand, but it is less flexible. From an architectural point of view, ADO is an OLE DB consumer which provides an Automation compatible interface (and appropriate object model presentation).

ADO is designed to be easy to learn and consequently keeps much of the familiar syntax and semantics of earlier MS data access technologies: **Remote Data Objects** – RDO (SQL Server optimized Automation compatible access) and **Data Access Objects** – DAO (Microsoft Access Jet Engine centric ODBC and Automation compatible access layer). ADO 2.0 defines a set of independent objects. They include:

- ❑ **Connection** – connect, logon and establish session with data source
- ❑ **Commands** – SQL command, potentially parameterized for execution; or for calling a stored procedure
- ❑ **Recordset** – typically a result from executing a command; provides a navigation capability through the set; provides data access to the fields of each record

The unique thing about ADO is that the ADO objects can be used independently of each other, and you do not have to navigate a hierarchy to go between them. For example, you can create a recordset by instantiating a recordset object. From this object, you can actually logon and execute a command. The net effect is that ADO is extremely simple to use in scripting languages, and ADO code is simpler and more direct than legacy RDO or DAO code which depends on more complicated object model hierarchies. Because ADO uses VARIANTs for Automation support and access through VARIANTs is not particularly efficient in Java, Microsoft have created the WFC/ADO native Java library classes for their Visual J++ product. These library classes use a similar object model to ADO.

RDS

Remote Data Service provides a remoting infrastructure for OLE DB data. It allows data from an OLE DB data source to be accessed and modified efficiently over low-speed connections (i.e. the Internet) or possibly in disconnected situations.

RDS provides ease of use through a familiar Visual Basic-like data binding facility for ActiveX controls hosted on a web page (through the RDS Data Control). In fact, the data set is marshaled across the network and hosted locally in an RDS-managed cache. Updates can be coordinated through a server-side business object which reflects the changes back to the OLE DB data source. RDS can make use either of the pure HTTP protocol for its operation, making it suitable for data access through firewalls, or a combination of HTTP and DCOM protocols.

OLE DB and Universal Data Access

The vision of Universal Data Access will be fulfilled with successive releases of OLE DB in future Microsoft operating systems.

OLE DB provides the 'trenchwork' in the lowest layer of the Microsoft Data Access picture. It provides a component-based access layer for all data access.

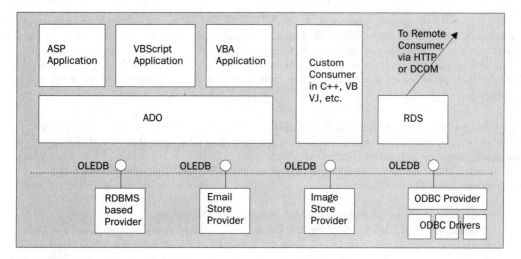

Consumers vs Providers

OLE DB providers are equivalent (in some senses) to ODBC drivers in the ODBC world. They are components which expose the basic set of OLE DB interfaces.

In the same way, OLE DB consumers are equivalent to ODBC clients. They are components or applications which make use of another component's exposed OLE DB interfaces.

Where the analogy breaks with the ODBC world is in the fact that a component can be both a consumer and provider at the same time. That is, these components make use of other components' exposed OLE DB interfaces and also expose their own. Thanks to COM, this is not only possible, but highly desirable. These are the service components. By composing different providers and service components, one can build custom data access stacks with made-to-order behaviors.

A scenario that often sparks the imagination is the use of a SQL query processor provider/consumer on top of different OLE DB providers. First on an **ISAM** (Indexed Sequential Access Method) storage, then a spreadsheet, then the symbol table output of a C++ compiler. In the first case, SQL queries can be performed on an ordinary ISAM database; in the second, we can use formal SQL on spreadsheet columns or zones; in the third, we can use existing tools that work with SQL to query for project information, variable names, class names or method names across all our development projects. In each case, the client is able to realize the added value provided by the query processor working against the corresponding data type.

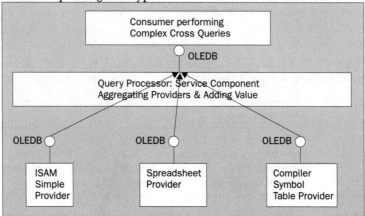

In most cases, we are only interested in writing OLE DB consumers. Microsoft is putting a lot of effort into providing tools for creating OLE DB providers. It is understandable since wide adoption of OLE DB depends on the availability of good third-party OLE DB providers. ATL 3 has a wizard for assisting in creating such a provider. Most business object implementations in the real world will be using OLE DB consumer templates and very few should require the development of custom providers. Interested readers are encouraged to study the MSDN documentation on custom provider development.

Factoring the Data Access Problems

With the experience gained from ODBC, Microsoft has factored the generic data access problem into the following interacting components.

- ❑ The client first needs to select a DataSource
- ❑ The client makes a connection through the DataSource, logs on, and establishes a Session
- ❑ The client works with the data by issuing Commands, either inside or outside transactions active within the scope of the Session
- ❑ The client accesses any data returned due to the execution of the Command through a rowset

This is a general model of how OLE DB components are factored. It is misleadingly simple. When we dig into the details, however, the picture is quite different. Catering for the eventuality of working with non-relational data, and adapting to the features and requirements of the many existing RDBMSes means that OLE DB components carry interfaces supporting a bewildering array of options.

The idea is that a minimal client should be able to interoperate with any OLE DB provider and do useful work. Microsoft has defined a minimal level of compliance for both the consumer and the provider to make sure that this is true.

OLE DB Objects and Interfaces

Let us now look at the OLE DB interfaces, the components expected to provide these interfaces, and how they are typically used. Do not worry if some of the description appear rather skimpy, we do not need to know all the details to use OLE DB effectively.

Root Enumerator

Provided with OLE DB SDK, this enumerator searches the registry for all the data sources known on a particular system. It can be instantiated through CLSID_OLEDB_ENUMERATOR.

Interface	Description
ISourcesRowset	With one single method called GetSourcesRowset(), this call will return a rowset object accessible through the IRowSet interface. The rowset will contain known data source information, or information on secondary enumerators.

Data Source Object

This object encapsulates the connection and the connection details to an actual data source. It serves as a session factory – that is, multiple sessions may be created from the same data source object.

Interface	Description
IDBProperties	An interface, exposed by the provider, for the consumer to set specific data source properties before initialization. It has three methods: GetProperties(), GetPropertyInfo(), and SetProperties(). Property settings at this level include the Server Name, the Login User Name, the Password, the database name, etc.
IDBInitialize	Contains two methods: Initialize() and Uninitialize(). These methods are called to initialize the data source with the properties set previously with IDBProperties interface, or to return the data source to an uninitialized state, respectively.
IDBCreateSession	Factory method for creating a new session. The sole CreateSession() method creates a new session object, and returns a requested interface from the object.
IPersistFile	Allows the persisting of a data source via IPersistFile::Save(). Only the data source and properties information is stored. The persisted data source can be re-instantiated by a call to IPersistFile::Load() with an uninitialized data source object.

Session Object

A session object creates and manages a connection to the data source. It is both a command factory and a rowset factory; and it manages local transactions.

Interface	Description
ISessionProperties	Two methods, GetProperties() and SetProperties(), may be used to obtain or change the current session properties.
IGetDataSource	Provides a backward link to the data source object from which this session is created. There is only one method, called GetDataSource().
IOpenRowset	A method called OpenRowset() can be used to create a rowset object containing all the records in a table or index within the data source.
ITransactionLocal	Contains two methods. GetOptionsObject() can be used to obtain an interface for setting transaction options. StartTransaction() starts a transaction on the session.
	Since it inherits from ITransaction, it also inherits Abort(), Commit(), and GetTransactionInfo() methods.
	If a session does not expose this interface, or if StartTransaction() is not called, then updates are automatically committed immediately.
IDBCreateCommand	Creates a new command object with its sole CreateCommand() method. Not all providers will support this, so you may need to access data from simpler providers through the IOpenRowset interface.
	Optionally, a session may also support the modification of tables and index information.
ITableDefinition	The AddColumn(), CreateTable(), DropColumn(), and DropTable() methods may be used to programmatically modify the table definition.
IIndexDefinition	The CreateIndex() and DropIndex() methods may be used to modify the index definition.

Command Object

This object typically encapsulates a SQL statement, a parameterized query, or a stored procedure.

Interface	Description
ICommandProperties	The GetProperties() and SetProperties() methods can be used to obtain or modify the command properties. You can also request special properties (such as insertable, deletable, or updatable) for the rowset that will be returned after executing the command.
ICommandText	The GetCommandText() and SetCommandText() methods can be used to obtain or set the text (i.e. the SQL code) of the command. Also contains methods of ICommand, described next.
ICommand	Contains three methods: Cancel() – used to cancel an executing command from another thread, Execute() – called to execute a command, and GetDBSession() – acts as a backward pointer and returns the session object that created the command.
ICommandWithParameters	Optionally exposed by the command object. Indicates that the command object supports parameterization. The GetParameterInfo() and SetParameterInfo() methods can be used to obtain or set the name and data type information of each parameter. MapParameterNames() can be used to obtain the ordinal number of a named parameter.
IConvertType	The single CanConvert() method can be used to find out whether the resulting rowset object from the command will support a specified data type conversion.
IAccessor	This is an optional interface – see following description of accessor objects.

Accessor Object

Accessor objects are data-transfer mapping objects; creatable from either command or rowset objects, both of which expose IAccessor to make this possible. It is vital to understand the role of an accessor object, so we will spend a little time here explaining the two most common uses for accessors in OLE DB.

For a command object, an accessor maps C++ variables in your code to parameters in a parameterized SQL statement, and manages the binding/type conversion required when the command is executed. Here is how it may look:

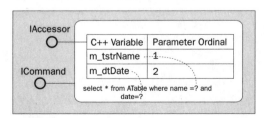

For a `rowset` object, the `accessor` maps C++ variables in your code to columns returned from each row of the rowset and it manages the binding/type conversion necessary when you are traversing through the rowset. Here is a diagram of such an `accessor`:

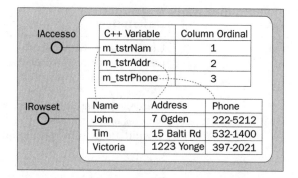

Once created, these objects are managed by their respective containers (either a `command` or a `rowset` for now) – the consumer only gets a handle to the object. Each `accessor` defines the mapping of memory locations (typically C++ class members) within the consumer, and contains datatype, offset, scale and precision information.

`Accessors`, as illustrated above, are typically used in parameterized commands to pass in parameters when `ICommand::Execute()` is called, or in rowsets to perform data binding when `IRowset::GetData()` or `IRowsetChange::SetData()` are called. A `command` with an `accessor` that creates a `rowset`, will actually pass on a copy of that `accessor` to the `rowset`. Both `accessors` continue to exist independently. `Accessor` objects are subject to standard COM reference counting rules, but reference counting must be performed through special methods provided by the `IAccessor` interface (since the lifetime of the `Accessor` object is managed by its host container).

Interface	Description
`IAccessor`	This interface is exposed by `rowset` objects, and optionally by `Command` objects. It has four methods. `CreateAccessor()` creates a new accessor object with reference count 1. Binding information is passed in during this call. `AddRefAccessor()` and `ReleaseAccessor()` peform reference counting on the host-managed accessor object. `GetBindings()` retrieves binding information from an existing accessor.

Rowset Object

`Rowset` objects are central to OLE DB. Each `rowset` contains a tabular buffer of data. You typically get a `rowset` by:

- ❑ Executing a `Command` via `ICommand::Execute()`
- ❑ Opening a `Table` or `Index` via `IOpenRowset::OpenRowset()` from a `Session` object

A `rowset` manages a collection of row objects internally and also any `accessor` objects that may be used. These managed objects are accessible from the consumer through handles. The `rowset` properties are set via `ICommandProperties::SetProperties()` prior to `rowset` creation – this will allow a provider to honor requests for `rowset` interfaces above and beyond the basics (i.e. for updatability through `IRowsetUpdate`).

Interface	Description
IRowset	Contains five methods. AddRefRows() and ReleaseRows() are used to perform reference counting on managed rows. GetData() is used to transfer data from a row to an accessor object. GetNextRows() performs the actual fetching of rows from the data source, creating internally managed row objects and returning handles to the rows. RestartPosition() causes the rowset to 'rewind' to an initial position during the next row fetch.
IAccessor	See description of accessor objects above.
IRowsetInfo	This interface provides information about the rowset to a consumer. A consumer can use this interface (along with the IColumnInfo interface) to 'discover' the rowset at runtime. This may be necessary if an unknown command and/or stored procedure is executed. It has three methods: GetProperties() returns the properties associated with the rowset; GetSpecifications() is used to move up the creation chain to either a Session object or Command object (the creator of the rowset) where more information can be obtained; GetReferencedRowset() is used to obtain a referenced rowset in bookmark or chapter handling (we will have more on this later).
IConvertType	Please refer to the IConvertType coverage in the command object description.
IColumnsInfo	This interface contains two methods. GetColumnInfo() provides metadata on the column, giving name, size, type, scale, and precision information. In addition, it also provides row ordinal and updatability information.
	This provides for runtime discovery by the consumer. MapColumnIDs() provides a rowset-specific mapping between column IDs and ordinal numbers. Column IDs are unique numbers defined by the data schema in GUID form; ordinal numbers are rowset-dependent offsets that represent a specific column. Ordinal numbers are used in most rowset operations to enhance access speed.
IRowsetIdentity	The single method, IsSameRow(), is provided by a rowset to determine if two row handles refer to the same row. Not all consumers will need this interface.

Other specializations of rowset can support additional interfaces. A list of the most common set of additional interfaces found in rowsets is shown below. This list is by no means exhaustive.

Interface	Description
IRowsetLocate	An optional interface exposed by a rowset. It indicates that the rowset supports bookmarks. Bookmarks allow arbitrary positioning of the fetch position. This interface has four methods: Compare() will compare two bookmarks to see if they are equal, or if one is further into the data than the other; Hash() provides a hash value for a bookmark based on its underlying row; GetRowsAt() allows row fetching starting at a bookmark plus a specified offset; GetRowsByBookmark() fetches rows underlying a set of bookmarks.
IRowsetFind	Optional interface exposed by a rowset. Allows a consumer to find a row within a rowset satisfying criteria based on a single column value. FindNextRow() is the method which does the search.
IRowsetChange	Optional interface exposed by a rowset. Allows the addition and deletion of rows in a rowset. It has three methods: InsertRow() adds a new row to the rowset; DeleteRows() deletes an existing row in a rowset; SetData() modifies the field values in a row. The action of SetData() is very similar to that which IRowsetUpdate provides, and when both exist, SetData() will not immediately update the underlying rowset. Instead, any changes will only be reflected when IRowsetUpdate::Update() is called.
IRowsetUpdate	Optional interface exposed by a rowset. It inherits from IRowsetChange and allows column values of a rowset to be changed. Modifications made using this interface are buffered within the rowset until Update() is called. The interface has five methods: GetOriginalData() retrieves the most recently fetched value for a row – ignoring recently made modifications; GetPendingRows() returns a list of rows with changes pending for update; GetRowStatus() returns the state that a set of rows is in (i.e. pending update); Undo() will undo any pending modifications and restore the rowset back to the state of the last fetch or Update() call; Update() reflects changes made to the rowset back to the data source.

Schema Access

A schema is a blueprint for a particular database. It contains meta-information on every aspect of the database, including information on all the tables, indexes, views, stored procedures and other database objects. While different providers may supply very different schema information, OLE DB specifies a minimum set that all providers exposing schema information should support. Schema information is typically useful for vendors of programming tools, having to work with the end-user's defined database.

We will not go into schema access in any depth here; it is enough that you know that metadata information exists for the discovery of an entire database through OLE DB at runtime.

Interface	Description
IDBSchemaRowset	This interface is optionally exposed by a session object. It has two methods: GetSchemas() return a list of schema rowsets obtainable through the interface; GetRowset() returns a specific schema rowset to the consumer.

Typical Consumer Uses of OLE DB Interfaces

The overview of OLE DB interfaces has hopefully prepared us for some data access scenarios. To give you a taste of how OLE DB is used in working with data sources, we will go through five very common scenarios of data access:

- ❏ Reading records from a table
- ❏ Obtaining results of a query
- ❏ Obtaining results of a parameterized query
- ❏ Adding a record to a table
- ❏ Deleting a record from a table

We will describe, on a high level, the code that needs to be written for each scenario. If we were to include actual, functional, raw C/C++ OLE DB code, some of our readers may faint. Such code is typically bulky, complex, and, for any moderately significant example, almost impossible to digest. To spare you any unpleasant consequences, we will stick to the pseudo-code level, and refer interested readers to the sample raw OLE DB code provided with the Visual Studio 6 Platform SDK. Later, we will be coding these scenarios using ATL 3 OLE DB Consumer Templates. The code will be much more concise, manageable and comprehensible.

Now, let's look at the scenarios.

Reading Records from a Table

In this scenario, we have a table whose records we want to access sequentially.

1. Assuming we know the CLSID of our provider, we first create the data source object, QueryInterface() (QI) for IDBProperties.

2. Set the properties for proper authentication with the provider via IDBProperties::SetProperties().

3. QI for IDBInitialize, and call IDBInitialize::Initialize().

4. QI for IDBCreateSession, and call CreateSession() to get a session object by its IOpenRowset interface.

5. Call `IOpenRowset::OpenRowset()` to create a `rowset` based on the table desired, returning `IRowset`.

6. QI the `rowset` for `IAccessor`.

7. Call `IAccessor::CreateAccessor()`, passing in our binding information, indicating where the row values should be stored.

8. Loop on calls to `IRowset::GetNextRows()` and `IRowset::GetData()` passing in the accessor handle to obtain data.

9. Call `IAccessor::ReleaseAccessor()` to free the accessor

10. Release the remaining objects.

Obtaining Results of a Query

In this scenario, we are executing a SQL query that returns a set of records, and we want to traverse the returned set of records one at a time.

1. Assuming we know the CLSID of our provider, we first create the data source object, QI for `IDBProperties`.

2. Set the properties for proper authentication with the provider via `IDBProperties::SetProperties()`.

3. QI for `IDBInitialize`, and call `IDBInitialize::Initialize()`.

4. QI for `IDBCreateSession`, and call `CreateSession()` to get a session object by its `IDBCreateCommand` interface.

5. Call `IDBCreateCommand::CreateCommand()` to create a new command object.

6. QI the command object for `ICommandText` and call `ICommandText::SetCommandText()` to set your query command. .

7. QI the command object for `ICommandProperties` and call `ICommandProperties::SetProperties()` to configure the interface you want from the `rowset` returned by command execution.

8. Call `ICommand::Execute()` to execute the query, returning a `rowset`.

9. QI the `rowset` for `IAccessor`.

10. Call `IAccessor::CreateAccessor()`, passing in our binding information, indicating where the row values should be stored.

11. Loop on calls to `IRowset::GetNextRows()` and `IRowset::GetData()`, passing in the accessor handle to obtain data.

12. Call `IAccessor::ReleaseAccessor()` to free the accessor

13. Release the remaining objects.

Obtaining Results of a Parameterized Query

As in the previous scenario, we are executing a SQL query that will return a set of records. However, this is a parameterized query, and we can submit arbitrary values to the query during runtime. The result is a set of records that we will traverse sequentially.

1. Assuming we know the CLSID of our provider, we first create the data source object and then QI for `IDBProperties`.

2. Set the properties for proper authentication with the provider via `IDBProperties::SetProperties()`.

3. QI for `IDBInitialize`, and call `IDBInitialize::Initialize()`.

4. QI for `IDBCreateSession`, and call `CreateSession()` to get a session object by its `IDBCreateCommand` interface.

5. Call `IDBCreateCommand::CreateCommand()` to create a new command object.

6. QI the command object for `ICommandText` and call `ICommandText::SetCommandText()` to set your query command.

7. QI the command for `IAccessor` and call `IAccessor::CreateAccessor()`, passing in binding information for the parameters as well as the returned `rowset`.

8. QI the command object for `ICommandWithParameters`, and call `ICommandWithParameters::SetParameterInfo()` with information associating the parameters with the accessor.

9. QI the command object for `ICommandProperties` and call `ICommandProperties::SetProperties()` to configure the interfaces you want from the `rowset` returned by command execution.

10. Call `ICommand::Execute()` to execute the query, returning a `rowset`.

11. Loop on calls to `IRowset::GetNextRows()` and `IRowset::GetData()`, passing in the accessor handle (from the command) to obtain data.

12. Call `IAccessor::ReleaseAccessor()` to free the accessor.

13. Release the remaining objects.

Adding a Record to a Table

This is the first scenario where modification is made to the database. Here, we will be adding a new record to a table within the database.

1. Assuming we know the `CLSID` of our provider, we first create the data source object and then QI for `IDBProperties`.

2. Set the properties for proper authentication with the provider via `IDBProperties::SetProperties()`.

3. QI for `IDBInitialize`, and call `IDBInitialize::Initialize()`.

4. QI for `IDBCreateSession`, and call `CreateSession()` to get a session object by its `IOpenRowset` interface.

5. Call `IOpenRowset::OpenRowset()` to create a `rowset` based on the table desired, returning `IRowset`.

6. QI the `rowset` for `IAccessor`.

7. Call `IAccessor::CreateAccessor()`, passing in our binding information, indicating where the row values should be stored.

8. Fill in the variables in the `IAccessor` binding with values for the new record.

9. QI the `rowset` for `IRowsetChange`, call `IRowsetChange::InsertRow()` to add the row to the table – passing in the accessor handle.

10. Call `IAccessor::ReleaseAccessor()` to free the accessor.

11. Release the remaining objects.

Deleting a Record from a Table

In our final scenario, we will be deleting a record from a table, based on a specific criterion. In fact, we will be traversing the rows of the table until we find the row that corresponds to the criterion, and then delete it.

1. Assuming we know the CLSID of our provider, we first create the data source object, QI for `IDBProperties`.

2. Set the properties for proper authentication with the provider via `IDBProperties::SetProperties()`.

3. QI for `IDBInitialize`, and call `IDBInitialize::Initialize()`.

4. QI for `IDBCreateSession`, and call `CreateSession()` to get a session object by its `IOpenRowset` interface.

5. Call `IOpenRowset::OpenRowset()` to create a `rowset` based on the table desired, returning `IRowset`.

6. QI the `rowset` for `IAccessor`.

7. Call `IAccessor::CreateAccessor()`, passing in our binding information, indicating where the row values should be stored.

8. Fill in the variables in the `IAccessor` binding with values for the record you want to delete.

9. Loop on calls to `IRowset::GetNextRows()` and `IRowset::GetData()` passing in the accessor handle to obtain data, stopping at the row you want to delete.

10. QI the `rowset` for `IRowsetChange`, call `IRowsetChange::DeleteRow()` — passing in the desired row handle.

11. Call `IAccessor::ReleaseAccessor()` to free the accessor.

12. Release the remaining objects.

This concludes our high level discussion of the typical data access scenarios. We will see some ATL code implementing them shortly. These scenarios should provide insights into how you can combine procedures or use similar techniques to solve your own specific data access problems.

OLE DB as a Work In Progress

At the time of writing, OLE DB 2.0 has been released but still has unimplemented functionality in the areas of security and remote data access.

While OLE DB is certainly usable in its current form with SQL server or Microsoft Access based data access programming (as we are doing with SQL server in our A&W project), general usage involving interoperation with other vendors' products requires careful planning and experimentation. Most native OLE DB providers for most other vendors' products are not available at the time of writing (although some may argue that since OLE DB supports ODBC, it can work with any RDBMS supported by ODBC).

Painfully Tedious OLE DB Programming

After seeing the typical consumer usage of OLE DB and the multitude of interfaces that need to be queried and accessed, one can imagine the sheer complexity of the actual code. All the method calls will involve complex parameters, and error conditions need to be anticipated. Even for the most rudimentary task, raw OLE DB programming is a tedious and highly error-prone task. There must be a better way, and, of course, there is! ATL 3 provides OLE DB templates.

Making OLE DB Programming Easier

As promised, we will now use the OLE DB consumer templates from ATL 3 to make OLE DB programming real easy. Instead of working with some arbitrary examples illustrating the scenarios we have explored earlier, we will actually create portions of the middle-tier business objects that reside on the departmental and centralized server for the A&W project.

We will focus on the database access portion of these business objects in this chapter, and will defer the discussion of their overall design and construction to the next chapter. Do not be alarmed if you find certain interfaces and/or methods alien to you at this time; as long as you understand the OLE DB template operations we present, the rest of the business object design should become crystal clear in the next chapter.

Setting Up the SQL Server Data

First, we must get the data source itself set up properly. Assuming that you may only have one server running Windows NT 4 to try all of this out, we will define both the departmental and central server tables in the same physical database.

> **You will need an installation of SQL Server 6.5 with Service Pack 4 or later to work with the sample code.**

Using whatever method is convenient, define the following tables in your SQL Server. We have provided two SQL files, called makecent.sql (for central server DB creation), and makedept.sql (for departmental server DB creation) in the \sql distribution directory for your convenience. The following is a breakdown of the different tables and views being set up.

First, there are the central server's tables. We have actually created this in its own database called proa2. The first table consolidates the event count for any particular day, for any particular department. This table acts as a cache, providing rapid centralized access to information on which departments have events, and how many, for a particular month. Here is the SQL table definition:

```
if exists (select * from sysobjects where id = object_id('dbo.EventCount')
                                          and sysstat & 0xf = 3)
      drop table dbo.EventCount
GO
CREATE TABLE dbo.EventCount
(
      Dept int NOT NULL ,
      DateOnly datetime NOT NULL ,
      CountEvent int NOT NULL ,
      CONSTRAINT PK___1__15 PRIMARY KEY  CLUSTERED
      (
            Dept,
            DateOnly
      )
)
GO
```

The second table contains details of the departments that had posted events.

```
if exists (select * from sysobjects where id = object_id('dbo.EvtDepts')
                                          and sysstat & 0xf = 3)
      drop table dbo.EvtDepts
GO
CREATE TABLE dbo.EvtDepts
(
      Name char (50) NOT NULL ,
      ID int NOT NULL ,
      CanRead bit NOT NULL ,
      CanPostNew bit NOT NULL ,
      Symbol char (1) NOT NULL ,
      Color int NOT NULL ,
```

```
    Host char (20) NOT NULL ,
    CONSTRAINT PK___2__15 PRIMARY KEY  CLUSTERED
    (
        ID
    )
)
GO
```

Here is what the `proa2` database looks like, if you open up a new database project on it from Visual Studio:

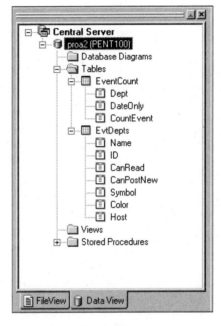

We use another database called `engevt` to simulate the (Engineering) departmental server. On the departmental server there are two tables The first is a table of the department details:

```
if exists (select * from sysobjects where id = object_id('dbo.Dept')
                                        and sysstat & 0xf = 3)
    drop table dbo.Dept
GO
CREATE TABLE dbo.Dept
(
    Name char (50) NOT NULL ,
    Number int NOT NULL ,
    CanRead bit NOT NULL ,
    CanPostNew bit NOT NULL ,
    Symbol char (1) NOT NULL ,
    Color int NOT NULL ,
    CONSTRAINT PK___1__15 PRIMARY KEY  CLUSTERED
    (
        Number
    )
)
GO
```

The second is a table of the events for that department:

```
if exists (select * from sysobjects where id = object_id('dbo.Events')
                                          and sysstat & 0xf = 3)
      drop table dbo.Events
GO
CREATE TABLE dbo.Events
(
      EvntID int NOT NULL ,
      Date datetime NOT NULL ,
      DateTime datetime NOT NULL ,
      Heading char (50) NOT NULL ,
      Hlink char (50) NOT NULL ,
      Location char (50) NOT NULL ,
      Organizer char (50) NOT NULL ,
      Details char (200) NOT NULL ,
      CONSTRAINT PK___2__15 PRIMARY KEY  CLUSTERED
      (
            EvntID
      )
)
GO
```

On the same departmental server, we also need to create two views, facilitating our queries via OLE DB. The first one, called FindTotal, gets the total count of events grouped by date.

```
if exists (select * from sysobjects where id = object_id('dbo.FindTotal')
                                          and sysstat & 0xf = 2)
      drop view dbo.FindTotal
GO
CREATE VIEW FindTotal AS
SELECT Events.Date AS Date, Count(*) AS Total
FROM Events
GROUP BY Events.Date
GO
```

The second one, called MaxEvent, obtains the maximum event ID in the table at any time. We will be using this whenever we need to add a new event to the Events table.

```
if exists (select * from sysobjects where id = object_id('dbo.MaxEvent')
                                          and sysstat & 0xf = 2)
      drop view dbo.MaxEvent
GO
CREATE VIEW MaxEvent AS
SELECT Max(EvntID) AS MaxID
FROM Events
GO
```

Here is what the final `engevt` database will look like, if you open up a database project on it within Visual Studio:

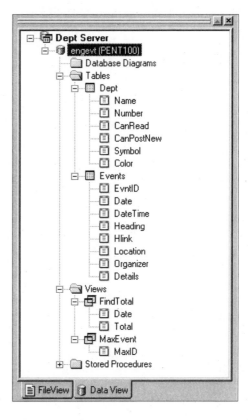

Setting up ODBC Data Sources

Next, we need to set up the two ODBC data sources, with one connection to each of the servers. We will be using the OLE DB provider for ODBC, in order to take advantage of the automatic transaction capabilities and connections pooling offered by the ODBC resource dispenser/manager. We will learn a lot more about what this means in the next chapter. For now, set up the first ODBC data source as follows.

Select the ODBC (32 bit) applet from the Control Panel, and then select the System DSN tab. From this tab, click the Add button.

- ❑ From the Create New Data Source dialog, double click the SQL Server driver, making sure that you have at least version 3.60.0315, or later.
- ❑ In the Configuration dialog, enter the following values:

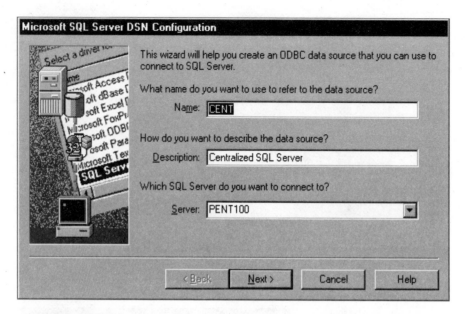

Replace the server name above with the server name where the tables are stored, and then press
Next>:

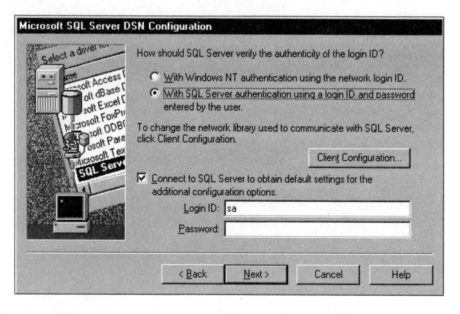

Enter the appropriate authentication information. In our case, we are using the default `sa` account with a blank password. Press Next>.

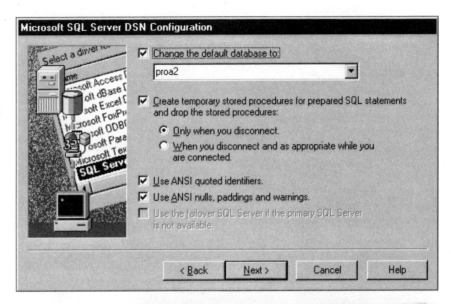

Make sure you have the database representing the central server selected here. In our case it was `proa2`. Take the default for the rest of the options. Press Next> twice and then press Finish on the last dialog, taking the defaults for the rest of the setup. You should then see the summary dialog:

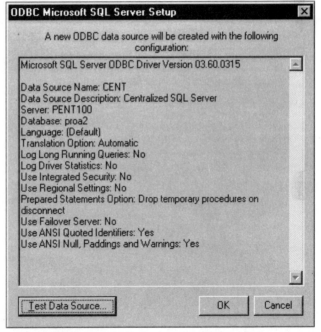

If everything is configured properly, you should be able to press the Test Data Source... button and get a reassuring response. If you do not get a successful response, make sure you have set the server name, database name, and authentication information correctly.

This completes the setup of the CENT system data source, simulating the centralized server. Repeat the procedure to create the ENG system data source. On the Configuration dialog, use 'Engineering Department SQL Server' as the description. This data source should point to the server and database where the departmental tables are kept. For now, in our code, we'll put the engevt database on the same server as the rest of the code.

Creating the Business Object Skeletal Projects

We will now create the skeletal projects for our business objects. Before we move on, though, one question constantly surfaces amongst designers of three-tiered component based systems: all these 'business objects' actually access databases directly – so, architecturally, are they really 'third-tier' data objects?

The answer is no, and the reason why will become clear when we examine Microsoft Transaction Server object states in Chapter 9. Briefly, these are actually objects that facilitate, or enforce, business rules above and beyond accessing the simple data stored in the database. The reason why they are bound to database access has to do with their need to maintain 'durable' state information. That is, they need to recover from machine and/or network crashes, and not lose any information that they were working with. The only reliable, easily accessible means to store durable state information is, currently, via databases.

A good example of a business object with durable state is our centralized server that maintains a consolidated, cached list of departments that currently have events posted – and the associated event count. The state that this business object maintains is architecturally dynamic (i.e. departments can add new events at any time). However, in order to keep this information durable (system crash survivable), we have used OLE DB to maintain the state within a SQL Server table.

Let us now get back to Visual Studio and create some projects for our business objects. We will be creating two DLLs, one for the central server, and one for the departmental server. Here is a brief tabulation and description of the components within each DLL and their functions.

DLL	Component	Comment
CentBusObj		This is the central server DLL containing all components for the central server.
	BoCentDeptsAdmin – cached event count update object	This is the count consolidator. It provides a method for the departmental server to update the event count information, in order to reflect the latest state of the system.
	BoDeptsFinder – access object to cached information, customized for ATLFinder mapping object	This object is used by ATLFinder.exe (object model presenter) to discover the departments that have events posted for a particular month.

Table Continued on Following Page

DLL	Component	Comment
DeptBusObj		This is the departmental server DLL containing all components running on the departmental server.
	BoDeptEvent – departmental event administration	Provides interface and methods to add and delete events for the department. Will co-ordinate with centralized server to ensure the cached centralized count is accurate and up-to-date. Also supports methods for getting all the events for the department (used for testing and debugging), and for getting all the events for the department in a specified month (used by CViscal clients).
	LocalDeptAdmin – DB configuration support	This is not implemented in our case, but can be implemented to support modification of department information in the departmental database.

We will have class diagrams, and more in-depth coverage of these business objects in the next chapter. The above tabulation should be enough to let us proceed with building the OLE DB data access code required by each component.

First, we will create the DLL for the two business objects:

1. From the File menu, select **New...**
2. From the **Project** tab, choose **ATL COM AppWizard** and call the new project `CentBusObj`.
3. In the **ATL COM AppWizard** dialog box, select **DLL** for Server Type, and make sure the **Support MTS** box is checked. This will add the MTS required headers and libraries to your code and will also generate the appropriate code for MTS support. We will have a lot more to say about MTS support in the next chapter.
4. Generate the skeletal project.

Repeat the above to create the departmental server object, calling the project `DeptBusObj`.

With the `DeptBusObj` workspace open, add a new ATL object by selecting **Insert** from the menu, and **New ATL Object...**
From the **Objects** selection box, select **MS Transaction Server**:

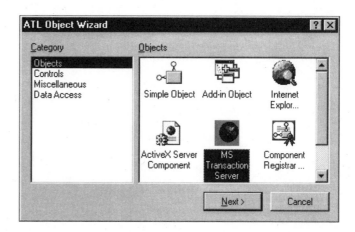

Press the <u>N</u>ext> button. We
will call this first component
`BoDeptEvent`:

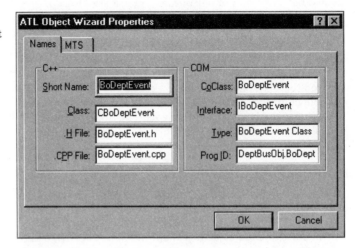

Select the MTS tab, and
check the following:

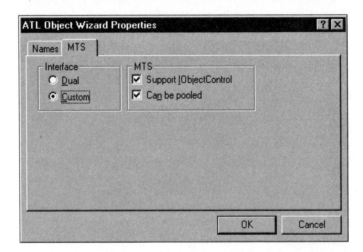

We will be using non-Automation compatible interfaces for their additional performance (we already
have `ATLFinder` and `ATLDept` layer to provide the Automation compatible access layer) and
therefore we have selected Custom rather than Dual. Regarding the MTS checkboxes, we will have
much more to say about `IObjectControl` and object pooling in the next chapter. Please bear with
me for now. Press OK and let the wizard generate the skeleton code for the component.

Now, repeat the same steps and generate the skeleton code for another component called
`LocalDeptAdmin` in the `DeptBusObj` workspace.

Finally, close the `DeptBusObj` workspace and open the `CentBusObj` workspace. In this project,
add two MTS components, one called `BoCentDeptAdmin` and another one called `BoDeptsFinder`.
When you are creating the `BoDeptsFinder` component, override the default interface name
(`IBoDeptsFinder`) and call it `IBoDeptCache` instead.

This completes the generation of our business object skeletons. If you had trouble with this, you can download the code. Simply open the workspace under the \DeptBusObj and \CentBusObj to gain access to all the files of the projects.

Putting OLE DB Templates to work

We have created the SQL Server databases, set up the ODBC data sources, and created two skeleton MTS-compatible components. We are ready now for some OLE DB coding. We will proceed to add data access ability to the business components. The order we follow will be the same as in the earlier *Typical Consumer Uses of OLE DB* section; this will allow us to contrast the steps required and the effort saved.

Understanding ATL 3 OLE DB Consumer Templates

ATL 3 provides a very thin, yet timesaving layer over the basic OLE DB objects. There are no new object models to learn. Every one of the OLE DB objects and its full functionality is still available. However, the ATL 3 wrapping will provide reasonable defaults wherever feasible; when setting properties or making method calls. It will also attempt to provide implementations for the most frequently used actions when working with these objects. Here is a high-level diagram of the major OLE DB template classes and their relationships:

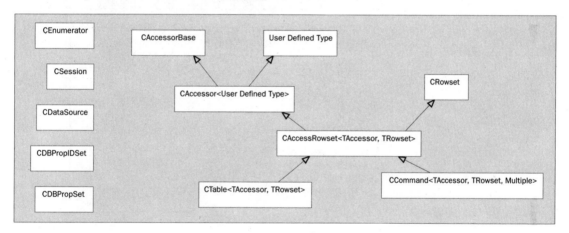

For simplicity, not all classes are shown in the above diagram. What is shown, however, should be familiar from our previous discussion of OLE DB. These classes are also sufficient for us to complete our data access coding.

The User Defined Type in the hierarchy allows us to define the user record (a C++ class with member variables) that will be used within the CAccessor class (via the IAccessor interface) to transfer field values, or command parameters, to and from the rowset, or parameterized commands.

At the bottom of the chart, the factoring between CTable<> and CCommand<> reflects the usage of OLE DB where we may be dealing either with the resulting rowset from IOpenRowset (a table/index) or from ICommand (a query). The CAccessorBase concrete class provides much of the implementation to simplify accessor handling. We simply define our class variables in the user-defined class, and call the appropriate mapping macros to get the inherited functionality.

The combination of the ATL OLE DB Consumer wizard and the template implementation makes the coding of most common tasks straightforward and concise. The next few sections will provide evidence for this claim.

Revisiting Data Access Scenarios with OLE DB Templates

It is time to fulfill our promise, and show how the complex scenarios, detailed earlier using raw OLE DB, can be simplified via ATL 3 OLE DB templates and the associated wizards. Along the way, we will fill in vital durable state functionality for our business objects. You may want to contrast the raw operations necessary by comparing the two lists. Here again, as a refresher, are the common access scenarios that we will be covering, – this time using ATL 3 OLE DB templates:

❑   Reading records from a table
❑   Obtaining results of a query
❑   Obtaining results of a parameterized query
❑   Adding a record to a table
❑   Deleting a record from a table

Reading Records from a Table

Let us implement a method for the departmental server which will read, and return to the caller, all records in the Events table.

In the DeptBusObj ClassView, select the IBoDeptEvent interface and add the following method:

```
HRESULT getAllEvents([out] long * lNumEvents, [out,size_is(,*lNumEvents)]
                    EVTDETAIL ** pevtDet);
```

Translated, what this IDL says is that the component being called will return an array of EVTDETAIL structures, of size *lNumEvents, to the caller. The caller will supply the storage for the single EVTDETAIL* pointer, and the component will allocate all the storage for the array members. The caller must freethe storage upon receiving the array data. As usual, the memory allocation is done via CoTaskMemAlloc() calls, which are also used by the marshaler.

To make sure the IDL compiles OK, we must add the following structure to the top of the DeptBusObj.idl file:

```
typedef struct {
long lEvtID;
DATE dtDateTime;
BSTR Heading;
BSTR Hlink;
BSTR Location;
BSTR Organizer;
BSTR Details;
} EVTDETAIL;
```

We notice immediately that `getAllEvents()` is definitely not an Automation compatible method – the default Automation marshaler definitely does not have the knowledge to marshal the `EVTDETAIL**` structure. This means that we must provide our own proxy/stub (more on this later) for marshaling and ensure that the proxy/stub is registered properly.

Next, we will create the OLE DB consumer code to get the data. From the open `DeptBusObj` workspace, select **Insert** from the menu and select **New ATL Object...**

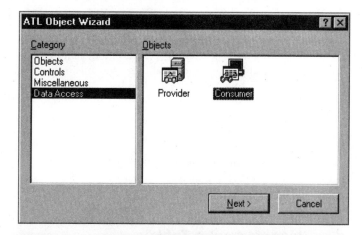

Now, in the **Category** selection box, select **Data Access** and in the **Objects** box, select **Consumer**. You should be greeted with this screen:

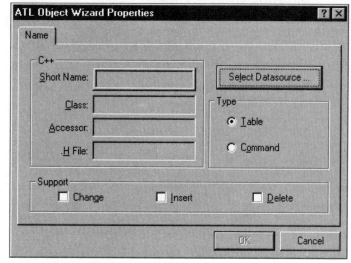

Select **Table** for the type to use `IOpenRowset` functionality.

Note the **Change, Insert** *and* **Delete** *checkboxes. These will generate code to requested properties of the final* `rowset` *if we check them; in this case we are only interested in read access. For example, if* **Insert** *or* **Delete** *is checked, a* `rowset` *supporting* `IRowsetChange` *will be requested.*

Press the Select Datasource button:

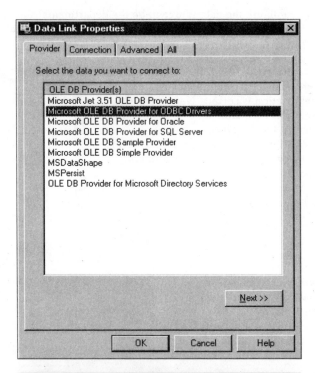

You can select the appropriate provider from this box. We will select the OLE DB Provider for ODBC Drivers. Press the Next>> button or the Connection tab:

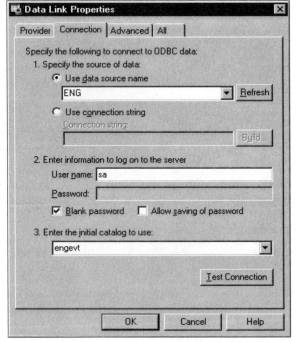

Here we configure the data source to be the departmental source called ENG. We will be authenticating using the default sa account, and the initial catalog will be engevt, our departmental database.

You can also press **Test Connection** to verify that the connection is functional and all parameterization is correct. Next, press **OK**, and then select the table for IOpenRowset from the list that appears:

In our case, we select dbo.Events as this is where the events we are interested in are stored.

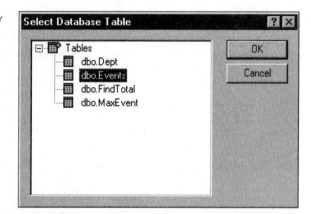

Press **OK** to continue. Change the default **Short Name** of the consumer class to dboAllEvents, and press **OK** to start code generation.

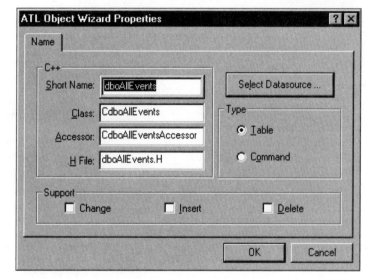

That's it! All the code required in the ten steps in the *Reading Records from a Table* section has been generated flawlessly. We are ready to use it to send data back to our client.

Examining the Generated Code

Taking a look at the generated code will give us some idea of how the OLE DB templates work. The two classes generated are:

- ☐ CdboAllEventsAccessor – the user-defined class (user record)
- ☐ CdboAllEvents – a CTable-templated class, parameterized by an accessor based on the user record

Both classes are completely defined in the generated dboAllEvents.h file.

Here is what the generated user record class looks like:

```
class CdboAllEventsAccessor
{
public:
     LONG m_EvntID;
     DBTIMESTAMP m_Date;
     DBTIMESTAMP m_DateTime;
     TCHAR m_Heading[51];
     TCHAR m_Hlink[51];
     TCHAR m_Location[51];
     TCHAR m_Organizer[51];
     TCHAR m_Details[201];
```

Notice the member variables are automatically created (based on metadata available from the database) for use by IAccessor when transferring data to and from rows in the owset.

```
BEGIN_COLUMN_MAP(CdboAllEventsAccessor)
     COLUMN_ENTRY(1, m_EvntID)
     COLUMN_ENTRY(2, m_Date)
     COLUMN_ENTRY(3, m_DateTime)
     COLUMN_ENTRY(4, m_Heading)
     COLUMN_ENTRY(5, m_Hlink)
     COLUMN_ENTRY(6, m_Location)
     COLUMN_ENTRY(7, m_Organizer)
     COLUMN_ENTRY(8, m_Details)
END_COLUMN_MAP()
```

This set of macros map the column ordinal number to the member variables. The CAccessor-derived class will use this information to handle the accessor and create binding to the variables.

The remaining function in this class is a convenient function for zeroing the member variables.

```
     void ClearRecord()
     {
          memset(this, 0, sizeof(*this));
     }
};
```

Here is the definition of the CTable template class. Notice the inheritance of accessor functionality through nested templates.

```
class CdboAllEvents : public CTable<CAccessor<CdboAllEventsAccessor> >
{
public:
     HRESULT Open()
     {
          HRESULT  hr;
```

```
        hr = OpenDataSource();
        if (FAILED(hr))
            return hr;

        return OpenRowset();
    }
```

This is the 'do everything' Open() method. If you do not need any special handling, using this class is reduced to a two-step process: instantiate it, and call Open()!

Internally, we can see that it is doing a lot of the work behind the scenes, including initializing the data source, creating a session through a call to OpenDataSource() and then opening the rowset via IOpenRowset. Here is what OpenDataSource() looks like.

```
    HRESULT OpenDataSource()
    {
        HRESULT  hr;
        CDataSource db;
        CDBPropSet  dbinit(DBPROPSET_DBINIT);

        dbinit.AddProperty(DBPROP_AUTH_PASSWORD, OLESTR(""));
        dbinit.AddProperty(DBPROP_AUTH_PERSIST_SENSITIVE_AUTHINFO,
                                                    false);
        dbinit.AddProperty(DBPROP_AUTH_USERID, OLESTR("sa"));
        dbinit.AddProperty(DBPROP_INIT_DATASOURCE, OLESTR("ENG"));
        dbinit.AddProperty(DBPROP_INIT_PROMPT, (short)4);
        dbinit.AddProperty(DBPROP_INIT_LCID, (long)1033);
        dbinit.AddProperty(DBPROP_INIT_CATALOG, OLESTR("engevt"));
```

The existence of the CDBPropSet class greatly simplifies (and makes it humanly possible to understand) the setting of database properties. Most properties above are self-explanatory.

```
        hr = db.Open(_T("MSDASQL"), &dbinit);
```

The ODBC driver for SQL Server is called MSDASQL, and it is asked for by name here.

```
        if (FAILED(hr))
            return hr;

        return m_session.Open(db);
    }
```

The member m_session implements the required opening of the session.

Here is OpenRowset(). The CTable<>::Open() call will invoke IOpenRowset on the dbo.Events table:

```
        HRESULT OpenRowset()
        {
return CTable<CAccessor<CdboAllEventsAccessor>>
                                    ::Open(m_session, _T("dbo.Events"));
        }
```

The CSession member contains the session object. This object is useful for creating commands (via IDBCreateCommand), opening rowsets on a table (via IOpenRowset), or managing local transactions (via ILocalTransaction).

```
        Csession  m_session;
    };
```

This generated code is sufficent for a surprisingly large number of data access scenarios. Even if you do not use the generated code, it provides some insight into how the ATL 3 OLE DB template classes are meant to be used together.

Implementing the getAllEvents() Method

Now we have a consumer object, we need to provide an implementation for the getAllEvents() method we added earlier – it is in the BoDeptEvent.cpp file from the DeptBusObj project. The method will simply obtain, and return to the caller, all the events within a department, regardless of date.

The first thing to notice is that we restrict the maximum number of events returned to 20 here, for testing purposes.

```
#define MAX_EVENTS 20

STDMETHODIMP CBoDeptEvent::getAllEvents(long* lNumEvents,
                                        EVTDETAIL** pevtDet)
{
      ATLTRACE(_T("CBoDeptEvent::getAllEvents called..."));
      USES_CONVERSION;
```

We will be doing some TCHAR to BSTR conversions later, and this macro allows us to use the great conversion routines in Atlconv.h.

```
        (*pevtDet) = reinterpret_cast<EVTDETAIL *>(
                        CoTaskMemAlloc(sizeof(EVTDETAIL) * MAX_EVENTS));

        if ((*pevtDet) == NULL)
        {
            ATLTRACE(_T("CBoDeptEvent::CoTaskMemAlloc FAILED!!..."));
            m_spObjectContext->SetAbort();
            return E_OUTOFMEMORY;
        }
```

Here, we are allocating the memory to hold the events to be returned. `CoTaskMemAlloc()` is used so the proxy can free it after marshalling.

```
long evtCount = 0;
CdboAllEvents  tpEvents;
if( tpEvents.Open() != S_OK)
{
      // not necessary for read, but do for good form
      m_spObjectContext->SetAbort();
      return E_FAIL;
}
```

Here's our 'instantiate and open' object, replacing all the complex and tedious steps of raw OLE DB coding. Ignore the `SetAbort()` MTS calls for now, we will talk about them in the next chapter.

```
while((tpEvents.MoveNext() == S_OK) && (evtCount < MAX_EVENTS))
      {
      // copy into the return array for marshalling
      (*pevtDet)[evtCount].lEvtID = tpEvents.m_EvntID;
      CDateTime tpDateTime(tpEvents.m_DateTime);
      (*pevtDet)[evtCount].dtDateTime = tpDateTime.ConvertToDATE();
      BSTR a = (*pevtDet)[evtCount].Heading =
                  T2BSTR(tpEvents.m_Heading);    // these are TCHARs
      BSTR b = (*pevtDet)[evtCount].Hlink = T2BSTR(tpEvents.m_Hlink);
      (*pevtDet)[evtCount].Location = T2BSTR(tpEvents.m_Location);
      (*pevtDet)[evtCount].Organizer = T2BSTR(tpEvents.m_Organizer);
      (*pevtDet)[evtCount].Details = T2BSTR(tpEvents.m_Details);
      evtCount++;
      }
```

Here, we loop through the rowset and fetch data, one row at a time, to put into the member variables of our user-defined class (through an accessor, internally). For each record, we copy the value over to the buffer just allocated. We need to convert the BSTR parameters from the TCHAR member variables (actually doing a `SysAllocString()` underneath) using the `Atlconv.h` macros.

You may recognize the `CDateTime` class from the last chapter — we'll come back to that in a moment.

```
*lNumEvents = evtCount;
```

Finally, we set the count of elements so that the marshaler will know the size of the marshaled array, and the caller will know the size of the returned data stream.

```
m_spObjectContext->SetComplete();
tpEvents.Close();
return S_OK;
}
```

Finally, we need to add a simplified version of `CalUtils.h` and `CalUtils.cpp` from the `Cviscal` project. They provide conversion routines for date variables through the `CDateTime` class. Add the files to the project and make the following changes...

In `CalUtils.h,` **comment out** `Stdafx.h, CalDefs.h` **and** `Int2TString()`

```
#ifndef       _CALUTILS_H
#define _CALUTILS_H
//#include "StdAfx.h"
//#include "CalDefs.h"
#include <time.h>
#include <math.h>

//tstring Int2TString( int i );
```

Add the following method definitions, and comment out a few as shown, for good measure:

```
class CDateTime
{
public:

...

    CDateTime(const DBTIMESTAMP& sysTime);

...

    // operator tstring() const;            // convert to tstring
    // tstring Format( LPCTSTR fmt ) const; // pass format string as
                                            // per strftime()
    bool ConvertToDBTIMESTAMP(DBTIMESTAMP * pDbTime);

...

    // TCHAR      m_buf[BUFSIZ];            // for debugging
};
```

Then comment out every class definition apart from `CDateTime` and `CDateTimeDiff`.

In `CalUtils.cpp,` **again comment out** `CalDefs.h`, **and the implementation of the** `Int2TString()` **method. All** `wsprintf()` **statements need to be commented out as well.**

Add the following constructor:

```
CDateTime::CDateTime(const DBTIMESTAMP& sysTime)
{
    *this = CDateTime(sysTime.year, sysTime.month, sysTime.day,
            sysTime.hour, sysTime.minute, sysTime.second);
}

...

/*CDateTime::operator tstring() const
{
    return tstring( (t == (time_t)-1) ? "" : _tasctime(localtime( &t )) );
}
```

```
tstring CDateTime::Format( LPCTSTR fmt ) const
{
    struct tm* pt;

    if ( (t == (time_t)-1) || (pt =localtime( &t )) == NULL )
        return tstring( NULL );
    else {
        TCHAR buf[100];
        memset( buf, 0, sizeof(buf) );
        size_t n = _tcsftime( buf, sizeof(buf), fmt, pt );
        return tstring( buf );
    }
}*/

    ...

bool CDateTime::ConvertToDBTIMESTAMP(DBTIMESTAMP * pDbTime)
{
    struct tm*     tm_t = localtime( &t );

    if ( ! tm_t )
        return false;

    pDbTime->year        = tm_t->tm_year + 1900;
    pDbTime->month     = tm_t->tm_mon + 1;
    pDbTime->day         = tm_t->tm_mday;
    pDbTime->hour         = tm_t->tm_hour;
    pDbTime->minute     = tm_t->tm_min;
    pDbTime->second     = tm_t->tm_sec;
    pDbTime->fraction = 01;
    return true;
}
```

Then, comment out the `CMonthInfo` and `CRect` implementations. Finally, add these lines to the `BoDeptEvent.cpp` file:

```
#include "dboAllEvents.h"
#include "CalUtils.h"
```

Obtaining Results from a Query

The steps for creating code that obtains results from a query are exactly the same as those for a table. The only difference is in selecting **Command** instead of **Table** in the wizard selection screen.

The ATL 3 wrapping makes the subtle differences in actual interface calls a non-issue. This is true as long as the resulting rowset will be used for read-only purposes. If you need to change, insert, or delete capabilities from the rowset; there may be differences in behavior between a table-based rowset or query-based rowset depending on the provider, data source, and nature of the query.

Obtaining a Result from a Parameterized Query

Working with parameterized queries is a little more interesting.

First, add a method to the `IBoDeptCache` interface on the `CentBusObj` with the following specifications:

```
HRESULT getEventDepts([in] DATE dtMonthYear,
                      [out] long* lNumDepts,
                      [out, size_is(,*lNumDepts)] EVTDEPT** pevtDept);
```

This method fetches department records from the `dbo.EvtDepts` table, but only for departments with events occurring in the month specified in the input. This calls for a relatively complex parameterized query. The query we will be using is:

```
SELECT * FROM dbo.EvtDepts
WHERE ID IN (SELECT DISTINCT Dept FROM dbo.EventCount
WHERE datepart(year,DateOnly)= ? AND datepart(month,DateOnly)=?)
```

Notice that not only is the query complicated, it is also quite specific to the SQL Server dialect of the SQL language. We can see two parameters for the query, one for the year and another one for the month.

To deal with this query, you'll first need to add this structure definition to the `CentBusObj.idl` file:

```
typedef struct
{
    long lDeptID;
    BSTR bstrName;
    BSTR bstrSymbol;
    OLE_COLOR clrColor;
    BSTR bstrHost;
    VARIANT_BOOL vbCanRead;
    VARIANT_BOOL vbCanPostNew;
} EVTDEPT;
```

To implement the method, we need to first generate our OLE DB code. Here are the steps:

1. Ensure the `CentBusObj` workspace is open.

2. Select **Insert** from menu and select **New ATL Object...**

3. Select **Data Access** in the **Category** box, and **Consumer** in the **Objects** box.

4. In the **ATL Object Wizard Properties** dialog, select **Command** as **Type** and press the **Select Datasource** button.

5. Choose **Microsoft OLE DB Provider for ODBC Drivers** as the provider, press **Next >>**

6. Select the data source to be the central server – in our case, **CENT** – and then enter the authentication information – in our case, sa – leaving the password blank. Select the initial catalog, proa2 here. Finally test the connection by pressing the **Test Connection** button.

7. Press the **OK** button .

8. From the list of tables, select `dbo.EvtDepts`.

9. Back in the **ATL Object Wizard Properties** box, accept the short name `dboEvtDepts`.

10. Click **OK** to generate the code.

Examining and Modifying the Generated Code

Here is the generated code, in dboEvtDepts.h, with modifications highlighted.

```
class CdboEvtDeptsAccessor
{
public:
      TCHAR m_Name[51];
      LONG m_ID;
      VARIANT_BOOL m_CanRead;
      VARIANT_BOOL m_CanPostNew;
      TCHAR m_Symbol[2];
      LONG m_Color;
      TCHAR m_Host[21];
      LONG m_ParamYear;
      LONG m_ParamMonth;
```

The user-defined class (user record) begins as usual, with the generated member variables to hold the values to be transferred from the rows. However, we add in the two parameter values we'll need shortly. We will be using the same accessor for parameter input and row data output.

```
BEGIN_COLUMN_MAP(CdboEvtDeptsAccessor)
      COLUMN_ENTRY(1, m_Name)
      COLUMN_ENTRY(2, m_ID)
      COLUMN_ENTRY_TYPE(3, DBTYPE_BOOL, m_CanRead)
      COLUMN_ENTRY_TYPE(4, DBTYPE_BOOL, m_CanPostNew)
      COLUMN_ENTRY(5, m_Symbol)
      COLUMN_ENTRY(6, m_Color)
      COLUMN_ENTRY(7, m_Host)
END_COLUMN_MAP()
```

The standard column map, gives information to the accessor implementation for data binding. We now need to add a **parameter map**, this is an accessor mapping between the C++ member variables and the parameters in the parameterized SQL query:

```
// add our parameter map here
BEGIN_PARAM_MAP(CdboEvtDeptsAccessor)
      SET_PARAM_TYPE(DBPARAMIO_INPUT)
      COLUMN_ENTRY(1, m_ParamYear)
      SET_PARAM_TYPE(DBPARAMIO_INPUT)
      COLUMN_ENTRY(2, m_ParamMonth)
END_PARAM_MAP()
```

The parameter map notifies the accessor implementation that there are two input parameters and they map to the two member variables respectively. Next, make the following changes to the generated SQL command:

```
DEFINE_COMMAND(CdboEvtDeptsAccessor, _T(" \
      SELECT  *  \
      FROM dbo.EvtDepts where ID in \
      (select distinct Dept from dbo.EventCount WHERE  \
      datepart(year,DateOnly)= ? and datepart(month,DateOnly)=?)"))
```

We must define the command text which the command object implementation will use to call ICommandText. The generated code just provides a dummy 'select all' statement. That's all the changes we need to make to the accessor object.

The second generated class is now Ccommand based rather than Ctable based:

```
class CdboEvtDepts : public CCommand<CAccessor<CdboEvtDeptsAccessor> >
{
public:
    HRESULT Open()
    {
        HRESULT hr;

        hr = OpenDataSource();
        if (FAILED(hr))
            return hr;

        return OpenRowset();
    }
    HRESULT OpenDataSource()
    {
        HRESULT hr;
        CDataSource db;
        CDBPropSet dbinit(DBPROPSET_DBINIT);

        dbinit.AddProperty(DBPROP_AUTH_PASSWORD, OLESTR(""));
        dbinit.AddProperty(DBPROP_AUTH_PERSIST_SENSITIVE_AUTHINFO,
                                                        false);
        dbinit.AddProperty(DBPROP_AUTH_USERID, OLESTR("sa"));
        dbinit.AddProperty(DBPROP_INIT_DATASOURCE, OLESTR("CENT"));
        dbinit.AddProperty(DBPROP_INIT_MODE, (long)1);
        dbinit.AddProperty(DBPROP_INIT_PROMPT, (short)4);
        dbinit.AddProperty(DBPROP_INIT_LCID, (long)1033);
        dbinit.AddProperty(DBPROP_INIT_CATALOG, OLESTR("proa2"));
        hr = db.Open(_T("MSDASQL"), &dbinit);
        if (FAILED(hr))
            return hr;

        return m_session.Open(db);
    }
    HRESULT OpenRowset()
    {
        return CCommand<CAccessor<CdboEvtDeptsAccessor> >
                                            ::Open(m_session);
    }
    CSession m_session;
};
```

In general, we see the same coding above as in the CTable<> case, allowing for 'instantiate and open' usage. In this case, we must also initialize the two variables used as parameters after instantiation, before calling Open(). Let us put this into the BoDeptsFinder::getEventDepts() method implementation.

Implementing the getEventDepts() method

Since the general data flow is identical to the `getAllEvents()` method shown earlier, you will see a very similar coding pattern here.

First, add the data accessor includes and constant defines to `BoDeptsFinder.cpp`:

```
#include "stdafx.h"
#include "CentBusObj.h"
#include "BoDeptsFinder.h"
#include "dboEvtDepts.h"
#include "CalUtils.h"
#define MAX_EVENTCOUNTS 100
#define MAX_DEPTS 5
```

Next, allocate the buffer to be used for transferring the array of structures.

```
STDMETHODIMP CBoDeptsFinder::getEventDepts(DATE dtMonthYear,
                                           long *lNumDepts, EVTDEPT **pevtDept)
{
    ATLTRACE(_T("CBoDeptsFinder::getEventDepts called..."));

    (*pevtDept) = reinterpret_cast<EVTDEPT *>(
                        CoTaskMemAlloc(sizeof(EVTDEPT) * MAX_DEPTS));
    if ((*pevtDept) == NULL)
    {
        ATLTRACE(_T("CBoDeptsFinder::CoTaskMemAlloc FAILED!!..."));
        m_spObjectContext->SetAbort();
        return E_OUTOFMEMORY;
    }
```

We store the input date in a `CDateTime` variable, this means that we must include the modified `Calutils.cpp` and `Calutils.h` as before.

```
    USES_CONVERSION;
    // Set the current record
    CDateTime dtWorkDate(dtMonthYear);
```

Next, we set the query parameters and call the `Open()` method.

```
    // fill the department table up
    CdboEvtDepts tpDept;
    long deptCount = 0;
    tpDept.m_ParamYear = dtWorkDate.GetYear();
    tpDept.m_ParamMonth = dtWorkDate.GetMonth();
    if( tpDept.Open() != S_OK)
    {
        m_spObjectContext->SetAbort();
        tpDept.Close();
        return E_FAIL;
    }
```

Finally, we loop through and transfer the data from the rowset, through the accessor, into the marshaling memory buffer.

```
while( ( tpDept.MoveNext() == S_OK) && (deptCount < MAX_DEPTS))
    {
     // copy into the return array for marshaling

    (*pevtDept)[deptCount].bstrName = T2BSTR(tpDept.m_Name);
    (*pevtDept)[deptCount].lDeptID = tpDept.m_ID;
    (*pevtDept)[deptCount].vbCanRead = tpDept.m_CanRead;
    (*pevtDept)[deptCount].vbCanPostNew = tpDept.m_CanPostNew;
    (*pevtDept)[deptCount].bstrSymbol = T2BSTR(tpDept.m_Symbol);
    (*pevtDept)[deptCount].clrColor = tpDept.m_Color;
    (*pevtDept)[deptCount].bstrHost = T2BSTR(tpDept.m_Host);
    deptCount++;
    }
```

Setting the number of departments completes our code.

```
    *lNumDepts = deptCount;
    tpDept.Close();

    m_spObjectContext->SetComplete();
    return S_OK;
}
```

So far, all our activity has centered around read-only OLE DB rowsets. Let us look at a couple of examples that change data.

Adding a Record to a Table

Add a method to the IBoDeptEvent interface in the DeptBusObj project with the following signature:

```
HRESULT addEvent([in] DATE dtOnDate,
                 [in] BSTR bstrHeading,
                 [in] BSTR bstrHlink,
                 [in] BSTR bstrLocation,
                 [in] BSTR bstrOrganizer,
                 [in] BSTR bstrDetails,
                 [out, retval] long * plID);
```

This method will allow the insertion of a new record into the dbo.Events table. All the values for the new record are passed as parameters of the method call.

For this we need to create an OLE DB rowset, based on the dbo.Events table, that can be used to insert new records.

This part of the puzzle is actually trivial. Follow the same procedure as in the *Reading Records from a Table* section, but in the **ATL Wizard Property Dialog**, make sure the **Insert** box is checked. When you are going through the wizard, make sure you give the new accessor stack the name of dboEventsTbl.

In fact, the only difference in the generated code is in the `OpenRowset()` method of the generated `CTable<>` template class:

```
HRESULT OpenRowset()
    {
    // Set properties for open
    CDBPropSet  propset(DBPROPSET_ROWSET);
    propset.AddProperty(DBPROP_IRowsetChange, true);
    propset.AddProperty(DBPROP_UPDATABILITY, DBPROPVAL_UP_INSERT);

    return CTable<CAccessor<CdboEventsTblAccessor> >
                        ::Open(m_session, _T("dbo.Events"), &propset);
    }
```

This shouldn't be surprising. The only additional work that we need to do, even if we code manually, would be to set the desired properties of the rowset when `IOpenRowset` is called. This is exactly what the code above accomplishes.

Now for the hard part. As with any data modification or deletion task, the toughest part is to ensure the integrity of the remaining data. This will become more obvious when we implement the method.

Implementing the addEvent() Method

We need to answer one question: what event number will the new record have? In situations where there may be concurrent users calling the `addEvent()` method, there may be no simple answer. In our case, however, we are assuming a single departmental administrator performing updates – this problem is much easier to solve.

This is the purpose of the `dbo.MaxEvent` view. It will provide us with the current largest event ID. This will be used to provide a unique ID for each newly added event (assuming no contention, as there is only one departmental administrator per department). To implement the `addEvent()` method, we must create one more OLE DB accessor stack – this time, a read-only `command`, based on the query:

```
SELECT * from dbo.MaxEvent
```

Make sure you name this new stack `dboMaxEvent`.

With the new accessor stack defined, here is the code to implement the `addEvent()` method:

```
STDMETHODIMP CBoDeptEvent::addEvent(DATE dtOnDate, BSTR bstrHeading,
                                    BSTR bstrHlink, BSTR bstrLocation,
                                    BSTR bstrOrganizer, BSTR bstrDetails,
                                    long *plID)
{
        USES_CONVERSION;
        ATLTRACE(_T("CBoDeptEvent::addEvent called..."));

        CdboEventsTbl evtTblWork;
        CdboMaxEvent evtMaxID;
```

```
if (evtTblWork.Open() != S_OK)
{
     m_spObjectContext->SetAbort();
     evtTblWork.Close();
     return E_FAIL;
}
// locate the current max ID
if(evtMaxID.Open() != S_OK)
{
     m_spObjectContext->SetAbort();
     evtMaxID.Close();
     return E_FAIL;
}
```

The above code instantiates and opens both of our accessors, one for the event table itself, the other one for locating the maximum ID.

```
evtMaxID.MoveFirst();

// use ID that is 1 larger than MAX
evtTblWork.m_EvntID = evtMaxID.m_MaxID + 1;
evtMaxID.Close();   // that's all we need this for
```

We extract the maximal ID, add one, and store it in the table accessor as the new ID.

```
// set data into the current record
CDateTime dtWorkDate(dtOnDate);
DBTIMESTAMP dbtsWorkTimestamp;
dtWorkDate.ConvertToDBTIMESTAMP(&dbtsWorkTimestamp);
evtTblWork.m_DateTime = dbtsWorkTimestamp;
dbtsWorkTimestamp.hour = 0;
dbtsWorkTimestamp.minute = 0;
dbtsWorkTimestamp.second = 0;
evtTblWork.m_Date = dbtsWorkTimestamp;

_tcscpy(evtTblWork.m_Details, OLE2T(bstrDetails));
_tcscpy(evtTblWork.m_Heading, OLE2T(bstrHeading));
_tcscpy(evtTblWork.m_Hlink, OLE2T(bstrHlink));
_tcscpy(evtTblWork.m_Location, OLE2T(bstrLocation));
_tcscpy(evtTblWork.m_Organizer, OLE2T(bstrOrganizer));
```

We then stuff the rest of the fields into the table accessor.

```
if (evtTblWork.Insert() != S_OK)
{
     m_spObjectContext->SetAbort();
     evtTblWork.Close();

     return E_FAIL;
}
```

Finally, we call `Insert()`, essentially an `IRowsetChange::InsertRow()`, completing the request.

```
    evtTblWork.Close();
    m_spObjectContext->SetComplete();
    return S_OK;
}
```

Make sure you have added the #includes for the OLE DB accessors at the top of the file:

```
#include "stdafx.h"
#include "DeptBusObj.h"
#include "BoDeptEvent.h"
#include "dboAllEvents.h"
#include "dboMaxEvent.h"
#include "dboEventsTbl.h"
```

Next, let us take a look at how to delete a record from a table.

Deleting a Record from a Table

Add a method with the following signature to the `IBoDeptEvent` interface in the `DeptBusObj` project:

```
HRESULT delEvent([in] long lEventID, [out,retval] long * lSuccess);
```

This method provides for the deletion of an existing event, given its event ID number.

Again, we could follow the step in the *Reading Records from a Table* section and create another accessor stack. However, there is an easier way. Since we know that the generated code will only have very minor modifications from the `dboEventsTbl` stack, we will instead change `dboEventsTbl` to work with our deletion.

This involves the following one line change in the properties setting, found in the `dboEventsTbl.h` file:

```
HRESULT OpenRowset()
    {
    // Set properties for open
    CDBPropSet  propset(DBPROPSET_ROWSET);
    propset.AddProperty(DBPROP_IRowsetChange, true);
    propset.AddProperty(DBPROP_UPDATABILITY, DBPROPVAL_UP_INSERT |
                                             DBPROPVAL_UP_DELETE );

    return CTable<CAccessor<CdboEventsTblAccessor> >
                        ::Open(m_session, _T("dbo.Events"), &propset);
    }
```

Implementing the delEvent() Method

The only complexity in implementing event deletion is locating the event to be deleted. In our case, we simply loop through the rowset until we find the event with the matching ID.

Here is the method implementation:

```
STDMETHODIMP CBoDeptEvent::delEvent(long lEventID, long *lSuccess)
{
        CdboEventsTbl evtTblWork;
        if( evtTblWork.Open() != S_OK)
        {
              m_spObjectContext->SetAbort();
              evtTblWork.Close();
              return E_FAIL;
        }
```

First, we instantiate and open the accessor stack.

```
        bool tpDeleteFlag = false;

        while( evtTblWork.MoveNext() == S_OK)
              {
                    if (evtTblWork.m_EvntID  == lEventID)
                    {
                    evtTblWork.Delete();   // delete the row
                    tpDeleteFlag = true;
                    break;
                    }
              }
```

We reset a delete flag, then loop through the rowset until we find the required event ID. If we find it, we call `Delete()`, really `IRowsetChange::DeleteRows()`, set the flag, and break from the loop.

```
        if( tpDeleteFlag == false)
        {
              m_spObjectContext->SetAbort();
              evtTblWork.Close();
              return E_FAIL;
        }
```

If we don't find the row, the operation fails.

```
        m_spObjectContext->SetComplete();
        return S_OK;
}
```

We ask you to hold your urge to compile and test the project at this time! It is incomplete. In the next chapter, we will be adding several new methods to the interfaces, and more OLE DB accessor stacks for them. You can find the code for the complete project (including additional code from the next chapter) in the \DeptBusObj and \CentBusObj directories of the source code distribution.

The Exciting Road Ahead

In this chapter, we have coded two middle-tier objects that will present an Automation compatible object model for scripting and for our Visual Calendar clients. We then examined Microsoft's data access technologies and saw how they are rapidly migrating to Universal Data Access using OLE DB. Programming in raw OLE DB is not fun, but we've seen how ATL 3's OLE DB templates come to the rescue. We have thus been able to implement various methods in our middle tier business objects.

Unfortunately, we cannot test the new OLE DB components at the moment. This is because they have been created as MTS components and will require a configured MTS system for proper operation. And that's the subject of the next chapter, where we'll complete the coding of the business objects.

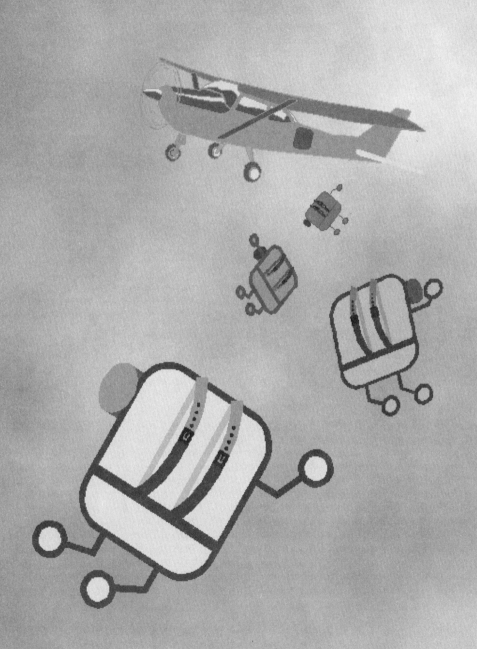

Microsoft Transaction Server and Distributed Objects with DCOM

In this chapter, we will be adding distributed transaction support to our middle-tier business object in the A&W Distributed Calendar system. Along the way, we will learn about the versatility of MTS for deploying distributed components in a manageable and scalable manner. Specifically, we'll learn about:

- ❑ Using MTS as a component deployer
- ❑ Using MTS as a super surrogate
- ❑ Using MTS as a scalable transaction monitor
- ❑ Working with just-in-time activation
- ❑ Declarative programming and automatic transactions
- ❑ Resource dispensers and resource managers
- ❑ The Distributed Transaction Coordinator (DTC)
- ❑ Connection pooling
- ❑ MTS object pooling
- ❑ MTS extension to Threading Model: Activity
- ❑ Using ATL 3 MTS support to create MTS components

However, before we can embark on this journey, we need some basic understanding of Distributed COM, along with some details about how things were done before MTS was available.

Distributed COM

Thus far, our discussion of COM has been restricted to COM components that either work in-process or locally (in a separate EXE). We're about to experience one of the major benefits of designing component objects based on COM technology. Our objects are network-ready without any extra work!

Making COM Objects work over Networks

Here's one explanation of what DCOM is which originated in Microsoft:

> **DCOM is just COM with a longer wire**

This is a great way to describe how DCOM provides extension to basic COM that we have grown to know and love. By examining how COM operates when a client interacts with object instances served through a local EXE server, we'll be able to see how DCOM actually does its job.

Obtaining DCOM

DCOM is a standard part of the Windows NT 4.0 and Windows 98 distribution, but is an add-on for Windows 95. The latest DCOM for Windows 95 add-on is called DCOM98. You will find DCOM98 on your Visual Studio 6 distribution CD (or with IE 4.01 SP 1).

Even if you've installed Windows NT 4.0 release distribution, it's important that you have applied the latest Service Pack for the operating system. As of the time of writing, Service Pack 3 for Windows NT 4.0 is available. This Service Pack fixes several DCOM related bugs and is vital for the proper function of our sample code. You can also find the Service Pack on the Visual Studio 6 distribution CD.

Once you have all the above pieces assembled and installed on your system, you're ready to explore the capabilities of DCOM by following the next example.

After installation, the only directly user accessible application is a configuration utility called DCOMCnfg.exe. When you run it, it looks like this:

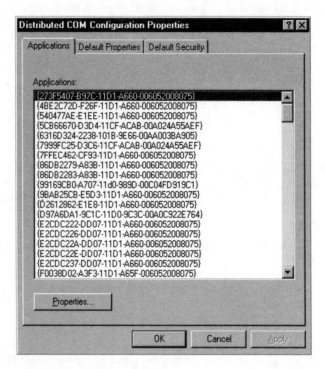

DCOM also includes other system EXEs: `Rpcss.exe` and `Dllhost.exe`. `Rpcss.exe` is the DCOM enhanced **System Control Manager** (SCM), the `Dllhost.exe` utility surrogate, which allows in-process COM servers to be executed out-of-process or remotely across the network.

DCOM Enabling Our ActiveX Controls: A Preview

To help us gain a better understanding of DCOM, we'll now get our hands wet with a quick demonstration. Since our ActiveX control and the back-end objects are already communicating across processes (the Calendar control running inside the Visual Basic or Test Container process and the Finder object running inside `Atlfinder.exe`), it should be an easy matter to make them run across machine boundaries over the network. In fact, it's quite simple, with the help of DCOM.

First, we'll need machines connected over a TCP/IP network with DCOM enabled. In our example, we'll be using two Windows NT 4.0 machines. Make sure both machines have Service Pack 3 or later installed, are connected, and can see each other over the network. If you are working with Windows 98, the procedures should be very similar. In either case, we will assume that DCOM security has not been explicitly enabled after initial installation. If your installation is already security enabled, you may need to read Chapter 11 and the security information on your MSDN CD first.

Installing the Software Components

Now, we're ready to move the `Atldept.dll` and `Atlfinder.exe` over to the remote machine. This 'server' machine is called `PENT100` in our case.

Log on to the server machine as the same user as the client machine. Next, create a directory called `C:\Test` directory on the server machine and copy the following files into the directory:

Log on to the server machine as the same user as the client machine. Next, create a directory called C:\Test directory on the server machine and copy the following files into the directory:

- ❑ Atldept.dll
- ❑ Atlfinder.exe

Now change directory to C:\Test and type in the following:

```
regsvr32 AtlDept.dll
Atlfinder /RegServer
```

Each of these operations should complete successfully. Now start up oleview.exe. Check under the All Objects or Automation Objects list and find **ATLFinder1 Class** and **ATLDept1 class**. Double-click each one to ensure that you can create an instance of each class. Release the instances.

Launching the Server

If you are running on Windows 98, you will need to type in ATLFINDER /Server. This will start the Atlfinder.exe COM server listening for incoming COM requests. Windows 98 DCOM doesn't support remote server launching, so all remote servers must be started manually. On a Windows NT 4.0 system, however, you'll not need to manually enter the above command. Atlfinder.exe will be automatically launched on-demand under Windows NT DCOM.

Now the server machine is completely configured for operations. Go back to the client machine. I assume that this machine has been properly configured, and that you've logged on with the same user ID as on the server machine. Now, start up oleview.exe and click on the **ATLFinder1 Class** under All Objects or Automation Objects. On the right-hand pane, you'll see a set of tabs. Click on the Implementation tab. If you click on Local Server, you should see a path to the Atlfinder.exe on your system. Remove this path and leave the edit box empty. This effectively removes the content of the LocalServer32 key from the registry. Now, we need to tell the client machine that the ATLFinder1 class is to be instantiated remotely.

To do this, click on the Activation tab, and then on Launch As Interactive User and key in the host name of the server machine:

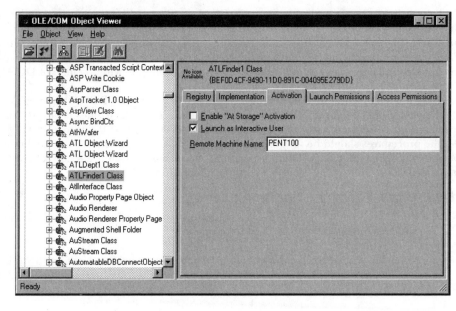

Now go back to the left-hand pane and click on the **ATLFinder1 Class** entry to instantiate an object. If this is successful (it may take a little while), you'll see the interfaces listed – you've created an object across the network.

To put the entire scenario to work now, open `Tstcon32.exe` and instantiate a Visual Calendar instance. After a moment the calendar should start and display all the events. Try selecting a cell with events to get the details. Notice the response. Next, try changing months: notice again the significantly slower response. The ActiveX control is now working over the network via DCOM. The exact same interaction is happening across machine boundaries, with data transfer speed limited only by the bandwidth of the network.

The significant note to make here is that we haven't specifically programmed any DCOM server or DCOM client. The binary code (Win32/Intel) hasn't actually changed at all. It's the same in-process `Atldept.dll` server, the same `Atlfinder.exe` local server, and the same ActiveX control. All we did was some external configuration, and our COM objects started to communicate with each other over the network. This is significant because it shows the fact that:

> **DCOM *is* COM**

Almost all legacy COM applications (ones designed with no consideration for DCOM) can be configured to work with DCOM. Of course, new 'from-scratch' applications can take specific advantage of the new features available in DCOM by programming directly to it or, more importantly, being designed specifically for it. DCOM delivers added value to COM by network enabling COM components transparently, and supplying a robust security model for COM components. We'll have further discussion on Security in Chapter 11.

The following diagram depicts the interaction between the ActiveX control and the remote DCOM server components:

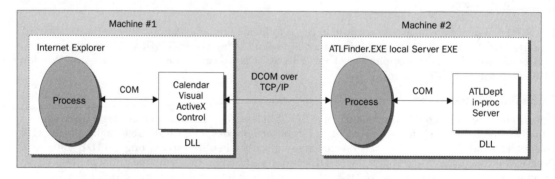

Making Calls Across Processes

Let's now take a closer look at how DCOM works. When a client creates an object instance supported by a local EXE server, this is what happens:

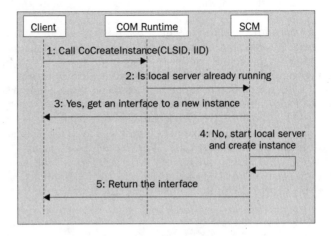

- ❑ The client calls CoCreateInstance() on a CLSID supported by a local server.
- ❑ The DCOM runtime, working together with the Service Control Manager (SCM), determines if the requested local server is already running and whether a connection to it can be established. The SCM is a part of the OS on Windows NT
- ❑ If the local server is up and running, the client is provided with a pointer to an **interface proxy** (more on this later)
- ❑ If no connectable instance of the class requested exists, a new instance of the object is created by launching the local server if necessary
- ❑ An interface proxy representing the requested interface from the newly created object is returned to the client

The SCM is a process whose sole purpose in life is to locate implementations or specific instances of requested COM classes. Because of this, it's a close friend of the system registry, where all the CLSID-to-implementation mappings are kept. This SCM is typically named Rpcss.exe on Windows 98/95 and Windows NT systems.

Interface Proxies and Stubs

Once a client is connected to an instance of a DCOM class, the interface pointer that it holds is actually provided by an interface **proxy object**. Interface proxies (and stubs) are actually small COM objects. The code for these objects is created automatically when we run our original IDL (Interface Description Language) file through the MIDL compiler. Based on the data type of the method arguments and return values, the MIDL compiler creates these marshaling proxy/stub pairs for communicating between processes. One pair of proxy/stub classes is created for each interface. In our project, for the local server called ATLFinder.exe, you'll find in the project directory a file called Atlfinderps.mk. At the command prompt, you can type:

```
nmake -f Atlfinderps.mk
```

This creates the proxy/stub DLL for marshaling the interfaces supported by the ATLFinder.exe local server. To register that DLL, you'll need to call Regsvr32, as usual. To satisfy your curiosity, look in your Chapter 7 working directory for the ATLFinder.exe project and find the ATLFinder_p.c file to see what MIDL generated proxy/stub code physically looks like.

Back to Inter-process Calls

With this interface proxy, the client may obtain other interface pointers using QueryInterface() or call methods of the interface directly. When such methods are invoked, the COM runtime must send all the arguments for the method from the client process to the local server process. This requires the use of a type of inter-process communication supported by the underlying operating system. In the case of COM, the mechanism used is DCE RPC (Distributed Computing Environment Remote Procedure Calls). DCE RPC has several nice features:

- It works in the same way across processes on the same machine or across machines on a network
- It handles procedure calls and parameter passing across two machines with dissimilar hardware architectures and operating systems
- It provides security support that allows the identity of the client process to be passed over to the server
- It's basically network-transport protocol independent, as it's currently able to work over TCP, UDP, IPX/SPX, or Named Pipes
- It's a time-tested mechanism widely deployed in both Windows NT and UNIX-based network programming

COM and DCOM rely heavily on these capabilities.

Note that COM actually will attempt to use lightweight RPC (LRPC) whenever possible when the two communicating objects/components reside on the same machine and OS. LRPC is a Microsoft-proprietary variant of RPC which has the same calling syntax as the DCE RPC runtime (thus the seamless interchangeability) but is optimized to reduce data copying and eliminate access to the networking code altogether.

When we put the RPC layer into the picture during a method invocation, the situation becomes a bit more complex – the call is now 'cross-process' or 'cross-machine'. The actual call is delivered to the interface proxy. The following diagram shows the activities that will occur:

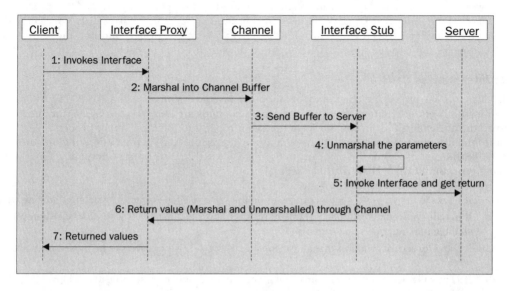

- ❑ The client invokes the interface through the interface proxy
- ❑ The interface proxy **marshals** the parameters into a buffer provided by a **channel**.
- ❑ The channel forwards the data to the server
- ❑ An interface stub on the server receives the buffer from the channel and **unmarshals** the data from the buffer
- ❑ The interface stub calls the associated interface on the server object
- ❑ The interface stub sends return values back to the interface proxy
- ❑ The interface proxy returns the values to the client

The channel is supplied by the RPC runtime system and is an abstraction above the different transports. The channel can operate in shared memory spanning two processes on the same machine, or could be operating over a network protocol stack across two machines. It can be viewed as a virtual tunnel connecting the two communicating processes (regardless of their location). Data going into the tunnel on Process A is said to have been marshaled, and will come out the same way (be unmarshaled) at the other end of the tunnel on Process B. Loosely speaking, marshaling means packing the data into the channel's buffer in a well-defined format – for DCE RPC, this well defined format is called the Network Data Representation or NDR. NDR is an agreed format for transmitting different data types between dissimilar machines so that the same data can be reconstructed exactly at the destination machine.

Note that there are many more subtleties associated with marshaling than this simple description implies. For example, if a pointer to a data item is marshaled across two processes, just sending the value of the pointer itself is useless since the receiver resides in a completely separate process/address space. Instead, the actual data item itself must be sent across the wire and a pointer to it reconstructed within the receiver process in order for the marshaling to work.

So far we've focused on the conceptual view of providing proxy and stub code for interface method invocation across processes, and indeed, this was the way that COM worked for a period of time. With DCOM, though, Microsoft introduced automatic type library based marshaling. Automatic type library marshaling will build these proxy and stub objects *on the fly* using type library information obtained from an interface. What we see here is actually a reuse of the marshaling technology Microsoft had been using for Automation. As long as the data type that needs to be marshaled is compatible with Automation (which essentially means all the data types that a VARIANT can hold), you don't even need the MIDL generated proxy/stub code.

Calling COM Methods between Machines

Now that we have a basic understanding of how an interface method call is transmitted across two communicating processes on the same machine or across a network, the next logical question is: how is the object at the destination created in the first place? Simply put, the SCM will locate or create the object instance across the network whenever necessary. (If there are no object instances which can service the call, the SCM will launch the required object server on the remote machine, subject to security constraints detailed in Chapter 11.) In the case where the caller and called party are both on the same machine under the same OS, the channel is typically working over shared memory and LRPC will be used. In the case where the caller and called party are on different machines over a network, the channel uses the DCE RPC over a layer of network software called the protocol stack (usually TCP/IP, but IPX and NETBEUI are also supported by RPC on Windows platforms).

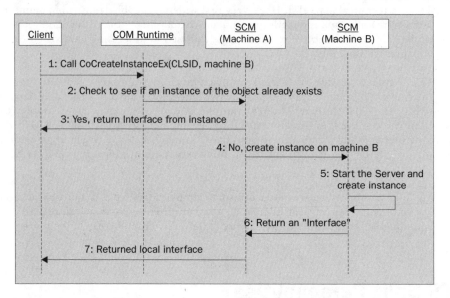

Of course, there's low-level sanity checking and connection management work that DCOM must do because of the added network connection. All this work, though, is completely hidden from you as an application developer, and you can develop components without worrying about where they may be executed.

A Potential Problem

One thing that you may already be pondering over is the amount of manual work involved in just getting two components talking across the network. What if we have tens of components and hundreds of clients that need to establish connection dynamically during normal operation? The configuration chore alone would be a nightmare. We need an automated configuration and deployment tool for DCOM components! This is one of the roles fulfilled by the Microsoft Transaction Server (MTS), which we will now examine in detail.

Object Deployment using MTS

The **Microsoft Transaction Server** (**MTS**), currently part of the NT 4.0 Option Pack installation, is a cornerstone of the DNA architecture and will be vital in the future world of COM+.

What is MTS? Pretending for a moment that we are aliens from space looking at our deployment problem, MTS is an EXE that will run your DLLs in strange yet comforting ways and has a slightly set of weird rules and nuances. Such is the physical essence of MTS. Why, then, would we ever want to program with MTS?

Physically totally unremarkable, once we understand its logical function and reason for its existence, we see that MTS is a technical marvel. It is the very first widely available **transaction monitor** to be available on a mainstream computing platform. So mainstream, in fact, that it is within reach of every working developer. This is incredible. Previously, true transaction processing has existed only in the domain of companies with big budgets.

Microsoft's MTS architects, though, have tried to solve a much more complex problem than simply re-inventing the transaction monitor (something many of them have already done) and slapping it onto Windows NT. They also needed to fit MTS into the DCOM component-based strategy for building applications, and use it to simplify aspects of development with DCOM. The MTS designers have done an incredible job of meeting these objectives. So much so that I would argue within the next five years, it would be silly for a programmer doing server applications on Windows NT not to use MTS.

Since it is going to be so important, we better pay some attention to what it is and what it can do. In fact, MTS has several personalities, each addressing a rather different domain – all related to distributed computing. It is rather like a Swiss Army knife – the more you use it, the more you'll need it.

The MTS Split Personalities

MTS is not just another transaction monitor; instead it is a 3-in-1 Titan server with tremendous versatility. Let us look briefly at the three personalities of MTS.

MTS as Component Deployer

Even non-MTS components can make use of some of MTS's ability to systematically distribute sets of components. The very same tedious task of copying over DLLs, configuring registry entries, registering components, registering proxy stubs, and so on, can be done quickly with MTS. The component packaging and distribution features include these abilities:

❑ Combines multiple components into a physically distributable, self-installing **package**, greatly simplifying DCOM components distribution. Ultimately, all components in the same package will run within the same MTS executive process.

❑ Allows server components to be moved between different Windows NT servers running MTS via simple graphical operations from a single location, and without affecting client applications. No more running around with DLLs!

❑ Generates a standalone client executable for installing everything necessary for a client workstation (typically a bundle of proxy/stub DLLs) – Windows 98 or Windows NT, with or without MTS – to access an MTS package executing on a server via DCOM. This enables controlled deployment on a massive scale.

MTS's deployment capabilities are delivered directly through its Transaction Explorer, making it relatively easy for system administrator (often non-developer) to learn and use. We will see first-hand how this is done later when we package our business objects up for migration between two servers.

MTS as Super Surrogate

MTS enables the execution of in-process servers remotely. These sorts of special purpose executables are commonly called **surrogates**.

The Dllhost.exe that comes with the basic DCOM distribution (and on Windows 98) is a standard surrogate for running in-process components out-of-process. Such surrogates are 'dumb' – that is, they simply aggregate the DLL component's interfaces and present them as an out-of-process client. With Dllhost.exe, there is also the restriction of one running instance (process) per directly hosted component.

Therefore, MTS can be considered a super-surrogate, because it not only provides the surrogate hosting function, but also adds tremendous value for the components being hosted.

As with other surrogates, one additional advantage of running MTS is its 'fault isolation' property that leverages the process isolation of Windows NT. This allows MTS users to partition each related group of components to run within their own process. If one of the components crashes within a process, only the related components in the process will be affected; operations of non-related components in other independently running processes will not be affected. This grouping of components, as we saw in the previous section, is called a **package**.

MTS as Scalable Transaction Monitor

This is the most valuable contribution of MTS. A transaction monitor traditionally provides a runtime environment for applications that are designed in terms of individual transactions. MTS does this and much more. Simply put:

> **MTS enables you to quickly create great servers – if you follow the rules!**

In fact, the reason why you will be able to create highly functional and scalable applications quickly is that most of the complex code has already been written for you. When programming with MTS, you simply supply the missing parts that vary from server to server. The code you create (in component form, they're physically DLLs) simply plugs into MTS. The parts of the code that you write invariably deal with some core business function that you would like to perform on the server on behalf of the clients – making every MTS component a business object. It should also be obvious, then, that the code you typically write for your business objects is miniscule compared to the code that Microsoft has already written for MTS. This is the very reason why you need to code by some very well defined rules – in order to fit into the architecture properly. If you play by the rules, your server application will enjoy the optimization and scalability features that MTS has designed in.

Just to reinforce the point, take a look at what MTS does for you:

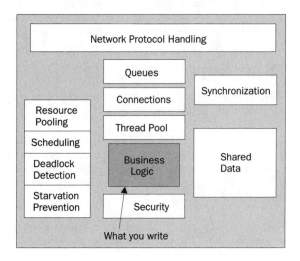

Properly-designed MTS based applications can scale across processor boundaries (that is, in Symmetric Multiprocessing (SMP) systems) and across machine boundaries (in networked distributed servers), allowing your business logic to serve a very large client base. You get all this without coding a single line of networking code.

In future versions of MTS, it may even be possible to make dynamic intelligent decisions about where, when and how many instances of a component to create, enabling almost perfect load balancing. Most importantly, MTS today allows a developer to focus on what is crucial to the application – the business logic – rather than trying to become a systems programming expert.

The Pieces of MTS

The MTS distribution consists of these user-visible executables:

- Transaction Explorer
- Executive
- mtxrereg.exe

The Transaction Explorer

The Transaction Explorer is a tool for configuring MTS components, controlling the operation of MTS, and creating self-installing packages and client executables. The Transaction Explorer is a Microsoft Management Console (MMC) snap-in.

*In case you are not familiar with MMC, it is a new initiative by Microsoft to consolidate the administration of enterprise computer systems through a single application. The vision is that a system administrator will be able to configure and control every service running on every system (for which she or he has privileges) from that one console. The MMC acts as a standard container framework within which services (well known or otherwise) can plug administration DLLs named **snap-ins**.*

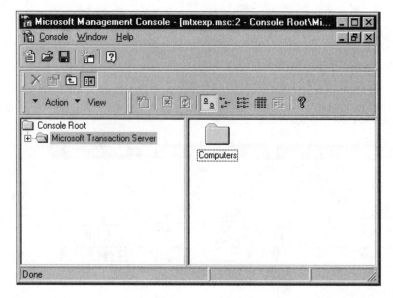

MTS explorer on Windows 9x has a slightly different user interface, though many of the options are available through it. Be aware, however, of serious limitations when using MTS on Windows 9x – see the section below, *Caveat: MTS on Windows 9x.*

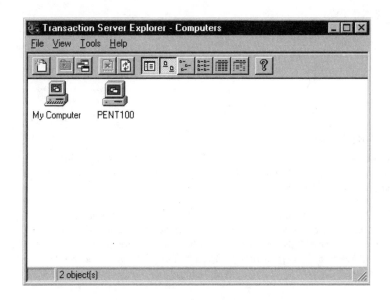

Executive

This is the surrogate host for MTS components, and the gateway to most of MTS runtime functionality. It is located in the `Windows\System` directory and is called `Mtx.exe`. Each running `Mtx.exe` represents a package running on a server.

Tracking instances of components that are being created and activated, rather than packages, is best done by looking at the Transaction Explorer. Here, we can see how the Transaction Explorer shows status of the central server components.

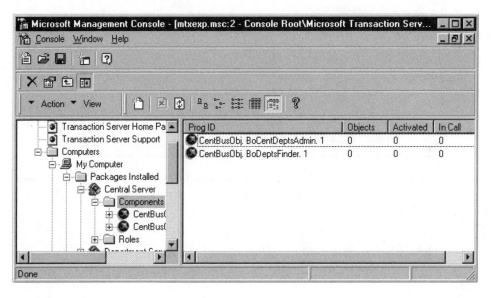

Instead of having instances of `Mtx.exe` loading and unloading packages as their components are being utilized, typical package configurations include a time-out value. An idle executive process will 'hang-around' with the package loaded for the timeout value before unloading. This enhances performance and avoids 'process creation thrashing'. You can access this timeout parameter by right clicking on the package and selecting **Properties**.

If you need to terminate an executive process before its timeout, you can either right click on the package and select **S**hut down, or you can highlight the computer on which they are running, right click and select **Shutdown Server Processes...**. This is especially handy when you are debugging components (that is, when you want the `Mtx.exe` to reload the most recently compiled version of your components).

MTXReReg.exe

This is a command line executable used to update information on all the installed components in the current MTS server. As we will find out shortly, MTS works by intercepting object creation calls. This means that MTS must modify the registry entries of an MTS component (a COM DLL) to point to its own executive/surrogate EXE (which in turn loads the component). If a component has been recompiled and reregistered, the registry will contain information on how to create the component directly. Specifically, `mtxrereg.exe` will clear the value of the `{CLSID}\InprocServer32` key, and set the `{CLSID}\LocalServer32` key to point to the `mtx.exe` executable. You can see this replacement in action by examining the keys, before and after running `mtxrereg.exe`, using `oleview.exe`.

It's therefore essential to call `mtxrereg.exe` each time a component has been recompiled and reregistered with the system. When using the Transaction Explorer, you can highlight the Computer icon and right click to get an option called **Refresh all components...**. Selecting this option is equivalent to running `mtxrereg.exe`.

Caveat: MTS on Windows 9x

Before proceeding any further, a disclaimer must be made regarding MTS on Windows 9x. While the installation of Windows NT Options Pack Client Support will install a version of MTS on your system, you should be aware that this version of MTS (at the time of writing) is not to be relied upon for distributed transaction operation. This information may save you endless hours of debugging to see why something would not work properly on these platforms.

The Windows 9x MTS can be safely used for building experimental components and/or programs making the appropriate MTS calls. However, testing and actual deployment of components making use of distributed transactions *must* be made on Windows NT. For our code, the version of Windows NT must have Service Pack 3 or later applied.

This restriction may not be as drastic as it first appears. Windows 9x as an operating system simply lacks the plumbing to support a properly functioning, distributed transaction system – an occasionally working or improperly working distributed transaction system is not worth a penny to anyone. Here is a short list of pieces that are missing in Windows 9x:

❏   Security – All processes running on an Windows 9x system are in the context of the interactively-logged-on user. The OS has no provision for any other scheme.

- ❑ Robustness – Windows 3.1 and DOS compatibility has forced Windows 9x to share critical system structure between different processes. This is detrimental to fault isolation and robustness requirement of MTS.
- ❑ Survivability – SQL Server on Windows NT provides journaling and recovery (surviving system reboots). Windows NT itself has an auto-recovering file system, NTFS, (surviving media level error). More complete fault tolerant features are available through Cluster Server (surviving any single point of catastrophic hardware failure). None of these exist for Windows 9x.

Retrofitting Windows 9x with the above capabilities would require an effort akin to rewriting Windows NT. It is therefore likely that MTS on Windows 9x will never be updated to the level of its Windows NT cousin.

How Does MTS Work?

What you want to do when working with MTS is to think in terms of **transactions**. This is quite contrary to the linear style of programming we have learnt to love with languages like C/C++, Basic and Java. Instead, we must think about a logic flow consisting of discrete isolated units of work.

Transactions as the Unit of Work

Sitting around dreaming about the future shape of computing, you might imagine an innovative, non-conventional computing language where every statement is independent of every other. In this world, we could submit a 5000 line program to an SMP machine with 5000 CPUs and have the result of the computation back in the time it takes to execute the most complex program line. How's that for a programmer's utopia?

Before you laugh out loud and throw away this book, please appreciate that the essence of this concept is fundamental to transactional computing.

Transactions are isolated units of work, pretty much like the lines of code above. The discipline of coding with transactions is the art of breaking up your server business logic code into these units of work. Transactions are usually not as independent as the lines of source code in our utopian vision. One transaction may depend on the outcome of another, while others may be totally independent. Totally independent groups of transactions can be scheduled in parallel, and MTS facilitates this parallelism (as long as you have the computing resources) much as we described above. For dependent groups, MTS tries to achieve maximal resource usage, while minimizing resource contention – allowing the server logic to scale with the available hardware resources as much as possible. Proper system design and independent grouping is therefore key to the effectiveness of MTS based system.

You will find many textbooks that rehash the definitions of the four ACID properties of a transaction:

- ❑ **Atomic** – The entire unit of work is either completed or it is not. There is no room for 'maybe completed' or 'partially completed'.
- ❑ **Consistent** – Whether you perform your piece of work one time or one thousand times, it isn't going to break the system. The unit of work does not violate any system constraints or change system states in a non-deterministic fashion.

❑ **Isolated** – While the unit of work is being performed, there is no impact whatsoever on other people simultaneously performing their unit of work.

❑ **Durable** – When the unit of work is completed, its effect on the system lasts ad infinitum, come hell or high water.

When a transaction completes its work successfully, a **commit** operation is performed. If a transaction is unable to complete its work, an **abort,** or **rollback**, operation is performed. A commit makes the effect of the completed unit of work permanent. An abort or rollback restores the system to the state it had before you attempted the unit of work, leaving no trace whatsoever.

Transactions may be 'nested' – within the execution of one transaction, one may start another transaction. In this case, all nested (inner) transactions must have successfully committed before the outer one commits successfully. If any nested transaction aborts, the entire group of transaction must abort. This behavior maintains the ACID properties of the outer transaction.

Once your business logic is broken down in terms of transactions, and coded according to MTS conventions, MTS carries out parallel instances of your orchestration of these transactions, at runtime, to give your server application close to optimal usage of resources, while providing application scalability.

MTS Context Object: Your Shadow Object

In MTS, within the coding of your unit of work (the transaction), you can call `SetComplete()` to cause MTS to commit the transaction on your behalf, or you can call `SetAbort()` to tell MTS something has gone wrong and it should abort the transaction on your behalf. You will see mention of these two method calls again and again, and the proper use of these calls is your gateway to much of MTS's functionality. Note the relatively passive role your component plays, always letting MTS do things on your behalf. This is exactly how you will interact with MTS – you yield control and it does all the work (but reserves the right to refuse should you ask it to do something foolish).

The `SetComplete()` and `SetAbort()` methods are part of the `IObjectContext` interface, provided by a **context object** that MTS creates for you. MTS creates a 'shadowing' context object whenever an instance of an MTS component is created. This context object maintains MTS specific state information on behalf of your MTS component instance; it does this in a transparent fashion. Some of the information maintained by the context object includes:

❑ Transaction
❑ Activity (see the later section on this)
❑ Security

The context object is also instrumental to just-in-time activation, another topic that we will discuss shortly.

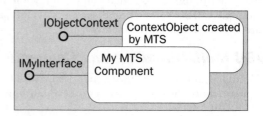

Carefree Transactional Programming

When you get used to thinking about server applications as composed of transactions, you will begin to wonder why in the world people have ever coded server-side business logic in any other way. The bottom line is that coding the flow of business logic as transactional components is much easier than conventional linear style of programming. Why? Two words: error handling.

Once you have defined your transactions, things will only change between transaction boundaries as far as you are concerned. Any problem that occurs between transaction boundaries simply isn't your business any more. MTS will deal with them all.

What exactly can happen? Wow, glad you asked. Your program or some other running program may crash, the executing program may run out of resource, someone may kick the server power-cord, the hard disk head may decide to do a tango on the platter, your network may be spammed by some hacker – the list goes on, but you get the idea. The lesson in all of this is that once you've broken up your business logic into transactions and settled in the warm embrace of MTS, you no longer have to worry about Armageddon... again, you get the idea.

Transactional system design definitely requires a fresh look at first principles, to re-evaluate accepted conventional linear programming language wisdom. The rewards in terms of increased developer productivity, system maintainability, scalability, and robustness are well worth the effort.

Resource Managers and Resource Dispensers

MTS does not rule the world alone. It needs the help of software modules called **resource dispensers** and **resource managers** to provide efficient resource sharing amongst the concurrently executing components. The essential difference between managers and dispensers is:

❑ Resource managers manage the allocation of durable resources
❑ Resource dispensers manage the allocation of temporary resources

The acid test (no pun intended) is to turn off the server. Resources that continue to exist (for example, database information) are what resource managers manage. Currently, there are resource managers available for SQL Server and Microsoft Message Queue (which is covered in the next chapter).

Resource dispensers manage things that disappear when you turn the system off. This includes database connections and shared in-memory 'global' variables. MTS currently supports an ODBC connections resource dispenser, and a Shared Properties Manager (SPM) for the global variables.

Managers and dispensers provide efficient sharing of the resources through whatever algorithm is necessary to minimize actual contention, while maximizing throughput and scalability. Taking as an example ODBC connection dispensers, techniques such as multithreading and connections pooling are used to achieve the objective.

ODBC Multi-threading and Connections Pooling

Multithreading allows more concurrency within the ODBC driver software. This concurrency can squeeze more throughput from an SMP multiprocessor system when working with database servers via ODBC.

Connection pooling allows ODBC itself to manage and cache a pool of recently used open database connections. This caching provides for efficient handling of repeated open and close requests from higher level software to the same set of data sources. ODBC can return database connections in this way without incurring the heavy performance hit associated with an actual connection opening. More specifically, ODBC connection pooling enables MTS components to repeatedly acquire and release database connections with fine granularity, with little or no performance disadvantage. MTS components should grab database connections as late as possible and release them as soon as possible after use.

Automatic Transaction Enlistment

While you do not absolutely have to use any of the resource dispensers or managers when programming MTS components, not to do so would be foolish. You will leave yourself an awful lot of coding and even more concurrency testing.

Being a bona-fide MTS component, a resource dispenser knows about transactions. This is another area of code saving – the dispenser can pass a transactional context to a resource manager. What this literally means is that, simply by using the service of a dispenser like the ODBC connections dispenser, your business logic and the underlying database changes all roll into one single transaction! What happens underneath is a complex enlistment process between the manager and dispenser that you do not have to code. With this ability alone, programming logic that formerly could only be done using cryptic unmanageable stored procedures and/or triggers can now be extracted to easier C/C++, Basic, or even Java.

What MTS and the resource dispensers/manager do is even more amazing when one considers distributed transactions – that is, transactions which occur across the network between multiple machines.

Tight Integration with DTC

The MTS executive does not handle distributed transactions by itself; instead it enlists the service of the Distributed Transaction Coordinator (DTC) to perform the task. The DTC is so closely integrated with the MTS executive that it is hard to think of them as separate entities.

> *In the Transaction Explorer, when you right click on the computer icon, you have the option of stopping or starting DTC. You should really never turn it off. However, if you are convinced that what you do will never run a transaction across the network (i.e. you only have one machine), then you can save some memory turning off the DTC.*

What the DTC does is to orchestrate something called a **two-phase commit protocol**. If you refer back to our brief discussion on nested transactions, the two-phase commit protocol enables participants on multiple machines to participate in the same transaction. Multiple DTCs, one per machine, are involved in enlisting local participants (i.e. resource managers), while one specifically designated DTC is the 'master co-ordinator' for the distributed transaction. All participants are asked if they are prepared for the transaction – this is the first phase. Only if they all agree do they go on to the second phase. Here, the participants are all asked to commit. If any one of them aborts, then they all abort. It is really a protocol 'internal' to DTC when working with MTS in a distributed fashion, although hard core system programmers can program directly to the DTC protocol – and become a participant (i.e. a resource manager).

DTC can work with participants using OLE transactions (Microsoft MTS and its resource managers). DTC can also work with resource managers compliant with an industry standard called XA. XA is owned by the X/Open DTP group (predominately UNIX). Most existing, competing TP monitors on the market are XA compliant. This compatibility allows other resource mangers, such as ORACLE, Informix or IBM DB/2 databases to participate in DTC transactions.

The Object and Transaction Clash

So, if COM is all about object-oriented and component-based software system design, and MTS is all about breaking up business logic flow into transactional units of work – what do they have to do with each other?

The answer is a lot, and soon it'll be even more!

As we have seen already, the transactional style of computing is invaluable for simplifying the coding of server-based business logic.

COM, on the other hand, is the component technology of choice for programming anything and everything that is Microsoft, especially on the client desktop. In this desktop environment, speed and responsiveness are king and everything else plays second fiddle. COM objects are predominately in-process (to save context switching time) and they hold state wherever and whenever convenient in the name of increased performance and speed. Designs range from the mildly object-oriented to fanatically object loyal. It is a largely undisciplined 'anything' goes pragmatic world.

There's a problem here. Pure object-orientation, transactional programming and concurrency management are basically orthogonal concepts. Decades of research have failed to turn out a generally acceptable and comprehensible model to accommodate them all. Indeed, there may be no convergence!

So what does all this mean to you and me? If you are already used to the purity of almost OO programming provided by desktop COM, be prepared to do some yoga-like twisting and bending when attacking server based MTS. Rest assured that once you've done it enough times, there'll be light at the end of the tunnel.

MTS is designed to bridge the two worlds. Existing transaction gurus from the mainframe and minicomputer world, who may never have heard of the concept of an object in their entire life, can immediately dive into it with Visual Basic or a script language and have a field day. COM developers who have learnt to recite the COM specification and OO manifestos may have a slightly harder time. In fact, some of them may never make the transition, because for them their core business centers around a client/desktop world (the simple fact that Microsoft has moved on to focus on client/server does not mean the world of desktop development vanishes overnight). Taking the leap of faith, developers can start to tinker and get used to this paradigm of server program construction, with a little relearning pain.

Meanwhile, who knows, with enough heads put into the problem, an acceptable conversion of concepts may one day be discovered, and COM and MTS can live happily ever after. COM+, due from Microsoft shortly beyond the Windows NT 5 timeframe, promises to integrate MTS into the COM support fabric, taking us one step further in this direction. (Unfortunately, the technical approach MS intends to take is still sketchy at the time of writing).

Coping with Changing Paradigms

'Junk encapsulation! Trash inheritance! Burn polymorphism!

This chant is certainly bad for your personal health if recited amongst a group of OO or COM developers. Yet, transactional system design requires us to re-evaluate our OO prejudices. Before we go any further, a disclaimer: you can, and you definitely should, continue to practice all that is OO (encapsulation, inheritance, polymorphism and so on) with the coding and design of the *components within* the transactional system, nothing has changed here. When designing the system as a whole, MTS requires us to be completely 'state-conscious'. On this system design level, and only at this level, the partitioning of work amongst the MTS components should always try to:

❑ Minimize the need for maintaining non-durable, component internal, state information between method invocations
❑ Call SetAbort() or SetComplete() within each method whenever possible
❑ Maintain durable states only through MTS resource managers
❑ Maintain shared non-durable states only through the SPM resource dispenser

None of these guidelines are particularly OO friendly, they all require you to manage state explicitly, but following them will ensure that your system design will 'play well' with the MTS architecture.

MTS Details

MTS, even though complex on the inside, is quite easy to work with. Most of its magic is done transparently through **interception**. After you have run mtxrereg.exe (or selected Refresh All Components... in Transaction Explorer), MTS actually makes mtx.exe the component's local server (replacing the existing in-process entry). Here is the entry from one of the Central Server component as viewed through Oleview.exe:

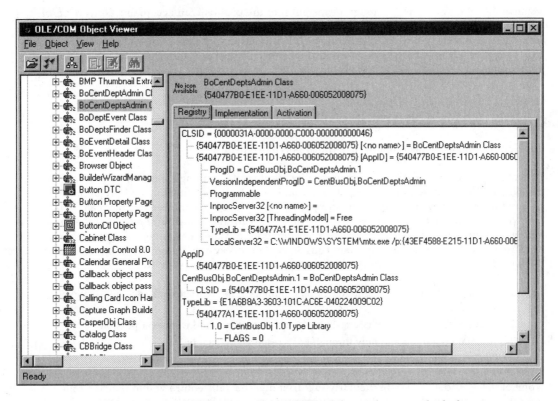

In the `LocalServer32` key, the GUID after `/p:` is the ID of the package in which the component resides.

Now, when the client (the base client in MTS jargon) creates an instance of the object, it is actually an instance of `mtx.exe` for that package, if it is not already started. In any case, a new MTS object (the context object that we mentioned earlier) is created, and the reference of this context object is returned to the caller.

What happens here is that MTS actually intercepts the call to create an instance, and returns something that is *not* actually the object that you have requested. Let's examine this further:

❑　MTS must know how to create an instance of your object eventually, which means you must follow some standard instance factory convention. The convention used in MTS is the `IClassFactory` interface. All MTS components must support this interface for instance creation.

❑　Before MTS actually creates your component, it must provide an identical set of interfaces to the base client, so that the base client cannot tell that MTS is working in the middle. This means that type library information must be available for MTS to create the proxy (for objects supporting automation compatible interfaces) or an actual 'standard MIDL generated' proxy/stub DLL must be available to be aggregated. Furthermore, this also implies that MTS can only work with components that use standard marshalling – MTS will not work with components implementing custom marshalling.

❑　Somewhere along the way, MTS will have to create the actual object.

Let us examine the last point in some detail and find out when MTS actually creates the object instance.

Just-in-time Activation

An actual instance of your component is created during the first 'activation' (see the object pooling section later to see why we do not call this instance creation). This activation is postponed until a call is actually made to one of the methods of a supported interface (except IUnknown). In other words, the actual component is created as late as possible – *just in time* to do useful work.

Assume that our component instance actually consumes significant resources when it is created (we will say more about this later). From the client point of view, it is now OK to create the object instance as early as possible and hold onto a reference of the object. Why? Because the object is not actually created – and therefore no resources are consumed – while the client is holding the reference. Resources are consumed only when the object is actually used, at which time it is unavoidable to take the hit.

> **When working with MTS objects, grab references to them as early as you want. Just-in-time activation eliminates the penalty.**

And the savings continue. The object can go through the a converse 'deactivation' process whenever IObjectContext::SetAbort() or IObjectContext::SetComplete() is called by your component. Deactivation releases the last reference on your object instance – and it dies the natural COM way. Note that again the client is still happily holding a reference to the object context, and using minimal resources.

You can view MTS as the invisible object liberator; it liberates object instances whenever possible, in order to reduce resource consumption and resource contention – both of which are enemies of a scalable system. At the same time, the client is happily holding onto a re-connectable reference that they think is the actual object instance. One problem with client/server computing is the case when hundreds of clients are intermittently using a server, but all keep active references. This places heavy burden on server resources. MTS disconnects the two but provides a place to re-connect, effectively solving the problem.

Object Pooling

The reason why a new terminology set (activation and deactivation) was invented was not only to improve MTS's usefulness, but also because activation and deactivation may not map to instance creation and instance release in the near future.

In the future, MTS will support object pooling, further enhancing system throughput. In the object-pooling scenario, MTS creates object instances only once – on the first activation, the instances are then kept around after deactivation in a pool. When another object context receives a call, an object instance is fetched from this pool, saving the computing time involved in instance creation. This scenario gives activation and deactivation their true meaning. It also implies that an activated object from the pool must be totally indistinguishable from a newly created instance of the same object (i.e. it must not have any non-durable, component internal state that persists after deactivation), otherwise inconsistency in the system will be introduced.

The reason why object pooling is not here today has to do with MTS's evolving internal threading model. At this present time, the internal threading model of MTS (an apartment-like model) takes an expensive toll in terms of overhead on any pooling implementation.

MTS Components and Threading Model

The only advice I have on becoming a master of MTS threading models is: don't!

The whole essence of MTS is to make server-side logic programming simple. Consideration of threading models (especially changing ones) just isn't simple. If you find yourself toiling to figure out MTS threading models in order to get your application to work, the best approach is to re-examine the transaction factoring of your business logic and eliminate the problem. The problem is most likely a design one.

And if your application requires intricate footwork between threads and components, then may be MTS isn't your best bet. You should consider rolling your own object pooler with bare COM. This way, you will have much better control over your execution environment.

The bottom line is, the internal threading model of MTS is subject to change, and the properly designed and coded MTS component shouldn't care.

> **In MTS components, you should always try to code as if you are programming for one client on a single thread**

Activity

Having said that you are not supposed to know too much about MTS threading models, let me tell you now that any new MTS component should be created as apartment threaded in-process server. Even though MTS supports single-threaded components as well, there is no advantage in creating new ones this way.

The apartment model as we know it has been extended for MTS to include the notion of an **activity**. Simply put, an activity is a trace through the set of components as a client method call executes.

Imagine a chained creation (through `IObjectContext::CreateInstance()` calls) of six components by one client. The first two are within the same package, the third and fourth ones created in a different package on the same system, and the fifth and sixth on a remote computer, and you will get the idea.

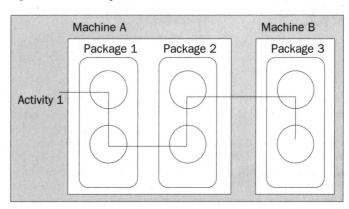

Assuming all of the components are apartment threaded, we can see that the first pair of component instances are in the same apartment within the package, the second pair are in the same apartment within another package, and the last pair are in the same apartment within a remote package. Yet all of these component instances belong to the same activity. The simple rule enforced by MTS is that no two component instances in the same activity can execute concurrently on the same machine. This allows you to create MTS components without worrying about protecting your class variables against concurrent access.

An activity is often viewed as a *logical* thread of execution, since it transcends process and machine boundaries. The activity of a component is a property of its object context and can be obtained as a GUID.

By definition, each `CoCreateInstance()` on an MTS component creates a new activity. This is because a `CoCreateInstance()` call is a non-MTS aware COM API call. If you are creating other MTS objects from inside an MTS component, always use `IObjectContext::CreateInstance()` or `ITransactionContextEx::CreateInstance()` instead. This will not only ensure that the new components participate in the calling object's activity, but will also ensure the transaction attributes are passed on properly. If you use the classic `CoCreateInstance()` or `CoCreateInstanceEx()`, there is no reliable way for MTS to accomplish this.

Doing Things Declaratively

Microsoft's upcoming COM+ technology is one of the forces pushing us closer to the world of **declarative programming**. The promise is that the tedious and rigid programming style we are used to will soon be history.

Declarative programming allows us to set certain attributes or properties of programming constructs (for example, declaring a function to be an interface method in the source code). The development and execution environment would do all the tedious work for us (such as creating and maintaining the IDL and header files, compiling and maintaining the type library and the proxy stub, etc.). A parallel exists today in MTS, and that is the notion of **automatic transactions**.

Automatic Transactions

Automatic transactions work declaratively. We set some properties, and MTS does all the hard work for us.

To set an MTS's component's transaction properties declaratively, right click on the component and select Properties:

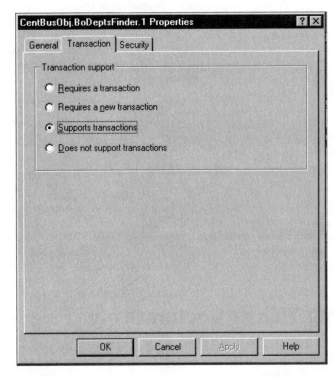

Here is a tabulation of the properties and what MTS will do for you.

Property	Action
Requires a transaction	MTS knows that this component requires a transaction, and will create a new one if the calling object is not already in a transaction.
Requires a new transaction	MTS knows that this component always requires a new transaction, and will create a new one for the object regardless of who creates it.
Supports transactions	MTS knows that this component supports transactions, and will execute within the creator's transaction if there is one. Otherwise, this component will execute without transactions.
Does not support transactions	MTS knows this object does not participate in any transaction regardless of who creates it. It will be created without participation in any transactions.

This set of properties allows for the actual assignment of an object's transaction properties as late as possible, that is, right up to the time of deployment. Two extremely desirable effects result:

❑ Enhanced reuse of components through composition
❑ Drastically simpler coding for each component

You can flexibly combine (compose) a complex transaction out of a set of transaction supporting components that each do a small piece of work. Reuse is encouraged here, because each component can now essentially do the job of several if the attributes had to be hard-coded. When your code composes the operations of multiple components, even more permutations of reuse are allowed. In all cases, no recompile is required.

Coding is much simpler since many hard-coded transactional relationships between components can be eliminated. This reduces complex logic flow. Each component could be made as fine grained as possible, performing only one simple task.

Explicit Transactions

Explicit transactions are caller-managed transactions, which we start manually via `ITransactionContextEx::CreateInstance()`. The `ITransactionContextEx` interface is obtained from a standalone MTS component called a transaction context. You can create such an object using:

```
CoCreateInstance(CLSID_TransactionContextEx, NULL,
                 CLSCTX_INPROC, IID_ITransactionContextEx,
                 reinterpret_cast<void**>(&m_pTC));
```

Once you have created obtained the `ITransactionContextEx` interface, any new object creation or method invocation will be in the same transaction (unless the object being created is declaratively overriden – see the previous section). By creating new MTS objects and calling their methods, you can 'compose' their work into one transaction. In these explicit transactions, you can control the transaction boundary by calling `ITransactionContextEx::Commit()` or `ITransactionContextEx::Abort()`.

Be aware that even though the client creating the transaction context controls the transaction, it never enters the transaction itself. This means that any work it performs outside of the components created by the transaction context object cannot participate in commit or abort. The source for this type of explicit transaction management is frequently very confusing and hard to maintain.

Automatic transactions should be used whenever possible in preference to explicit ones because of their flexibility and ease of maintenance.

Strategies in MTS Programming

Let us do a quick re-cap of the MTS programming strategies that we have talked about so far. Following these strategies ensures that our server will behave within the MTS environment.

Call SetComplete() and SetAbort()

Always strive for a transactional factoring of your business logic where your component can call `SetComplete()` or `SetAbort()` within every method call. This allows MTS to function with maximum efficiency. If there is some reason why you can't do this, you can call the other two methods of `IObjectContext`, `DisableCommit()` and `EnableCommit()`, but you must do so cautiously. Improper use of these two methods can severely hamper the overall server throughput and scalability.

Grab MTS Object References as Early as you Wish

There is no penalty in creating MTS components early in your code and keeping them around until the end. Just-in-time activation will ensure that no unnecessary object instances actually get created. This is really counter-intuitive and takes some getting used to, especially when you know the component you are creating is a resource hog. So get used to it!

There is a caveat: if you are creating an MTS component within another MTS component, the above may not necessarily be true. The lifetime of the client (calling) component itself may be highly dynamic and intermittent; this will be especially common before true object pooling is implemented in MTS. In this case, it makes almost no difference whether you create other MTS object references early or before use.

Grab Resources for as Short a Time as Possible

This is common sense and easy to understand. The sooner you release shared resources (e.g. database connections), the sooner others can use them. Think of resource acquisition as holding locks on the resources (even though MTS and your resource dispenser/manager take care of the details). You always want to hold locks for as short a time as possible. So, acquire your resources as late as possible and release them as early as possible.

Make Your Components Composable

Automatic transactions make the task of composing components into transactions simple. Try to factor your components, so that each one does one small unit of work. More complex operations can then be performed by composing one or more of these components in a transaction. The code should then be straightforward, easy to maintain and the transaction boundary can be set declaratively before use. We will see how this is done for the A&W business objects in the next section.

From MTS Theory to Practice

That was more than a mouthful of MTS theory. We need to put these concepts into practice and start writing some MTS component code.

We will be testing the MTS and OLE DB components created in the last chapter shortly. First, let us recap what these components are supposed to do. Remember that we have a set of departmental server business objects and a set of central server business objects.

Components on Departmental Server

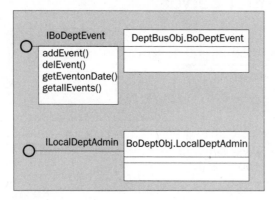

There are two components on the departmental server. On this server, we keep track of all the events occurring at the department.

The DeptBusObj.LocalDeptAdmin Object

This object is meant for local departmental administration (i.e. setting the actual identity of the department) and has no relevant interface implemented for our purposes.

The DeptBusObj.BoDeptEvent Object

This is the local events administrator object, providing an IBoDeptEvent interface. The following table lists the methods of this interface and their function.

Method	Description
addEvent()	Adds an event to the department's event database. It should also update the central servers' event count to reflect the newly added event.
delEvent()	Deletes an event from the department's event database. It should also update the central servers' event count to reflect the recently deleted event.
getAllEvents()	Retrieves all available events for this department currently in the event database.
getEventOnDate()	Retrieves all available events from this department occurring within the input specified month. This method was not defined on the interface in the last chapter, but we will be adding it in this chapter.

Components on Central Server

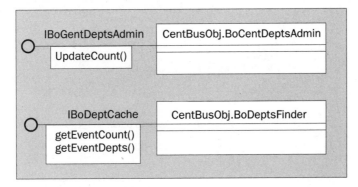

There are also two components on the central server. This server acts mainly as a consolidator and cache. It maintains a running count of all the events available from all departments. It is the department's responsibility to ensure that the count maintained at the central server is accurate and up-to-date.

CentBusObj.BoCentDeptsAdmin Component

This component is used by departmental servers in maintaining an up-to-date running count. It has only one interface, IBoCentDeptsAdmin, whose single method is:

Method	Description
updateCount()	Given a department, date, time, and an event count, this method will update the count database to reflect the change. If a record matching the department and time is not found, a new one is created. This method was not defined in the last chapter, but we will be implementing it in this chapter.

CentBusObj.BoDeptsFinder Component

This component provides a cached running count of all events happening across all departments. It's only interface, IBoDeptCache, is defined as:

Method	Description
getEventDepts()	Returns all the departments that have events for a specified month.
getEventCount()	Returns all the event count entries for a particular month across all departments. Also returns the department details. We will be adding this method in this chapter.

The Need for Distributed Transactions

Whenever our departmental business object adds or deletes a row in the event table, the total count of events occurring on the affected date will change. Since we keep a running count cached at the central server, we need to make sure that the total is also updated appropriately.

Let's take another look at this problem. First we need to coordinate the update of two databases, each situated on a different server. Second, we need the updates to be atomic – to either all happen successfully, or not happen at all. We are already used to the notion of a transaction whenever we need to update multiple tables atomically within a database. In this case, what we need is support for distributed transactions.

We will, of course, use MTS and DTC for our distributed transaction. Using the ODBC connections dispenser will ensure that the SQL server resource managers on both machines are enlisted in the transaction automatically.

Note that some RDBMS (noticeably ORACLE) systems coordinate distributed transactions completely within the database. Essentially, tables from remote servers appear locally with a host prefix. Creating distributed transactions in these systems is as straightforward as creating a local transaction.

ATL 3 Support for MTS Components

Let us look back at our business object code. When we created these components, we told the ATL wizard that we wanted them to be MTS components. For example, the BoDeptEvent object in the departmental server has the following header file:

```
#include "resource.h"        // main symbols
#include <mtx.h>

/////////////////////////////////////////////////////////////////////////////
// CBoDeptEvent
class ATL_NO_VTABLE CBoDeptEvent :
    public CComObjectRootEx<CComSingleThreadModel>,
    public CComCoClass<CBoDeptEvent, &CLSID_BoDeptEvent>,
    public IObjectControl,
    public IBoDeptEvent
```

Here, being a custom interface (non-Automation compatible) we inherit directly from
IBoDeptEvent.

The object also inherits from IObjectControl. This interface, if implemented by an MTS object,
will cause the MTS runtime to call our component after activation via
IObjectControl::Activate(), before deactivation via IObjectControl::Deactivate(),
and to check if we support pooling via IObjectControl::CanBePooled(). These calls allow us
to hook into the activation and deactivation process. They will become important when object
pooling becomes supported in the future. For now, the ATL Object Wizard generates stubs for us as
well as we shall see.

```
public:
    CBoDeptEvent()
    {
    }

DECLARE_REGISTRY_RESOURCEID(IDR_BODEPTEVENT)

DECLARE_PROTECT_FINAL_CONSTRUCT()
```

MTS components cannot be aggregated for obvious reasons: namely, that it is actually the object
context that the client gets, not the component itself.

```
DECLARE_NOT_AGGREGATABLE(CBoDeptEvent)
```

Note also that our two custom interfaces are declared for QI in the COM_MAP here.

```
BEGIN_COM_MAP(CBoDeptEvent)
    COM_INTERFACE_ENTRY(IBoDeptEvent)
    COM_INTERFACE_ENTRY(IObjectControl)
END_COM_MAP()
```

Next are the methods of IObjectControl, which we talked about earlier.

```
// IObjectControl
public:
    STDMETHOD(Activate)();
    STDMETHOD_(BOOL, CanBePooled)();
    STDMETHOD_(void, Deactivate)();
```

Finally, we have a smart pointer for our object context member. It is through this pointer that we will
be calling our SetComplete() and SetAbort(). It can be also be used to create new MTS objects
for execution within the same transaction later on.

```
CComPtr<IObjectContext> m_spObjectContext;
```

In the corresponding `BoDeptEvent.cpp` file, here is what ATL generates for us:

```
// BoDeptEvent.cpp : Implementation of CBoDeptEvent
#include "stdafx.h"

//////////////////////////////////////////////////////////////////////////
// CBoDeptEvent
```

During activation, we grab a pointer to our object context using the MTS helper `GetObjectContext()` call.

```
HRESULT CBoDeptEvent::Activate()
{
    HRESULT hr = GetObjectContext(&m_spObjectContext);
    if (SUCCEEDED(hr))
        return S_OK;
    return hr;
}
```

`CanBePooled()` is implemented, trivially indicating our object can always be pooled. Until MTS supports true object pooling, this coding should be satisfactory for most purposes.

```
BOOL CBoDeptEvent::CanBePooled()
{
    return TRUE;
}
```

`Deactivate()` releases that object context.

```
void CBoDeptEvent::Deactivate()
{
    m_spObjectContext.Release();
}
```

All this is very straightforward and simple, and it is all that is needed to create MTS components using ATL.

Preparing our Components for Compilation

Before compiling our MTS components, we must add the required methods for our business object interfaces. Even though we will actually be coding these methods later on in this chapter, we will add stubs for the new methods now to avoid changing the interface later.

Using the class view, add the following methods to the `IBoDeptEvent` interface of the `\DeptBusObj` project:

Method	Parameters	Return Type
getEventOnDate	[in] DATE dtOnDate, [out] long * lNumEvents, [out,size_is(,*lNumEvents)] EVTDETAIL ** pevtDet	HRESULT

Make sure the event record structure definition is at the top of the IDL file in the `\DeptBusObj` directory:

```
import "oaidl.idl";
import "ocidl.idl";
typedef struct {
    long lEvtID;
    DATE dtDateTime;
    BSTR Heading;
    BSTR Hlink;
    BSTR Location;
    BSTR Organizer;
    BSTR Details;
} EVTDETAIL;
```

The rest of the IDL file in `\DeptBusObj` should be:

```
[
    object,
    uuid(5721C361-E1D1-11D1-A660-006052008075),

    helpstring("IBoDeptEvent Interface"),
    pointer_default(unique)
]
interface IBoDeptEvent : IUnknown // IDispatch
{
    [helpstring("method getAllEvents")] HRESULT getAllEvents(
                [out] long * lNumEvents,
                [out,size_is(,*lNumEvents)] EVTDETAIL * * pevtDet);
    [helpstring("method addEvent")] HRESULT addEvent(
                [in] DATE dtOnDate,
                [in] BSTR bstrHeading,
                [in] BSTR bstrHlink,
                [in] BSTR bstrLocation,
                [in] BSTR bstrOrganizer,
                [in] BSTR bstrDetails,
                [out, retval] long * plID);
    [helpstring("method delEvent")] HRESULT delEvent(
                [in] long lEventID,
                [out,retval] long * lSuccess);
    [helpstring("method getEventOnDate")] HRESULT getEventOnDate(
                [in] DATE dtOnDate,
                [out] long * lNumEvents,
                [out,size_is(,*lNumEvents)] EVTDETAIL ** pevtDet);
```

```
    };
    [
        object,
        uuid(D2612861-E1E8-11D1-A660-006052008075),
        helpstring("ILocalDeptAdmin Interface"),
        pointer_default(unique)
    ]
    interface ILocalDeptAdmin : IUnknown //IDispatch
    {
    };

[
    uuid(D5972B01-E004-11D1-A660-006052008075),
    version(1.0),
    helpstring("DeptBusObj 1.0 Type Library")
]
library DEPTBUSOBJLib
{
    importlib("stdole32.tlb");
    importlib("stdole2.tlb");

    [
        uuid(5721C362-E1D1-11D1-A660-006052008075),
        helpstring("BoDeptEvent Class")
    ]
    coclass BoDeptEvent
    {
        [default] interface IBoDeptEvent;
    };
    [
        uuid(D2612862-E1E8-11D1-A660-006052008075),
        helpstring("LocalDeptAdmin Class")
    ]
    coclass LocalDeptAdmin
    {
        [default] interface ILocalDeptAdmin;
    };
};
```

Add the following methods to the IBoDeptCache interface of the \CentBusObj project:

Method	Parameters	Return Type
getEventCount	[in] DATE dtMonthYear, [out] long* lNumEntry, [out, size_is(,*lNumEntry)] EVTCOUNTENTRY** pevtCount, [out] long* lNumDepts, [out, size_is(,*lNumDepts)] EVTDEPT * * pevtDept	HRESULT

We also have a method to add to the interface called `IBoCentDeptsAdmin` in the `\CentBusObj` project:

Method	Parameters	Return Type
updateCount	[in] long lDeptID, [in] long lNumEntry, [in, size_is(lNumEntry * sizeof(EVTCOUNTENTRY))] EVTCOUNTENTRY * pevtCount	HRESULT

Add the structure definition for a department, and an event count entry (we will discuss these later) to the top of the IDL file in `\CentBusObj` directory:

```
import "oaidl.idl";
import "ocidl.idl";

typedef struct {
    long lDeptID;
    BSTR bstrName;
    BSTR bstrSymbol;
    OLE_COLOR clrColor;
    BSTR bstrHost;
    VARIANT_BOOL vbCanRead;
    VARIANT_BOOL vbCanPostNew;
} EVTDEPT;

typedef struct {
    DATE dtEvtDay;
    long lDeptID;
    long lEvtCount;
} EVTCOUNTENTRY;
```

The rest of the IDL should look like this:

```
[
    object,
    uuid(540477AD-E1EE-11D1-A660-006052008075),
    helpstring("IBoDeptCache Interface"),
    pointer_default(unique)
]
interface IBoDeptCache : IUnknown
{
        [id(1), helpstring("method getEventDepts")]
        HRESULT getEventDepts([in] DATE dtMonthYear,
                [out] long * lNumDepts,
                [out, size_is(,*lNumDepts)] EVTDEPT * * pevtDept);
        [id(2), helpstring("method getEventCount")]
        HRESULT getEventCount([in] DATE dtMonthYear,
                [out] long * lNumEntry,
                [out, size_is(,*lNumEntry)] EVTCOUNTENTRY * * pevtCount,
                [out] long * lNumDepts,
                [out, size_is(,*lNumDepts)] EVTDEPT * * pevtDept);
```

```
};
[
      object,
      uuid(540477AF-E1EE-11D1-A660-006052008075),
      helpstring("IBoCentDeptsAdmin Interface"),
      pointer_default(unique)
]
interface IBoCentDeptsAdmin : IUnknown
{
      [id(1), helpstring("method updateCount")]
      HRESULT updateCount([in] long lDeptID,
                 [in] long lNumEntry,
                 [in, size_is(lNumEntry * sizeof(EVTCOUNTENTRY))]
                                     EVTCOUNTENTRY * pevtCount);
};


[
   uuid(540477A1-E1EE-11D1-A660-006052008075),
   version(1.0),
   helpstring("CentBusObj 1.0 Type Library")
]
library CENTBUSOBJLib
{
   importlib("stdole32.tlb");
   importlib("stdole2.tlb");

   [
      uuid(540477AE-E1EE-11D1-A660-006052008075),
      helpstring("BoDeptsFinder Class")
   ]
   coclass BoDeptsFinder
   {
      [default] interface IBoDeptCache;
   };
   [
   uuid(540477B0-E1EE-11D1-A660-006052008075),
      helpstring("BoCentDeptsAdmin Class")
   ]
   coclass BoCentDeptsAdmin
   {
      [default] interface IBoCentDeptsAdmin;
   };
};
```

Both the \DeptBusObj and \CentBusObj should now be ready, so go ahead and build the projects.

Installing our MTS Packages

Now let's put the components into their respective MTS packages.

Make sure that you have compiled the departmental business objects in the \DeptBusObj directory, and the central server business objects in the \CentBusObj directory. Furthermore, make sure that you have compiled and registered the proxy/stubs DLL for both projects.

Here's a quick reminder on how to compile the proxy/stubs:

1. Make sure the Visual C++ 6 environment variables have been set for command line console. You may need to run vcvars32.bat in \vc98\bin\ directory.

2. Go to the \DeptBusObj directory.

3. type NMAKE -f DeptBusObjps.mk

4. After the compile, type REGSVR32 DeptBusObjps.dll

5. Repeat steps 3 and 4 in the \CentBusObj directory.

To install our packages, start up the Transaction Explorer. Then:

1. Right click on the Packages Installed folder for My Computer, and select New|Package

2. Select Create an empty package from the popup dialog and click Next>

3. Name the package Central Server

4. Set the Account to Interactive User and click Finish

5. Open up the components folder on the new package

6. Open up a file explorer window and locate the CentBusObj.dll under the \CentBusObj\Debug directory

7. Drag and drop the DLL into the new empty package

Repeat the above process to create another new package called Departmental Server, and add the file \DeptBusObj\Debug\DeptBusObj.dll.

Here is what the
Transaction
Explorer will
end up looking
like.

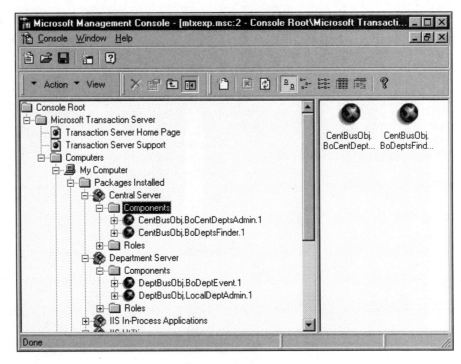

This completes our installation of the MTS components and we are now ready to run some tests against them.

Testing Our MTS Components

As a first step in testing the basic functionality of our MTS component, we will create a test harness program for each business object. Each and every method supported by a business object will be tested with the harness program.

Departmental Server

You will find code to test the Departmental Server objects in the \TestDept distribution directory. It's a Win32 console application with the file TestDept.cpp, which has the following source:

```
#include "stdafx.h"
#include "comdef.h"
#include "..\DeptBusObj\DeptBusObj.h"
#define IID_DEFINED
#include "..\DeptBusObj\DeptBusObj_i.c"
```

We are using raw COM calls for this test program, so we need to include the appropriate interface and GUID definitions for the DeptBusObj project.

```
DATE CreateADate(short year, short month, short day, short hour, short minute,
hort second)
{
   SYSTEMTIME s;
   DATE d;
   memset( &s, 0, sizeof(s) );
   s.wYear = year;
   s.wMonth = month;
   s.wDay = day;
   s.wHour = hour;
   s.wMinute = minute;
   s.wSecond = second;

   if ( SUCCEEDED(SystemTimeToVariantTime( &s, &d)) )
      return d;
   else
      return 0;
}
```

This is a short routine to construct a DATE value. It is converted from one of the CalUtils.cpp functions and we will see it frequently.

```
void ClearAnEvent(EVTDETAIL* pEvt)
{
   ::SysFreeString(pEvt->Heading);
   ::SysFreeString(pEvt->Hlink);
   ::SysFreeString(pEvt->Location);
   ::SysFreeString(pEvt->Organizer);
   ::SysFreeString(pEvt->Details);
}
```

Given an EVTDETAIL structure passed back from the business object, this function frees all the BSTRs within the structure. As a caller receiving an output buffer, we are obliged to do this.

```
#define MAX_EVENTS   20

int _tmain(int argc, _TCHAR * argv[])
{
   IUnknown * pM;
   IClassFactory * pCF;
   IBoDeptEvent * pCI;
   HRESULT hRes;
        EVTDETAIL  *pmyEvent = NULL;
   EVTDETAIL **ppmyEvent = &pmyEvent;

   CoInitialize(NULL);

   hRes = CoGetClassObject(CLSID_BoDeptEvent, CLSCTX_ALL, NULL,
                    IID_IClassFactory, reinterpret_cast<void **>( &pCF));
   hRes = pCF->CreateInstance(NULL, IID_IUnknown,
                         reinterpret_cast<void **>( &pM));
   hRes = pM->QueryInterface(IID_IBoDeptEvent,
                         reinterpret_cast<void **>( &pCI));
```

We have initialized for the apartment model, created an instance of the `BoDeptEvent` object and got `IBoDeptEvent` from it. No sign whatsoever of MTS. This shows how transparent an MTS component is to the base client.

```
long DummyVal;
if (argc > 1)
  {
    if (!_tcscmp(argv[1], _T("DEL")))
    {
    _tprintf(_T("** DELETING ONE EVENT ***\n"));

    long eventNo;
    eventNo = _ttol(argv[2]);
    hRes =pCI->delEvent(eventNo, &DummyVal);
    }
```

This bit tests the `delEvent()` call. The calling syntax is: `TESTDEPT DEL <event ID>`

```
if (!_tcscmp(argv[1], _T("SHOW")))
{
    long numElements = MAX_EVENTS;
    hRes =pCI->getAllEvents(&numElements, ppmyEvent);
    _tprintf(_T("*** There are %d events.***\n"),numElements);
    for (int i =0; i<numElements; i++)
    {
        _tprintf(_T("Event No# %d,%ls\n"),
                            (pmyEvent + i)->lEvtID,
                            (pmyEvent + i)->Heading);
        ClearAnEvent(pmyEvent); // free the BSTRs
    }
    CoTaskMemFree(pmyEvent);
}
```

This portion tests the `getAllEvents()` call. It will print out the ID and heading of each event in the departmental database. Notice the freeing of BSTRs per event record, and the freeing of the basic buffer using `CoTaskMemFree()`. It is useful for ensuring that the `delEvent()` and `addEvent()` methods work properly. The syntax is: `TESTDEPT SHOW`

```
if (!_tcscmp(argv[1], _T("ADD")))
{
    _tprintf(_T("** ADDING ONE EVENT ***\n"));

    short inYear = 1991;
    short inMonth = 1;
    short inDay = 1;
    _bstr_t inHeading = _T("Dummy Heading");
    if(argc == 6)
    {
        short tp = _ttoi(argv[2]);
        if ((tp !=0) &&(tp>1990) && (tp<2030)) inYear = tp;
        tp = _ttoi(argv[3]);
        if ((tp !=0) && (tp>0) && (tp<13)) inMonth = tp;
```

```
            tp = _ttoi(argv[4]);
            if ((tp !=0) && (tp>0) &&(tp<32)) inDay = tp;
            inHeading = argv[5];
        }

        hRes =pCI->addEvent(CreateADate(inYear,inMonth,inDay,0,0,0),
                        inHeading, _bstr_t(_T("My Hlink")),
                        _bstr_t(_T("My Location")),
                        _bstr_t(_T("My Organizer")),
                        _bstr_t(_T("My Details")), &DummyVal);
    }
```

This portion tests the addEvent() call, and takes a date and heading in the parameter. The syntax is: TESTDEPT ADD <year> <month> <day> <"heading">

```
    }
    else _tprintf(_T("invalid usage\n"));

    pCI->Release();
    pM->Release();
    CoUninitialize();
    return 0;
}
```

Since the server should be properly installed, you can go ahead and compile the program.

Before you can test the departmental server, you must seed the database with some initial event information. Using msqry32.exe supplied with SQL Server 6.5, or the database project editor of Visual Studio Enterprise edition, add the following records to the dbo.Events table of ENG data source (the engevt database):

EvntID:	1
Date:	10/11/99
DateTime:	10/11/99 14:00:00
Heading:	United Way Kickoff
Hlink:	http://awi/unitedkick/
Location:	Lunch room
Organizer:	Jack Dormer
Details:	Come to this event for a treat

EvntID:	2
Date:	11/2/99
DateTime:	11/2/99 09:15
Heading:	An Event
Hlink:	http://awi/test/
Location:	Test Location
Organizer:	Test Organizer
Details:	This is a test event
EvntID:	3
Date:	11/15/99
DateTime:	11/15/99 07:30
Heading:	World's First
Hlink:	http://awi/first/
Location:	Main Hall
Organizer:	Martin Thomas
Details:	See the world very first five headed manager

You are now ready to run tests against your business object. To use the test harness, the test commands are summarized as follows:

Action	Parameters
DEL	EventID
SHOW	
ADD	Year, Month, Day, Heading in quotes

Here is a sample run we have completed:

```
Command Prompt                                                    _ □ ×
*** There are 3 events.***
Event No# 1,United Way Kickoff
Event No# 2,An Event
Event No# 3,World's First

G:\proa2\TestDept\Debug>testdept ADD 1999 12 15 "Super Party"
** ADDING ONE EVENT ***

G:\proa2\TestDept\Debug>testdept SHOW
*** There are 4 events.***
Event No# 1,United Way Kickoff
Event No# 2,An Event
Event No# 3,World's First
Event No# 4,Super Party

G:\proa2\TestDept\Debug>testdept DEL 4
** DELETING ONE EVENT ***

G:\proa2\TestDept\Debug>testdept SHOW
*** There are 3 events.***
Event No# 1,United Way Kickoff
Event No# 2,An Event
Event No# 3,World's First

G:\proa2\TestDept\Debug>
```

Other than the slight delay in starting up (MTS executive has to start), there should be no clue that MTS is actually involved for these servers.

Central Server

To test the central server business object, we have created a test program called `TestCent.exe`. You can find the source in the distribution in the `\TestCent` directory.

The code is written to use the Visual C++ compiler COM support that we have discussed in earlier chapters. This again shows that you can use whatever COM technique to create your client using MTS components. It also means that you could in fact, retrofit an existing COM-based system with MTS components without any effect on the client.

`TestCent.cpp` looks like this:

```
#include "stdafx.h"
#import "..\CentBusObj\CentBusObj.tlb" no_namespace
```

Since, Visual C++ COM compiler support is used here, we only need the type library.

```
DATE CreateADate(short year, short month, short day, short hour, short minute,
short second)
{
...
}
```

```
void ClearADept(EVTDEPT * pCount)
{

    ::SysFreeString(pCount->bstrName);
    ::SysFreeString(pCount->bstrSymbol);
    ::SysFreeString(pCount->bstrHost);
}
```

Next we have our DATE creation function. ClearADept() is used to free the BSTRs in an EVTDEPT structure passed back from the component (actually allocated by the proxy).

```
int _tmain(int argc, _TCHAR * argv[])
{
    EVTDEPT * pDept = NULL;
    EVTDEPT * * ppDept = &pDept;
    CoInitialize(NULL);

    try
    {
        IBoCentDeptsAdminPtr  pCI(__uuidof(BoCentDeptsAdmin));
        IBoDeptCachePtr pBC(__uuidof(BoDeptsFinder));
```

Creating objects and performing QueryInterface() for interfaces requires less code here thanks to COM compiler support.

```
        if (argc > 1)
        {
          if (!_tcscmp(argv[1], _T("GETDATEDEPT")))
          {
            _tprintf(_T("** INSIDE GETDATEDEPT***\n"));

            long numDepts;
            short inYear = 1991;
            short inMonth = 1;
            short inDay = 1;
            if(argc == 5)
            {
            short tp = _ttoi(argv[2]);
            if ((tp !=0) && (tp>1990) && (tp<2030)) inYear = tp;
            tp = _ttoi(argv[3]);
            if ((tp !=0) && (tp>0) && (tp<13)) inMonth = tp;
            tp = _ttoi(argv[4]);
            if ((tp !=0) && (tp>0) &&(tp<32)) inDay = tp;

            }

            pBC->getEventDepts(CreateADate(inYear,inMonth,inDay,0,0,0),
                                     &numDepts, ppDept);
            _tprintf(_T("On %d/%d/%d... \n"), inMonth, inDay, inYear);
            _tprintf(_T("Number of departments with events = %d \n"),
                    numDepts);
            _tprintf(_T("They are...\n"));
```

```
        for (int i =0; i<numDepts; i++)
        {
            _tprintf(_T("%ls\n"),    (pDept + i)->bstrName);
            ClearADept(pDept + i);   // free the BSTRs
        }
        CoTaskMemFree(pDept);
    }
}
```

This section of code is similar to that of `TestDept.exe`. The syntax of the test program is quite simple: `TESTCENT GETDATEDEPT <year> <month> <day>`

This will get you all the departments that have event on the specified date. If you do not enter any year, month, day on the command line, a default date of 1/1/1991 will be used instead.

```
    else
        _tprintf(_T("invalid usage\n"));

    }
    catch(_com_error e)
    {
        _tprintf(_T("%08x : %s\n"), e.Error(), e.ErrorMessage());

    }
    CoUninitialize();
    return 0;
}
```

To run this test program effectively, you must get some data manually into the table. We used `msqry32.exe` to do this, but you may use MS Access or your favorite data access tool.

We will have the central server tracking events from Engineering and Accounting departments. Here is some sample data you can add to the table named `EvtDepts`:

Name	ID	Can Read	CanPost New	Symbol	Color	Host
Engineering	21240	1	1	E	16711680	192.168.23.15
Accounting	23240	1	1	A	65280	192.168.23.14

Note that the `Host` field should contain the IP address of the actual machine with the departmental server installed.

To start off with some event counts, we will add the following rows to the `EvtCount` table:

Dept	DateOnly	CountEvent
21240	10/11/99	1
21240	11/2/99	1
21240	11/15/99	1
23240	11/2/99	1
23240	11/15/99	2

Here is our result of a test run using the `TestCent` program:

```
G:\proa2\TestCent\Debug>testcent GETDATEDEPT 1998 7 1
** INSIDE GETDATEDEPT ***
On 7/1/1998...
Number of departments with events = 1
They are...
Engineering

G:\proa2\TestCent\Debug>testcent GETDATEDEPT 1991 1 1
** INSIDE GETDATEDEPT ***
On 1/1/1991...
Number of departments with events = 1
They are...
Accounting

G:\proa2\TestCent\Debug>testcent GETDATEDEPT
** INSIDE GETDATEDEPT ***
On 1/1/1991...
Number of departments with events = 1
They are...
Accounting

G:\proa2\TestCent\Debug>
```

As you can see, creating and running MTS components isn't so bad when you've got Visual C++ and ATL 3. If you're running into problems with the components, you may need to debug them – something we will try now to provide some tips for.

Tips for Debugging MTS Components

Debugging MTS components is similar to debugging any DLL hosted by an EXE, but with a few caveats. We will try to discuss them here to save you some aggravation.

Use /p:<package ID>

To debug an MTS component, go to the Project | Settings... menu selection in Visual Studio 6 and select the Debug tab. The Executable field should be:

```
\<path to windows>\system32\mtx.exe
```

And the Program arguments field should be:

```
/p:<package ID>
```

Where `<path to windows>` is your path to the Windows NT directory, and `<package ID>` is the GUID representing the package where the component is installed.

To obtain this ID, you can highlight the package in Transaction Explorer and right-click, selecting Properties. You can then cut and paste this ID into Visual Studio 6 (or alternatively, you can find the ID from OLEVIEW by examining the component's associated registry entries.

Set Timeout to Zero

If you pause for a time while debugging MTS components (they are usually so simple that this should never be the case), that instance of `Mtx.exe` may timeout on you. This timeout is adjustable as we have discussed earlier, and you can set it to 0, in which case `Mtx.exe` won't shutdown until you do so explicitly. For the thinking programmer, this can be a handy feature.

Remember those Proxy Stubs!

The most common problem facing MTS component programmers is forgetting to recompile and re-register proxy/stub DLLs. On desktop COM, almost everything is in-process and most modern clients are apartment threaded, so proxy/stubs are not strictly necessary for STA components (although it is a good practice to include one). With MTS, you must always remember your proxy/stubs, unless all the interfaces on your component are automation compatible.

Every time you make a change to any interface details, you must manually recompile and re-register the proxy/stub DLLs. Try to get used to:

```
nmake -f <my project>ps.mk
regsvr32 <myproject>ps.dll
```

Anything can happen if you forget to register your proxy/stub DLL. Typical symptoms are calls failing, MTS rejection of the component when adding it to a package or giant cryptic message boxes complaining about changed call syntax.

MTXReReg needs to be Run after each Recompile

After you have recompiled your component, remember to run `mtxrereg.exe`, or Refresh All Components... from the Transaction Explorer. Otherwise, the default in-process registration will be in the registry, and running the component will probably crash when `SetComplete()` or `SetAbort()` is called.

Shutdown and Restart Server when Things Get Weird

If you find something unexplainable happening after a component has been working for a long time, try the command line `mtxstop.exe` or **Shutdown Server Processes...** from the Transaction Explorer. Frequently, you may just be running with slightly out-of-date components inside stale servers that have hung around.

MTS, the Great Deployer

For a change of pace, we shall take a tour on using MTS for deployment.

So far, we have been running our tests with both business components running on the same server machine (and this is a valid testing strategy). Let us now move the central server to another Windows NT machine, using Transaction Explorer. The operation is pretty much drag-and-drop, and allows you to easily move middle-tier objects around different servers for load balancing and/or problem isolation.

Both systems must be running Windows NT 4.0 (with Service Pack 3 or later), and must have MTS installed.

Here is our configuration:

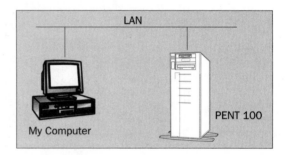

Our working system so far has been MYCOMPUTER, and the remote server is called PENT100. To be able to see the remote computer in MTS explorer, we must first add the computer to the **Computers** folder.

To add the PENT100 server:

- ❑ Click on the **Computers** folder in the left pane of the explorer so that **My Computer** shows up on the right pane
- ❑ From the menu click **Action**, and select **New Computer...**
- ❑ Enter the name of the computer

As viewed from the MTS explorer, we now have the following packages installed on the two servers:

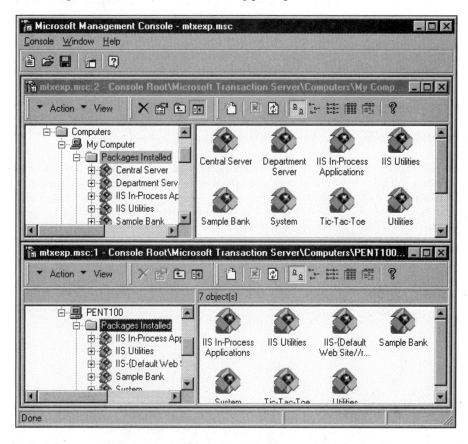

You can see that Central Server and Departmental Server are both running on the local server, called My Computer.

Next, we need to export the Central Server package. This can be accomplished by highlighting the package, clicking the right button, and then selecting Export. A dialog box will prompt you for a location of the resulting PAK package file.

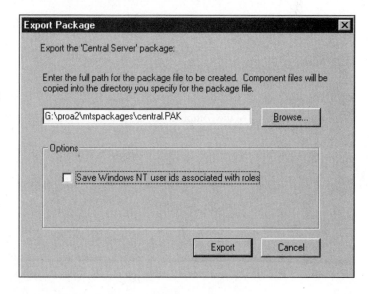

For us, we will store it in a file called `central.PAK` under an `mtspackages` directory that we have created for it. Ideally, this directory should be on a shared volume between the two servers. If not, you need to copy the content of the directory to the other server. Ignore the Options group box for now, it is used to preserve role security assignments, we will discuss role-based security at length in Chapter 11.

Exporting the package puts the following files in your shared directory:

- `central.pak`
- `CentBusObj.dll`
- `CentBusObjps.dll`

Now we need to install the package on the `PENT100` server. From the MTS explorer (still local), highlight the Packages Installed folder of the `PENT100` server and right click, selecting New | Package:

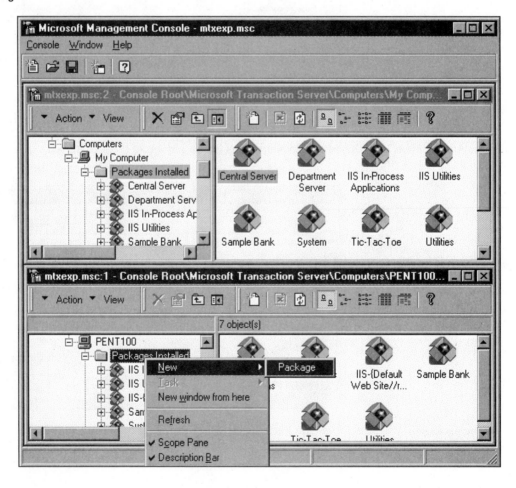

The wizard will now start, and we can select the Install pre-built packages button.

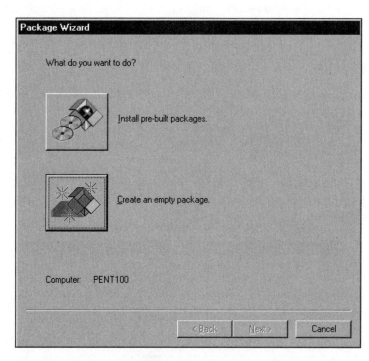

Press the Add... button from the Select Package Files dialog and locate the PAK file we exported earlier. Then press Open:

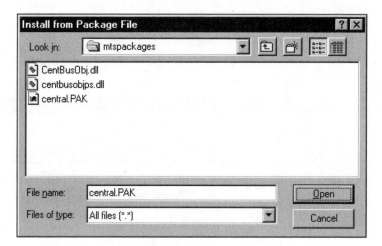

Select the package in the Select Package Files dialog and press the Next> button.

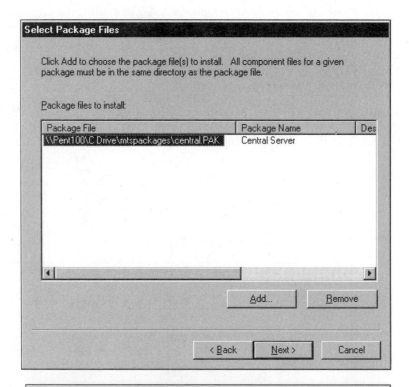

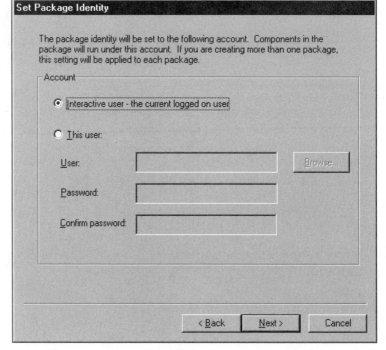

In the Set Package Identity dialog, leave the selection as Interactive user. In production installations, you would specify the identity (account) that you want the package to be running under – adding the appropriate access rights to resources, etc. Press Next>.

Leave all the options in the Installation Options dialog at default, and press the Finish button.

If all goes
well, the
Central
Server will
now be
installed at
the remote
server
(PENT100
in our
case).

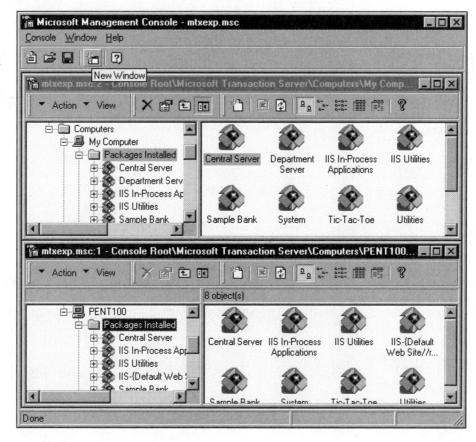

Now, all that remains to do is:

- ❑ Remove the local Central Server package
- ❑ Configure the local server to use the remote Central Server package
- ❑ Set up the ODBC System DSN on the remote server so that the business object can function properly
- ❑ Transfer the proa2 database between the two SQL servers

To remove the local Central Server package, simply highlight the package, right-click, and select Delete. Confirm the removal.

To gain access to the remote package, highlight the Remote Components folder of the local computer, right-click and select New | Remote Component.

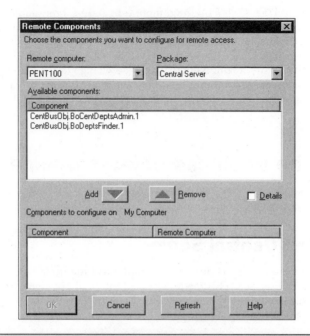

In the **Remote Components** dialog, select the remote computer, PENT100, and the package, **Central Server**. From the **Available** components list, select the components and press the **Add** button. Finally, press OK. You should now see the components from the **Central Server** package under your **Remote Components** folder.

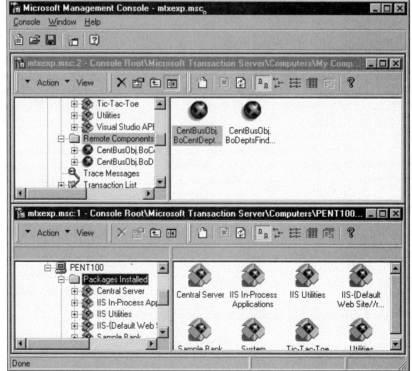

Set up the ODBC System DSN CENT on the remote PENT100 server, and we are ready to rock. As a rule,you should highlight each computer and right click select **Shutdown Server Processes** before and after the procedure, which should prevent any surprises during the procedure.

We can now try out TestCent again. Note that with no change to the client, we have moved a business object from one server to another relatively easily. This same procedure can be used to move middle-tier components between any two servers on a network, as long as they both running MTS.

Completing the Business Objects Coding

Now, we need to implement the methods that we have added to the interface earlier in the chapter, which will complete our business objects coding.

Fleshing Out the Central Server

To update our central business object, we need to implement the updateCount() method of the IBoCentDeptsAdmin interface. This method is used internally by departmental business objects, within a distributed transaction, to update the cached count of events for the department for a certain day. This method has the following signature:

```
HRESULT updateCount([in] long lDeptID,
                    [in] long lNumEntry,
                    [in, size_is(lNumEntry * sizeof(EVTCOUNTENTRY))]
                    EVTCOUNTENTRY * pevtCount);
```

Use **Class View** in Visual Studio 6 to add the method definition. We also need to create two more **OLE DB** consumer accessors, dboEventCount and dboEvtCntTbl. dboEventCount's properties are summarized as follows:

Short Name	dboEventCount
Data source	CENT
Type	Command
Table	dbo.EventCount
Command	SELECT * FROM dbo.EventCount WHERE Dept = ?
Parameter	LONG m_ParamDept;
Properties	Insert and Change

After the OLE DB wizard generation, make sure you remember to manually:

❑ Add the parameter member variable shown above to the header file
❑ Add a PARAM_MAP for that variable
❑ Modify the command text with the SQL above

The other OLE DB accessor required is:

Short Name	dboEvtCntTbl
Data source	CENT
Type	Table
Table	dbo.EventCount
Properties	Insert and Change

Review the last chapter if the procedure is not yet clear. If you have not followed along, you can find source code to this method in the \CentBusObj.2\BoCentDeptsAdmin.cpp directory. Here is the actual code of the method:

```
STDMETHODIMP CBoCentDeptsAdmin::updateCount(long lDeptID, long lNumEntry,
EVTCOUNTENTRY *pevtCount)
{
    ATLTRACE(_T("CBoCentDeptsAdmin::updateCount called...\n"));
    CdboEventCount evtcntWork;
    bool bBadUpdate = false;

    for (int i=1; i<=lNumEntry; i++)
    {
```

The calling client may pass in a whole bunch of event count entries at a time. We want to see if something matching the date and time already exists. If it does not, we will add the entry, but if it does, we will simply update it.

```
        evtcntWork.m_ParamDept = lDeptID;
        DBTIMESTAMP tpTimeStamp;
        CDateTime tpDate(pevtCount[i-1].dtEvtDay);
        tpDate.ConvertToDBTIMESTAMP(&tpTimeStamp);

        if( evtcntWork.Open() != S_OK)
        {
            m_spObjectContext->SetAbort();
            return E_FAIL;
        }
        bool bRowFound = false;
```

This opens a rowset on the event count table with only those entries that match the department of this current incoming entry.

```
        // SQL date is not easily done in SELECT, do manually
        while( evtcntWork.MoveNext() == S_OK)
        {
            if (memcmp(&(evtcntWork.m_DateOnly),
            &tpTimeStamp, sizeof(tpTimeStamp))==0)
            {
```

519

```
            bRowFound = true;
            break;
            }
        }
```

We loop through the rowset looking for a matching date and time.

```
        if(!bRowFound)
        {
            // insert
            evtcntWork.Close();
            CdboEvtCntTbl tblWork;
            tblWork.Open();
            tblWork.m_Dept = lDeptID;
            tblWork.m_DateOnly = tpTimeStamp;
            tblWork.m_CountEvent = pevtCount[i-1].lEvtCount;
            if (tblWork.Insert() != S_OK)
            {
                tblWork.Close();
                bBadUpdate = true;
                break;
            }
            tblWork.Close();
        }
```

If a matching row is not found, we perform an insert using the `CdboEvtCntTbl` accessor stack.

```
        else
        {
            // modify
            evtcntWork.m_Dept = lDeptID;
            evtcntWork.m_DateOnly = tpTimeStamp;
            evtcntWork.m_CountEvent = pevtCount[i-1].lEvtCount;

            if(   evtcntWork.SetData(0) != S_OK)
            {
                evtcntWork.Close();
                bBadUpdate = true;
                break;
            }
```

If a matching row is found, we simply update the entry using `SetDate()` call after filling in the accessor.

```
            evtcntWork.Close();
        }
        // of else rowFound

    } // of for (i)

    if(bBadUpdate)
    {
```

```
        m_spObjectContext->SetAbort();
        return E_FAIL;
    }
    else
    {
        m_spObjectContext->SetComplete();
        return S_OK;
    }
} //of UpdateCount();
```

Check the header files, and make sure all the includes for the OLE DB accessors are in place:

```
#include "stdafx.h"
#include "CentBusObj.h"
#include "BoCentDeptsAdmin.h"
// Database
#include "dboEventCount.h"
#include "dboEvtCntTbl.h"
#include "CalUtils.h"
```

Before we proceed further, remember to recompile and reregister the proxy/stub DLL!

The second method we need to implement is from the `IBoDeptCache` interface, and is called `getEventCount()`. This method has the following signature:

```
HRESULT getEventCount([in] DATE dtMonthYear,
                      [out] long * lNumEntry,
                      [out, size_is(,*lNumEntry)]
                          EVTCOUNTENTRY** pevtCount,
                      [out] long* lNumDepts,
                      [out, size_is(,*lNumDepts)]
                          EVTDEPT** pevtDept);
```

For this method, we need to create one more OLE DB consumer accessor. This accessor, `DboCntOnDate`, will be used to locate all the event counts matching a specified month from the `dbo.EventCount` table. To define this accessor, you need the following information:

Short Name	DboCntOnDate
Data Source	CENT
Type	Command
Table	dbo.EventCount
Command	.SELECT * FROM dbo.EventCount WHERE datepart(year,DateOnly)=? and datepart(month,DateOnly)=?
Parameters	LONG m_ParamYear; LONG m_ParamMonth;

Here is the implementation code of the method. You can find it in the
\CentBusObj.2\BoDeptsFinder.cpp file. Given a month, this method will return all the
consolidated event count entries to the client. In addition, to save the client another network round-
trip, it will also supply all the department information for the departments having events in that
month.

```
STDMETHODIMP CBoDeptsFinder::getEventCount(DATE dtMonthYear,
                                            long *lNumEntry,
                                            EVTCOUNTENTRY **pevtCount,
                                            long *lNumDepts,
                                            EVTDEPT **pevtDept )
{
    ATLTRACE(_T("CBoDeptsFinder::getEventCount called..."));
    (*pevtCount) = reinterpret_cast<EVTCOUNTENTRY*>
                (CoTaskMemAlloc(sizeof(EVTCOUNTENTRY) * MAX_EVENTCOUNTS));
    (*pevtDept) = reinterpret_cast<EVTDEPT*>
                (CoTaskMemAlloc(sizeof(EVTDEPT) * MAX_DEPTS));
    if (((*pevtCount) == NULL) || ((*pevtDept) == NULL))
    {
        ATLTRACE(_T("CBoDeptsFinder::CoTaskMemAlloc FAILED!!..."));
        m_spObjectContext->SetAbort();
        return E_OUTOFMEMORY;
    }
```

Allocate the two buffers for returned data.

```
    USES_CONVERSION;
```

The code in ATLConv.h for converting TCHAR from the accessor to BSTR that we need to use for
returned records is enabled by this macro.

```
    CdboCntOnDate tpCount;
    tpCount.ClearRecord();

    // set the current record
    CDateTime dtWorkDate(dtMonthYear);
    long t = tpCount.m_ParamYear = dtWorkDate.GetYear();
    long u = tpCount.m_ParamMonth = dtWorkDate.GetMonth();
    long evtCount = 0;

    if( tpCount.Open() != S_OK)
    {
        // not necessary for read, but do for good form
        m_spObjectContext->SetAbort();
        tpCount.Close();
        return E_FAIL;
    }
```

We parameterize the query with the month desired and open the rowset on the event count table.

```
    while( tpCount.MoveNext() == S_OK) && (evtCount < MAX_EVENTCOUNTS))
    {
        // copy into the return array for marshalling
```

```
            CDateTime tpDateTime(tpCount.m_DateOnly);
            (*pevtCount)[evtCount].dtEvtDay = tpDateTime.ConvertToDATE();
            (*pevtCount)[evtCount].lDeptID = tpCount.m_Dept;
            (*pevtCount)[evtCount].lEvtCount = tpCount.m_CountEvent;
            evtCount++;
        }

        *lNumEntry = evtCount;
        tpCount.Close();
```

Looping through the returned rowset, we copy each entry into the buffer and finally set the count for the marshaller and the client.

```
        // fill the department table up
        CdboEvtDepts tpDept;
        long deptCount = 0;
        tpDept.m_ParamYear = dtWorkDate.GetYear();
        tpDept.m_ParamMonth = dtWorkDate.GetMonth();

        if( tpDept.Open() != S_OK)
        {
            // not necessary for read, but do for good form
            m_spObjectContext->SetAbort();
            tpDept.Close();
            return E_FAIL;
        }
```

Here, we parameterize the department table query in the exact same way.

```
        while( ( tpDept.MoveNext() == S_OK) && (deptCount < MAX_DEPTS))
        {
            // copy into the return array for marshalling
            (*pevtDept)[deptCount].bstrName = T2BSTR(tpDept.m_Name);
            (*pevtDept)[deptCount].lDeptID = tpDept.m_ID;
            (*pevtDept)[deptCount].vbCanRead = tpDept.m_CanRead;
            (*pevtDept)[deptCount].vbCanPostNew = tpDept.m_CanPostNew;
            (*pevtDept)[deptCount].bstrSymbol = T2BSTR(tpDept.m_Symbol);
            (*pevtDept)[deptCount].clrColor = tpDept.m_Color;
            (*pevtDept)[deptCount].bstrHost = T2BSTR(tpDept.m_Host);
            deptCount++;
        }
```

Finally, we loop through the rowsets returned from the department table and stuff them into the buffer as well.

```
        *lNumDepts = deptCount;
        tpDept.Close();

        m_spObjectContext->SetComplete();
        return S_OK;
    }
```

Make sure the include headers and defines are in place:

```
#include "stdafx.h"
#include "CentBusObj.h"
#include "BoDeptsFinder.h"
#include "dboEvtDepts.h"
#include "CalUtils.h"

#include "dboCntOnDate.h"
#define MAX_EVENTCOUNTS 100
#define MAX_DEPTS 5
```

This is all the work we need to perform on the central server, you can now save the project and compile it.

You can find the completed project in the \CentBusObj.2 directory. In either case, remember to recompile the proxy/stubs, and to run mtxrereg.exe!

Finishing up the Departmental Server

Let's take a look at the Departmental Server, where we need to implement a new method called getEventOnDate() on the IBoDeptEvent interface with the following signature:

```
HRESULT getEventOnDate([in] DATE dtOnDate,
                       [out] long * lNumEvents,
                       [out,size_is(,*lNumEvents)] EVTDETAIL** pevtDet);
```

This method returns all the events for a particular month from the departmental database.

We will need to create three more OLE DB consumer accessors:

❑ DboFindTotal
❑ DboEvtOnDate
❑ DboWorkDept

Let's take a look at these now. The first one will obtain the total number of events in the table:

Short Name	DboFindTotal
Data Source	ENG
Type	Command
Table	dbo.FindTotal
Command	SELECT * FROM dbo.FindTotal

The second accessor obtains all events for a specified month:

Short Name	DboEvtOnDate
Data Source	ENG
Type	Command
Table	dbo.Events
Command	SELECT * FROM dbo.Events WHERE datepart(year,Date)=? and datepart(month,Date)=?
Parameters	LONG m_ParamYear; LONG m_ParamMonth;

The third provides detailed information for the department itself:

Short Name	DboWorkDept
Data source	ENG
Type	Command
Table	dbo.Dept
Command	SELECT * FROM dbo.Dept

Here is the `getEventOnDate()` method implementation, you can find the source in
`\DeptBusObj.2\BoDeptEvent.cpp`:

```
STDMETHODIMP CBoDeptEvent::getEventOnDate(DATE dtOnDate, long *lNumEvents,
EVTDETAIL **pevtDet)
{
    ATLTRACE(_T("CBoDeptEvent::getEventOnDate called..."));

    (*pevtDet) = reinterpret_cast<EVTDETAIL *>
                        (CoTaskMemAlloc(sizeof(EVTDETAIL) * MAX_EVENTS));
    USES_CONVERSION;
```

Here, we allocate the memory for the return buffer, and declare our use of `AtlConv.h` conversions.

```
    CdboEvtOnDate   tpEvents;
    tpEvents.ClearRecord();
    // set the current record
    CDateTime dtWorkDate(dtOnDate);

    tpEvents.m_ParamYear = dtWorkDate.GetYear();
    tpEvents.m_ParamMonth = dtWorkDate.GetMonth();
```

```
    long evtCount = 0;
    if( tpEvents.Open() != S_OK)
    {
        // not necessary for read, but do for good form
        m_spObjectContext->SetAbort();
        tpEvents.Close();
        return E_FAIL;
    }
```

Next, we parameterize the query on the Events table with the required month and open it to get a return rowset.

```
    long maxEvents    = *lNumEvents;

    while((tpEvents.MoveNext() == S_OK) && (evtCount < MAX_EVENTS))
    {
        // copy into the return array for marshalling
        (*pevtDet)[evtCount].lEvtID = tpEvents.m_EvntID;
        CDateTime tpDateTime(tpEvents.m_DateTime);
        (*pevtDet)[evtCount].dtDateTime = tpDateTime.ConvertToDATE();
        BSTR a = (*pevtDet)[evtCount].Heading = T2BSTR(tpEvents.m_Heading);
        BSTR b = (*pevtDet)[evtCount].Hlink = T2BSTR(tpEvents.m_Hlink);
        (*pevtDet)[evtCount].Location = T2BSTR(tpEvents.m_Location);
        (*pevtDet)[evtCount].Organizer = T2BSTR(tpEvents.m_Organizer);
        (*pevtDet)[evtCount].Details = T2BSTR(tpEvents.m_Details);
        evtCount++;
    }

    *lNumEvents = evtCount;
    m_spObjectContext->SetComplete();
    tpEvents.Close();
    return S_OK;
}
```

Finally, we loop through the rowset and stuff the entries into the return buffer, and set the size appropriately.

Make sure the OLE DB accessor header and constant definition is included at the top of the file:

```
#include "stdafx.h"
#include "DeptBusObj.h"
#include "BoDeptEvent.h"
#include "dboAllEvents.h"
#include "dboMaxEvent.h"
#include "dboEventsTbl.h"
#include "CalUtils.h"

#include "dboFindTotal.h"
#include "dboEvtOnDate.h"
#include "dboWorkDept.h"
#define MAX_EVENTS 20
```

We have completed all our required methods. However, the addEvent() and delEvent() methods currently don't yet use distributed transaction to update the central server's count. Let's add this functionality now.

Adding the Distributed Transaction Support

Still in \DeptBusObj.2\BoDeptEvent.cpp, here is the code we have to add for the addEvent() method to implement distributed transaction support:

```
STDMETHODIMP CBoDeptEvent::addEvent(DATE dtOnDate,
                                    BSTR bstrHeading,
                                    BSTR bstrHlink,
                                    BSTR bstrLocation,
                                    BSTR bstrOrganizer,
                                    BSTR bstrDetails,
                                    long *plID)
{
    IBoCentDeptsAdmin* pCentDeptsAdmin;
    EVTCOUNTENTRY evtcntWork;

    USES_CONVERSION;
    ATLTRACE(_T("CBoDeptEvent::addEvent called..."));
```

This new section of code allows us to find out which department this server is for and stores the ID in m_myDeptID. This is configurable via the Dept table.

```
    CdboWorkDept tpDept;
    if( tpDept.Open() != S_OK)
    {
        m_spObjectContext->SetAbort();
        tpDept.Close();
        return E_FAIL;
    }
    tpDept.MoveFirst();
    m_myDeptID = tpDept.m_Number;
    tpDept.Close();


    CdboEventsTbl evtTblWork;
    CdboMaxEvent evtMaxID;

    if (evtTblWork.Open() != S_OK)
    {
        m_spObjectContext->SetAbort();
        evtTblWork.Close();
        return E_FAIL;
    }

    // locate the current max ID
    if(evtMaxID.Open() != S_OK)
    {
```

```
      m_spObjectContext->SetAbort();
      evtMaxID.Close();
      return E_FAIL;
   }
   evtMaxID.MoveFirst();

   // use ID that is 1 larger than MAX
   evtTblWork.m_EvntID = evtMaxID.m_MaxID + 1;
   evtMaxID.Close();   // that's all we need this for

   // set data into the current record
   CDateTime dtWorkDate(dtOnDate);
   DBTIMESTAMP dbtsWorkTimestamp;
   dtWorkDate.ConvertToDBTIMESTAMP(&dbtsWorkTimestamp);
   evtTblWork.m_DateTime = dbtsWorkTimestamp;
   dbtsWorkTimestamp.hour = 0;
   dbtsWorkTimestamp.minute = 0;
   dbtsWorkTimestamp.second = 0;
   evtTblWork.m_Date = dbtsWorkTimestamp;

   _tcscpy(evtTblWork.m_Details, OLE2T(bstrDetails));
   _tcscpy( evtTblWork.m_Heading, OLE2T(bstrHeading));
   _tcscpy( evtTblWork.m_Hlink, OLE2T(bstrHlink));
   _tcscpy( evtTblWork.m_Location, OLE2T(bstrLocation));
   _tcscpy(evtTblWork.m_Organizer, OLE2T(bstrOrganizer));

   if (evtTblWork.Insert() != S_OK)
   {
     m_spObjectContext->SetAbort();
     evtTblWork.Close();
     return E_FAIL;
   }

   evtTblWork.Close();
```

Here, we obtain the event count associated with the date.

```
   // get the latest event count for the day
   CdboFindTotal evtTotal;

   // set up parameter
   dbtsWorkTimestamp.second = 0;

   // perform query
   if (evtTotal.Open() != S_OK)
   {
      m_spObjectContext->SetAbort();
      evtTotal.Close();
      return E_FAIL;
   }

   while( evtTotal.MoveNext() == S_OK)
   {
```

```
            if (memcmp(&(evtTotal.m_Date), &dbtsWorkTimestamp,
                               sizeof(dbtsWorkTimestamp))==0)
            {
                break;
            }
        }
```

We create and stuff a single event count entry to pass as input parameter.

```
        evtcntWork.dtEvtDay = CDateTime(dbtsWorkTimestamp).ConvertToDATE();
        evtcntWork.lEvtCount = evtTotal.m_Total; // assign total
        evtcntWork.lDeptID = m_myDeptID;
```

Coding the Distributed Transaction

The next line of code is the crux of creating distributed transactions via composition. By simply using
the CreateInstance() method from the context object, we ensure that any transaction that we are
in will be passed onto the object being composed (in this case, it is the central server business object).
Notice that we are not creating this object as early as possible, but our object's lifetime is rather
temporary – until object pooling is implemented by MTS.

```
        // compose - pass on the transaction context
        m_spObjectContext->CreateInstance(CLSID_BoCentDeptsAdmin,
                          IID_IBoCentDeptsAdmin,
                          reinterpret_cast<void **>( &pCentDeptsAdmin));
```

Finally, we call updateCount() and then call SetAbort() if there are any problems:

```
        if( pCentDeptsAdmin->updateCount(m_myDeptID, 1, &evtcntWork) != S_OK)
        {
            m_spObjectContext->SetAbort();
            evtTotal.Close();
            pCentDeptsAdmin->Release();
            return E_FAIL;
        }
```

This is a nice segment of code that we can uncomment to cause a call to SetAbort() and observe
the result on the two databases. But then again, you could simply disconnect the networking cable.

```
//**** INDUCE an error for testing
/* {
        m_spObjectContext->SetAbort();
        evtTotal.Close();
        pCentDeptsAdmin->Release();
        return E_FAIL;
    }
*/
```

If everything is fine, then we call `SetComplete()`:

```
    m_spObjectContext->SetComplete();
    evtTotal.Close();
    pCentDeptsAdmin->Release();
    return S_OK;
}
```

For the `delEvent()` method, also found in `\DeptBusObj.2\BoDeptEvent.cpp`, the modification to the source is:

```
STDMETHODIMP CBoDeptEvent::delEvent(long lEventID, long *lSuccess)
{
    IBoCentDeptsAdmin* pCentDeptsAdmin;
    EVTCOUNTENTRY evtcntWork;
    USES_CONVERSION;
```

As in `addEvent()`, this is the department discovery code.

```
    CdboWorkDept tpDept;
    if( tpDept.Open() != S_OK)
    {
        m_spObjectContext->SetAbort();
        tpDept.Close();
        return E_FAIL;
    }
    tpDept.MoveFirst();
    m_myDeptID = tpDept.m_Number;
    tpDept.Close();

    CdboEventsTbl evtTblWork;
    if( evtTblWork.Open() != S_OK)
    {
        m_spObjectContext->SetAbort();
        evtTblWork.Close();
        return E_FAIL;
    }
    bool tpDeleteFlag = false;
    DBTIMESTAMP dbtsWorkTimestamp;
```

We keep the date and time of the event we deleted here. It will be used later to update the count.

```
    while( evtTblWork.MoveNext() == S_OK)
    {
        if (evtTblWork.m_EvntID  == lEventID)
        {
            dbtsWorkTimestamp = evtTblWork.m_Date;
            evtTblWork.Delete();  // delete the row
            tpDeleteFlag = true;
            break;
        }
    }
```

Unlike the previous version, we are interested in the case if a record has been deleted.

```
if( tpDeleteFlag == true)
{
    // get the latest event count for the day
    CdboFindTotal evtTotal;

    // set up parameter
    dbtsWorkTimestamp.second = 0;

    // perform query
    if (evtTotal.Open() != S_OK)
    {
        m_spObjectContext->SetAbort();
        evtTblWork.Close();
        evtTotal.Close();
        return E_FAIL;
    }
}
```

We actually deleted a row, so we use the saved timestamp to find the new event count for that date and time.

```
while( evtTotal.MoveNext() == S_OK)
{
    if (memcmp(&(evtTotal.m_Date), &dbtsWorkTimestamp,
                            sizeof(dbtsWorkTimestamp))==0)
    {
        break;
    }
}
```

We stuff an event count entry for input to `updateCount()` shortly.

```
evtcntWork.dtEvtDay = CDateTime(dbtsWorkTimestamp).ConvertToDATE();
evtcntWork.lEvtCount = evtTotal.m_Total; // assign total
evtcntWork.lDeptID = m_myDeptID;
```

Again, we create the central server within our transaction, and then call update count. Finally, we call `SetComplete()` or `SetAbort()` accordingly.

```
// compose - pass on the transaction context
m_spObjectContext->CreateInstance(CLSID_BoCentDeptsAdmin,
                    IID_IBoCentDeptsAdmin,
                    reinterpret_cast<void **>( &pCentDeptsAdmin));
if(pCentDeptsAdmin->updateCount(m_myDeptID, 1, &evtcntWork) != S_OK)
{
    m_spObjectContext->SetAbort();
    evtTblWork.Close();
    evtTotal.Close();
    pCentDeptsAdmin->Release();
    return E_FAIL;
}
```

```
//**** INDUCE an error for testing
/*      {
            m_spObjectContext->SetAbort();
            evtTblWork.Close();
            evtTotal.Close();
            pCentDeptsAdmin->Release();
            return E_FAIL;
        }
*/

        m_spObjectContext->SetComplete();
        evtTblWork.Close();
        evtTotal.Close();
        pCentDeptsAdmin->Release();
    }
    else
    {
        m_spObjectContext->SetAbort();
        evtTblWork.Close();
        return E_FAIL;
    }
    m_spObjectContext->SetComplete();
    return S_OK;
}
```

For this project, we need a reference to the central department object, so add the following line to
stdafx.h:

```
#include "..\CentBusObj.2\CentBusObj.h"
```

And the following to stdafx.cpp:

```
#include "..\CentBusObj.2\CentBusObj_i.c"
```

This completes all our modifications for these middle tier components. You can compile and link
both \CentBusObj.2 and \DeptBusObj.2 directories. Make sure you have also recompiled the
proxy/stubs and reregistered them on your system:

```
nmake -f DeptBusObjps.mk
regsvr32 DeptBusObjps.dll

nmake -f CentBusObjps.mk
regsvr32 CentBusObjps.dll
```

Setting up Automatic Transactions

Now, remove the Central Server from the Remote Components folder and reinstall it locally for
more testing.

Using the Transaction Explorer, make sure you have set the declarative transaction properties for the components properly:

Component	Transaction Property
DeptBusObj.BoDeptEvent	Requires a transaction
DeptBusObj.LocalDeptAdmin	Supports transactions
CentBusObj.BoDeptsFinder	Supports transactions
CentBusObj.BoCentDeptsAdmin	Supports transactions

The departmental business object, BoDeptEvent, handles the addEvent() and delEvent() methods to always start with a transaction. Since the updateCount() handling central object supports transactions, they will both execute under the same transaction. If we also set the DeptBusObj.BoDeptEvent property to Supports transactions, no transaction will be started. Such dynamic configuration is the real strength of declarative automatic transaction.

Adding Testcases to the Testing Harness

You can find new testing programs in the \TestDept.2 and \TestCent.2 directories. These programs have been enhanced to support the new methods on the two servers.

You can now use TestCent to try out updateCount(). The code we added is:

```
if (!_tcscmp(argv[1], _T("UPDATECOUNT")))
{
    short inYear = 1991;
    short inMonth = 1;
    short inDay = 1;
    long inDept = 22322;
    long inCount = 10;

    if(argc == 7)
    {
        short tp = _ttoi(argv[2]);
        if ((tp !=0) &&(tp>1990) && (tp<2030))
            inYear = tp;

        tp = _ttoi(argv[3]);
        if ((tp !=0) && (tp>0) && (tp<13))
            inMonth = tp;

        tp = _ttoi(argv[4]);
        if ((tp !=0) && (tp>0) &&(tp<32))
            inDay = tp;

        tp = _ttoi(argv[5]);
        if ((tp !=0) && (tp>20000) &&(tp<30000))
            inDept = tp;
```

```
            tp = _ttoi(argv[6]);
            if ((tp !=0) && (tp>0) &&(tp<50))
                inCount = tp;
        }
        anEntry.dtEvtDay = CreateADate(inYear,inMonth,inDay,0,0,0);
        anEntry.lDeptID = inDept;
        anEntry.lEvtCount = inCount;
        pCI->updateCount(anEntry.lDeptID, 1, &anEntry);
    }
```

The syntax for use is:

```
TestCent UPDATECOUNT <year> <month> <day> <deptID> <count>
```

If a count exists for the department on the date specified, it is updated; otherwise a new record is created in the table. Try this out with `msqry32.exe` running and you'll see the table being updated.

To test out the `getEventCount()` method, we have added the following code to `TestCent.cpp`:

```
    if (!_tcscmp(argv[1], _T("GETEVENTCOUNT")))
    {
        EVTCOUNTENTRY * pEvt = NULL;
        EVTCOUNTENTRY * * ppEvt = &pEvt;
        EVTDEPT * pDept = NULL;
        EVTDEPT * * ppDept = &pDept;
        short inYear = 1991;
        short inMonth = 1;
        short inDay = 1;
        long  numElements ;
        long numDepts ;
        int i;

        if(argc == 5)
        {
            short tp = _ttoi(argv[2]);
            if ((tp !=0) &&(tp>1990) && (tp<2030)) inYear = tp;
            tp = _ttoi(argv[3]);
            if ((tp !=0) && (tp>0) && (tp<13)) inMonth = tp;
            tp = _ttoi(argv[4]);
            if ((tp !=0) && (tp>0) &&(tp<32)) inDay = tp;
        }

        _tprintf(_T("** INSIDE GETEVENTCOUNT ***\n"));

        pBC->getEventCount(CreateADate(inYear,inMonth,inDay,0,0,0),
                                            &numElements,
                                            ppEvt, &numDepts, ppDept);
        _tprintf(_T("Number of Event Count Entries = %d\n"),numElements);
        for ( i =0; i<numElements; i++)
        {

            _tprintf(_T("Dept # %d, Events Count = %d\n"),
                                            (pEvt + i)->lDeptID,
                                            (pEvt + i)->lEvtCount);
```

```
    }
    _tprintf(_T("Number of Departments = %d \n"), numDepts);
    for ( i=0; i<numDepts; i++)  // free all the BSTRs
    {
        _tprintf(_T("Dept # %d  is %ls\n"),
                                (pDept + i)->lDeptID,
                                (pDept + i)->bstrName  );

        ClearADept(pDept + i);
    }
    CoTaskMemFree(pEvt);
    CoTaskMemFree(pDept);
}
```

The syntax for use is:

```
TestCent GETEVENTCOUNT <year> <month> <day>
```

This will fetch all the event count entries associated with the specified date. TestCent will print out all the entries, plus the department details that is also supplied by the method upon return. Here is an example test run of the program:

On the departmental server side, the distributed transaction can now be tested with the ADD and DEL operations of the TestDept.exe testing harness. Try adding an event on the department server and observe that the central server's count is updated. Use TestDept SHOW and TestCent GETEVENTCOUNT <date> to see this. Try deleting the event and see how the count is decremented. Try simulating an error by disabling access to the central server (or uncommenting the error injection code in the AddEvent() method) and see the transaction abort. Both the local and central server's tables should be unchanged, and an aborted transaction should appear in the Transaction Explorer's Transaction Statistics.

`TestDept.exe`, found in `\TestDept.2`, also has support for the new `getEventOnDate()` method. Here's the additional code:

```
if (!_tcscmp(argv[1], _T("GETEVENTONDATE")))
{
    _tprintf(_T("** GET EVENT ON DATE ***\n"));

    short inYear = 1991;
    short inMonth = 1;
    short inDay = 1;
    if(argc == 5)
    {
        short tp = _ttoi(argv[2]);
        if ((tp !=0) &&(tp>1990) && (tp<2030)) inYear = tp;
        tp = _ttoi(argv[3]);
        if ((tp !=0) && (tp>0) && (tp<13)) inMonth = tp;
        tp = _ttoi(argv[4]);
        if ((tp !=0) && (tp>0) &&(tp<32)) inDay = tp;
    }
    long numElements = MAX_EVENTS;
    hRes =pCI->getEventOnDate(CreateADate(inYear,inMonth,inDay,0,0,0),
                                        &numElements, ppmyEvent);
    _tprintf(_T("*** On %d/%d/%d, there are %d events!***\n"),
                            inMonth, inDay, inYear, numElements);
    for (int i =0; i<numElements; i++)
    {
        _tprintf(_T("Event No# %d,%ls\n"),
                            (pmyEvent + i)->lEvtID,
                            (pmyEvent + i)->Heading);
        ClearAnEvent(pmyEvent); // free the BSTRs
    }
    CoTaskMemFree(pmyEvent);
}
```

You can call the method with this syntax:

```
TestDept GETEVENTONDATE <year> <month> <day>
```

This will print all the events available on the specified day for the local department.

While creating and maintaining command line test programs like `TestDept.exe` and `TestCent.exe` for business objects may appear to be a rather old-fashioned approach to testing, the strength lies in the fact that these test programs can be easily scripted. Ability to script these calls allows for automated testing and creation of regression test suites. In fact, one can even write a wizard to generate test scripts, making the testing process extremely flexible.

Updating the Object Model Presentation Components

Last but not least, we need to modify the middle tier, Automation-compatible objects that present the object model to the calendar. If we modify them to actually use the MTS components that we have just completed, the calendar client can be used to display real data from the distributed databases!

You can find the modified version of these objects in the \ATLFinder.2 and \ATLDept.2 directories. We will quickly go through the necessary modifications here.

In ATLFinder1.cpp, we need to include the GUID and typelib definitions from the central server project:

```
#include "ATLFinder.h"
#include "ATLDepts1.h"
#include "ATLFinder1.h"
#include "..\..\CentBusObj.2\CentBusObj_i.c"
```

Similarly in ATLFinder1.h:

```
#ifndef __ATLFINDER1_H_
#define __ATLFINDER1_H_

#include "resource.h"       // main symbols
#include "..\..\CentBusObj.2\CentBusObj.h"
```

A new m_spCentralServer member is declared in ATLFinder1.h as:

```
private:
    CComPtr<IATLDepts1> m_spEventfulDepts;
    DATE m_dCurStartDate;

    // Link to third tier objects
    CComPtr<IBoDeptCache> m_spCentralServer;
    bool m_bDateChanged;
protected:
    void ClearADept(EVTDEPT* pCount);
```

Notice the new ClearADept() member, this is the familiar free BSTR routine, in ATLFinder1.cpp:

```
void CATLFinder1::ClearADept(EVTDEPT *pCount)
{
    // free the BSTR members (embedded pointers) from struct
    ::SysFreeString(pCount->bstrName);
    ::SysFreeString(pCount->bstrSymbol);
    ::SysFreeString(pCount->bstrHost);
}
```

We need to know that date has been changed to reset the EventfulDepts collection. This is done in SetFindDate():

```
STDMETHODIMP CATLFinder1::SetFindDate(DATE inDate)
{
    HRESULT hRes;
    if (m_dCurStartDate != inDate)
    {
        m_dCurStartDate = inDate;
        m_bDateChanged = true; // get object ready for reset
    }
```

```
      if (!m_spCentralServer) // create backend object if necessary
      {
        hRes = m_spCentralServer.CoCreateInstance(
                            OLESTR("CentBusObj.BoDeptsFinder"));
        if (hRes != S_OK)
           return hRes;
      }
      return S_OK;
    }
```

The code above also creates the central server object if it has not yet been created.

Finally, when someone calls to get a reference for the EventfulDepts collection, we go to the central server and obtain all the departments with events in the month, via a call to getEventDepts(). This is done in the get_EventfulDepts() member:

```
STDMETHODIMP CATLFinder1::get_EventfulDepts(VARIANT * pVal)
{
    if (m_bDateChanged)
    {
        EVTDEPT * pDept = NULL;
        EVTDEPT * * ppDept = &pDept;
        HRESULT hRes;
        // get the department and event count
        long numDepts ;

        hRes = m_spCentralServer->getEventDepts(m_dCurStartDate,
                                        &numDepts, ppDept);

        if (hRes != S_OK)  // backend call failed
           return hRes;
```

We have got all the department information. Before we stuff the collection with the information, we'll empty it out.

```
        // clean up the eventful departments collection
        long tpCount;
        m_spEventfulDepts->get_Count(&tpCount);
        while( tpCount > 0)
        {
            m_spEventfulDepts->DeleteFirst();
            m_spEventfulDepts->get_Count(&tpCount);
        }
```

Now, we add departments one at a time from the central server list into the collection.

```
        // store the departments
        for (int i=0; i<numDepts; i++)
        {
            USES_CONVERSION;
            EVTDEPT * pTp = (pDept + i);
            TCHAR tpVal[20];
```

```
        _itot(pTp->lDeptID, tpVal, 10);
        m_spEventfulDepts->Add(pTp->bstrName,
                               T2BSTR(tpVal),
                               pTp->vbCanRead,
                               pTp->vbCanPostNew,
                               pTp->bstrSymbol,
                               pTp->clrColor,
                               pTp->bstrHost,
                               m_dCurStartDate);
        ClearADept(pTp);   // free the BSTRs
    }

    CoTaskMemFree(pDept);
    m_bDateChanged = false;
}

// get the IDispatch of the embedded collection and return it
VariantInit(pVal);
IDispatch* pDisp;
m_spEventfulDepts->QueryInterface(IID_IDispatch, (void**)&pDisp);
pVal->vt = VT_DISPATCH;
pVal->pdispVal = pDisp;
return S_OK;
}
```

This concludes the changes for `ATLFinder` project.

For the `ATLDept` project, we need to add this header to `ATLDept1.cpp`:

```
// ATLDept1.cpp : Implementation of CATLDept1
#include "stdafx.h"
#include "ATLDept.h"
#include "ATLCorpEvents1.h"
#include "ATLDept1.h"

#include "..\..\DeptBusObj.2\DeptBusObj_i.c"
```

And in `ATLDept1.h`, we add:

```
// ATLDept1.h : Declaration of the CATLDept1

#ifndef __ATLDEPT1_H_
#define __ATLDEPT1_H_

#include "resource.h"        // main symbols
#include "..\..\DeptBusObj.2\DeptBusObj.h"
```

When our date member is changed, we want to set the member flag to be the same as in the
`ATLFinder` case.

```
STDMETHODIMP CATLDept1::put_Date(DATE inDate)
{
    if( m_CurDate != inDate)
    {
        m_CurDate = inDate;
        m_bDateChanged = true;
    }
    return S_OK;
}
```

When the `KnownEvents` collection is accessed, we want to go to the departmental server, fetch all
the events within the month, and store them into the collection.

```
STDMETHODIMP CATLDept1::get_KnownEvents(VARIANT * pVal)
{
    if (m_bDateChanged)
    {
        EVTDETAIL* pmyEvent = NULL;
        EVTDETAIL** ppmyEvent = &pmyEvent;

        HRESULT hRes;
        // get the department and event count
        long numElements;
```

Notice that we create the back-end departmental server using the Host field of the department
information. This Host field typically contains the IP address of the departmental server. The
`CoCreateInstanceEx()` API call we use here allows us to create a remote COM server with one
single call.

*`CoCreateInstanceEx()` takes 6 arguments, the first 3 are identical to those of
`CoCreateInstance()`. The 4th argument is a COSERVERINFO structure, which can
contain the host name of the remote server, and associated security information (see Chapter 11).
The 5th argument is a count of the number of elements in a MULTI_QI array passed in the 6th
argument. A MULTI_QI structure array allows the remote server to perform multiple
QueryInterface() calls on behalf of the client. The client simply fills out the interfaces
that it is interested in, ship the MULTI_QI array across the network, and obtain pointers to the
relevant interfaces with one single network round-trip.*

```
    if (!m_spDeptServer) // create backend object if necessary
    {
        COSERVERINFO tpSvrInfo = {0,
                        reinterpret_cast<LPWSTR>(m_bstrHost.m_str),
                        NULL,
                        0};
        MULTI_QI tpQI[1] = {{&IID_IBoDeptEvent, 0, 0}};
```

```
        CoCreateInstanceEx(
            CLSID_BoDeptEvent,        //CLSID of the object to be created
            NULL,                      //Controlling Unknown
            CLSCTX_REMOTE_SERVER,      //CLSCTX values
            &tpSvrInfo,                //Machine where object is instantiated
            1,                         //Number of MULTI_QI structures in pResults
            tpQI);                     //Array of MULTI_QI structures

        hRes = tpQI[0].hr ;
        if(hRes != S_OK)
            return hRes;
        m_spDeptServer.Attach(
                    reinterpret_cast<IBoDeptEvent *>(tpQI[0].pItf));
    }

    hRes =m_spDeptServer->getEventOnDate(m_CurDate, &numElements,
                                                          ppmyEvent);

    if (hRes != S_OK)  // backend call failed
        return hRes;
```

We have got the list from the departmental server, so we clean up our collection and stuff it with the newly available data.

```
        // clean up the events list first
        long tpCount;
        m_spKnownEvents->get_Count(&tpCount);
        while( tpCount > 0)
        {
            m_spKnownEvents->DeleteFirst();
            m_spKnownEvents->get_Count(&tpCount);
        }

        for (int i =0; i<numElements; i++)
        {
            EVTDETAIL * pTp = (pmyEvent + i);
            m_spKnownEvents->Add(pTp->dtDateTime,
            pTp->Location, pTp->Heading, pTp->Organizer,
            m_bstrName, // this department organizes
            pTp->Details, pTp->Hlink);
            ClearAnEvent(pTp);
        }

        CoTaskMemFree(pmyEvent);
        m_bDateChanged = false;
    }
    // get the IDispatch of the embedded collection and return it
    VariantInit(pVal);
    IDispatch* pDisp;
    m_spKnownEvents->QueryInterface(IID_IDispatch, (void**)&pDisp);
    pVal->vt = VT_DISPATCH;
    pVal->pdispVal = pDisp;
    return S_OK;
}
```

We also have a BSTR cleanup routine here for cleaning an event record:

```
void CATLDept1::ClearAnEvent(EVTDETAIL *pEvt)
{
    ::SysFreeString(pEvt->Heading);
    ::SysFreeString(pEvt->Hlink);
    ::SysFreeString(pEvt->Location);
    ::SysFreeString(pEvt->Organizer);
    ::SysFreeString(pEvt->Details);
}
```

These are the new members declared in ATLDept1.h:

```
    HRESULT FinalConstruct();
    HRESULT FinalRelease();
protected:
    void ClearAnEvent(EVTDETAIL * pEvt);
    CComBSTR m_bstrName;
    CComBSTR m_bstrNumber;
    VARIANT_BOOL m_bCanPostNew;
    VARIANT_BOOL m_bCanRead;
    CComBSTR m_bstrSymbol;
    long m_ulColor;
    CComPtr<IATLCorpEvents1> m_spKnownEvents;
    // Link to third tier objects
    CComPtr<IBoDeptEvent> m_spDeptServer;
    CComBSTR m_bstrHost;
    DATE m_CurDate;
    bool m_bDateChanged;
```

Build the projects, and remember to recompile the proxy/stub for ATLFinder.exe and reregister the DLL.

Testing the Automation Compatible Objects in Visual Basic 6

In the \TestMid directory, we have a Visual Basic 6 fully automation-driven test program. This program presents a user interface with three buttons:

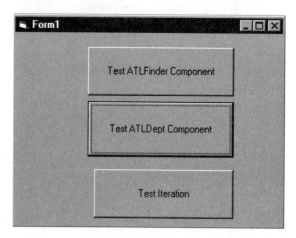

Each button will test a different facet of the three-tier system through the automation compatible object model mapping layer. Here is a tabulation of what each button tests:

Button	Comments
Test ATLFinder Component	Creates an ATLFinder object instance and set its start date to a hard-coded date. Next, iterates through the EventfulDepts collection and prints out the department names. This essentially finds all the departments that have events in a specified month. This tests the basic functionality of ATLFinder.exe and the central caching server.
Test ATLDept Component	Creates an ATLDept object instance, and set its date property to a hard-coded date. Next, iterates through its KnownEvents collection and prints out the event heading and location for each event found. This tests the basic functionality of a local ATLDept component and that of the departmental server.
Test Iteration	Creates an ATLFinder object instance, and set its start date to a hard-coded one. Next, iterates through the EventfulDepts collection and prints out the first the department name. For each department, iterate through its KnownEvents collection and print out the heading and location of each event. This tests the complete calendaring system back-end, both the central caching server, and all the departmental servers in the network. It is equivalent to testing the data requirements of our visual calendar control.

You can change the date in the source, and try the various tests on the object model mapping components. This program allows you to test the back-end system easily without having the adding complexity of the visual calendar control in the way. If the **Test Iteration** case works properly, you should have good confidence that the visual calendar will work with the system as well. Here is an excerpt from the **Test Iteration** code:

```
Dim aFinder As Object
Dim manyDepts As Variant
Dim aDept As Object

Dim manyEvents As Variant
Dim anEvent As Object

Set aFinder = CreateObject("ATLFinder.ATLFinder1")
aFinder.SetFindDate CDate("1999/7/10")
```

We create an ATLFinder object, and set the month we are interested in.

```
Set manyDepts = aFinder.EventfulDepts
```

Next, we get the Finder's `EventfulDepts` collection and enumerate through.

```
For Each aDept In manyDepts
    Debug.Print Trim(aDept.Name)
    Set manyEvents = aDept.KnownEvents
```

We get each department's `KnownEvents` collection and iterate through.

```
    For Each anEvent In manyEvents
        Debug.Print CStr(anEvent.DateTime) + Trim(anEvent.Heading) + _
                    "," + Trim(anEvent.Location)
    Next
    Set manyEvents = Nothing
Next
Set manyDepts = Nothing
Set aDept = Nothing
Set aFinder = Nothing
```

Notice the extensive use of enumeration through the `For Each...` construct in the above code. The very same syntax may be used when the components are used in ASP or a Windows Scripting host. This allows our stack of business objects to be used for many other web applications, so they are just limited to the visual calendar that we have created.

Testing the Entire System with Visual Calendar

Now, for the ultimate moment. We haven't seen our visual calendar control for a while. You can find the most evolved version, with both OC96 windowless support and deferred activation, in the `Ch09\viscal` directory.

The modifications we have to make are minor. All of `viscal`'s data access routines, by design, are isolated to the model of the MVC pattern, and modifications will be restricted to the data management class, residing in `CDataMgr.h` and `CDataMgr.cpp`. Previously, these classes stuffed test data into the backend. Now that the middle-tier objects are in place and fully tested, we only need modify these two files in order to call the backend properly.

First, we must update the location of the backend code. In `CDataMgr.h`, we set the COM compiler support to point to the desired type library:

```
#ifndef __CDATAMGR_H_
#define __CDATAMGR_H_
#import "..\new\ATLFinder.2\ATLFinder.tlb" rename_namespace( "Finder" )
```

Do the same thing in `CDataMgr.cpp`:

```
#include "stdafx.h"
#include "CalDefs.h"
#include "CalUtils.h"

#import "..\new\ATLDept.2\ATLDept.tlb" rename_namespace( "Dept" )

#include "CDataMgr.h"
```

The only other thing we need to do is comment out the old code that fed the backend with fake data. This was in `CDataMgr::SetEventMonth()`.

```
void CDataMgr::SetEventMonth( const CDateTime& inMonth )
{
    ATLTRACE( _T("CDataMgr::SetEventMonth\n") );

    if ( ! m_MyFinder )
        return;

    // get rid of hh:mm:ss information
    (*m_MyFinder)->SetFindDate(inMonth.ConvertToDATE());
/*
    Finder::IATLDepts1Ptr    tmpDepts( (*m_MyFinder)->GetEventfulDepts() );
    if ( tmpDepts->GetCount() == 0 ) {
        // if none, add a couple of depts

... commented off old stuffing code ....

    tpEvents->Add(   tmpDate.ConvertToDATE(), _T("Toronto Campus"),
            _T("Hammer the IBM370 Fest"), _T("Joanne Rogers"),
            _T("Support"),
            _T("$5 for each punch with a sledgehammer on the retired  370,
proceed goes to United Way."),
            _T("http://www.anw.com/events"));
*/
}
```

Make sure you have recompiled before testing. You can use the ActiveX Control Test Container `Tstcon32.exe` to test it out. Since the version of the visual calendar control that we used is the OC96 compliant version supporting windowless operations and deferred activation, you must remember to:

❑ Be sure that the test container is in user mode, not design mode

❑ Make sure you move the mouse cursor over the calendar grid to activate the calendar

❑ Make sure that the month displayed actually has some event data

❑ Wait sufficient amount of time (watch disk lights on machines) for the data acquisition across the network to occur

To get live data displayed, you can use the `TestDept.exe` to add some events to the month being displayed and the months after that. Notice that they show up in real-time on the calendar as you move forward and backwards through the month. A fully functional three-tier DNA application at your fingertips!

A Word on Staging our DNA Sample Project

In the architectural design of our three-tiered DNA system for this book, we have aimed to make the final system deployable on as few physical machines as possible. Realizing that some readers may not have more than a couple of server machines for testing and experimentation, the system is designed so that it can be staged on a minimum of two Windows NT Server systems.

To make the system work within this minimal configuration, we had to make certain design trade-offs that would not normally occur in a production environment. In this section, we'll examine what these trade-offs and the implication of them. In production scenarios, there typically should not be a restriction on the availability of testing machines.

If you have the minimum configuration, the table below shows how you must configure each machine:

	Machine 1	Machine 2
Operating System	Windows NT 4.0 Server (SP 3 or later)	Windows NT 4.0 Server (SP 3 or later)
Further installations	SQL Server 6.5 SP 4 or later	SQL Server 6.5 SP 4 or later
	Windows NT Options Pack (MTS, MSMQ)	Windows NT Options Pack (MTS, MSMQ)
Role(s) of Server	Central Server	Department Server 2
	Department Server1	

Note that it is not possible, with our design, to stage two departmental servers on one single machine. This is because each departmental business object discovers its own identity during runtime. This identity is stored in the dbo.Dept table of the departmental database. This table should always only contain one row – the identity of the department.

For simplicity of discussion in earlier chapter, we have also called own ODBC data source name ENG and our SQL database engevt. In production, we should call both the DSN and the SQL database by a more generic name (for example, DEPT and deptevt). If you should make this change, you will also need to change the appropriate OLE DB consumer template access code in the business object as well.

Summary

In this chapter, we have examined how DCOM works and showed that most of the tedious work involved can be done easily using MTS. We learnt that MTS is not only a transaction server, but also a surrogate and a great distributed components deployment tool. We went through the new transactional programming paradigm and have shown how it is slightly short of a natural evolution from desktop COM.

We then started using MTS and got the business objects from the last chapter up and running. We wrote a couple of test harnesses and tested them. Next, we used MTS to move a component from one server to another without leaving a seat. Finally, we completed the coding of all the business objects and tested them with the visual calendar control that we had previously created.

In the next chapter, we will create an administrative utility that will facilitate adding events to the system. Of all the ways of fabricating an ActiveX control, we will use the simplest – Dynamic HTML within a control. We'll also be examining one of the most recent additions to the BackOffice family – the Microsoft Message Queue Server (MSMQ). We will see how it will let our remote administrator add events to the system, even when they are disconnected and working on a notebook at home.

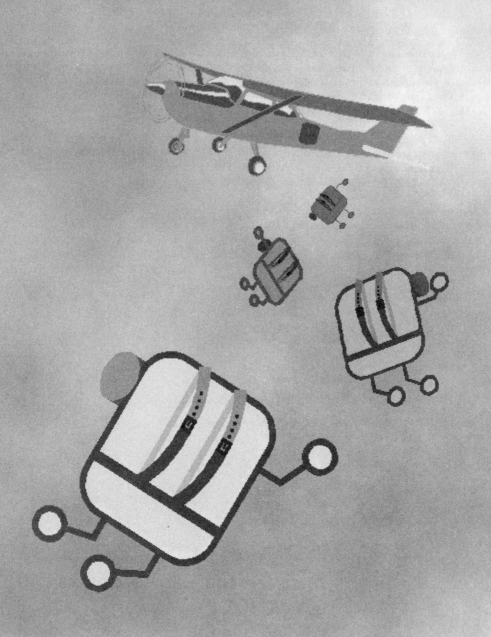

10

Administering the Events Calendar

In this chapter, in providing basic administration support for our Events Calendar, we'll look at two new and exciting technologies – hybrid controls and Microsoft's Message Queue server (MSMQ).

Most of the excitement surrounding hybrid controls, where Dynamic HTML is the user interface for an ActiveX control, is that the merging of two user interface technologies makes the most of their strengths while counteracting their weaknesses. Plus, ATL 3 makes the creation of such controls very easy.

We will tap into this to create an Administrator control for the A&W distributed calendar, which will allow administrators to add new events for their department over the intranet.

The Microsoft Message Queue (MSMQ) is a brand new, rapidly evolving member of the BackOffice server family. It provides a reliable and durable queuing infrastructure within the DNA whenever you require basic store and forward communication. As with transactional system design, we will discover that designing MSMQ applications requires us to make fundamental changes in our approach to system design.

In this chapter, we will be taking a look at the implications of using MSMQ , how we can program it, and then we'll enhance our Administrator control to use it. The new Administrator control will then be suitable for administrators who don't have constant access to the intranet. Finally, we will examine some features planned for future releases of MSMQ that will further simplify the construction of COM controls.

Creating User Interfaces Rapidly

Dynamic HTML, for those who may not be familiar with it, is an enhanced HTML dialect supported by Microsoft Internet Explorer 4.x products. Among many other interactive features, it enables:

- ❑ Precise placement of user interface elements
- ❑ Multimedia, animation
- ❑ Dynamic page rendering capabilities

For further information, interested readers may want to take a look at Instant Dynamic HTML and Professional IE4 Programming from Wrox Press.

The overwhelming advantage of using Dynamic HTML for creating user interfaces is its ease of construction. HTML can be created easily and rapidly using any text editor. To test any Dynamic HTML page, simply load it up in Internet Explorer 4 and try it. Any mistakes or enhancements can be made immediately using the text editor and the page rendered again – allowing highly iterative development of sophisticated user interfaces. Couple this with the many eye-candy features of Dynamic HTML and you will appreciate why it is so popular.

Unfortunately, Dynamic HTML residing on the disk as a file, can only be accessed directly by Internet Explorer 4.x or be 'served' by an HTTP server over a network, and this severely restricts the possibility of using the Dynamic HTML facility for 'regular' user interfaces.

ActiveX controls, on the other hand, are completely self contained. Once an ActiveX control had been downloaded and installed, its user interface is immediately available without accessing the disk or the network. Unfortunately, as we have seen in the earlier part of this book, designing even simple user interface elements in an ATL-based ActiveX control is non-trivial.

No problem! ATL 3 to the rescue... again. Its support for the Dynamic HTML based control allows you to rapidly create an ActiveX control, where the user interface is actually a Dynamic HTML page! The page itself is stored as a compiled resource in the DLL, making the control one self-contained package. The resource-based page can be easily modified by the programmer/creator and is much less vulnerable to abuse by the end-user.

How's that for the best of both worlds!

Bridging Scripts and Compiled Code

The simple act of using Dynamic HTML for the user interface of an ActiveX control is already a great feature for control designers. However, it would be nice if we could also partition the logic of the control so that a portion of it can be handled by scripting within the Dynamic HTML page, and the rest reside in the ActiveX control as compiled C++. One candidate for scripting may be validation code for data entry, while more involved data formatting or communications code can be done more effectively in C++.

This is exactly what the ATL 3 Dynamic HTML Control offers. The diagram below shows how our ATL-based ActiveX control can interact with its container, the embedded web control hosting the Dynamic HTML page, and the scripting code within the Dynamic HTML page.

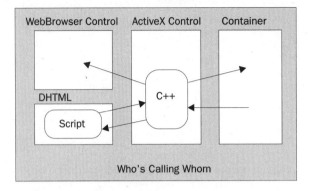

To be more precise, the Dynamic HTML Control provides:

- ❑ The ability to use a Dynamic HTML page for the user interface of an ActiveX control
- ❑ The ability for scripts within the Dynamic HTML page to call compiled C++ code within the control
- ❑ The ability for the compiled C++ code within the control to interact with the Dynamic HTML control – accessing every aspect of the Dynamic HTML object model

If the importance of this last point is not immediately apparent to you, then the next section should persuade you.

A Comprehensive Object Model

The elements on a Dynamic HTML page are part of a comprehensive object model, within which every aspect of each element may be changed programmatically. The effect of any changes are immediately rendered to the end user.

So, the page that is the user interface of our ActiveX control may be changed at runtime in any arbitrary fashion by the C++ code within the control. The object model is large and moderately complex. Coverage of the model is beyond the scope of this chapter, but readers who are interested in further details are encouraged to read the excellent *Professional IE4 Programming* book from Wrox Press.

The diagram here provides a graphical analogy to what we have been talking about so far. It depicts a web page where every element on the page is a component accessible to COM.

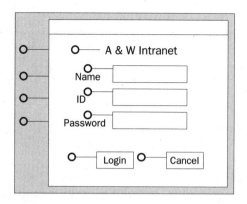

In Dynamic HTML, every element on the page exposes COM interfaces, so you can change them within your C++ code by calling methods on these interfaces.

The Dynamic HTML ActiveX control also has direct access to the 'web browser component' which hosts the displayed page. This 'web browser component' is essentially Internet Explorer 4,without the navigation frame (toolbar, menus, status bar, etc.). Having control over this component means that we can make use of many of IE 4's capabilities, including navigation to any arbitrary URL and rendering it within the control's frame.

Using Dynamic HTML for a Control's UI

How is this amazing feat accomplished? Unsurprisingly, COM makes it all possible. Microsoft's Internet Explorer 4 is a completely componentized application rather than the monolithic whole that it appears. From the top, we have a container (or frame – iexplore.exe) hosting a web browser control (shdocvw.dll). The web browser control knows how to interpret and render Dynamic HTML, navigate to another URL, and so on. Internally, the shdocvw.dll web browser control actually uses another component, mshtml.dll (the Microsoft HTML render), to render the web page. The container frame simply provides user interface elements – like a back button on the cool-bar – to control the action of the web browser control.

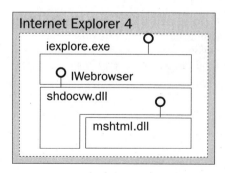

ATL 3 enables you to harness the web browser control − the very same one used by Internet Explorer 4 − within the display area of your ActiveX control.

ATL 3 for Instant ActiveX Control

Dynamic HTML ActiveX controls are not only easy to create under ATL 3, they are also quite easy to understand.

The Elusive CAxWindow Class

One ATL class, CAxWindow, single-handedly accounts for this super UI flexibility. Furthermore, the way to use the class is to include an instance of it as a child window. Exactly like the two CContainedWindows that we had in the Viscal control we created in Chapter 6, the code generated by ATL 3 for a Dynamic HTML ActiveX control intercepts the WM_CREATE message of the control's window and creates a child window/control of the CAxWindow class.

You'll see this very shortly when we create a Dynamic HTML ActiveX control using the ATL wizards. For now, just take a look at the code that is generated for you:

```
LRESULT OnCreate(UINT /*uMsg*/, WPARAM /*wParam*/,
                 LPARAM /*lParam*/, BOOL& /*bHandled*/)
{
    CAxWindow wnd(m_hWnd);
    HRESULT hr = wnd.CreateControl(IDH_DHTMLCLNT);
    if (SUCCEEDED(hr))
        hr = wnd.SetExternalDispatch(static_cast<IDhtmlClntUI*>(this));
    if (SUCCEEDED(hr))
        hr = wnd.QueryControl(IID_IWebBrowser2, (void**)&m_spBrowser);
    return SUCCEEDED(hr) ? 0 : -1;
}
```

We see here that the instance of CAxWindow, wnd, is created as a child of our control's window. The control's constructor sets the m_bWindowOnly flag to ensure active-when-visible behavior. The CAXWindow's CreateControl() member takes a resource ID as a parameter, this is the Dynamic HTML page to be displayed, and calls AtlAxCreateControl() which itself creates the ActiveX control and hosts it within the associated window.

The SetExternalDispatch() method is akin to the SetClientSite() function of the OC94/96 specification. This method allows us to pass in a pointer to our object, so that the child control can call back out. In this particular case, the IDhtmlClntUI interface is where we will be implementing our custom functionality to call the middle-tier objects for adding events. The scripts executing within the control (in our Dynamic HTML page) can then call back out to our C++ ActiveX control implementation.

Finally, QueryControl() calls QueryInterface() on the associated control and returns a pointer to an IWebBrowser2 interface. This interface is exposed by the web browser control that we talked about earlier. Having this interface in a smart pointer member allows us full control over how the embedded web browser will behave.

This is what the final hookup looks like:

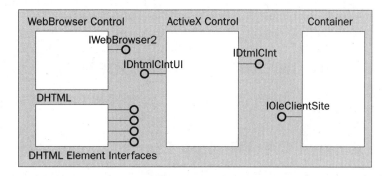

If you are really curious, you may want to check out the source code of the `CAxWindow` class in the `Atlwin.h` file under the `\VC98\Atl\include` directory.

In practice, you don't even have to know that the `CAxWindow` class exists. The ATL 3 wizard will generate enough usable code that you can concentrate on designing your Dynamic HTML user interface, and hooking this up to any custom C++ functionality.

Let's try out the wizard by fulfilling the Add Events Use Case for our A&W Administrators. The final product will be an Administrative ActiveX control which can be used by the Administrators to add new events to their own department. This control can be accessed within a web page from anywhere over the intranet.

A&W Calendar: Adding an Administrative Control

In this section, we will:

- ❑ Use the ATL 3 wizard to generate the skeleton code for our control
- ❑ Add the Dynamic HTML user interface code
- ❑ Add custom C++ code to call the business objects on the departmental server

An ActiveX Administrator Control

Before we get stuck in, let's have a look at what the final control will look like, hosted inside Internet Explorer 4:

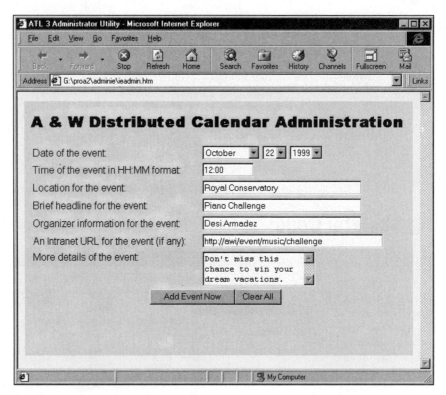

The user can select the month, day, and year from the drop down boxes at the top of the control, and enter the rest of the event's details below. Data validation will be performed via scripting within the Dynamic HTML page itself. Once the data is validated, the script will 'call out' to the C++ code within our ActiveX control, which will then send the event data to the actual departmental business objects (in `DeptBusObj`). Finally, these objects will update the departmental and central databases via a distributed transaction, as we saw in Chapter 9.

To summarize:

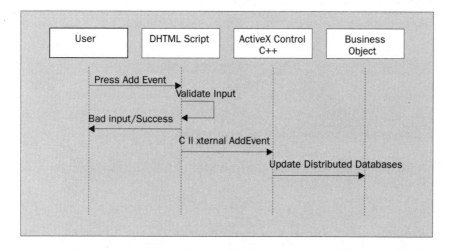

Generating Skeletal Code

Create a DLL-based ATL COM project and call it called `AdminClnt`. This is going to be a visual ActiveX control, so there is no need to support MTS. After the basic files have been generated, select **Insert ATL Object...** as usual. From the selection screen, chose the **HTML Control** from the **Controls** category:

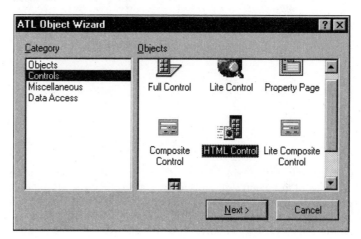

Press Next> and then fill in the names as follows:

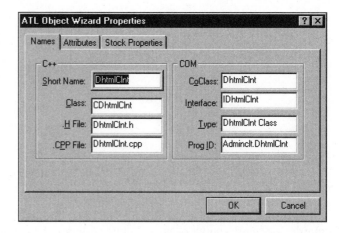

Take a look at the Attributes tag. We're simply going to keep these default attributes, so just press OK and have the wizard generate the skeletal code. That is all we need to do for now. The generated code already has a sample Dynamic HTML page and associated code in place. First, we will replace the Dynamic HTML page.

The Dynamic HTML Code

Here is the Dynamic HTML code that renders and manages the user interface. You should be able to follow this even if you are not an HTML expert. This entire HTML file is actually compiled into a resource within the DLL. You can access the file independently from the File View pane of Visual C++ IDE.

You can find the complete HTML file in the source code that accompanies this book, in \AdminClnt\DhtmlClntUI.htm.

```
<HTML>
<script language="VBScript">
```

The <script> tag starts our scripting section. We could have placed the <script> tag almost anywhere, but by convention, doing it before the <body> section, is preferred for maintenance purposes.

The first routine is the OnClick() handler for a button that we have named ClearForm. Event handlers like this are automatically 'found' by the Dynamic HTML rendering engine, and will be hooked up with the associated element on the actual user interface.

```
Sub ClearForm_OnClick()

    InTime.value = ""
    Heading.value = ""
    Hlink.value = ""
    Loc.value = ""
    Organizer.value = ""
    Details.value = ""

end sub
```

This handler simply goes to the five input fields and one text area to set their values to a null string. This effectively clears all the input fields on the screen (except for the drop-down list boxes, of course).

The next routine is another OnClick() handler, this time for the AddEvent button. This handler is considerably more complex, but still quite understandable if we take it one step at a time:

```
Sub AddEvent_OnClick()

    ' verify date time input here
    tpTime = InTime.value
```

We grab the user's input from the InTime entry field. This field is expected to be in the HH:MM format, so it must have five characters.

```
    if (Len(tpTime)<>5) then
        MsgBox "Sorry, time must be in HH:MM format."
```

Here, we're simply checking the format of the time entry and notifying the user if it is incorrect.

```
    else
        inHour = CInt(Left(tpTime,2))
        inMin = CInt(Mid(tpTime,4))
```

If it does contain five characters, we extract the two numbers, corresponding to the hour and the minutes, and store them as numeric values in inHour and inMin respectively.

```
        if (inHour <0) or (inHour >23) or _
           (inMin <0) or (inMin > 59) then
            MsgBox "Sorry, the time you have entered is invalid."
            'If they violate these basic consistency check,
            'we notify the    user.
        else
            tpDate = CStr(inMonth.value) & "/" & CStr(inDay.value) & _
                    "/" & CStr(inYear.value) & " " & tpTime & ":00"
```

If the time entered is valid, we go on to convert the date and the time entered into a string taking the form MM/DD/YY HH:MM:00.

```
tpHeading = Heading.value
tpHlink = Hlink.value
tpLoc = Loc.value
tpDetails = Details.value
tpOrganizer = Organizer.value
```

We grab the rest of the user's input from the form and set put it into temporary variables. These variables will be used in calling the C++ code. Finally, we call the C++ method, AddEvent() (which we'll go on to write in a moment as part of our C++ implementation):

```
        window.external.AddEvent ClearForm,tpDate,tpHeading, _
                            tpHlink,tpLoc,tpOrganizer,tpDetails
    end if
  end if

end sub
</script>
```

Calling any C++ method exposed through the control's IDhtmlClntUI interface is as easy as calling:

```
window.external.<method name>(<method parameters>)
```

In order to call methods like this from our script, we just need to make sure that the interface defined is Automation compatible (that is, no user-defined structure as parameters, etc). We'll construct this as a dual interface.

That's all the script we need. The rest is pretty standard HTML coding:

```
<body style="background:yellow;
      font-family:Arial;
      font-size:10pt">
<H1 style="font-family:Arial Black,Arial;
      font-size:18pt">A & W Distributed Calendar Administration</H1>
```

Dynamic HTML allows control over the use of fonts on every element via the style attribute.

```
<table width=600><tr><td>
Date of the event:</td><td>

<select id=inMonth>
<option value=1>January<option value=2>February
<option value=3>March<option value=4>April
<option value=5>May<option value=6>June
<option value=7>July<option value=8>August
<option value=9>September<option value=10>October
<option value=11>November<option value=12>December
</select>
```

This is what a standard `<select>` tag looks like – all the choices are explicitly specified. A little bit tedious, wouldn't you say? Well in the next `<select>`, it'll get worse, because we need to give a choice from 1 to 31 for the selection of days in the month. In order to simplify this a little, we'll take advantage of Dynamic HTML's capability to generate code in-line from a script, and have the generated code created all in one single sweep:

```
<select id=inDay>
<script language='VBScript'>
for i=1 to 31
    document.writeln "<option value=" & Cstr(i) & ">" & CStr(i)
next
</script>
</select>
```

Now, that is significantly simpler than coding a thirty-one way `<select>`. The next one is simple, so we'll code it direct. We allow a selection for the current and the next two years and 2010 for good measure.

```
<select id=inYear><option value=1998>1998<option value=1999>1999
<option value=2000>2000<option value=2010>2010</select>
```

Now for the rest of the entry fields:

```
</td></tr><tr><td>
Time of the event in HH:MM format:
</td><td>
<input type="text" size=10 id=InTime>
</td></tr><tr><td>

Location for the event:
</td><td>
<input type="text" size=35 id=Loc>
</td></tr><tr><td>

Brief headline for the event:
</td><td>
<input type="text" size=35 id=Heading>
</td></tr><tr><td>

Organizer information for the event:
</td><td>
<input type="text" size=35 id=Organizer>
</td></tr><tr><td>

An Intranet URL for the event (if any):
</td><td>
<input type="text" size=40 id=Hlink>
</td></tr><tr><td valign=top>

More details of the event:
</td><td>
<textarea rows=3 columns=60 id=Details></textarea>
</td></tr><tr><td colspan=2>
```

```
<center>
<button id=AddEvent>Add Event Now</button>
<button id=ClearForm>Clear All</button>
</center>

</td></tr></table>
</BODY>
</HTML>
```

Towards the end, we create the two buttons, `AddEvent` and `ClearForm`. The only thing we need to be careful about is that the ID or name attributes we assign them match the ones we have coded earlier in the handlers. Mismatch in IDs is a frequent source of puzzling problems in Dynamic HTML coding.

That is all there is to our user interface coding. We can even create this interactively and iteratively, using any of a large number of drag-and-drop web page design tools.

Coding the C++ Layer

First, in the generated header `DhtmlClnt.h`, we must add the following line at the top of the file:

```
#ifndef __DHTMLCLNT_H_
#define __DHTMLCLNT_H_

#include "resource.h"        // main symbols
#include "..\DeptBusObj\DeptBusObj.h"
#include <atlctl.h>
```

Close to the bottom of the file, we should add a declaration for a smart pointer to the department server object that we will use:

```
    ...
    CComPtr<IWebBrowser2> m_spBrowser;
    CComQIPtr<IBoDeptEvent> m_spDeptServer;
};

#endif //__DHTMLCLNT_H_
```

Now, let us code the C++ helper function. First, go to the **ClassView** pane, and add a new method to the `IDhtmlClntUI` interface with the following signature:

```
HRESULT AddEvent([in] IDispatch* pdisp,
                 [in] DATE DateTime,
                 [in] BSTR Heading,
                 [in] BSTR Hlink,
                 [in] BSTR Location,
                 [in] BSTR Organizer,
                 [in] BSTR Details);
```

The `IDhtmlCltntUI` interface was the one that was passed into the `CAxWindow` instance, as we saw earlier, in the `OnCreate()` method:

```
hr = wnd.SetExternalDispatch(static_cast<IDhtmlClntUI*>(this));
```

It is to the `IDhtmlClntUI` interface that you add all your additional functionality provided for the Dynamic HTML script. The `AddEvent()` method shown above will be called by the Dynamic HTML code when the administrator clicks the `AddEvent` button. You can find the skeleton implementation of the method in `DhtmlClnt.cpp`. We will need an instance of the departmental object that we created in the last chapter, so we include its definition here:

```
#include "stdafx.h"
#include "Adminclt.h"
#include "DhtmlClnt.h"
#define IID_DEFINED
#include "..\DeptBusObj\DeptBusObj_i.c"
```

The implementation for the `AddEvent()` method is shown below:

```
STDMETHODIMP CDhtmlClnt::AddEvent(IDispatch* pdisp, DATE DateTime,
                                  BSTR Heading, BSTR Hlink,
                                  BSTR Location, BSTR Organizer,
                                  BSTR Details)
{
    HRESULT hRes;
    long DummyVal;
```

If the departmental server object has not been created yet, we should create it now. The server object is actually an MTS reference, so we'll create it and won't let it go until the user exits the page. Just-in-time activation will ensure that there are no inefficiencies.

```
    if (!m_spDeptServer)
    {
        hRes = m_spDeptServer.CoCreateInstance(
                            OLESTR("DeptBusObj.BoDeptEvent"));
        if (hRes != S_OK) return hRes;
    }
```

To add the event, we call right through to the corresponding method on the department server object with parameters we got from the calling Dynamic HTML code. Note that this code is almost identical to what we used in our testing program in the last chapter, `TestDept.exe`.

```
    hRes = m_spDeptServer->addEvent(DateTime, Heading, Hlink,
                            Location, Organizer, Details, &DummyVal);
```

If the `addEvent()` call fails for some reason (remember that it was actually a distributed transaction, and could fail), we simply show a message box. We return the user back to the entry so he can try again shortly, without re-entering all the data.

```
    if (hRes != S_OK)
    {
        ::MessageBox(NULL, "Distributed Cal Problem",
            "Sorry, the system is not functional at this time.", MB_OK);
    }
```

If the addEvent() call succeeds, we also prompt with a dialog indicating success. Next, we call back into the Dynamic HTML scripting code from the C++ code. The way we do it is to take the IDispatch pointer that was passed in with the call, which we know is an HTML element, the ClearForm button, on the Dynamic HTML page. Our smart pointer QIs IDispatch for IHTMLElement interface. This interface contains many common properties and methods that all Dynamic HTML elements have. There are numerous methods of this interface, and interested readers should look in the MSDN library for more details.

```
    else
    {
        ::MessageBox(NULL, "Distributed Cal Add Event",
                "The event has been successfully added.", MB_OK);
        // clear the screen
        CComQIPtr<IHTMLElement> spButton(pdisp);
        if (spButton != NULL)
            spButton->click();
    }
    return S_OK;
}
```

The single method we are interested in is IHTMLElement::click(). By calling this method, it is equivalent to the end user pressing the ClearForm button. Since our Dynamic HTML code has a handler for this button, calling click() actually clears the form.

Note that this is actually a very powerful technique. Just look at all the IHTMLElement methods; and that is just for the generic element! If you examine the platform SDK documentation in your MSDN CD, you can see all the other interfaces that all sorts of Dynamic HTML elements expose. Using this technique, you can gain control of every element on the user interface, and gain the ability to control them completely within the C/C++ environment. The user interface innovations that you can create are left to your imagination!

That's it – we have completed all the code for DhtmlClnt.cpp!

'I'm sure you'll agree that this is very simple and direct. If you were not following along with code, you can find it all in the \AdminClnt directory of the source distribution. You can compile and link the project there.

Now, call up the ActiveX Control Container (`Tstcon32.exe`) and insert an instance of `DhtmlClnt` class into the page. Your screen will look like this:

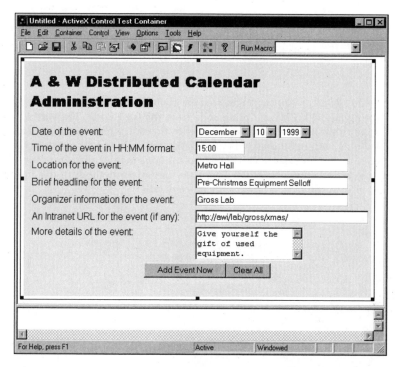

Enter in a new event and press **Add Event Now**. Next, open up an instance of `Msqry32.exe` displaying the department server's events table, and you should see your newly added event there. Similarly, if you look in the central server's `EvtCount` table, and notice that the count is updated.

> *Of course, you could equally well use the test programs that we created in the last chapter,* `TestDept.exe` *and* `TestCent.exe`, *to dump the data as well.*

That was record time for creating a functional ActiveX control! Compare that to what we had to do back in Chapter 7 for the `Viscal` control. And this one even updates distributed databases!

Our Dynamic HTML control is now ready for deployment. You can embed it into a web page and put the page on the intranet for administrator access. Here is the source for such a page. (Remember that if you have created this control yourself, you'll need to replace the CLSID with that of your own `CDhtmlClnt` class):

```
<html>
<head>
<title>ATL 3 Administrator Utility</title>
</head>
<body bgcolor="#f0f3f8">
<center>
<object id="DhtmlClnt"
    classid="CLSID:79FFF224-1807-11D2-A7D8-006052008075"
    align="baseline" border="0"
```

```
        width="630" height="400">
</object>
</p>
<center>
</body>
</html>
```

Administrators now have a friendly graphical interface to enter new events. However, we must remember our promise to cater for administrators who may be working from notebook computers at home and not connected to the network or the Internet. What can we do about them? Well, we will now turn our attention to MSMQ. Using MSMQ, we will be replacing the implementation of the C/C++ addEvent() method. The new method will work equally well while connected to the network, as well as when disconnected. The big bonus is that, with MSMQ, it is actually quite easy to do.

Microsoft Message Queue Server

Before we can understand MSMQ, we must first get acquainted with MOM.

Your MOM or my MOM

MSMQ is Microsoft's MOM. This is not to say that Mrs. Gates Senior has anything to do with coding MSMQ, but rather, MSMQ is Microsoft's **message-oriented middleware**. MOM is just another one of those interesting industry acronyms.

In the world of message-oriented middleware, pieces of a system communicate purely through messages. Messages are passed between collaborating applications in a manner akin to email. Also like email, the sender and receiver do not have to be connected all the time. As a matter of fact, they may never ever be connected together at the same time. Please read that last statement again – that is the power of a MOM.

> **MOMs like MSMQ allow systems that may never be connected together communicate and interwork with each other.**

This is not as surprising as it sounds once you realize that you receive email daily from people whose systems are never directly connected to yours. But, as an application architecture it's arresting.

Store and Forward Communications

The magic of MOMs in general, and MSMQ, in particular, is worked through a scheme of durable caches. All this means is that the message sent is stored somewhere permanently until the receiver can pick it up. If multiple applications are using the MOM, messages should be delivered in a First-in-First-out (FIFO) basis, so the caches are actually queues – hence the moniker **message queues**.

In fact, if the sender and receivers are actually several network hops away from each other, the system managing the queues must also handle the required routing of the message. This assumes that all intermediate nodes have some version of the service installed.

The combination of storing messages in queues, and forwarding them between nodes from source sender to destination is often called 'store and forward' communication.

Systems in an Imperfect World

Now if all that is required for a MOM is what we have mentioned above, the Internet with its SMTP and POP can become the pervasive World Wide MOM. Unfortunately, life in an imperfect world is not so simple.

The problem of using an email system as a MOM is that there is no guarantee of anything. When you send an email to Bill over the Internet, there is no guarantee that Bill will receive it. Most of the time he will get it, but sometimes the message may be lost. He may also receive multiple copies of the same message. Worst yet, another Bill altogether may actually receive the message. Imagine programming your applications on top of such a system! We'd be better off giving up before we try.

It should be clear, then, the features that distinguish a MOM from another store and forward communication system like email are:

❏ There are some guarantees
❏ When you send a message, you know it will be delivered, or you will be notified of the problem
❏ When you send one single message, you know the receiver will only get one single message
❏ When you send a message to a recipient, you know your message will never be misrouted to another recipient

With these guarantees in place, a MOM is certainly useful for writing applications. Microsoft's Message Queue makes these guarantees, plus more. It is also capable of interworking with our new friend MTS, which means that more substantial guarantees can be made. With MSMQ , we can guarantee:

❏ If the server picks up the message, the sales figures are guaranteed to be updated in the database
❏ If the data center picks up your message before 3pm, the order is guaranteed to be shipped by 7pm
❏ If our data center discover charge discrepancies of greater than $5, the debit card plugged in on your notebook is guaranteed to be credited the next time you connect to our service; otherwise we will mail you the check

In each of these cases, MSMQ can participate as part of a larger, potentially distributed, transaction. This is all made possible by the fact that MSMQ is a bona-fide MTS resource manager, just like the SQL Server resource manager that we saw in the last chapter.

At first glance, MOMs might appear to be quite easy to design and write. When you sit back and analyze the bewildering permutations of potential failures in such a system, however, it will be clear that a MOM project is a non-trivial undertaking. It took Microsoft no less than seven years, with sizable project teams, to get MSMQ to the state it is today – you may want to consider saving some effort, and start using MSMQ instead of creating your own store-and-forward system.

MSMQ Fundamentals

Unlike email, MSMQ uses queues as destinations for messages. A 'client' application sends messages to a destination queue to be picked up by another 'server' application. Typically, the destination queue is a remote one to the client and is closer to the server.

This diagram depicts the function of a MOM like MSMQ. The sender sends the message through MSMQ, MSMQ takes care of ensuring the delivery of the message to the destination queue (at its leisure), and the server picks up the message from the destination queue and performs its work.

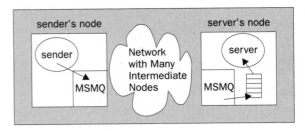

Before going further with MSMQ, we need to have a quick look at system administration.

Administrators vs Developers

The installation of MSMQ-based systems requires significant planning, administration, and maintenance efforts. Recognizing the responsibilities of the administrator versus those of the developer is the first step in creating a successful installation. As developers, we must understand a significant amount of what the administrator does, without actually needing to know how he does it.

MSMQ Server Types

In MSMQ, our applications send messages using client APIs to a destination service or application (running on another client or on a server). The client we work with connects to one of the servers, and the network of servers will route the message to the corresponding server where the message can be retrieved.

There are basically five types of MSMQ server installations:

Server type	Description
Primary Enterprise Controller (PEC)	This is where knowledge about the enterprise configuration resides. There must be one and only one of these per enterprise. It doubles as a Primary Site Controller (see next). Runs an information service in a minimal installation of SQL Server.
Primary Site Controller (PSC)	Caches information for the site. One of these per site in the enterprise. Does routing.
Backup Site Controller (BSC)	Maintains backup information for a PEC or PSC. Does routing. May or may not exist per installation
Routing Server	Servers for routing messages, no database function.
Connector Server	Bridging servers with non-Microsoft queuing systems.

Enterprise in the above description refers to a business enterprise consisting of many sites (divisions). The sites are islands of networks with high bandwidth connections amongst the machines within a site, but narrower bandwidth connecting between sites.

Setting up and configuring enterprise, sites, and servers is the domain of MSMQ administrators. For our coding and testing purposes, you will need to put on the administrator's hat and install MSMQ on two Windows NT Server machines. On the first one, you should install at least one PEC/PSC combo. The second Windows NT system can be configured as an independent client, of which more later.

MSMQ Client Types

When you install MSMQ clients, there are two choices:

❑   Dependent Client – Has no storage capabilities and no local queues. Relies on connection to a server for proper operation. Multiple dependent clients (up to 15) can be hosted by one server.

❑   Independent Client – These clients maintain queues. They can work in a disconnected fashion, allowing applications to send messages even if not connected to any servers. They do not, however, route messages or contain the information service.

Of interest to us is the independent client installation. We want to simulate disconnected operations, because our A&W administrators may be running their admin client from a notebook at home. The second server mentioned above will simulate this.

MSMQ Information Store

The **MSMQ Information Store** (**MQIS**) is a distributed database that stores configuration, system and queue information. It is distributed because the PEC and every PSC and BSC contain the same database. Replication is used to keep them consistent.

> *Currently, the MQIS depends on an installation of SQL Server on the PEC and PSC. Soon, however, this entire service should migrate to the unifying Active Directory Service that Windows NT 5 will supply. One way of thinking about the MQIS (or the upcoming Active Directory) is as special 'persistent shared memory over the network'.*

As developers, we need to be aware of this service, because it will be used frequently for lookup of queues. Furthermore, many APIs in MSMQ implicitly connect to MQIS to do lookup. Since MQIS is not available from an independent client when it is disconnected from the network, we must be careful not to make the assumption that MQIS is always available when using API calls.

Queues Types

Not all queues in MSMQ are application message queues. In fact, much of the operation of MSMQ itself relies on queues. Here are the different types of queues you will find in MSMQ 1.0:

Queue Type	Description
Message	These are the queues that are created, deleted, and used by applications. Each message queue can be public or private. Public means that MQIS knows about it, and others can find it. A private queue is more efficient, but users must get its name via some back door before using it.
Administration	Actually a message queue, but it's used to hold an ACK or NACK acknowledge message generated when a message arrives at the destination queue. If you want this behavior, you have to explicitly specify in the message you send.
Response	Like administration queues, but they receive messages generated when an application actually retrieved the message from MSMQ. You also have to explicitly ask for this behavior in the messages you send.
Journal	A machine journal queue is created by MSMQ for each machine. There is also a 'queue journal' queue for each user-created message queue. When journaling is turned on, a copy of every message that goes through the queue (or the machine) is logged in this queue by MSMQ. You can only read from this queue. These queues are ideal for auditing purposes.
Dead Letter	Holds a copy of messages that cannot be delivered. For non-transactional messages, the node that fails to send ends up with the message. You also have to explicitly request this behavior.

With transactional messages, it is always the originating sender's node that will have the undeliverable message in its dead letter queue (not the intermediate node where transmission failed). |
| Report | Typically used for message tracing and reporting purposes, this queue is created by an administrator to hold MSMQ report messages. |

Message Delivery Modes

When you send messages to a queue, you can control how the message will be delivered by manipulating the properties of the message. One important property is the **delivery mechanism**, indicated by PROPID_M_DELIVERY. It can have values of either:

- ❏ MQMSG_DELIVERY_RECOVERABLE
- ❏ MQMSG_DELIVERY_EXPRESS

In the express mode, which is the default with non-transactional queues, message delivery is done 'in memory'. This results in fast delivery, but the message will not survive a server crash while the message is en-route to the destination. We'll look at the recoverable mode in the next section.

Message Recoverability and Disconnected Mode Operations

If you set the `PROPID_M_DELIVERY` property to `MQMSG_DELIVERY_RECOVERABLE`, MSMQ will guarantee that you will not lose a message, even if an intermediate node crashes during delivery. This is more costly, using more memory movements and disk writes during the delivery process. However, this is the appropriate mode to use in many situations. For example, in a disconnected operating environment (say, on a notebook), you definitely want the recoverable mode, since the delivery will not be successful initially (because you're not connected to the server), and the message must survive the notebook being switched off. Note that all messages delivered into a transactional queue are recoverable by default.

Another important point about disconnected operations is that the MQIS will not be available. This means no 'look-ups' of queues. Any operation that involves a look up directly or indirectly will not work – and may lock the machine while waiting for a timeout. One has to be very careful when designing and coding for a disconnected environment. We will see how we can do this later in this chapter with our 'at home' administrators on their notebook computers.

One operation that may indirectly trigger a look up is the simple action of opening a queue. When you open a queue, you supplied the queue name and the system returns a handle if the open succeeds. The API you call may or may not do a look up, depending on the name you give it.

Three Ways to Name A Queue

Here are the three ways of naming a queue, and whether or not they trigger a lookup:

Queue Name	Description
Format Name	No immediate look up. Can be used in disconnected operations. Lookup happens only after re-connection with MQIS.
Direct Format Name	No lookup ever. Can be used in disconnected operations, but highly discouraged because it bypasses any lookup checks.
Pathname	Lookup immediately. Should not be used in disconnected information. Requires MQIS to be online.

A **format name** is the 'raw' identity of the queue entity. As with any other system entities in the Microsoft world, it is actually a UUID. A public queue may have format name:

```
"PUBLIC=40752CED-1CAA-11D2-ACF7-0020AF11BC7D"
```

And a private queue may be named:

```
"PRIVATE=30352ACE-3CAA-11D2-ACF7-0020EE11BAAC"
```

A **direct format name** is analogous to a URL for the web. You spell out everything explicitly:

❑ Protocol
❑ Address
❑ Local pathname to the queue

Here is an example direct format name:

```
"DIRECT=TCP:192.168.23.15\MyQueue"
```

Use of the direct format name is discouraged, because you are bypassing all levels of indirection and talking to the physical queue at the remote directly. All the nice things that MSMQ gives you in terms of store and forward routing are lost. In many situations, it may not even be possible to use direct format name – if the destination node is not connected, for example.

A **pathname** is the most intuitive way to name a queue:

```
"MYMACHINE\AdminQueue"
"MYMACHINE\PRIVATE$\MyPrivateQ"
```

Below are some examples of pathnames for system managed queues, such as journal and dead letters queues:

```
"MYMACHINE\AdminQueue;JOURNAL"
"MYMACHINE;DEADLETTER"
```

Pathnames are the most 'human friendly', but the least 'machine friendly', because of their potential ambiguity, dependency on locales, etc. In fact, MSMQ doesn't use them directly – they are stored as a property called PROPID_Q_PATHNAME.

You can open a queue using any of the three ways of naming it. In each case, you get back an MSMQ-managed handle after the queue is opened. It is this handle that you use for send/receive operations.

Programming MSMQ

What? No ATL 3 Support!

That's correct, there is no wizard support for MSMQ in ATL 3. It is not by accident. The plain truth is that MSMQ as we know it today will very likely be quite different in COM+. We will have much more to say about why and how at the end of this chapter. For now, we will just have to be satisfied with programming directly to the MSMQ APIs, of which there are two:

❑ The raw API layer
❑ The Automation-compatible COM components layer (often called the ActiveX control layer)

Deceptively Simple APIs

What would you ever want to do with a queue? Open or close it. What would you ever want to do with a message? Send it or read it. MSMQ provides a set of API calls for you to directly do what you want to do with each of its objects. They are not COM-based, but they do look simple. The table below shows a list of the APIs, together with a brief description of what they do:

API Function	Description
MQOpenQueue()	Opens a queue for sending or receiving messages. You can specify the type of access you need, and the call returns a handle to the queue.
MQCloseQueue()	Close a queue given a handle
MQSendMessage()	Send a message to a destination queue. To call this, you need a queue handle, the message, and optionally a transaction context. You can control how the message is sent, whether acknowledge or response messages are triggered, etc., by modifying the message property before sending it.
MQReceiveMessage()	Receive a message from a queue (local or remote). This can be called synchronously or asynchronously. For synchronous calls, you can specify a maximum wait timeout. When it is asynchronous, you can register a callback, wait on an event, or wait on an IO completion port. Transacted queues can be read only using synchronous calls – which presents a dilemma because transactions can get 'stuck' this way. Some fancy coding can alleviate this problem, and we will be doing this later in our code.
MQCreateQueue()	Create a queue and assign it certain properties that you specify. The pathname of the queue is set as the PROPID_Q_PATHNAME property, which must be specified. This call will also register the queue with MQIS if it is public. You get the format name (UUID) back if the create call is successful.
MQDeleteQueue()	Delete a queue given its format name. Also unregister the queue with MQIS if it is public. Note that it is possible for other users to still hold handles to the queue after it has been deleted. It is also possible for MQIS to take significant time to reflect (propagate) the deletion. Again, the design of asynchronous disconnected systems needs to be quite different from those of tightly-coupled, highly-concurrent ones.
MQCreateCursor()	Create a cursor for an open queue. You pass in a queue handle and get back a cursor handle. The cursor is a movable pointer into a message inside the queue. Cursors are for random access into the queue.
MQCloseCursor()	Close a cursor, logically delete it, given a cursor handle.

API Function	Description
MQSetQueueProperties()	Given a format name of a queue and a properties array, set the properties of a queue. The queue does not need to be opened.
	Some properties, such as whether or not a queue is transactional, can only be set when the queue is first created.
MQSetQueueSecurity()	Given a format name and security descriptor information, set the access control properties of a queue.
MQGetQueueProperties()	Get the properties of a queue given its format name. This API queries the MQIS. Private queue properties are local to a machine and not stored in MQIS – you just have to know their value.
MQGetQueueSecurity()	Get the access control information of a queue.
MQGetMachineProperties()	Given either the textual machine name, or the machine's GUID, get its properties via a query to MQIS.
MQLocateBegin() MQLocateEnd() MQLocateNext()	These functions work together to give an LDAP-like interface into the MQIS for locating a queue within an enterprise. When Active Directory arrives with Windows NT 5, these location functions may be replaced.
MQGetSecurityContext()	Called to retrieve security information associated with the certificate being passed in. It returns a security context handle, which can be used repeatedly in supplying messages with the information required for their authentication.
MQFreeSecurityContext()	Frees the security context object specified by the handle, created by the previous call.
MQBeginTransaction()	Used to create a transaction object for internal (non-DTC) MQIS transactions. It returns a pointer to the transaction object which can be used in MQSendMessage() or MQReceiveMessage() calls.
MQFreeMemory()	Used to free MQIS-allocated memory buffers ([out] marshaled structure arrays) typically associated with the MQGetxxxProperties() series of API calls.
MQPathNameToFormatName()	Queries the MQIS to convert a pathname (a queue property) to its format name (true UUID name of queue).
MQInstanceToFormatName()	Finds the format name of a queue, given its identifier, stored as PROPID_Q_INSTANCE. This identifier is what you get back when you use the MQLocateXXX() series of APIs to find a queue.
MQHandleToFormatName()	Given a queue's currently open handle, finds its format name.

There are many properties associated with MSMQ objects, such as queues and messages, and several of the methods shown above deal solely with manipulating these properties. Programming using the MSMQ API is quite a laborious process, involving many complex structures. The large variations in the parameters, many of them system structures, make API-based code rather difficult both to write and maintain.

One of the main reasons why the programming interface for MSMQ is non-COM based is to woo existing queuing applications developers to switch their applications over to the Microsoft platform. To this end, you will find an almost one-to-one correspondence between this MSMQ API and the product from the leading competitor (IBM's MQ/Series).

Automation compatible COM Components

Just as we have done with ATLFinder and ATLDept, Microsoft has created a layer of Automation compatible COM servers for programming MSMQ. This layer of components presents an object model that makes MSMQ programming easier than pi. This opens up the use of MSMQ in ASP, scripting languages, Visual Basic or Visual J++. The fact that these COM servers provide the encapsulation of complex APIs, and reasonable defaults when parameters aren't explicitly specified, makes programming of simple MSMQ applications much easier in any programming language.

MSMQ Automation components present a very simple object model consisting of only ten different objects. The objects accessible through Automation are shown in the table below:

Object	Description
MSMQQueueInfo	Encapsulates an unopened queue. You can use this object to create and delete the queue, or set its properties one at a time. Performing an Open() on this object will return an MSMQQueue object, covered next.
MSMQQueue	Encapsulates an opened queue (the handle). You use this object to peek at or receive messages. It can also manage asynchronous event handlers upon receipt of a message. Upon successful receipt of a message, you get back a MSMQMessage object.
MSMQMessage	Encapsulates a message. You can get and set their properties one at a time, attach a security context to them, and also send them.
MSMQQuery	Query object to simplify the search of public queues via MQIS. This object and the next encapsulate the MQLocateXXX() series.
MSMQQueueInfos	Works together with MSMQQuery to encapsulate the MQLocateXXX() series of directory lookup calls. Presented in the form of a collection, like our EventfulDepts collection.
MSMQEvent	Used for configuring an event handler for message arrival and error conditions.
MSMQTransaction	Encapsulates a transaction object obtained from either one of the two objects below.

Object	Description
`MSMQCoordinated TransactionsDis penser`	Encapsulation used to obtain a DTC (external) transaction object. This object can then be used in send and receive operations to and from transactional queues.
`MSMQTransaction Dispenser`	Encapsulation used to obtain an MSMQ (internal) transaction object. This object can then be used in send and receive operations to and from transactional queues.
`MSMQApplication`	Provides a method to get the machine identifier.

Only the objects that you actually need have to be instantiated by your application. The most frequently used objects are at the top of this list. All objects have built in behaviors that facilitate the most commonly required operations, making typical code for sending and receiving messages trivial to write.

We will be using this approach in creating our MSMQ client and server code. The compiler COM support in Visual C++ 6 really shines here. Programming in C++ with the MSMQ components becomes *almost* as easy as programming Visual Basic.

Data in Messages as BLOBs Only

As a generic queuing service, MSMQ cannot assume too much about the data transmitted in messages sent by client applications. Unfortunately, MSMQ does not provide rich data type handling for message properties. This literally means that one can only use the BODY property of the message to transfer application data and must send the data as a binary blob. This property can take one single VARIANT as parameter. However, since a VARIANT can contain an array of bytes (we will see how later), it can carry any arbitrary BLOB. If it sounds a little like performing custom marshaling to you, you've hit the nail on the head. Programming MSMQ feels very much like coding custom marshallers.

Transactional Queue ≠ Queued Transaction

The moment someone mentions 'transactional queue', some of us retreat quietly into the pipe dream of being able to use MSMQ to extend a transaction not simply through space (as the DTC does today), but also through time. Heed this warning:

> **A transactional queue is not a queued transaction.**

Think of it this way and the confusion may dissipate – you cannot use transacted queues to extend a transaction over two systems that may never connect directly to each other.

Programming with asynchronous disconnected systems often requires thought that may seem to be a little counter-intuitive. The ability to pass a transaction through a queue, or to nest two transactions at the queue boundary is not typically useful. After all, the two systems connected by the queue are assumed to be occasionally disconnected, and can in fact be turned on and off independently.

What is useful, though, is the ability to establish a transaction boundary at the queue – and have the queue's transactional property guarantee the ACID transfer of overall system state between the client and the server systems. Then, the message gets from the client to the queue and from the queue to the server, whenever the server can take the message

This implies that work is done on both sides of the queue in separate transactions. However, the completion order of these transactional units of work is controlled by the way they use the queues. The time when each piece of work is actually performed is flexible, thanks to the durable queues. This is the essence of what is sometimes called a **workflow**.

Individual transactions in this workflow always involve either a message-send or message-receive operation. Additionally, they can also include other resource managers. Given that the most frequently-used resource is inevitably a database, this means that you can combine the action of database update and message sending/receiving into one transaction. The commit/abort scenarios of the individual transaction become something like:

> *Pick up message and update database with it, but if database cannot be updated, leave the message in the queue.*

Or:

> *Update database and send message with the new data, but if the database update fails do not send any message.*

In a workflow, generally you do not want to lose work that you have completed, because it took significant time and effort. Typically, when a transaction in the workflow aborts, the desired behavior is to keep trying until it succeeds – up to a reasonable limit. MSMQ facilitates this by placing the message back in the queue for the server to process again if the transaction is aborted. The `PROPID_M_TIME_TO_BE_RECEIVED` property can limit the time taken in retries. The notification message, which is sent when a message fails to be received, can also be used upstream in the workflow to divert the flow. In extreme cases, human intervention can track down the problem by tracing through the MSMQ journaling, and reporting information.

No Asynchronous Message Receipt when Using Transacted Queues

This is a real bummer. Asynchronous message receipt is a great feature that allows your program to be 'notified' either via a callback function or the Windows message-passing mechanism when a message arrives in a queue. The means that the mainline business logic can proceed within a queueing component, and logic for dequeueing message and message processing can be coded in an event-driven manner. When using the Automation compatible components for MSMQ, this 'message arrival' event can be handled via a connection point incoming interface supplied by the client.

Unfortunately, when you are using transacted queues, all bets are off. One cannot use any asynchronous message receive mechanism for receiving transacted queues. This is the chief reason why we have implemented the seemingly awkward 'polling peek' mechanism in our MSMQ server example.

In a full system, we would probably use a service to poll the queue. For detailed information on service programming and MSMQ , check out Professional NT Services, from Wrox Press.

A&W Calendar: Adding Support for Mobile Administrator

Time to put our knowledge to work and code up an MSMQ storm. The Automation compatible components for MSMQ are contained in a DLL called `mqoa.dll`. You should find this in your `System32` directory.

Retrofitting the Dynamic HTML Client

We are going to modify the Dynamic HTML ActiveX control we created earlier in the chapter. Instead of calling the business objects directly, this new version will send a message to a queue.

We then implement a server that waits for messages on that queue. For each message, this server will decode it and call the corresponding `addEvent()` method on the department server object. Here is a component diagram of the system:

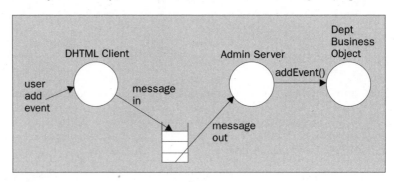

Our first iteration will simply replace the functionality of the existing client. Later, we will try disconnected operations, and finally we'll use transacted queues.

The MSMQ Explorer: Creating the Queue

MSMQ has its own Explorer tool, which you can use to examine all the queues in the enterprise. Almost every aspect of a queue and its contained messages can be queried using this tool. You can also perform administration tasks, such as creating queues, deleting queues, or purging queues of messages. Unfortunately, the MSMQ Explorer is not created as an MMC snap-in. This means that you will need MMC/MTS opened as well as the MSMQ Explorer when working with transacted queues. The MSMQ Explorer is shown here:

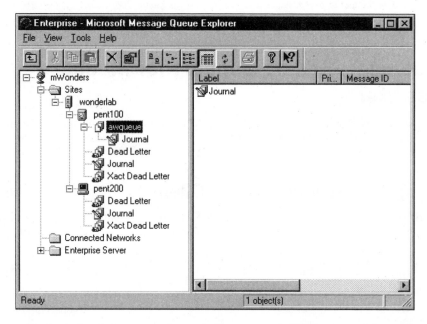

Using it is quite simple, right click on any object and you can get actions that can be performed on it.

Using this MSMQ Explorer, create a public queue called AWQueue on the machine where the PEC (Primary Enterprise Controller) is installed. Make this queue non-transactional for now – we'll be looking at transactional queues later on.

In our specific case, the PEC machine is called PENT100. Our testing topology consists of two machines, connected in this fashion:

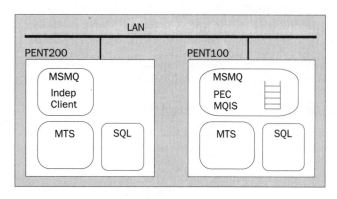

Coding the Message Sender

To modify the client control, we work with the DhtmlClnt.cpp file:

```cpp
#include "stdafx.h"
#include "Adminclt.h"
#include "DhtmlClnt.h"
#define IID_DEFINED
```

```
#include "..\DeptBusObj\DeptBusObj_i.c"
```

```
#import "mqoa.dll" no_namespace
```

We need to add an `#import` directive for the type library information of the MSMQ Automation compatible components.

Next, we're need to define a `struct` to contain information that will go into the body of the message:

```
struct {
    DATE datetime;
    OLECHAR Heading[50];
    OLECHAR Hlink[50];
    OLECHAR Location[50];
    OLECHAR Organizer[50];
    OLECHAR Details[200];
} anEvent;
```

This structure will form the body of the message as an array of bytes. There is a one-for-one correspondence with the database record that it will ultimately update. Note that in order to reconstitute the structure, we must ensure that both the client and the server side use the same structure packing settings for the compiler. Structure misalignment can cause hard-to-find intermittent bugs. This is why the type-aware marshaling provided by COM is so useful – it frees us from concerns of these details.

The modified `AddEvent()` method of `CDhtmlClnt` is shown below:

```
STDMETHODIMP CDhtmlClnt::AddEvent(IDispatch* pdisp, DATE DateTime,
                                  BSTR Heading, BSTR Hlink,
                                  BSTR Location, BSTR Organizer,
                                  BSTR Details)
{
    VARIANT aVar;
    anEvent.datetime = DateTime;
    wcscpy(anEvent.Heading, Heading);
    wcscpy(anEvent.Hlink, Hlink);
    wcscpy(anEvent.Location, Location);
    wcscpy(anEvent.Organizer, Organizer);
    wcscpy(anEvent.Details, Details);
```

The first thing we do is to stuff the structure that we declared above with the incoming values from the call (which is made from the scripting in the HTML page). We also define a VARIANT that will eventually hold this structure as an array of bytes.

```
    MakeASafeArrayOfBytes(&aVar, sizeof(anEvent), &anEvent);
```

We make this array of bytes using a helper function, `MakeASafeArrayOfBytes()`. We'll see the implementation of this function shortly. The first parameter is the VARIANT to hold the final array, the second parameter is the size of the array, and the third is the data to be placed into the array. For now, just remember that the VARIANT, aVar, will be holding the array after this call.

```
try
{
    IMSMQQueueInfoPtr pQInfo(_T("MSMQ.MSMQQueueInfo"));
    IMSMQMessagePtr pMsg(_T("MSMQ.MSMQMessage"));
```

Here we immediately use the MSMQ Automation components to create an `MSMQQueueInfo` object and an `MSMQMessage` object.

```
    pQInfo->put_PathName(CComBSTR("PENT100\\AWQueue"));
```

We set the `PathName` property of the `MSMQQueueInfo` object to the queue we want to open. Remember that you'll need to update this line with the name of the computer that you are using as the PEC.

```
    IMSMQQueuePtr pQueue = pQInfo->Open(MQ_SEND_ACCESS, MQ_DENY_NONE);
```

The queue is opened here is send the message and non-exclusive access.

```
    pMsg->put_Label(CComBSTR("admin-addevent"));
```

Now, we start preparing our message, first by giving it a label to identify it.

```
    pMsg->put_Body(aVar);
```

This is the important part, where we assign our array to the body of the message. Notice the simplicity of the call. Compiler COM support really makes client code simple.

```
    pMsg->Send(pQueue);
```

The message is fully prepared, so we send it with a call to `Send()`.

```
    pQueue->Close();
}
```

Everything completed, we close our instance of the queue. Going out of scope here will clean up all our objects, thanks to the smart pointers. We need a catch-all block:

```
catch(_com_error e)
{
    ATLTRACE(_T("%08x : %s\n"), e.Error(), e.ErrorMessage());
}
```

After the message is sent, we clear the screen by calling back our `ClearForm` handler in the Dynamic HTML script code, as before.

```
        // clear the screen
        CComQIPtr<IHTMLElement> spButton(pdisp);
        if (spButton != NULL)
            spButton->click();

        return S_OK;
    }
```

Using the `mqao.dll` really simplifies MSMQ coding. API-based coding would be at least twice as long.

Let's now turn our attention to the array-making process. The declaration for this helper function needs to be added to the header file for `DhtmlClnt` as follows:

```
    protected:
        void MakeASafeArrayOfBytes(VARIANT* inVar,
                                   long inLength, void* inPointer);
```

The helper function is listed below:

```
    void CDhtmlClnt::MakeASafeArrayOfBytes(VARIANT* inVar,
                                           long inLength, void* inPointer)
    {
        SAFEARRAY * pArray;
```

The `SAFEARRAY` is a structure describing an array, used in early Visual Basic interpreters. Since Automation has its origins in Visual Basic, this type (together with others like `BSTR` and `VARIANT`) has lingered on to the present day. The `SAFEARRAY` manages a descriptor, in addition to the streams of data representing the array. The descriptor gives the number of elements in the array and the upper bound, as well as the lower bound. Readers familiar with the `OPTION BASE` statement in Visual Basic will understand why the bounds needs to be stored with the array. Not only does this help to prevent out-of-bound access, but also allows the array to start at an offset other than 0 or 1.

A `SAFEARRAY` can contain members consisting of almost any one of the `VARIANT` supported types. A pointer to a `SAFEARRAY` is itself a `VARIANT`-supported type. This means that the Automation marshaler actually knows how to marshal this automatically without requiring any proxy/stub. So, why didn't we use it for passing back custom structures in our business objects?

True, using a `SAFEARRAY` of bytes would have allowed us to eliminate the need of proxy/stubs for our business objects, but only at a cost – more cryptic code, plus the need to pack and unpack the structures ourselves. The most severe limitation, however, is the subtle dependence of structure alignment and packing on compilation switches. Since our business objects must work with many clients, this sort of subtle dependency can cause a lot of compatibility problems.

Now, let see how we stuff a structure into the `SAFEARRAY`.

```
        VariantInit(inVar);
```

First, we zero the incoming VARIANT.

```
pArray = ::SafeArrayCreateVector(VT_UI1, 1, inLength);
```

Here, we use a call to SafeArrayCreateVector(), created specifically for this purpose. This call creates a SAFEARRAY of type VT_UI1 (a byte), with lower bound 1, and a length of inLength elements. The useful thing about this call is that it also allocates memory for storing the data at the same time.

```
unsigned char* tp;
SafeArrayAccessData(pArray, reinterpret_cast<void**>( &tp));
```

Even though the SAFEARRAY structure has a direct member pointing to the array's data area, you should not access the pointer directly. Using the SafeArrayAccessData() call is the preferred way to get at this pointer. The SafeArrayAccessData() function essentially performs a Lock() call to prevent concurrent access to the array data area before returning the pointer.

```
if (tp)
{
    memcpy(tp, inPointer, inLength);
}
SafeArrayUnaccessData(pArray);
```

Finally, we copy the structure into the data area and unlock the array.

```
inVar->vt = VT_ARRAY | VT_UI1;
inVar->parray = pArray;
}
```

The last couple of lines set the type flag and the VARIANT to contain the SAFEARRAY.

Now, build the control, and try it out – you can also find code in the \AdminClt.2 directory. Adding an event now should send a message to the AWQueue queue. You can use the MSMQ Explorer to verify that the message has been delivered. If you double click on the message, you'll see the Properties window and you can view the message and see the information you have added in the body.

Architecture of the Server Side

The server side of our administration application, running on the departmental server, must retrieve the message from the queue, decode the event, and add the event to the departmental database using the departmental business objects created in the last chapter. This will also cause the cached event count at the central server to change, thanks to the distributed transaction from the last chapter.

At first glance, a server can be written simply with the following pseudo-code:

```
while msg = queue.receive(wait_infinite)
    decode message into event
    call deptobject.addEvent()
end while
```

However, since we eventually want to use transacted queues, we must make sure our server contains an MTS component. It will be inside the component that we perform the work of reading from the queue, decoding, and updating the database (all within a transaction).

One design possibility might be simply to put the above pseudo-code into an MTS component. Let's say that it is exposed through an interface method called IAdminServer::StartService().

```
IAdminServer::StartService()
{
    while msg = queue.receive(wait_infinite)
        decode message into event
        call deptobject.addEvent()
    end while
}
```

In this case, we would need to create a host program with this pseudo-code:

```
create MTS component and get IAdminServer interface
call IAdminServer::StartService()
```

There is one problem with this, however. If we set the MTS component declaratively to 'require transactions', the component will be waiting for message inside a transaction – holding it open! This is very bad and defeats the purpose of using transaction in the first place. We don't want to start the transaction until there is a message in the queue, so the final host program has the following pseudo-code:

```
while msg = queue.peek(wait_infinite)
    IAdminServer::StartService()
end while
```

This means that the host program waits on the queue, peeking at it continuously until a message arrives. Once a message is detected, it calls the MTS component. The MTS component can be described by the pseudo-code:

```
IAdminServer::StartService()
{
    msg = queue.receive(0)
    decode message into event
    call deptobject.addEvent()
}
```

At this point, the transaction begins. Since we know for sure that a message is in the queue, the MTS component quickly retrieves the message, decodes it, and calls addEvent() on the business object. It then immediately exits the transaction and returns control to the host program. Here is what the final architecture of the server side piece looks like:

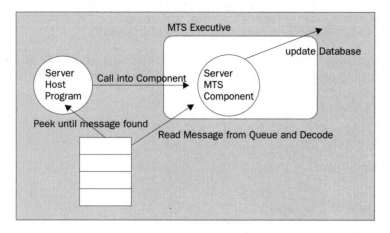

We can see above that the server host program will peek in the message queue, outside of transaction, until a message is found. Once a message is found, it will call into an MTS component – starting a transaction.

This means that we will have two discrete pieces of coding to do. First we will code the server-side MTS component, and then we will code the server-side host program.

Coding the Server Side MTS Component

First, we create an ATL project called MqRmtServer, and add a skeleton MTS server component using the ATL Objects AppWizard. Just like our business objects in earlier chapters, select **Custom interface**, **Supports IObjectControl**, and **Can be Pooled** in the wizard. Call the object AdminSvr, and the interface IAdminSvr.

Next, we modify the generated header file and add some new include/class members to the generated header file: AdminSvr.h. #include the DeptBusObj.h file:

```
#include "resource.h"        // main symbols
#include <mtx.h>
#include "..\DeptBusObj\DeptBusObj.h"
```

Add the type library information from the Automation compatible MSMQ support component.

```
#import "mqoa.dll" no_namespace
```

Also, we add a smart pointer for holding a pointer to the departmental business object (used in adding event to the departmental database) as a member of the CAdminSvr class:

```
CComPtr<IObjectContext> m_spObjectContext;
CComQIPtr<IBoDeptEvent> m_spDeptServer;
```

These are all the changes necessary for the AdminSvr.h file.

Next, we add one single method to `IAdminSvr`:

```
HRESULT StartService();
```

As we saw in the previous section, the implementation of `StartService()` needs to check the message queue to see if there is an event waiting, and, if so, call the `addEvent()` method of the department server object. You can find the code for this method in the `\MqRmtSvr\AdminSvr.cpp` file. We will be using `Atlconv.h` routines to convert between `OLECHAR[]` and `BSTR`s.

```
STDMETHODIMP CAdminSvr::StartService()
{
    USES_CONVERSION;
```

For holding the details of the event, we have a structure, `QEVENT`, which is the same as the sending client. Make sure you copy the `anEvent` structure from the client, and rename it `QEVENT`.

```
    QEVENT anEvent;
```

Here, we set a maximal timeout for testing purposes. In practice, this timeout should never be reached, since the server host program ensures that a message is available in the queue before calling this method.

```
    bool bAbort = false;
    long longTime = 600; // 10 minutes
```

We open our message queue, specifying receive access. You will need to change the machine name that is part of the `PathName` to match your server.

```
    try
    {
        IMSMQQueueInfoPtr pQInfo(_T("MSMQ.MSMQQueueInfo"));
        pQInfo->put_PathName(CComBSTR("PENT100\\AWQueue"));

        IMSMQQueuePtr pQueue = pQInfo->Open(MQ_RECEIVE_ACCESS,
                                            MQ_DENY_NONE);
```

We set the parameters of the `Receive()` method here to wait up to one second, and use the MTS based transaction if one is available. This is done by setting the `varTransaction` parameter to `MQ_MTS_TRANSACTION`.

```
        CComVariant varTransaction, varWantDest, varWantBody, varTimeout;
        varTransaction = MQ_MTS_TRANSACTION;
        varWantDest = false;
        varWantBody = true;
        varTimeout = 1000;

        IMSMQMessagePtr pMsg = pQueue->Receive(&varTransaction,
                    &varWantDest, &varWantBody, &varTimeout);
```

We expect this always to be true, since the host program already knows that a message is in the queue before this method is called.

Here, we reverse what we did on the client and get the data out of the SAFEARRAY and back into our event structure.

```
if (pMsg)
    {
        BSTR tpVar;
        VARIANT tpBody;
        pMsg->get_Label(&tpVar);
        pMsg->get_Body(&tpBody);
        SAFEARRAY * tpArray = tpBody.parray;
        void * tp;
        SafeArrayAccessData(tpArray, reinterpret_cast<void**> (&tp));
memcpy(&anEvent, tp, sizeof(anEvent));
        SafeArrayUnaccessData(tpArray);
```

We create an instance of the departmental server business object if it is not already available.

```
        HRESULT hRes;
        long DummyVal;
        if (!m_spDeptServer)
        {
            hRes = m_spDeptServer.CoCreateInstance(
                    OLESTR("DeptBusObj.BoDeptEvent"));
            if (hRes != S_OK) return hRes;
        }
```

Next, we call the addEvent() method on the department server object with the parameters in the message.

```
        hRes = m_spDeptServer->addEvent(anEvent.datetime,
            OLE2BSTR(anEvent.Heading),
            OLE2BSTR(anEvent.Hlink),
            OLE2BSTR(anEvent.Location),
            OLE2BSTR(anEvent.Organizer),
            OLE2BSTR(anEvent.Details), &DummyVal);
```

Finally, we call SetComplete(), or SetAbort() if we get an error.

```
        if (SUCCEEDED(hRes))
        {
            if (m_spObjectContext)
            m_spObjectContext->SetComplete();
        }
        else
        {
            if (m_spObjectContext)
            m_spObjectContext->SetAbort();
            Error(OLESTR("Create event failed"),IID_IAdminSvr);
        }
    }
    else
    {
        if (m_spObjectContext)
        m_spObjectContext->SetAbort();
        Error(OLESTR("No message received"),IID_IAdminSvr);
    }
```

If we get an error, we will pass back a COM error message to the host program.

```
        pQueue->Close();
    }
    catch(_com_error e)
    {
        ATLTRACE(_T("%08x : %s\n"), e.Error(), e.ErrorMessage());
        if (m_spObjectContext)
        m_spObjectContext->SetAbort();
        Error(e.ErrorMessage(),IID_IAdminSvr);
        return e.Error();
    }

    return S_OK;
}
```

Compile the MTS component, and install it inside a new package called Admin Server on your PEC computer. In our case, the computer is called PENT100. Do not set the component to Requires a transaction at this time.

Coding the Server Side Host Program

Now is time to code the server-side host program. This is a console application, it will peek into the queue until it finds a message, once a message is located, it will call the MTS component to do the transacted work. For simplicity, we will be doing this in an infinite loop in our implementation.

You can use Visual Studio to create a console application, and start with a simple application. Alternatively, you will find the source for the host program under the Ch10\admin directory – called admin.cpp:

At the top of the file, we add two #import directives to get the type library of the MSMQ Automation component, plus the type library of our MTS component.

```
#include "stdafx.h"
#import "mqoa.dll" no_namespace
#import "..\MqRmtSvr\MqRmtSvr.tlb" no_namespace

int _tmain(int argc, _TCHAR * argv[])
{

    CoInitialize(NULL);

    try
    {
```

Firstly, we create the MTS component, as well as an MSMQQueueInfo component.

```
        IAdminSvrPtr  pCI(__uuidof(AdminSvr));
        IMSMQQueueInfoPtr pQInfo(_T("MSMQ.MSMQQueueInfo"));
```

With the call to `Open()`, we open the queue for peeking access.

```
pQInfo->put_PathName(_bstr_t("PENT100\\AWQueue"));

IMSMQQueuePtr pQueue = pQInfo->Open(MQ_PEEK_ACCESS, MQ_DENY_NONE);
```

Then we loop forever – waiting sixty seconds each time before checking for new messages. If a message is found, close the queue and call the MTS component we created earlier to process the message, and finally open the queue again.

```
      while (true)
      {
          IMSMQMessagePtr pMsg = NULL;
          _variant_t varWantDest = false;
          _variant_t varWantBody = true;
          _variant_t varTimeout = 600001;
          pMsg = pQueue->Peek(&varWantDest, &varWantBody, &varTimeout);

          if (pMsg)
          {
              pQueue->Close();
              // transactional read
              pCI->StartService();
              pQueue = pQInfo->Open(MQ_PEEK_ACCESS, MQ_DENY_NONE);
          }
      }
  }
  catch(_com_error e)
  {
      _tprintf(_T("%08x : %s\n"), e.Error(), e.ErrorMessage());
  }

  CoUninitialize();
  return 0;
}
```

Compile this program and copy it over to the PEC computer.

Testing Connected Operations

Enough coding, for now, it's time we tested some connected operations. This should work in the same way as the Dynamic HTML ActiveX control before we modified it for MSMQ. Make sure you have the following installed and running:

On the PEC, you should have the following:

- ❑ The Department Server package in MTS
- ❑ The Admin Server package in MTS
- ❑ The admin host program running
- ❑ The Central Server running as a Remote Component in MTS

And on the independent client:

- ❑ The Central Server package in MTS
- ❑ The Dynamic HTML ActiveX Control

We choose to configure our testing network this way in anticipation of testing the transacted case later. A transacted queue requires the de-queuing server to be running on the same server as the queue (the departmental server). We also want to make sure that the distributed data update transaction is still occurring across the network. Our configuration fits all these requirements and uses only two machines. It basically reuses the central server as a departmental administrator's machine.

Here is a diagram of the configuration for testing:

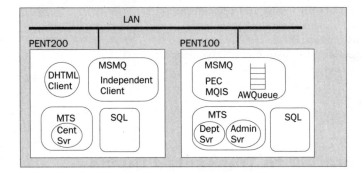

Add an event using the ActiveX Control, and check the database for the new event. Use `Msqry32`, `TestDept`, or `TestCent` to make sure the distributed transaction is working.

Testing Disconnected Operations

Now, for our mobile administrators, we need to make our system work even when the network is down. To make this happen, we need to make a change in the Dynamic HTML ActiveX Control. In the `DhtmlClnt.cpp` file, for the `AddEvent()` method, we must open the queue with its format name (GUID) instead of its path name.

Since the MQIS is not available in a disconnected environment, we cannot lookup a path name. Here is the change:

```
STDMETHODIMP CDhtmlClnt::AddEvent(IDispatch* pdisp, DATE DateTime,
                                  BSTR Heading, BSTR Hlink,
                                  BSTR Location, BSTR Organizer,
                                  BSTR Details)
{

    ...

try {
        IMSMQQueueInfoPtr pQInfo(_T("MSMQ.MSMQQueueInfo"));
        IMSMQMessagePtr pMsg(_T("MSMQ.MSMQMessage"));

        pQInfo->put_FormatName(
                CComBSTR("PUBLIC=40752CED-1CAA-11D2-ACF7-0020AF11BC7D"));
IMSMQQueuePtr pQueue = pQInfo->Open(MQ_SEND_ACCESS, MQ_DENY_NONE);
    ...
```

Note that you will need to alter the GUID here to correspond to the one for your queue, which you can easily obtain, using the MSMQ Explorer. Highlight the queue, right-click, and select Properties. You can highlight, copy, and past the GUID into your source code.

Restart all MTS services and the admin host program. Then, disconnect the LAN connection between the two servers. Now, start the ActiveX control on the independent client and add a few messages. Note that nothing unusual appears to happen, the messages are accepted normally.

If you now try reconnecting the LAN connection, you should notice how the Admin Server immediately empties the queue and adds all the pending events to the distributed databases. This is exactly how our remote administrators will be using the system.

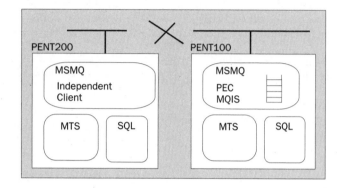

Migrating to Transacted Queues

Finally, we are ready to see transacted queues in action. In our case, transacted queues will provide the following added value:

- ❑ On the client side, the message will be sent atomically. Either the message is sent to the destination queue or it will be sent to the originating server's dead letter queue. It will not be lost or partially sent.
- ❑ On the server side, if the database operation fails, the message will be restored back to the queue as if it had never been removed and the system will retry until the message timeout is reached

The following diagram illustrates the two transactions, one on the DHTML client, the other one on the server. Both sides are connected via the transacted queue – which can be viewed as a third long-duration transaction.

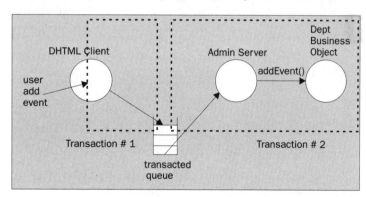

To work with transacted queues, we must:

- ❑ Delete the orginal AWQueue and create a new one with transaction enabled
- ❑ Use Transaction Explorer to set the AdminSvr object's properties to **Requires a Transaction**
- ❑ Make several modifications to the client program to send the message within a transaction
- ❑ Update the client source code with the new format name of the transacted queue

The modifications to the client source code (in DhtmlClnt.cpp) are shown below. First, we need to update the format name with the new one from the transacted queue.

```
STDMETHODIMP CDhtmlClnt::AddEvent(IDispatch* pdispButton, DATE DateTime,
                                  BSTR Heading, BSTR Hlink,
                                  BSTR Location, BSTR Organizer,
                                  BSTR Details)
{

    ...

    try {
        IMSMQQueueInfoPtr pQInfo(_T("MSMQ.MSMQQueueInfo"));
        IMSMQMessagePtr pMsg(_T("MSMQ.MSMQMessage"));
        pQInfo->put_FormatName(
                CComBSTR("PUBLIC=40752CED-1CAA-11D2-ACF7-0020AF11BC7D"));
        IMSMQQueuePtr pQueue = pQInfo->Open(MQ_SEND_ACCESS, MQ_DENY_NONE);
```

Remember from our discussions earlier in the chapter that transacted messages must use recoverable delivery.

```
        pMsg->put_Delivery(MQMSG_DELIVERY_RECOVERABLE);
        pMsg->put_Label(CComBSTR("admin-addevent"));
        pMsg->put_Body(aVar);
```

We need to ask to use an MSMQ local transaction when sending the message. This is done by passing MQ_SINGLE_MESSAGE as the second argument of the Send() call. This is required; as the send to a transacted queue must done be within a transaction.

```
        CComVariant tpV = MQ_SINGLE_MESSAGE;
        pMsg->Send(pQueue, &tpV);
        pQueue->Close();
    }
```

This final transacted client code is the source code found in AdminClnt.4 directory in the source distribution. You can compile it and test it from there.

If you try the client again, you will see that it is functional like the original client except it is a little bit slower. You can try modifying the code of the business object to make it abort the transaction and watch the retries at the server.

Debugging MSMQ Applications

In an attempt to save you potentially hours or days of agony debugging applications for this sparsely documented technology, we will pass on a few tips that we have learnt the hard way.

You Need Several Machines, Period!

Testing and debugging on one machine is not really feasible when working with MSMQ applications. It is not possible to stage typical MSMQ testing scenarios on just one machine. You should have access to at least two fully loaded networked development systems, one with Windows NT 4 Server with Service Pack 3 or later, NT 4.0 Option Pack, and full Visual Studio install. If you have more than two machines, make the additional ones Windows 98 machines to test some minimal client behaviors.

Decide if You need Transacted Queues Up-front

Applications coded with non-transacted queues are significantly different from those with transacted queues. There are subtle error conditions that can occur when transacted queues are used, which may not normally occur with non-transacted queues. Writing code that will work flexibly with both types of queues is possible, but will increase code complexity. In most designs, you should be able to decide up-front what type of queue you need. It is best to make this decision as early as possible.

Rules are Rules, Follow Them!

The MSMQ Reference, the SDK Reference, the Administrator's Guide, and the Programmer's Guide should be your friends. They are available in both HTML and WINHELP form with the Windows NT Option Pack release. Study them and have them handy when coding.

The rules cited in the above documentation regarding transacted queues are real, so follow them closely. The two most important ones are:

❑ All message sends to a transacted queue must be transacted; this could mean either an MSMQ internal transaction or a DTC-coordinated transaction

❑ Receives from a transacted queue do not have to be transacted, but if they are, they must be from a local transacted queue – implying the server user that transacted queue must be on the same machine

Transacted queues work with the current MSMQ release (1.0 at the time of writing), but you do have to make sure the rules are followed carefully.

There is a confirmed bug with MSMQ 1.0 when working with transacted queues on an independent client in disconnected mode. If you need to work in disconnected mode and need transacted queues, you may have to wait for a new service pack.

Be Fluent with Transaction Explorer and MSMQ Explorer

This is an absolute prerequisite. If you are not comfortable with either tool, debugging distributed transacted queuing applications can get a lot more complex than it actually is.

Test other MTS Components First

If you are doing transactional queues, and the transactions involve other MTS components, test those thoroughly first. One good way of testing MTS components is to write command line drivers for the APIs that they offer (as we did with `TestDept` and `TestCent` in the last chapter). This way, you can script the testing in batch files and perform regression tests quickly after each update.

Once you have the additional MTS components fully tested, the only problem that you will have to deal with will be with the new MSMQ component and debugging with be significantly easier.

The Very Handy Mqoai.h File

Under the `\Microsoft Visual Studio\Vc98\include` directory, you will find the mqoai.h file. If you are using the Automation compatible components to program your MSMQ application (as we do in our example), you may find the definitions in this file quite useful. The error code definition in this file should help you understand what is going on when a method call returns an error.

The Future of MSMQ

One immediately notices the oddball nature of MSMQ compared to other new BackOffice servers – it has a complete C-based programmatic interface. Whatever happened to Microsoft's indomitable commitment to COM? It turns out that the MSMQ 'interim' API interface serves three very important marketing functions:

❑ It has a call-for-call functional equivalence to IBM's MQ/Series, allowing rapid migration of software formerly using this technology

❑ It is easy to learn and use, tremendously lowering the barrier of entry during this early adopter's phase of the technology

❑ MSMQ may in time become so tightly integrated with COM that explicit call to the infrastructure may no longer be necessary

The last point deserves some additional explanation. Unlike MTS's transactional model, the asynchronous messaging model of MSMQ and DCOM's distributed components model do not clash. Heck, they even complement each other! Asynchronous reliable messaging can become a viable transport mechanism for COM components. This means, instead of using MS RPC over UDP or TCP, COM calls will be relayed via MSMQ.

For an idea of how you might use MSMQ as an asynchronous marshaling layer, see Professional DCOM Application Development *from Wrox Press.*

This is very close to a marriage made in heaven; the only regret of the architects was, 'Why didn't we think of that earlier?' Retrofitting the infrastructure at this level of maturity of the technology will require meticulous design and substantial effort. The fruit of this labor may not even arrive in time for the first phase of COM+.

Of course, the combination of COM and MSMQ would require some new conventions in handling COM method calls. Currently, all COM method calls are synchronous – they perform the function and then return to the caller. In the MSMQ-enabled world, the call must be asynchronous, the caller must be released immediately, and if return values are desired, a mechanism needs to be established to re-synchronize with the call. Since MSMQ also functions in a totally disconnected manner, the machine hosting the caller may actually shutdown before the reply arrives. This means that the calling convention must also be modified to cater for a 'call and forget' scenario. In this case, the caller simply makes the call, and will not expect any return value.

At the most recent technical conference hosted by Microsoft, they confirmed that work is being performed internally on all of the above. We should be using one shiny new MSMQ in the not too distant future. Rest assured, however, that the current API for MSMQ will probably be supported indefinitely, as long as there are non-COM based queuing applications remaining in this world.

Summary

In this chapter, we have demonstrated how user interfaces for an ActiveX control can be designed rapidly using Dynamic HTML. Thanks to the new Dynamic HTML Control support built into ATL 3, creating these ActiveX controls is extremely easy. The flexibility of these controls allow us to manipulate and change the displayed HTML elements with our C++ code within the control, use scripting code within the Dynamic HTML page to call C++ based extension, or use C++ code to interact with scripts within the Dynamic HTML page. Using this exciting new technology, we quickly built an ActiveX control for the A&W administrators for them to add events to their department's database.

In order to enable the remote administrators (ones on notebook computers) to participate, we modified the administrative control to use MSMQ. Before we started coding, we covered the basics of Message Oriented Middleware (MOM), store-and-forward communications, and disconnected system operations. Next, we took a look at Microsoft Message Queues (MSMQ) as a MOM. We learnt about how MSMQ operates, the types of MSMQ servers available, and the APIs available to program MSMQ applications. We also discovered transacted queues and the subtleties of transactions in MSMQ. Finally, we modified the administration ActiveX control to use MSMQ through the Automation compatible object model mapping layer provided with MSMQ.

This completes our examination into the multi-tiered DNA system for A&W Intranet. It also concludes our examination of how COM, DCOM, and ActiveX technologies can be applied in practical and productive ways. Furthermore, it wraps up our examination of the new features in ATL 3 and Visual C++ 6.0 that ease development of COM components, ActiveX controls, and DNA business components.

In the next chapter, we will discuss one final subject that we have consciously stayed away from so far – Security.

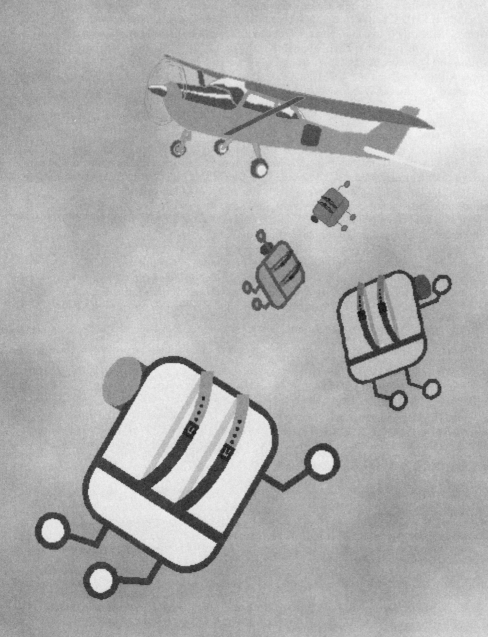

11
Security

Overview

Throughout this book, while we've been looking at ActiveX, COM, DCOM, DNA and component software, we have avoided the issue of security. This is not because security is an unimportant topic, of course, but because security is of paramount importance, and can't be treated lightly in a 'by the way' fashion within sections embedded in other chapters. With this in mind, and in order to do it justice, we've opted to focus on security in its own independent chapter.

The sheer complexity of security issues means that they don't mix easily with other technical subjects which require their own focus. Furthermore, the implementation of security measures in a distributed computing environment is far from simple. The situation is further aggravated by the new terminology, jargon and acronyms that the security industry employs. In this chapter, we'll demystify many of the concepts, and discover the available APIs, system objects and built-in system features, which facilitate the implementation of secure distributed computing systems.

On the other side of the coin, we'll also be looking at the roadblocks and harassment that a DNA business object has to live and deal with, in order to carry out its chores in a secured environment.

The branches of security on which we'll be focusing in this chapter are those related to distributed component computing (COM and DCOM security), as well as DNA services (MTS and MSMQ security). We will discover that most of these security schemes use the foundation security built into the Windows NT operating system kernel.

The Need for Network Security

Throughout the history of multi-user computing, there has always been a need to protect and secure the information or resources of one user from access by another. Security violations can be intentional or unintentional, malicious or benign. In all cases they're highly undesirable and best prevented, if at all possible. Now that networking machines and sharing of resources and information has become enterprise-wide (in the intranet) and global (in the Internet), the need for sound and robust security measures is more important than ever before.

The security industry is a 'fear' driven one, and deservedly so. The sensational cases that occasionally surface, with employees or demonic individuals bringing down entire enterprises through electronic attack or espionage, is enough to drive any executive into committing major resources to prevention measures.

There are many reasons why you should secure a web server or distributed software components in an intranet environment. Most of them revolve around the need to protect the information and/or resources belonging to one party against access or tampering from other unauthorized parties. In order to achieve this, one typically has to provide means for:

❑ Restricting access
❑ Providing positive identification and authentication
❑ Ensuring data integrity (against embedding of a virus into a program, or data tampering during network transmission, for example)
❑ Ensuring privacy (for example, against 'unauthorized peeks' into secret data)

We'll start by examining the above points and seeing how they all fit together.

Restricting Access

Let's try to clarify the definition of **access**. Access is the ability of an **accessing entity** to interact with an object. What we mean by 'object' in this sense is not an ActiveX object or a COM object, but rather any logical or physical entity in the computing environment (i.e. a process or a file). The accessing entity isn't necessarily a person sat at a keyboard and could quite easily be another object (for example, an ActiveX component running as an unattended service).

There are different types of access too. Some examples are:

❑ List – the accessing entity is aware of the existence of the object in question (i.e. can see it), but can't do anything with it
❑ Read – allows the accessing entity to view the actual content of the object, but not change that content
❑ Change – the contents can be updated by the accessing entity
❑ Create – the accessing entity can create a new instance of the object
❑ Delete – the object can be deleted by the accessing entity
❑ Execute – this is possibly the most 'dangerous' as the object itself may have access to other objects to which the accessing entity normally has no access rights, potentially allowing a breach of security

Access rights

There is a need to assign different levels of access to objects in a system. **Access rights** are the mechanism by which security-conscious operating systems achieve this (for example, Windows NT). Access rights specify what the accessing entity has the right to do with an object. Objects in the system have associated with them a list of access rights that specify which accessing entities have which rights.

This brings us to the issue of how to ensure that the accessing entity is what it claims to be, so that it can be allowed to exercise only those rights that it may have. That is, the accessing entity must be **authenticated**.

Identification and Authentication

In most computer systems that support security mechanisms, the notion of a **user** or **account** is used to associate an accessing entity with certain access rights to the objects managed by the system. Any programs running on such systems run 'on behalf of' or 'in the context of' a user or an account.

The first security issue that arises, as a consequence of this, is that when an entity presents its credentials as user 'A' to the system, there needs to be a mechanism to check whether or not it is, in fact, 'A'.

Authentication is the mechanism of ensuring or verifying the identity of the entities requiring access to a computer system, and it is based on the secure exchange of identity information.

Integrity

In the context of security, **integrity** doesn't cover the alteration of data or interactions due to non-malicious, unintentional errors. Taking care of these is the job of error recovery on a local or network scale. Instead, integrity means ensuring that data or communications aren't tampered with. For example:

❏   A user has accessed certain system resources. Preserving integrity means that they can't claim that they didn't. History can't be rewritten. Support for auditing the exercising of access rights ensures this.

❏   A user has sent a message. Preserving integrity means that they can't claim it wasn't them; actions can be uniquely attributed to the entity that initiated them. Signatures are valid. The technical name for this issue is **non-repudiation**.

❏   A user sends data that gets modified en route to the receiving party. Preserving integrity means that the modification can't go unnoticed. You can't change somebody else's letter with impunity! 'Message tampering' activities are detected.

In this context, even authentication can be construed as an aspect of integrity. It preserves the integrity of presenting an identity.

Privacy

We define **privacy** as the right to disallow access to one's private data, or communications with another party.

If there are no 'third parties', that is, in a totally isolated system, this requirement is vacuously true.

In reality, however, the world is much more interesting than that and there is more to ensuring privacy than setting access rights for known users. The need to use insecure communication channels may mean that you have eavesdroppers who can gain access to the information passing between trusted users, without needing to impersonate one of the users.

The fundamental mechanism that provides solutions to the issue of privacy is **encryption,** a process of transforming the data to be protected into a form that only the trusted parties have the ability to interpret.

Fitting the Pieces Together

The following table shows how all these elements fit together in a typical security implementation:

Security Issue	Security mechanism
Controlled access	Access rights, authenticated identities
Right for privacy	Encryption
Integrity	Authentication

In the following pages, we'll be examining the security implementations of Windows NT, and Windows 98/95, in the context of ActiveX components and distributed computing in an intranet environment. We'll be revisiting each of the above security elements, as appropriate, and showing how you can implement and reuse them.

ActiveX and Windows NT Server Network

Thankfully, when dealing with ActiveX based technology in a Windows NT Server network, there is a lot that can be done. The Windows NT Server product was, from the conceptual stage, designed to provide a secure computing environment.

Security isn't something that can be added to an operating system as an afterthought. It has to be designed into the core of the system from day one. In particular, Windows NT (from the earliest version) was designed to meet the C2 security guidelines set out by the U.S. government. Even though certified compliance with the C2 guidelines may only be required for deployment in government organizations, the enhanced security that compliant systems offer is very important for businesses generally.

The main requirements for C2 compliance are:

- ❏ *User identification and authentication* – the system requires users to prove their identity before they are allowed access.
- ❏ *Auditing* – user actions and object access can be logged by the system.
- ❏ *Discretionary access control* – Objects on the system have owners who can grant or restrict (at various levels) access to the resources.
- ❏ *Object reuse* – the system guarantees that discarded or deleted objects are not accessible by other entities. This holds true, for example, for deleted files and de-allocated memory.
- ❏ *System integrity* – the system protects resources that belong to one entity from being read or written to by other entities. For example, the memory that's been allocated to a process isn't accessible by other processes.

The C2 guidelines refer to standalone systems only, and are published in an orange book, aptly called the *Orange Book*. Guidelines for networking aspects of security are covered in the *Red Book*.

NT 3.5 with SP 3 received C2 certification in July 1995, while NT 3.51 received C2 certification in September 1996. NT 4.0 is still undergoing networking and C2 certification, both in US and in Europe, at the time of writing.

With such robust security support in place, network software, application software, and distributed components (networked application software pieces) can use these system features to extend the secure computing environment. We'll see how this is done throughout the rest of the chapter.

Where We Need Security In An Intranet

Other than controlling and administering access to the individual machines in an intranet (this is the function of the network operating system), we may want to restrict access to certain intranet-accessible information to only a selected group of users. For example, we may want everybody to be able to access the general Accounting Department web server, but we want only people in the Accounting Department to access a draft annual report that is linked to the home page.

Controlled Access To Web Pages

In many ways, this type of protection is very similar to the access control that's supplied by the network operating system, such as Windows NT Server. What's different, though, is that the user may not be currently 'logged in' to the network serving the page. He or she may be totally remote, may not be using an ActiveX-enabled browser, and may even be running on a Macintosh computer. Yet, we still want to be able to enforce the same access control.

It's easy enough to protect specific web pages, or other files, from casual access. Simply use Explorer and disable read access (assuming you're in a secured installation using the NTFS file system). This, however, will prevent *all* users from accessing the protected pages.

Whatever the solution may be in this kind of situation, the web server must somehow obtain the capability of identifying who the user is at the other end of the connection (sitting behind the browser), in order for it to work. This, of course, boils down to the ability of the server to authenticate the identity of a remote user. How could such authentication be performed? Even if we obtain the true identity of the user, what happens if the network hosting the web server doesn't know about the user at all? There might be no account information on the user.

In addition, a web server typically runs unattended and must have an identity associated with it for access checks. User requests must not be handled using this server identity in order to avoid security breaches. Instead, the server typically 'assumes the user's identity' during the access of protected resources. This process is called **impersonation**.

Let's consider a hypothetical case where Joe Belmont of Accounting is trying to access the secured draft report (to which he has access rights) from Italy, via a modem, using a Unix machine at a trade show. We'll take a look at the different ways in which this authentication can be performed in the next section.

Secure Intranet and Internet Interactions

Ensuring orderly controlled access, data integrity and user privacy in an intranet environment requires careful analysis of the access scenarios and access patterns of a typical intranet application (or Active web site). If access control is designed too tightly, the user may end up with an impression of a highly restrictive, and rather frustrating experience. Repeated requests for passwords and user IDs can have this effect. Designed too loosely, and the system/application may be subjected to security abuse and malicious attacks.

Before we look at how to secure DCOM, MTS and MSMQ, let's look at the state-of-the-art with respect to security in the 'normal' web page access scenario. This access pattern is fundamental to our later discussions.

Let's briefly outline, once again, the scenario we're looking at here. We need to authenticate a remote user, who is accessing a web server, in order to restrict access to certain web pages. We'll look at three specific cases and see how the problem is solved:

- ❑ The first case will be the general case where both the browser and the server may not be a Microsoft product
- ❑ Next, we'll look at the case where we have a Microsoft browser and a Microsoft server, over a private intranet
- ❑ The final case also features a Microsoft browser and a Microsoft server, but this time over the public Internet

As you'll soon realize, even though everything looks very similar on the surface, major differences in security implementation exist under the covers.

A Non-Microsoft Scenario

If you've surfed the Internet at all, you've probably encountered sites or web pages that require a password and user ID before you can access them. When such a page is reached, the browser pops up a little password entry dialog box. The interesting thing here is that there seems to be something built into the browser-server combination that provides this authentication capability. Yet, if you were to look into the documentation for the browser (and sometimes even for the server), you may be surprised to find that this capability is often not well described. At any rate, there seems to be no standard way to follow for authenticating a remote user using a random browser and server combination. How exactly is this done?

The secret, it turns out, lies in the transmitted HTTP packet's header information.

The series of events that occur during this scenario are summarized below:

1. The client clicks on a link on the browser display, which attempts to access some protected resource

2. The browser, having no way to tell that a requested resource is protected, formats a normal HTTP request packet asking for the resource and transmits it to the server

3. The server attempts to access the resource and faces an 'access denied' situation

4. The server sends an access denied HTTP response packet back to the client, but in the header indicates the authentication schemes that the server will support, in order of preference

5. The browser receives the 'access denied' packet, looks into the header to find what the authentication schemes supported by the server are, and matches them against what it would support

6. If the highest common level of authentication support provided by both the browser and the server is basic authentication, then the browser will pop up the dialog box asking the user for a user ID and password

7. The user keys in the user ID and password

8. The browser retries the request packet, this time including the desired authentication method, the user ID, and the base 64-encoded (totally unsecured) password in the header

9. The server receives the request packet with authentication information, impersonates the client if authentication is successful, and accesses the protected resource on behalf of the remote user

10. If the server can access the requested resource under impersonation, it sends the content of the requested resource back to the browser which promptly displays it

We should notice a few distinguishing points about the above scenario:

❑ Nothing about it is specific to Microsoft or ActiveX: the situation can be handled with any browser supporting basic authentication, and any server running on any operating system which supports authentication capabilities

❏ If the user were to access a series of protected pages, the above scenario might repeat itself, asking the user to repeatedly enter his or her user ID and password (although some form of caching, by the browser, of the most recently used user ID/password can eliminate this).

❏ The password of the user is sent over the wire with minimal encoding, leaving it vulnerable to interception

The form of authentication detailed above is called **basic authentication** and is the most widely used form over the Internet, since most combinations of browser, web server and operating system will support it.

Internet Explorer with IIS over an Intranet

Now let's switch some details of the previous scenario. We're on a private intranet that is controlled under one Windows NT domain (we'll cover Windows NT security in the next section). In this case, an IIS 4 server is running on a departmental server machine and is accessed from a Windows 98 client, logged on as an Accounting department user, and running Internet Explorer 4.

The first three steps are exactly the same as the above example. Picking up from step 4 above, we now have a greatly improved situation:

4. The server sends an access denied HTTP response packet back to the client, but in the header indicates the authentication schemes that the server will support, in order of preference. At the top of the list is NTLM challenge/response authentication. (NTLM stands for NT LAN Manager, and is discussed in the section on basic NT security.)

5. IE 4 receives the 'access denied' packet, looks into the header to find the authentication schemes supported by the server, and matches them against what it would support. It supports the NTLM challenge/response authentication.

6. IE 4 will actually initiate the challenge/response authentication process by informing the NTLM Security Support Provider (NTLMSSP, also discussed in a later section). The user will not be asked for the user ID and password, because IE 4 can cause the local user logon details to be passed to NTLMSSP (the user ID and password is cached by the system, as long as the user remains logged on).

7. NTLM-based challenge/response authentication takes place over the network across the two nodes using a proprietary (non-HTTP) protocol. See the next section for details of how NTLM challenge/response works.

8. The challenge/response sequence terminates with the server impersonating the client, if authentication is successful, and retries the access to the protected resource on behalf of the remote user (under impersonation).

9. If the user has permission to access the requested resource, the server sends the content of the requested resource back to the browser, which promptly displays it.

Note the great improvements of this scenario over the previous one:

❏ The password of the user is never transmitted over the network; there's no risk of password capture.

❑ The user is never prompted for user ID and password. To the user, the protected web pages were accessible just like unprotected pages.

This improvement certainly makes intranet surfing (and intranet resource access control) much simpler to manage. However, there's one potential drawback: everything, from the desktop OS to the network OS, from the desktop browser to the web server, is from Microsoft.

Internet Explorer with IIS over the Internet

Finally, let's take a look at a situation similar to the one described above, but taking place over the Internet instead. Here, we still have everything from Microsoft. However, since the user logged on is authorized against a domain that's separate and unconnected from the server machine, one can't enjoy the cached user ID and password capability.

In this case, the IE 4 and IIS combination will still try the NTLM challenge/response sequence first, using the cached user ID and password at the client end. This attempt will fail, however, because the user is unknown to the server domain. IE 4 will then pop up a dialog box prompting the user for an ID and password. Next, it will reattempt the NTLM challenge/response authentication using this new set of user ID and password.

Since the user will enter a user ID and password that can be authenticated in the IIS's domain, this will succeed, and the server will reply with the protected data (after passing access control checks). From this point on, if the server requests any further authentication, IE 4 will use the user-entered user ID and password to authenticate the request.

The end result is somewhere between the transparent, all-Microsoft intranet situation, and the any browser/any server situation:

❑ The user's password is never transmitted over the wire
❑ The user only has to enter his or her user ID and password once for the entire session, accessing multiple protected objects

Best Method for Secured Intranet

We can see from this that there is a range of ways in which a web browser and server combination could react in a secured environment. It's interesting to observe that a fully homogeneous Microsoft installation in the intranet scenario can make security control completely transparent to the end user. This is obviously done by design rather than by accident, and is often a consideration when IS departments consider new intranet implementations.

Basic Windows NT Security

Before bravely diving into the specifics of DCOM, MTS, and MSMQ security, it's essential that we give a brief coverage to basic Windows NT security. This is the security framework upon which all DCOM and application services security implementations are built. An understanding of the basic framework will go a long way in ensuring that our later discussions can proceed without hindrance.

The Security Model

The security model prescribed by the Windows platform is a client-server one. The model is pervasive in that a network need not be involved; we could be talking about client and server processes running on the same machine. In this situation, the partitioning is between the application space that the client is running in and the (usually) kernel mode protected space that the server is running in.

Under this model, clients should only access objects through servers, and they should never access objects directly. This means that access to files, devices, other servers, and so on must be arbitrated and 'passed through' by an intermediary server.

Servers, on the other hand, must manage the access to an object and enforce access control. This can be done by the server with assistance from the operating system, or the server may decide to 'roll its own' access control mechanism. Specifically, under Windows NT, servers typically don't actually maintain and verify access rights directly. To make life simpler (and more secure) for server writers, servers impersonate the identity of the client and attempt access to objects under such impersonation. In this way, unauthorized access would be prevented by the operating system without the server maintaining elaborate access verification schemes.

Windows NT provides such an impersonation capability for server applications through Win32 APIs.

The Elements of Security: Domains, Users, SIDs, And Security Descriptors

From the operating system point of view, everything creatable on Windows NT is securable. By 'creatable' we mean any object (excuse our overloaded usage of the word object again) that either the system can create or the programmer may create using programmatic means. This includes the standard files and devices, processes, threads, and even more mundane things like semaphores, shared memory or a registry key. By 'securable' we mean that specific access rights can be associated with the object, and those rights can be verified by the OS when it is accessed.

The implementation for such security handling is buried deep in the kernel space. Essentially, every new object created gets a handle, which can have a **security descriptor** associated with it. We'll talk about the composition of this security descriptor shortly.

Domains

A **domain** is an administrative grouping of networked machines, together with all the users and resources associated with those machines. The **domain controller** machine stores and authenticates all users in the domain for network resource access. This means that the user and password database is stored and managed by the domain controller. The domain implementation in Windows NT allows for a **Primary Domain Controller** (**PDC**) and a **Backup Domain Controller** (**BDC**). The BDC sits on the network and gets a replication of all modifications and changes to the PDC. If and when the PDC should go out of commission, the BDC can take over in the place of the PDC, ensuring continued network operation. Note that it isn't currently possible to perform any administrative operations on the BDC while the PDC is still alive and operating (multi-master replication of the Active Directory in Windows NT 5 will make this possible).

For properly secured operations, every machine within a domain should authenticate user IDs and passwords against its domain controller.

For every large installation, it's possible to organize multiple domains in one or more 'trusted relationships'. This basically allows all users in one domain to access resources on another, provided that they have the requisite access rights. Operationally, a domain controller will authenticate a user against a trusted domain, should it fail to authenticate the user locally. This gives a degree of separation between the functions of user-account administration and shared resource management.

Authentication Authority

Each and every time a user on a secured Windows network is authenticated, three pieces of information are required: the authentication authority (the domain that the user belongs to), the user ID and the password.

For example:

UserID: WRXDOMAIN\JULIAN
Password: xyzzy

This indicates that the authentication authority is the domain controller of WRXDOMAIN, the user ID is JULIAN, and the password is xyzzy.

If the authentication authority isn't explicitly named, it will always default to the local authentication authority, which is the local registration database on a non-domain controller Windows machine, and the domain registration database on a domain controller machine.

Users and Groups

To make administration and assignments of access rights somewhat easier, Windows NT Server-based networking allows the assignment of users to groups. A user is considered to be a 'member' of a group if the group is defined to be containing the user. Access rights can then be assigned to the object, allowing or denying access to a group instead of spelling out all its members.

Groups that contain only users from a single domain are called **global groups**; these groups are assigned and tracked on the domain controller. Groups that are administered local to a machine are called **local groups** and can contain users on the local machine, users from trusted domains, or global groups.

Security Identifier

Each user on a secured Windows network has an account, which contains information such as:

❑ password
❑ groups that the user belongs to
❑ profile-specific items
❑ hours allowed to logon

It also contains something called a **Security ID** (or **SID**). A SID uniquely identifies the user in both space and time. What this means is that no two SIDs will ever be the same, due to the generation algorithm. It contains information which can be used to uniquely locate the user's account information on a registration database. Note that a group can also have its own SID.

Security Descriptors

Earlier, you may remember that we said that every elementary operating system object created by the OS (either by itself or on behalf of the user) can be associated with a security descriptor. This descriptor contains the following important pieces:

Information Contained	Description
Owner	Owner of the object, qualified by authentication authority
Group	Group that the owner belongs to, qualified by authentication authority
Discretionary Access Control List (DACL)	A set of access rights set by owner or administrator
System Access Control List (SACL)	A set of access rights set by the system for system operations

The **discretionary access control list**, or **DACL**, can be used specifically either to allow or deny access to the object by certain user and/or groups. The OS provides set and query operations to this descriptor. It also provides APIs to assist in manipulation of access lists, perform access checking, or assist in generating operating system based audits.

Let's take a look now at access control lists.

Access Control Lists

An access control list consists of zero or more **Access Control Entries** (**ACEs**). Each ACE will contain the following information:

❑   The type of entry – either an ACCESS_ALLOWED_ACE_TYPE or an ACCESS_DENIED_ACE_TYPE

❑   The access rights to control (read, write, delete, etc.)

❑   The user or group (global or local) as represented by its SID

The access control list within a security descriptor that can be changed programmatically by applications or users is called the discretionary access control list (DACL). All security descriptors and their associated ACLs are stored in compact binary form.

> Note that an object which has a security descriptor with a DACL containing no ACEs is deemed to be explicitly inaccessible to everyone, while an object that has a security descriptor with no DACL (i.e. set to NULL) is accessible by everyone.

Historically, programmatic modification of ACLs was a very complex procedure, which required painstakingly careful coding (and testing, since you can easily lock up a machine or a domain with faulty ACL modification code). Windows NT 4.0 Service Pack 2 (and later) has fixed this problem through the implementation of a well-tested body of code, which takes the form of a reusable COM based software component! This provides an interface called `IAccessControl`, which ActiveX/COM programmers can readily reuse in situations requiring modifications to ACLs. The `IAccessControl` interface is well documented in Visual Studio 6 MSDN, and is quite straightforward to use.

Security Access Tokens

ACLs are associated with static objects such as files, devices and users. Dynamic objects in the operating system (things that come and go relatively quickly), such as processes and threads, have associated with them something called a **security access token**. It's this security access token that enables a server to impersonate a client after authentication. The security access token contains the following very important information:

- ❏ The user SID, used for matching against ACLs
- ❏ The SID of the groups that the user belongs to, used for matching against ACLs
- ❏ The default ACL for creating new objects
- ❏ Default owner SID for creating new objects
- ❏ Special token privileges, such as reboot, settime, logout, etc. These are used in very special cases only

Since it's always servers (or more precisely, threads within a server process) which actually access protected resources, it's important that threads can carry with them a context for security. The security access token is such a context.

By switching security access tokens, a thread of execution can assume an alternative personality – it impersonates others. A security access token used for impersonation is sometimes called an **impersonation token**. The same thread can later revert to its original identity by switching back to the base process's security access token.

Client Credential

Client credential refers to the set of user ID and password information maintained by a server on behalf of a calling client. This is often required, in addition to an impersonation token, to access networked resources on other networked nodes.

SSPI and NTLMSSP Authentication

So far, we've talked about authentication as if it just magically happens between the client seeking authentication and the server performing the authentication. If the client simply sends the textual user ID and password over the network to the server, the system can't be totally secure, because other nodes on the network can easily capture the user ID and password, and wreak havoc on the server with this information.

Since so much of the Windows security implementation rests on dependably robust and secure authentication, the simple scenario described above can't be relied upon for proper authentication.

Instead, Microsoft has designed an elaborate architecture for handling authentication. This architecture allows the actual method of authentication to be abstracted away from the user of the authentication service. As a side benefit, it allows arbitrary extensibility through the 'plug-in' of new authentication providers. This architecture is frequently referred to as the **Security Service Provider Interface** (**SSPI**).

The following diagram shows how the SSPI fits in with the rest of the security implementation:

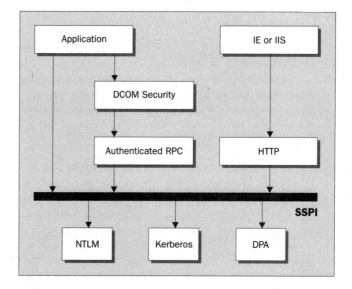

This architecture clearly separates the user of the security services from the provider of the services, and allows newer service providers to 'plug-in', and function with, an existing application using the SSPI services.

While the architecture is indeed elegant, the only easily usable default security provider for Windows NT 4 is the NT Lan Manager Security Support Provider (or NTLMSSP). As a bonus, the client portion of the NTLMSSP is also implemented on Windows 98/95, which means that Windows 98/95 client workstations can participate in the network.

Since this is all we've got today, it is worthwhile understanding how NTLM works. The key element here is that the user's password is never transmitted across the wire during authentication. This proves to be both NTLM's strong point (for security) and its weakness. We'll cover the weakness part later, but first let's see how this works. When a client application supplies the authentication authority (domain), user ID, and password triplet to the client portion of the NTLMSSP, the following things happen:

1. The client NTLMSSP sends the domain, user ID and machine information to the server NTLMSSP

2. The server NTLMSSP uses this information to generate a unique challenge sequence (of binary bits)

3. The client NTLMSSP receives this sequence and encrypts it using the user's password as a key – this forms the response

4. The client NTLMSSP sends the encrypted response to the server NTLMSSP

5. The server NTLMSSP calls the authentication authority with the user ID, the challenge sequence and the response sequence

6. The authentication authority uses the password associated with the user ID to encrypt the challenge sequence and verify it against the response sequence, authenticating the user in the process

7. If successful, the authentication is completed, and the server NTLMSSP will allow the server to impersonate the client

So far so good – only an encrypted response is sent across the wire, but not the actual password. However, since the server actually never receives the password, it will have no way of using the password to access other resources that the user would have access to. Specifically, these may be other networked servers (in a three-tiered or n-tiered client/server system) that the user would normally be able to access. This is one weakness of NTLMSSP, significantly reducing the number of possible tasks that the server can perform on behalf of the client.

A Kerberos security provider will be available with Windows NT 5. It is based on a mature public standard, called MIT Kerberos V5, which originated from MIT and has been endorsed by the Internet Engineering Task Force for interoperability. This new security provider is expected to provide improved performance, scalability and flexibility over the NTLM implementation. Most important of all, it will eliminate the problem with the NTLM provider described above.

NTFS

The format of the NT File System (NTFS), although not new, is an essential piece of the Windows NT security jigsaw. While NT supports alternative file format for hard disk, such as FAT and HPFS, one must make use of NTFS to enable a fully secured system. Besides offering higher performance and less fragmentation with large disks, it is the only NT-supported disk format which allows ACLs to be associated and stored with files and folders. This capability is vital to the proper operation of a secured Windows network.

As a bonus, NTFS also supports optional journalization of all disk transactions (i.e. a record of all disk-changing transactions is kept), allowing the file system to be totally recovered in the event of a disk failure.

Authenticated RPC

Take a careful look at the diagram from the previous section, and you'll notice a box called 'Authenticated RPC' under the 'DCOM Security' box. This implies that authenticated RPC, whatever this might be, is the foundation upon which DCOM security is built. It would be wise, then, for us to take a look at what authenticated RPC is about.

> You'll frequently see **Secure RPC** mentioned as well. Both terms actually refer to basically the same thing.

DCOM (or COM for that matter) is based on RPC (or LRPC) as the interprocess communications mechanism. RPC can operate over a variety of network transports, including TCP/IP, IPX and named pipes. The named pipe protocol provided authenticated connections across networks long before the arrival of RPC. Unfortunately, other TCP/IP or IPX based protocols don't offer this authentication feature.

By building-in code which will call the SSPI services and bundle additional security information 'on-the-wire' in the runtime implementation of RPC, Microsoft has created authenticated RPC which can operate over all transports supported by the raw RPC implementation.

This can be viewed as a layer of software on top of RPC, which provides a secured channel for intermachine procedure calls (but since it's implemented in the RPC runtime code, it can be treated just as a variant of RPC). The specification for Secure RPC has five levels of security:

Security Level	Description
NONE (1)	This is regular RPC with no security ramifications
CONNECT (2)	Authenticate the client connection during the connection phase (when the initial TCP/IP socket is established under TCP/IP)
CALL (3)	Authenticate the request for each and every interface call
INTEGRITY (4)	Authenticate and verify that the request packets received have not been modified
PRIVACY (5)	Perform all of the above *and* encrypt the data packets for transmission along the wire

Obviously, level 5 security would be very CPU-intensive when performed on a packet level. For performance reasons, only the CONNECT level of security is implemented on Windows 98/95 clients. The symmetric nature of RPC connections requires both ends to be at the same security level. This means that most applications or software components must work on the CONNECT level of security, or below, if they are ever to accommodate Windows 98/95 clients.

From what we have seen so far, Windows NT appears to be far more secure than Windows 98/95. We have always been saying '...but Windows 98/95 cannot do this...' or '...except for Windows 98/95...'. Is Windows 98/95 really a security 'wimp'? You bet your CDROMs! Let's take a good look at what's missing.

Windows NT versus Windows 98/95

It's important to realize that Windows 98/95 plays a purely 'client' role in the overall Windows network security picture. This was necessary to fulfill several other non-security related objectives in the design of Windows98/95:

- ❑ To be 100% compatible with 16-bit Windows 3.1 applications
- ❑ To require a very small memory and disk footprint, lowering the cost of platforms required to run it
- ❑ To run with excellent performance even in low-end processors and configurations
- ❑ To be easy to configure and use

Unfortunately, every one of these objectives runs against the goals and requirements of a fully secured system. And this is aside from the fact that the heritage evolution for Windows 98/95 (from DOS to Windows 3.1 to Windows 98/95) is one with a desktop focus, with little consideration for security.

Security Features in Windows 98/95

There are various provisions made in Windows 98/95 for it to be 'compatible' with Windows NT system APIs. What this means in practice is that applications that are written to be secure (using the various security APIs) will run without difficulty under Windows 98/95. However, almost all of these APIs don't actually perform a useful task, they simply call empty stubs that do nothing and let the application carry on with its chores.

The client side of all network based security measures is implemented, however. For example, a Windows 98/95 client can participate in authenticated RPC exchange with a server over any network transport (although secured RPC link with full encryption isn't yet supported). A Windows 98/95 machine can securely authenticate against a Windows NT domain controller, using the SSPI and the NTLM security provider, without transmitting the password over the wire. It's important to note, though, that such logons are valid only for further network based resource access (access through servers as per Windows security model). Access to local resources on the Windows 98/95 workstation does not conform to the Windows NT security model and is essentially unsecured.

The **Client for Microsoft Networks** component of Windows 98/95 enables something called **User Level Resource Sharing**. Sharing of resources (printers, directories, disk volumes, but not files) can be specified on a user-by-user basis, with custom permissions. The actual authentication of the user, in this case, will be performed by the authentication authority, such as a Windows NT domain controller.

What this means is that if all you ever do after logon is access network drives and interact with distributed remote software components on a secured server, then you'll be operating in a secured environment. If you start using the local disk on the Windows 98/95 workstation and working with locally executing applications, however, then there's no security protection.

In summary, Windows 98/95 is a secure client partner in the Windows security model, but it is not a secure desktop platform.

What Is Not There

Almost everything that makes Windows NT secure is missing from Windows 98/95.

System enforced secured access to system resources is nonexistent on Windows 98/95. Not only does it not support the NTFS securable file system, anyone with an access to a Windows 98/95 workstation can access all the files and data (and devices) residing on the workstation.

More specifically:

- No ACLs are maintained with system resources, files, etc. – nothing is protected by the OS
- User login and authentication is done via unsecured databases in either standalone or peer-to-peer configurations (when the system is not part of a Windows NT domain or the user does not logon using a domain qualified user ID)
- All processes running on an entire Windows 98/95 machine are considered to be in the context of the currently logged on user

❑ There's no documented way to run a process on a Windows 98/95 system with no current user logon (if you disable logon and/or press Cancel on the logon box, the 'default user' will own the current session)

❑ No hardware-enforced isolation between running processes, leaving system corruption as a definite possibility after an application crash (this is a major blow to the robustness requirement of any typical server platforms)

In any case, gaining physical access to a Windows 98/95 workstation means gaining complete access to all the data contained on that workstation. There are tricky ways of configuring Windows 98/95 so that it looks as though the system is secure, but there are a variety of methods to thwart all such attempts. This fact alone is driving many corporations to switch to its secured elder brother: the Windows NT Workstation operating system.

In fact, Windows NT Workstation is a fully-fledged Windows NT operating system, with full security implementation, but specially configured and tuned for interactive workstation operation (leaving out most server-specific functionality in order to maintain a smaller memory footprint, as well as creating a market differentiation).

What Is Possible

Just because the Windows 98/95 operating system doesn't enforce security on behalf of its applications doesn't mean that the operating system can't be used for secured computing. First, as a client accessing networked servers, Windows 98/95 has all the bells and whistles built in to maintain security. Second, it's possible to build a secure server infrastructure on top of the unsecured operating system, and implement what is missing from the underlying OS. (Indeed, some vendors have done so: WebSite Server from O'Reilly and FastTrack Server from Netscape).

Another nontrivial example of a security infrastructure implementation is Microsoft's own User Level Resource Sharing that we mentioned earlier. It provides an 'ACL-like' capability for controlling access to resources down to a directory level (not file level), but only when such resources are accessed through the Microsoft network client layer (not the OS kernel, as with Windows NT). This application-level security infrastructure is proprietary in implementation. In our discussions that follow, however, we'll view Windows 98/95 – without enhancement – as a capable secured client platform, but as an unsecured server platform.

DCOM Security

Now let's look at security issues which are specific to DCOM operations and programming.

We've seen in the *Authenticated RPC* section that the DCOM security implementation is based on authenticated RPC. Authenticated RPC uses the security support providers that are available through the Win32 Security Support Provider Interface (SSPI). At the time of writing, authenticated RPC uses the NTLMSSP exclusively.

Security can be configured externally, that is, without either the client or the server having to include security specific code. This is suitable for both legacy and simple COM applications. If the security needs of the application are more sophisticated, then a variety of functions and interfaces are available to both clients and servers to configure security programmatically, as we'll see shortly.

DCOM Security Blankets

The set of services and parameters that can be configured in order to specify the security settings for a DCOM component is called the **security blanket**. This is essentially a packaging of security parameters. By bundling security parameters in a package, the negotiation process between the client and the server can be made 'network efficient'. Instead of negotiating each parameter across the network with multiple round-trips, only a single round-trip is required to complete the negotiation. We'll see how this is possible in the next section.

The parameters contained in the security blanket are shown in the table below:

Parameter	Description
Authentication service	The SSPI to use for authentication, e.g. NTLM.
Authorization service	The authorization service to be used in order to check client access rights, e.g. DCE.
Server Principal Name	The user security context under which the COM server is running.
Authentication level	The degree to which the access to the object is authenticated to ensure the privacy of the communications over the connection. These are identical to the security levels of authenticated RPC.
Impersonation level	The degree to which the COM server is allowed to impersonate the client during execution. For example, it is possible to restrict the COM server so that it has only query rights to security information, and cannot actually impersonate the client.
Authentication identity	The identification of the client, as seen by the server. Usually a user name.

Security Blanket Negotiation

During a security blanket negotiation, the client supplies a security blanket, which indicates the maximum level of security that the client can support. When the server receives this security blanket, it matches it against what it would accept. The server decides the minimum level of security that it will accept. If the client's security blanket levels are all above those expected by the server, then the negotiation succeeds.

This approach reduces network traffic down to a single round trip. This low overhead allows security negotiation on a very fine-grain level – for example, it can be performed on a 'per remote interface instance' level.

DCOM Security Categories

The following security categories are important in DCOM:

Category	Description
Access security	Specifies which clients have the right to connect with a running object. Clients might not have the right to launch a server, but might be allowed to connect to one if it is already running.
Launch (activation) security	Specifies which clients can start the execution of the server process on the remote machine.
Call security	Allows for security blanket negotiation on a 'per interface instance' level. More precisely, it enables the client to set the security blanket for each server interface proxy object, which allows the server to check the security blanket per call, when it arrives.
	It is important to have call level security in DCOM. After a successful launch, the client might pass a remote interface pointer (actually a proxy) to another unauthorized client. If security isn't provided on a per call level, the system could be compromised.

Security Level Configuration

Let's see now how we can configure the system for launch and call security. These activities can be performed through the Dcomcnfg.exe tool that provides a user-friendly interface for modifying the corresponding registry entries. If, like me, editing ACLs in binary in the registry editor isn't your idea of fun, then Dcomcnfg is indispensable!

Launch Security

Launch security is automatically applied by the COM runtime whenever a server application is started up due to a remote object creation request. After the request has been received from a client, the COM runtime obtains all the necessary security parameters from the registry (if the creating process doesn't specify any security parameters).

There are two default activation settings in the registry that have machine-wide effect. They are both named values under the same key.

```
HKEY_LOCAL_MACHINE\Software\Microsoft\OLE
   EnableDCOM = <value>
```

The value is a string (REG_SZ) and can be a Y or an N. A value of Y enables remote activation of COM servers on this machine, and any other value disables it. Even when remote activation is disabled, local activation is still allowed. It is governed by the specific permissions in the LaunchPermission key of each class and the default settings in the DefaultLaunchPermission key.

```
HKEY_LOCAL_MACHINE\Software\Microsoft\OLE
    DefaultLaunchPermission = <value>
```

The DefaultLaunchPermission value is of type REG_BINARY and consists of a binary ACL of the principals (accounts or groups) that can launch COM servers on this system. The value can be overridden by specifying a LaunchPermission value in the registry for a particular COM object. By default, the following principals are given 'allow launch' permissions:

- ❑ Administrators – the administrator group
- ❑ System – the local system-privileged account
- ❑ Interactive – corresponding to the user currently logged on at the console

On a per-class basis, security configuration settings are stored as a set of named values under the following key:

```
HKEY_LOCAL_MACHINE\Software\Classes\AppID\{AppID_value}\<named_value> = <value>
```

For a class, the AppID_value is a GUID that appears, as a string, under the AppID named value which is under the CLSID key of the class. The string {AppID_value} is used as a subkey under ...\Classes\AppID.

For an executable, the AppID_value is the name of the module (e.g. myapp.exe). Under the {myapp.exe} key there's a REG_SZ named value AppID with the AppID associated with the executable.

The launch permissions are set in the named value LaunchPermission. The type and content of the value is the same as in the DefaultLaunchPermission. Other named values under the same key are:

- ❑ AccessPermission – specifies permissions to access running instances of the class. It's used only if the client doesn't call CoInitializeSecurity()
- ❑ RunAs – specifies that the server should run with the security context of the specified user.
- ❑ LocalService – specifies that the server is a Windows NT service.
- ❑ ServiceParameters – specifies the parameters to be passed to the service on invocation.
- ❑ RemoteServerName – specifies the remote machine on which the server will be activated by default provided that the client hasn't programmatically requested otherwise (by specifying, for example, a COSERVERINFO parameter to CoCreateInstanceEx()).

You can change the default settings through the Dcomcnfg utility, so let's take a look at that now. You can start Dcomcnfg.exe located in your \windows\system or \winnt\system32 directory. If you go to the **Default Security** tab, you can edit the default launch permissions:

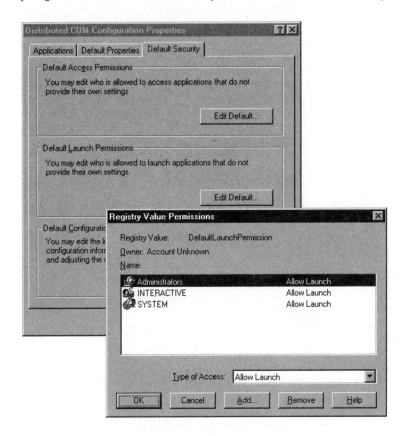

The procedure is similar for setting the security parameters of a specific application. You can find these under the Applications tab:

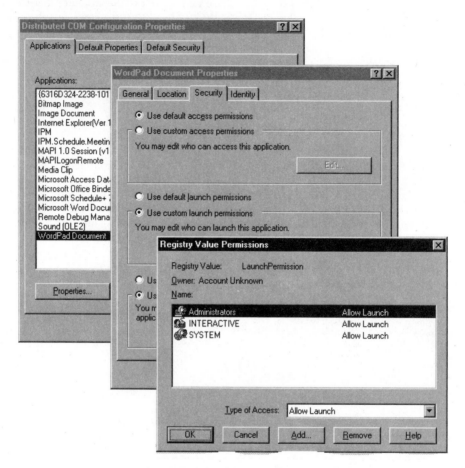

Other than configuring DCOM security parameters through registry editing, it's also possible to have fine-grain control over these parameters using programmatic means. Let's take some time now to examine some of the Win32 APIs and COM object interfaces associated with DCOM security control.

DCOM Security API

The CoCreateInstanceEx() call can be used to create COM servers, just like the CoCreateInstance() call. We have seen this API in action back in Chapter 8. However, it has one additional parameter, COSERVERINFO, which is quite interesting. The COSERVERINFO parameter allows us to specify a remote machine on which to create the new instance. The support for multiple QueryInterface() calls in a single round-trip keeps everything fast and efficient.

CoCreateInstanceEx() and Client Security Blanket

If we take a look at the COSERVERINFO structure, there's a member of the structure that we didn't cover at any length in our earlier examination. It was the COAUTHINFO structure, which is the actual client security blanket.

```
typedef struct _COSERVERINFO
{
    DWORD         dwReserverd1;
    LPWSTR        pwszName;
    COAUTHINFO*   pAuthInfo;
    DWORD         dwReserved2;
} COSERVERINFO;
```

pAuthInfo is the security blanket which gets passed through the COM runtime to the server for negotiation. Setting this to NULL will force the COM runtime to use the application default (registry values under the AppID entry at HKLM\SOFTWARE\Classes\AppID\{}) or the system default values for authentication settings (i.e. NTLMSSP will be used, with the client's identity). You may find it quite instructive to look at the details of the COAUTHINFO structure, since some fields are identical to the ones for the CoInitializeSecurity() call that we'll be covering later. You can find this definition in Wtypes.h:

```
typedef struct  _COAUTHINFO
{
    DWORD               dwAuthnSvc;
    DWORD               dwAuthzSvc;
    LPWSTR              pwszServerPrincName;
    DWORD               dwAuthnLevel;
    DWORD               dwImpersonationLevel;
    COAUTHIDENTITY *    pAuthIdentityData;
    DWORD               dwCapabilities;
} COAUTHINFO;
```

dwAuthnSvc signifies the authentication service. It's a value from the enumeration RPC_C_AUTHN_xxx:

dwAuthnSvc **Value**	**Description**
RPC_C_AUTHN_DCE_PRIVATE	Distributed Computing Environment (DCE) private key authentication.
RPC_C_AUTHN_DCE_PUBLIC	DCE public key authentication.
RPC_C_AUTHN_DEC_PUBLIC	DEC public key authentication.
RPC_C_AUTHN_DEFAULT	A (planned to be supported) value for Windows NT 5. This value enables the security blanket negotiation process between the client and server to select the best authentication service.
RPC_C_AUTHN_WINNT	The NTLM Security Support Provider. This is the only supported authentication service for Windows NT 4.

dwAuthnSvc **Value**	Description
RPC_C_AUTHN_NONE	No authentication.
RPC_C_AUTHN_GSS_KERBEROS, RPC_C_AUTHN_GSS_NEGOTIATE, RPC_C_AUTHN_GSS_SCHANNEL, RPC_C_AUTHN_DPA, RPC_C_AUTHN_MSN, RPC_C_AUTHN_MQ	Other possible values for this enumeration, selecting other security support providers. Many of these new providers are scheduled to be available with Windows NT 5.

dwAuthzSvc signifies the authorization service. In other words, this indicates what the server should use in order to check the access rights it should have on behalf of the client. The values are from the RPC_C_AUTHZ_xxx enumeration:

dwAuthzSvr **Value**	Description
RPC_C_AUTHZ_NONE	Server performs no authorization.
RPC_C_AUTHZ_NAME	Server performs authorization using the client's name.
RPC_C_AUTHZ_DCE	Server performs authorization using the client's DCE privileges.
RPC_C_AUTHZ_DEFAULT	A (planned to be supported) value for Windows NT 5. This enables the security blanket negotiation process between the client and the server to select an authorization service.

The pwszServerPrincName member of the COAUTHINFO structure points to a wide character string, which indicates the principal name to use on the server with the authentication name. If the service chosen is RPC_C_AUTHN_WINNT, the value should be NULL.

dwAuthnLevel specifies the level of authentication required, ranging from once when connecting, to packet-level authentication and encryption. It takes a value from RPC_C_AUTHN_LEVEL_XXX:

dwAuthnLevel **Value**	Meaning
RPC_C_AUTHN_LEVEL_NONE	No authentication.
RPC_C_AUTHN_LEVEL_CONNECT	Authenticates only when a client establishes a connection.
RPC_C_AUTHN_LEVEL_CALL	Authenticates at the beginning of each remote procedure call.
RPC_C_AUTHN_LEVEL_PKT	Authenticates origin of all data. Used by datagram transports.

Table Continued on Following Page

dwAuthnLevel **Value**	Meaning
RPC_C_AUTHN_LEVEL_PKT_INTEGRITY	Authenticates origin and integrity of data.
RPC_C_AUTHN_LEVEL_PKT_PRIVACY	Authenticates origin and integrity of data, and encrypts remote procedure call arguments.
RPC_C_AUTHN_LEVEL_DEFAULT	It is equivalent to RPC_C_AUTHN_LEVEL_CONNECT in Windows NT 4. Under Windows NT 5, this will be used to let the security blanket negotiation process, between the client and the server, to select the authentication level.

dwImpersonationLevel specifies the impersonation level. It corresponds to the levels of impersonation specified in NT 4.0, which are shown in the table below:

dwImpersonationLevel **Value**	Meaning
RPC_C_IMP_LEVEL_ANONYMOUS	The server doesn't get any information about the client identification and doesn't attempt to impersonate the client. This value is not supported by Windows NT 4.
RPC_C_IMP_LEVEL_IDENTIFY	The server can get security information about the client – for example, security identifiers and privileges – but it can't impersonate the client. The significance of this is that the server can make decisions about whether the client has the right to access resources. However, it can't use system resources or access objects 'as the client'. This is supported by Windows NT 4, but is buggy. See MSDN documentation for more details.
RPC_C_IMP_LEVEL_IMPERSONATE	The server can impersonate the client's security context. Note that this is valid *only* on the server's local systems and it is *not* supported on remote systems. In other words, the server can't access resources over the network as if it were the client. This is the only level reliably supported by Windows NT 4.
RPC_C_IMP_LEVEL_DELEGATE	This level allows the server to impersonate the client over a network across two or more nodes. It isn't currently supported by the default SSP (NTLM) on NT 4. It will, however, be supported by the Kerberos SSP, which will be the default for Windows NT 5.

dwImpersonationLevel **Value**	**Meaning**
RPC_C_IMP_LEVEL_DEFAULT	A (planned to be supported) value for Windows NT 5. This enables the security blanket negotiation process between the client and the server to select an acceptable impersonation level.

Finally, the pAuthIdentityData member of the COAUTHINFO structure is specific to the authentication service, and is usually left as NULL. dwCapabilities provides for extra capabilities which are yet to be defined. It must be set to EOAC_NONE.

The CoIntializeSecurity() Call

If the client or server calls CoInitializeSecurity(), the default security blanket for the process is set. This only needs to be called once per process. If a DCOM client or server doesn't call CoInitializeSecurity(), the COM runtime will use the configured default security blanket in the registry. The call is typically made immediately after a call to CoInitializeEx(). The CoInitializeSecurity() settings can be overridden on a per-class basis by setting the COSERVERINFO parameter in a call to CoCreateInstanceEx().

Let's examine the calling syntax of the CoInitializeSecurity() API:

```
HRESULT CoInitializeSecurity( PSECURITY_DESCRIPTOR pVoid,
                              LONG cAuthSvc,
                              SOLE_AUTHENTICATION_SERVICE* asAuthSvc,
                              void* pReserved1,
                              DWORD dwAuthnLevel,
                              DWORD dwImpLevel,
                              SOLE_AUTHENTICATION_LIST * pAuthList,
                              DWORD dwCapabilities,
                              void* pReserved3 );
```

The parameters for this function are shown in the table below:

Parameter	Description
pVoid	If this is NULL, then all callers are allowed to communicate with the process. Otherwise it specifies those principals that are allowed to communicate with the process and those that are not.
cAuthSvc	This is the size of the array asAuthSvc. If 0 is passed, no authentication service is registered. 1 tells COM to choose for itself which service to use.

Table Continued on Following Page

Parameter	Description
asAuthSvc	Specifies an array of structures, each containing a principal name as well as an authentication and authorization service ID. These are the initial values used. The actual services to be used for each connection are negotiated and may be different.
dwAuthnLevel	Default authentication level for proxies. The available values are as in the CoCreateInstanceEx() call.
dwImpLevel	Default impersonation level for proxies. The available values are the same as those in the CoCreateInstanceEx() call.
pAuthList	Must be NULL on Windows NT 4. It is reserved for specifying the default authentication information in Windows NT 5.
dwCapabilities	Flag value from the EOLE_AUTHENTICATION_CAPABILITIES enumeration. Specifies additional capabilities of the client or server. See MSDN for more details on the allowed values. Typically EOAC_NONE under Windows NT 4.

IClientSecurity for Call Security Control

If the client calls CoInitializeSecurity(), the security values for authentication and authorization for the process are set. If a fine-grain security control is required on the calls to individual interfaces, the client can achieve this by invoking security functions on each of the interface proxies. The main security interface to achieve this on the client side is IClientSecurity. You can obtain a pointer to this interface by doing a QueryInterface() for IID_IClientSecurity on an interface from the remote object. In reality, every remote object method invocation goes through a proxy, managed by a proxy manager (which actually aggregates the proxy object). The diagram below shows a remote interface called IRemoteItf. This means that it is the proxy manager that intercepts and provides this IClientSecurity interface:

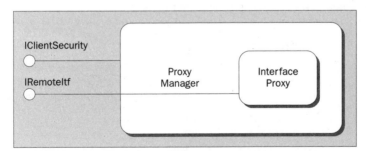

Once the IClientSecurity interface is obtained, the client can change the security blanket for this single proxy instance by using two method calls on this interface. First, it creates a new instance of the proxy using the IClientSecurity::CopyProxy() method, and then alters the blanket using IClientSecurity::SetBlanket(). It's important to make a copy of the proxy first, in order to avoid contention with other portions of the process that may be setting the security blanket to other values. We will have more to say on this in the next section.

There are wrapper functions available which call the `IClientSecurity` methods. These include:

- ❑ `CoSetProxyBlanket()` — sets a new security blanket on a proxy
- ❑ `CoQueryProxyBlanket()` — inquires about the existing security blanket on a proxy
- ❑ `CoCopyProxy()` — obtains a proxy copy on which a security blanket can be set without contention

Client-Side Proxy Copying

Occasionally, a client may want to ensure that a specific security blanket is set on a particular interface proxy instance when the blanket is presented to the server for security negotiation. Directly changing the security blanket on the default proxy (returned by the initial `QueryInterface()` call) will affect all other users of the proxy, who may have different security requirements. The way out of this predicament is to make a private copy of the proxy (with a call to `CoCopyProxy()`), on which to set the desired security blanket.

> **You should beware when making a copy of the proxy, because a `QueryInterface()` on a proxy copy will return a pointer to an interface on the original proxy, with the original's security blanket.**

The `CoCopyProxy()` function encapsulates several steps. First, it does a `QueryInterface()` on the original proxy for `IID_IClientSecurity`, then invokes `IClientSecurity::CopyProxy()` on this interface before finally releasing it.

```
HRESULT CoCopyProxy(IUnknown* pProxy,    // original
                    IUnknown** ppCopy );  // pointer to copy pointer
```

The client can now set the security blanket on the proxy copy obtained from the above function by calling `CoSetProxyBlanket()`:

```
IUnknown pCopy;      // copy proxy

CoCopyProxy(pProxy, &pCopy );
CoSetProxyBlanket(pCopy,
        RPC_C_AUTHN_WINNT,
        RPC_C_AUTHZ_NONE,
        L"HOST",
        RPC_C_AUTHN_LEVEL_CONNECT,
        RPC_C_IMP_LEVEL_IMPERSONATE,
        NULL,
        0);
// use the proxy
...
pCopy->Release();
```

Here's the exact declaration:

```
HRESULT CoSetProxyBlanket( IUnknown* pProxy,
                           DWORD dwAuthnSvc,
                           DWORD dwAuthzSvc,
                           OLECHAR* pServerPrincName,
                           DWORD dwAuthnLevel,
                           DWORD dwImpLevel,
                           RPC_AUTH_IDENTITY_HANDLE* pAuthInfo,
                           DWORD dwCapabilities );
```

We've seen most of the arguments before, and they are summarized in the table below:

Parameter	Description
pProxy	Pointer to a copy proxy on which this blanket will be set.
dwAuthnSvc	An RPC_C_AUTHN_xxx value.
dwAuthzSvc	An RPC_C_AUTHZ_xxx value.
pServerPrincName	A wide character string with server's principal name to be used for authentication.
dwAuthnLevel	An RPC_C_AUTHN_LEVEL_xxx value.
dwImpLevel	An RPC_C_IMP_LEVEL_xxx value.
pAuthInfo	Authentication service specific. NULL for default.
dwCapabilities	Extra capabilities for the proxy – a flag built from the EOLE_AUTHENTICATION_CAPABILITIES enumeration; set this to EOAC_NONE for Windows NT 4.

Working with IServerSecurity

On the server side, the server needs to obtain the parameters contained in the client's security blanket for the interface being used and perform manipulation based on these parameters (such as impersonating the client). The main interface for this purpose is the IServerSecurity. This also provides control over the security level while the server is executing on behalf of the client.

IServerSecurity Interface

The server obtains the IServerSecurity interface by invoking CoGetCallContext(). This is the easiest way for the server to work with successfully negotiated security parameters from the client.

```
IServerSecurity*   pSS;
CoGetCallContext(IID_IServerSecurity, (void **)&pSS);
```

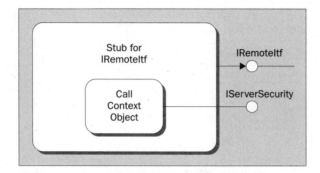

Once the `IServerSecurity` interface is obtained, the server has the option to:

- Get specific security level information from the blanket by making the `IServerSecurity::QueryBlanket()` method call
- Impersonate the client's security level and identification while carrying out resource access by calling `IServerSecurity::ImpersonateClient()` and `IServerSecurity::RevertToSelf()`
- Determine if the server thread is currently impersonating the client using `IServerSecurity::IsImpersonating()`

As with the `IClientSecurity` interface, there are wrapper APIs to make the use of the `IServerSecurity` interface somewhat simpler. These include:

- `CoQueryClientBlanket()`
- `CoImpersonateClient()`
- `CoRevertToSelf()`

A call to `CoQueryClientBlanket()` enables the server to get more information on the security blanket from the client:

```
HRESULT CoQueryClientBlanket( DWORD* pAuthnSvc,
                              DWORD* pAuthzSvc,
                              OLECHAR** pServerPrincName,
                              DWORD* pAuthnLevel,
                              DWORD* pImpLevel,
                              RPC_AUTHZ_HANDLE* pPrivs,
                              DWORD* pCapabilities );
```

One of the interesting new fields here is the `pPrivs` (the type is really a `void**`), which is set to point to a Unicode string identifying the client. The caller must not modify the string in any way. The default NTLMSSP will return a `Domain\\User` value.

In order to access resources with the client's security context, the server can impersonate the client of this call and then revert to its own security context when done. You can use the wrapper functions for the `IServerSecurity` interface for this:

```
CoImpersonateClient();
//access resources
...
CoRevertToSelf();
```

MTS Security

Unlike DCOM, MTS is, architecturally, a higher level NT application service. In theory, such a service can choose to expose whatever security model it wishes to extensions running within the service. For MTS, of course, these architectural service extensions are the very MTS components that we are now familiar with. MTS security evolves around providing access control to objects that the component based MTS server application manages. It is also the aim of the MTS security implementation to make it easy to plan, implement, and maintain application specific security schemes.

MTS Components as Service Extensions

MTS as an NT service must abide by the Windows NT security model. To refresh our memory, the model specifies:

- ❑ clients access objects (files, devices, other servers) only through servers
- ❑ servers enforce access control to objects
- ❑ servers should impersonate clients before accessing resources

At the same time, MTS's security enforcement operations are meant to be transparent to both clients and writers of components. The client thinks that it is using a regular DCOM component. To fulfill this requirement, MTS exposes the same Windows NT security model to the writer of MTS components. This will also allow MTS to one day disappear into the OS, and become a part of the basic system services, without requiring the rewrite of components or client applications. This is illustrated by the diagram below.

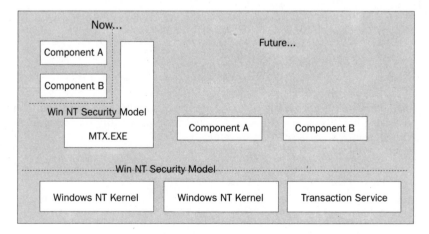

The designers of MTS have worked very hard to make the life of server components easy by performing all the tough work. We saw this back in Chapter 9. When it comes to the matter of security, MTS has added major value by taking the complexity out of the equation. MTS provides a higher level model of security management that is simpler to understand and implement, but is fully compliant and compatible with the underlying NT security model.

This value-added model is a role-based security model. In addition, MTS also allows security to be implemented and managed declaratively (as opposed to programmatically). Here is a summary of the possible security implementations with MTS:

Security Implementation	Comments
Declarative Role Based	Simplest to plan, manage, and maintain. Should use this whenever possible with an application.
Programmatic Role Based	Next best choice to pure declarative role based – many business components will require this.
Programmatic DCOM Based	Best to avoid since it does not take advantage of the MTS security implementation at all.

Role Based Security

MTS provides a role based security model that is consistent with the underlying Windows NT security model. Here is a simple synopsis:

1. The developer defines a set of roles for a package, typically representing real-world groupings of users with differing security requirements (for example: executives, managers, individual contributors or administrator, users, casual users).

2. The developer also assigns a set of roles to each package, each component within the package, and each interface within a component. This is a type of Access Control List (ACL), maintained by MTS and based on roles. MTS ensures that only the roles specified on the list can access the specific element.

3. The developer *or* the MTS administrator assigns real Windows NT users or groups to the role at deployment time.

4. The MTS executive can handle all of the security checking during runtime, according to the declarative specification (declarative role-based security)

5. The developer may program the secure components and packages by checking access against roles within the code (using programmatic role-based security).

Essentially, MTS provides an additional level of indirection in mapping between security principals and programmatic access checking. This additional 'roles' layer enables late binding of access list membership, as well as flexibility in deployment and composition.

Working with Role Based Security

If the transactional properties of a component can be declaratively specified long after the completion of coding for an MTS component, then why can't security? The answer is, of course, that it can.

The declarative assignment of roles can be performed through the MTS Transaction Explorer. By right-clicking in the roles folder associated with a package, you can readily add new roles to the package. A role must be defined at the package level before it can be assigned to a specific component or interface within the package. This makes sense, since one must have access to a package (running EXE), before gaining access to its component or interfaces (loaded DLLs).

Because of straight enforcement of roles by MTS and the Transaction Explorer, the role of Administrator in the MTS's own system package is an important one. Before you turn on security, you must add yourself to this role, and turn on authorization checking in the system package.

Programmatic Role Based Security

Programmatic role based security refers to a security implementation that takes advantage of MTS's definition of roles, but performs its own access verifications programmatically.

Two methods provided by the `IObjectContext` interface are useful in implementing programmatic role based security (we saw how to obtain and work with this interface through ATL in Chapter 9):

❑ `IObjectContext::IsSecurityEnabled()` will let a component know whether security checking is being performed by the MTS at any time. Note that the security check is not enabled when the caller originates from within the same package, or if the client loads the MTS component in-process.

❑ `IObjectContext::IsCallerInRole()` will determine if the direct caller of the method is in a particular role. This can be used for programmatic access checks within the MTS component coding. By default, this will return TRUE, even if security is not enabled. Therefore, one should always call `IObjectContext::IsSecurityEnabled()` before interpreting the result from this call

`IObjectContext` also supports other methods for detailed auditing, please refer to the MSDN API description for more information.

Programmatic DCOM Security

Of course, being a DLL running within an application service EXE, there is nothing preventing an MTS component from creating its own security model by calling the relevant Win32 APIs. As a matter of fact, all of the DCOM security APIs are at your disposal. After all, an MTS component is simply a specially coded DCOM component.

This form of security programming, however, should not be necessary for MTS components. It really should only be used as a last resort if the MTS approach to security is not appropriate for your needs. The crux of the matter is, MTS can handle much of the complex programming for you up-stream, before your component is actually called.

Packages, Processes and Security Boundaries

MTS packages run as independent processes within Windows NT, and all components within a package run inside the same process. As a result, calls between such components are direct and not subject to any of MTS's authorization checks. This is done, by design, to enable components that 'trust' each other to execute in an efficient environment. Since fault-isolation also occurs at a process boundary, this partitioning also makes sense for tightly coupled inter-dependent components. You can use this to your advantage when designing the security infrastructure for your DNA application. Features that you can benefit from include:

- ❑ High efficiency calls between trusted components within a package
- ❑ Robust security checks between packages
- ❑ Late binding offered by role based security

Granularity of Authorization

Using role-based security, the MTS developer can secure a package down to the granularity of an interface offered by a component inside a package. This is also the maximum level that a raw DCOM security API developer can hope to establish. The only value that raw DCOM coding will afford you is extra flexibility in negotiating the security level with the client proxy. If you actually require this fine grain access control, which should be rare in the design of DNA business objects, you must code raw DCOM to achieve it.

MSMQ Security

Microsoft Message Queues, typically operated in an asynchronous, disconnected, store-and-forward fashion, have security concerns quite unlike any other server in the DNA family. MSMQ networks can span many separate NT domains and can even incorporate foreign (non-Microsoft) queuing systems (i.e. IBM MQ/Series). The dynamic nature of network level authentication and authorization, critical to DCOM, is less critical to MSMQ than the following aspects:

- ❑ Static object (queue) creation
- ❑ Static object (queue) access control
- ❑ Message authentication
- ❑ Message delivery integrity
- ❑ Message encryption.

Object Creation and Access Security

For creating and accessing queue objects, MSMQ offers standard Windows NT based security. This means that a security descriptor can be supplied during queue creation, with a DACL for access control. Every restricted operation on the queue can then be checked to ensure that the caller has been granted access rights. Interestingly, such checking cannot occur with the depositing of a message into a queue.

Due to the store-and-forward nature of MSMQ, the actual depositor of the message is almost always a routing server in the MSMQ network. Getting the access token of the depositor to determine the depositor's identity is useless in this case.

Instead, MSMQ relies on an embedded SID (a SID associated with the actual sender) coming along with the message to determine the identity of the sender. MSMQ will use this SID to check against the access control list for granted access rights. If you think this may make forgery possible, read on!

Authentication of Messages

MSMQ supports the authentication of messages through public-key technology digital signatures. Both internal (MSMQ only) certificates and external (third party Certificate Authority managed) certificates are supported.

In the internal case, a pair of keys is required by MSMQ. One of these is the private key, which is kept secret by MSMQ, and the other is a public key, which is distributed widely through MQIS.

The SID, from which MSMQ can determine the sender's identity, is sent with the message digitally signed using the public key of the destination queue. This allows the destination queue server to verify that the SID content has not been tampered with during transmission. The destination queue server uses its own private key to verify the digital signature. MSMQ can then validate the SID to verify the sender's identity and proceed with access checking.

External certificate support requires a third party Certificate Authority (CA). In this scenario, MSMQ will participate in the signing of, and authenticating of, the digital signature, but the MSMQ service at the receiving queue level cannot possibly validate the content of the certificate – it doesn't know anything about it – only the message receiving application can do that. This is typically used when the receiving application needs more information than simply the identity of the sender, or when the application is inter-working with non-MSMQ systems.

Encryption of Messages

The body of a message sent using MSMQ can be encrypted for privacy purposes. It is in an encrypted form during its entire passage through the store-and-forward network.

The default encryption algorithm is RC2. You can set the encryption of a message body by setting the PROPID_M_PRIV_LEVEL and PROPID_M_ENCRYPTION_ALG properties of the message (see the MSDN for more details). When using the automation compatible components, the PrivLevel and EncryptAlgorithm of the MSMQMessage object also allow you to encrypt the message body.

Note that a receiving application participating in the encrypted message sequence will always receive a decrypted message, even though it is always encrypted during transit. It can, however, determine that a message was previously transferred in encrypted form by examining the above properties. Here is a sequence diagram showing what happens en-route:

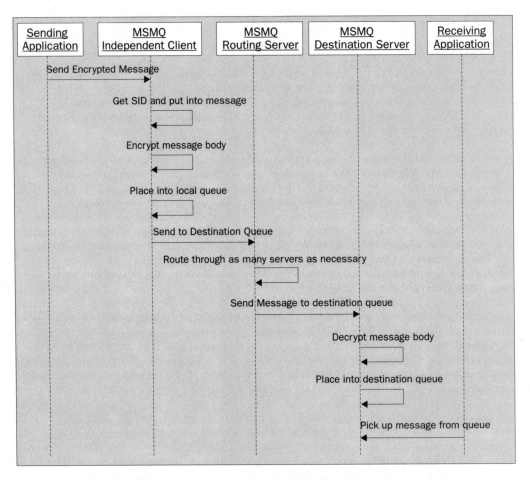

In the design of some systems, it may be desirable to ensure that all messages transferred between the client and the receiving application are sent encrypted. This can be configured by setting the receiving queue to handle only encrypted messages, which can be done by setting the PROPID_Q_PRIV_LEVEL of the receiving queue to MQ_PRIV_LEVEL_BODY. Equivalently, for the automation compatible components, you can set the PrivLevel property of the corresponding MSMQQueueInfo object.

Summary

In this chapter, we've given the vast topic of security a fair shake. We began by examining what security means in the intranet context. Narrowing it down to interactions between a web browser and a web server, we examined the specifics of where security measures should be implemented. We found that authentication of the client is a big and essential issue in intranet security. While simple on the surface, this is a complex task underneath, and no standard implementation exists today. However, an all-Microsoft solution in an intranet/Internet environment can provide a secured environment with security features that are transparent to an authorized end-user.

Laying the foundation for a more in-depth coverage of security, we examined all the fundamentals of Windows NT security. We covered the basic client/server security model, and stressed the importance of impersonation. We discovered the built-in and designed-in nature of Windows NT security and resolved many of the definitions involved in security-specific terminology.

In our DCOM security coverage, we examined the DCOM security blanket, which significantly optimizes the security negotiation process. We discussed access security, launch security, and call security. The importance of fine-grain security control was stressed during our discussion, and we concluded with a comprehensive discussion of the APIs and COM interfaces available that enable both clients and servers to set, discover and manipulate security parameters.

MTS and MSMQ both provide a unique transformation of the basic security model to fulfill their own specialized needs. MTS strives to simplify both the programming and administration of network security, through its own management of a declarative, role based model of component security. MTS components designed to use this higher level security model can enjoy simplicity in programming, late binding to security principals, and flexibility in deployment. For MTS components that 'must touch the bare metal', the entire set of DCOM security APIs is also at its disposal.

The security concerns of MSMQ are unique in that dynamic network access checking is not important in a store-and-forward based system. Instead, MSMQ utilizes exactly the same ACL based access model as Windows NT for access checking on static objects such as queues. Other concerns of MSMQ include authenticating the identity of a message sender, and ensuring privacy of the message sent through the store-and-forward system. MSMQ provides digital signature and encryption services to address these two concerns.

The message is clear in this chapter. Security for a DNA system, or in the wider distributed component computing context, is a nontrivial matter. A functional, secure computing environment requires careful planning and design. The Windows NT security model gives a solid and robust foundation upon which we can build more elaborate security schemes appropriate for our intranet project, using many of the new Win32 API and COM interfaces available.

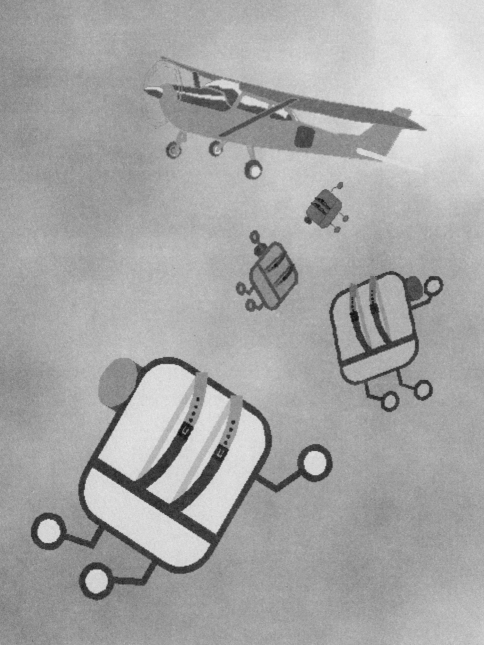

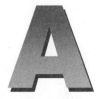

A Quick Tour of the System Registry

Even though we have only examined two COM interfaces in detail, it's clear that the System Registry plays a very important part in the proper functioning of COM. Furthermore, since the system and application configurations, the user preferences and the security database (under NT) are all stored in the registry, the registry is vital to the health and well being of the system as a whole.

In this appendix, we'll introduce the registry editor, and we'll cover how to use it in order to examine and modify many of the vital entries related to COM object operations.

The registry editor may be used to:

❑   View registry entries
❑   Add, delete and modify registry entries
❑   Backup a portion of or the entire registry
❑   Batch update the registry through a script file

We won't go into the intricate details of how to use the tool, since you either already know or can learn it quickly. Instead, we'll use the tool immediately, as a viewer, to take a look at how the COM runtime hides away the essential information. In the next chapter, we'll visit the registry editor again when we create custom entries for our very own from-scratch ActiveX control.

Find the registry editor on your system and run it. In Windows 95/8, it's called **Regedit.exe**. There are six subtrees that are displayed in the left pane, each of which has associated keys and information.

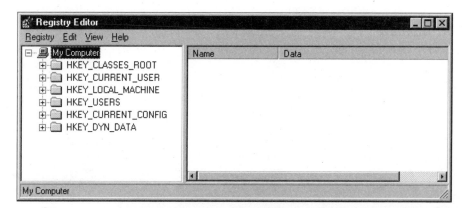

In Windows NT 4.0, it is called **Regedt32.exe**. On running it, you'll find that only five subtrees are displayed and this time, each subtree has its own window.

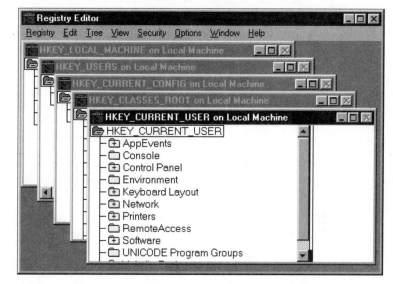

The one we're most interested in is, not surprisingly, the **HKEY_CLASSES_ROOT** subtree. When we expand this subtree, we'll typically find a very large list of keys. One interesting key is the **CLSID** key. Try expanding this one.

You'll be greeted with a large list of CLSIDs, remember them? These, as we know, are actually 'names' or 'keys' for classes of COM objects. If you expand any one of them, you'll see that they have additional subkeys (attributes) which describe the class further. Typically, you may see a key called `InprocServer32`. This key indicates to the COM runtime that the CLSID represents an in-proc server. The server is a 32-bit implementation (remember there exists still a very large base of 16-bit software out there). The named values under this subkey typically include a `(Default)` and a `ThreadingModel`. COM runtime looks into the `(Default)` value to find out where the in-proc server implementation DLL is located. The `ThreadingModel` value gives COM an indication of what sort of threading model the server will support – we've covered the various threading models and what they do in Chapter 2. For COM objects that are local server based, you'll find a `LocalServer32` key that will provide the COM runtime with a path to find the server EXE. The following table summarizes many of the keys that you'll find under `\HKEY_CLASSES_ROOT\CLSID\{-----}`

Key Name	Applies To	Comment
InprocServer	16/32-bit servers	Path to 16/32-bit DLL on same machine. Implements an in-proc server.
InprocServer32	32-bit servers	Path to 32-bit DLL on same machine. Implements an in-proc server.
InprocHandler32	32-bit servers	An object handler is nothing more than a piece of code that implements the interfaces expected by a container when an object is in its loaded state (i.e. it isn't running yet). In other words, it's a glue object that provides the interfaces but doesn't necessarily provide the full functionality. It's typically used in cases where bringing up the local server (where the full functionality is implemented) would be too inefficient.
LocalServer32	32-bit servers	Path to 32-bit EXE on same machine. Implements a local server running in a separate process.
Insertable	32-bit servers	Indicates that the 32-bit server can be used by existing 16-bit applications.
MiscStatus		Object status information, usually stored in the registry when the object isn't running; that is, at creation, and when loading. Interfaces exist so that interested applications can check on an object's status at all times.

Table Continued on Following Page

Key Name	Applies To	Comment
ProgId		A programmatic identifier. The default value of the key is a human readable string uniquely (but not universally) identifying a class that can appear in an Insert Object dialog box. It can also serve as the identifier in a macro programming language to identify the class. APIs are available to convert from/to the corresponding CLSID.
VersionIndependent ProgId		A server must register a second, version-independent programmatic identifier that's guaranteed to remain constant across all versions. A client application accessing the object through this key in, for example, a scripting language, will have access to the current version installed.
Verb	OLE objects	Verbs are specific actions the object can execute that are meaningful to the end user. A container (client app) looks at this key in the registry to find out what verbs the object supports, in order to present them to the user, typically in a pop-up menu.
Control		If the key is present, the object is a control.
Typelib		Type library ID for the object.
MainUserType		The constant name referring to the currently installed version of the server.
AuxUserType		Auxiliary names, for example, a short name for the class, a real-world name for the application when necessary to present to the user, etc.
DataFormat		Lists the default and main data formats supported by the application.
DefaultIcon		Contains icon information for iconic representations of the object. It includes the full path to module (DLL or EXE) where the icon resides and the index of the icon within the executable.

This list is certainly not exhaustive, and any particular pair of COM objects can establish their own private use of keys associated with the CLSID. What we attempt to cover here are the most common ones that we may encounter in our ActiveX programming activities. This explains how COM can know so much about a class given a CLSID. The `ProgId` entry above, for example, is an interesting entry – it gives a human readable string for locating a CLSID. This makes it unnecessary to use and remember CLSIDs in most programming activities. If we know the `ProgID`, we can get the CLSID by invoking the API `CLSIDFromProgID()`. Conversely, from the CLSID, we can get the associated `ProgID` by invoking `ProgIDFromCLSID()`. Given a `ProgID`, it's possible to call `CoCreateInstance()` with the following syntax:

```
CoCreateInstance("ABC.1" )
```

In this case, all we have is a text based name of the class to create. How does `CoCreateInstance()` create the object instance without a CLSID?

The answer, again, lies within the registry. Any COM classes that are registered with a text name are doubly linked back to the CLSID entry with a key right under `HKEY_CLASSES_ROOT`. For example, the `MyObject.1` class with CLSID `{xxxxxxx}` will have the registry entries:

```
\HKEY_CLASSES_ROOT\Myobject.1\CLSID\(Default) = "{xxxxxx}"
```

```
\HKEY_CLASSES_ROOT\CLSID\{xxxxxxx}\ProgID\(Default) = "Myobject.1"
```

```
\HKEY_CLASSES_ROOT\CLSID\{xxxxxxx}\InProcServer32\(Default) =
"C:\DLLDIR\MYOBJECT.DLL"
```

This should completely demystify how the COM runtime does much of its job during object creation. Other keys that are also quite interesting include:

Key Name	Comment
\HKEY_CLASSES_ROOT \TypeLib	All the type libraries registered with the system, ordered by their LIBID.
\HKEY_CLASSES_ROOT \Interface	All the registered interfaces, ordered by their IID. Since you can use `QueryInterface()` during runtime between objects to discover interfaces, this set doesn't cover all the interfaces exposed by all the objects in the system.
	The `(Default)` value contains the text name of the interface (i.e. `"IUnknown"`).
	The `BaseInterface` subkey contains the IID of the interface upon which this interface is based. (Not directly enforced.)
	The `NumMethods` subkey contains a count of the number of methods contained in this interface.
	The `ProxyStubClsid32` subkey contains the CLSID of the proxy/stub object used in marshaling parameters and arguments across process or machine boundaries for the local and remote servers.

Bear in mind that what we've examined are very Win32-specific implementation details. COM residing on another non-Win32 platform will have alternative representation and storage for the same object information.

Object Browsing Made Easier: The Object Viewer Tool

After working with the registry editor for a while during COM programming and debugging, you'll wish you had a more intelligent tool available. The problem with the registry editor is that it isn't specific to COM or OLE, and relies on you as the intelligent filter to get to the information you need.

Microsoft has released an excellent tool that practically makes the registry editor obsolete as a viewer. The tool is called the Object Viewer, in the form of `Oleview.exe`. This tool combs the entire registry, looking up all the OLE objects and controls, stores and sorts all the relevant object information entries, and then presents the compiled information in a browseable, easy-to-use format.

> `Oleview.exe` *is now a standard item including with distributions of Visual C++ 6.*
> *However, you can still download the latest version of it from its original home on the Internet.*
> *The URL is:*

`http://www.microsoft.com/com/resource/oleview.htm`

Sounds too good to be true? You can try Object Viewer for yourself. Once started, Object Viewer displays all its collected information on two panes.

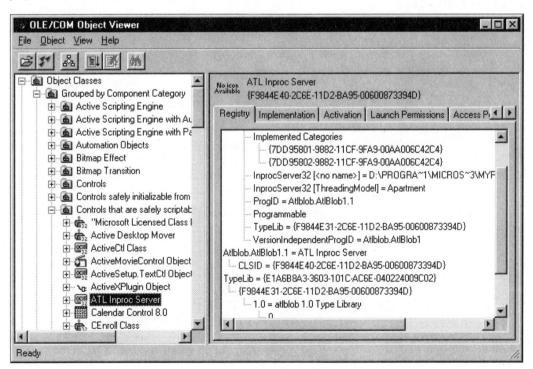

The left pane is a tree view displaying all the various COM objects that are installed on the system. The information available includes:

Information	Comment
ActiveX and OLE Controls by category	The OC96 specification recommended the classification of OCXs (including ActiveX controls) using UUID based component categories (CATIDs). We'll cover this further in Chapter 5. These classifications will allow clients to determine the set of services provided or conventions followed by objects before actually creating them.
COM objects regardless of type	This is a complete list of all the COM objects registered with the system. Different icons represent different type of COM objects.
Type Libraries	A type library provides the client with information on the interfaces, methods and parameters that a particular object supports without actually requiring the client to load the object. Originally only used in OLE/ActiveX Automation, the type library is now extended to apply to all ActiveX objects regardless of the server characteristics or binding mechanism.
Interfaces	The interfaces registered with the system, including their interface ID, type libraries if available, as well as location of marshaling proxy/stub for local server and DCOM operations.

By expanding any of the information categories, information from individual COM objects can be viewed on the right-hand pane. Furthermore, if you expand any of the individual object entries, the type library information will be displayed. Double-clicking on the object entry will cause Object Viewer to actually create an instance of your object, and to fire `QueryInterface()` calls into your object to determine what sort of known and standard interfaces the selected object supports.

Unfortunately, Object Viewer is just that, a viewer. If you want to adjust and tweak object registry setting directly, you'll still need to use the registry editor. Therefore, you will frequently find instances of Visual Studio, Object Viewer, and the registry editor all opened on the typical COM developer's desktop (and the manager asks why COM developers need at least 64MB of memory, and a 21-inch monitor!)

Programmatic Access to the System Registry

It's fine to be able to view the COM related entries of the registry using either the registry editor or the OLE Viewer. COM object servers, however, are required to register themselves with the registry (adding all the relevant entries) under various circumstances. It would be quite an inconvenience to have to spawn Regedit.exe every time in order to make the necessary changes.

Instead, Win32 offers a standard set of registry manipulation APIs that the application may use to add, delete, or modify the registry entries. These APIs are quite straightforward; the following table summarizes them and provides some usage examples.

Function	Comments
RegCreateKeyEx()	Create a new key in the registry (or open an existing one). Specify options for the key as well as the kind of access allowed.
RegOpenKeyEx()	Open the specified key. A subkey can be specified as well as options denoting the kind of access the user wants. The key must exist otherwise the call will fail.
RegCloseKey()	Release an open key.
RegDeleteKey()	Deletes a specified key from the registry.
RegEnumKeyEx()	Enumerates subkeys of a given key.
RegEnumValue()	Enumerates values of a given key. A key can hold many named values of different data types as well as an unnamed value – the default.
RegQueryValueEx()	Retrieve a particular value for a key.
RegSetValueEx()	Set a key to a particular value. All types of values are supported.
RegDeleteValue()	Deletes a value from a key.

Now you've had a little time to ingest these calls, it's time for an example. We can add the value **"C:\DLLDIR\MYOBJECT.DLL"** of the in-proc server DLL to the key **\HKEY_CLASSES_ROOT\CLSID\{xxxxxxx}\InprocServer32** in the following manner:-

```
HKEY    hKey;
char    *path =  "C:\\DLLDIR\\MYOBJECT.DLL";
LONG    rc;

rc = RegOpenKey( HKEY_CLASSES_ROOT,                     // predefined symbol
                "CLSID\\{xxxxxxx}\\InprocServer32", // sub-key
                &hKey                                  // handle to the key
            );

if  ( rc != ERROR_SUCCESS )
    // handle errors

rc = RegSetValueEx( hKey,
                    NULL,          // no value name - sets the (Default)
                    0L,            // reserved, must be 0
                    REG_SZ,        // value type is null-terminated string
                    (CONST BYTE *) path, // address of data
                    lstrlen(path)+1 // size of data
                );
```

```
if ( rc != ERROR_SUCCESS )
    // handle errors

rc = RegCloseKey( hKey );

if ( rc != ERROR_SUCCESS )
    // handle errors
```

Further information on the usage of these registry APIs can be found in the MSDN Library under **Platform SDK/Windows Base Services/General Library/Registry/Registry Reference.**

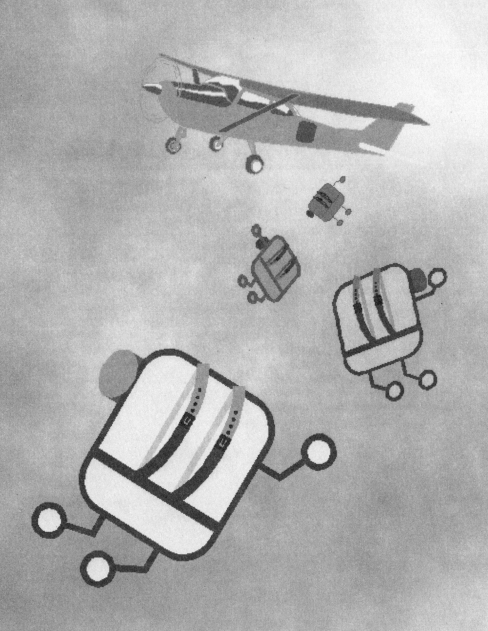

B

UML Notation

Classes and Objects

A class is represented in the UML like this:

Class
attribute1   attribute2
MethodA()   MethodB()

The rectangle representing the class is divided into three compartments, the top one showing the class name, the second showing the attributes and the third showing the methods.

If the class is abstract, then the class name in the first compartment is italicized.

An object looks very similar to a class, except that its name is underlined:

<u>AnObject</u>
attribute1   attribute2
MethodA()   MethodB()

Relationships

Relationships between classes are generally represented in class diagrams by a line or an arrow joining the two classes. UML can represent the following, different sorts of object relationships.

Dependency

If A depends on B, then this is shown by a dashed arrow between A and B, with the arrowhead pointing at B:

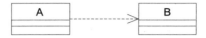

Association

An association between A and B is shown by a line joining the two classes:

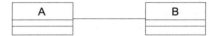

If there is no arrow on the line, the association is taken to be bidirectional. A unidirectional association is indicated like this:

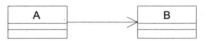

Aggregation

An aggregation relationship is indicated by placing a white diamond at the end of the association next to the aggregate class. If B aggregates A, then A is a part of B, but their lifetimes are independent:

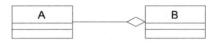

Composition

Composition, on the other hand, is shown by a black diamond on the end of association next to the composite class. If B is composed of A, then B controls the lifetime of A.

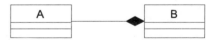

Multiplicity

The multiplicity of a relationship is indicated by a number (or *) placed at the end of an association.

The following diagram indicates a one-to-one relationship between A and B:

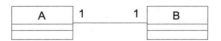

This next diagram indicates a one-to-many relationship:

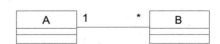

A multiplicity can also be a range of values. Some examples are shown in the table below:

`1`	One and only one
`*`	Any number from 0 to infinity
`0..1`	Either 0 or 1
`n..m`	Any number in the range n to m inclusive
`1..*`	Any positive integer

Naming an Association

To improve the clarity of a class diagram, the
association between two objects may be named:

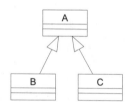

Inheritance

An inheritance (generalization/specialization) relationship is indicated in the UML by an arrow with a
triangular arrowhead pointing towards the generalized class.

If A is a base class, and B and C are classes derived from A, then this would
be represented by the following class diagram:

Multiple Inheritance

The next diagram represents the case where class C is derived from
classes A and B:

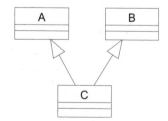

States

States of objects are represented as rectangles with rounded corners. The *transition* between different states is represented as an arrow between states, and a *condition* of that transition occurring may be added between square braces. This condition is called a guard.

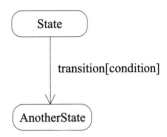

Object Interactions

Interactions between objects are represented by interaction diagrams – both sequence and collaboration diagrams. An example of a collaboration diagram is shown here:
Objects are drawn as rectangles and the lines between them indicate links – a link is an instance of an association. The order of the messages along the links between the objects is indicated by the number at the head of the message.

Sequence diagrams show essentially the same information, but concentrate on the time-ordered communication between objects, rather than their relationships. An example of a sequence diagram is shown here:
The dashed vertical lines represent the lifeline of the object (starting at the top).

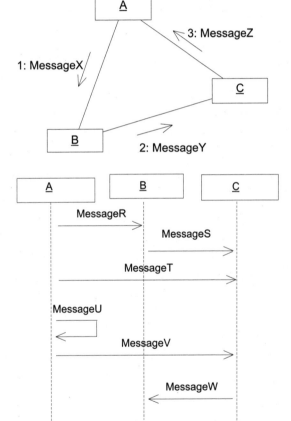

Use Cases

A use case is a description of an interaction between an actor (person or external system) and system under design. In UML it is denoted like this:

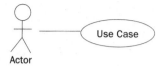

Design Patterns

Design patterns are represented in the UML notation by collaborations (shown as dotted elipses) between classes. Each class that is part of the pattern is joined to it by a dotted line labeled with the particular role played by the class:

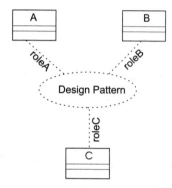

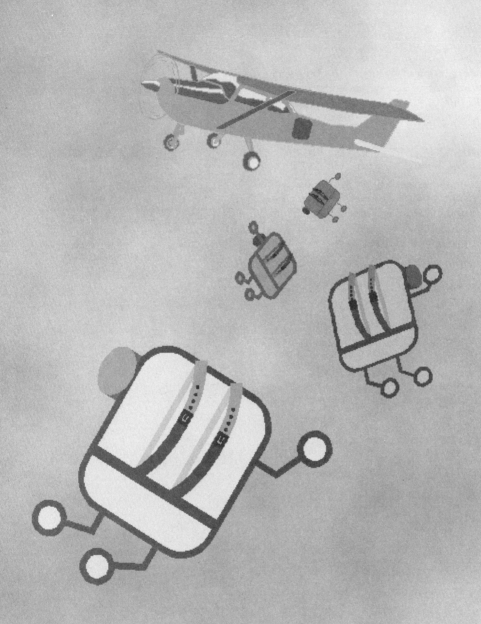

A Template Quickie

If you've been using the new STL (**Standard Template Library**) support in Visual C++ 6, you're probably already familiar with C++ templates and what they can do. For those who aren't so familiar with templates, as well as for those who want a quick refresher, we'll breeze right through a quick introduction to templates over the next few pages. We will cover the basics, plus a couple of advanced features of C++ templates – just enough so that you will not be overwhelmed when going through the ATL 3 source code.

As C/C++ programmers, we're fully familiar with the macro preprocessor's function. We also know that the good old #define can be used for parameterized macros, as in:

```
#define GREATER_THAN(x,y)      ((x) > (y))
```

Which allows us to use:

```
if ( GREATER_THAN(my_value,100) ){
    printf("greater\n");
}
```

Here's the actual code generated after the source has been preprocessed:

```
if ( ((my_value) > (100)) )
{
    printf("greater\n");
}
```

In the past, this was the only way one could easily define constants and write inline functions. Today, however, with `const` keyword and `inline` qualified functions, there's no excuse for using preprocessor macros for this purpose. The macros perform textual substitution without any knowledge of the underlying language. As a result, nasty side effects are possible, and the lack of any type checking makes for some recurring debugging nightmares. Nonetheless, they are still extremely useful in helping manage the project build process, by hiding some system dependencies and facilitating conditional header file inclusion and compilation.

Until a few years ago, macros were the only way one could get something like a 'type variable' or 'parameterized type'. In languages like C/C++ typing is static, that is, the compiler must know the type of an object at compile time. This makes it impossible to write generic pieces of code that would work equally well for a variety of data types. The only way to do this is to create a base class and derive all data types as subject to the generic operation from this base. This ties data type, and the generic operations that operate on them — two orthogonal concepts — tightly into the C++ inheritance hierarchy. The old pre-template MFC list management classes are a good example of this approach (the base class is `CObject`, and the generic operations operate on `CObject`). Typical usage of such classes involves a lot of class upcasting and downcasting, which isn't exactly a trivial task.

Enter templates!

Behaviors Parameterized by Datatype

The advantage of templates is that they enable parameterization of generic operations using data types. Templates operate at compile time and obey scope, access and type rules. Essentially, one can write C++ classes for generic data types, and then be able to substitute the data type into this class definition 'skeleton' whenever needed. Take the following trivial class example:

```
template < class T >
class ComparableObject
{
public:
    ComparableObject(T aVal): m_var(aVal) {}
    BOOL GreaterThan(T comp) { return (m_var > comp); }
    BOOL LessThan(T comp){ return (m_var < comp); }

private:
    T m_var;
};
```

Once we have this template class defined, we may use it in the following fashion:

```
ComparableObject<int> aVal(10);

if (aVal.GreaterThan(100))
    printf("greater\n");
```

Instead of working on a text substitution level, templates work via parameterized code generation. Essentially, a new class has been defined for you above, which 'looks like' the `ComparableObject` that you've defined, but operates specifically on the `int` data type. The following code was effectively generated into your executable:

```
class ComparableObjectInt
{
public:
    ComparableObjectInt(int   aVal):m_var(aVal) {}
    BOOL  GreaterThan(int comp) { return (m_var > comp); }
    BOOL  LessThan(int comp)  { return (m_var < comp); }

private:
    int m_var;
};

ComparableObjectInt aVal(10);
if (aVal.GreaterThan(100))
    printf("greater\n");
```

Notice how one single instantiation of the template (in the line: `ComparableObject<int>` `aVal(10);`) actually caused the creation of new class, based on the parameterized type.

We could have other lines like this:

```
ComparableObject<float> aFloat(3.14195);
ComparableObject<String> aString("starter");
ComparableObject<CMytype> aVal( CMytype());
```

Here, each instantiation with a new data type in the parameter will actually create another class definition for us, as if we'd written the classes ourselves for each of the data types. In our case, the only assumption that we make is that our data type will support the less than (<) and greater than (>) operators. If the data type that we supplied as an argument to the template instantiation doesn't support the required operator, then the linker will complain about undefined function references. This is exactly what would happen if we'd defined the classes ourselves with a type that didn't have the required operators.

Template Signatures

Template signatures refer to the parameterization of a template instantiation (i.e. what parameters are inside the angled brackets). Template instantiation can be very powerful when used in combination with inheritance and virtual functions. Note that it's also possible to parameterize a template with multiple class arguments, as well as non-class and default arguments. For example:

```
template < class MappedKey, class MappedItem, long HashType = 3 >
class MagicList
{
...
};
```

In this case, `MappedKey` and `MappedItem` represents two data types or classes which are parameters to the template class. The class definition itself will make use of these two types, in our example, maybe to create a hash value from arbitrary data type `MappedKey` to another arbitrary data type `MappedItem`. The third value may be used to cause the final instantiated class to behave slightly differently. In our example, the instantiated class may use a different hash algorithm in the lookup depending on the value of `HashType`. If `HashType` isn't supplied, the default value of 3 will be assumed.

It's important to realize that every unique parameterization of a template class generates another unique class. This applies to all cases, including:

```
#define HASH_SPARSE 3
#define HASH_DENSE 4

MagicList<String, Mytype, HASH_SPARSE> FirstMap();
MagicList<String, Mytype, HASH_DENSE> SecondMap();
```

In this case, even though the class parameterization of `FirstMap` and `SecondMap` is identical, the difference in the non-class argument causes the two signatures (consisting of the template class name and its parameters) to be unique, and two mutually exclusive classes will be generated through the instantiation.

Exploiting Template Functions

A member function of a template class can also be defined separately (outside of the template) from the class definition. For example, we could have defined the `LessThan()` method from the `ComparableObject<>` class in this way (assuming we have removed the body of `LessThan()` from the original declaration):

```
template < class T >
BOOL ComparableObject<T>::LessThan(T comp)
{
    return (m_var < comp);
}
```

To illustrate another important point, let's add one more function declaration to our template. Suppose `ComparableObject` came from some library we've purchased for in-house development, and the definition of the template includes the declaration of a function that is not included in the template library:

```
template < class T >
class ComparableObject
{
public:
    ComparableObject(T aVal): m_var(aVal)
    {}
    BOOL GreaterThan(T comp) { return (m_var > comp); }
    BOOL LessThan(T comp);
    BOOL SuperOp(T comp);
```

```
private:
   T m_var;
};

template <class T>
BOOL ComparableObject<T>::LessThan(T comp)
{
   return (m_var < comp);
}
```

The point to notice here is that even though SuperOp() isn't implemented, the library is *not* considered incomplete. This is because no problem will arise until someone actually attempts to instantiate the template. Even then, as long as you've defined a SuperOp() function for your template instantiation parameter signature, the compiler will be completely happy. For example, if we were to instantiate ComparableObject for our own type called MyType, we would need to have:

```
BOOL ComparableObject<MyType>::SuperOp(MyType inVal)
{
   return MyType.CheckValidity();
}

ComparableObject<MyType> aValue();
```

Consider the real power here: you've actually augmented the function of the class at design time based on your own requirements. Though object-oriented design purists will frown upon this practice (since the template class definition isn't complete and there's a chance that our last minute supplement may completely break the other behavior of the template class), I've seen this technique used quite successfully in many in-house development projects.

Notational Complexity

Frequently, a very complex template construct can be lurking behind a simple symbolic representation, courtesy of the friendly typedef operator. For example:

```
typedef   ARealMessyTemplateClass<int, long, char *, \
          MyClass, \
          AnotherMessyTemplateClass<long, MyClass>, \
          51123> \
          ReallySimpleType ;

ReallySimpleType SoSimple(1, 2, "3");
```

Note that the template class isn't instantiated at typedef time (there's no code generated by the typedef, only a new symbol table is created by the compiler), but occurs at the time that the SoSimple variable is defined. This is clear when you remember that, although ARealMessyTemplateClass<> is completely and specifically parameterized by <int, long, char *, MyClass,...>, the actual code generation for the parameterized class doesn't occur until the compiler hits the declaration of ReallySimpleType.

Note also that the `SoSimple(1,2,"3")` portion isn't template parameterization, but rather a constructor defined for the templated class (which we haven't shown above) which takes (`long, long, char *`) for parameters. The syntax may well look quite ugly to you, but it does happen often in real life template coding, and you'll find plenty of examples in the ATL source code.

A template based class becomes an actual data type when instantiated, and as such, can be used as a class type parameter in another template. Template libraries like ATL do tend to use this construct. Pay particular attention to the extra space between the pair of the closing angle brackets. This space is vital; it's the only thing that the compiler has to distinguish the templates from the operator >>.

```
template < class T >
class A
{...};

template < class S, class A< int > >    // notice the space between > >
class B
{...};
```

Class Bridging

Unlike the ordinary classes in binary class libraries, template classes generate code, so the final relationship between a library's classes and the user defined class is not determined until template instantiation. In other words, it is not necessary for a user implemented class to always be the most derived. This may be surprising for some new template users. A binary class library might have an inheritance hierarchy like the one shown here:

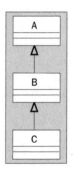

In this situation, the developer can choose to inherit from class A, B, or C, and obtain the use of the public and protected members of the class, plus all its base classes. In every one of these cases, the user-defined class will become the most derived class in the hierarchy (or a leaf of the tree).

A template library, on the other hand, might have a class hierarchy like this:

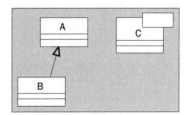

For those of you unfamiliar with the UML notation, the box in the upper right hand corner of class C indicates that it is a template class. There's more info on UML in Appendix B.

In this kind of situation, the actual final instantiation can become:

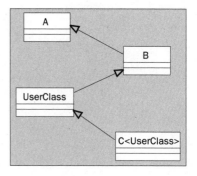

The code that makes this happen is shown below:

```
class A  // not templated
{...}

class B: public A  // not templated
{...}

template< class T >
class C: public T
{...}

class myClass: public B // not templated
{...}

C<myClass> anInstance;
```

Note that class C now derives from myClass, and can access public or protected members of A, B, and myClass. Class C can collaborate with A and B to perform tasks transparent to the user defined myClass.

This technique is precisely how ATL handles the variations in IUnknown implementation for COM components.

Explicit Specialization

Consider the following templated code:

```
template< class T >
class S
{... implementation 1 ...};

template <> class S<int>   // specialization
{... implementation 2 ...};
```

The funny looking template<> syntax allows you to specify a *specialization* of the template defined. This basically means that if the class S<int> is ever instantiated in the code, the specialization (implementation 2) will be used instead. On the other hand, for all other typed instantiation of class S (for example, S<char>, S<float>), the regular specification (implementation 1) will be used.

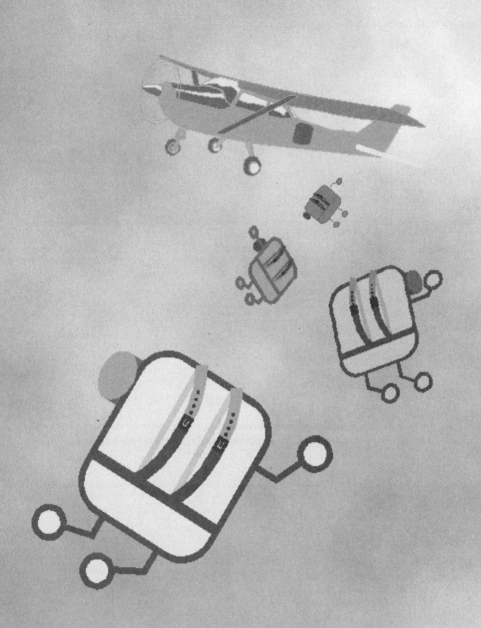

D

Bibliography

UML

UML Toolkit,
Hans Erikson and Magnus Penker, 1997, ISBN 0-471-19161-2

Instant UML,
Pierre-Alain Muller, Wrox Press, 1997, ISBN 1-861-00087-1

Design Patterns

Design Patterns - Elements of Reusable Object-Oriented Software,
Erich Gamma, Richard Helm, Ralph Johnson and John Vlissides,
Addison-Wesley, 1995, ISBN 0-201-63361-2

COM / ATL

Professional DCOM Programming,
Richard Grimes, Wrox Press, 1997, ISBN 1-861-00060-X

Essential COM,
Don Box, Addison-Wesley, 1998, ISBN 0-201-63446-5

Beginning ATL COM Programming,
Richard Grimes, Alex Stockton, Julian Templeman and George Reilly,
Wrox Press, 1998, ISBN 1-861-00011-1

Professional COM Applications with ATL

Professional ATL COM Programming,
Richard Grimes, Wrox Press, 1998, ISBN 1-861-00140-1

Professional DCOM Application Development,
Jonathan Pinnock, Wrox Press, 1998, ISBN 1-861-00131-2

Dynamic HTML

Instant IE4 Dynamic HTML Programmer's Reference,
Alex Homer and Chris Ullman, Wrox Press, 1997, ISBN 1-861-00068-5

Professional IE4 Programming,
Mike Barta, Jon Bonnell, Andrew Enfield, Dino Esposito, Brian Francis, Richard Harrison, Alex
Homer, Stephen Jakab, Sing Li, Shawn Murphy and Chris Ullman,
Wrox Press, 1997, ISBN 1-861-00070-7

Windows

Professional NT Services,
Kevin Miller, Wrox Press, 1998, ISBN 1-861-00130-4

Advanced Windows,
Jeffrey Richter, Microsoft Press, 1997, ISBN 1-572-31548-2

Database Programming

An Introduction to Database Systems,
Chris Date, Addison Wesley, 1994, ISBN 0-201-54329-X

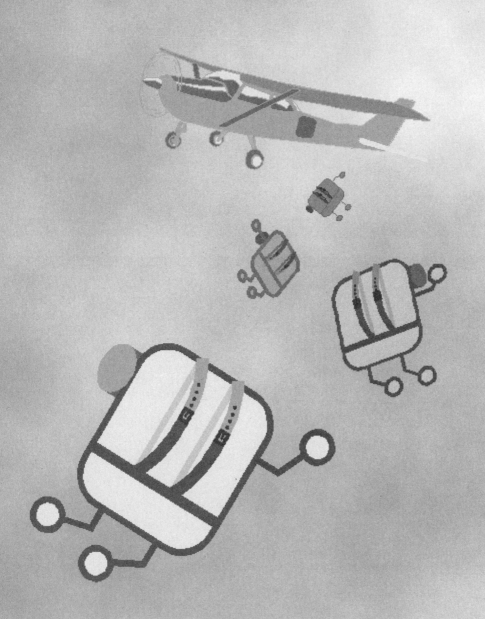

Support Classes for the Viscal Project

In this appendix, we will give listings for the final versions of the following support classes. Detailed listings in Chapter 7 would have detracted from the discussion. Where we have shown the structure, class definition or method implementation in the chapter, we'll note that.

The files are:

- ❏ CalDefs.h
- ❏ CalUtils.h
- ❏ CalUtils.cpp
- ❏ CCellMgr.h
- ❏ CCellMgr.cpp
- ❏ CDataMgr.h
- ❏ CDataMgr.cpp
- ❏ CEvents.h
- ❏ CEvents.cpp
- ❏ EventListDlg.h
- ❏ EventListDlg.cpp
- ❏ OneEventDlg.h
- ❏ OneEventDlg.cpp
- ❏ CalButton.h
- ❏ CalButton.cpp

CalDefs.h

```
#ifndef _CALDEFS_H
#define _CALDEFS_H

typedef basic_string<TCHAR> tstring;

// Common definitions
const kDaysInWeek = 7;
const kMontshInYear = 12;
const kSecondsInADay = 24 * 60 * 60;

const kShortNameLen = 3;              // # of chars in month/day short names

// Constants related to the visual display of the information
const kRowsDisplayed = 6;            // how many rows to display in Calendar
const kMinTitleFontSize = 6;
const kMaxTitleFontSize = 48;

// Constants related to the amount of information available
const kMaxCellAttachments = 3;

// Limits for sample program
const kMaxEvents = 10;
const kMaxDepts = 3;

const kCalTopMargin = 3;
const kCalLeftMargin = 2;
const kButSizeToHeightRatio = 8;  // button size is 1/8 of height

// have the control respond to inquisitive containers that they are safe
#define CTL_IS_SAFE

#endif // _CALDEFS_H
```

CalUtils.h

```
#ifndef _CALUTILS_H
#define _CALUTILS_H

#include "CalDefs.h"
#include <time.h>

tstring Int2TString(int i);

////////////////////////////////////////////////////////////////////////
//    CDateTimeDiff class
//    Shown in Chapter 7

////////////////////////////////////////////////////////////////////////
//    CDateTime class
//    Encapsulate a date and time
//    Shown in Chapter 7
```

```
//////////////////////////////////////////////////
//   CDatesList - collection of CDateTime entries
class CDatesList : public vector<CDateTime>
{
};

//////////////////////////////////////////////////
//   CMonthInfo class
//     Shown in Chapter 7

//////////////////////////////////////////////////
//   CRectangle struct
//     Shown in Chapter 7

ostream& operator << (ostream& os, const CRectangle& cell);

#endif // _CALUTILS_H
```

CalUtils.cpp

```cpp
#include "stdafx.h"
#include "CalDefs.h"
#include "CalUtils.h"

tstring Int2TString(int i)
{
    TCHAR buf[BUFSIZ];
    _itot(i, buf, 10);
    return tstring(buf);
}

/////////////////////////////////////////////////////////////////////////////
//   CDateTimeDiff implementation
CDateTimeDiff::CDateTimeDiff(int year, int month, int day, int hours,
                            int minutes, int seconds)
{
    tm_t.tm_year = year + 1970 - 1900;
    tm_t.tm_mon = month;
    tm_t.tm_mday = day;
    tm_t.tm_hour = hours;
    tm_t.tm_min = minutes;
    tm_t.tm_sec = seconds;

    tm_t.tm_wday = 0;    // ignored
    tm_t.tm_yday = 0;    // ignored
    tm_t.tm_isdst = 0;   // ignored - it's not absolute time
}

CDateTimeDiff::operator time_t() const
{
    // mktime is showing its age - it doesn't take a const parm
    return mktime(const_cast<struct tm*>(&tm_t));
}
```

```
///////////////////////////////////////////////////////////////////////
//   CDateTime implementation
CDateTime::CDateTime() : t((time_t)-1)
{
    wsprintf(m_buf, _T(""));
}

CDateTime::CDateTime(int year, int month, int day,
                     int hours, int minutes, int seconds)
{
    struct tm tm_t;

    _ASSERTE(year > 1970 && year < 2036);
    tm_t.tm_year = year - 1900;

    _ASSERTE(month >= 1 && month <= 12);
    tm_t.tm_mon   = month - 1; // struct tm takes 0 - 11 for the month

    _ASSERTE(day >= 1 && day <= 31);
    tm_t.tm_mday = day;

    _ASSERTE(hours >= 0 && hours <=23);
    tm_t.tm_hour = hours;

    _ASSERTE(minutes >= 0 && minutes <= 59);
    tm_t.tm_min = minutes;

    _ASSERTE(seconds >= 0 && seconds <= 59);
    tm_t.tm_sec = seconds;

    tm_t.tm_wday = 0;      // ignored
    tm_t.tm_yday = 0;      // ignored
    tm_t.tm_isdst = -1;    // required - ask the library to find out

    t = mktime(&tm_t);
    _ASSERTE(t != (time_t)(-1));

    wsprintf(m_buf, _T("%s"), ((tstring)(*this)).c_str());
}

CDateTime::~CDateTime()
{
}

CDateTime::CDateTime(const CDateTime& other)
{
    t = (time_t)other;
    wsprintf(m_buf, _T("%s"), ((tstring)(*this)).c_str());
}

CDateTime::CDateTime(const time_t other)
{
    t = other;
    wsprintf(m_buf, _T("%s"), ((tstring)(*this)).c_str());
}

CDateTime::CDateTime(const SYSTEMTIME& sysTime)
{
```

```
        if (sysTime.wYear < 1970)
            *this = (time_t)0L;
        else
            *this = CDateTime(sysTime.wYear, sysTime.wMonth, sysTime.wDay,
                              sysTime.wHour, sysTime.wMinute, sysTime.wSecond);
    }

    CDateTime::CDateTime(const DATE date)
    {
        SYSTEMTIME sysTime;

        if (SUCCEEDED(VariantTimeToSystemTime((double)(date), &sysTime)))
            *this = CDateTime(sysTime);
        else
            *this = (time_t)0L;
    }

    CDateTime& CDateTime::operator=(const CDateTime& other)
    {
        t = (time_t)other;
        wsprintf(m_buf, _T("%s"), ((tstring)(*this)).c_str());
        return *this;
    }

    CDateTime& CDateTime::operator=(time_t other)
    {
        t = other;
        wsprintf(m_buf, _T("%s"), ((tstring)(*this)).c_str());
        return *this;
    }

    CDateTime CDateTime::operator+(const CDateTimeDiff diff) const
    {
        time_t newT = (time_t)-1;
        struct tm tm_t, *pt;

        if (t != (time_t)-1 && (pt =localtime(&t)) != NULL)
        {
            tm_t = *pt;
            tm_t.tm_year += diff.tm_t.tm_year - (1970 - 1900);
            tm_t.tm_mon  += diff.tm_t.tm_mon;
            if (tm_t.tm_mon < 0)
            {
                int m = tm_t.tm_mon;
                tm_t.tm_year -= 1 + (-m) / 12;
                tm_t.tm_mon   = 12 - (-m) % 12;
            }
            tm_t.tm_mday += diff.tm_t.tm_mday;
            tm_t.tm_hour += diff.tm_t.tm_hour;
            tm_t.tm_min  += diff.tm_t.tm_min;
            tm_t.tm_sec  += diff.tm_t.tm_sec;
            newT = mktime(&tm_t);
        }
        return  CDateTime(newT);
    }

    int CDateTime::GetYear() const
    {
        // year in tm stored minus 1900
        return (t == (time_t)-1) ? t : localtime(&t)->tm_year + 1900;
    }
```

```
int CDateTime::GetMonth() const
{
    // month in tm is in [ 0, 11 ]
    return (t == (time_t)-1) ? t : localtime(&t)->tm_mon + 1;
}

int CDateTime::GetDay() const
{
    return (t == (time_t)-1) ? t : localtime(&t)->tm_mday;
}

int CDateTime::GetHours() const
{
    return (t == (time_t)-1) ? t : localtime(&t)->tm_hour;
}

int CDateTime::GetMinutes() const
{
    return (t == (time_t)-1) ? t : localtime(&t)->tm_min;
}

int CDateTime::GetSeconds() const
{
    return (t == (time_t)-1) ? t : localtime(&t)->tm_sec;
}

int CDateTime::GetDayOfWeek() const
{
    return (t == (time_t)-1) ? t : localtime(&t)->tm_wday;
}

int CDateTime::GetDayOfYear() const
{
    return (t == (time_t)-1) ? t : localtime(&t)->tm_yday;
}

CDateTime& CDateTime::Clear(void)
{
    t = (time_t)-1;
    return *this;
}

CDateTime::operator time_t() const
{
    return t;
}

CDateTime::operator tstring() const
{
    return tstring((t == (time_t)-1) ? "" : _tasctime(localtime(&t)));
}

tstring CDateTime::Format(LPCTSTR fmt) const
{
    struct tm* pt;

    if ((t == (time_t)-1) || (pt =localtime(&t)) == NULL)
        return tstring(NULL);
    else
        {
```

```
        TCHAR buf[100];
        memset(buf, 0, sizeof(buf));
        size_t n = _tcsftime(buf, sizeof(buf), fmt, pt);
        return tstring(buf);
    }
}

CDateTime CDateTime::CurrentTime(void)
{
    return CDateTime(::time(NULL));
}

DATE CDateTime::ConvertToDATE() const
{
    SYSTEMTIME    s;
    double        d;
    struct tm*    tm_t = localtime(&t);

    if (! tm_t)
        return 0;

    memset(&s, 0, sizeof(s));
    s.wYear = tm_t->tm_year + 1900;
    s.wMonth = tm_t->tm_mon + 1;
    s.wDay = tm_t->tm_mday;
    s.wHour = tm_t->tm_hour;
    s.wMinute = tm_t->tm_min;
    s.wSecond = tm_t->tm_sec;

    if (SUCCEEDED(SystemTimeToVariantTime(&s, &d)))
        return d;
    else
        return 0;
}

////////////////////////////////////////////////////////////////////////////
// CMonthInfo CMonthInfo::months[]
// Shown in Chapter 7

////////////////////////////////////////////////////////////////////////////
// tstring CMonthInfo::dayNames[] =
// Shown in Chapter 7

const tstring CMonthInfo::GetMonthLongName(const CDateTime& d) const
{
    return tstring(months[ d.GetMonth() - 1 ].monthName.c_str());
}

const tstring CMonthInfo::GetMonthShortName(const CDateTime& d) const
{
    return tstring(GetMonthLongName(d), 0, 3);
}

int CMonthInfo::GetDaysInMonth(const CDateTime& d) const
{
    int month = d.GetMonth();
    int nDays = months[ month - 1 ].daysInMonth;
    if (month == 2)
{
        int year = d.GetYear();
```

```
               if (year % 4 == 0 && year % 100 != 0 || year % 400 == 0)
                  ++nDays;    // leap year
         }
         return nDays;
}

// return short names
const tstring CMonthInfo::GetDayOfWeekName(const int i) const
{
   _ASSERTE(i >= 0 && i <= kDaysInWeek);
   tstring& s = dayNames[i];
   return tstring(s.begin(), s.begin() + 3);
}

//////////////////////////////////////////////////////////////////////
//    CRectangle implementation
CRectangle CRectangle::LPtoDP(HDC hdc) const
{
   CRectangle dp = (*this);
   ::LPtoDP(hdc, (LPPOINT)&dp.r, 2);
   return dp;
}

CRectangle CRectangle::DPtoLP(HDC hdc) const
{
   CRectangle lp = (*this);
   ::DPtoLP(hdc, (LPPOINT)&lp.r, 2);
   return lp;
}

CRectangle CRectangle::Center(const SIZE& size)
{
   CRectangle   c;
   RECT&    cr = c.r;
   RECT&    rr = this->r;

   if (size.cx >= Width() && size.cy >= Height())
      c = *this;
   else if (size.cx >= Width() && size.cy < Height())
   {
      cr.left     = rr.left;
      cr.top      = rr.top + (Height() - size.cy) / 2;
      cr.right    = rr.right;
      cr.bottom   = cr.top + size.cy;
   }
   else if (size.cx < Width() && size.cy >= Height())
   {
      cr.left     = rr.left + (Width() - size.cx) / 2;
      cr.top      = rr.top;
      cr.right    = cr.left + size.cx;
      cr.bottom   = cr.top + Height();
   }
   else
   {
      // totally contained
      cr.left     = rr.left + (Width() - size.cx) / 2;
      cr.top      = rr.top + (Height() - size.cy) / 2;
      cr.right    = cr.left + size.cx;
      cr.bottom   = cr.top + size.cy;
   }
   return c;
```

```
}

bool CRectangle::PtInRect(const POINT& pt) const
{
    return ::PtInRect(&r, pt) != 0;
}

ostream& operator << (ostream& os, const CRectangle& cell)
{
    if (os)
    {
        RECT r = (RECT)cell;
        os    << _T("(L,T,R,B)=(")
            << r.left << _T(",")
            << r.top << _T(",")
            << r.right << _T(",")
            << r.bottom << _T(")");
    }
    return os;
}
```

CCellMgr.h

```
#include "CalDefs.h"
#include "CalUtils.h"

class CellAttachment
{
public:
    CellAttachment(ULONG num = 0) : item(num) {}
    void Clear() { item = 0; }

    ULONG item;
};

//////////////////////////////////////////////////////////////////////////
// CCalCell class
// Shown in Chapter 7

ostream& operator << (ostream& os, const CCalCell& cell);

//////////////////////////////////////////////////////////////////////////
// CCellMgr class
// Shown in Chapter 7
```

CCellMgr.cpp

```
#include "Stdafx.h"
#include "CCellMgr.h"

CCellMgr::CCellMgr() : m_CellPressed(-1)
{
    m_NumCells = sizeof(m_Cells) / sizeof(CCalCell);
    ClearCellContents();
}
```

```
CCellMgr::~CCellMgr()
{
}

//   CCellMgr::ClearCells
//   Clear all cells managed by this instance of CCellMgr
void CCellMgr::ClearCellContents()
{
    ATLTRACE(_T("CCellMgr::ClearCells\n"));

    for (CCalCell* pCell = m_Cells; pCell < m_Cells + m_NumCells; pCell++)
        pCell->ClearContent();
}

ULONG CCellMgr::GetNumCells(void) const
{
    return m_NumCells;
}

///////////////////////////////////////////////////////////////////////////
// void CCellMgr::SetCellCoords(int i, const CRectangle& rect)
// Shown in Chapter 7

bool CCellMgr::CellCoordsHaveBeenSet(void) const
{
    return m_Cells[0].rect != CRectangle();
}

void CCellMgr::SetCellHasEvent(int i, bool hasEvent)
{
    _ASSERTE(i >= 0 && i <= m_NumCells);
    m_Cells[i].hasEvent = hasEvent;
}

bool CCellMgr::GetCellHasEvent(int i) const
{
    _ASSERTE(i >= 0 && i <= m_NumCells);
    return m_Cells[i].hasEvent;
}

///////////////////////////////////////////////////////////////////////////
// void CCellMgr::SetDate(const CDateTime& d)
// Shown in Chapter 7

void CCellMgr::SetMonthYearLabel(const CDateTime& d)
{
    TCHAR buf[BUFSIZ];
    wsprintf(buf, _T("%s %d"), CMonthInfo().GetMonthLongName(d).c_str(),
            d.GetYear());
    // erase() returns a reference to *this
    m_MonthYearLabel.erase() = tstring(buf);
}

const tstring& CCellMgr::GetMonthYearLabel(void) const
{
    return m_MonthYearLabel;
}

const tstring& CCellMgr::GetCellLabel(int i) const
{
```

```
    _ASSERTE(i >= 0 && i <= m_NumCells);
    return m_Cells[i].label;
}

const tstring& CCellMgr::GetCellDayNumber(int i) const
{
    _ASSERTE(i >= 0 && i <= m_NumCells);
    return m_Cells[i].dayNumber;
}

const CDateTime& CCellMgr::GetCellDate(int i) const
{
    _ASSERTE(i >= 0 && i <= m_NumCells);
    return m_Cells[i].date;
}

void CCellMgr::OnLMouseButtonDown(const POINT& pt)
{
    // keep track of cell just pressed, iff it has events
    if (! CellHitTestWithEvents(pt, &m_CellPressed))
        m_CellPressed = -1;
}

bool CCellMgr::OnLMouseButtonUp(const POINT& pt, int* pCellIndex)
{
    // if cell just hit was the one pressed before, we have a click
    bool rc = pCellIndex != NULL
            && m_CellPressed != -1
            && CellHitTestWithEvents(pt, pCellIndex)
            && m_CellPressed == *pCellIndex;
    // reset
    m_CellPressed = -1;
    return rc;
}

bool CCellMgr::CellHitTestWithEvents(const POINT& pt, int* pi) const
{
    ATLTRACE(_T("CCellMgr::CellHitTestWithEvents\n"));

    return (pi && CellHitTest(pt, pi) && GetCellHasEvent(*pi));
}

bool CCellMgr::CellHitTest(const POINT& pt, int* pi) const
{
    TCHAR buf[BUFSIZ];
    wsprintf(buf, _T("- x=%3d [ %3d %3d ]   y=%3d [ %3d %3d ]\n "),
            pt.x, m_Cells[0].rect.Left(), m_Cells[6 ].rect.Right(),
            pt.y, m_Cells[0].rect.Top(),  m_Cells[41].rect.Bottom()
            );
    ATLTRACE(_T("CCellMgr::CellHitTest "));
    ATLTRACE(buf);

    for (int i = 0; i < GetNumCells(); i++)
        if ( m_Cells[i].rect.PtInRect(pt))
        {
            if (pi)
                *pi = i;
            return true;
```

```
        }
    return false;
}

///////////////////////////////////////////////////////////
//   CCalCell class implementation
CCalCell::CCalCell()
{
    ClearContent();
    rect.SetRectEmpty();
}

CCalCell::~CCalCell()
{
}

void CCalCell::ClearContent()
{
    // erase content but not the coordinates.
    // These are (re)set explicitly and separately
    date.Clear();
    dayNumber.erase();
    hasEvent = false;
    label.erase();
    for (int i = 0; i < kMaxCellAttachments; i++)
        attach[i].Clear();
}

ostream& operator << (ostream& os, const CCalCell& cell)
{
    os << _T("[") << (cell.label.size() != 0 ? cell.label : _T("")) << _T("]")
        << _T(" ") << cell.dayNumber
        << _T(" D=") << cell.date << _T(" ")
        << (cell.hasEvent? _T("HAS EVENTS") : _T("NO EVENT"))
        << _T(" Rect=") << cell.rect << endl;
    return os;
}
```

CDataMgr.h

```
#ifndef __CDATAMGR_H_
#define __CDATAMGR_H_

#import "..\ATLFinder\ATLFinder.tlb" rename_namespace("Finder")
#include "CEvents.h"

///////////////////////////////////////////////////////////////////////////
//   CDataMgr class
//   Shown in Chapter 7

#endif //__CDATAMGR_H_
```

CDataMgr.cpp

```cpp
#include "stdafx.h"
#include "CalDefs.h"
#include "CalUtils.h"

#import "..\ATLDept\ATLDept.tlb" rename_namespace("Dept")

#include "CDataMgr.h"

#pragma warning(disable: 4800)    // long to bool conversion

/////////////////////////////////////////////////////////////////
//    CDataMgr implementation
CDataMgr::CDataMgr(void) : m_MyFinder(NULL), m_InfoAvail(FALSE)
{
}

CDataMgr::~CDataMgr(void)
{
}

bool CDataMgr::CreateFinder(void)
{
   try
   {
      m_MyFinder = new Finder::IATLFinder1Ptr(__uuidof(Finder::ATLFinder1));
   }
   catch (const _com_error& err)
   {
      m_MyFinder = NULL;

      TCHAR buf[BUFSIZ];
      wsprintf(buf, _T("CDataMgr::CreateFinder:
                  Could not create Finder.\n"
                  "COM Error: 0x%x"), err.Error());
      ATLTRACE(buf);
   }
   return m_MyFinder != NULL;
}

void CDataMgr::ReleaseFinder(void)
{
   delete m_MyFinder;
}

bool CDataMgr::InfoAvail(void)
{
   return m_InfoAvail;
}

const CCalDept& CDataMgr::GetDept(ULONG idx) const
{
   return m_DeptEventList[ idx ].Dept;
}

ULONG CDataMgr::GetDeptCount(void) const
{
   return m_DeptEventList.size();
}
ULONG CDataMgr::GetNumDeptEventsInMonth(const ULONG inDept) const
```

```
    {
        return m_DeptEventList[ inDept ].OnDates.size();
    }

    void CDataMgr::GetDeptEventsOnDate(const ULONG inDept,
                                       const CDateTime& inDate,
                                       CCalEventList& events) const
    {
        _ASSERTE(inDept >= 0 && inDept < GetDeptCount());

        for (int i = 0; i < GetNumDeptEventsInMonth(inDept); i++)
          {
          CCalEvent ev;
          GetAnEvent(inDate, inDept, i, ev);
          if (inDate.GetYear() == ev.DateTime.GetYear()
             && inDate.GetMonth() == ev.DateTime.GetMonth()
             && inDate.GetDay() == ev.DateTime.GetDay())
          {
              events.push_back(ev);
          }
        }
    }

    void CDataMgr::ResetState(void)
    {
        m_InfoAvail = false;
    }

    //////////////////////////////////////////////////////////////////////
    //   on return, the i-th entry in the output vector<ULONG>& parameter
    //   contains the number of events, on the inDate, of the i-th department
    void CDataMgr::GetNumEventsOnDate(const CDateTime& inDate,
                                      vector<ULONG>& eventCount) const
    {
        CDeptEventList::const_iterator ci;

        // iterate through all deparments in the list
        // append a ULONG to eventCount for each one of them.
        for(ci = m_DeptEventList.begin(); ci < m_DeptEventList.end(); ci++)
            eventCount.push_back(ci->GetNumEventsOnDate(inDate));
    }

    void CDataMgr::GrabActiveDepts(void)
    {
        ATLTRACE(_T("CDataMgr::GrabActiveDepts\n"));

        if (! m_MyFinder)
            return;

        // clear up existing department list, if any
        m_DeptEventList.erase(m_DeptEventList.begin(), m_DeptEventList.end());

        // NOTE:  m_MyFinder is a ptr to an object which has the operator ->()
        // defined.  Consequently, we have to get at the object first,
        // before we can apply the -> operator. Ergo, (*objPtr)->
        // The invocation of GetEventfulDepts returns a  _variant_t which must be
        // cast in order to get the actual value.  In this case, it is a IDispatch*
        // (of course, we don't need the explicit cast, but it makes it clearer)
        IDispatch* finderDepts = static_cast<IDispatch*>
                                            ((*m_MyFinder)->GetEventfulDepts());
        Finder::IATLDepts1Ptr tmpDepts(finderDepts);
```

```
   for (int i = 1; i <= tmpDepts->GetCount(); i++)
   {
      // get a smart com pointer to the current department
      Dept::IATLDept1Ptr tpDept(tmpDepts->GetItem(i));

      // get the department info
      CDeptEvents    dptEvents;
      dptEvents.Dept.DeptName     = tpDept->GetName();
      dptEvents.Dept.DeptNumber   = tpDept->GetNumber();
      dptEvents.Dept.CanRead      = tpDept->GetCanRead();
      dptEvents.Dept.CanPostNew   = tpDept->GetCanPostNew();
      dptEvents.Dept.Symbol       = tpDept->GetSymbol();
      dptEvents.Dept.Color        = tpDept->GetColor();
      dptEvents.Dept.DeptNumber   = tpDept->GetNumber();
      dptEvents.Dept.DeptNumber   = tpDept->GetNumber();
      dptEvents.Dept.DeptNumber   = tpDept->GetNumber();

      // get a smart com pointer to the event collection for current
      //   department
      Dept::IATLCorpEvents1Ptr tpEvents(tpDept->GetKnownEvents());
      for (int j = 1; j <= tpEvents->GetCount(); j++)
      {
         // get a com ptr to the current event
         Dept::IATLCorpEvent1Ptr tpEvent(tpEvents->GetItem(j));
         // add event to list of events for current department
         dptEvents.OnDates.push_back(CDateTime(tpEvent->GetDateTime()));
      }
      // add to the department list
      m_DeptEventList.push_back(dptEvents);
   }
   m_InfoAvail = true;
}

///////////////////////////////////////////////////////////////////////////
//   Get an event given a date, a department and an event index
void CDataMgr::GetAnEvent(const CDateTime & inDate, ULONG inDept, ULONG idx,
                          CCalEvent& anEvent) const
{
   ATLTRACE(_T("CDataMgr::GetAnEvent\n"));

   if (! m_MyFinder)
      return;

   Finder::IATLDepts1Ptr tmpDepts((*m_MyFinder)->GetEventfulDepts());
   Dept::IATLDept1Ptr tpDept(tmpDepts->GetItem(inDept + 1));
   Dept::IATLCorpEvents1Ptr tpEvents(tpDept->GetKnownEvents());
   Dept::IATLCorpEvent1Ptr tpEvent(tpEvents->GetItem(idx + 1));

   // demonstrate the power of the new wrapper classes
   // e.g. use
   //            tpEvent->Property
   // rather than
   //            tpEvent->GetProperty()

   anEvent.DateTime = CDateTime(tpEvent->DateTime) ;
   anEvent.Details = tpEvent->Details;
   anEvent.Heading = tpEvent->Heading;
   anEvent.Hlink = tpEvent->Hlink;
   anEvent.Location = tpEvent->Location;
```

```
        anEvent.Organizer = tpEvent->Organizer;
        anEvent.OrgDept = tpEvent->OrgDept;
}

void CDataMgr::SetEventMonth(const CDateTime& inMonth)
{
    ATLTRACE(_T("CDataMgr::SetEventMonth\n"));

    if (! m_MyFinder)
        return;

    // get rid of hh:mm:ss information
    CDateTime workDate = CDateTime(inMonth.GetYear(), inMonth.GetMonth());

    Finder::IATLDepts1Ptr tmpDepts((*m_MyFinder)->GetEventfulDepts());
    if (tmpDepts->GetCount() == 0)
    {
        // if none, add a couple of depts
        tmpDepts->Add( _T("Accounting"), _T("23240"), TRUE, FALSE,
                    _T("A"), RGB(255,0,0), _T("192.168.1.1"), (DATE)inMonth);
        tmpDepts->Add( _T("Engineering"), _T("21204"), TRUE, FALSE,
                    _T("E"), RGB(0,0,255), _T("192.168.1.2"), (DATE)inMonth);
    }

    (*m_MyFinder)->SetFindDate((DATE)inMonth);

    // first delete all items in the event list
    for (int i = 1; i <= tmpDepts->GetCount(); i++)
    {
        Dept::IATLDept1Ptr       tpDept(tmpDepts->GetItem(i));
        Dept::IATLCorpEvents1Ptr tpEvents(tpDept->GetKnownEvents());
        for (int j = 1; j <= tpEvents->GetCount(); j++)
        {
            tpEvents->DeleteFirst();
        }
    }

    // fill them up again
    CDateTime tmpDate;
    Dept::IATLDept1Ptr tpDept(tmpDepts->GetItem(1));
    Dept::IATLCorpEvents1Ptr tpEvents(tpDept->GetKnownEvents());
    tmpDate = workDate + CDateTimeDiff(0, 0, 5, 14, 30, 1);
    tpEvents->Add( tmpDate.ConvertToDATE(), _T("Toronto Campus"),
                _T("Super Christmas Celebration"),
                _T("Ray Neveda"), _T("Armanda"),
                _T("everybody welcomed to this terrific party"),
                _T("http://www.anw.com/events"));

    tmpDate = workDate + CDateTimeDiff(0, 0, 17, 15, 0, 1);
    tpEvents->Add( tmpDate.ConvertToDATE(), _T("San Jose Site"),
                _T("New Hire Training"), _T("Ray Neveda"),
                _T("Armanda"),
                _T("See your training calendar for more details"),
                _T("http://www.anw.com/events"));

    tpDept.Detach()->Release();
    tpEvents.Detach()->Release();

    // next department

    // previous Release shouldn't be necessary
```

```
        // TO DO: Check following assignment carefully, whether
        //        it does the right thing with the interface pointers.
        tpDept = tmpDepts->GetItem(2);
        tpEvents = tpDept->GetKnownEvents();

        tmpDate = workDate + CDateTimeDiff(0, 0, 5, 10, 0, 1);
        tpEvents->Add( tmpDate.ConvertToDATE(), _T("Toronto Campus"),
                    _T("United Way Kickoff"), _T("Jack Lateman"),
                    _T("Toledo"),
                    _T("Come donate to this great charity."),
                    _T("http://www.anw.com/events"));

        tmpDate = workDate + CDateTimeDiff(0, 0, 8, 19, 30, 1);
        tpEvents->Add( tmpDate.ConvertToDATE(), _T("Toronto Campus"),
                    _T("Farewell Dinner for John Monroe"),
                    _T("Jack Lateman"), _T("Toledo"),
                    _T("Sorry to see John go after 40 years of service."),
                    _T("http://www.anw.com/events"));

        tmpDate = workDate + CDateTimeDiff(0, 0, 17, 9, 0, 1);
        tpEvents->Add( tmpDate.ConvertToDATE(), _T("Toronto Campus"),
                    _T("Internet Training"), _T("Jack Lateman"), _T("Toledo"),
                    _T("Free to all employees, take advantage of it!"),
                    _T("http://www.anw.com/events"));

        tmpDate = workDate + CDateTimeDiff(0, 0, 17, 12, 0, 1);
        tpEvents->Add( tmpDate.ConvertToDATE(), _T("Toronto Campus"),
                    _T("Dim Sum Breakfast"), _T("Joanne Rogers"),
                    _T("Support"), _T("Dare to try something new?"),
                    _T("http://www.anw.com/events"));

        tmpDate = workDate + CDateTimeDiff(0, 0, 20, 16, 0, 1);
        tpEvents->Add( tmpDate.ConvertToDATE(), _T("Toronto Campus"),
                    _T("Hammer the IBM370 Fest"), _T("Joanne Rogers"),
                    _T("Support"),
                    _T("$5 for each punch with a sledgehammer on the retired 370,
                      proceed goes to United Way."),
                    _T("http://www.anw.com/events"));
}
```

CEvents.h

```
#ifndef _CEVENTS_H
#define _CEVENTS_H

#include "CalUtils.h"

//////////////////////////////////////////////////////////////////////////////
//   CCalDept class
//   Shown in Chapter 7

//////////////////////////////////////////////////////////////////////////////
//   CDeptEvents class
//   Shown in Chapter 7
```

```
//////////////////////////////////////////////////////////////////////////////
//    CCalEvent struct
//    Shown in Chapter 7

//////////////////////////////////////////////////////////////////////////////
//    CDeptEventList class
//    Shown in Chapter 7

class CCalEventList: public vector<CCalEvent>
{
};

//////////////////////////////////////////////////////////////////////////////
//    CDeptEventInfo
//    the set of events of a particular department that we're interested in

struct CDeptEventInfo
{
   CCalDept Dept;
   CCalEventList Events;
};

//////////////////////////////////////////////////////////////////////////////
//    CDeptEvents
//    a collection of departments and their event sets

class CDeptEventInfoList : public vector<CDeptEventInfo>
{
};

#endif    // _CEVENTS_H
```

CEvents.cpp

```
#include "stdafx.h"
#include "CEvents.h"

//////////////////////////////////////////////////////////////////////
//    CDeptEvents implementation

ULONG CDeptEvents::GetNumEventsOnDate(const CDateTime& inDate) const
{
   ULONG count = 0;

   for(CDatesList::const_iterator ci = OnDates.begin();
          ci < OnDates.end(); ci++)
   {
      if (  ci->GetYear() == inDate.GetYear()
         && ci->GetMonth() == inDate.GetMonth()
         && ci->GetDay() == inDate.GetDay())
      {
         count++;
      }
   }
   return count;
}
```

EventListDlg.h

```
#include "resource.h"
#include "CalUtils.h"
#include "viscal1.h"
#include "viscal.h"
#include "CEvents.h"

//////////////////////////////////////////////////////////////////////////
//    CEventListDlg class
//    Shown in Chapter 7
```

EventListDlg.cpp

```
#include "stdafx.h"
#include "EventListDlg.h"
#include "OneEventDlg.h"

//////////////////////////////////////////////////////////////////////////
// CEventListDlg
CEventListDlg::CEventListDlg() : m_pCalCtl(NULL)
{
}

CEventListDlg::~CEventListDlg()
{
}

LRESULT CEventListDlg::OnInitDialog(UINT uMsg, WPARAM wParam, LPARAM lParam,
                                    BOOL& bHandled)
{
    FillEvents(m_DateToShow);
    return 1;   // Let the system set the focus
}

LRESULT CEventListDlg::OnOK(WORD wNotifyCode, WORD wID, HWND hWndCtl,
                            BOOL& bHandled)
{
    EndDialog(wID);
    return 0;
}

LRESULT CEventListDlg::OnCancel(WORD wNotifyCode, WORD wID, HWND hWndCtl,
                                BOOL& bHandled)
{
    EndDialog(wID);
    return 0;
}

void CEventListDlg::SetDateToShow(const CDateTime& d)
{
    m_DateToShow = d;
}

void CEventListDlg::SetParent(const Cviscal& ctl)
{
```

```
        m_pCalCtl = &ctl;
}

/////////////////////////////////////////////////////////////////////////////
// LRESULT CEventListDlg::OnDblClickList(WORD wNotifyCode, WORD wID,
//                                       HWND hWndCtl, BOOL& bHandled)
// Shown in Chapter 7

void CEventListDlg::FillEvents(const CDateTime& inDate)
{
    // set the label

    // Remove the hh:mm:ss designation. Formatting of CDateTime is fixed,
    // so we can do it as follows.
    tstring header = _T("Events for: ")
                     + tstring(inDate).replace(10, 9, _T(","), 1);
    SetDlgItemText(IDC_EVENTLISTDATE, header.c_str());

    const CDataMgr& dm = m_pCalCtl->GetDataMgr();

    // get the # of events per department for this date
    vector<ULONG> evCount;
    dm.GetNumEventsOnDate(inDate, evCount);

    // iterate through all departments and gather event info
    for (int dept = 0; dept < evCount.size(); dept++)
    {
        if (evCount[ dept] != 0)
        {
            CDeptEventInfo evInfo;
            // add department info
            evInfo.Dept = dm.GetDept(dept);
            // add events in current department
            dm.GetDeptEventsOnDate(dept, inDate, evInfo.Events);
            m_Events.push_back(evInfo);
        }
    }

    // Display the info.  We could have equally well used [] since
    // the STL vector class has operator[] defined.
    for (CDeptEventInfoList::const_iterator di = m_Events.begin();
            di < m_Events.end(); di++)
    {
        for (CCalEventList::const_iterator ei = di->Events.begin();
                ei < di->Events.end(); ei++)
        {
            tstring evStr (ei->DateTime.Format(_T("%I:%M %p")));
            evStr += _T(", ");
            evStr += di->Dept.DeptName;
            evStr += _T(" - ");
            evStr += ei->Heading;
            SendDlgItemMessage(IDC_EVENTLIST, LB_ADDSTRING, 0,
                        (LPARAM)evStr.c_str());
        }
    }
}
```

OneEventDlg.h

```cpp
#include "CEvents.h"

//////////////////////////////////////////////////////////////////////////
//    COneEventDlg class
//    Shown in Chapter 7
```

OneEventDlg.cpp

```cpp
// OneEventDlg.cpp : Implementation of COneEventDlg
#include "stdafx.h"
#include "resource.h"
#include "OneEventDlg.h"

//////////////////////////////////////////////////////////////////////////
// COneEventDlg
COneEventDlg::COneEventDlg()
{
}

COneEventDlg::~COneEventDlg()
{
}

LRESULT COneEventDlg::OnInitDialog(UINT uMsg, WPARAM wParam, LPARAM lParam,
                                   BOOL& bHandled)
{
   InitListbox();
   FillDetails();

   return 1;   // Let the system set the focus
}

LRESULT COneEventDlg::OnOK(WORD wNotifyCode, WORD wID, HWND hWndCtl,
                           BOOL& bHandled)
{
   EndDialog(wID);
   return 0;
}

LRESULT COneEventDlg::OnCancel(WORD wNotifyCode, WORD wID, HWND hWndCtl,
                               BOOL& bHandled)
{
   EndDialog(wID);
   return 0;
}

COneEventDlg& COneEventDlg::SetCalEvent(const CCalEvent& ev)
{
   m_Event = ev;
   return const_cast<COneEventDlg&>(*this);
}
void COneEventDlg::InitListbox(void)
{
```

```
    // The listbox has been created with the WS_HSCROLL style.
    // However, in order to enable horizontal scroll we need to
    // define the horizontal extent.  Ideally, we need to find out
    // the extent (and set it) only if the items added to the listbox
    // exceed its width.  Here, for simplicity, we will just set it
    // so that all items can be exhibited.
    SendDlgItemMessage(IDC_EVENTDETAILS, LB_SETHORIZONTALEXTENT, 500, 0);

    // The listbox has been created with the LBS_USETABSTOPS style.
    // here we set the tab stops in dialog units.
    INT   i = 45;
    SendDlgItemMessage(IDC_EVENTDETAILS, LB_SETTABSTOPS, 1, (LPARAM)&i);
}

void COneEventDlg::AddLine(const tstring& s)
{
    SendDlgItemMessage (IDC_EVENTDETAILS, LB_ADDSTRING, 0, (LPARAM)s.c_str());
}

void COneEventDlg::FillDetails(void)
{
    tstring details;

    details = _T("Date:\t");
    details += m_Event.DateTime.Format(_T("%B %d, %Y"));
    AddLine(details);

    details = _T("Time:\t");
    details += m_Event.DateTime.Format(_T("%I:%M %p"));
    AddLine(details);

    details = _T("Location:\t");
    details += m_Event.Location;
    AddLine(details);

    details = _T("Event:\t");
    details += m_Event.Heading;
    AddLine(details);

    details = _T("Organizer:\t");
    details += m_Event.Heading;
    details += _T(",");
    details += m_Event.OrgDept;
    AddLine(details);

    details = _T("Description:\t");
    details += m_Event.Details;
    AddLine(details);
}
```

CCalButton.h

```
#include "resource.h"

/////////////////////////////////////////////////////////////////////
//    CCalButton class
//    Shown in Chapter 7
```

CCalButton.cpp

```
// CCalButton.cpp : Implementation of CCalButton
#include "stdafx.h"
#include "CCalButton.h"

CCalButton::CCalButton(long ID) : m_ID(ID), m_bClicked(FALSE),
                                  m_bVisible(TRUE)
{
}

CCalButton::~CCalButton()
{
}

// This is the rectangle where the button is wrt to hitTest

void CCalButton::ResetHitTestSize(const CRectangle& hitRect)
{
   m_hitrect = hitRect;
}

// this is the rectangle where the button is wrt painting and repainting
// IE4 Windowless operation requires this

void CCalButton::ResetSize(const CRectangle& winRect)
{
   m_rect = winRect;
}

void   CCalButton::Show(BOOL visible)
{
   if (m_bVisible != visible)
      m_bVisible = visible;

}

void CCalButton::ReDraw(HDC hdc)
{
   if (m_bClicked)
      DrawClicked(hdc);
   else
      DrawNormal(hdc);
}

void CCalButton::DrawClicked(HDC hdc)
{
   ::DrawEdge(hdc, &m_rect.r, EDGE_SUNKEN, BF_RECT | BF_SOFT);
   m_bClicked = TRUE;

}

void CCalButton::DrawFlash(HDC hdc)
{
}

void CCalButton::DrawNormal(HDC hdc)
{
   ::DrawEdge(hdc, &m_rect.r, EDGE_RAISED, BF_RECT | BF_SOFT);
```

```
        m_bClicked = FALSE;
}

void CCalButton::DrawClear(HDC hdc)
{
}

bool CCalButton::HitTest(const POINT& pt) const
{
    return m_hitrect.PtInRect(pt);
}
```

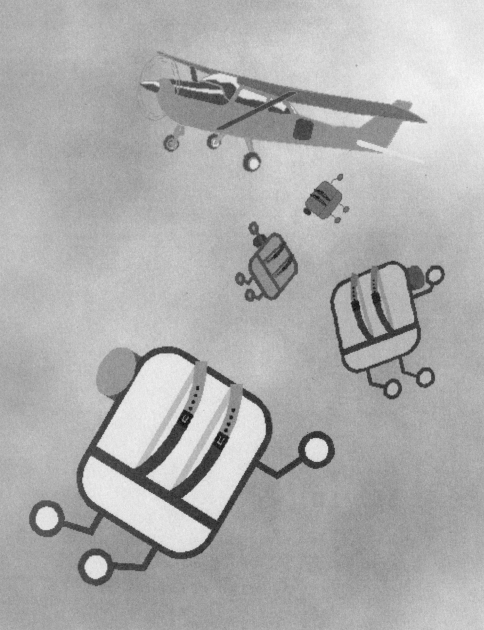

Index

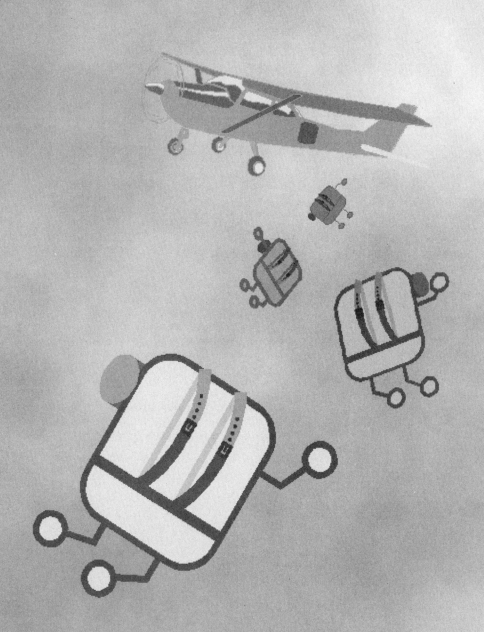

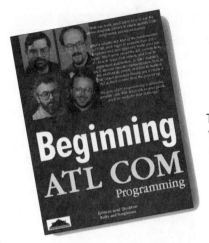

Beginning ATL COM Programming

Authors: Various
ISBN: 1861000111
Price: $39.95 C$55.95 £36.99

This book is for fairly experienced C++ developers who want to get to grips with COM programming using the Active Template Library. The Beginning in the title of this book refers to COM and it refers to ATL. It does not refer to Programming.

We don't expect you to know anything about COM. The book explains the essentials of COM, how to use it, and how to get the most out of it. If you do already know something about COM, that's a bonus. You'll still learn a lot about the way that ATL works, and you'll be one step ahead of the COM neophytes.

Neither do we expect you to know anything about ATL. ATL is the focus of the book. If you've never touched ATL, or if you've been using it for a short while, but still have many unanswered questions, this is the book for you.

Professional DCOM Application Development

Author: Jonathan Pinnock
ISBN: 1861001312
Price: $49.99 C$69.95 £45.99

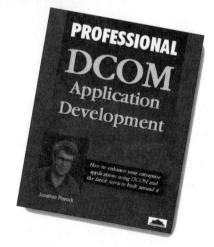

Jonathan Pinnock writes:

"When you start building systems that stretch over an entire enterprise, things get complicated, and it gets more and more difficult to deliver flexible, reliable and timely solutions to your end users. Any tools that can simplify and standardize the process of developing enterprise-wide systems are therefore of immense significance. My view is that COM and DCOM and all the technologies that are based around them provide us with just that toolkit. I want to show you how to put them to use in building real solutions to real problems."

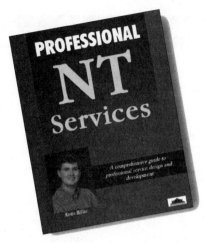

Professional NT Services

Author: Kevin Miller
ISBN: 1861001304
Price: $59.99 C$83.95 £55.49

Professional NT Services teaches developers how to design and implement good NT services using all the features and tools supplied for the purpose by Microsoft Visual C++. The author develops a set of generic classes to facilitate service development, and introduces the concept of usage patterns — a way of categorizing the roles that services can fulfil in the overall architecture of a system. The book also gives developers a firm grounding in the security and configuration issues that must be taken into account when developing a service.

To date, the treatment of NT services has been sketchy and widely scattered. This book is aimed at bringing the range of relevant material together in an organized way. Its target readership is C/C++ Windows programmers with experience of programming under Win32 and basic knowledge of multithreaded and COM programming. At an architectural level, the book's development of usage patterns will be invaluable to client-server developers who want to include services as part of a multi-tiered system.

Professional ATL COM Programming

Author: Richard Grimes
ISBN: 1861001401
Price: $59.99 C$89.95 £55.49

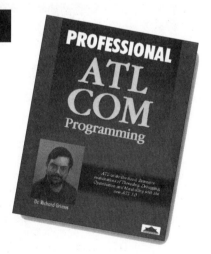

Richard Grimes writes:

"If you've ever looked at Wizard-generated ATL code and wondered exactly how it works, why it was implemented in that way, and what options are available to you for customizing and extending it, you should find the answers in these pages. I've explored the plumbing of the Active Template Library to see how everything fits together, and this book is a dossier of my discoveries.

At the same time, I've tried to make the order of presentation into a description of the process of building a COM server from the ground up, so each new piece of information is provided in the context of a particular consideration in that procedure. In that way, I aim to give you the knowledge about ATL and COM server design that you need to create robust components with confidence."

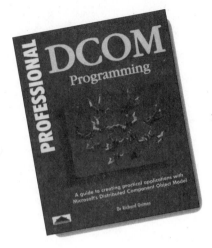

Professional DCOM Programming

Author: Dr. Richard Grimes
ISBN: 186100060X
Price: $49.95 C$69.95 £46.99

This book is for Win32 programmers taking up the challenge of building applications using the distributed component object model. There is a strong emphasis on the practicalities of distributed object design and use, and the text is also a complete examination of COM programming. The code is described and developed using Visual C++ 5, MFC and ATL.

Instant UML

Authors: Pierre-Alain Muller
ISBN: 1861000871
Price: $34.95 C$48.95 £32.49

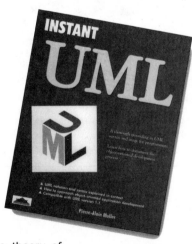

UML is the Unified Modeling Language. Modeling languages have come into vogue with the rise of object-oriented development, as they provide a means of communicating and recording every stage of the project. The results of the analysis and design phases are captured using the formal syntax of the modeling language, producing a clear model of the system to be implemented.

Instant UML offers not only a complete description of the notation and proper use of UML, but also an introduction to the theory of object-oriented programming, and the way to approach object-oriented application development. This is UML in context, not a list of the syntax without rhyme or reason.

This book is relevant to programmers of C++, VB, Java and other OO-capable languages, users of Visual Modeler (which comes with the Enterprise Edition of Microsoft's Visual Studio) and novice users of Rational Rose and similar UML-compliant tools.